Pathophysiology of Disease

An Introduction to Clinical Medicine

third edition

Edited by

Stephen J. McPhee, MD
Professor of Medicine
University of California, San Francisco

Vishwanath R. Lingappa, MD, PhD
Professor of Physiology and Medicine
University of California, San Francisco

William F. Ganong, MD
Jack and DeLoris Lange Professor
of Physiology Emeritus
University of California, San Francisco

Jack D. Lange, MD (deceased)
(Formerly) Clinical Professor
of Medicine Emeritus
University of California, San Francisco

Lange Medical Books/McGraw-Hill
Health Professions Division

New York   St. Louis   San Francisco   Auckland   Bogotá   Caracas   Lisbon   London
Madrid   Mexico City   Milan   Montreal   New Delhi   San Juan
Singapore   Sydney   Tokyo   Toronto

McGraw-Hill
*A Division of The **McGraw·Hill** Companies*

Pathophysiology of Disease: An Introduction to Clinical Medicine, 3/e

Copyright © 2000 by The **McGraw-Hill Companies,** Inc. All rights reserved. Printed in the United States of America. Except as permitted under the United States Copyright Act of 1976, no part of this publication may be reproduced or distributed in any form or by any means, or stored in a data base or retrieval system, without the prior written permission of the publisher.

Previous editions copyright © 1997, 1995 by Appleton & Lange

1234567890DOWDOW99

International Edition

Copyright ©2000

Exclusive rights by The **McGraw-Hill Companies,** Inc., for manufacture and export. This book cannot be re-exported from the country to which it is consigned by McGraw-Hill.

When ordering this title, use ISBN 0-7-112004-1

Notice

Medicine is an ever-changing science. As new research and clinical experience broaden our knowledge, changes in treatment and drug therapy are required. The editors and the publisher of this work have checked with sources believed to be reliable in their efforts to provide information that is complete and generally in accord with the standards accepted at the time of publication. However, in view of the possibility of human error or changes in medical sciences, neither the editors nor the publisher nor any other party who has been involved in the preparation or publication of this work warrants that the information contained herein is in every respect accurate or complete, and they are not responsible for any errors or omissions or for the results obtained from use of such information. Readers are encouraged to confirm the information contained herein with other sources. For example and in particular, readers are advised to check the product information sheet included in the package of each drug they plan to administer to be certain that the information contained in this book is accurate and that changes have not been made in the recommended dose or in the contraindications for administration. This recommendation is of particular importance in connection with new or infrequently used drugs.

This book was set in Times Roman by Pine Tree Composition.
The editors were David Barnes, Jim Ransom, and Harriet Lebowitz.
The production supervisor was Frank Del Vecchio.
The production service was Pine Tree Composition.
The cover designer was Elizabeth Schmitz.
The art manager was Eve Siegel.
The art coordinator was Becky Hainz-Baxter.
The illustrators were Teshin Associates.
The index was prepared by Kathy Pitcoff.

R. R. Donnelley was printer and binder.

This book is printed on acid-free paper.

Dedication

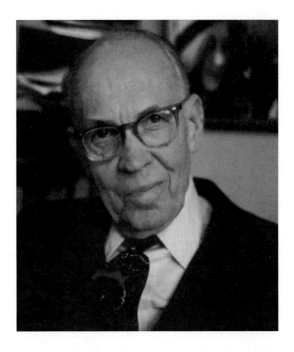

The editors and contributors wish to dedicate this third edition of *Pathophysiology of Disease* to Dr. Jack Damgaard Lange, who died at age 92 while this revision was under way. Jack was the president and one of the founding partners—with his wife DeLoris—of Lange Medical Publications. He retired in 1986 but maintained an active interest in medical book publishing with the goal of making inexpensive medical texts of high quality available to students and practitioners in the health science professions in all parts of the world. One of his goals late in life was to add a pathophysiology textbook to the Lange series. This book is the result.

Contents

Preface	vii
Authors	ix
1. Introduction *Jack D. Lange, MD*	1
2. Genetic Disease *Gregory Barsh, MD, PhD*	2
3. Disorders of the Immune System *Richard S. Shames, MD, & Jeffrey L. Kishiyama, MD*	28
4. Infectious Diseases *Karen C. Bloch, MD, MPH*	50
5. Neoplasia *Debasish Tripathy, MD*	79
6. Blood Disorders *J. Ben Davoren, MD, PhD*	98
7. Nervous System Disorders *Robert O. Messing, MD*	124
8. Diseases of the Skin *Timothy H. McCalmont, MD*	166
9. Pulmonary Disease *Thomas J. Prendergast, MD, & Stephen J. Ruoss, MD*	184
10. Cardiovascular Disorders: Heart Disease *Fred Kusumoto, MD*	222
11. Cardiovascular Disorders: Vascular Disease *William F. Ganong, MD*	258
12. Disorders of the Adrenal Medulla *Stephen J. McPhee, MD*	282
13. Gastrointestinal Disease *Vishwanath R. Lingappa, MD, PhD*	293
14. Liver Disease *Vishwanath R. Lingappa, MD, PhD*	327

15. **Disorders of the Exocrine Pancreas** 362
Stephen J. McPhee, MD

16. **Renal Disease** 382
Vishwanath R. Lingappa, MD, PhD

17. **Disorders of the Parathyroids & Calcium Metabolism** 405
Dolores M. Shoback, MD, & Gordon J. Strewler, MD

18. **Disorders of the Endocrine Pancreas** 432
Kenneth R. Feingold, MD, & Janet L. Funk, MD

19. **Disorders of the Hypothalamus & Pituitary Gland** 459
Vishwanath R. Lingappa, MD, PhD

20. **Thyroid Disease** 481
Stephen J. McPhee, MD, & Douglas C. Bauer, MD

21. **Disorders of the Adrenal Cortex** 500
Stephen J. McPhee, MD

22. **Disorders of the Female Reproductive Tract** 529
Vishwanath R. Lingappa, MD, PhD

23. **Disorders of the Male Reproductive Tract** 556
Stephen J. McPhee, MD

24. **Inflammatory Rheumatic Diseases** 576
Eric L. Greidinger, MD, & Antony Rosen, MD

25. **Illustrative Case Studies** 584
Eva M. Aagaard, MD

Index 610

Preface

WHAT THE BOOK IS

This is a text designed to present an orientation to disease considered as disordered physiology. It is intended to enable the student and practitioner to understand how and why the symptoms and signs of various conditions occur. In approaching disease as disordered physiology, this text analyzes the mechanism of production of the symptoms and signs of different diseases and syndromes. In so doing, it recognizes the student's and practitioner's need to understand the mechanisms underlying the disease and its clinical manifestations so that rational therapies can be offered.

WHAT THE BOOK IS NOT

We do not offer a standard textbook of medicine that proceeds in conventional sequence from etiology, pathology, symptoms and signs, laboratory findings, diagnosis, and differential diagnosis to treatment and prognosis. Nor is *Pathophysiology of Disease* intended to serve as a standard textbook of physiology, pathology, or physical diagnosis. Furthermore, the text is not intended to be all-encompassing in the disordered physiologic mechanisms or disease states taken up for discussion. Rather, the authors have selected examples of disordered physiology and disease states which seemed most relevant to the clinical practice of medicine.

INTENDED AUDIENCE

Medical students in basic pathophysiology courses will find that this text makes a useful contribution to their understanding of how disordered physiology produces common diseases and syndromes. Students taking courses on the introduction to clinical medicine or engaged in basic internal medicine and surgery clerkship rotations will find this work helpful in comprehending how and why the symptoms and signs of various disease states appear. House officers will find the concise, up-to-date descriptions of disease mechanisms, with citations to the current literature, of use in devising proper patient management. Practitioners (internists, family physicians, and other specialists who provide generalist care) will find *Pathophysiology of Disease* useful as a refresher text, designed to update their understanding of the mechanisms underlying disease. Nurses and other health practitioners will find that the concise format and broad scope of the book facilitate their understanding of basic disease entities.

ORGANIZATION OF THE BOOK

Pathophysiology of Disease is divided into 25 chapters, developed chiefly by organ system. Each chapter is divided into sections emphasizing normal structure and function, pathology and disordered physiology, common clinical presentations, and mechanisms underlying symptoms and signs. Text review questions are provided in boxes throughout the chapters. A list of pertinent recent references is provided at the end of each chapter as suggestions for further reading.

NEW TO THIS EDITION

The third edition of *Pathophysiology of Disease* contains two new chapters. One is on inflammatory rheumatic diseases. The other provides 38 illustrative cases with a brief discussion of each. Other chapters have been updated and revised, and recent references have been substituted.

San Francisco, California
November, 1999

Stephen J. McPhee, MD
Vishwanath R. Lingappa, MD, PhD
William F. Ganong, MD
Jack D. Lange, MD

Authors

Eva M. Aagaard, MD
Research Fellow, Division of Internal Medicine, University of California, San Francisco

Gregory Barsh, MD, PhD
Assistant Professor of Pediatrics and Genetics; Assistant Investigator, HHMI, Stanford University School of Medicine, Stanford, California

Douglas C. Bauer, MD
Assistant Professor of Medicine, Epidemiology and Biostatistics, University of California, San Francisco

Karen C. Bloch, MD, MPH
Assistant Professor, Infectious Diseases and Preventative Medicine, Vanderbilt University School of Medicine, Nashville, Tennessee

J. Ben Davoren, MD, PhD
Assistant Clinical Professor of Medicine, San Francisco Veterans Affairs Medical Center, San Francisco

Kenneth R. Feingold, MD
Professor of Medicine and Dermatology, University of California, San Francisco; Staff Physician, Veterans Affairs Medical Center, San Francisco

Janet L. Funk, MD
Assistant Professor of Clinical Medicine, University of Arizona, Tucson

William F. Ganong, MD
Jack and DeLoris Lange Professor of Physiology Emeritus, University of California, San Francisco

Eric L. Greidinger, MD
Assistant Professor of Internal Medicine and Pathology, University of Missouri Health Sciences Center; Staff Physician, VMAC, Columbia, Missouri

Jeffrey L. Kishiyama, MD
Director, Clinical Allergy and Immunology, Assistant Clinical Professor of Medicine, University of California, San Francisco

Fred Kusumoto, MD
Director, Electrophysiology and Pacing Service, Lovelace Medical Center, Albuquerque; Assistant Clinical Professor of Medicine, University of New Mexico, Albuquerque

Jack D. Lange, MD (deceased)
(Formerly) Clinical Professor of Medicine Emeritus, University of California, San Francisco

Vishwanath R. Lingappa, MD, PhD
Professor of Physiology and Medicine, University of California, San Francisco

Timothy H. McCalmont, MD
Assistant Professor of Pathology and Dermatology, University of California, San Francisco

Stephen J. McPhee, MD
Professor of Medicine, University of California, San Francisco

Robert O. Messing, MD
Associate Professor of Neurology, University of California, San Francisco, Assistant Director, Ernest Gallo Clinical and Research Center

Thomas J. Prendergast, MD
Assistant Professor of Medicine, Dartmouth Medical School; Chief, Pulmonary Section, Veterans Affairs Medical Center, White River Junction, Vermont

Antony Rosen, MD
Associate Professor of Medicine; Deputy Director, Division of Rheumatology, Johns Hopkins University School of Medicine, Baltimore

Stephen J. Ruoss, MD
Assistant Professor, Division of Pulmonary and Critical Care Medicine, Stanford University Medical Center, Stanford, California

Richard S. Shames, MD
Assistant Professor of Pediatrics (Allergy and Clinical Immunology), Stanford University Medical Center, Stanford, California

Dolores M. Shoback, MD
Staff Physician, San Francisco Department of Veterans Affairs Medical Center; Associate Professor of Medicine, University of California, San Francisco

Gordon J. Strewler, MD
Chief, Department of Medicine, Brockton/West Roxbury Veterans Affairs Medical Center, Professor of Medicine, Harvard Medical School, Boston, Massachusetts

Debasish Tripathy, MD
Associate Clinical Professor of Medicine, University of California, San Francisco

Introduction 1

Jack D. Lange, MD

WHAT IS PATHOPHYSIOLOGY?

Pathophysiology may be defined as the physiology of disease, of disordered function, or derangement of function seen in disease that is produced by the action of an etiologic agent (eg, bacteria) on susceptible tissues or organs. The term "pathophysiology" emphasizes alterations in function—as distinguished from "pathology," which emphasizes structural changes. Pathophysiology includes also the study of the mechanisms underlying disease. The study of pathophysiology is an essential introduction to clinical medicine and serves as a bridge between the basic sciences and disease.

Pathophysiology differs from pathogenesis. Pathogenesis is the mode of origin or development of any disease process (eg, development of autoimmunity to the thyroid-stimulating hormone receptor). Pathophysiology describes the resulting disordered physiology and clinical consequences (eg, release of excess thyroid hormone, producing the syndrome of hyperthyroidism).

WHY IS PATHOPHYSIOLOGY IMPORTANT?

An orientation to disease as disordered physiology can enable the student and practitioner to understand how and why the symptoms and signs of various conditions appear. A pathophysiologic approach to disease as disordered physiology enables the clinician to analyze the mechanism of production of the symptoms and signs of different disease syndromes. In so doing, it recognizes the student's and practitioner's need to understand the mechanisms underlying the disease and its clinical manifestations so that rational therapies can be devised.

This book was written with the principles described above in mind. It summarizes the normal structure and function of each organ system, then discusses a number of the major diseases of each system, showing how symptoms and signs of the selected diseases are produced by disordered physiology. It also provides an introduction to clinical medicine by analyzing in the same way the broad topics of genetic abnormalities, neoplasia, and infectious disease.

2

Genetic Disease

Gregory Barsh, MD, PhD

Mechanisms of cellular and tissue dysfunction in genetic diseases are as varied as the organs they affect. To some extent, these mechanisms are similar to those that occur in nonheritable disorders. For example, a fracture due to the decreased bone density in osteoporosis heals in the same fashion as one caused by a defective collagen gene in osteogenesis imperfecta, and the response to coronary atherosclerosis in most individuals does not depend on whether they have inherited a defective LDL receptor. Thus, the pathophysiology of genetic diseases relates not so much to the affected organ system as to the mechanisms of mutation, inheritance, and molecular pathways from genotype to phenotype.

This chapter begins with a discussion of the terminology used to describe inherited conditions, the prevalence of genetic disease, and some major principles and considerations in clinical genetics. Important terms and key words used throughout the chapter are defined in Table 2–1.

Next, a group of disorders caused by mutations in collagen genes is discussed, ie, **osteogenesis imperfecta.** Though osteogenesis imperfecta is often considered a single entity, different mutations and different genes subject to mutation lead to a wide spectrum of clinical phenotypes. The different types of osteogenesis imperfecta exhibit typical patterns of autosomal dominant or autosomal recessive inheritance and are therefore examples of so-called **mendelian conditions.**

Recently, several genetic conditions have been found to depend not only on the gene being inherited but also on the phenotype or the sex of the parent. As an example of a condition that exhibits nonclassic inheritance, the **fragile X-associated mental retardation syndrome** is discussed. This syndrome is not only the most common inherited cause of mental retardation but also illustrates a recently discovered principle of molecular and cellular biology.

One of the most common types of human genetic disease that does not affect DNA structure per se is **aneuploidy,** or a change in the normal chromosome content per cell. The example that is considered, **Down's syndrome,** has had a major impact on reproductive medicine and reproductive decision making and serves to illustrate general principles that apply to many aneuploid conditions.

Finally, to show how environmental factors can influence the relationship between genotype and phenotype, we shall discuss **phenylketonuria,** which serves as the paradigm for newborn screening programs and treatment of genetic disease.

UNIQUE ASPECTS OF GENETIC PATHOPHYSIOLOGY

Although the phenotypes of genetic diseases are diverse, their causes are not. The primary cause of any genetic disease can be defined as a discrete event that affects gene expression in a group of cells related to each other by lineage. Most genetic diseases are caused by an alteration in DNA sequence that alters the synthesis of a single gene product. However, some genetic diseases are caused (1) by chromosome rearrangements that result in deletion or duplication of a group of closely linked genes or (2) by mistakes during mitosis or meiosis that result in an abnormal number of chromosomes per cell. In most genetic diseases, every cell in an affected individual carries the mutated gene or genes as a consequence of its inheritance via a mutant egg or sperm **(gamete).** However, mutation of the gametic cell may have arisen during its development, in which case somatic cells of the parent do not carry the mutation and the affected individual is said to have a "new mutation." In addition, some mutations may arise in somatic cells during early embryogenesis, in which case tissues of the affected individual contain a mixture, or **mosaic,** of mutant and nonmutant cells (Figure 2–1).

One must bear in mind the distinctions between gene, locus, and allele and between mutation, polymorphism, and phenotype since confusion about the terminology of genetics and genetic diseases can

Table 2–1. Glossary of terms and keywords.

Term	Definition
Acrocentric	Pertaining to the terminal location of the centromere on chromosomes 13, 14, 15, 21, and 22, which contain so-called satellite DNA on their short arms that encodes for ribosomal RNA genes.
Allele	Alternative forms of a gene that occupy the same locus on a specific chromosome.
Allelic heterogeneity	The state in which multiple alleles at a single locus can produce a disease phenotype or phenotypes.
Amorphic	Refers to a mutation that results in a complete loss of function.
Aneuploidy	A general term used to denote any unbalanced chromosome complement.
Antimorphic	Refers to a mutation which, when present in heterozygous form opposite a nonmutant allele, results in a phenotype similar to homozygosity for loss-of-function alleles.
Ascertainment bias	The problem that arises when individuals or families in a genetic study are not representative of the general population because of the way in which they are identified.
Autosomal	Located on chromosomes 1–22 rather than X or Y.
CpG island	A segment of DNA that contains a relatively high density of 5′-CG-3′ dinucleotides. Such segments are frequently unmethylated and located close to ubiquitously expressed genes.
Dictyotene	The end of prophase during female meiosis I in which fetal oocytes are arrested prior to ovulation.
Dominant	A pattern of inheritance or mechanism of gene action in which the effects of a variant allele can be observed in the presence of a nonmutant allele.
Dominant negative	Mutant alleles that give rise to structurally abnormal proteins that interfere with the normal function of the nonmutant gene products.
Dosage compensation	Mechanism by which a difference in gene dosage between two cells is equalized; for XX cells, decreased expression from one of the two X chromosomes results in a concentration of gene product similar to that of an XY cell.
End product deficiency	A pathologic mechanism in which absence or reduction in the product of a particular enzymatic reaction leads to disease.
Epigenetic	Refers to a phenotypic effect that does not depend on genotype. DNA methylation that occurs during gametogenesis can affect gene expression in zygotic cells, but the pattern of methylation can also be reversed in subsequent generations and thus does not affect genotype.
Expressivity	The extent to which a mutant genotype affects phenotype. A quantitative measure of a disease state that may vary from mild to severe but is never completely absent.
Fitness	The likelihood that an individual who carries a particular mutant allele will produce progeny that also carry the allele.
Founder effect	One of several possible explanations for an unexpectedly high frequency of a deleterious gene in a population. If the population was founded by a small ancestral group, it may have, by chance, contained a large number of carriers for the deleterious gene.
Gamete	The egg or sperm cell that represents a potential reproductive contribution to the next generation. Gametes have undergone meiosis and so contain half the normal number of chromosomes found in zygotic cells.
Gene dosage	The principle that the amount of product expressed for a particular gene is proportionate to the number of gene copies present per cell.
Genetic anticipation	A clinical phenomenon that occurs when the phenotype observed in individuals carrying a deleterious gene appears more severe in successive generations. Possible explanations include ascertainment bias or a multistep mutational mechanism such as expansion of triplet repeats.
Genetic heterogeneity	A situation in which mutations of different genes produce similar or identical phenotypes. Also referred to as locus heterogeneity.
Haplotype	A set of closely linked alleles that are not easily separated by recombination. Often refers to DNA sequence alterations such as restriction fragment length polymorphisms.
Heterochromatin	One of two alternative forms of chromosomal material (the other is euchromatin) as determined by the way in which chromosomal DNA is bound to proteins and condensed. Heterochromatin is highly condensed and usually does not contain genes that are actively transcribed.

(*continued*)

Table 2–1. Glossary of terms and keywords. (continued)

Term	Definition
Heterozygote advantage	One way to explain an unexpectedly high frequency of a recessively inherited mutation in a particular population. During recent evolution, carriers (ie, heterozygotes) are postulated to have had a higher fitness than homozygous nonmutant individuals.
Hypermorphic	Refers to a mutation that has an effect similar to increasing the number of normal gene copies per cell.
Hypomorphic	Refers to a mutation that reduces but does not eliminate the activity of a particular gene product.
Imprinting	As applied most commonly, the process whereby expression of a gene depends on whether it is transmitted through a female or male gamete.
Linkage disequilibrium	The situation occuring when certain combinations of closely linked alleles are present in a population at frequencies not predicted by their individual frequencies.
Monosomy	A reduction in zygotic cells from two to one in the number of copies for a particular chromosomal segment or chromosome.
Mosaicism	A situation in which a genetic alteration is present in some but not all cells of a single individual. In germline or gonadal mosaicism, the alteration is present in germ cells but not in somatic cells. In somatic mosaicism, the genetic alteration is present in some but not all of the somatic cells (and is generally not present in the germ cells).
Neomorphic	Refers to a mutation that imparts a novel function to its gene product and thus results in a phenotype distinct from an alteration in gene dosage.
Nondisjunction	Failure of two homologous chromosomes to separate, or disjoin, at metaphase of meiosis I; or the failure of two sister chromatids to disjoin at metaphase of meiosis II or mitosis.
Penetrance	In a single individual of a variant genotype, penetrance is an all-or-none phenomenon determined by the absence or presence of defined phenotypic criteria. In a population, reduced penetrance implies that an individual of a variant genotype is less likely to be recognized according to the same phenotypic criteria.
Phenotypic heterogeneity	The situation occurring when mutations of a single gene produce multiple different phenotypes.
Polymorphism	An allele that is present in 1% or more of the population.
Postzygotic	Refers to a mutational event that occurs after fertilization, and that commonly gives rise to mosaicism.
Premutation	A genetic change that does not itself result in a phenotype but has a high probability of developing a second alteration—a full mutation—that does cause a phenotype.
Primordial germ cells	The group of diploid cells set aside early in development that go on to give rise to gametes.
Recessive	A pattern of inheritance or mechanism of gene action in which a particular mutant allele gives rise to a phenotype only in the absence of a nonmutant allele. Thus, for autosomal conditions, the variant or disease phenotype is manifest when two copies of the mutant allele are present. For X-linked conditions, the variant or disease phenotype is manifest in cells, tissues, or individuals in which the nonmutant allele is either inactivated (a heterozygous female) or not present (a hemizygous male).
RFLP	Restriction fragment length polymorphism, a type of DNA-based allele variation in which different alleles at a single locus are recognized and followed through pedigrees based on the size of a restriction fragment. The locus is defined by the segment of DNA that gives rise to the restriction fragment; the different alleles are generally (not always) caused by a single change in DNA sequence that creates or abolishes a site of restriction enzyme cleavage.
Robertsonian translocation	A type of translocation in which two acrocentric chromosomes are fused together with a single functional centromere. A carrier of a Robertsonian translocation with 45 chromosomes has a normal amount of chromosomal material and is said to be euploid.
Substrate accumulation	A pathogenetic mechanism in which deficiency of a particular enzyme causes disease because the substrate of that enzyme accumulates in tissue or blood.
Triplet repeat	A three-nucleotide sequence that is tandemly repeated many times, ie, $(XYZ)_n$. Alterations in length of such simple types of repeats (dinucleotide and tetranucleotide as well) occur much more frequently than most other kinds of mutations; however, alterations in the length of trinucleotide repeats is the molecular basis for several heritable disorders.
Trisomy	An abnormal situation in which there are three instead of two copies of a chromosomal segment or chromosome per cell.

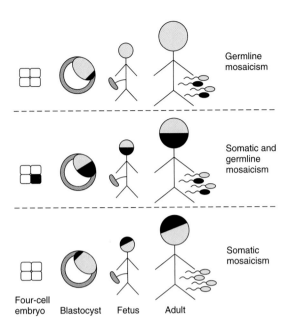

Figure 2–1. Cellular origin of mutations can lead to somatic mosaicism, germline mosaicism, or both. The effects of a mutation on mosaicism depend on the cell and the developmental stage in which the mutation occurs. The early blastocyst is composed of two different tissues: the inner cell mass (light-colored), which mostly gives rise to embryonic tissues, including somatic and germ cells; and the trophoblast (dark-colored), which gives rise to extraembryonic tissues cells such as the placenta. If a mutation (black) occurs in a portion of the inner cell mass whose daughter cells contribute exclusively to the germline, the adult will not exhibit phenotypic features of the mutation in somatic tissues but may produce germ cells both with and without the mutation (germline mosaicism; upper panel). However, if a mutation occurs in the four-cell embryo, the adult may also exhibit phenotypic features of the mutation in some but not all somatic tissues (somatic and germline mosaicism; middle panel). Finally, a mutation that occurs in a portion of the blastocyst or fetus that does not give rise to germ cells results only in somatic mosaicism (lower panel). (Adapted from Thompson MW et al: *Genetics in Medicine,* 5th ed. Saunders, 1991.)

have unfortunate consequences for patients and their families. Although genes were recognized and studied long before the structure of DNA was known, it has become common usage to regard a **gene** as a short stretch of DNA (usually but not always < 100 kb in length) that encodes a product (usually protein) responsible for a measurable trait. The **locus** is the place where a particular gene lies on its chromosome. A gene's DNA sequence nearly always shows slight differences when many unrelated individuals are compared, and the variant sequences are described as **alleles.** A **mutation** is a biochemical event such as a nucleotide change, deletion, or insertion that has produced a new allele. Many changes in the DNA sequence of a gene, such as those within introns or at the third "wobble" position of codons for particular amino acids, do not affect the structure or expression of the gene product; therefore, although all mutations result in a biochemical or molecular biologic phenotype—ie, a change in DNA—only some result in a clinically abnormal phenotype. The word **polymorphism** denotes an allele that is present in 1% or more of the population. At the biochemical level, polymorphic alleles are usually recognized by their effect on the size of a restriction fragment (**restriction fragment length polymorphism [RFLP]**), or the length of a short but highly repetitive region of DNA. On the other hand, at the clinical level, polymorphic alleles are recognized by their effect on a phenotype such as HLA type or hair color. The HLA system is an example where there are many polymorphic alleles; therefore, most individuals are heterozygous.

Finally, this discussion helps to illustrate the use of the word **phenotype,** which refers simply to any characteristic that can be described by an observer. Hair color is a phenotype readily apparent to a casual observer, whereas RFLPs are a phenotype that can only be detected with a laboratory test.

PENETRANCE & EXPRESSIVITY

It is an important principle of human genetics that two individuals with the same mutated gene may have different phenotypes. For example, in the autosomal dominant condition called type I osteogenesis imperfecta, pedigrees may occur in which there is both an affected grandparent and an affected grandchild even though the obligate carrier parent is asymptomatic (Figure 2–2). Given a set of defined criteria, recognition of the condition in individuals known to carry the mutated gene is described as **penetrance.** In other words, if seven out of ten individuals over age 40 with the type I osteogenesis imperfecta mutation have an abnormal bone density scan, the condition is said to be 70% penetrant by that criterion. Penetrance may vary both with age and according to the set of criteria being used; for example, type I osteogenesis imperfecta may be 90% penetrant at age 40 when the conclusion is based on a bone density scan in conjunction with laboratory tests for abnormal collagen synthesis. **Reduced penetrance** or **age-dependent penetrance** is a common feature of dominantly inherited conditions that have a relatively high **fitness** (likelihood of reproduction by the individual with the mutant allele), such as Huntington's disease or polycystic kidney disease.

Although the presence of a mutated gene can be observed in many individuals, their phenotypes may still be different. For example, blue scleras and lower than normal height may be the only manifestations of type I osteogenesis imperfecta in a particular individ-

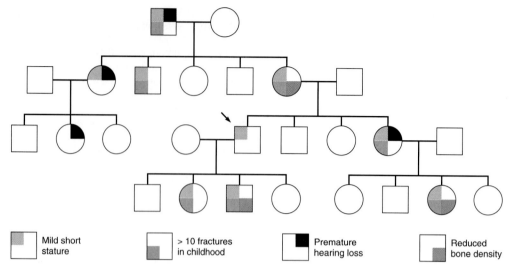

Figure 2–2. Penetrance and expressivity in type I osteogenesis imperfecta. In this schematic pedigree of the autosomal dominant condition type I osteogenesis imperfecta, nearly all of the affected individuals exhibit different phenotypic features that vary in severity (variable expressivity). As is shown, type I osteogenesis imperfecta is fully penetrant, since every individual who transmits the mutation is phenotypically affected to some degree. However, if mild short stature in the individual indicated with the arrow had been considered to be a normal variant, then the condition would have been nonpenetrant in this individual. Thus, in this example, judgments about penetrance or nonpenetrance depend on the criteria for normal and abnormal stature.

ual, while a sibling who carries the identical mutation may be confined to a wheelchair as a result of multiple fractures and deformities. The phenomenon of different phenotypes in these individuals is referred to as **variable expressivity.** Both reduced penetrance and variable expressivity occur in related individuals who carry the exact same mutated allele; therefore, phenotypic differences between these individuals must be due to the effects of other "modifier" genes, to environmental interactions, or to chance.

MECHANISMS OF MUTATION & INHERITANCE PATTERNS

Mutations can be characterized both by their molecular nature—nucleotide deletion, insertion, substitution—or by their effects on the gene product, ie, no effect (neutral), complete loss-of-function (amorphic), partial loss of function (hypomorphic), gain of function (hypermorphic), or acquisition of a new property (neomorphic). Geneticists who study experimental organisms frequently use specific deletions to ensure that a mutated allele causes a loss of function, but human geneticists rely on biochemical or cell culture studies. Amorphic and hypomorphic mutations are probably the most frequent type of mutation in human genetic disease because there are many ways to interfere with a protein's function.

For autosomal genes (those that lie on chromosomes 1–22), the fundamental difference between dominant and recessive inheritance is that with dominant inheritance, the disease state or trait being measured is apparent when one copy of the mutated allele and one copy of the normal allele are present. With recessive inheritance, two copies of the mutated allele must be present for the disease state or trait to be apparent. For genes that lie on the X chromosome, the same definitions apply to females (with two X chromosomes): A phenotype caused by one copy of a mutant gene is X-linked dominant; a phenotype caused by two copies is X-linked recessive. Because most mutations are amorphic or hypomorphic, however, one copy of an X-linked mutant allele in males is not "balanced" with a nonmutant allele, as it would be in females; therefore, one copy of an X-linked recessive gene is sufficient to produce a mutant phenotype in males.

Recessive Inheritance & Loss-of-Function Mutations

As mentioned above, most recessive mutations are due to a loss of function of the gene product, which can occur by a variety of different pathways, including failure of the gene to be transcribed or translated or failure of the translated gene product to function correctly. There are two general principles to keep in mind when considering loss-of-function mutations. First, because expression from the nonmutant allele usually does not change (ie, there is no **dosage com-**

pensation), gene expression in a heterozygous carrier of a loss-of-function allele is reduced to 50% of normal. Second, for most biochemical pathways, a 50% reduction in enzyme concentration is not sufficient to produce a disease state. Thus, most diseases due to enzyme deficiencies such as phenylketonuria (Table 2–2) are inherited in a recessive fashion.

Dominant Inheritance & Loss-of-Function Mutations

If 50% of a particular product is not enough for the cell or tissue to function normally, then a loss-of-function mutation in this gene will produce a dominantly inherited phenotype. Such mutations usually occur in structural proteins; the example we will consider below is type I osteogenesis imperfecta. Most dominantly inherited phenotypes are really **semi-dominant,** which means that two copies of the mutant allele produce a phenotype more severe than one mutant and one normal copy. However, for most dominantly inherited conditions, homozygous mutant individuals are rarely observed. For example, inheritance of achondroplasia, the most common genetic cause of very short stature, is usually described as autosomal dominant. However, rare matings between two affected individuals have a 25% probability of producing offspring with two copies of the mutant gene. This results in homozygous achondroplasia, a condition that is very severe and usually fatal in the perinatal period. Huntington's disease, a dominantly inherited neurologic disease, is the only known human condition in which the homozygous mutant phenotype is identical with the heterozygous mutant phenotype (sometimes referred to as a "true dominant").

Dominant Negative Mutations

A special kind of mutation referred to as a dominant negative occurs frequently in human diseases that involve polymeric structural proteins. In these disorders, the mutant allele gives rise to a structurally abnormal protein that interferes with the function of the normal allele. The presence of a dominant negative allele can be proved in experimental organisms by showing that one copy of the putative dominant negative allele has an effect similar to two copies of a loss-of-function allele. Such a mutation is said to

Table 2–2. Phenotype, genetic mechanism, and prevalence of selected genetic disorders.

Disorder	Phenotype	Genetic Mechanism	Prevalence
Down's syndrome	Mental and growth retardation, dysmorphic features, internal organ anomalies	Chromosomal imbalance caused by trisomy 21	≈ 1:800; increased risk with advanced maternal age
Fragile X-associated mental retardation	Mental retardation, characteristic facial features, large testes	X-linked; progressive expansion of unstable DNA causes failure to express gene encoding RNA-binding protein	≈ 1:1500 males; can be manifest in females; multistep mechanism
Sickle cell anemia	Recurrent painful crises, increased susceptibility to infections	Autosomal recessive; caused by a single missense mutation in beta globin	≈ 1:400 blacks
Cystic fibrosis	Recurrent pulmonary infections, exocrine pancreatic insufficiency, infertility	Autosomal recessive; caused by multiple loss-of-function mutations in a chloride channel	≈ 1:2000 whites; very rare in Asians
Neurofibromatosis	Multiple café au lait spots, neurofibromas, increased tumor susceptibility	Autosomal dominant; caused by multiple loss-of-function mutations in a signaling molecule	≈ 1:3000; about 50% are new mutations
Duchenne's muscular dystrophy	Muscular weakness and degeneration	X-linked recessive; caused by multiple loss-of-function mutations in a muscle protein	≈ 1:3000 males; about 33% are new mutations
Osteogenesis imperfecta	Increased susceptibility to fractures, connective tissue fragility	Phenotypically and genetically heterogeneous	≈ 1:10,000
Phenylketonuria	Mental and growth retardation	Autosomal recessive; caused by multiple loss-of-function mutations in phenylalanine hydroxylase	≈ 1:10,000

be "antimorphic." Note that any molecular lesion—eg, deletion, nonsense, missense, or splicing—can produce a loss-of-function allele. However, only molecular lesions that yield a protein product—eg, splicing, missense, or nonsense mutations—can result in a dominant negative allele. Type II osteogenesis imperfecta, described below, is an example of a dominant negative mutation.

The words "dominant" and "recessive" are sometimes used imprecisely. Mutations are simply molecular alterations in a strand of DNA and therefore, strictly speaking, are not in themselves dominant or recessive. The terms are instead appropriate to the *effect of a mutation* on a particular trait. Therefore, when a particular mutation is characterized as "recessive," one is referring to the effect of this mutation on the trait being studied.

THE PREVALENCE OF GENETIC DISEASE AND THE HUMAN GENOME PROJECT

Estimates of the total number of genes in the human genome are on the order of 60,000–80,000. However, only 5000 or so single-gene disorders have been recognized to cause a human disease. In considering possible explanations for this disparity, it seems likely that mutations of many single genes are lethal very early in development and thus not clinically apparent, whereas mutations in other genes do not cause an easily recognizable phenotype. In the general population, the overall frequency of disease attributable to defects in single genes—ie, mendelian disorders—is approximately 1%. However, because many genetic conditions are recessively inherited and because the rate for new deleterious mutations is relatively high—approximately 10^{-6}–10^{-5} per locus per generation—every individual in the population is estimated to carry four or five deleterious genes.

Table 2–2 lists the major symptoms, genetic mechanisms, and prevalence of the diseases considered in this chapter as well as of several others. The most common conditions, such as neurofibromatosis, cystic fibrosis, and fragile X-associated mental retardation syndrome, will be encountered at some time by most health care professionals regardless of their field of interest. Other conditions such as Huntington's disease and adenosine deaminase deficiency, while of intellectual and pathophysiologic interest, are unlikely to be seen by most practitioners.

Many common conditions such as atherosclerosis and breast cancer that do not show strictly mendelian inheritance patterns have a genetic component evident from familial aggregation or twin studies. These conditions are usually described as **multifactorial,** which means that the effects of one or more mutated genes and environmental differences all contribute to the likelihood that a given individual will manifest the phenotype.

The major goal of the Human Genome Project is to determine the entire 3 billion nucleotide sequence of the human genome by the year 2003. This collaborative international effort should provide a "dictionary" that lists every gene and will also provide valuable information about genetic differences in human populations that could influence susceptibility to multifactorial diseases. Genetic differences are likely to be a major determinant of susceptibility to conditions such as diabetes, hypertension, and schizophrenia. Genetic differences may also help identify subgroups of patients whose course is likely to be more or less severe and who may respond to a particular treatment. A useful analogy is the application of sophisticated histologic and pathologic techniques to categorization of types of leukemia, which helps to determine the best therapeutic regimen for a particular subtype. An important objective of the Human Genome Project is to identify ways of classifying common diseases based on underlying genetic differences and to use this information to guide treatment.

ISSUES IN CLINICAL GENETICS

Most patients with genetic disease present during early childhood with symptoms that ultimately give rise to a diagnosis such as fragile X-associated mental retardation or Down's syndrome. The major clinical issues at presentation are arriving at the correct diagnosis and counseling the patient and family regarding the natural history and prognosis of the condition. One of the most important questions is the likelihood that the same condition will occur again in the family and whether it can be diagnosed prenatally. These issues are the subject matter of genetic counseling by a medical geneticist and a trained genetic counselor.

Currently, only a few genetic conditions such as phenylketonuria and some forms of maple syrup urine disease can be treated effectively. Efforts are under way, however, to develop treatments for some of the more common single-gene disorders such as Duchenne's muscular dystrophy, cystic fibrosis, and hemophilia. Some forms of therapy are directed at replacing the mutant protein, while others are directed at ameliorating its effects.

---

1. Define gene, locus, allele, mutation, polymorphism, and phenotype.
2. How is it possible for two individuals with the same mutated gene to have differences in penetrance and expressivity?
3. How many genes are in the human genome? How many single gene disorders have been recognized clinically?

PATHOPHYSIOLOGY OF SELECTED GENETIC DISEASES

OSTEOGENESIS IMPERFECTA

Osteogenesis imperfecta is a condition inherited in a mendelian fashion that illustrates many principles of human genetics. It is a heterogeneous and pleiotropic group of disorders characterized by a tendency toward fragility of bone. Advances in the last decade demonstrate that virtually every case is caused by a mutation of the *COL1A1* or *COL1A2* genes, which encode the subunits of type I collagen, $\alpha 1(I)$ and $\alpha 2(I)$, respectively. More than 100 different mutant alleles have been described for osteogenesis imperfecta; the relationships between different DNA sequence alterations and the type of disease (genotype-phenotype correlations) illustrate several pathophysiologic principles in human genetics.

Clinical Manifestations

The clinical and genetic characteristics of four clinical subtypes of osteogenesis imperfecta are summarized in Table 2–3. The timing and severity of fractures, the radiologic findings, the presence of additional clinical features, and the family history are used to discriminate among the different subtypes. Individuals with type I or type IV osteogenesis imperfecta present in early childhood with one or a few fractures of long bones in response to minimal or no trauma; x-rays reveal mild osteopenia, little or no bony deformity, and often evidence of earlier subclinical fractures. However, most individuals with type I or type IV osteogenesis imperfecta do not have fractures in utero. Type I and type IV osteogenesis imperfecta are distinguished by the severity (less in type I than in type IV) and by scleral hue, which indicates the thickness of this tissue and the deposition of type I collagen. Individuals with type I osteogenesis imperfecta have blue scleras, while the scleras of those with type IV are normal or slightly gray. In type I, the typical number of fractures during childhood is 10–20; fracture incidence decreases after puberty, and the main features in adult life are mild short stature, a tendency toward conductive hearing loss, and occasionally dentinogenesis imperfecta. Individuals with type IV osteogenesis imperfecta generally experience more fractures than those with type I and have significant short stature due to a combination of long bone and spinal deformities, but they often are able to walk independently. Approximately one-fourth of the cases of type I or type IV osteogenesis imperfecta will represent new mutations; in the remainder, the history and examination of other family members will reveal findings consistent with autosomal dominant inheritance.

Type II osteogenesis imperfecta presents at or before birth (diagnosed by prenatal ultrasound) with multiple fractures, bony deformities, increased fragility of nonbony connective tissue, and blue scleras and usually results in death in infancy. Two typical radiologic findings are the presence of isolated "islands" of mineralization in the skull (wormian bones) and a beaded appearance to the ribs. Nearly all cases of type II osteogenesis imperfecta represent a new dominant mutation, and there is no family history. Death usually results from respiratory difficulties.

Table 2–3. Clinical and molecular subtypes of osteogenesis imperfecta.

Type	Phenotype	Genetics	Molecular Pathophysiology
Type I	Mild: Short stature, postnatal fractures, little or no deformity, blue scleras, premature hearing loss	Autosomal dominant	Loss-of-function mutation in pro$\alpha 1(I)$ chain resulting in decreased amount of mRNA; quality of collagen is normal; quantity is reduced twofold
Type II	Perinatal lethal: Severe prenatal fractures, abnormal bone formation, severe deformities, blue scleras, connective tissue fragility	Sporadic (autosomal dominant)	Structural mutation in pro$\alpha 1(I)$ or pro$\alpha 2(I)$ chain that slows heterotrimer assembly; quality of collagen is abnormal; quantity often reduced also
Type III	Progressive deforming: Prenatal fractures, deformities usually present at birth, very short stature, usually nonambulatory, blue scleras, hearing loss	Autosomal dominant (rare cases autosomal recessive)	Structural mutation in pro$\alpha 1(I)$ or pro$\alpha 2(I)$ chain that has mild or no effect on heterotrimer assembly; quality of collagen is mildly abnormal; quantity can be normal
Type IV	Deforming with normal scleras: Postnatal fractures, mild to moderate deformities, premature hearing loss, normal or gray scleras, dentinogenesis imperfecta	Autosomal dominant	Structural mutation in pro$\alpha 2(I)$ chain that has little or no effect on heterotrimer assembly; quality of collagen is mildly abnormal; quantity can be normal

Type III osteogenesis imperfecta presents at birth or in infancy with progressive bony deformities, multiple fractures, and blue scleras. It is intermediate in severity between types II and IV; most affected individuals will require multiple corrective surgeries and lose the ability to ambulate by early adulthood. Unlike other forms of osteogenesis imperfecta, which are nearly always due to mutations that act dominantly, type III can be inherited in either a dominant or recessive fashion. From a biochemical and molecular perspective, type III osteogenesis imperfecta is the least well understood form.

Although different subtypes of osteogenesis imperfecta can often be distinguished biochemically, the classification presented in Table 2–3 is clinical rather than molecular, and the disease phenotypes for each subtype show a spectrum of severities that overlap one another. For example, a few individuals diagnosed with type II osteogenesis imperfecta based on the presence of severe bony deformities in utero will survive for many years and thus overlap the type III subtype. Similarly, some individuals with type IV osteogenesis imperfecta may have fractures in utero and develop deformities that lead to loss of ambulation. Distinguishing this presentation from type III osteogenesis imperfecta may only be possible if other affected family members exhibit a milder course.

This discussion illustrates that clinical classifications are often somewhat arbitrary. Nonetheless, this approach is helpful for most affected individuals in predicting the course and inheritance pattern of the illness and can serve also as a framework within which to correlate molecular abnormalities with disease phenotypes.

Pathophysiology

Osteogenesis imperfecta is a disease of type I collagen, which constitutes the major extracellular protein in the body. It is the major collagen in the dermis, the connective tissue capsules of most organs, and the vascular and gastrointestinal adventitia and is the only collagen in bone. A mature type I collagen fibril is a rigid structure that contains multiple type I collagen molecules packed in a staggered array and stabilized by intermolecular covalent cross-links. Each mature type I collagen molecule contains two $\alpha1$ chains and one $\alpha2$ chain, encoded by the COL1A1 and COL1A2 genes, respectively (Figure 2–3). These chains are synthesized as larger precursors with amino and carboxyl terminal "propeptide" extensions, assemble with each other inside the cell, and are ultimately secreted as a heterotrimeric type I procollagen molecule. During intracellular assembly, the three chains wind around each other in a triple helix which is stabilized by interchain interactions between hydroxyproline and adjacent carbonyl residues. There is a dynamic relationship between the posttranslational action of prolyl hydroxylase and assembly of the triple helix, which begins at the carboxyl terminal end of the molecule. Increased levels of hydroxylation result in a more stable helix, but helix formation prevents further prolyl hydroxylation.

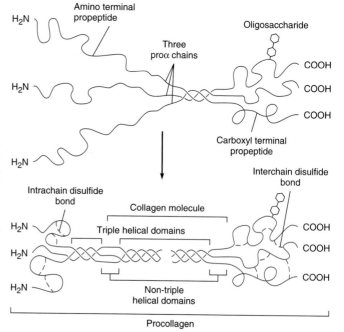

Figure 2–3. Molecular assembly of type I procollagen. Type I procollagen is assembled in the endoplasmic reticulum from three proα chains that associate with each other beginning at their carboxyl terminals. An important requirement for proper assembly of the triple helix is the presence of a glycine residue at every third position in each of the proα chains. After secretion, the amino and carboxyl terminal propeptides are proteolytically cleaved, leaving a rigid triple helical collagen molecule with very short non-triple helical domains at both ends. (Reproduced, with permission, from Alberts BA: *Molecular Biology of the Cell,* 3rd ed. Garland, 1994.)

The nature of the triple helix causes the side chain of every third amino acid to point inward, and steric constraints allow only a proton in this position. Thus, the amino acid sequence of virtually all collagen chains in the triple helical portion is $(Gly-X-Y)_n$, where Y is proline about one-third of the time.

The fundamental defect in nearly all individuals with type I osteogenesis imperfecta is reduced synthesis of type I collagen due to loss-of-function mutations in *COL1A1*. Biochemical measurements of chain synthesis show that the mutant *COL1A1* allele produces little or no detectable proα1(I) mRNA, corresponding to a hypomorphic or amorphic mutation, respectively. Because the nonmutant *COL1A1* allele continues to produce mRNA at a normal rate (ie, there is no dosage compensation), an amorphic mutation results in a 50% reduction in the rate of proα1(I) mRNA synthesis, while a hypomorphic mutation results in a less severe reduction. Although three proα1(I) peptide chains can assemble into a stable trimer, molecules that contain one proα1(I) and two proα2(I) chains do not assemble. Thus, a reduced concentration of proα1(I) chains limits the production of type I procollagen, and the consequences of a hypomorphic or amorphic *COL1A1* mutation are (1) a reduced amount of structurally normal type I collagen and (2) an excess of unassembled proα2(I) chains, which are degraded inside the cell (Figure 2–4).

The molecular defects responsible for *COL1A1* mutations in type I osteogenesis imperfecta have not been identified. By analogy with other systems, possible lesions include alterations in a regulatory region leading to reduced transcription or splicing abnormalities leading to reduced steady state levels of RNA. Deletion of the entire *COL1A1* gene would also cause an amorphic mutation, but this possibility has been ruled out in every case of type I osteogenesis imperfecta examined to date.

In contrast to type I osteogenesis imperfecta, type I collagen produced by patients with perinatal lethal (type II) osteogenesis imperfecta is structurally ab-

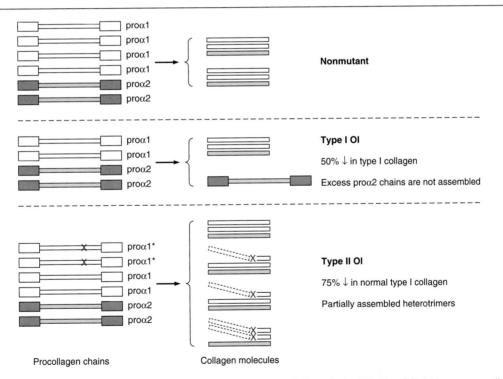

Figure 2–4. Molecular pathogenesis of type I and type II osteogenesis imperfecta (OI). The *COL1A1* gene normally produces twice as many proα chains as the *COL1A2* gene. Therefore, in nonmutant cells, the ratio of proα1 to proα2 chains is 2:1, which corresponds to the ratio of α1 and α2 chains in intact collagen molecules. In type I osteogenesis imperfecta, a mutation in one of the *COL1A1* alleles results in failure to produce proα1 chains, leading to a 50% reduction in the total number of proα1 chains, a 50% reduction in the production of intact type I collagen molecules, and an excess of unassembled proα2 chains, which are degraded inside the cell. In type II osteogenesis imperfecta, a mutation in one of the *COL1A1* alleles results in a structural alteration that blocks triple helix formation and secretion of partially assembled collagen molecules containing the mutant chain. (Adapted from Thompson MW et al: *Genetics in Medicine,* 5th ed. Saunders, 1991.)

normal and can be caused by defects in both *COL1A1* and *COL1A2*. Most of the actual mutations are simple DNA sequence alterations, but the effects on the peptide chain fall into two very different categories. Some type II osteogenesis imperfecta mutations affect the protein-coding sequence, in which case they usually result in an amino acid substitution at one of the conserved glycine residues within the triple helix (Figure 2–5). Other type II osteogenesis imperfecta mutations lie at intron-exon borders, in which case splicing abnormalities usually cause several internal exons to be excluded from the mature mRNA, leading to a severely shortened peptide chain.

An important principle apparent from biochemical studies of type II osteogenesis imperfecta is that in every case, the mutant peptide chain can bind to normal chains in the initial steps of trimer assembly (Figure 2–4). However, triple helix formation is ineffective, either because amino acids with large side chains are substituted for glycine or because alterations in the length of the mutant chain lead to abnormal interchain interactions. Ineffective triple helix formation leads to increased posttranslational modification by prolyl hydroxylase and a reduced rate of secretion. These appear to be critical events in the cellular pathogenesis of type II osteogenesis imperfecta, since glycine substitutions toward the carboxyl terminal end of the molecule are generally more severe than those at the amino terminal (Figure 2–5).

A second important principle apparent from these studies is that the effects of an amino acid substitution in a proα1(I) peptide chain are amplified at the levels of both triple helix assembly and fibril formation. Because every type I procollagen molecule has two proα1(I) chains, only 25% of type I procollagen molecules will contain two normal proα1(I) chains even though only one of the two *COL1A1* alleles is mutated. Furthermore, because each molecule in a fibril interacts with several others, incorporation of an abnormal molecule can have disproportionate effects on fibril structure and integrity. Because this phenotype is similar to that predicted for a homozygous *COL1A1* loss-of-function mutation, type II osteogenesis imperfecta provides a clinical example of "dominant negative" gene action.

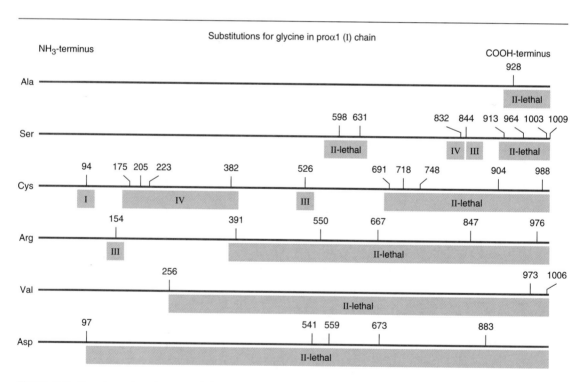

Figure 2–5. Genotype phenotype correlations for glycine substitutions in osteogenesis imperfecta. Many cases of osteogenesis imperfecta are caused by missense mutations in *COL1A1* that result in substitutions of the glycine residue conserved at every third position in the triple helix. In general, substitutions of amino acids with bulky side chains like Asp and Arg are more severe than substitutions of amino acids with smaller side chains like Ser and Ala. Because assembly of the triple helix proceeds from the carboxyl terminal, the phenotypic effect of substitutions generally correlates with their distance from the amino terminal. (Reproduced, with permission, from Thompson MW et al: *Genetics in Medicine,* 5th ed. Saunders, 1991.)

Collagen mutations that cause type III and type IV osteogenesis imperfecta are diverse and include glycine substitutions in the amino terminal portion of the collagen triple helix, a few internal deletions of *COL1A1* and *COL1A2* that do not significantly disturb triple helix formation, and some unusual alterations in the non-triple helical extensions at the amino and carboxyl terminals of proα chains.

Genetic Principles

Inheritance of type I and type IV osteogenesis imperfecta is autosomal dominant. However, the high frequency of new mutations (approximately 25%) and the multitude of molecular lesions that can produce a hypomorphic or an amorphic allele suggest that most families with type I osteogenesis imperfecta will have different molecular lesions in *COL1A1*. As a practical consequence of **allelic heterogeneity,** molecular diagnosis based on a particular DNA sequence abnormality is unfeasible, since both *COL1A1* alleles would need to be sequenced in every individual at risk. Some attempts have been made to develop an efficient test for type I osteogenesis imperfecta based on measurements of *COL1A1* mRNA levels. In some situations, a diagnostic approach based on linkage analysis is possible. For example, in a family in which type I osteogenesis imperfecta is known to segregate based on clinical and biochemical studies, it is usually possible to distinguish between chromosomes that carry the mutant and nonmutant alleles using closely linked DNA-based polymorphisms even though the actual *COL1A1* molecular defect is not known. Once this information is established for a particular family, inheritance of the mutant allele can be predicted in future pregnancies. A similar approach is more difficult to apply for type IV osteogenesis imperfecta. In contrast to type I, in which nearly all cases are caused by defective *COL1A1* alleles, mutations of both *COL1A1* and *COL1A2* can cause type IV osteogenesis imperfecta. As a consequence of this **genetic heterogeneity,** the type IV osteogenesis imperfecta phenotype could be linked to two different chromosomal locations.

For both type I and type IV osteogenesis imperfecta, the most important question in the clinical setting often relates to the natural history of the illness. For example, reproductive decision making in families at risk for osteogenesis imperfecta is influenced greatly by the relative likelihood of producing a child who will never ambulate and require multiple orthopedic operations versus a child whose major problems will be a few long bone fractures and an increased risk of hearing loss. As evident from the discussion above, both different mutant genes and different mutant alleles—as well as other genes that modify the osteogenesis imperfecta phenotype—can all contribute to this **phenotypic heterogeneity.** When allelic rather than genetic heterogeneity is op-

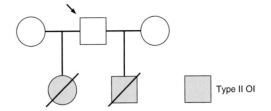

Figure 2–6. Gonadal mosaicism for type II osteogenesis imperfecta. In this idealized pedigree, the phenotypically normal father (indicated with the arrow) has had two children by different mates, each of whom is affected with autosomal dominant type II osteogenesis imperfecta. Analysis of the father showed that some of his spermatozoa carried a *COL1A1* mutation, indicating that the explanation for this unusual pedigree is germline mosaicism. (Adapted from Cohn DH et al: Recurrence of lethal osteogenesis imperfecta due to parental mosaicism for a dominant mutation in a human type I collagen gene [*COL1A1*]. Am J Hum Genet 1990;46:591.)

erative, as in type I osteogenesis imperfecta, comparison of interfamilial to intrafamilial variability allows one to assess the relative contribution of different mutant alleles to phenotypic heterogeneity. For most genetic diseases, including type I osteogenesis imperfecta, intrafamilial variability is less than interfamilial variability.

In type II osteogenesis imperfecta, a single copy of the mutant allele causes the abnormal phenotype and therefore has a dominant mechanism of action. Although the type II phenotype itself is never inherited, there are rare situations in which a phenotypically normal individual will harbor a *COL1A1* mutant allele among his or her germ cells. These individuals with so-called **gonadal mosaicism** can produce multiple offspring with type II osteogenesis imperfecta (Figure 2–6), a pattern of segregation that can be confused with recessive inheritance. In fact, many other mutations, including Duchenne's muscular dystrophy, which is X-linked, and type 1 neurofibromatosis, which is autosomal dominant, also occasionally show unusual inheritance patterns explained by gonadal mosaicism.

---

4. When and how does type II osteogenesis imperfecta present? To what do these individuals succumb?
5. What are two typical radiologic findings in type II osteogenesis imperfecta?
6. Describe the pathophysiology of type II osteogenesis imperfecta and explain how it is an example of "dominant negative" gene action.

FRAGILE X-ASSOCIATED MENTAL RETARDATION

Fragile X-associated mental retardation syndrome produces a unique combination of phenotypic features that affect the central nervous system, the testes, and the cranial skeleton. These features were recognized as a distinct clinical entity more than 50 years ago. A laboratory test for the syndrome was developed during the 1970s, when it was recognized that most affected individuals exhibit a cytogenetic abnormality of the X chromosome—failure of the region between bands Xq27 and Xq28 to condense at metaphase. Instead, this region appears in the microscope as a thin constriction that is subject to breakage during preparation, which accounts for the designation "fragile X." Advances in the past decade have helped to explain both the presence of the fragile site and the unique pattern of inheritance exhibited by the syndrome. In some respects, fragile X-associated mental retardation syndrome is similar to other genetic conditions caused by X-linked mutations—affected males are impaired more severely than affected females, and the condition is never transmitted from father to son. However, the syndrome "breaks the rules" of mendelian transmission in that at least 20% of carrier males manifest no signs of it. Daughters of these nonpenetrant but "transmitting males" are themselves nonpenetrant but produce affected offspring, male and female, with frequencies close to mendelian expectations (Figure 2–7). About a third of "carrier" females (those with one normal and one abnormal X chromosome) exhibit a significant degree of mental retardation. These unusual features of the syndrome were explained when the subchromosomal region spanning the fragile site was isolated and shown to contain a segment in which the triplet sequence CGG was repeated many times, $(CGG)_n$. Slight amplification in the number of triplet repeats is a rare occurrence but does not cause a clinical phenotype or a cytogenetic fragile site and therefore is described as a "premutation." However, after transmission through the female germline, this slightly lengthened segment nearly always exhibits additional amplification to a "full mutation," which results in the typical features of the syndrome (Figures 2–8 and 2–9).

Clinical Manifestations

Fragile X-associated mental retardation (FMR) syndrome is usually recognized in affected boys because of developmental delay apparent by 1–2 years

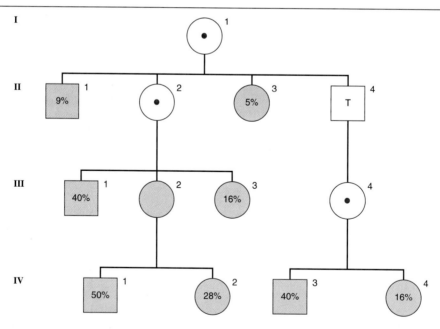

Figure 2–7. Likelihood of fragile X-associated mental retardation syndrome in an artificial pedigree. The percentages shown indicate the likelihood of clinical manifestation according to position in the pedigree. Because individuals carrying the abnormal X chromosome have a 50% chance of passing it to their offspring, penetrance is twice that of the values depicted. Penetrance increases with each successive generation owing to the progressive expansion of a triplet repeat element (see text). Expansion is dependent on maternal inheritance of the abnormal allele; thus, daughters of normal transmitting males (indicated with a T in II-4) are nonpenetrant. (Reproduced, with permission, from Scriver CR et al [editors]: *The Metabolic and Molecular Bases of Inherited Disease,* 7th ed. McGraw-Hill, 1995.)

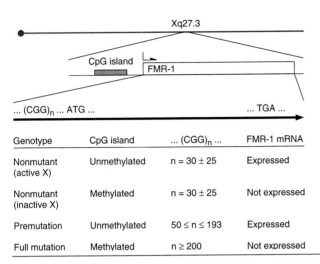

Figure 2–8. Molecular genetics of fragile X-associated mental retardation syndrome. The cytogenetic fragile site at Xq27.3 is located close to a small region of DNA that contains a CpG island (see text) and the *FMR1* gene. Within the 5′ untranslated region of the *FMR1* gene lies an unstable segment of repetitive DNA 5′-(CGG)$_n$-3′. The table shows the methylation status of the CpG island, the size of the triplet repeat, and whether the FMR1 mRNA is expressed depending on the genotype of the X chromosome. Note that the inactive X chromosome in nonmutant females has a methylated CpG island and does not express the FMR1 mRNA. The methylation and expression status of *FMR1* in premutation and full mutation alleles applies to males and to the active X chromosome of females; premutation and full mutation alleles on the inactive X chromosome of females will exhibit methylation of the CpG island and fail to express the FMR1 mRNA.

of age, small joint hyperextensibility, mild hypotonia, and a family history of mental retardation in maternally related males. Affected females generally have either mild mental retardation or only subtle impairments of visuospatial ability, and the condition may not be evident or diagnosed until it is suspected following identification of an affected male relative.

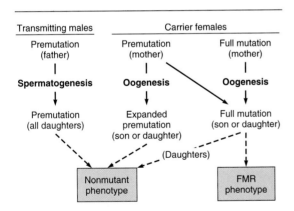

Figure 2–9. Transmission and amplification of the fragile X-associated mental retardation triplet repeat. The heavy arrows show expansion of the triplet repeat, which is thought to occur postzygotically after the premutation or full mutation is transmitted through the female germline. The dashed arrows represent potential phenotypic consequences. Daughters with the full mutation may not express the fragile X-associated mental retardation phenotype, depending on the proportion of cells in which the mutant allele happens to lie on the inactive X chromosome. (Adapted from Tarleton JC, Saul RA: Molecular genetic advances in fragile X syndrome. J Pediatr 1993;122:169.)

In late childhood or early adolescence, affected males begin to exhibit large testes and characteristic facial features that include mild coarsening, large ears, a prominent forehead and mandible, a long face, and relative macrocephaly (considered in relation to height). The syndrome is extremely common and affects about 1:1500–1:1000 males. Virtually all affected males are born to females who are either affected or carry the premutation, and there are no well-recognized cases of new premutations in males or females.

The inheritance of FMR syndrome exhibits several unusual features and is most easily described in terms of empiric risk figures (Figure 2–9). In particular, the likelihood that an individual carrying an abnormal chromosome will manifest clinical features depends on the number of generations through which the abnormal chromosome has been transmitted and the sex of the transmitting parent. For example, nonpenetrant "transmitting" males tend to occur in the same sibship with each other and with nonpenetrant carrier females. This is reflected in low risk figures for brothers and sisters of transmitting males—9% and 5%, respectively, compared with 40% and 8% for their maternal grandsons and granddaughters. This latter observation, in which the penetrance or expressivity (or both) of a genetic disease seems to increase in successive generations, is sometimes referred to more generally as **genetic anticipation.**

Genetic anticipation in fragile X-associated mental retardation is caused by progressive expansion of the triplet repeat. A similar phenomenon occurs in several neurodegenerative disorders such as Huntington's disease and spinocerebellar ataxia, ie, grandchildren are affected more severely than grandparents. The neurodegenerative disorders are caused by production of abnormal proteins; fragile X-associated mental retardation is caused by failure to produce a normal protein. Although the biochemical mechanisms are different, the underlying molecular causes of genetic anticipation are identical and involve progressive expansion of an unstable triplet repeat.

In addition to triplet repeat expansion, genetic anticipation can be caused by **bias of ascertainment,** which occurs when a mild or variably expressed condition first diagnosed in grandchildren from a three-generation pedigree is then easily recognized in siblings of the grandchildren who are available for examination and testing. In contrast to genetic anticipation caused by expansion of a triplet repeat, anticipation caused by bias of ascertainment affects the *apparent* rather than the actual penetrance.

Pathophysiology

Amplification of the $(CGG)_n$ repeat at the fraXq27.3 site affects both methylation and expression of the *FMR1* gene. This gene and the unstable DNA responsible for the expansion were isolated on the basis of their proximity to the cytogenetic fragile site in Xq27.3. *FMR1* encodes an RNA-binding protein that is one of a large group of related proteins involved in the processing or transport of nuclear mRNA precursors. It is possible that the FMR1 protein fulfills a general role in the cellular metabolism of nuclear RNA, but only in the tissues in which it is primarily expressed—the central nervous system and the testes.

The $(CGG)_n$ repeat is located in the 5′ untranslated region of the *FMR1* gene (Figure 2–8). This segment is highly variable in length; the number of repeats, n, is equal to about 30 ± 25 in individuals who are neither affected with nor carriers for the FMR syndrome. In transmitting males and in unaffected carrier females, the number of repeats may range from 52 to 193 and is usually between 70 and 100. Remarkably, alleles with less than 50 repeats are very stable and almost always transmitted without a change in repeat number. However, alleles with more than 52 repeats are unstable and often exhibit expansion after maternal transmission; thus, individuals with 52–193 repeats do not exhibit the FMR phenotype but are said to carry a **premutation.** The degree of expansion is related to the number of repeats; premutation alleles with a repeat number less than 60 rarely are amplified to a full mutation, but premutation alleles with a repeat number greater than 90 are almost always amplified to a full mutation. The number of repeats in the full mutation—observed both in affected males and in affected females—is always greater than 200 but is generally heterogeneous, suggesting that once this threshold is reached, additional amplification occurs frequently in somatic cells.

Expansion from a premutation to a full mutation has two important effects: *FMR1* gene transcription is shut off, and DNA surrounding the transcriptional start site of the *FMR1* gene becomes methylated. The clinical phenotype is caused by failure to produce *FMR1;* in addition, methylation of surrounding DNA has important implications for molecular diagnosis. Methylation occurs in a so-called **CpG island,** a several hundred base-pair segment just upstream of the FMR1 transcriptional start site that contains a high frequency of 5′CpG3′ dinucleotides compared with the rest of the genome. Methylation of the CpG island and expansion of the triplet repeat can be easily detected with molecular biologic techniques and are the basis of the common diagnostic tests for individuals at risk.

Genetic Principles

In addition to the tendency of $(5'CGG3')_n$ premutation alleles to undergo further amplifications in length, the molecular genetics of fragile X-associated mental retardation syndrome exhibits several unusual features. As described above, each phenotypically affected individual carries a full mutation defined by a repeat number greater than 200, but the exact repeat number exhibits considerable heterogeneity in different cells and tissues.

For example, diagnostic testing for the number of CGG repeats is usually performed on approximately 10^7 lymphocytes taken from a small amount of peripheral blood. In individuals who carry a repeat number less than 50, each of the 10^7 cells has the same number of repeats. However, in phenotypically affected males or females, ie, those with a repeat number greater than 200, many of the 10^7 cells may have a different number of repeats. This situation, often referred to as **somatic mosaicism,** indicates that at least some of the amplification is **postzygotic,** meaning that it occurs in cells of the developing embryo after fertilization. Surprisingly, when the repeat number present in sperm DNA was examined in several affected individuals, only premutation alleles were found—even though each individual had a range of full mutation alleles present in their lymphocytes. Mature spermatozoa do not arise until after puberty, but their precursors—the **primordial germ cells**—are allocated early in development around the time of implantation and are segregated from other cells of the embryo. Thus, it is possible that expansion from a premutation to a full mutation is exclusively postzygotic and occurs only in parts of the embryo that do not give rise to primordial germ cells. In this case, the difference between individuals who carry premutation and those who carry full mutation alleles would derive not from the number of repeats on the allele they inherit but from what happens to that allele after fertilization.

In addition to the DNA methylation associated with an abnormal *FMR1* gene, methylation of many genes is a normal process during development and differentiation that helps to regulate gene expression. Cells in which a particular gene should not be expressed frequently shut off that gene's expression by methylation. For example, globin should be expressed only in reticulocytes; albumin should be expressed only in hepatocytes; and insulin should be expressed only by pancreatic B cells. During gametogenesis and immediately following fertilization, specific patterns of methylation characteristic of differentiated cells are erased, only to be reestablished in fetal development. Thus, methylation provides a reversible change in gene structure that can be inherited during mitosis of differentiated cells yet erased during meiosis and early development. This type of alteration—a heritable phenotypic change that is not determined by DNA sequence—is broadly referred to as **epigenetic.**

Analysis of FMR pedigrees reveals that one of the most important factors influencing whether a premutation allele is subject to postzygotic expansion is the sex of the parent who transmits the premutation allele (Figures 2–7 and 2–9). As discussed above, a premutation allele transmitted by a female expands to a full mutation with a likelihood proportionate to the length of the premutation. Premutation alleles with a repeat number between 52 and 60 rarely expand to a full mutation, and those with a repeat number greater than 90 nearly always expand. In contrast, a premutation allele transmitted by a male rarely if ever expands to a full mutation regardless of the length of the repeat number. The concept that alleles of the same DNA sequence can behave very differently depending on the sex of the parent who transmitted them is an example of **parental imprinting.** It is thought to be caused by biochemical modifications to the chromosome such as methylation that occur during gametogenesis and that do not affect the actual DNA sequence but which can be stably transmitted for a certain number of cell divisions.

The high incidence of the fragile X-associated mental retardation syndrome—approximately 1:1000 males—is paradoxic given that affected individuals almost never reproduce. From the standpoint of population genetics, the relative probability—compared with the general population—of transmitting one's genes to the next generation is called **fitness.** For this syndrome, fitness is almost nil. Reduced fitness exhibited by many genetic conditions such as Duchenne's muscular dystrophy or type 1 neurofibromatosis is balanced by an appreciable **new mutation rate,** so that the incidence of the condition remains constant in successive generations. In fragile X-associated mental retardation syndrome, however, family studies have failed to identify any cases of a new premutation. For recessive conditions (both autosomal and X-linked), another factor that can influence disease incidence is whether heterozygous carriers experience a selective advantage or disadvantage compared with homozygous nonmutant individuals. For example, the relatively high incidence of sickle cell anemia in West Africa is thought to be due in part to **heterozygote advantage** conferring resistance to malaria. It is possible that the high incidence of fragile X-associated mental retardation syndrome is due in part to a selective advantage of premutation carriers. A final alternative likely to contribute to the high incidence of the syndrome is the **founder effect,** ie, the high frequency of a premutation allele that occurs by chance in a population founded by a small number of ancestors. Evidence for a founder effect in the fragile X-associated mental retardation syndrome is based on the observation that rare molecular polymorphisms close to the *FMR1* gene are found in association with premutation alleles more frequently than expected by chance. This situation is called **linkage disequilibrium** and is said to occur when the frequency of chromosomes that carry two distinct but genetically linked loci at the same time is significantly different from the product of their individual frequencies. Stated another way, fragile X-associated mental retardation syndrome and a closely linked locus A are in linkage disequilibrium if the frequency distribution of alleles at locus A is different depending on whether or not the chromosome carries an *FMR1* mutation.

---

7. How common is fragile X syndrome, and what is the phenotype of patients with fragile X syndrome?
8. What is genetic anticipation? What are two explanations for it?
9. What are the roles of parental imprinting and linkage disequilibrium in the molecular pathophysiology of fragile X syndrome?

DOWN'S SYNDROME

The clinical features of Down's syndrome were described over a century ago. Although the underlying cause—an extra copy of chromosome 21—has been known for more than 3 decades, the relationship of genotype to phenotype is just beginning to be understood, and many questions about the molecular pathophysiology of the condition have not yet been answered. Down's syndrome is broadly representative of **aneuploid** conditions, or those that are caused by a deviation from the normal chromosome complement (**euploidy**). Chromosome 21, which contains a little less than 2% of the total genome, is one of the **acrocentric** autosomes (the others are 13, 14, 15, and 22), which means one in which nearly all the DNA lies on one side of the centromere. In general, aneuploidy may involve part or all of an autosome or sex chromosome. Most individuals with Down's syndrome have 47 chromosomes (ie, one extra chromosome 21, or **trisomy 21**) and are born to parents with normal karyotypes. This type of aneuploidy is usu-

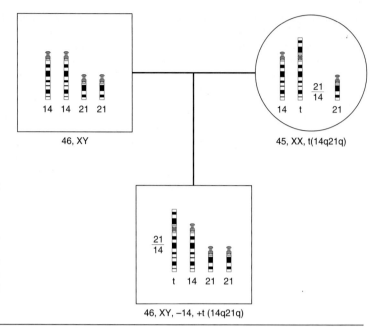

Figure 2–10. Mechanisms leading to Down's syndrome. A pedigree in which the mother is phenotypically normal yet is a balanced carrier for a 14;21 Robertsonian translocation. She transmits both the translocation chromosome and a normal chromosome 21 to her son, who also inherits a normal chromosome 21 from his father. Three copies of chromosome 21 in the son cause Down's syndrome. (Adapted from Thompson MW et al: *Genetics in Medicine,* 5th ed. Saunders, 1991.)

ally caused by **nondisjunction** during meiotic segregation, which means failure of two homologous chromosomes to separate (disjoin) from each other at anaphase. In contrast, aneuploid conditions that affect part of an autosome or sex chromosome must, at some point, involve DNA breakage and reunion. DNA rearrangements are an infrequent but important cause of Down's syndrome and are usually evident as a karyotype with 46 chromosomes in which one chromosome 21 is fused via its centromere to another acrocentric chromosome. This abnormal chromosome is described as a **Robertsonian translocation** and can sometimes be inherited from a carrier parent (Figure 2–10). Thus, Down's syndrome may be caused by a variety of different karyotypic abnormalities, which have in common a 50% increase in **gene dosage** for nearly all of the genes on chromosome 21.

Clinical Manifestations

Down's syndrome occurs approximately once in every 700 live births and accounts for approximately one-third of all cases of mental retardation. The likelihood of conceiving a child with Down's syndrome is related exponentially to increasing maternal age. However, screening programs detect most Down's syndrome pregnancies in pregnant women over 35 years of age (Figure 2–11). This fact, combined with the inverse relationship of maternal age to overall birth rate, means that most children with Down's syndrome are now born to women under 35 years of age. The condition is usually suspected in the perinatal period from the presence of characteristic facial and dysmorphic features such as brachycephaly, epi-

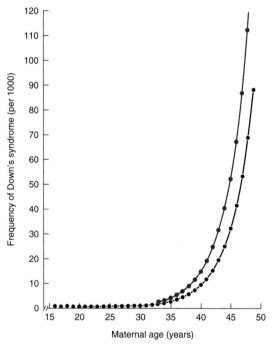

Figure 2–11. Relationship of Down's syndrome to maternal age. The frequency of Down's syndrome rises exponentially with increasing maternal age. The frequency at amniocentesis (brown symbols) is slightly higher than in liveborn infants (black symbols) because miscarriages are more likely in fetuses with Down's syndrome. (Data from Scriver CR et al [editors]: *The Metabolic and Molecular Bases of Inherited Disease,* 7th ed. McGraw-Hill, 1995.)

canthal folds, small ears, transverse palmar creases, and hypotonia (Table 2-4). Approximately 50% of affected children have congenital heart defects that come to medical attention in the immediate perinatal period because of cardiorespiratory problems. Strong suspicion of the condition on clinical grounds is usually confirmed by karyotyping within 2–3 days.

A great many minor and major abnormalities occur with increased frequency in Down's syndrome, yet two affected individuals rarely have the same set of abnormalities, and many single abnormalities can be seen in unaffected individuals. For example, the incidence of a transverse palmar crease in Down's syndrome is about 50%, ten times that in the general population, yet most individuals in whom transverse palmar creases are the only unusual feature do not have Down's syndrome or any other genetic disease.

The natural history of Down's syndrome in childhood is characterized mainly by developmental delay, growth retardation, and immunodeficiency. Developmental delay is usually apparent by 3–6 months of life as failure to attain age-appropriate developmental milestones and affects all aspects of motor and cognitive function. The mean IQ is between 30 and 70 and declines with increasing age. However, there is a considerable range in the degree of mental retardation in adults with Down's syndrome, and many affected individuals can live semi-independently. In general, cognitive skills are more limited than affective performance, and only a minority of affected individuals are severely impaired. Retardation of linear growth is moderate, and most adults with Down's syndrome have statures 2–3 standard deviations below that of the general population. In contrast, weight growth in Down's syndrome exhibits a mild proportionate increase compared with that of the general population, and most adults with Down's syndrome are overweight. Although increased susceptibility to infections is a common clinical feature at all ages, the nature of the underlying abnormality is not well understood, and laboratory abnormalities can be detected in both humoral and cellular immunity.

One of the most prevalent and dramatic clinical features of Down's syndrome—premature onset of Alzheimer's disease—is not evident until adulthood. Although frank dementia is not clinically detectable in many adults with Down's syndrome, the incidence of typical neuropathologic changes—senile plaques and neurofibrillary tangles—is nearly 100% by age 35. The major causes of morbidity in Down's syndrome are congenital heart disease, infections, and leukemia. Life expectancy depends to a large extent on the presence of congenital heart disease; survival to ages 10 and 30 years is approximately 60% and 50%, respectively, for individuals with congenital heart disease and approximately 85% and 80%, respectively, for individuals without congenital heart disease.

Pathophysiology

The advent of molecular markers for different portions of chromosome 21 has provided much information about when and how the extra chromosomal material arises in Down's syndrome. In contrast, much less is known about why increased gene dosage for chromosome 21 should produce the clinical features of Down's syndrome.

For trisomy 21 (47,XX+21 or 47,XY+21), cytogenetic or molecular markers that distinguish between the maternal and paternal copies of chromosome 21 can be used to determine whether the egg or the sperm contributed the extra copy of chromosome 21. There are no obvious clinical differences between these two types of trisomy 21 individuals, which suggests that parental imprinting does not play a significant role in the pathogenesis of Down's syndrome. If both copies of chromosome 21 carried by each parent can be distinguished, it is usually possible to determine whether the nondisjunction event leading to an abnormal gamete occurred during anaphase of meiosis I or meiosis II (Figure 2–12). Studies such as these show that approximately 75% of cases of trisomy 21 are caused by an extra maternal chromosome; that approximately 75% of the nondisjunction events (both maternal and paternal) occur in meiosis I; and that both maternal and paternal nondisjunction events increase with advanced maternal age.

Several theories have been proposed to explain why the incidence of Down's syndrome increases with advanced maternal age (Figure 2–11). Most germ cell development in females is completed before birth; oocytes arrest at prophase of meiosis I (the **dictyotene** stage) during the second trimester of gestation. One proposal suggests that biochemical abnormalities that affect the ability of paired chromosomes to disjoin normally accumulate in these cells

Table 2–4. Phenotypic features of trisomy 21.[1]

Feature	Frequency
Upslanting palpebral fissures	82%
Excess skin on back of neck	81%
Brachycephaly	75%
Hyperextensible joints	75%
Flat nasal bridge	68%
Wide gap between first and second toes	68%
Short, broad hands	64%
Epicanthal folds	59%
Short fifth finger	58%
Incurved fifth finger	57%
Brushfield spots (iris hypoplasia)	56%
Transverse palmar crease	53%
Folded or dysplastic ear	50%
Protruding tongue	47%

[1]Data from Scriver CR et al (editors): *The Metabolic and Molecular Bases of Inherited Disease*, 7th ed. McGraw-Hill, 1995.

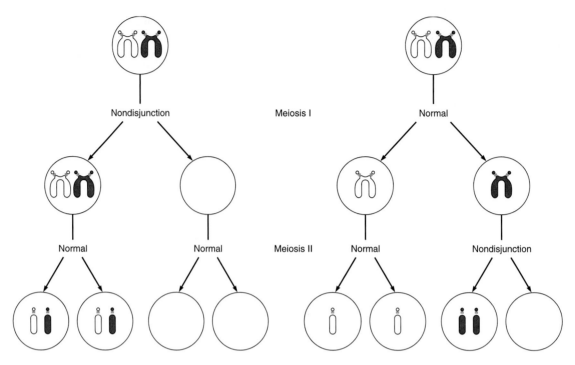

Figure 2–12. Nondisjunction has different consequences depending on whether it occurs at meiosis I or meiosis II. The abnormal gamete has two copies of a particular chromosome. When nondisjunction occurs at meiosis I, each of the copies originates from a different chromosome; but when nondisjunction occurs at meiosis II, each of the copies originates from the same chromosome. Both cytogenetic and molecular polymorphisms can be used to determine the stage and the parent in which nondisjunction occurred. (Reproduced, with permission, from Thompson MW et al: *Genetics in Medicine,* 5th ed. Saunders, 1991.)

over time and that without a renewable source of fresh eggs, the proportion of eggs that undergo nondisjunction increases with maternal age. However, this hypothesis does not explain why the relationship between the incidence of trisomy 21 and advanced maternal age holds for *paternal* as well as maternal nondisjunction events.

Another hypothesis proposes that structural, hormonal, and immunologic changes that occur in the uterus with advanced age produce an environment less able to reject a developmentally abnormal embryo. Thus, an older uterus would be more likely to support a trisomy 21 conceptus to term regardless of which parent contributed the extra chromosome. This hypothesis can explain why paternal nondisjunction errors increase with advanced maternal age. However, it does not explain why the incidence of Down's syndrome due to chromosomal rearrangements (see below) does not increase with maternal age.

These and other hypotheses are not mutually exclusive, and it is possible that a combination of factors is responsible for the relationship between the incidence of trisomy 21 and advanced maternal age. A number of environmental and genetic factors have been considered as possible causes for Down's syndrome, including exposure to caffeine, alcohol, tobacco, radiation, and the likelihood of carrying one or more genes that would predispose to nondisjunction. Although it is difficult to exclude all of these possibilities from consideration as minor factors, there is no evidence that any of these factors play a role in Down's syndrome.

The recurrence risk for trisomy 21 is not altered significantly by previous affected children. However, approximately 5% of Down's syndrome karyotypes are not trisomy 21 and instead are caused by Robertsonian translocations that usually involve chromosomes 14 or 22. As described above, this type of abnormality is not associated with increased maternal age; but in about 30% of such individuals, cytogenetic evaluation of the parents will reveal a so-called balanced rearrangement such as 45,XX,+t(14q;21q). Because the Robertsonian translocation chromosome can pair with both of its component single acrocentric chromosomes at meiosis, the likelihood of segregation leading to unbalanced gametes is significant (Figure 2–13), and the recurrence risk to the parent with the abnormal karyotype is much higher than for trisomy 21 (Table 2–5). Approximately 1% of

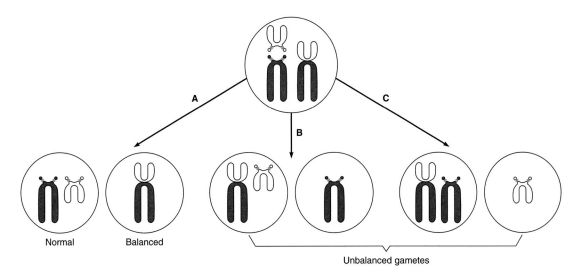

Figure 2–13. Types of gametes produced at meiosis by a carrier of a Robertsonian translocation. In a balanced carrier for a Robertsonian translocation, different types of segregation at meiosis lead to several different types of gametes, including ones that are completely normal (A), ones that would give rise to other balanced translocation carriers (B), and ones that would give rise to aneuploid progeny (C).

Down's syndrome karyotypes show mosaicism in which some cells are normal and some abnormal. Somatic mosaicism for trisomy 21 or other aneuploid conditions may initially arise either pre- or postzygotically, corresponding to nondisjunction in meiosis or mitosis, respectively. In the former case (one in which a zygote is conceived from an aneuploid gamete), the extra chromosome is then presumably lost mitotically in a clone of cells during early embryogenesis. The range of phenotypes seen in mosaic trisomy 21 is great, ranging from mild mental retardation with subtle dysmorphic features to "typical" Down's syndrome, and does not correlate with the proportion of abnormal cells detected in lymphocytes or fibroblasts. Nonetheless, on average, mental retardation in mosaic trisomy 21 is generally milder than in nonmosaic trisomy 21.

Genetic Principles

A fundamental question in understanding the relationship between an extra chromosome 21 and the clinical features of Down's syndrome is whether the phenotype is caused by abnormal gene expression or an abnormal chromosomal constitution. An important principle derived from studies directed at this question is that of **gene dosage,** which states that the amount of a gene product produced per cell is proportionate to the number of copies of that gene present. In other words, the amount of protein produced by all or nearly all genes that lie on chromosome 21 is 150% of normal in trisomy 21 cells and 50% of normal in monosomy 21 cells. Thus, unlike the X chromosome, there is no mechanism for dosage compensation that operates on autosomal genes.

Experimental evidence generally supports the view that the Down's syndrome phenotype is caused by increased expression of specific genes and not by a nonspecific detrimental effect of cellular aneuploidy. Rarely, karyotypic analysis of an individual with Down's syndrome reveals a chromosomal rearrangement (usually an unbalanced reciprocal translocation) in which only a very small portion of chromosome 21 is present in three copies per cell (Figure 2–14). These observations suggest that there

Table 2–5. Risk for Down's syndrome depending on parental sex and karyotype.[1]

Karyotype of Parent	Risk of Abnormal Liveborn Progeny	
	Female Carrier	Male Carrier
46,XX or 46,XY	0.5% (at age 20) to 30% (at age 30)	<0.5%
Rb(Dq;21q) (mostly 14)	10%	<2%
Rb(21q;22q)	14%	<2%
Rb(21q;21q)	100%	100%

[1]Data from Scriver CR et al (editors): *The Metabolic and Molecular Bases of Inherited Disease,* 7th ed. McGraw-Hill, 1995.

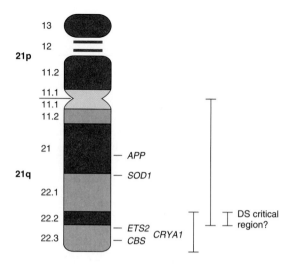

Figure 2–14. Down's syndrome (DS) critical region. Rarely, individuals with Down's syndrome will have chromosomal rearrangements that cause trisomy for just a portion of chromosome 21. The *APP, SOD1, ETS2, CRYA1,* and *CBS* genes encode proteins (amyloid precursor, superoxide dismutase, the ets1 transcriptor factor, crystallin, and cystathionine beta-synthase, respectively, that may play a role in the pathogenesis of Down's syndrome. Analysis of two sets of individuals (indicated by the two vertical lines) suggests that the genes responsible for Down's syndrome lie in the region of overlap. (Reproduced, with permission, from Thompson MW et al: *Genetics in Medicine,* 5th ed. Saunders, 1991.)

fant with Down's syndrome is higher than for other aneuploid conditions, in part because embryos with other types of aneuploidies are likely to result in miscarriages early in development. Thus, the consequences of trisomy for embryonic and fetal development are proportionate to the number of genes expressed to 150% of their normal levels. Because monosomy for chromosome 21 (and other autosomes) is virtually never seen in liveborn infants, a similar line of reasoning suggests that a 50% reduction in gene expression is more severe than a 50% increase. Finally, female Robertsonian translocation carriers exhibit much higher empiric recurrence risks than male carriers, which suggests (1) that selective responses against aneuploidy can operate on gametic as well as somatic cells, and (2) that spermatogenesis is more sensitive to aneuploidy than oogenesis.

---

10. What are the common features of the variety of different karyotypic abnormalities resulting in Down's syndrome?
11. What are the major categories of abnormalities in Down's syndrome, and what is their natural history?
12. Explain why trisomy 21 is associated with such a wide range of phenotypes from mild mental retardation to that of "typical" Down's syndrome.

---

may be a "critical region" of chromosome 21 which, when present in triplicate, is both sufficient and necessary to produce Down's syndrome. Genes that lie within or close to this critical region are candidates for contributing to the Down's syndrome phenotype and include the gene that encodes the amyloid protein found in senile plaques of Alzheimer's disease and the gene that encodes the cytoplasmic form of superoxide dismutase, which plays an important role in free radical metabolism.

The idea that altered gene dosage of a group of closely linked genes can produce a distinct clinical phenotype is also supported by the observation that several multiple congenital anomaly syndromes are due to small interstitial deletions of particular autosomes. These deletions, which often are detectable only with special cytogenetic or molecular techniques, result in monosomy for the genes located within the deleted segment. Such **contiguous gene syndromes,** described in Table 2–6, are generally rare, but they have played important roles in understanding the pathophysiology of aneuploid conditions.

Carriers for Robertsonian translocations that involve chromosome 21 can produce several different types of unbalanced gametes (Figure 2–13). However, the empiric risk for such a carrier bearing an in-

Table 2–6. Phenotype and karyotype (deletion) of some contiguous gene syndromes.

Disorder	Phenotype	Deletion
Langer-Gideon syndrome	Mental retardation, microcephaly, bony exostoses, redundant skin	8q24.11 to q24.3
WAGR syndrome	Wilms' tumor, aniridia, gonadoblastoma, mental retardation	11p13
Prader-Willi syndrome	Mental and growth retardation, hypotonia, obesity, hypopigmentation	15q11 to q13
Angelman's syndrome	Mental and growth retardation, seizures, hypertonia, paroxysmal laughter	15q11 to q13
Williams' syndrome	Mental retardation, hypercalcemia, supravalvular aortic stenosis	7q11.2
Miller-Dieker syndrome	Severe mental retardation, absence of cortical gyri (lissencephaly) and corpus callosum	17p13.3
DiGeorge-velocardiofacial syndrome	Parathyroid and thymic hypoplasia, congenital heart disease	22q11

PHENYLKETONURIA

Phenylketonuria presents one of the most dramatic examples of how the relationship between genotype and phenotype can depend on environmental variables. Phenylketonuria was first recognized as an inherited cause of mental retardation in 1934, and systematic attempts to treat the condition were initiated in the 1950s. Treatment outcomes have been hailed, perhaps prematurely, as the pinnacle of success in applying biochemistry and molecular biology to societal problems that stem from inherited disease. The term "phenylketonuria" denotes elevated levels of urinary phenylpyruvate and phenylacetate, which occur when circulating phenylalanine levels, normally between 0.06 and 0.1 mmol/L, rise above 1.2 mmol/L. Thus, the primary defect in phenylketonuria is **hyperphenylalaninemia,** which itself has a number of distinct genetic causes.

The pathophysiology of phenylketonuria also illustrates a number of important principles in human genetics, including the rationale for and application of population-based newborn screening programs for inherited disease. More than 10 million newborn infants per year are tested for phenylketonuria, and the focus today in treatment has shifted in several respects. First, "successful" treatment of phenylketonuria by dietary restriction of phenylalanine is, in general, accompanied by subtle neuropsychologic defects that have been recognized only in the last decade. Thus, current investigations focus on alternative treatment strategies such as somatic gene therapy as well as on the social and psychologic factors that affect compliance with dietary management. Second, a generation of females treated for phenylketonuria are now bearing children, and the phenomenon of **maternal phenylketonuria** has been recognized, in which in utero exposure to maternal hyperphenylalaninemia results in congenital abnormalities regardless of fetal genotype. The number of pregnancies at risk has risen in proportion to the successful treatment of phenylketonuria and represents a challenge to public health officials, physicians, and geneticists in the next decade.

Clinical Manifestations

The incidence of hyperphenylalaninemia varies among different populations. In American blacks it is about 1:50,000; in Yemenite Jews, about 1:5000; and in most Northern European populations, about 1:10,000. Postnatal growth retardation, moderate to severe mental retardation, recurrent seizures, hypopigmentation, and eczematous skin rashes constitute the major phenotypic features of untreated phenylketonuria. However, with the advent of widespread newborn screening programs for hyperphenylalaninemia, the major phenotypic manifestations of phenylketonuria today occur when treatment is partial or terminated prematurely during late childhood or adolescence. In these cases, there is usually a slight but significant decline in IQ, an array of specific performance and perceptual defects, and an associated increased frequency of learning and behavioral problems.

Newborn screening for phenylketonuria is performed on a small amount of dried blood obtained at 24–72 hours of age. Most screening programs are administered by state or regional governments, and the actual measurements of phenylalanine levels are performed at one or a few central laboratories. From the initial screen, there is about a 1% incidence of positive or indeterminate test results, and a more quantitative measurement of plasma phenylalanine is then performed before 2 weeks of age. In neonates who undergo a second round of testing, the diagnosis of phenylketonuria is ultimately confirmed in about 1%, providing an estimated phenylketonuria prevalence of 1:10,000, though there is great geographic and ethnic variation (see above). The false-negative rate of phenylketonuria newborn screening programs is approximately 1:70; these unfortunate individuals are usually not detected until developmental delay and seizures during infancy or early childhood prompt a systematic evaluation for an inborn error of metabolism.

Infants in whom a diagnosis of phenylketonuria is confirmed are usually placed on a dietary regimen in which a semisynthetic formula low in phenylalanine can be combined with regular breast feeding. This regimen is adjusted empirically to maintain a plasma phenylalanine concentration at or below 1 mmol/L, which is still several times greater than normal but similar to levels observed in so-called **benign hyperphenylalaninemia** (see below), a biochemical diagnosis which is not associated with phenylketonuria and has no clinical consequences. Phenylalanine is an essential amino acid, and even individuals with phenylketonuria must consume small amounts to avoid protein starvation and a catabolic state. Most children require 25–50 mg/kg/d of phenylalanine, and these requirements are met by combining natural foods with commercial products designed for phenylketonuria treatment. When dietary treatment programs were first implemented, it was hoped that the risk of neurologic damage due to the hyperphenylalaninemia of phenylketonuria would have a limited window and that treatment could be stopped after childhood. However, it now appears that even hyperphenylalaninemia greater than 1.2 mmol/L in adults is associated with neuropsychologic and cognitive deficits; therefore, dietary treatment of phenylketonuria should probably be continued indefinitely.

As an increasing number of treated females with phenylketonuria reach childbearing age, a new problem—fetal hyperphenylalaninemia via intrauterine exposure—has become apparent. Newborn infants in such cases exhibit microcephaly and growth retardation of prenatal onset, congenital heart disease, and

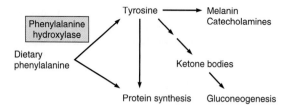

Figure 2–15. Metabolic fates of phenylalanine. Because catabolism of phenylalanine must proceed via tyrosine, the absence of phenylalanine hydroxylase leads to accumulation of phenylalanine. Tyrosine is also a biosynthetic precursor for melanin and certain neurotransmitters, and the absence of phenylalanine hydroxylase causes tyrosine to become an essential amino acid.

Pathophysiology

The normal metabolic fate of free phenylalanine is incorporation into protein or hydroxylation by phenylalanine hydroxylase to form tyrosine (Figure 2–15). Because tyrosine but not phenylalanine can be metabolized to produce fumarate and acetoacetate, hydroxylation of phenylalanine can be viewed both as a means of making tyrosine a nonessential amino acid and as a mechanism for providing energy via gluconeogenesis during states of protein starvation. This may explain why in humans the tissue distribution of phenylalanine hydroxylase is restricted primarily to the liver. Transamination of phenylalanine to form phenylpyruvate normally does not occur unless circulating concentrations exceed 1.2 mmol/L, but the pathogenesis of central nervous system abnormalities in phenylketonuria is related more to phenylalanine itself than to its metabolites. Besides a direct effect of elevated phenylalanine levels on energy production, protein synthesis, and neurotransmitter homeostasis in the developing brain, phenylalanine can also inhibit the transport of neutral amino acids across the blood-brain barrier, leading to a selective amino acid deficiency in the cerebrospinal fluid. Thus, the neurologic manifestations of phenylketonuria are felt to be due to a general effect on central nervous system metabolism. The pathophysiology of the eczema seen in untreated or partially treated phenylketonuria is not well understood, but eczema is a common feature

severe developmental delay regardless of the fetal genotype. Rigorous control of maternal phenylalanine concentrations from before conception until birth reduces the incidence of fetal abnormalities in maternal phenylketonuria, but the level of plasma phenylalanine that is "safe" for a developing fetus is 0.12–0.36 mmol/L, significantly lower than what is considered acceptable for phenylketonuria-affected children or adults on phenylalanine-restricted diets.

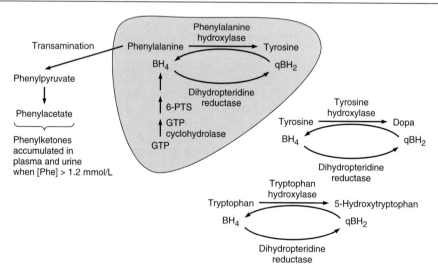

Figure 2–16. Normal and abnormal phenylalanine metabolism. Tetrahydrobiopterin (BH_4) is a cofactor for phenylalanine hydroxylase, tyrosine hydroxylase, and tryptophan hydroxylase. Consequently, defects in the biosynthesis of BH_4 or its metabolism result in a failure of all three hydroxylation reactions. The absence of phenylalanine hydroxylation has phenotypic effects due to substrate accumulation, but the absence of tyrosine or tryptophan hydroxylation has phenotypic effects due to end-product deficiency. (6-PTS, 6-pyruvoyltetrahydrobiopterin synthetase; qBH_2, quinonoid dihydrobiopterin.)

Haplotype	BglII	EcoRI	MspI	EcoRV	Frequency
1	−	−	+	−	35
2	−	−	+	+	5
3	−	+	−	−	3
4	−	+	−	+	32
5	+	+	+	+	11
6	+	+	+	−	< 1
7	+	+	−	−	11
8	−	+	+	+	2
% − of total	77	40	46	49	
% + of total	22	59	53	50	

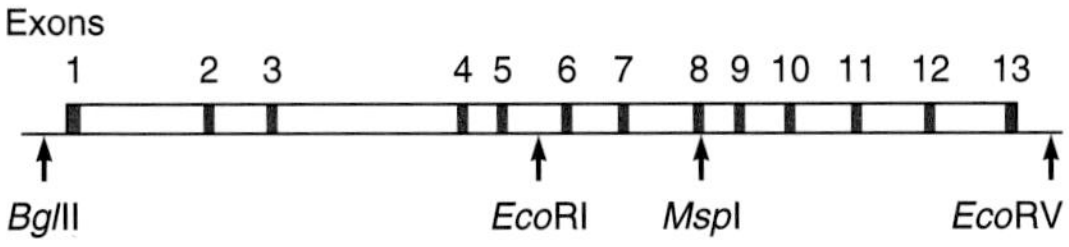

Exons

Figure 2–17. Linkage disequilibrium for phenylalanine hydroxylase haplotypes. Different haplotypes are defined by a particular combination of RFLPs whose locations are indicated relative to exons within the phenylalanine hydroxylase gene. For example, haplotype 1 is an allele that contains an MspI site but not a BglII, EcoRI, or EcoRV site at the locations indicated. Shown are 8 of 12 haplotypes described initially in a large analysis of Danish families. Linkage disequilibrium is said to occur when the frequency of each haplotype differs from that predicted by the frequency of individual RFLPs. For example, 59% or 53% of all chromosomes contain EcoRI or MspI sites, respectively. The predicted frequency of all chromosomes that contain both sites at the same time is 31% (0.59 × 0.53), which differs substantially from the observed frequency of 14%. (Adapted from Scriver CR et al: *The Metabolic and Molecular Bases of Inherited Disease,* 7th ed. McGraw-Hill, 1995.)

of other inborn errors of metabolism in which plasma concentrations of branched-chain amino acids are elevated. Hypopigmentation in phenylketonuria is probably caused by an inhibitory effect of excess phenylalanine on the production of dopaquinone in melanocytes, which is the rate-limiting step in melanin synthesis.

Approximately 90% of infants with persistent hyperphenylalaninemia detected by newborn screening have typical phenylketonuria caused by a defect in phenylalanine hydroxylase (see below). Of the remainder, most have benign hyperphenylalaninemia, in which circulating levels of phenylalanine are between 0.1 and 1 mmol/L. However, approximately 1% of infants with persistent hyperphenylalaninemia have defects in the metabolism of tetrahydrobiopterin (BH_4), which is a stoichiometric cofactor for the hydroxylation reaction (Figure 2–16). Because hydroxylation of tyrosine and of tryptophan also requires BH_4 as a cofactor, defects in its metabolism lead not only to phenylketonuria but also to deficiencies of catecholaminergic and serotonergic neurotransmitters that in early childhood result in a severe neurologic disorder manifested by hypotonia, inactivity, and developmental regression. Infants affected with defects in BH_4 metabolism are treated not only with dietary restriction of phenylalanine but also with dietary supplementation with BH_4, dopa, and 5-hydroxytryptophan.

Shortly after the gene for phenylalanine hydroxylase was isolated in 1982, many polymorphic restriction sites at or close to the gene were identified that did not by themselves affect phenylalanine hydroxylase expression or structure. However, analysis of these RFLPs in pedigrees and in populations indicated that phenylketonuria was associated with a limited number of **haplotypes**, or certain groups of RFLPs held in linkage disequilibrium with each other. For example, the initial analysis of Danish families demonstrated 12 different RFLP haplotypes (of 1152 theoretically possible), of which four were associated with phenylalanine hydroxylase mutations (Figure 2–17; Table 2–7). The distribution of these four haplotypes among phenylalanine hydroxylase mutant chromosomes was significantly different compared with nonmutant chromosomes (Table 2–7). Comparison of haplotype data with hyperphenylalaninemia phenotypes suggested that allelic heterogeneity accounted for benign hyperphenylalaninemia as well as for phenylketonuria. For example, haplotype 1 in homozygous form or as a heterozygous compound with other haplotypes is usually associated with benign hyperphenylalaninemia or mild phenylketonuria, but haplotypes 2 or 3 in homozygous form are associated with severe phenylke-

Table 2–7. Linkage disequilibrium for phenylketonuria.[1]

Haplotype	Frequency on Nonmutant Chromosomes	Frequency on Phenylketonuria Chromosomes	Molecular Basis of Phenylalanine Hydroxylase Mutation
1	35%	18%	R261Q
2	5%	20%	R408W
3	3%	38%	G→A(IVS12)
4	32%	14%	R158Q

[1]Adapted from Thompson MW et al: *Genetics in Medicine,* 5th ed. Saunders, 1991.

Table 2–8. Phenylalanine hydroxylase (PAH) activity (%) and phenylketonuria (PKU) phenotypes for different combinations of PAH alleles.[1]

Haplotype (Mutation)	3 (IVS12)	2 (R408W)	4 (R158Q)	1 (R261Q)
3(IVS12)	0% Classic PKU	0% Classic PKU	5% Classic PKU	15% Intermediate or mild
2(R408W)		0% Classic PKU	5% Classic PKU	15% Intermediate or mild
4(R158Q)			10% Classic PKU	20% Mild PKU
1(R261Q)				30% Benign hyperphenylalaninemia

[1]Adapted from Okano Y et al: Molecular basis of phenotypic heterogeneity in phenylketonuria. N Engl J Med 1991; 324:1232.

tonuria (Table 2–8). Measurements of phenylalanine hydroxylase activity in liver biopsy specimens correlate with these findings and demonstrate that individuals with phenylketonuria have levels of enzyme activity less than 1% of normal, while those with benign hyperphenylalaninemia generally have activity levels that are 5–30% of normal.

Most of the phenylalanine hydroxylase mutations affect the protein-coding sequence by a missense mechanism, including the one associated with benign hyperphenylalaninemia and haplotype 1, an Arg to Gln change at residue 261 (Table 2–8). A notable exception, however, is a point mutation in the noncoding splice donor sequence immediately following exon 12 (Figure 2–18). This mutation, which was the first to be identified at a molecular level, causes exon 12 to be "skipped" from the mature mRNA and leads to production of a truncated protein associated with severe phenylketonuria.

For the 1% of infants affected with phenylketonuria in which the underlying defect is not in phenylalanine hydroxylase but in metabolism of BH_4, at least three different genetic defects have been identified. All of these are inherited in an autosomal recessive fashion and can be distinguished from each other and from phenylalanine hydroxylase deficiency by direct analysis of enzyme activity in liver biopsy samples.

Genetic Principles

Because the fitness of individuals affected with phenylketonuria has until recently been very low, the relatively high incidence of the condition could only be explained by a high mutation rate, founder effects, heterozygote advantage, or a combination of these mechanisms. New mutations of phenylketonuria are exceedingly rare, but population genetic studies provide evidence for both a founder effect and heterozygote advantage. As in the case of fragile X-associated mental retardation syndrome, linkage disequilibrium between phenylalanine hydroxylase mutations and closely linked RFLPs supports a founder effect. However, the presence of multiple phenylalanine hydroxylase mutations at relatively high frequencies and the variation in phenylketonuria prevalence between different populations suggests that reduced levels of phenylalanine hydroxylase activity in heterozygotes may have provided a selective advantage under certain environmental or geographic conditions.

The effect of dietary phenylalanine on the phenylketonuria phenotype illustrates how manipulation of an environmental variable can alter expressivity of a particular genotype. Factors that influence the expressivity of phenylalanine hydroxylase deficiency have been relevant not only to the treatment of phenylketonuria but also to public health, since aspartame, a widely used artificial sweetening agent that becomes hydrolyzed to phenylalanine and aspartic acid, can affect phenylalanine concentrations in phenylketonuria heterozygotes. Although phenylketonuria heterozygotes who consume large amounts of aspartame are not at risk of developing phenylketonuria, these considerations underscore the impor-

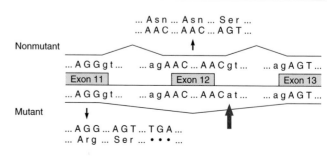

Figure 2–18. A phenylalanine hydroxylase splice donor mutation causes exon skipping in a common phenylketonuria allele. A **g** to **a** mutation in the intron sequences following exon 12 (large arrow) causes the preceding exon 12 to be skipped during processing of the nuclear RNA and results in production of a truncated protein with no phenylalanine hydroxylase activity. (Adapted from Scriver CR et al [editors]: *The Metabolic and Molecular Bases of Inherited Disease,* 7th ed. McGraw-Hill, 1995.)

tance of genotypic diversity in the population when evaluating the effects of pharmaceutical, cosmetic, or dietary agents.

The different genetic forms of phenylketonuria illustrate two important pathophysiologic mechanisms by which inborn errors of metabolism can cause disease: **end-product deficiency** and **substrate accumulation.** The mental retardation in phenylalanine hydroxylase deficiency is caused not by deficiency of tyrosine or its metabolites but by accumulation of the substrate for phenylalanine hydroxylase. In contrast, the progressive hypotonia and developmental regression seen in disorders of BH_4 metabolism are caused by a decrease in the metabolic products of tryptophan hydroxylase and tyrosine hydroxylase.

Finally, a thorough understanding of the pathophysiology of phenylketonuria is a prerequisite for the development of gene therapy. For example, since most phenylalanine hydroxylation occurs in the liver, attempts to deliver a normal phenylalanine hydroxylase gene to affected individuals have focused on strategies to express the gene in hepatocytes. However, since individuals with benign hyperphenylalaninemia have phenylalanine hydroxylase activities that may be as low as 5% of normal, successful gene therapy of phenylketonuria might be accomplished by expressing phenylalanine hydroxylase in only a small proportion of hepatic cells.

---

13. What is the primary defect in phenylketonuria?
14. Why is dietary modification a less than satisfactory treatment of this condition? What might be a better therapeutic approach and why?
15. What is the false-negative rate for neonatal screening, and how do these individuals come to medical attention?
16. Explain the phenomenon of "maternal phenylketonuria."

REFERENCES

General

Scriver C et al (editors): *The Metabolic and Molecular Bases of Inherited Disease,* 7th ed. McGraw-Hill, 1995.

Thompson MW, McInnes RR, Willard HF: *Genetics in Medicine,* 5th ed. Saunders, 1991.

Vogel F, Motulsky AG: *Human Genetics,* 3rd ed. Springer, 1996.

Osteogenesis Imperfecta

Cole WG, Dalgleish R: Perinatal lethal osteogenesis imperfecta. J Med Genet 1995;32:284.

Lund AM et al: Parental mosaicism and autosomal dominant mutations causing structural abnormalities of collagen I are frequent in families with osteogenesis imperfecta type III/IV. Acta Paediatr 1997;86:711.

Prockop DJ, Kivirikko KI: Collagens: Molecular biology, diseases, and potentials for therapy. Annu Rev Biochem 1995;64:403.

Raghunath M et al: Genetic counselling on brittle grounds: Recurring osteogenesis imperfecta due to parental mosaicism for a dominant mutation. Eur J Pediatr 1995;154:123.

Willing MC et al: Osteogenesis imperfecta type I is commonly due to a *COL1A1* null allele of type I collagen. Am J Hum Genet 1992;51:508.

Fragile X-Associated Mental Retardation

de Vries BB et al: The fragile X syndrome. J Med Genet 1998;35:579.

Feng Y et al: Translational suppression by trinucleotide repeat expansion at *FMR1.* Science 1995;268:731.

Nelson DL: The fragile X syndromes. Semin Cell Biol 1995;6:5.

O'Donnell DM, Zoghbi HY: Trinucleotide repeat disorders in pediatrics. Curr Opin Pediatr 1995;7:715.

Reddy PS, Housman DE: The complex pathology of trinucleotide repeats. Curr Opin Cell Biol 1997;9:364.

Siomi H et al: The protein product of the fragile X gene *FMR1* has characteristics of an RNA-binding protein. Cell 1993;74:291.

Sutherland GR, Richards RI: Unusual inheritance patterns due to dynamic mutation in fragile X syndrome. Ciba Found Symp 1996;197:119.

Down's Syndrome

Epstein CJ: Down syndrome. In: *The Metabolic and Molecular Bases of Inherited Disease,* 7th ed. Scriver CR et al (editors). McGraw-Hill, 1995.

Phenylketonuria

Eisensmith RC et al: Multiple origins for phenylketonuria in Europe. Am J Hum Genet 1992;51:1355.

Eisensmith RC et al: Recurrence of the R408W mutation in the phenylalanine hydroxylase locus in Europeans. Am J Hum Genet 1995;56:278.

Matalon R, Michals K: Phenylketonuria: screening, treatment and maternal PKU. Clin Biochem 1991;24:337.

Scriver CR et al.: The hyperphenylalaninemias of man and mouse. Annu Rev Genet 1994;28:141.

Waters PJ et al: In vitro expression analysis of mutations in phenylalanine hydroxylase: linking genotype to phenotype and structure to function. Hum Mutat 1998;11:4.

3

Disorders of the Immune System

Richard S. Shames, MD, & Jeffrey L. Kishiyama, MD

ABBREVIATIONS AND ACRONYMS USED IN THIS CHAPTER

ADCC	Antibody-dependent cell-mediated cytotoxicity
ADA	Adenosine deaminase
BTK	Bruton's tyrosine kinase
cAMP	Cyclic adenosine monophosphate
CD4	T helper cell subset
CD8	T suppressor cell subset or cytotoxic T cell subset
F(ab)	Antigen-binding fragment
Fc	Crystallizable fragment
FcεRI	High-affinity IgE receptor
FcγR	Fc gamma receptor
GM-CSF	Granulocyte macrophage colony-stimulating factor
HPV	Human papillomavirus
HSV	Herpes simplex virus
HZV	Herpes zoster virus
ICAM-1	Intercellular adhesion molecule 1
IFN-γ	Gamma interferon
IL-1, IL-2, etc	Interleukin-1, interleukin-2, etc
LAK cell	Lymphokine-activated killer cell
LPS	Lipopolysaccharide
MHC	Major histocompatibility complex
NK cells	Natural killer cells
PAF	Platelet-activating factor
PGD	Prostaglandin D
PNP	Purine nucleoside phosphorylase
RAG	Recombination-activating gene
RANTES	Chemokine regulated on activation normal T expressed and secreted
RAST	Radioallergosorbent test
SCID	Severe combined immunodeficiency disease
TH1	T helper 1 subset
TH2	T helper 2 subset
TNF	Tumor necrosis factor
TSH	Thyroid-stimulating hormone
V-CAM-1	Vascular cell adhesion molecule 1
VIP	Vasoactive intestinal peptide
ZAP-70	Protein tyrosine kinase ZAP-70

The function of the immune system is to protect the host from invasion of foreign organisms by distinguishing "self" from "nonself." Such a system is necessary for survival. A well-functioning immune system not only protects the host from external factors such as microorganisms or toxins but also prevents and repels attacks by endogenous factors such as tumors or autoimmune phenomena. Dysfunction or deficiency of components of the immune system leads to a variety of clinical diseases of varying expression and severity, ranging from atopic disease to rheumatoid arthritis, severe combined immunodeficiency, or cancer. This chapter introduces the intricate physiology of the immune system and abnormalities which lead to diseases of hypersensitivity and immunodeficiency.

NORMAL STRUCTURE & FUNCTION OF THE IMMUNE SYSTEM

ANATOMY

Cells of the Immune System

The immune system consists of both specific and nonspecific components that have distinct yet overlapping functions. The antibody-mediated and cell-mediated immune systems provide specificity and memory of previously encountered antigens. The nonspecific cellular component consists of phagocytic cells, whereas the complement proteins constitute the primary nonspecific plasma factors. Despite their lack of specificity, these components are essential because they are largely responsible for natural immunity to a vast array of environmental microorganisms. Knowledge of the components and physiology of normal immunity is essential for understanding the pathophysiology of diseases of the immune system.

The major cellular components of the immune system consist of monocytes and macrophages, lymphocytes, and the family of granulocytic cells, including neutrophils, eosinophils, and basophils.

Monocytes and **macrophages** play a central role in the immune response. Macrophages are derived from blood monocytes. These cells leave the circulation to become active tissue macrophages. In response to antigenic stimulation, macrophages engulf the antigen (phagocytosis), then process and present that antigen in a form recognizable to T lymphocytes. Activated macrophages secrete proteolytic enzymes, active metabolites of oxygen (including superoxide anion and other oxygen radicals), arachidonic acid metabolites, cyclic adenosine monophosphate (cAMP), and cytokines such as interleukin-1 (IL-1), IL-6, IL-8, and tumor necrosis factor (TNF), among others. Many tissue-specific cells are of macrophage lineage, and function to process and present antigen (Langerhans' cells, oligodendrocytes, etc).

Lymphocytes are responsible for the initial specific recognition of antigen. They are functionally and phenotypically divided into B lymphocytes and T lymphocytes. Structurally, B and T lymphocytes cannot be distinguished visually from each other under the microscope, though about 70–80% of circulating blood lymphocytes are T lymphocytes and 10–15% B lymphocytes; the remainder are neither B nor T lymphocytes and are often referred to as "null cells."

Null cells probably include a number of different cell types, including a group called **natural killer (NK) cells.** These cells appear distinct from other lymphocytes in that they are slightly larger, with a kidney-shaped nucleolus, and have a granular appearance (large granular lymphocytes). NK cells are capable of binding IgG because they have a membrane receptor for the IgG molecule (FcγR). Antibody-dependent cell-mediated cytotoxicity (ADCC) occurs when an organism or a cell is coated by antibody and undergoes NK cell-mediated destruction. Alternatively, NK cells can destroy virally infected cells or tumor cells without involvement of antibody. Other characteristics of NK cells include recognition of antigens without major histocompatibility restrictions, lack of immunologic memory, and regulation of activity by cytokines and arachidonic acid metabolites.

Polymorphonuclear leukocytes (neutrophils) are granulocytic cells that originate in the bone marrow and circulate in blood and tissue. Their primary function is antigen-nonspecific phagocytosis and destruction of foreign particles and organisms. The presence of Fcγ receptors on the surface of neutrophils also facilitates the clearance of opsonized microbes through the reticuloendothelial system.

Eosinophils are often found in inflammatory sites or at sites of immune reactivity and play a crucial role in the host's defense against parasites. Despite many shared functional similarities to neutrophils, eosinophils are considerably less efficient than neutrophils at phagocytosis. Eosinophils exhibit modulatory or regulatory functions in various types of inflammation. However, in the airway inflammatory response in asthma, eosinophil-derived cytotoxic proteins, including major basic protein, lipid mediators (eg, leukotriene C4), oxygen radicals, and cytokines (eg, IL-3) can induce damage to airway epithelium and potentiate the allergic response.

Basophils play an important role in both immediate and late phase allergic responses. These cells release many of the potent mediators of allergic inflammatory diseases, including histamine, leukotrienes, prostaglandins, and platelet-activating factor (PAF), all of which have significant effects on the vasculature and on the inflammatory response. Basophils are present in the circulation, possess high-affinity receptors for IgE (FcεRI), and mediate immediate hypersensitivity (allergic) responses.

The **epithelium,** like the skin, has long been considered merely a barrier between the external and internal environments. The epithelium lining the upper and lower airways, for instance, contains cilia that remove surface secretions, preventing penetration of foreign matter. Recent evidence has shown that the epithelium can also serve immunologic functions: presenting antigen and producing cytokines such as GM-CSF, IL-6, and IL-8. Some of these cytokines can recruit neutrophils and prolong eosinophil survival. Epithelial cells can produce nitric oxide, which has vasodilating and bronchodilating effects, and play a role in neurotransmission, immune defense, cytotoxicity, ciliary beat frequency, and mucus secretion.

Organs of the Immune System

Several tissues and organs play roles in host defenses and are functionally classified as the immune system. In mammals, the primary lymphoid organs are the thymus and the bone marrow.

All cells of the immune system are originally derived from **bone marrow.** Pluripotent stem cells differentiate into lymphocyte, granulocyte, monocyte, erythrocyte, and megakaryocyte populations. In humans, B lymphocytes, which are the antibody-producing cells, undergo early antigen-independent maturation into immunocompetent cells in the bone marrow. Deficiency or dysfunction of the pluripotent stem cell or the various cell lines developing from it can result in immune deficiency disorders of varying expression and severity.

The **thymus,** derived from the third and fourth embryonic pharyngeal pouches, functions to produce T lymphocytes and is the site of initial T lymphocyte differentiation. Its reticular structure allows a significant number of lymphocytes to migrate through it to become fully immunocompetent thymus-derived cells. A large number of cells undergo **clonal deletion** in the thymus by a mechanism in which autoreactive lymphocyte clones (ie, clones of cells that react with self antigens) are eliminated. The thymus also regulates immune function by secretion of multiple hormones that promote T lymphocyte differentiation and are essential for T lymphocyte-mediated immunity.

In mammals, the **lymph nodes, spleen,** and **gut-associated lymphoid tissue** are secondary lymphoid organs connected by blood and lymphatic vessels. Through these vessels, lymphocytes circulate and recirculate, respond to antigen, and spread the specific experience of this antigen exposure to all parts of the lymphoid system.

Lymph nodes are strategically dispersed throughout the vasculature and are the principal organs of the immune system that localize and prevent the spread of infection. Lymph nodes have a framework of reticular cells and fibers that are arranged into a **cortex** and **medulla.** B lymphocytes, the precursors of antibody-producing cells, or **plasma cells,** are found in the cortex (the follicles and germinal centers) as well as in the medulla. T lymphocytes are found chiefly in the medullary and paracortical areas of the lymph node (Figure 3–1).

The spleen is functionally and structurally divided into B lymphocyte and T lymphocyte areas similar to those of the lymph nodes. The spleen filters and processes antigens from the blood.

Gut-associated lymphoid tissue includes the tonsils, Peyer's patches of the small intestine, and the appendix. Similar to the lymph nodes and spleen, these tissues exhibit similar separation into B lymphocyte-dependent and T lymphocyte-dependent areas. Many lymphocytes are also seen within the lamina propria of the small intestinal villi and between the epithelial cells of the intestinal mucosal surface.

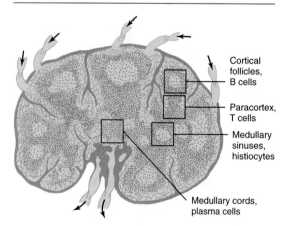

Figure 3–1. Anatomy of a normal lymph node. (Reproduced, with permission, from Chandrasoma P, Taylor CR: *Concise Pathology,* 3rd ed. Appleton & Lange, 1997.)

Neuronal pathways, including the sympathetic, parasympathetic, and peripheral sensory nerves, can serve roles in inflammation. Sympathetic and parasympathetic responses in the nasal airway and lungs have been recognized for decades. The role of **neuropeptides** such as neuropeptide Y, substance P, calcitonin gene-related peptide, and vasoactive intestinal peptide (VIP) in affecting vascular tone, airway smooth muscle activity, vascular permeability, nasal airway resistance, cellular chemotaxis, cytokine expression, epithelial and fibroblast growth, and mucus secretion has emerged more recently.

It is this network of dispersed immune organs that facilitates the rapid and efficient response to antigenic assaults on the host organism.

---

1. What are the specific and nonspecific components of the cellular and noncellular limbs of the immune system?
2. What is the role of macrophages in the immune system, and what are some of the products they secrete?
3. What are the categories of lymphocytes, and how are they distinguished?
4. What is the role of lymphocytes in the immune system, and what are some of the products they secrete?
5. What is the role of eosinophils in the immune system, and what are some of the products they secrete?
6. What is the role of basophils in the immune system, and what are some of the products they secrete?
7. What is the role of epithelial cells in the immune system, and what are some of the products they secrete?
8. What are the primary and secondary lymphoid organs, and what roles do they play in the proper functioning of the immune system?

PHYSIOLOGY

1. INNATE & ADAPTIVE IMMUNITY

Living organisms exhibit two levels of response against external invasion: an **innate system** of natural immunity and an **adaptive system** that is acquired. Innate immunity is present from birth and is nonspecific in its activity. The skin surface serves as the first line of defense of the innate immune system, while enzymes, the alternative complement system pathway, acute phase proteins, natural killer cells, and certain cytokines provide additional layers of protection. Higher organisms have evolved the adaptive immune system, which is triggered by encounters with foreign agents that have evaded or penetrated the innate immune defenses. The adaptive immune system is characterized both by **specificity** for individual foreign agents and by **immunologic memory,** which makes possible an intensified response to subsequent encounters with the same or closely related agents. The introduction of a stimulus into the adaptive immune system triggers a complex sequence of events initiating the activation of lymphocytes, the production of antibodies and effector cells, and ultimately the elimination of the inciting organism.

2. ANTIGENS (Immunogens)

Foreign substances that can induce an immune response are called **antigens,** or **immunogens.** Antigenicity (immunogenicity) implies that the substance has the ability to react with products of the adaptive immune system (ie, antibodies). Complex foreign agents possess distinct and multiple immunogenic components. Most antigens are proteins, though pure carbohydrates may be antigenic as well. The immune response to a particular antigen may depend on the route of entry of the foreign substance. Blood-borne substances are normally removed by the spleen. Antigens entering through the skin may provoke a local inflammatory response involving afferent lymphatic channels and regional lymph nodes. Entry of agents through mucosal surfaces (respiratory or gastrointestinal systems) stimulates the production of local antibodies. Activated lymphocytes are then carried to other lymphoid organs to amplify the initial response.

3. THE IMMUNE RESPONSE (Figure 3–2)

The primary role of the immune system is to discriminate self from nonself and to eliminate the foreign substance. A complex network of specialized cells, organs, and biologic factors is necessary for the recognition and subsequent elimination of foreign antigens. The major pathways of antigen elimination include the direct killing of target cells by a subset of T lymphocytes called **cytotoxic T lymphocytes (cellular response)** and the elimination of antigen through antibody-mediated events arising from T and B lymphocyte interactions **(humoral response).** The series of events that comprise the immune response includes antigen processing and presentation, lymphocyte recognition and activation, cellular or humoral immune responses, and antigenic destruction or elimination.

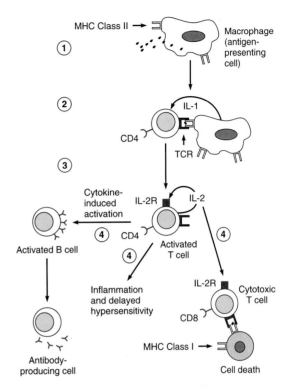

Figure 3–2. The normal immune response. ① Antigen processing and presentation by antigen-presenting cells. ② Recognition of antigen-MHC complex by CD4 T lymphocytes induces IL-1 secretion by antigen-presenting cells and subsequent cellular activation. ③ Activated T lymphocytes express IL-2 receptors and secrete IL-2, which up-regulates IL-2 receptor expression in an autocrine fashion. ④ Activated CD4 T lymphocytes can stimulate CD8 cytotoxic T lymphocytes to mediate cellular cytotoxicity, B lymphocyte activation, and differentiation into antibody-producing plasma cells, which mediate humoral immunity or mediate delayed hypersensitivity and other inflammatory reactions.

Antigen Processing & Presentation

Most foreign immunogens are not recognized by the immune system in their native form and require capture and processing by specialized **antigen-presenting cells.** Antigen-presenting cells include macrophages, dendritic cells in lymphoid tissue, Langerhans cells in the skin, Kupffer cells in the liver, microglial cells in the nervous system, and B lymphocytes. Antigens are recognized in their native form by B cells that can act as antigen-presenting cells. Following encounter with immunogens, the antigen-presenting cells internalize the foreign substance by phagocytosis or pinocytosis, modify its parent structure, and display antigenic fragments of the native protein on its surfaces in association with MHC class II molecules (see below).

T Lymphocyte Recognition & Activation

The recognition of processed antigen by specialized T lymphocytes known as **T helper (CD4) lymphocytes** constitutes the critical event in the immune response. The T helper lymphocytes orchestrate the many cells and biologic signals that are necessary to carry out the immune response. T helper lymphocytes recognize processed antigen displayed by antigen-presenting cells only in association with polymorphic cell surface proteins called the **major histocompatibility (MHC) complex.** The process of dual recognition is referred to as **MHC restriction.** Exogenous foreign antigens that require an antibody-mediated response are expressed in association with **MHC class II** structures. Only the specialized antigen-presenting cells can express MHC class II.

The antigen-MHC class II complex forms the epitope that is recognized by antigen-specific **T cell receptors** on the surface of the CD4 molecules. This interaction is accompanied by the binding of two additional cell surface molecules: B7, expressed on antigen presenting cells, and CD28, expressed on T helper cells. Intracellular signaling within the T cell receptor complex thereby activates the CD4 cells. This signaling induces the transcription, translation, and expression of **CD40 ligand** protein on the surface of the CD4 cell. The CD40 ligand binds to the **CD40 receptor** on the surface of the antigen-presenting cells. The antigen-presenting cells are subsequently activated to release **interleukin 1 (IL-1)**, which induces the release of both **IL-2** and **gamma interferon (IFN-γ)** from CD4 cells. IL-2 then feeds back to stimulate the expression of **IL-2 receptors** on the surface of the CD4 cells as well as the production of various cell growth and differentiation factors **(cytokines)** by the activated CD4 cells. The binding of secreted IL-2 to receptor-positive T cells induces clonal T cell proliferation. The requirement for both IL-2 production and IL-2 receptor expression for T cells to proliferate ensures that only T cells specific for the antigen inciting the immune response will become activated. Activated CD4 T lymphocytes subsequently trigger the **effector cells** that mediate the cellular and humoral arms of the immune response.

Activation of Cytotoxic T Lymphocytes (Cellular Immune Response)

Cytotoxic T lymphocytes (CD8 T lymphocytes) eliminate target cells (virally infected cells, tumor, or foreign tissues), thus constituting the cellular immune response. Cytotoxic T lymphocytes differ from helper T lymphocytes in their expression of the surface antigen CD8 and by the recognition of antigen complexed to cell surface proteins of **MHC class I.** Pathogenic microorganisms whose proteins gain access to the cell cytoplasm (eg, malarial parasites) or by de novo gene expression in the infected cell cytoplasm (eg, viruses) stimulate CD8 class I MHC restricted T cell responses. All somatic cells can express MHC class I molecules. Cytotoxic T lymphocytes become activated (1) by binding to the MHC class I antigen complex and (2) following stimulation by IL-2 elaborated by helper T lymphocytes. Activated cytotoxic T lymphocytes then release substances linked to cytolytic effector activity that lead to the killing of infected target cells. Once the lethal hit has been delivered to the target cell, the cytotoxic T lymphocyte can detach from the target cell. The target cell then undergoes programmed cell death by increasing cell membrane permeability, which leads to cell disintegration and, by apoptosis, a form of cell death characterized by vesicular blebbing from the cytoplasmic membrane and rapid destruction of DNA.

Activation of B Lymphocytes (Humoral Immune Response)

Activated T helper cells may also induce the growth and differentiation of B lymphocytes, which mediate the humoral or **antibody-mediated response.** Release of cytokines with growth and differentiation activity by CD4 T lymphocytes promotes the proliferation and terminal differentiation of B cells into high-rate antibody-producing cells called plasma cells, which secrete antigen-specific antibody. B lymphocytes may also bind and internalize foreign antigen directly, process that antigen, and present it to CD4 T lymphocytes. A pool of activated B lymphocytes may differentiate to form **memory cells,** which respond more rapidly and efficiently to subsequent encounters with identical or closely related antigenic structures.

Antibody Structure & Function

The primary function of B lymphocytes is to make antibodies. Antibodies are **immunoglobulins** directed toward specific antigens. Antibodies are proteins that combine specifically with antigens to initiate the humoral (antibody-mediated) immune response. Circulating immunoglobulins have specificity that enables them to combine with one particular antigenic structure. Humoral immune responses result in the production of a diverse repertoire of antibodies that makes them able to combine with a broad range of antigens. This diversity is a function of complex DNA rearrangements and RNA processing within B lymphocytes early in ontogenetic development.

All immunoglobulin molecules share a four-chain polypeptide structure consisting of two heavy and two light chains (Figure 3–3). Each chain includes an amino terminal portion, containing the **variable (V) region,** and a carboxyl terminal portion, containing four or five **constant (C) regions.** V regions are highly variable structures that form the antigen-binding site, while the C domains support effector functions of the molecules. The five classes (**isotypes**) of immunoglobulins are **IgG, IgA, IgM, IgD,** and **IgE** and are defined on the basis of differences in the C region of the heavy chains. Digestion of an immunoglobulin molecule by the enzyme papain produces two antigen-binding F(ab) fragments and the Fc (crystallizable) fragment. Pepsin digestion of the immunoglobulin molecule results in a single F(ab)$_2$ fragment joined by a disulfide bond. Immunoglobulins serve a variety of secondary biologic roles, including complement fixation, transplacental passage, and facilitation of phagocytosis (**opsonization**), all of which participate in host defenses against disease.

The IgE molecule is a monomeric structure of molecular weight 190,000. It constitutes only 0.004% of the total serum immunoglobulins and binds with very high avidity via its Fc region to the high-affinity Fcε receptor on mast cells and basophils. IgE specifically mediates the release of chemical mediators from mast cells and basophils in allergic hypersensitivity diseases as well as in the host defense against parasites.

Humoral Mechanisms of Antigen Elimination

Antibodies may induce the elimination of foreign antigen through a number of different mechanisms. Binding of antibody to bacterial toxins or foreign venoms promotes elimination of these antigen-antibody complexes through the reticuloendothelial system. Antibodies may also coat bacterial surfaces, allowing clearance by macrophages in a process known as opsonization. Some classes of antibodies may complex with antigen and activate the complement system of cascading components, culminating in lysis of the target cell. Finally, the major class of antibody, IgG, can bind to natural killer cells that subsequently complex with target cells and release cytotoxins (see antibody-dependent cellular cytotoxicity, above).

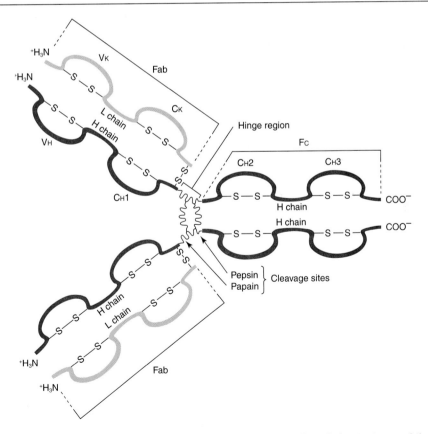

Figure 3–3. Structure of a human IgG antibody molecule. Depicted are the four-chain structure and the variable and constant domains. (V, variable region; C, constant region. The sites of pepsin and papain cleavage are shown.) (Reproduced, with permission, from Stites DP, Terr AL, Parslow TG: *Basic & Clinical Immunology,* 9th ed. Appleton & Lange, 1997.)

Hypersensitivity Immune Responses

Gell and Coombs classified the mechanisms of immune responses to antigen into four distinct types of reactions to allow for clearer understanding of the immunopathogenesis of disease.

A. Type I: Anaphylactic or immediate hypersensitivity reactions occur after binding of antigen to preformed IgE antibodies attached to the surface of the mast cell or basophil and result in the release of inflammatory mediators (see Mechanisms of Inflammation, below) that produce the clinical manifestations. Examples of type I-mediated reactions include anaphylactic shock, allergic rhinitis, allergic asthma, and acute allergic reactions to drugs.

B. Type II: Cytotoxic reactions involve the binding of either IgG or IgM antibody to antigens covalently bound to cell membrane structures. Antigen-antibody binding activates the complement cascade and results in destruction of the cell to which the antigen is bound. Examples of tissue injury by this mechanism include immune hemolytic anemia and Rh hemolytic disease in the newborn. Another example of the type II-mediated disease process without cell death is autoimmune hyperthyroidism, a disorder in which thyroid-stimulating antibodies stimulate thyroid tissue or TSH-binding inhibitory antibodies inhibit binding of TSH to its receptor. Similarly, in myasthenia gravis, antibodies are directed to the acetylcholine receptor, blocking this neuromediator from interacting with its receptor.

C. Type III: Immune complex-mediated reactions occur when immune complexes are formed by the binding of antigens to antibodies. Complexes are usually cleared from the circulation by the phagocytic system. However, deposition of these complexes in tissues or in vascular endothelium can produce immune complex-mediated tissue injury by leading to complement activation, anaphylatoxin generation, chemotaxis of polymorphonuclear leukocytes, phagocytosis, and tissue injury. Serum sickness, certain types of nephritis, and certain features of infective endocarditis are clinical examples of type III-mediated diseases.

D. Type IV: Delayed hypersensitivity reactions are mediated not by antibody but by T lymphocytes (cell-mediated immunity). Classic examples are tuberculin skin test reactions and contact dermatitis.

Mechanisms of Inflammation

Elimination of foreign antigen by cellular or humoral processes is integrally linked to the inflammatory response, in which cytokines and antibodies trigger the recruitment of additional cells and the release of endogenous vasoactive and proinflammatory enzymatic substances (**inflammatory mediators**).

Inflammation may have both positive and deleterious effects. Tight control of inflammatory mechanisms promotes efficient elimination of foreign substances and prevents uncontrolled lymphocyte activation and unregulated antibody production. However, uncontrolled inflammation can lead to tissue damage and organ dysfunction. Inflammation is responsible for hypersensitivity reactions and for many of the clinical effects of autoimmunity. The major type of immunologic inflammation—important in allergic diseases—involves the type I IgE-directed release of chemical mediators from mast cells and basophils (immediate-type hypersensitivity). Clinical allergy represents a hypersensitivity response arising from deleterious inflammation in response to the presence of normally harmless environmental antigens. Other pathways of immunologic inflammation include cell-mediated immunity and immune complex-mediated inflammation. Cell-mediated immunity is responsible for host defenses against intracellular pathogenic organisms, though abnormal regulation of this system may result in allergic contact dermatitis (eg, type IV delayed-type hypersensitivity responses). Similarly, immune complex-mediated (type III) inflammation is an important aspect of complement-mediated processes in normal host defenses, including opsonization and antibody-dependent cell-mediated cytotoxicity (ADCC), while hypersensitivity of immune complex-mediated immunity is responsible for the cutaneous Arthus reaction, systemic serum sickness, and some aspects of clinical autoimmunity. Imbalances in the inflammatory system may result from genetic defects, infection, neoplasms, and hormonal disturbances, though precise mechanisms that promote abnormal regulation and persistence of inflammatory processes are complex and poorly understood.

Synthesis of IgE in Allergic Reactivity

Allergic hypersensitivity results from the inappropriate production of IgE in response to allergen. Induction of B lymphocytes to synthesize IgE is primarily a function of the interaction of IL-4, IL-13, and gamma interferon (IFN-γ). The cytokine IL-4 is a critical factor for isotype switching to IgE and is sufficient to initiate germ line transcription of IgE. IL-13 has about 30% structural homology with IL-4 and shares much of IL-4's activities on mononuclear cells and B lymphocytes. IL-4 tends to be an earlier and more transient signal compared with IL-13. Recent sibling pair studies suggest that five markers on chromosome 5 at 5q31.1 are linked with a gene modulating total serum IgE concentration. Evidence was found for the linkage of 5q31.1 and the IL-4 gene, suggesting that IL-4 or a nearby gene in this chromosome locale regulates overall IgE production. Additional B lymphocyte activation and differentiation factors triggered through the B cell membrane receptor CD40 are required for the expression of mature mRNA and subsequent IgE synthesis. In humans, a variety of secondary signals work in concert with IL-

4 to promote IgE synthesis, including IL-2, IL-5, and IL-6. In contrast, gamma interferon (IFN-γ) inhibits IL-4-dependent IgE synthesis in humans. Thus, an imbalance favoring IL-4 over IFN-γ may induce IgE formation. In one study, reduced interferon gamma at birth was associated with clinical atopy at age 12 months. A defect in IFN-γ secretion may be due to a posttranscriptional defect in secretion.

Helper (CD4) T lymphocytes play a central role in the induction of normal immune responses. In allergic inflammatory processes, T lymphocytes represent a source of IL-4 as well as of secondary signals necessary to drive the production of IgE by B lymphocytes. Two subsets of CD4 helper T lymphocytes have been identified, differing in their phenotypic patterns of cytokine synthesis and release. **TH1** cells elaborate IFN-γ and TNFβ (tumor necrosis factor β) but not IL-4 and IL-5, and have been found to participate in type IV delayed hypersensitivity reactions. **TH2** cells secrete IL-4, IL-5, and IL-9 but not IFN-γ and TNFβ, and have been implicated in allergic and inflammatory responses. As mentioned, IL-4 is critical to isotype switch to IgE. IL-5 promotes maturation, activation, and chemotaxis of eosinophils, and IL-9 is a mast cell and T cell growth factor. Activated T lymphocytes exhibiting TH2-characteristic cytokines have been demonstrated at sites of inflammation in allergic airway disease and are believed to direct the immune response toward allergic inflammation. The demonstration of allergen-specific T cell lines that proliferate and secrete large amounts of IL-4 on exposure to relevant antigen in vitro further supports the existence of specific TH2-like clones. It is not known what drives undifferentiated CD4 T lymphocytes to become either TH1 or TH2 cells, though the specific cytokine milieu in which the TH cell differentiation occurs appears to be an important element in determining the direction of differentiation. The major determinant of TH2 differentiation is the cytokine IL-4, while the cytokine IL-12 appears to drive the differentiation to TH1 cells. Mononuclear phagocytes are the major source of IL-12, suggesting a mechanism whereby antigens more likely to be processed by macrophages, including bacterial antigens and intracellular pathogens, produce TH1 responses. The original source of the IL-4 responsible for TH2 differentiation is unclear, though the milieu of allergic inflammation would appear to drive the continued TH2 response.

Since the discovery of IgE over 2 decades ago, scientists have considered various therapeutic strategies to selectively inhibit IgE antibody production and action. Research has focused on understanding the mechanisms controlling IgE production, including the molecular events of B cell switching to IgE synthesis, IL-4 and IL-13 signaling, T and B cell surface receptor interactions, and the mechanisms driving TH2 differentiation. IL-4 antagonists and IL-4 neutralizing antibodies, anti-CD23 (FcεRII) antibodies, allergen modification, oligonucleotides that inhibit IgE binding to FcεRI, soluble FcεRI proteins, and FcεRI-IgG fusion proteins have been used in treatment with limited success. Perhaps the most promising strategy is the neutralization of IgE by antibodies directed against the region of IgE involved in the interaction with IgE receptors. Animal models have shown that such anti-IgE antibodies can inhibit IgE activity by preventing binding of IgE to its receptor as well as down-regulating new IgE antibody production. Early clinical trials in humans have shown that these antibodies are well tolerated and can reduce rhinitis symptoms and early and late phase bronchoconstriction.

---

9. What are the components of and distinctions between the innate and adaptive forms of immunity?
10. Indicate the primary role of the immune system and the major classes of events by which this is accomplished.
11. What is the phenomenon of MHC restriction?
12. What signals are necessary for activation of helper T lymphocytes?
13. What two signals are necessary for activation of cytotoxic T lymphocytes?
14. What are the common structural features of antibodies?
15. Name four different mechanisms by which antibodies can induce the elimination of foreign antigens.
16. What are the four types of immune reactions in the Gell and Coombs classification scheme, and what are some examples of disorders in which each is involved?
17. What is the critical factor in switching Ig synthesis to the IgE isotype? What are some secondary factors which contribute to, or inhibit, IgE synthesis?

PATHOPHYSIOLOGY OF SELECTED IMMUNE DISORDERS

ALLERGIC RHINITIS

Clinical Presentation

Allergic airway disease, such as allergic rhinitis and allergic asthma, is characterized by local tissue damage and organ dysfunction arising from an abnormal hypersensitivity immune response to normally harmless and ubiquitous environmental allergens. Allergens that cause airway disease are predominantly seasonal tree, grass, and weed pollens or perennial inhalants (eg, house dust mite antigen, cockroach, mold, animal dander, and other protein antigens). Occasionally, food or drug allergens may produce allergic airway disease. Allergic disease is a common cause of pediatric and adult acute and chronic airway problems. Both allergic rhinitis and asthma account for significant morbidity, and asthma has increased in prevalence, severity, and mortality since the 1970s. The diagnosis of allergic airway disease is based on the history and physical examination confirmed by the demonstration of allergen-specific IgE in the serum or at the tissue level. Because asthma is considered elsewhere in this book (Chapter 9), allergic rhinitis will be discussed here as a model for the pathophysiology of IgE-mediated allergic airway disease.

Etiology

Upper airway disease may be acute or chronic. Acute (nonallergic) rhinitis arises from infectious causes or, in children, occasionally as a result of nasal foreign body obstruction. Chronic rhinitis occurring episodically or continuously is often a result of allergic hypersensitivity, though other causes may underlie this syndrome.

Allergic rhinitis implies the existence of hypersensitivity to environmental allergens that impact the upper respiratory mucosa physically and directly. Particles larger than 5 mm are filtered almost completely by the nasal mucosa. Since most pollen grains are at least this large, few intact particles would be expected to penetrate the lower airway when the nose is functioning normally. Gases affect primarily the lower airway except for some amount partially cleared in the nasal vault. Heating and humidification of inspired particles reduce hypersensitivity responses in the upper airway, presumably as a result of temperature and osmolar effects on the nasal mucosa. In allergic individuals, antigen absorbed through the nasal airway mucosa can induce a type I immediate hypersensitivity response. The allergic or atopic state is characterized by an inherited tendency to generate IgE antibodies to specific environmental allergens and the inflammatory response that ensues from the interaction of allergen with cell-bound IgE. The clinical presentation of allergic rhinitis includes nasal, ocular, and palatal pruritus, paroxysmal sneezing, rhinorrhea, and nasal congestion. A personal or family history of other allergic diseases such as asthma or atopic dermatitis supports a diagnosis of allergy. Physical stigmas that support the diagnosis include bilateral infraorbital edema ("allergic shiners"), a horizontal nasal crease, pale and boggy nasal mucosa, nasal obstruction, and eczema involving the flexural surfaces of the extremities. Evidence of tissue eosinophilia or basophilia by nasal smear or scraping may support the diagnosis also. Confirmation of allergic rhinitis requires the demonstration of specific IgE antibodies to common allergens by in vitro tests such as the radioallergosorbent test (RAST) or in vivo (skin) testing.

Pathology & Pathogenesis

The clinical and laboratory manifestations of allergic rhinitis are due to local tissue inflammation and organ dysfunction of the upper airway arising from type I, IgE-mediated immune response. The inflammatory response mediated by the interaction of antigen with IgE bound to mast cells and basophils triggers the release of vasoactive, enzymatic, and chemotactic mediators. Activation of mast cells and basophils induces both the release of preformed mediators (histamine, chemotactic factors, and enzymes) and the synthesis and release of newly generated mediators (prostaglandins, leukotrienes, and platelet activating factor). Mast cells and basophils also have the ability to synthesize and release proinflammatory cytokines, growth and regulatory factors that interact in complex networks.

The interaction of mediators with various target organs and cells of the upper airway can induce a biphasic response: an early effect on blood vessels, smooth muscle, and secretory glands marked by vascular leakiness, smooth muscle constriction, and mucus hypersecretion; and a late response characterized by mucosal edema and the influx of inflammatory cells. Early phase events are mediated chiefly by histamine, while late phase events are induced by cytokines, preformed chemotactic mediators, arachidonic acid metabolites (leukotrienes), and platelet-activating factor.

The **early phase response** occurs within minutes after exposure to an antigen. Following intranasal challenge or ambient exposure to relevant allergen, the allergic patient begins sneezing and develops an increase in nasal secretions. After approximately 5 minutes, the patient develops mucosal swelling leading to reduced airflow. These changes are accompanied by release of vasoactive and smooth muscle constrictive mediators, including histamine,

N-α-p-tosyl-L-arginine methylester-esterase (TAME), leukotrienes, prostaglandin D_2 (PGD_2), and kinins and kininogens from mast cells and basophils. The **early phase response** is marked grossly by erythema, localized edema, and pruritus resulting largely from the interaction of histamine with target tissues of the upper airway. Histologically, the early response is characterized by vasodilation, edema, and a mild cellular infiltrate of mostly granulocytes.

The **late phase response** may follow the early phase response (dual response) or may occur as an isolated event. Late phase reactions begin 2–4 hours following initial exposure to antigen, reach maximal activity at 6–12 hours, and usually resolve within 12–24 hours. The late phase response appears to be antigen dose-dependent. Patients who manifest a late response have primarily nasal obstruction as a result of reduced airflow. Mediators of the early phase response—except for PGD_2—reappear during the late phase response in the absence of antigen rechallenge. Absence of PGD_2, an exclusive product of mast cell release, suggests that basophils and not mast cells are an important source of mediators in the late phase response. The late phase response is characterized grossly by erythema, induration, local heat, burning, and itching and microscopically by an influx of mainly eosinophils and mononuclear cells. There is strong circumstantial evidence that eosinophils are important proinflammatory cells in allergic airway disease (particularly asthma). Eosinophils are frequently found in secretions from the nasal mucosa of patients with allergic rhinitis and in the sputum of asthmatics. Products of activated eosinophils such as major basic protein and eosinophilic cationic protein, which are destructive to airway epithelial tissue and predispose to persistent airway reactivity, have also been localized to the airways of patients with allergic disease. Epithelial disruption is a feature in patients with both atopic dermatitis and asthma. The recruitment of eosinophils and other inflammatory cells to the airway is largely a product of activated **chemokines**. These chemotactic cytokines are 7–16 kDa proteins that attract and activate lymphocytes, granulocytes, and monocytes. Two subfamilies of chemokines differ in the cells they primarily attract and in the chromosome location of their genes. The C-C chemokines, including RANTES, MCP-1, MCP-3, and eotaxin, are located on chromosome segment 7q11-q21 and selectively recruit eosinophils. Leukocytes recruited into the airway attach to vascular endothelial cells through receptor-ligand interaction of cell surface **adhesion molecules** of the integrin, selectin, and immunoglobulin supergene family. Endothelial cell adhesion molecule receptors, including ICAM-1, VCAM-1, and E-selectin, are up-regulated by IL-1, TNF-α, and LPS. The interaction of these receptors with ligands present on the surface of leukocytes mediates a sequence of events that includes margination of leukocytes along the walls of the microvasculature, adhesion of leukocytes to the epithelium, transmigration of leukocytes through vessel walls, and migration along a chemotactic gradient to reach tissue compartments. Inflammatory cells infiltrating tissues in the late response may further elaborate cytokines and histamine-releasing factors that may perpetuate the late phase response, leading to a sustained hyperresponsiveness and disruption of the target tissue (eg, bronchi, skin, or nasal mucosa). Release of proinflammatory mediators and cytokines can thus precipitate a sustained inflammatory response, resulting in localized edema, mucus secretion, epithelial disruption, and influx of eosinophils, neutrophils, and mononuclear cells. Pathophysiologic events of the late phase response characterize a persistent inflammatory state thought to most closely mimic clinical allergic disease. Indeed, late phase reactivity has been described in naturally occurring allergic conditions, including allergic rhinitis and conjunctivitis, asthma, food-sensitive atopic dermatitis, and anaphylaxis. Inflammatory changes in the airways are recognized as critical features of both allergic rhinitis and chronic asthma. Therefore, therapeutic interventions that prevent or reverse inflammatory processes are most effective in the control of chronic and severe allergic disease.

Clinical Manifestations

The clinical manifestations of allergic airway disease (Table 3–1) arise from the interaction of mast cell and basophil mediators with target organs of the upper and lower airway. The symptoms of allergic rhinitis appear immediately following exposure to a relevant allergen (early phase response), though many patients experience chronic and recurrent symptoms on the basis of the late phase response. Complications of severe or untreated allergic rhinitis include sinusitis, auditory tube dysfunction, dysosmia, sleep disturbances, and chronic mouth breathing.

A. Sneezing, Pruritus, Mucus Hypersecretion: Allergic rhinitis is characterized by chronic or episodic paroxysmal sneezing; nasal, ocular, or palatal pruritus; and watery rhinorrhea triggered by

Table 3–1. Clinical manifestations of allergic rhinitis.

Symptoms and signs
Sneezing paroxysms
Nasal, ocular, palatal itching
Clear rhinorrhea
Nasal congestion
Pale, bluish nasal mucosa
Transverse nasal crease
Infraorbital cyanosis ("allergic shiners")
Serous otitis media
Laboratory findings
Nasal eosinophilia
Evidence of allergen-specific IgE by skin or RAST testing

exposure to a specific allergen. Patients may demonstrate signs of chronic pruritus of the upper airway, including a horizontal nasal crease from frequent nose rubbing ("allergic salute") and palatal "clicking" from rubbing the itching palate with the tongue. These symptoms often occur immediately following allergen exposure, though the symptoms may occur during the late phase in patients with chronic or severe disease when early phase mediators may reappear. Sneezing is caused by stimulation of local irritant nerve endings, initiating central neural reflexes. Mucus hypersecretion results primarily from excitation of parasympathetic-cholinergic pathways. Pruritus results from the actions of histamine secreted by mast cells and basophils during the early response. Early phase symptoms are best treated with avoidance of relevant allergens and oral antihistamines, which competitively antagonize H_1 receptor sites in target tissues. Effective treatment of late phase or chronic symptoms requires the use of topical anti-inflammatory medications (nasal cromolyn or nasal steroids) with or without allergen-specific immunotherapy (hyposensitization). Anti-inflammatory treatment appears to reduce cellular inflammation during the late phase. The mechanisms of action of allergen immunotherapy in reducing symptoms and airway inflammation are diverse and include reducing levels of allergen-specific IgE while inducing the formation of allergen-specific IgG (blocking antibodies) and the formation of T cell clones that may inhibit IgE formation. Indeed, specific allergen immunotherapy has been found to decrease the production of IL-4 in vitro in response to a specific allergen.

B. Nasal Stuffiness: Nasal congestion results from swelling of the mucus membranes of the nose following secretion of mast cell mediators of inflammation and from the physical barrier caused by increased viscid secretions. **Acoustic rhinometry** can quantitatively assess changes in nasal airway caliber that correlate with nasal congestion and release of inflammatory mediators. Acoustic rhinometry uses the reflection of sound waves transmitted into the anterior nares to estimate geometry of the nasal passages. The measurement is noninvasive, rapid, and simple to perform and may ultimately have direct clinical application. Symptoms of nasal obstruction frequently occur during the late phase response and are characteristic of chronic perennial allergic rhinitis. Nasal mucosal membranes may appear pale blue and boggy. Children frequently show signs of obligate mouth breathing, including long facies, narrow maxillae, flattened malar eminences, marked overbite, and high-arched palates. These symptoms are not mediated by histamine and are poorly responsive to antihistamine therapy. Oral sympathomimetics that induce vasoconstriction by stimulation of alpha-adrenergic receptors are often used in conjunction with antihistamines to treat nasal congestion. Topical decongestants have limited value in patients with allergic rhinitis, as frequent use results in rebound vasodilation and the syndrome of rhinitis medicamentosa. Chronic nasal stuffiness in allergic rhinitis requires allergen avoidance, often in combination with anti-inflammatory agents or allergen immunotherapy.

C. Airway Hyperresponsiveness: Late phase inflammation induces a state of nasal airway hyperresponsiveness to both irritants and allergens in patients with chronic allergic rhinitis. Airway hyperreactivity can cause heightened sensitivity to both environmental irritants such as tobacco smoke and noxious odors as well as to allergens such as pollens. The phenomenon of heightened nasal sensitivity to allergen following initial exposures to the allergen is known as "priming." Airway hyperresponsiveness is also a hallmark of allergic asthma and has been correlated with disease severity and medication requirements. There are no standardized clinical tools to accurately assess late phase hyperresponsiveness in allergic rhinitis. Bronchial provocation with antigen or pharmacologic bronchoconstrictors may be used to assess airway hyperresponsiveness in asthma. Bronchial airway hyperresponsiveness appears to result from late phase cellular infiltration and mucosal edema. Eosinophil by-products may inflict airway epithelial damage, which in turn can predispose to airway hyperreactivity in asthma. Mechanisms contributing to nasal airway hyperresponsiveness are unclear. The increased sensitivity to allergen is related to inflammation but not necessarily linked to it, since inflammation can occur in the absence of priming.

Evidence is accumulating that there is a relationship between allergic rhinitis and asthma. Recent epidemiologic findings correlate worsening asthma with the presence of severe rhinitis, and therapies to control rhinitis have shown beneficial effects on the treatment of asthma. In patients with allergies who have both rhinitis and asthma, seasonal exposure to pollen can increase methacholine responsiveness in the lower airway. This lower airway responsiveness can be reduced by the use of topical steroids in the upper airway. The mechanisms underlying the relationship between the upper and lower airways are unclear. Putative mechanisms suggest the existence of a neural nasal-bronchial reflex, postnasal drip of inflammatory cells and mediators from the nose into the lower airways, absorption of inflammatory cells and mediators into the systemic circulation and ultimately to the lung, and nasal blockage and subsequent mouth breathing, which may facilitate the entry of asthmagenic triggers to the lower airway. Effective treatment of late phase airway responsiveness requires allergen avoidance and the use of anti-inflammatory medications with or without immunotherapy.

D. Nasal Eosinophilia: Infiltration of nasal mucosa with eosinophils is a characteristic finding in patients with allergic rhinitis. Release of IL-5 and GM-CSF and mast cell mediators (PAF and leukotrienes) induces the development and accumulation of eosinophils in late phase reactions. Basophils may occasionally appear in both early and late phases. Examination of nasal secretions for eosinophils can be a useful adjunct to the evaluation of patients with suspected allergic rhinitis. Specimens from patients with atopic disease frequently show moderate to large numbers of eosinophils, while nonatopic patients demonstrate an absence of these cells. The degree of nasal eosinophilia is related to the extent of allergic exposure and symptomatology, so that findings may vary in and out of allergy season. Specimens may be collected by instructing patients to blow their nose into wax paper or by scraping the medial third of the inferior turbinate with a plastic curette. The secretions are applied to a glass slide and stained with Wright's or Hansel's stain. Both techniques have approximately 70% sensitivity and 95% specificity in the diagnosis of allergic rhinitis. Because the eosinophil is primarily a tissue-dwelling cell, quantification of peripheral blood eosinophils to diagnose allergic disease is of limited value.

E. In Vivo or in Vitro Measurement of Allergen-Specific IgE: This is the primary tool for the confirmation of suspected allergic disease. In vivo skin testing with allergens suspected of causing hypersensitivity constitutes an indirect bioassay for the presence of allergen-specific IgE on tissue mast cells or basophils. Percutaneous or intradermal administration of dilute concentrations of specific antigens elicits an immediate wheal and flare response in a sensitized individual. This response marks a "local anaphylaxis" resulting from the controlled release of mediators from activated mast cells. Positive skin tests for inhalant allergens, combined with a history and examination suggestive of allergy, strongly implicate the allergen as a cause of the patient's symptoms. Negative skin tests with an unconvincing allergy history argue strongly against an allergic origin. Major advantages to skin testing include simplicity, rapidity of performance, and low cost.

In vitro tests provide quantitative assays of allergen-specific IgE in the serum. In these assays, patient serum is reacted initially with antigen bound to a solid phase material and then labeled with a radioactive or enzyme-linked anti-IgE antibody. These immunoallergosorbent tests show a 70–80% correlation with skin testing to pollens, dust mites, and danders and are useful in patients receiving chronic antihistamine therapy who are unable to undergo skin testing and in patients with extensive dermatitis.

F. Impaired Health-Related Quality of Life: Recently, there has been increasing awareness of the important role of health-related quality of life in the clinical assessment of patients with allergic rhinitis and asthma. A number of questionnaires now available focus on functional effects of the illness and its treatments as perceived by the patient. Most conventional clinical measures of airway status can define morbidity but do not often correlate with overall well-being. Patients with allergic rhinitis are often bothered by sleep disruption, limitations in daily activity, irritability, daytime fatigue, and nonnasal symptoms such as thirst, poor concentration, and headache.

G. Serous Otitis Media and Sinusitis: Serous otitis and acute and chronic sinusitis are the major morbidity in patients with allergic rhinitis. Both conditions occur secondary to the obstructed nasal passages and sinus ostia in patients with chronic allergic or nonallergic rhinitis. Complications of chronic rhinitis should be considered in patients with protracted rhinitis unresponsive to therapy, refractory asthma, or persistent bronchitis. Serous otitis results from auditory tube obstruction by mucosal edema and hypersecretion. Children with serous otitis media can present with conductive hearing loss, delayed speech, and recurrent otitis media associated with chronic nasal obstruction. Sinusitis may be acute, subacute, or chronic depending on the duration of symptoms. Obstruction of osteomeatal drainage in patients with chronic rhinitis predisposes to bacterial infection in the sinus cavities. Patients manifest symptoms of persistent nasal discharge, cough, sinus discomfort, and nasal obstruction. Examination may reveal chronic otitis media, infraorbital edema, inflamed nasal mucosa, and purulent nasal discharge. Radiographic diagnosis by x-ray or CT scan reveals sinus opacification, membrane thickening, or the presence of an air-fluid level. Effective treatment of infectious complications of chronic rhinitis requires antibiotics, systemic antihistamine and decongestants, and perhaps intranasal corticosteroids.

---

18. What are the major clinical manifestations of allergic rhinitis?
19. What are the major etiologic factors in allergic rhinitis?
20. What are the pathogenetic mechanisms in allergic rhinitis?

PRIMARY IMMUNODEFICIENCY DISEASES

There are many potential sites where developmental aberrations in the immune system can lead to abnormalities in immunocompetence (Table 3–2). When these defects are genetic in origin, they are referred to as the primary immunodeficiency disorders. This is in contrast to compromised immunity secondary to pharmacologic therapy, human immunodeficiency virus, malnutrition, or systemic illnesses

Table 3–2. Primary immunodeficiency disorders.

Functional Abnormality	Disease Category	Primary Cellular Component	Stage of Defect
Abnormal maturation	SCID (Swiss type)	Progenitor cell	Early
	X-linked agammaglobulinemia	B lymphocyte	Early
	DiGeorge's syndrome	T lymphocyte	Early
Abnormal proliferation and differentiation	Common variable immunodeficiency	B lymphocyte[1]	Late[1]
	Selective IgA deficiency	B lymphocyte	Late
	Hyper-IgM immunodeficiency	B lymphocyte	Late
	Ataxia-telangiectasia	T lymphocyte	Early
Abnormal regulatory cell function	Common variable immunodeficiency	T lymphocyte, B lymphocyte, macrophage	Late
	Chronic mucocutaneous candidiasis	T lymphocyte, macrophage	Late
Enzyme defect	SCID-ADA deficiency	B and T lymphocytes	Late
	PNP deficiency	T lymphocyte	Late
Abnormal cytokine response	Hyper-IgE syndrome	B lymphocyte	Late

Key: ADA = adenosine deaminase; PNP = purine nucleoside phosphorylase; SCID = severe combined immunodeficiency disease.
[1]Variable defects, though the most common is in terminal differentiation of B lymphocytes.

such as systemic lupus erythematosus or diabetes mellitus.

Clinical investigations of various congenital defects have helped characterize many aspects of normal immune physiology. The very nature of a defect in host immune responses places the susceptible individual at high risk for the development of a variety of infectious, malignant, and autoimmune diseases and disorders. The nature of the specific functional defect will significantly influence the type of infection that affects the host. Table 3–3 lists some of the typical organisms causing infection in patients with various immunodeficiency disorders. The T lymphocyte plays a central role in inducing and coordinating immune responses; thus, any immunopathogenic mechanism that impairs T lymphocyte function, or **cell-mediated immunity,** predisposes the host to the development of serious chronic and potentially life-threatening infections with viruses, mycobacteria, fungi, and protozoa involving any or all organ systems. Similarly, immunopathogenic dysfunction of B lymphocytes resulting in **antibody deficiency** will predispose the host to pyogenic sinopulmonary and mucosal infections.

Immunodeficiency disorders characterized by antibody deficiency or complement system deficiency are associated with an increased incidence of autoimmune phenomena, including diseases clinically similar to rheumatoid arthritis, systemic lupus erythematosus, autoimmune hemolytic anemia, and immune thrombocytopenic purpura. The underlying pathogenetic mechanisms have not been clearly elucidated. Patients with impaired immune responses are also at greater risk for certain malignancies than the general population. The occurrence of cancer may be related to an underlying impairment of immune surveillance, a theory which suggests that neoplastic changes occur frequently in cells but are manifested as malignant neoplasms only if they escape recognition and destruction by the immune system. There has been speculation also that chronic immune stimulation of an inadequate immune system may result in unregulated cellular proliferation and the subsequent development of malignancy (eg, B cell lymphomas).

Traditionally, the primary immunodeficiencies are classified according to which component of the immune response is principally compromised: the humoral response, cell-mediated immunity, complement, or phagocytic cell function. To facilitate clearer insights into underlying pathogenesis and potential therapies for these disorders, it is perhaps more useful to conceptualize these disorders according to their pathophysiologic abnormalities than according to their morphologic characteristics (Table 3–2). The physiology of the normal immune response to antigen is summarized in Figure 3–2. There are distinct developmental stages that characterize the maturation and differentiation of the cellular components of the immune system. The primary immunodeficiency disorders discussed below will include those characterized by (1) early developmental

Table 3–3. Relationship of various pathogens to infection in primary immunodeficiency disorders.

	Pyogenic Bacteria	Mycobacteria	Fungi		Viruses	Parasites		
			Pneumocystis carinii	Other Fungi		Giardia lamblia	Toxoplasma gondii	Cryptosporidium, Isospora
SCID	+	+	+	+	+	–	–	–
Thymic hypoplasia	–	+	–	+	+	–	–	–
X-linked agammaglobulinemia	+	–	–	–	–	+	–	–
Common variable immunodeficiency	+	–	–	–	–	+	–	–
Complement deficiency	+	–	–	–	–	–	–	–
Phagocytic defects	+	–	–	–	–	–	–	–

Key: SCID = severe combined immunodeficiency disease; + = association; – = no association.

defects in cellular maturation, (2) specific enzyme defects, (3) abnormalities in cellular proliferation and functional differentiation, (4) abnormalities in cellular regulation, and (5) abnormal responses to cytokines.

DISORDERS WITH EARLY DEFECTS IN CELLULAR MATURATION

1. SEVERE COMBINED IMMUNODEFICIENCY DISEASE (SCID)

Clinical Presentation

Clinically, many primary immunodeficiency disorders present early in the neonatal period. In patients with severe combined immunodeficiency, there is an absence of normal thymic tissue and the lymph nodes, spleen, and other peripheral lymphoid tissues are devoid of lymphocytes. In these patients, the complete or near-complete failure of development of both the cellular and humoral components of the immune system results in severe infections, and in untreated patients death usually occurs within the first year. Failure to thrive may be the initial presenting symptom, but mucocutaneous candidiasis, chronic diarrhea, and pneumonitis is common. The spectrum of infections is broad, as these patients may also suffer from overwhelming infection by opportunistic pathogens, disseminated viruses, and intracellular organisms. Without immune reconstitution by bone marrow transplantation, SCID is inevitably fatal within 1–2 years.

Pathology & Pathogenesis

SCID is a heterogeneous group of disorders characterized by reduced function of both B and T lymphocytes, hypogammaglobulinemia, and nonfunctioning circulating immature T lymphocytes. The genetic and cellular defects vary but in most cases can be traced to defective maturation of lymphoid stem cells. Identification of specific mutations allows for improved genetic counseling, prenatal diagnosis, and carrier detection. Moreover, specific gene transfer offers hope as a future therapy.

Two inheritance patterns have been identified: an autosomal recessive form, classically known as Swiss type and characterized by a lack of both T and B cells, and an X-linked form in which the maturation defect is mainly in the T lymphocyte lineage but humoral abnormalities result from dysfunctional T and B cell interactions. The two forms are clinically indistinguishable; however, the X-linked form is the most prevalent.

The genetic mutation causing X-linked SCID has been identified in the gamma chain of the trimeric interleukin-2 (IL-2) receptor. This defective gamma chain is shared by the receptors for IL-4 and IL-7 and leads to dysfunction of all of these cytokine receptors. Defective signaling through the IL-7 receptor appears to block normal maturation of T lymphocytes, and defective IL-2 responses inhibit proliferation of T, B, and NK cells.

The genetic defect for several forms of the autosomal recessive SCID has also been identified. Some patients have a deficiency of ZAP-70, a protein tyrosine kinase important in signal transduction through the T cell receptor. Deficiency of this kinase results in a total absence of CD8 T lymphocytes as well as functionally defective CD4 T lymphocytes that do not proliferate or differentiate normally. Other patients have defective recombination activating gene (*RAG-1* and *RAG-2*) products. RAG-1 and RAG-2 initiate recombination of antigen binding proteins, immunoglobulins, and T cell receptors. The failure to form antigen receptors leads to a quantitative and functional deficiency of T and B lymphocytes.

2. CONGENITAL THYMIC APLASIA (DiGeorge Syndrome)

Clinical Presentation & Pathogenesis

The clinical manifestations of DiGeorge syndrome reflect the defective embryonic development of organs derived from the third and fourth pharyngeal arches, including the thymus, the parathyroids, and the cardiac outflow tract. DiGeorge syndrome is classified as complete or partial depending on the presence or absence of immunologic abnormalities. In this syndrome, the spectrum of immunologic deficiency is wide, ranging from immune competency to conditions in which there are severe, life-threatening infections with organisms typically of low virulence. Patients affected by the complete syndrome have a profound T lymphocytopenia due to thymic aplasia with impaired T lymphocyte maturation, severely depressed cell-mediated immunity, and decreased suppressor T lymphocyte activity. B lymphocytes and immunoglobulin production are unaffected in most patients, though in rare instances patients may present with mild hypogammaglobulinemia and absent or poor antibody responses to neoantigens. In this subset of patients, inadequate "T helper function" due to dysfunctional T and B cell interaction and inadequate cytokine production leads to impaired humoral immunity.

DiGeorge syndrome is truly a developmental disorder and can be associated with structural abnormalities in the cardiovascular system such as truncus arteriosus or right-sided aortic arch. Parathyroid abnormalities may lead to hypocalcemia, presenting with neonatal tetany or seizures. In addition, it is common for patients to exhibit facial abnormalities such as micrognathia, hypertelorism, low-set ears with notched pinnae, and a short philtrum.

3. X-LINKED AGAMMAGLOBULINEMIA

Clinical Presentation

Formerly called Bruton's agammaglobulinemia, this condition is thought to be pathophysiologically and clinically more homogeneous than SCID. It is principally a disease of childhood, presenting clinically within the first 2 years of life with multiple and recurrent sinopulmonary infections caused primarily by pyogenic bacteria and, to a much lesser extent, viruses. Because encapsulated bacteria require antibody binding for efficient opsonization, these humorally immune-deficient patients suffer from sinusitis, pneumonia, pharyngitis, bronchitis, and otitis media secondary to infection with *Streptococcus pneumoniae* and other streptococci and *H influenzae*. Although infections due to fungal and opportunistic pathogens are rare, patients display a unique susceptibility to rare but deadly enteroviral meningoencephalitis.

Pathology & Pathogenesis

The patients are panhypogammaglobulinemic, with decreased levels of IgG, IgM, and IgA. They exhibit poor to absent responses to antigen challenge even though virtually all demonstrate normal functional T lymphocyte responses to in vitro as well as in vivo tests (ie, delayed hypersensitivity skin reactions). The basic defect in this disorder appears to be arrested cellular maturation at the pre-B lymphocyte stage. Indeed, normal numbers of pre-B lymphocytes can be found in the bone marrow, though B lymphocytes in the circulation are virtually absent. Lymphoid tissues lack fully differentiated B lymphocytes (antibody-secreting plasma cells), and lymph nodes lack developed germinal centers. The gene that is defective in X-linked agammaglobulinemia has been isolated. The defective gene product, BTK (Bruton's tyrosine kinase), is a B cell-specific signaling protein belonging to the cytoplasmic tyrosine kinase family of intracellular proteins. Gene deletions and point mutations in the catalytic domain of the *BTK* gene block normal BTK function, necessary for B cell maturation.

DISORDERS DUE TO DEFECTIVE ENZYME FUNCTION

1. ADENOSINE DEAMINASE (ADA) DEFICIENCY

About 20% of SCID cases are caused by a deficiency of ADA, which is an enzyme in the purine salvage pathway, responsible for the metabolism of adenosine. Absence of the ADA enzyme results in an accumulation of toxic adenosine metabolites within the cells (Figure 3–4). These metabolites inhibit normal lymphocyte proliferation and lead to extreme cytopenia of both B and T lymphocytes. The combined immunologic deficiency and clinical presentation of this disorder, known as SCID-ADA, are identical to that of the other forms of SCID. Skeletal abnormalities and neurologic abnormalities may be associated with this disease.

2. PURINE NUCLEOSIDE PHOSPHORYLASE (PNP) DEFICIENCY

In this very rare disorder, the enzymatic activity of PNP is severely depressed, resulting in the accumulation of intracellular purine metabolites (Figure 3–4), which in turn leads to severe functional abnormalities in T lymphocytes. Because T lymphocytes are primarily affected, patients with PNP deficiency develop severe opportunistic infections due to the cellu-

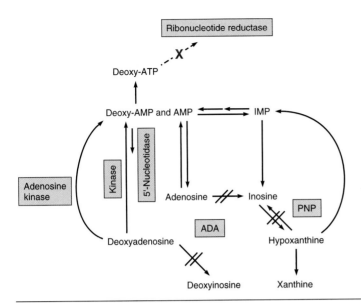

Figure 3–4. Simplified schema of the portion of the purine catabolic pathways affected by adenosine deaminase (ADA) deficiency and purine nucleoside phosphorylase (PNP) deficiency disorders. Lines across arrows indicate blocked reactions. (ATP, adenosine triphosphate; AMP, adenosine monophosphate; IMP, inosine monophosphate.) ADA catalyzes the metabolism of adenosine to inosine and deoxyadenosine to deoxyinosine. Similarly, PNP catalyzes the metabolism of inosine to hypoxanthine. In SCID-ADA, lymphocyte kinases rapidly convert deoxyadenosine to deoxy-AMP, though they are deficient in the 5'-nucleotidase that drives the reverse reaction. The result of the accumulation of deoxy-AMP and deoxy-ATP is inhibition of ribonucleotide reductase, an enzyme critical to purine and pyrimidine biosynthesis. Inhibition of this enzyme effectively shuts down DNA synthesis in the cell.

lar immune defects. Antibody production can remain intact. As many as two-thirds of affected individuals will develop such neurologic abnormalities as spastic diplegia, quadriparesis, hypotonia, or developmental delay. Autoimmunity can also be associated with PNP deficiency. This combined immune deficiency is highly lethal, though successful treatment with bone marrow transplantation has been reported.

3. CHRONIC GRANULOMATOUS DISEASE

Clinical Presentation

Chronic granulomatous disease is typically X-linked and characterized by impaired granulocytic function. This disorder of phagocytic cell function presents with recurrent skin infections, abscesses, and granulomas at sites of chronic inflammation. Abscesses can involve skin or viscera and may be accompanied by lymphadenitis. Catalase-positive organisms predominate; *S aureus* is thus the most common pathogen, though infections with gram-negative bacteria and aspergillus species also occur. Chronic granulomatous disease typically presents in childhood, though cases are occasionally reported into adulthood.

Pathology & Pathogenesis

Defects in the gene coding for NADPH oxidase inhibit oxidative metabolism and severely compromise neutrophil killing activity. NADPH oxidase catalyzes the conversion of molecular oxygen into superoxide. The oxidative burst relies on production of superoxide, which is later converted to hydrogen peroxide and sodium hypochlorite (bleach). In patients with chronic granulomatous disease, other neutrophil functions such as chemotaxis, phagocytosis, and degranulation remain intact but microbial killing is deficient.

DISORDERS WITH DEFECTIVE PROLIFERATION & DIFFERENTIATION RESPONSES

1. COMMON VARIABLE IMMUNODEFICIENCY

Clinical Presentation

This disorder is often referred to as acquired or adult-onset hypogammaglobulinemia. It is the most common serious primary immune deficiency disorder in adults. In North America, for example, it affects an estimated 1:75,000–1:50,000 individuals. The clinical spectrum is broad, and patients usually present within the first 2 decades of life. Affected individuals commonly develop recurrent sinopulmonary infections, including sinusitis, otitis, bronchitis, and pneumonia. Bronchiectasis can be the result of recurrent serious respiratory infections, and its development changes the long-term prognosis. A number of important noninfectious disorders are commonly associated with common variable immunodeficiency, including gastrointestinal malabsorption, autoimmune disorders, and neoplasms. The most frequently occurring malignancies are lymphoreticular, but gastric carcinoma and skin cancer also occur. Autoimmune disorders occur in 20–30% of patients and may precede the recurrent infections. Autoimmune cytopenias occur most frequently, but rheumatic diseases can also be seen. Serologic testing is unreliable in hypogammaglobulinemia. Monthly infusions of intravenous gamma globulin (IGIV) can reconstitute humoral immunity, decrease infections, and improve quality of life.

Pathology & Pathogenesis

Common variable immunodeficiency is a heterogeneous disorder in which the primary immunologic abnormality is a marked reduction in antibody production. The vast majority of patients will demonstrate an in vitro defect in terminal differentiation of B lymphocytes. Peripheral blood lymphocyte phenotyping demonstrates normal or reduced numbers of circulating B lymphocytes, but antibody-secreting plasma cells are conspicuously sparse in lymphoid tissues. In sharp contrast to X-linked agammaglobulinemia, no single gene defect can be held accountable for the multitude of defects noted to cause common variable immunodeficiency. In approximately 80% of patients, the defect is intrinsic to the B lymphocyte population. In the rest, a variety of T cell abnormalities lead to immune defects with subsequent impairment of B cell differentiation. These rare T lymphocyte abnormalities include increased suppressor T lymphocyte activity, decreased production of IL-2 and other cytokines, and defective synthesis of B lymphocyte growth factors such as IL-4 and IL-6. In some patients, there is also evidence of defective cytokine gene expression in T cells, decreased T cell mitogenesis, and deficient lymphokine-activated killer (LAK) cell function. Over half of patients also have some degree of T lymphocyte dysfunction as determined by absent or diminished cutaneous responses to recall antigens. Immune dysregulation may contribute to the morbidity and the myriad of autoimmune manifestations associated with common variable immunodeficiency.

2. SELECTIVE IgA DEFICIENCY

This is the most common primary immunodeficiency in adults, with a prevalence of 1:700–1:500 individuals. Most individuals with this defect have few or no clinical manifestations, but there is an increased incidence of upper respiratory tract infections, allergy, asthma, and autoimmune disorders. Whereas serum levels of the other immunoglobulin isotypes are typically normal, serum IgA levels in these individuals are markedly depressed and are often less than 5 mg/dL.

The primary functional defect is similar to the B lymphocyte differentiation defect in common variable immunodeficiency, ie, an inability of B cells to terminally differentiate to IgA-secreting B lymphocytes. An associated deficiency of IgG subclasses (mainly IgG2 and IgG4) and low-molecular-weight monomeric IgM is not uncommon. Because of the role of secretory IgA in mucosal immunity, patients with this immunodeficiency frequently develop significant infections involving the mucous membranes of the gut, conjunctiva, and respiratory tract. There is no specific treatment, but prompt antibiotic treatment is necessary in patients with recurrent infections. A subset of patients with selective IgA deficiency may develop abnormal immunologic responses, recognizing IgA as a foreign antigen. These patients are at risk for developing transfusion reactions to unwashed red blood cells or other blood products containing trace amounts of IgA.

3. HYPER-IgM IMMUNODEFICIENCY

Clinical Presentation

In patients with hyper-IgM immunodeficiency, serum levels of IgG and IgA are very low or absent but serum IgM (and sometimes IgD) levels are normal or elevated. The inheritance of this disorder may be autosomal, though it is most often X-linked. Clinically, this syndrome is manifested by recurrent pyogenic infections and an array of autoimmune phenomena such as Coombs-positive hemolytic anemia and immune thrombocytopenia.

Pathology & Pathogenesis

The principal abnormality is the defective expression of gp39, a T lymphocyte activation marker (also known as CD40-ligand). CD40-ligand interacts with CD40 on B cell surfaces during cellular activation, initiating proliferation and immunoglobulin isotype switching. Interference with receptor binding leads to a failure in isotype switching and subsequent production of IgM but no production of IgG or IgA.

DISORDERS DUE TO DEFECTIVE CYTOKINE RESPONSE

1. HYPER-IgE IMMUNODEFICIENCY

Clinical Presentation

This disorder is often referred to as "Job's syndrome" because affected individuals suffer from recurrent boils like the tormented biblical figure. The initial description of this immunodeficiency disorder was in two fair-skinned girls with recurrent staphylococcal "cold" skin abscesses associated with furunculosis, cellulitis, recurrent otitis, sinusitis, pneumatoceles, and a coarse facial appearance. The predominant organism isolated from sites of infection is *S aureus*, though other organisms such as *H influenzae*, pneumococci, gram-negative organisms, and *Candida albicans* are often identified also. Characteristically, patients have a chronic pruritic eczematoid dermatitis, growth retardation, and hyperkeratotic fingernails. Extremely high IgE levels (> 3000 IU/mL) have also been observed in patients' serum.

Pathology & Pathogenesis

The high IgE levels are thought to be a consequence of dysregulated immunologic responsiveness to cytokines, yet it is unclear if they contribute to the observed susceptibility to infection. Other immunopathologic states can be associated with elevated IgE levels, including graft-versus-host disease, AIDS, and Wiscott-Aldrich syndrome. Several immune defects have been described, but the primary defect remains unknown. Humoral immunodeficiency is suggested by poor antibody responses to neoantigens, deficiency of IgA antibody against *S aureus,* and low levels of antibodies to carbohydrate antigens. T lymphocyte functional abnormalities are suggested by decreased absolute numbers of suppressor T lymphocytes, poor in vitro proliferative responses, and defects in cytokine production. Several reports have also documented abnormalities in neutrophil chemotaxis.

---

21. What are the major clinical manifestations of each of the five categories of primary immune deficiency?
22. What are the major pathogenetic mechanisms in each category of primary immune deficiency?

ACQUIRED IMMUNODEFICIENCY SYNDROME (AIDS)

Clinical Presentation

AIDS is the most common immunodeficiency disorder in the world, and human immunodeficiency virus (HIV) infection is among the greatest epidemics in human history. AIDS is a disease defined by the presence of any of a variety of indicator diseases and serologic evidence of HIV infection. Table 3–4 lists the most recent criteria for defining and diagnosing AIDS. AIDS is the consequence of a chronic retroviral infection that produces severe, life-threatening CD4 helper T lymphocyte dysfunction and destruction. The disease is caused by the human retrovirus HIV and can be transmitted through parenteral exposure or sexual and perinatal contact.

Acute HIV infection may present as an acute, self-limited, febrile viral syndrome. Once an individual becomes infected with HIV, an initial viremic phase is followed by a period of clinical latency. Lymph tissues become centers for massive viral replication during a "silent" or asymptomatic stage of HIV infection despite an absence of detectable virus in the peripheral blood. Over time, there is a progressive decline in CD4 T lymphocytes, a reversal of the normal CD4:CD8 T lymphocyte ratio, and numerous other immunologic derangements. The clinical manifestations are directly related to HIV tissue tropism and defective immune function. Development of neurologic complications, opportunistic infections, or malignancy signal marked immune deficiency. The time course for progression of the disease varies, with the majority of individuals remaining asymptomatic for as long as 5–10 years. Typically, up to 70% of individuals will develop AIDS after a decade of subclinical HIV infection. Genetic, viral, and immunologic host factors affect both susceptibility to infection and progression of disease.

Pathology & Pathogenesis

Chemokine molecules are small cytokines characterized by significant homology which are functionally important in intercellular signaling. They have recently been discovered to play a significant role in the pathogenesis of HIV disease. During the initial stages of infection and viral proliferation, HIV surface proteins (gp120) bind to CD4 molecules on target lymphocytes and macrophages, facilitating cellular entry. The process also requires HIV-binding to chemokine co-receptors. A small percentage of individuals possessing nonfunctional alleles for the polymorphic chemokine receptor CCR5 appear to be highly resistant to HIV infection. Furthermore, macrophages, lymphocytes, and macrophage-derived microglia express different chemokine receptors, and changes in viral phenotype during the course of HIV infection may lead to changes in viral tissue tropism.

Mathematical models estimate that during HIV infection, 1 billion virions are produced per day. The reverse transcription step of HIV replication is error-prone, mutations are frequent and even within an individual patient, HIV heterogeneity develops rapidly. The development of antigenically and phenotypically distinct strains contributes to progression of disease, clinical drug resistance, and lack of efficacy of early vaccines.

Cellular activation is critical for viral infectivity and reactivation of integrated proviral DNA. Since only 2% of mononuclear cells are found peripherally, lymph nodes from HIV-infected individuals can contain large amounts of virus sequestered around infected follicular dendritic cells in the germinal centers. With HIV infection there is an absolute reduction of CD4 T lymphocytes, an accompanying deficit in CD4 T lymphocyte function, and an associated increase in CD8 suppressor or cytotoxic T lymphocytes, most of which have a cytotoxic phenotype. Cytotoxic lymphocyte activity is initially brisk and effective at inhibiting viral replication but ultimately fails. In addition to the cell-mediated immune defects, B lymphocyte function is altered such that many infected individuals have marked hypergammaglobulinemia but impaired specific antibody responses. HIV-infected patients with advanced disease (AIDS) fail to respond normally to immunization with neoantigens.

The increase in viral burden can be measured by

Table 3–4. 1993 revised classification system for HIV infection and expanded AIDS surveillance case definition for adolescents and adults.[1,2,3]

I. Clinical and lymphocyte categories:

	Clinical Categories		
CD4 T Cell Categories	(A) Asymptomatic, Acute (Primary) HIV or PGL[4]	(B) Symptomatic, Not (A) or (C) Conditions	(C) AIDS-Indicator Conditions
(1) ≥500/μL	A1	B1	C1
(2) 200–499/mL	A2	B2	C2
(3) <200/mL	A3	B3	C3

II. Conditions included in the 1993 AIDS surveillance case definition:

- Candidiasis of the esophagus, bronchi, trachea, or lungs
- Cervical cancer, invasive
- Coccidioidomycosis, disseminated or extrapulmonary
- Cryptococcosis, extrapulmonary
- Cryptosporidiosis, chronic intestinal (>1 month's duration)
- Cytomegalovirus disease (other than liver, spleen, or nodes); cytomegalovirus retinitis (with loss of vision)
- Encephalopathy, HIV-related
- Herpes simplex: chronic ulcers (>1 month's duration); or bronchitis, pneumonitis, or esophagitis
- Histoplasmosis, disseminated or extrapulmonary
- Isosporiasis, chronic intestinal (>1 month's duration)
- Kaposi's sarcoma
- Lymphoma, Burkitt's (or equivalent term); immunoblastic lymphoma (or equivalent term); primary brain lymphoma
- *Mycobacterium avium* complex or *Mycobacterium kansasii,* disseminated or extrapulmonary
- *Mycobacterium tuberculosis,* any site (pulmonary or extrapulmonary)
- *Mycobacterium,* other species or unidentified species, disseminated or extrapulmonary
- *Pneumocystis carinii* pneumonia
- Pneumonia, recurrent
- Progressive multifocal leukoencephalopathy
- *Salmonella* septicemia, recurrent
- Toxoplasmosis of brain
- Wasting syndrome due to HIV

III. Clinical Categories:

A. Category A consists of one or more of the conditions listed below in an adolescent or adult (>13 years) with documented HIV infection. Conditions listed in categories B and C must not have occurred.
- Asymptomatic HIV infection
- Persistent generalized lymphadenopathy
- Acute (primary) HIV infection with accompanying illness or history of acute HIV infection

B. Category B consists of symptomatic conditions in an HIV-infected adolescent or adult that are not included among conditions listed in clinical category C and that meet at least one of the following criteria: (a) the conditions are attributed to HIV infection or are indicative of a defect in cell-mediated immunity; or (b) the conditions are considered by physicians to have a clinical course or to require management that is complicated by HIV infection.

Examples of conditions in clinical category B include but are not limited to:
- Bacillary angiomatosis
- Oropharyngeal candidiasis (thrush)
- Vulvovaginal candidiasis, persistent, frequent, or poorly responsive to therapy
- Cervical dysplasia (moderate or severe) or cervical carcinoma in situ
- Constitutional symptoms, such as fever (38.5 °C) or diarrhea lasting >1 month
- Hairy leukoplakia
- Herpes zoster (shingles), involving at least two distinct dermatomes or more than one episode
- Idiopathic thrombocytopenic purpura
- Listeriosis
- Pelvic inflammatory disease, particularly if complicated by tubo-ovarian abscess
- Peripheral neuropathy

For classification purposes, category B conditions take precedence over those in category A. For example, someone previously treated for oral or persistent vaginal candidiasis (and who has not developed a category C disease) but who is now asymptomatic should be classified in clinical category B.

C. Category C includes the clinical conditions listed in the AIDS surveillance case definition (section II above). For classification purposes, once a category C condition has occurred, the person will remain in category C.

---

[1]Including the expanded AIDS surveillance case definition. Persons with AIDS-indicator conditions (category C) as well as those with AIDS-indicator CD4 T lymphocyte counts <200/μL (categories A3 or B3) have been reportable as AIDS cases in the United States and Territories since January 1, 1993.
[2]Modified from MMWR Morbid Mortal Wkly Rep 1992;41[RR-17].
[3]Sections II and III of this table are modified and reproduced, with permission, from Lawlor GL Jr, Fischer TJ, and Adelman DC (editors). *Manual of Allergy and Immmunology.* Little, Brown, 1994.
[4]PGL = persistent generalized lymphadenopathy. Clinical category A includes acute (primary) HIV infection.

plasma HIV-RNA levels. The development of assays to measure viral burden has led to a better understanding of HIV dynamics and provided a tool for assessing response to therapy. It is now well recognized that viral replication continues throughout the disease, and immune deterioration occurs despite clinical latency. The marked decline in CD4 T lymphocyte counts—characterizing HIV infection—is due to several mechanisms, including (1) direct HIV-mediated destruction of CD4 T lymphocytes, (2) autoimmune destruction of virus-infected T cells, (3) depletion by fusion and formation of multinucleated giant cells (syncytium formation), (4) toxicity of viral proteins to CD4 T lymphocytes and marrow suppression, and (5) induction of apoptosis (programmed cell death). Data from several large clinical cohorts have shown that there is a direct correlation between the CD4 T lymphocyte count number and the risk of AIDS-defining opportunistic infections. The viral load and the degree of CD4 T lymphocyte depletion serve as important clinical indicators of immune status in HIV-infected individuals. Prophylaxis for opportunistic infections such as pneumocystis pneumonia is started when CD4 T lymphocyte counts reach the 200–250 cells/µL range. Similarly, patients with HIV infection with fewer than 50 CD4 T lymphocytes/µL have a significantly increased risk of developing cytomegalovirus (CMV) retinitis and *Mycobacterium avium* complex (MAC) infection.

Cells other than CD4 T lymphocytes contribute to the pathogenesis of HIV infection. Monocytes and macrophages are infected with HIV and facilitate transfer of virus to sites in the central nervous system. Infected mononuclear cells also show functional defects, including reduced chemotaxis and nonspecific killing capability. HIV-infected monocytes will also release large quantities of the acute phase reactant cytokines, including IL-1, IL-6, and TNF. TNF can contribute to marked wasting and cachexia, which are noted in patients with advanced disease.

Clinical Manifestations

The clinical manifestations of AIDS are the direct consequence of the progressive and severe immunologic deficiency induced by HIV. Patients are susceptible to a wide range of atypical or opportunistic infections with bacterial, viral, protozoal, and fungal pathogens. Common nonspecific symptoms include fever, night sweats, and weight loss. Weight loss and cachexia can be due to nausea, vomiting, anorexia, or diarrhea and often portend a poor prognosis in patients with long-standing HIV infection.

As a direct consequence of HIV-induced immune dysfunction, the incidence of infection increases as the CD4 T lymphocyte number declines. **Lung infection** with *Pneumocystis carinii* is the most common opportunistic infection, affecting three-fourths of patients. Patients present clinically with fevers, cough, shortness of breath, and hypoxemia ranging in severity from mild to life-threatening. A diagnosis of pneumocystis pneumonia can be made by substantiation of the clinical and radiographic findings with Wright-Giemsa or silver methenamine staining of induced sputum samples. A negative sputum stain does not rule out disease in patients in whom there is a strong clinical suspicion of disease, and further diagnostic maneuvers such as bronchoalveolar lavage or fiberoptic transbronchial biopsy may be required to establish the diagnosis. Complications of pneumocystis pneumonia include pneumothoraces, progressive parenchymal disease with severe respiratory insufficiency, or, most commonly, adverse reactions to the medications used for treatment and prophylaxis. For reasons which are not clear, HIV-infected patients have an unusually high rate of adverse reactions to a wide variety of antibiotics and frequently develop severe debilitating cutaneous reactions.

As a consequence of chronic immune dysfunction, HIV-infected individuals are also at high risk for other pulmonary infections, including bacterial infections with *S pneumoniae* and *H influenzae* and mycobacterial infections with *Mycobacterium tuberculosis* or *Mycobacterium avium-intracellulare*, and fungal infections with *C neoformans*, *H capsulatum*, or *C immitis*. Clinical suspicion followed by early diagnosis and aggressive treatment are required.

The development of active tuberculosis is significantly accelerated in HIV infection due to compromised cellular immunity. The risk of reactivation is estimated to be 5–10% per year in HIV-infected patients compared with a lifetime risk of 10% in those without HIV. Furthermore, diagnosis may be delayed due to anergic skin responses. Extrapulmonary manifestations occur in up to 70% of HIV-infected patients with tuberculosis, and the emergence of multidrug resistance may compound the problem. MAC is a less virulent pathogen than *M tuberculosis,* and disseminated infections usually occur only with severe clinical immunodeficiency. Symptoms are nonspecific and typically consist of fever, weight loss, anemia, and gastrointestinal distress with diarrhea.

The presence on physical examination of **oral candidiasis (thrush)** and **hairy leukoplakia** is highly correlated with HIV infection and portends rapid progression to AIDS. Both oral infections result from the immunologic dysfunction associated with HIV infection. Abnormal outgrowth of candida from normal mouth flora is the cause of persistent oral candidiasis, while Epstein-Barr virus is the cause of hairy leukoplakia. HIV-infected individuals with oral candidiasis are at much greater risk for esophageal candidiasis, which may present as substernal pain and dysphagia. This infection and its characteristic clinical presentation are so common that most practitioners treat with empiric oral antifungal therapy. Should the patient not respond rapidly, other explanations for the esophageal symptoms should be explored, including herpes simplex and cytomegalovirus infections.

Persistent diarrhea, especially when accompanied by high fevers and abdominal pain, may signal **infectious enterocolitis.** The list of potential pathogens is long and includes bacteria, MAC, protozoans (cryptosporidium, microsporidia, *Isospora belli, Entamoeba histolytica, Giardia lamblia*), and even HIV itself. HIV-associated gastropathy and malabsorption are commonly noted in these patients and are associated with decreased gastric acid production. Because of their reduced gastric acid concentrations, patients have an increased susceptibility to infection with campylobacter, salmonella, and shigella.

Skin lesions commonly associated with HIV infection are typically classified as infectious (viral, bacterial, fungal), neoplastic, or nonspecific. Herpes simplex virus (HSV) and herpes zoster (HZV) may cause chronic, persistent or progressive lesions in patients with compromised cellular immunity. HSV commonly causes oral and perianal lesions but can be an AIDS-defining illness when involving the lung or esophagus. The risk of disseminated HSV or HZV infection appears to be correlated with the extent of immunoincompetence. Similarly, molluscum contagiosum is more likely to spread in severely immunocompromised patients. Seborrheic dermatitis due to *Pityrosporum ovale* and fungal skin infections (*Candida albicans,* dermatophyte species) are also commonly seen in HIV-infected patients. Staphylococcus can cause the folliculitis, furunculosis, and bullous impetigo commonly observed in HIV-infected patients and require aggressive treatment to prevent dissemination and sepsis. **Bacillary angiomatosis** is a potentially fatal dermatologic disorder of tumor-like proliferating vascular endothelial cell lesions, the result of infection by *Bartonella quintana* or *Bartonella henselae.* The lesions may resemble those of Kaposi's sarcoma but respond to treatment with erythromycin or tetracycline.

Central nervous system manifestations in HIV-infected patients include infections and malignancies. **Toxoplasmosis** frequently presents with space-occupying lesions, causing headache, altered mental status, seizures, or focal neurologic deficits. Cryptococcal meningitis commonly manifests as headache and fever. Up to 90% of patients with cryptococcal meningitis exhibit a positive serum test for *Cryptococcus neoformans* antigen.

HIV-associated cognitive-motor complex, or **AIDS dementia complex,** is the most frequently diagnosed cause of altered mental status in HIV-infected patients. Patients typically have difficulty with cognitive tasks, slowed motor function, personality changes, and waxing and waning dementia. Up to half of AIDS patients suffer from this disorder, perhaps caused by glial or macrophage infection by HIV resulting in destructive inflammatory changes within the central nervous system. The differential diagnosis can be broad, including metabolic disturbances and toxic encephalopathy due to drugs. Other causes of altered mental status include neurosyphilis, cytomegalovirus or herpes simplex encephalitis, lymphoma, and **progressive multifocal leukoencephalopathy,** a progressive demyelinating disease caused by a JC papovavirus.

Peripheral nervous system manifestations of HIV infection include sensory, motor, and inflammatory polyneuropathies. Almost a third of patients with advanced HIV disease develop peripheral tingling, numbness, and pain in their extremities. These symptoms are likely to be due to loss of nerve axons from direct neuronal HIV infection. Alcoholism, thyroid disease, syphilis, vitamin B_{12} deficiency, drug toxicity (ddI, ddC), CMV-associated ascending polyradiculopathy, and transverse myelitis also cause **peripheral neuropathies.** Less commonly, HIV-infected patients can develop an inflammatory demyelinating polyneuropathy similar to Guillain-Barré syndrome; but unlike the sensory neuropathies, this inflammatory demyelinating polyneuropathy typically presents before the onset of clinically apparent immunodeficiency. The origin of this condition is not known, though an autoimmune reaction is suspected because the disease typically responds favorably to treatment with plasmapheresis. **Retinitis** due to **cytomegalovirus** infection is the most common cause of rapidly progressive visual loss in HIV infection. The diagnosis can be difficult to make, since *Toxoplasma gondii* infection, microinfarction, and retinal necrosis can all cause visual loss.

HIV-related malignancies commonly seen in AIDS include Kaposi's sarcoma, non-Hodgkin's lymphoma, primary central nervous system lymphoma, invasive cervical carcinoma, and anal squamous cell carcinoma. The mechanism underlying the development of these malignancies may be similar to the mechanism responsible for the neoplasms seen in the primary immunodeficiency disorders.

Kaposi's sarcoma is the most common HIV-associated cancer. In San Francisco, 15–20% of HIV-infected homosexual men develop this tumor during the progression of their disease. Kaposi's sarcoma is uncommon in women and children for reasons which are not clear. Unlike "classic" Kaposi's sarcoma, which affects elderly men in the Mediterranean, the disease in HIV-infected patients may present with either localized cutaneous lesions or disseminated visceral involvement. It is often a progressive disease, and pulmonary involvement can be fatal. Histologically, the lesions of Kaposi's sarcoma consist of a mixed cell population that includes vascular endothelial cells and spindle cells within a collagen network. HIV appears to induce cytokines and growth factors that stimulate tumor cell proliferation rather than causing malignant cellular transformation. Clinically, cutaneous Kaposi's sarcoma typically presents as a purplish nodular skin lesion or painless oral lesion.

Sites of visceral involvement include the lung, lymph nodes, liver, and gastrointestinal tract. In the gastrointestinal tract, Kaposi's sarcoma can produce chronic blood loss or acute hemorrhage. In the lung it often presents as nodular coarse infiltrates bilaterally, frequently associated with pleural effusions. These infiltrates can be difficult to distinguish from opportunistic infections.

Non-Hodgkin's lymphoma is particularly aggressive in HIV-infected patients and usually indicative of significant immune compromise. The majority of these tumors are high-grade B cell lymphomas with a predilection for dissemination. The central nervous system is frequently involved, either as a primary site or an extranodal site of widespread disease.

Anal dysplasia and **squamous cell carcinoma** are also more commonly found in HIV-infected homosexual men. These tumors appear to be associated with concomitant anal or rectal infection with human papillomavirus (HPV). In HIV-infected women, the incidence of HPV-related **cervical dysplasia** is as high as 40%, and dysplasia can progress rapidly to **invasive cervical carcinoma.**

Other complications of HIV-infection include arthritides, myopathy, gastrointestinal syndromes, dysfunction of the adrenal and thyroid glands, hematologic cytopenias, and nephropathy. Since the disease was first described in 1981, medical knowledge of the underlying pathogenesis of AIDS has increased at a rate unprecedented in medical history. This knowledge has led to the rapid development of therapies directed at destroying or controlling HIV infection as well as the multitude of complicating opportunistic infections and cancers.

---

23. What are the major clinical manifestations of AIDS?
24. What are the major steps in development of AIDS following infection with HIV?

REFERENCES

General
Frank MM et al (editors): *Samter's Immunologic Diseases,* 5th ed. Little, Brown, 1995.

Leung DY: Molecular basis of allergic diseases. Mol Genet Metab 1998;63:157.

Middleton E et al (editors): *Allergy: Principles and Practice,* 5th ed. Mosby, 1998.

Allergic Rhinitis
Corren J: The impact of allergic rhinitis on bronchial asthma. J Allergy Clin Immunol 1998;101:S352.

Juniper EF: Impact of upper respiratory allergic diseases on quality of life. J Allergy Clin Immunol 1998; 101:S386.

Kita H, Gleich GJ: Chemokines active on eosinophils: Potential roles in allergic inflammation. J Exp Med 1996;183:2421.

Lim MC, Taylor RM, Naclerio RM: The histology of allergic rhinitis and its comparison to nasal lavage. Am J Respir Crit Care Med 1995;151:136.

Martin L et al: Eosinophils in allergy: Role in disease, degranulation, cytokines. Int Arch Allergy Immunol 1996;109:207.

Naclerio RM, Baroody F: Understanding the inflammatory processes in upper allergic airway disease and asthma. J Allergy Clin Immunol 1998;101:S345.

Naclerio RM, Solomon W: Rhinitis and inhalant allergens. JAMA 1997;278:1842.

Primary Immunodeficiency Diseases
Hassner A, Adelman DC: Biologic response modifiers in primary immunodeficiency disorders. Ann Intern Med 1991;115:294.

Lawton AR, Hummell DS: Primary antibody deficiencies. In: *Clinical Immunology, Principles and Practice.* Rich R et al (editors). Mosby, 1996.

Le Deist F, Fischer A: Primary T cell immunodeficiencies. In: *Clinical Immunology, Principles and Practice.* Rich R et al (editors). Mosby, 1996.

Stiehm ER (editor): *Immunologic Disorders in Infants and Children,* 4th ed. Saunders, 1996.

World Health Organization Scientific Group. Primary immunodeficiency diseases. Clin Exper Immunol 1997;109 (Suppl 1):1.

AIDS
Concorde Coordinating Committee: MRC/ANRS randomized double-blind controlled trial of immediate and deferred zidovudine in symptom-free HIV infection. Lancet 1994;343:871.

Hollander H, Katz M: HIV infection. In: *Current Medical Diagnosis and Treatment 1999.* Tierney LM Jr, McPhee SJ, Papadakis M (editors). Appleton & Lange, 1999.

Mellors JW et al: Quantification of HIV-1 RNA in plasma predicts outcome after seroconversion. Ann Intern Med 1995;122:573.

1993 revised classification system for HIV infection and expanded surveillance case definition for AIDS among adolescents and adults. MMWR Morbid Mortal Wkly Rep 1992;41(RR-17):1.

Projections of the number of persons diagnosed with AIDS and the number of immunosuppressed HIV-infected persons—United States, 1992–1994. MMWR Morbid Mortal Wkly Rep 1992;41(RR-18):1.

Stanley SK, Fauci AS: Acquired immunodeficiency syndrome. In: *Clinical Immunology, Principles and Practice.* Rich R et al (editors). Mosby, 1996.

4 Infectious Diseases

Karen C. Bloch, MD, MPH

Infectious diseases cause significant morbidity and mortality, especially in those individuals who are most vulnerable to illness: the very young, the elderly, the immunocompromised, and the poor.

An understanding of the pathogenesis of infectious diseases can begin by conceptualizing the relationships between the host, the infectious agent, and the environment. Figure 4–1 portrays a host-agent-environment paradigm for the study of infectious diseases. The infectious agent can be either **exogenous,** ie, not normally found on or in the body; or **endogenous,** ie, one which may be routinely cultured from a particular anatomic site but which does not normally cause disease in the host. An infection results when the host, the agent, and the environment interact in a way that favors host invasion by the agent. Clearly, host susceptibility plays an important role in this process.

The environment includes **vectors,** insects and other carriers that transmit infectious agents; and **zoonotic hosts,** animals that harbor infectious agents. For example, the white-footed mouse serves as an animal host for *Borrelia burgdorferi,* the bacterium that causes Lyme disease. The *Ixodes* tick serves as an insect vector. The tick larva feeds on a host mouse and becomes infected with *B burgdorferi.* The infected nymph form of the tick then feeds on humans, transmitting infection from the mouse to the human host.

The study of infectious diseases requires understanding of pathogenesis at the population and individual levels as well as the cellular and molecular levels. For example, at the population level, the spread of tuberculosis in the community is related to the social network of infectious human hosts. Outbreaks of tuberculosis have occurred in homeless shelters when an index case is housed in close quarters with susceptible persons. At the individual level, tuberculosis results from inhalation of respiratory droplets containing airborne tubercle bacilli. At the cellular level, these bacilli activate T cells, which play a critical role in containing the infection. Individuals with an impaired T cell response (eg, those infected with HIV) are at particularly high risk for primary or reactivation tuberculosis. Finally, at the genetic level, individuals with specific polymorphisms in a macrophage protein gene are at significantly higher risk for developing pulmonary tuberculosis.

Specific microorganisms have a tendency to cause certain types of infections: *Streptococcus pneumoniae* most commonly causes pneumonia, meningitis, bacteremia, and, rarely, endocarditis; *Escherichia coli* most commonly causes gastrointestinal and urinary tract infections; plasmodium species infect red blood cells and liver cells to cause malaria; *Entamoeba histolytica* causes amebic dysentery and liver abscesses, etc. Therefore, the specific diagnostic approach differs for each patient. Table 4–1 presents a clinical approach that incorporates knowledge of the microorganisms associated with specific clinical syndromes and the host-agent-environment paradigm in obtaining the history of the patient's illness.

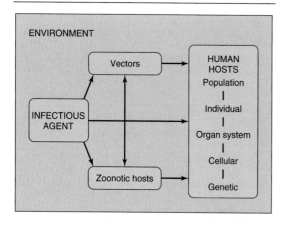

Figure 4–1. The fundamental relationships involved in the host-agent-environment paradigm. Note the role of zoonotic hosts and vectors in the environmental pathogenesis of infectious diseases. In the host, pathogenetic mechanisms extend from the level of populations (eg, person-to-person transmission) to the level of cellular and molecular processes (eg, genetic susceptibility).

Table 4–1. Obtaining a history in the diagnosis of infectious diseases.

Component of History	Host-Specific History	Environment-Specific History	Agent-Specific History

History of present illness	Demographics:
	  Age
	  Sex
	  Race/ethnicity
	Mild versus life-threatening
	Acute versus subacute versus chronic
	Relapse versus recurrent (reinfection)
	Pattern of symptoms (fevers, night sweats)
		Person-to-person transmission
		Animal-to-person transmission
		Vector-borne transmission
		Water-borne transmission
		Food-borne transmission
		Airborne transmission
		Nosocomial acquisition
		Community acquisition
		Occupational exposure
		Seasonal transmission
			Viral versus bacterial versus parasitic versus fungal. Infections or infectious agents associated with host-specific or environment-specific factors (eg, measles in a child; pelvic inflammatory disease in a female; salmonella infection in a black child with sickle cell disease; outbreak of food-borne hepatitis A infection; influenza epidemic in winter).

Past medical history (including medications, allergies, and immunization history)	Conditions predisposing to infections:
	  HIV infection
	  Chronic obstructive pulmonary disease
	  Diabetes mellitus
	  Sickle cell disease
	  Asplenia
	  Cancer
	  Pregnancy
	  Lack of immunizations
		Previous exposures to probable exogenous infectious agents:
		  Day-care centers
		  Nurseries
		  Schools
		  Correctional facilities
		  Hospitals
			Infections or infectious agents associated with host's predisposing comorbid or past medical conditions (eg, *Pneumocystis carinii* pneumonia in HIV-infected patients)

Habits	Substance use:
	  Smoking
	  Alcohol
	  Injection drug use
	  Cocaine (smoked or nasal)
		Sexual contacts (exchange of body fluids)
		Sharing of syringes or needles
		Outdoor exposure
		  Ticks
		  Mosquitoes
			Infections or infectious agents associated with host-specific habits (eg, HIV infection or *S aureus* endocarditis in injection drug users)

Social history	Socioeconomic status (lack of access to health care):
	  Occupation
	  Recent immigration
		Crowded housing
		Homelessness
		Congregated living facility:
		  Shelters, prisons
		  Nursing homes, hospitals
		Recent travel
			Infections or infectious agents epidemiologically associated with host-specific or environment-specific factors (eg, outbreak of tuberculosis in homeless shelter, prison, or hospital; typhoid fever or malaria in recent traveler)

Family history	Immune deficiency syndromes	Exposure to environment in severe combined immune deficiency (SCID)	Specific infections or infectious agents associated with inherited immune deficiency (Table 3–3)

Review of systems	Review by organ system:
	  Nonspecific constitutional symptoms (fever, chills, night sweats, weight loss)
	  Central nervous system (photophobia, confusion)
	  Cardiovascular system (light-headedness)
	  Lung (productive cough)
	  Kidney and urinary tract (dysuria)
	  Gastrointestinal system (diarrhea)
	  Hematologic system (easy bruisability)
	  Reproductive organs (genital discharge)
	  Skin and subcutaneous tissues (rash)
	  Muscle and bone (myalgia, bone pain)
		Organ-specific host-environment interaction (eg, penetrating CNS trauma; indwelling intravenous catheters; endotracheally intubated, mechanically ventilated patient; indwelling Foley catheter; contraceptive intrauterine device; postoperative wound; penetrating soft tissue injury)	Infections or infectious agents associated with organ-specific host-environment interaction (eg, intravenous catheter-related *S aureus* bacteremia; nosocomial *Pseudomonas* pneumonia; pelvic inflammatory disease; postoperative wound infection; osteomyelitis in injured bone)

HOST DEFENSES AGAINST INFECTION

NORMAL MICROBIAL FLORA

The human body normally harbors numerous species of bacteria, viruses, fungi, and protozoa. The great majority of these are **commensals,** or **"normal flora,"** defined as organisms that live on or within the human host but rarely cause disease. Common bacterial commensals and anatomic sites where they are normally found are listed in Table 4–2.

Differentiating normal flora from pathogens causing true infection is often difficult. Helpful clues include symptoms and signs of infection (eg, cough and fever) and the presence of inflammatory cells (eg, polymorphonuclear cells in the sputum). Isolation of an **obligate pathogen** (eg, *Mycobacterium tuberculosis*) from any site is diagnostic of infection. Fortunately, few microorganisms are absolute pathogens. For example, *Neisseria meningitidis,* a major bacterial cause of meningitis, can be cultured from the oropharynx of as many as 10% of asymptomatic individuals, in which case it represents transient normal flora. In this case, although the host is asymptomatic, he or she can serve as a **carrier,** potentially transferring bacteria to susceptible individuals. Infections caused by commensals that rarely cause disease (eg, *Candida albicans*) or organisms ubiquitous in the environment that are generally not considered human pathogens (eg, *Mycobacterium avium* complex; MAC) are termed **opportunistic infections.** These infections occur almost exclusively in **immunocompromised hosts** such as HIV-infected patients or transplant recipients. The agents are "opportunists" in that they take advantage of impaired host immunity to cause infection but are not significant pathogens in an immunocompetent host.

Isolation of an organism considered a commensal when cultured from a normally colonized site is diagnostic of infection when cultured from a normally sterile site. Sterile sites include blood, cerebrospinal fluid, synovial (joint) fluid, and deep tissues of the body. For example, bacteroides, the predominate species of bacteria in the colon, may cause intra-abdominal abscesses and sepsis when the integrity of the colonic mucosa is breached. *Staphylococcus epidermidis,* a common skin commensal, is the most common cause of bacteremia following intravascular catheter placement. Knowledge of the common endogenous flora may be useful in determining the cause of an infection and may allow institution of rational empiric antibiotic therapy.

When the delicate symbiosis between the commensal and the host is disturbed, the normal flora may be overgrown by exogenous, potentially pathogenic organisms. This phenomenon, which may be transient or persistent, is called **colonization.** When replacement of the normal flora occurs in the hospital environment, the colonizers are said to be **nosocomially acquired.** Nosocomial organisms are important pathogens because they are often resistant to multiple antibiotics. Not uncommonly, colonization will progress to symptomatic infection. For example, individuals hospitalized for extended periods often become colonized with gram-negative bacteria such as *Pseudomonas aeruginosa*. These individuals are then at increased risk for life-threatening infections such as pseudomonas pneumonia.

Host defense mechanisms that serve to inhibit colonization by pathogenic bacteria include (1) mechanical clearance, (2) phagocytic killing, and (3) depriving organisms of necessary nutrients. Successful colonizers have adapted to evade or overcome these defenses. For example, gonococci avoid excretion in the urine by adhering to the mucosal epithelium of the urogenital tract with pili. Pneumococci resist phagocytosis by encapsulation within a slimy capsule that impairs uptake by neutrophils. And some staphy-

Table 4–2. Examples of normal bacterial flora by body location.[1]

Location	Gram-Positive		Gram-Negative		Others
	Cocci	Rods	Cocci	Rods	
Skin	Staphylococci	Diphtheroids			
Oronasopharynx	Streptococci		Neisseria	Haemophilus Bacteroides	Spirochetes
Large intestine	Streptococci Enterococci	Clostridia Lactobacilli		Enteric bacilli Bacteroides	
Vagina	Streptococci	Lactobacilli		Bacteroides	Mycoplasma

[1]Modified and reproduced, with permission, from Eisenstein BI, Schaechter M: Normal microbial flora. In: *Mechanisms of Microbial Disease,* 2nd ed. Schaechter M, Medoff G, Eisenstein BI (editors). Williams & Wilkins, 1993.

lococci elaborate enzymes known as hemolysins that destroy host red blood cells, thus allowing them access to a needed source of iron.

Colonization of sites that are normally sterile or have very few microbes is generally easier because there are no competing endogenous flora. However, host defenses at these sites are often vigorous. For instance, the stomach is normally sterile because few microbes can survive at the normal gastric pH of 4.0. However, if antacids are used to decrease gastric acidity, detectable colonization of the stomach and trachea with gram-negative bacteria occurs. The deep tissues are normally sterile, and a vigorous host immune response limits invasive infections at these sites.

The normal flora prevents colonization through numerous mechanisms. These organisms often have a selective advantage over colonizers in that they are already established in an anatomic niche. This means that they are bound to receptors on the host cell and are able to metabolize local nutrients. Many species of normal flora are able to produce bacteriocins, proteins that are toxic to other bacterial strains or species. Finally, the normal flora promotes production of antibodies that may cross-react with colonizing organisms which the host has never previously encountered and thus to which it has never mounted an antibody response. For instance, an antibody produced against *E coli*, a gram-negative bacterium found in the large intestine, cross-reacts with the polysaccharide capsule of a meningitis-producing strain of *N meningitidis*. When the normal flora is altered—eg, by the administration of broad-spectrum antibiotics—one bacterial species may predominate, or pathogenic bacteria from the outside may colonize the site and predispose the host to infection.

CONSTITUTIVE DEFENSES OF THE BODY

Constitutive defenses of the human body are nonspecific barriers against infectious diseases that do not require prior contact with the microorganism. These defenses consist of simple physical and chemical barriers that prevent easy entry of microorganisms into the body. Some infectious agents utilize a vector (such as an insect) to bypass structural barriers and gain direct access to the blood or soft tissues of the body. Once an agent has entered the body, the major constitutive defenses are the acute inflammatory response and the complement system. These defenses can neutralize the agent, recruit phagocytic cells, and induce a more specific response through humoral and cell-mediated immunity. The constitutive defenses of the body are important from an evolutionary perspective in enabling humans to encounter and adapt to a variety of new and changing environments.

Physical & Chemical Barriers to Infection

The squamous epithelium of the skin is the first line of defense against microorganisms encountered in the outside world. As keratinized epithelial surface cells desquamate, the skin maintains its protective barrier by generating new epithelial cells beneath the surface. The skin is also bathed with oils and moisture from the sebaceous and sweat glands. These secretions contain fatty acids that inhibit bacterial growth. Poor vascular supply to the skin may result in skin breakdown and increased susceptibility to infection. For example, chronically debilitated or bedridden patients may suffer from decubitus ulcers due to constant pressure on dependent body parts, predisposing to severe infections by otherwise harmless skin flora.

The mucous membranes also provide a physical barrier to microbial invasion. The mucous membranes of the mouth, pharynx, esophagus, and lower urinary tract are composed of several layers of epithelial cells, whereas those of the lower respiratory tract, the gastrointestinal tract, and the upper urinary tract are delicate single layers of epithelial cells. These membranes are covered by a protective layer of mucus, which provides a mechanical and chemical barrier. The mucus traps foreign particles and prevents them from reaching the lining epithelial cells. Because the mucus is hydrophilic, many substances produced by the body easily diffuse to the surface, including enzymes with antimicrobial activity such as lysozyme and peroxidase.

Inflammatory Response

When a microorganism crosses the epidermis or the epithelial surface of the mucous membranes, it encounters other components of the host constitutive defenses. These responses are constitutive because they are nonspecific and do not require prior contact with the organism to be effective. Clinically, signs of inflammation (heat, erythema, pain, and swelling) are the characteristic features of localized infection, secondary tissue injury, and the body's response to this injury. Like fever, an elevated peripheral blood neutrophil count with an increased proportion of immature forms gives information about the presence and severity of infection. Blood supply to the affected areas increases in response to vasodilation, and the capillaries become more permeable, allowing antibodies, complement, and white blood cells to cross the endothelium and reach the site of injury. An important consequence of inflammation is that the pH of the inflamed tissues is lowered, creating an inhospitable environment for the microbe. The increased blood flow to the area allows continued recruitment of inflammatory cells as well as the necessary components for tissue repair and recovery.

When a microorganism enters host tissue, it activates the complement system and components of the coagulation cascade and induces the release of chemical mediators of the inflammatory response. These mediators result in the increased vascular permeability and vasodilation characteristic of inflammation. For example, the anaphylatoxins C3a, C4a, and C5a, produced by the activation of complement, stimulate the release of histamine from mast cells. Histamine dilates the blood vessels and increases their permeability. Bradykinin is also released, increasing vascular permeability.

Proinflammatory cytokines include interleukin-1, interleukin-6, tumor necrosis factor, and gamma interferon. These factors, singly or in combination, promote fever, stimulate hepatic acute phase responses, produce local inflammatory signs, and trigger catabolic responses.

During severe infection, hepatic synthesis of proteins is altered, changing the profile of serum proteins. This altered profile has been termed the **acute phase reaction.** Typically, serum albumin concentration is reduced while serum amyloid A protein, C-reactive protein, ferritin, and various proteinase inhibitors increase. Serum levels of zinc and iron decrease at the same time. A catabolic state is further augmented by simultaneous increases in levels of circulating cortisol, glucagon, catecholamines, and other hormones.

When mild to moderate in intensity, inflammatory responses serve important host defense functions. For example, elevated body temperature seems to accentuate lymphocyte responses and may inhibit viral replication. Inflammatory hyperemia and systemic neutrophilia optimize phagocyte delivery to sites of infection. The decreased availability of iron inhibits the growth of microbes that require this element as a nutrient. However, when the inflammatory responses become extreme, extensive tissue damage can result, as in the case of sepsis.

Complement System

The complement system is composed of a series of plasma protein and cell membrane receptors that are important mediators of host defenses and inflammation (Figure 4–2). Most of the biologically significant effects of the complement system are mediated by the third component (C3) and the terminal components (C5–9). The complement system is discussed in Chapter 3. In order to carry out their host defense and inflammatory functions, C3 and C5–9 must first be activated. Two pathways of complement activation have been recognized and have been termed the **classic** and **alternative** pathways. The classic pathway is activated by antigen-antibody complexes or antibody-coated particles, and the alternative pathway is activated by mechanisms independent of antibodies, usually by interaction with bacterial surface components. Both pathways form C3 convertase, which cleaves the C3 component of complement, a key protein common to both pathways. The two pathways then proceed in identical fashion to bind late-acting components to form a membrane attack complex (C5–9), which results in target cell lysis.

Once activated, complement functions to enhance the antimicrobial defenses in several ways: It makes invading microorganisms susceptible to phagocytosis; it lyses some of the infectious agents directly; it produces substances that are chemotactic for white blood cells; and it promotes the inflammatory response. Two of the activities of complement are specifically directed toward enhancing phagocytosis. In addition to the recruitment of white cells by chemotactic proteins, complement facilitates phagocytosis through proteins called **opsonins.** The membrane attack complex inserts itself into the membrane of a target cell, leading to increased permeability and subsequent lysis of the cell.

Inherited disorders of complement are associated with an increased risk of bacterial infection. The specific infections seen in complement-deficient patients relate to the biologic functions of the missing component (Figure 4–2). Typically, patients with a deficiency of C3 or of a component in either of the two pathways necessary for the activation of C3 have an increased susceptibility to infection by bacteria for which C3b-dependent opsonization is an important defense. For example, these patients are at increased risk for infections with encapsulated bacteria such as *S pneumoniae* and *Haemophilus influenzae*. In contrast, patients with deficiencies of C5–9 have normal resistance to *S pneumoniae* and *H influenzae* since C3b-mediated opsonization is intact, but they are unusually susceptible to life-threatening infections with *N meningitidis* and *Neisseria gonorrhoeae,* since they lack C5–9-mediated serum bactericidal activity, which serves to lyse the neisseria cell membrane. Complement deficiency diseases may be more common among patients with certain infectious diseases than was heretofore appreciated. For example, about 15% of patients with systemic meningococcal infections have a genetically determined deficiency of a terminal component of complement.

Phagocytosis

After the natural barriers of the skin or mucous membranes have been penetrated, the phagocytic cells—neutrophils, monocytes, and macrophages—constitute the next line of defense. The process of internalizing organisms by these cells (**phagocytosis**) involves attachment of the organism to the cell surface. This triggers extension of a pseudopod to enclose the bacterium in an endocytic vesicle, or **phagosome.** The circulating neutrophil or polymorphonuclear leukocyte is the best-studied and best-understood phagocyte. Before activation by chemoattractants, neutrophils circulate in a metabolically quiescent state. When chemotactic factors, arachidonic acid metabolites, or complement cleavage fragments interact with specific membrane receptors, the

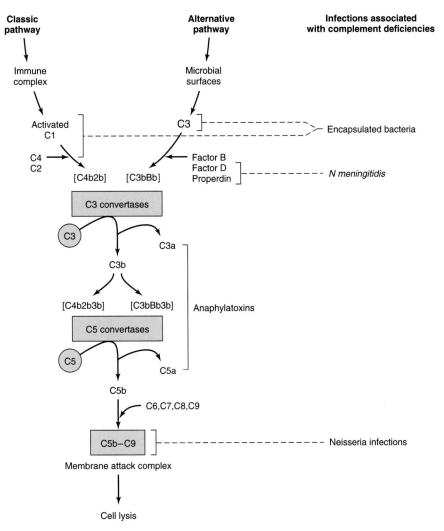

Figure 4–2. Complement reaction sequence and infections associated with deficiency states. (Modified and reproduced, with permission, from Nairn R: Immunology. In: *Jawetz, Melnick, and Adelberg's Medical Microbiology,* 21st ed. Brooks GF, Butel JS, Morse SA [editors]. Appleton & Lange, 1998.

neutrophil rapidly becomes activated and moves toward the chemoattractants. After phagocytosis, the mechanisms by which the phagolysosome kills the microorganism can be divided into oxygen-independent and oxygen-dependent processes. The former involves phagocytic killing of microbes in an anaerobic environment. In the oxygen-dependent process, neutrophils are triggered to produce hydrogen peroxide and other microbicidal oxidants. Functional or quantitative defects of neutrophils result in an increased incidence of infections with pyogenic bacteria.

Neutropenia—defined as an absolute neutrophil count < 1000 cells/μL—is a common predisposing factor for bacterial and fungal infections. The risk of infection rises significantly with neutrophil counts < 500 cells/μL and is especially high with counts < 100 cells/μL. The longer the duration of profound neutropenia, the higher the risk of infection. At the first sign of infection (eg, fever), these patients should immediately be given broad-spectrum antibacterial agents to cover the most life-threatening bacterial pathogens. Ironically, antibiotics are often so effective at killing a broad spectrum of bacteria that colonizing fungi, such as candida, have few competitors, allowing uninhibited growth. Patients with neutropenia consequently are at increased risk of fungal sepsis.

Several inherited disorders of neutrophil function have been described, including Chédiak-Higashi syndrome, myeloperoxidase deficiency, and chronic granulomatous disease. **Chédiak-Higashi syndrome** is a rare autosomal recessive hereditary disorder in which the neutrophils have a profound defect in the formation of intracellular granules. Opsonized bacteria, such as *S aureus,* are ingested normally, but viable bacteria persist intracellularly, presumably because of the inability of normal granules to fuse with phagosomes to form phagolysosomes. Patients with Chédiak-Higashi syndrome experience recurrent bacterial infections, most frequently involving the skin and soft tissues and the upper and lower respiratory tracts.

Myeloperoxidase deficiency is the most common neutrophil disorder, with a prevalence of 1:2000 individuals. In this disorder, phagocytosis, chemotaxis, and degranulation are normal, but microbicidal activity for bacteria is delayed. In general, these patients do not suffer from recurrent infections. In contrast, **chronic granulomatous disease** is a genetically heterogeneous group of inherited disorders with a common phenotype characterized by the failure of phagocytic cells to produce superoxides. The defect involves neutrophils, monocytes, eosinophils, and some macrophages. Oxygen-dependent intracellular killing is impaired, and these patients are susceptible to recurrent, often life-threatening infections. Patients with chronic granulomatous disease also tend to form granulomas in tissues, particularly in the lungs, liver, and spleen, and are particularly susceptible to infection with *S aureus* and aspergillus species.

INDUCED DEFENSES OF THE BODY

While constitutive host defenses against infectious agents are generally nonspecific and do not require prior exposure to the invading agent, induced defenses are highly specific for the invading infectious agent and are qualitatively and quantitatively altered by prior antigenic exposure. Details of the pathophysiology of the host immune system are covered in Chapter 3. Infections associated with common defects in the induced immune response are shown in Table 4–3.

ESTABLISHMENT OF INFECTIOUS DISEASES

An infectious disease occurs when a pathogenic organism causes signs or symptoms of inflammation or organ dysfunction. This may be caused directly by the infection itself, as when the etiologic agent multi-

Table 4–3. Infections associated with common defects in humoral and cellular immune response.[1]

Host Defect in Immune Response	Examples of Immune Defect States	Common Etiologic Agents of Infections
T lymphocyte deficiency or dysfunction	Thymic aplasia, hypoplasia Hodgkin's disease Sarcoid Pregnancy	*Listeria monocytogenes,* mycobacterium, candida, aspergillus, *Cryptococcus neoformans,* herpes simplex, herpes zoster
	AIDS	*Pneumocystis carinii,* cytomegalovirus, herpes simplex, *Mycobacterium avium* complex, *C neoformans,* candida
B cell deficiency or dysfunction	Bruton's X-linked agammaglobulinemia Agammaglobulinemia Chronic lymphocytic leukemia Multiple myeloma	*Streptococcus pneumoniae,* other streptococci, *Haemophilus influenzae, Neisseria meningitidis, Staphylococcus aureus, Klebsiella pneumoniae, Escherichia coli, Giardia lamblia, P carinii,* enteroviruses
	Selective IgM deficiency	*S pneumoniae, H influenzae, E coli*
	Selective IgA deficiency	*G lamblia,* hepatitis viruses, *S pneumoniae, H influenzae*
Mixed T and B cell deficiency or dysfunction	Common variable hypogammaglobulinemia	*P carinii,* cytomegalovirus, *S pneumoniae, H influenzae,* various other bacteria
	Ataxia-telangiectasia	*S pneumoniae, H influenzae, S aureus,* rubella virus, *G lamblia*
	Severe combined immunodeficiency	*S aureus, S pneumoniae, Candida albicans, P carinii,* varicella virus, rubella virus, cytomegalovirus
	Wiskott-Aldrich syndrome	Infections seen in T and B cell abnormalities

[1]Modified and reproduced, with permission, from Madoff LC, Kasper DL. Introduction to infectious diseases: Host-parasite interaction. In: *Harrison's Principles of Internal Medicine,* 14th ed. Fauci AS et al (editors). McGraw-Hill, 1998.

plies in the host, or indirectly from the host inflammatory response. Many infections are subclinical, not producing the usual manifestations of disease. To cause disease, all microorganisms must go through the following stages (Table 4–4): The microorganism must (1) **encounter** the host, (2) **gain entry** into the host, (3) **multiply and spread** from the site of entry, and (4) **cause host tissue injury,** either directly (eg, cytotoxins) or indirectly (inflammatory response). The severity of infection can be characterized along a spectrum from asymptomatic to life-threatening, and the course may be characterized as acute, subacute, or chronic. Whether infection is clinically evident or not, the outcome is either (1) eradication of the infecting agent (resolution), (2) chronic infection, (3) prolonged excretion of the agent (carrier state), (4) latency of the agent within host tissues, or (5) death (Figure 4–3).

Except for those with **congenital infections** (acquired in utero) caused by agents such as rubella, syphilis, and cytomegalovirus, human beings first encounter microorganisms at birth. During parturition, the newborn comes into contact with microorganisms present in the mother's vaginal canal and on her skin. Most of the bacteria that the newborn encounters do not cause harm, and for those that might cause infection, the newborn usually has antibodies that were acquired from the mother in utero. This phenomenon is termed **passive immunity.** For example, neonates are protected against infection with *H influenzae* by maternal antibodies for the first few months of life, until passive immunity wanes and the risk of infection with this bacterium rises. On the other hand, newborns whose mothers are colonized with group B streptococci at birth are at increased risk of serious infections such as sepsis and meningitis in the perinatal period.

Direct entry into the host—ie, bypassing the usual chemical and physical barriers—occurs via **penetration.** This may occur when (1) an insect vector directly inoculates the infectious agent into the host (mosquitoes transmitting malaria), (2) bacteria gain direct access to host tissues through loss of integrity of the skin or mucous membranes (trauma or surgical wounds), or (3) microbes gain access via instruments or catheters that allow communication between usually sterile sites and the outside world (eg, indwelling venous catheters). Invasion by **ingression** occurs when an infectious agent enters the host via an orifice contiguous with the external environment. This primarily involves inhalation of infectious aerosolized droplets *(M tuberculosis)* or ingestion of contaminated foods (salmonella, hepatitis A virus).

Other infectious agents directly infect the mucous membranes or cross the epithelia to cause infection. This commonly occurs in urinary tract infections and sexually transmitted diseases. The virus that causes AIDS, the human immunodeficiency virus (HIV), crosses mucous membranes by the penetration of virus-laden macrophages from semen. Such a mechanism of cell-mediated entry may function at other mucous membranes as well.

Following the initial encounter with the host, the infectious agent must successfully multiply at the site of entry. The process whereby microorganism successfully competes with normal flora and is able to multiply is termed colonization (eg, pneumococci colonizing the upper respiratory tract). When the microorganism multiplies at a usually sterile site, it is termed infection (eg, pneumococci multiplying in the alveoli, ie, causing pneumonia). Unless direct penetration occurs, agents must first successfully colonize the host to cause subsequent infection.

Factors that facilitate the multiplication and spread of infection include inoculum size (the quantity of infectious organisms introduced), host anatomic factors (eg, impaired ciliary function in children with cystic

Table 4–4. The establishment and outcome of infectious diseases.[1]

Stage of Infection	Factors Influencing Stage of Infection
Encounter	Host immune state Exogenous (colonization) Endogenous (normal flora)

Entry	Ingress
	  Inhalation
	  Ingestion
	  Mucous membrane entry
	Penetration
	  Insect bites
	  Cuts and wounds
	  Iatrogenic (intravenous catheters)

Multiplication and spread	Inoculum size Physical factors Microbial nutrition Anatomic factors Microbial sanctuary Microbial virulence factors

Injury	Mechanical
	Cell death
	Microbial product-induced
	Host-induced
	  Inflammation
	  Immune response
	    Humoral immunity
	    Cellular immunity

Course of infection	Asymptomatic versus life-threatening Acute versus subacute versus chronic

Outcome of infection	Resolution (self-limited)
	Chronic
	  Carrier state (saprophytic versus parasitic)
	  Latent → Reactivation
	Death

[1] Adapted in part, with permission, from Schaechter M, Medoff G, Eisenstein BI (editors): *Mechanisms of Microbial Disease,* 2nd ed. Williams & Wilkins, 1993.

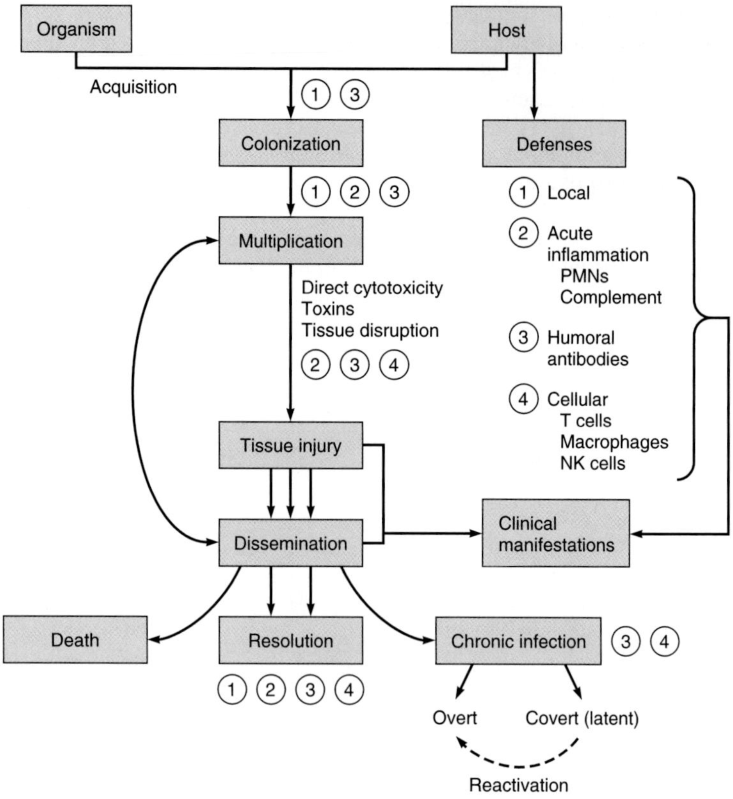

Figure 4–3. Schema of the establishment and outcome of infectious diseases. Note interplay between microorganisms and host factors that lead to infection, infectious disease, and resolution. The circled numbers indicate sites at which the designated host responses may interrupt or modify the pathogenesis of disease. (Modified and reproduced, with permission, from Heinzel FP, Root RK: Introduction to infectious diseases: Pathogenic mechanisms and host responses. In: *Harrison's Principles of Internal Medicine,* 12th ed. Wilson JD et al [editors]. McGraw-Hill, 1991.)

fibrosis), availability of nutrients for the microbe, physicochemical factors (eg, gastric pH), microbial virulence factors, and microbial sanctuary (eg, abscesses). An abscess is a special case where the host has contained the infection but is unable to eradicate it. The primary mode of therapy is surgical drainage. Infections that are not contained will spread. Infections can spread along the epidermis (impetigo), along the dermis (erysipelas), along subcutaneous tissue (cellulitis), along fascial planes (necrotizing fasciitis), into muscle tissue (myositis), along veins (suppurative thrombophlebitis), into the blood (bacteremia, fungemia, viremia, etc), along lymphatics (lymphangitis), and into organs (pneumonia, brain abscesses, hepatitis, etc).

Infections cause direct injury to the host through a variety of mechanisms. If organisms are present in sufficient numbers and are of sufficient size, **mechanical obstruction** can occur (eg, children with roundworm gastrointestinal infections may present with bowel obstruction). More commonly, pathogens cause an intense secondary **inflammatory response,** which may result in life-threatening complications (eg, children with *H influenzae* epiglottitis may present with mechanical airway obstruction secondary to intense soft tissue swelling). Some bacteria produce **neurotoxins** that affect cell metabolism rather than directly causing cell damage (eg, tetanus toxin antagonizes inhibitory neurons, causing unopposed motor neuron stimulation, manifested clinically as sustained muscle rigidity). Host cell death can occur by a variety of mechanisms. *Shigella* produces a **cytotoxin** that causes death of large intestine enterocytes, resulting in the clinical syndrome of dysentery. Poliovirus-induced cell lysis of the anterior horn cells of the spinal cord causes flaccid paralysis. Gram-negative bacterial **endotoxin** can initiate a cascade of cytokine release, resulting in sepsis syndrome and septic shock.

The time course of an infection can be characterized as **acute, subacute,** or **chronic,** and its severity may vary from asymptomatic to life-threatening. Many infections that begin as mild and easily treatable conditions readily progress without prompt treatment. Small, seemingly insignificant skin abrasions superinfected with toxic shock syndrome toxin (TSST-1)-producing *S aureus* can result in fulminant infection and death. Even infections that are indolent for weeks, such as subacute infective endocarditis, can be fatal unless they are recognized and appropriately treated.

There are three potential outcomes of infection: recovery, chronic infection, or death (Figure 4–3). Most infections **resolve,** either spontaneously (eg, rhinovirus, the leading cause of the common cold) or with medical therapy (eg, following treatment of streptococcal pharyngitis with penicillin). Chronic infections may be either **saprophytic,** in which case the organism does not adversely affect the health of the host; or **parasitic,** causing tissue damage to the host. An example of the former is *Salmonella typhi,* which may be harbored asymptomatically in the gallbladder of about 2% of individuals following acute infection. Chronic infection with the hepatitis B virus may be either saprophytic, in which case the human host is infectious for the virus but has no clinical evidence of liver damage; or parasitic, with progressive liver damage and cirrhosis. A final form of chronic infection is tissue **latency.** Varicella zoster, the virus causing chickenpox, survives in the dorsal root ganglia, with reactivation causing herpes zoster, commonly known as shingles. When the ability of the immune system to control either the acute or chronic infection is exceeded, the infection may result in **host death.** Table 4–5 summarizes some microbial strategies to overcome host immune defenses. A unifying theme is that all infectious agents, regardless of specific mechanisms, must successfully reproduce and evade host defense mechanisms (Tables 4–4 and 4–5). This knowledge helps the physician to plan intervention strategies to prevent infections; when infection occurs, to treat and cure; and when infection cannot be cured, to prevent further transmission, recurrence, or reactivation.

1. By what three general mechanisms do hosts resist colonization by pathogenic bacteria?
2. What are three ways in which the normal flora contributes to the balance between health and disease?
3. Which specific host defenses against infection do not require prior contact with the infecting organism?
4. What are the categories of outcomes from an infection?

PATHOPHYSIOLOGY OF SELECTED INFECTIOUS DISEASE SYNDROMES

INFECTIVE ENDOCARDITIS

Clinical Presentation

Infective endocarditis is a bacterial or fungal infection of the interior of the heart, most commonly involving the cardiac valves and less commonly the endocardial surface. Infection of extracardiac endothelium is termed endarteritis and can cause disease that is clinically similar to endocarditis. The most common predisposing factor for infective endocarditis is the presence of abnormal cardiac valves or structures. Consequently, patients with a history of rheumatic heart disease, congenital heart disease, mitral valve prolapse with valve leaflet redundancy or an audible murmur, a prosthetic heart valve, or a history of prior endocarditis are at increased risk of developing infective endocarditis.

Etiology

The most common infectious agents causing native valve infective endocarditis are gram-positive bacteria, including viridans streptococci, *S aureus,* and enterococcus. Infection involves the left heart (mitral and aortic valves) almost exclusively except in patients who are injection drug users or, less commonly, patients with valve injury from a pulmonary artery (Swan-Ganz) catheter, in whom infection of the right heart (tricuspid or pulmonary valves) occurs. Injection drug users most commonly develop *S aureus* tricuspid valve infective endocarditis; not uncommonly, they also have concomitant left-sided disease. Viridans streptococci and enterococci rarely infect the tricuspid valve. Risk factors for the former bacterial infection include oral lesions or recent dental work, while patients with the latter are more likely to have underlying genitourinary conditions. Patients with prosthetic heart valves are also at risk of developing infective endocarditis due to skin flora such as *S epidermidis* and fungi. Prior to the availability of antibiotics, infective endocarditis was a progressively debilitating, incurable, and fatal disease. Even with antibiotics, endocarditis continues to have a significant case fatality rate, and definitive cure often requires urgent or emergent surgery to replace damaged cardiac valves.

Pathogenesis

Hemodynamic factors that predispose patients to the development of endocarditis are the following: (1) a high-velocity jet stream causing turbulent blood flow, (2) flow from a high- to low-pressure chamber, and (3) a comparatively narrow orifice separating the two chambers that creates a pressure gradient. The lesions of infective endocarditis tend to form on the surface of the valve in the lower-pressure cardiac chamber—eg, they commonly form on the ventricular surface of an abnormal aortic valve and on the atrial surface of an abnormal mitral valve. Satellite lesions can also grow where the jet stream strikes the endocardium (Figure 4–4). The damaged endothelium promotes the deposition of fibrin and platelets, which form sterile vegetations (**nonbacterial thrombotic endocarditis**). Infective endocarditis occurs when microorganisms are deposited onto these sterile vegetations during the course of bacteremia. Not all bacteria adhere equally well to these sites. For example, *E coli,* a frequent cause of bacteremia, is rarely

Table 4–5. Selection of microbial strategies against host immune defenses.[1]

Host Defense Action	Microbial Counteraction	Example
Complement actions	Masking of complement activating substances	*Staphylococcus aureus*, surface capsule Meningococcus, coating with IgA
	Inhibition of surface complement activation	*Schistosoma mansoni*, decay accelerating factors
	Inhibition of action of membrane attack complex	*Salmonella*, long surface O antigen
	Inactivation of complement chemotaxin C5a	*Pseudomonas aeruginosa*
Phagocytic actions	Inhibition of phagocyte recruitment	*Bordetella pertussis*, toxin paralysis of chemotaxis
	Microbial killing of phagocytes	*P aeruginosa*, leukocidins
	Escape from phagocytosis	Staphylococci, surface protein A
	Survival following phagocytosis	Trypanosomes, enter cytoplasm Rickettsiae, enter cytoplasm *Mycobacterium tuberculosis*, inhibit lysosome fusion *Chlamydia psittaci*, inhibit lysosome fusion *Legionella*, inhibit lysosome fusion
	Inhibition of phagocyte oxidative pathway	Staphylococci, catalase production against H_2O_2
Cell-mediated immunity	CD4 T cell depletion	Human immunodeficiency virus (HIV)
	Decreased B cell immunoglobulin production	Measles virus
	Inhibition of lymphokine synthesis	Leishmania
Humoral-mediated immunity	Changing of surface antigens	Influenza virus *Neisseria gonorrhoeae* *Trypanosoma brucei*
	Proteolysis of antibodies	*Haemophilus influenzae*, IgA proteases
Humoral- and cell-mediated immunity	DNA incorporation into host genome	Herpes simplex Herpes zoster

[1]Modified and reproduced, with permission, from Plaut A: Microbial subversion of host defenses. In: *Mechanisms of Microbial Disease*, 2nd ed. Schaechter M, Medoff G, Eisenstein BI (editors). Williams & Wilkins, 1993.

implicated as a cause of endocarditis. Organisms that possess little inherent pathogenicity, such as viridans streptococci, usually implant only on damaged valves. However, more virulent organisms, such as *S aureus*, can infect apparently normal valves.

Once infected, these vegetations continue to enlarge through further deposition of platelets and fibrin, providing the bacteria a sanctuary from host defense mechanisms such as polymorphonuclear leukocytes and complement. Consequently, once infection takes hold, the infected vegetation continues to grow in a largely unimpeded fashion. For this reason, prolonged administration of bactericidal antibiotics is required to cure this disease. Bacteriostatic antimicrobial agents are inadequate to cure the infection. Operative intervention is sometimes required for cure, particularly for infections with gram-negative bacilli or fungi or in prosthetic valve infections.

A hallmark of infective endocarditis is persistent bacteremia, which stimulates both the humoral and cellular immune systems. A variety of immunoglobulins are expressed, resulting in immune complex formation, increased serum levels of rheumatoid factor, and nonspecific hypergammaglobulinemia. Immune complex deposition along the renal glomerular basement membrane may result in the development of glomerulonephritis and renal failure. Osler nodes—painful lesions of the pads of the fingers and toes—are thought to be caused by deposition of immune complexes in the skin.

Unless diagnosed and appropriately treated, the disease is uniformly fatal. Death is usually caused by hemodynamic collapse following valve rupture or by septic emboli to the central nervous system, resulting in brain abscesses or mycotic aneurysms and intracerebral hemorrhage. Because of its multisystem involvement, even with treatment the disease continues to have a high mortality rate, particularly with left-sided endocarditis.

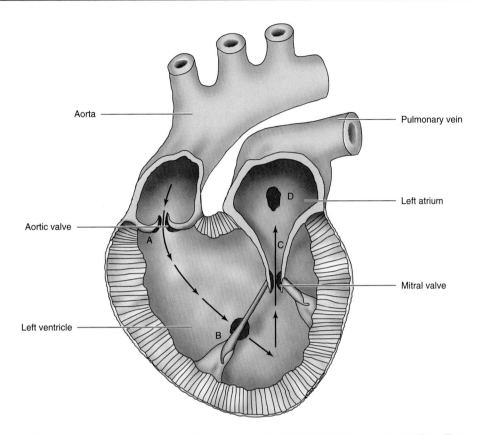

Figure 4–4. The location of endocarditic vegetations in relation to high-velocity regurgitant blood flow. The arrows indicate the high-velocity stream of blood. As a result of regurgitant flow through the orifice of the incompetent aortic valve, lesions form on the ventricular surface of the valve **(A)** or on the chordae tendineae of the anterior mitral leaflet **(B)**. Regurgitant flow across the incompetent mitral valve into the low-pressure left atrium allows a vegetation to form on the atrial surface of the mitral valve **(C)** or at the site of jet stream impact on the atrial wall **(D)**. (Modified and reproduced, with permission, from Karchmer AW: Intravascular infection. In: *Mechanisms of Microbial Disease,* 3rd ed. Schaechter M et al [editors]. Williams & Wilkins, 1998.)

Clinical Manifestations

Infective endocarditis is a multisystem disease with protean manifestations. For these reasons, the symptoms can be nonspecific and the diagnosis difficult to make. Table 4–6 summarizes the important features of the history, physical examination, laboratory data, and complications of infective endocarditis. The symptoms can be acute, subacute, or chronic. The clinical manifestations reflect primarily (1) hemodynamic changes from valvular damage, (2) end organ signs and symptoms from septic emboli (right-sided emboli to the lungs; left-sided emboli to the brain, spleen, kidney, gastrointestinal tract, and extremities), (3) end organ signs and symptoms from immune complex deposition, and (4) persistent bacteremia and distal seeding of infection (abscesses).

5. Which patients are at highest risk for infective endocarditis?
6. What are the leading etiologic agents of infective endocarditis?
7. What features characterize infective endocarditis in intravenous drug users? In patients with prosthetic heart valves?
8. What hemodynamic features predispose to infective endocarditis?
9. What are some of the range of clinical manifestations of untreated bacterial endocarditis?
10. What are the most common causes of death in untreated infective endocarditis?

Table 4–6. Diagnosis of infective endocarditis and its complications.

History	Physical Examination	Laboratory Data	Complications
Fever, chills, night sweats, fatigue, malaise (non-specific constitutional symptoms; can be acute, subacute, or chronic)	"Ill-appearing" Fever Tachycardia Hypotension Cardiac murmurs	Positive blood cultures ↑ White blood cell count ↑ Erythrocyte sedimentation rate ↑ Rheumatoid factor	**Systemic** Persistent bacteremia Sepsis syndrome (?)
Headaches Back pain Focal weakness	Papilledema Focal vertebral spinal tenderness Focal neurologic exam (weakness, hyperreflexia, positive Babinski's sign, etc)	Head CT Spinal MRI Cerebral arteriogram ↑ Erythrocyte sedimentation rate	**Central nervous system** Cerebral emboli Mycotic aneurysm (with or without hemorrhage) Vertebral osteomyelitis Epidural abscess
Dyspnea Orthopnea Pedal edema	↑ Jugular venous pressure Pathologic cardiac murmurs Quincke's pulses Water-hammer pulses Rales Hepatojugular reflux	Chest radiograph Electrocardiogram Transthoracic echocardiogram Transesophageal echocardiogram	**Cardiovascular (with left-sided endocarditis)** Mitral regurgitation Aortic regurgitation Congestive heart failure Valve ring abscess Pericarditis
Pleuritic chest pain, cough	Crackles Pleural rub	Chest radiograph	**Pulmonary (with right-sided endocarditis)** Septic pulmonary emboli
↓ Urine output Flank pain Discolored (brown) urine	Flank tenderness	↑ BUN, ↑ creatinine Pyuria Hematuria Renal sonogram	**Renal** Immune-complex glomerulonephritis Renal artery emboli Intrarenal abscess Perinephric abscess
Abdominal pain	Focal abdominal tenderness Hepatomegaly Splenomegaly	Abdominal sonogram Abdominal CT	**Gastrointestinal** Liver abscesses Splenic abscesses Intestinal artery emboli (intestinal ischemia)
Rashes Focal painful lesions Visual complaints	Janeway lesions (painless hemorrhagic macules on palms and soles) Splinter hemorrhages (nail beds) Petechiae Osler's nodes (painful nodules) Roth spots (funduscopic examination)	Skin biopsies (low yield for diagnosis)	**Skin, miscellaneous** Septic emboli Immune complex vasculitis

MENINGITIS

Clinical Presentation

Symptoms commonly associated with both bacterial and viral meningitis include acute onset of fever, headache, neck stiffness (**meningismus**), and confusion. Bacterial meningitis carries significant morbidity (neurologic sequelae, particularly sensorineural hearing loss) and mortality, and thus this infectious disease emergency requires immediate antibiotic therapy. With rare exceptions, only supportive care with analgesic is necessary for viral meningitis.

Because the clinical presentations of bacterial and viral meningitis may be indistinguishable, laboratory studies of the cerebrospinal fluid are critical in differentiating these two entities. Infection of the meninges is classified by hematologic characteristics of the cerebrospinal fluid into two main categories of meningitis: **neutrophil-predominant** (usually due to bacterial causes) and **lymphocyte-predominant** (sometimes called "aseptic meningitis"). Common causes of lymphocytic meningitis include viral infections (eg, enterovirus), fungal infections (eg, cryptococcus in HIV-infected persons), and spirochetal infections (eg, neurosyphilis or Lyme neuroborreliosis), as well as noninfectious causes such as cancer, connective tissue diseases, and hypersensitivity reactions to drugs. In addition to a neutrophilic pleocytosis, the cerebrospinal fluid in bacterial meningitis is generally characterized by marked elevations in pro-

Table 4–7. Common causes of bacterial meningitis by age group.[1]

Pathogen	< 3 months	3 months to < 18 years	18–50 years	> 50 years
Group B streptococci	•			
E coli	•			
Listeria monocytogenes	•			•
N meningitidis		•	•	•
S pneumoniae		•	•	•
H influenzae[2]		•		
Other gram-negative bacilli				•

[1]Modified and reproduced, with permission, from Quagliarello VJ, Scheld WM: Treatment of bacterial meningitis. N Engl J Med 1997;336:708.
[2]Pathogen among nonimmunized children.

tein concentration, an extremely low glucose level, and, in the absence of previous antibiotic treatment, a positive Gram stain for bacteria. However, there is often significant overlap between the cerebrospinal fluid findings in bacterial and nonbacterial meningitis, and differentiating these entities at presentation is a significant challenge for the clinician.

Etiology

The microbiology of bacterial meningitis in the United States has changed dramatically in the last decade as a result of introduction of the *Haemophilus influenzae* conjugate vaccine. The routine use of this vaccine in the pediatric population has essentially eliminated *H influenzae* as a cause of meningitis and has resulted in a 55% decrease in the total incidence of bacterial meningitis.

The distribution of the causative agents varies by age (Table 4–7). In infants less than 2 months old, *E coli* (and other enteric bacteria), listeria, and group B streptococci are the most common causes of meningitis. For children 2 months to 15 years of age, *S pneumoniae* and *N meningitidis* are the most common causes, with *H influenzae* remaining a concern in nonimmunized children. Among younger adults, *S pneumoniae* and *N meningitidis* remain the leading causes of meningitis, while the elderly are at risk for these pathogens as well as for listeria. Subacute or chronic meningitides are usually caused by *M tuberculosis*, *Borrelia burgdorferi* (the etiologic agent of Lyme disease), fungi (*Coccidioides immitis*, *Cryptococcus neoformans*), and syphilis (*Treponema pallidum*). The diagnosis of meningitis due to these organisms may be delayed because many of these pathogens are difficult to culture and require special serologic or molecular diagnostic techniques.

Pathogenesis

The pathogenesis of bacterial meningitis involves a sequence of events in which virulent microorganisms overcome the host's defense mechanisms (Table 4–8). Most of our knowledge of the pathogenesis of meningitis comes from studies of bacterial meningitis in animal models—inoculation of rats or rabbits with common bacterial pathogens associated with meningitis. The sequence of events is shown in Figure 4–5. First, bacteria colonize the host's nasopharynx, followed by local invasion of the mucosal epithelium and subsequent bacteremia. This is followed by cerebral endothelial cell injury, which increases blood-brain barrier permeability and facilitates meningeal invasion. The inflammatory response in the subarachnoid space, mediated by interleukins, tumor necrosis factor, and prostaglandins, results in cerebral edema, vasculitis, and infarction. The cascade of events leads to decreased cerebrospinal fluid outflow, hydrocephalus, worsening cerebral edema, increased intracranial pressure, and decreased cerebral blood flow.

Most cases of bacterial meningitis begin with host acquisition of a new organism by nasopharyngeal colonization. Pathogenic bacteria commonly associated with meningitis secrete an IgA protease that inactivates host antibody and facilitates mucosal at-

Table 4–8. Pathogenetic sequence of bacterial neurotropism.[1]

Neurotropic Stage	Host Defense	Strategy of Pathogen
1. Colonization or mucosal invasion	Secretory IgA Ciliary activity Mucosal epithelium	IgA protease secretion Ciliostasis Adhesive pili
2. Intravascular survival	Complement	Evasion of alternative pathway by polysaccharide capsule
3. Crossing of blood-brain barrier	Cerebral endothelium	Adhesive pili
4. Survival within CSF	Poor opsonic activity	Bacterial replication

[1]Reproduced, with permission, from Quagliarello V, Scheld WM: Bacterial meningitis: Pathogenesis, pathophysiology, and progress. N Engl J Med 1992;327:864.

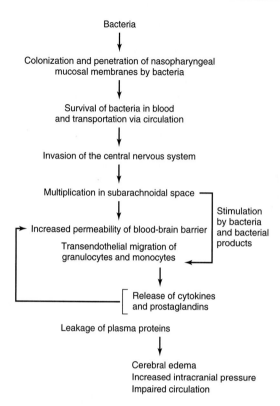

Figure 4–5. Pathogenesis of bacterial meningitis. (Reproduced, with permission, from Van Furth AM et al: Roles of proinflammatory and anti-inflammatory cytokines in pathophysiology of bacterial meningitis and effect of adjunctive therapy. Infect Immunol 1996;64:4883.)

tachment. Many of the causal pathogens possess surface characteristics that enhance mucosal colonization. *N meningitidis* binds to nonciliated epithelial cells by finger-like projections known as **pili.** For *H influenzae* and *S pneumoniae,* encapsulation may be important for nasopharyngeal colonization and systemic invasion.

Once the mucosal barrier is breached, bacteria gain access to the bloodstream, where they must overcome host defense mechanisms to survive and invade the central nervous system. The bacterial capsule, a feature of the above three bacteria, is the most important virulence factor in this regard. By inhibiting neutrophil phagocytosis and resisting complement-mediated bactericidal activity, the capsule enhances bacterial survival and replication. Host defenses counteract the antiphagocytic effects of the pneumococcal capsule by activating the alternative complement pathway, resulting in C3b activation, opsonization, phagocytosis, and intravascular clearance of the organism. This defense mechanism is impaired in patients who have undergone splenectomy. Such patients are predisposed to the development of overwhelming bacteremia and meningitis with encapsulated bacteria, particularly *S pneumoniae* and *H influenzae.* Activation of the complement system is an essential host defense mechanism against invasive disease by *N meningitidis,* and patients with deficiencies of the late complement components (C5–9) are at increased risk for invasive meningococcal disease.

The mechanisms by which bacterial pathogens gain access to the central nervous system are largely unknown. Experimental studies suggest that receptors for bacterial pathogens are present on cells in the choroid plexus, which may facilitate movement of these pathogens into the subarachnoid space. Invasion of the spinal fluid by a meningeal pathogen results in increased permeability of the blood-brain barrier, with leakage of albumin into the subarachnoid space.

Once the bacterial pathogen has accessed the subarachnoid space, local host defense mechanisms are inadequate to control the infection. Normally, complement components are minimal or absent in the cerebrospinal fluid. Meningeal inflammation leads to increased, but still low, concentrations of complement, inadequate for opsonization, phagocytosis, and removal of encapsulated meningeal pathogens. Immunoglobulin concentrations are also low in the cerebrospinal fluid, with an average blood:CSF IgG ratio of 800:1. While the absolute quantity of immunoglobulin in the cerebrospinal fluid increases with infection, the ratio of immunoglobulin in the cerebrospinal fluid relative to that in the serum remains low.

A hallmark of bacterial meningitis is the development of a neutrophilic pleocytosis—an increased number of polymorphonuclear cells—in the cerebrospinal fluid. However, despite the entry of leukocytes, host defense mechanisms in spinal fluid remain suboptimal because of the relative lack of opsonic and bactericidal activity.

The ability of meningeal pathogens to induce a marked subarachnoid space inflammatory response contributes to many of the pathophysiologic consequences of bacterial meningitis. Although the bacterial capsule is largely responsible for intravascular and cerebrospinal fluid survival of the pathogens, it is not responsible for the subarachnoid inflammatory response. In experimental infections, the subcapsular surface components (ie, the cell wall and lipopolysaccharide) of bacteria are more important determinants of meningeal inflammation than the bacterial surface components involved in cerebrospinal fluid invasion. The mediators of the inflammatory process are thought to be interleukin-1, interleukin-6, and tumor necrosis factor (TNF). Within 1–3 hours after intracisternal inoculation of meningococcal lipopolysaccharide in an animal model, there is a brisk release of TNF and IL-1 into the cerebrospinal fluid; their release precedes the development of inflammation or the exudation of protein. The most direct evidence that these cytokines are involved comes from experiments in which direct inoculation of TNF and IL-1 into the cerebrospinal fluid produces the same inflammatory response.

The development of cerebral edema contributes to an increase in intracranial pressure, potentially resulting in life-threatening cerebral herniation. **Vasogenic cerebral edema** is principally caused by the increase in blood-brain barrier permeability. **Cytotoxic cerebral edema** results from swelling of the cellular elements of the brain due to toxic factors from bacteria or neutrophils. **Interstitial cerebral edema** reflects obstruction of flow of cerebrospinal fluid, as in hydrocephalus. Recent literature suggests that oxygen free-radicals and nitric oxide may also be important mediators in cerebral edema. Other complications of meningitis include **cerebral vasculitis** with alterations in cerebral blood flow. The vasculitis leads to narrowing or thrombosis of cerebral blood vessels, resulting in ischemia and possible brain infarction. In combination with increased intracranial pressure, cerebral vasculitis may result in altered cerebral blood flow.

Understanding the pathophysiology of bacterial meningitis has therapeutic implications. Although bactericidal antibiotic therapy is critical for adequate treatment, rapid bacteriolysis can release high concentrations of inflammatory bacterial fragments, potentially exacerbating inflammation and abnormalities of the cerebral microvasculature. In animal models, antibiotic therapy has been shown to cause rapid bacteriolysis and release of bacterial endotoxin, resulting in increased cerebrospinal fluid inflammation and cerebral edema.

The importance of the immune response in triggering cerebral edema has led investigators to study the role of adjuvant anti-inflammatory medications for bacterial meningitis. The use of corticosteroids has been shown to decrease the risk of sensorineural hearing loss among children with *H influenzae* meningitis.

Clinical Manifestations

Among patients who develop community-acquired bacterial meningitis, an antecedent upper respiratory tract infection is common. Patients with a history of head injury or neurosurgery, especially those with a persistent cerebrospinal fluid leak, are at particularly high risk for meningitis. Manifestations of meningitis in infants may be difficult to recognize and interpret; therefore, a high index of suspicion must be maintained in the evaluation of any febrile neonate.

Most patients with meningitis have a rapid onset of fever, headache, lethargy, and confusion. Fewer than half complain of neck stiffness, but nuchal rigidity is noted on physical examination in more than 75%. Other clues include altered mental status, nausea, vomiting, photophobia, **Kernig's sign** (resistance to passive extension of the flexed leg with the patient lying supine), and **Brudzinki's sign** (flexion of the hip and knee occurring when the examiner passively flexes the patient's neck). About 50% of patients with meningococcemia develop a petechial or purpuric rash, predominantly on the extremities.

Although a change in mental status (lethargy, confusion) is common in bacterial meningitis, up to 30% of patients present with normal mentation. Ten to 20 percent of patients have cranial nerve dysfunction. Focal neurologic signs or seizures are seen in 10–30% of cases. When the cerebral swelling causes the brain to expand beyond the confines of the rigid cranium, herniation (brain displacement through the foramen magnum with brainstem compression) and death occur.

Any patient suspected of having meningitis requires emergent lumbar puncture for Gram stain and culture of the cerebrospinal fluid, followed immediately by the administration of antibiotics. Alternatively, if a focal neurologic process (eg, brain abscess) is suspected, antibiotics should be initiated immediately, followed by brain imaging (either CT or MRI) and lumbar puncture if there is no radiologic contraindication.

---

11. What is the typical presentation of bacterial meningitis?
12. What are the major etiologic agents of meningitis and how do they vary with age or other characteristics of the host?
13. What is the sequence of events in development of meningitis, and what features of particular organisms predispose to meningitis?
14. What are the diverse causes of cerebral edema in patients with meningitis?
15. Why is rapid bacteriolysis theoretically dangerous in therapy of meningitis?
16. What are the associated clinical manifestations of untreated bacterial meningitis?

PNEUMONIA

Clinical Presentation

The respiratory tract is the most common site of infection by pathogenic microorganisms. Pneumonia is the sixth leading cause of death in the United States and the commonest cause of death due to infectious disease. It is estimated that 2–3 million cases of community-acquired pneumonia occur each year in the United States, resulting in 1,000,000 physician visits, 500,000 hospitalizations, and 45,000 deaths.

Diagnosis and management of pneumonia requires knowledge of host risk factors, potential infectious agents, environmental exposures, and pathogenesis. Pneumonia can be caused by viruses, bacteria, atypical bacteria (mycobacteria, chlamydiae, mycoplasmas, legionellae), parasites, or fungi.

Pneumonia is an infection of the lung parenchyma leading to inflammation (alveolitis) and the accumulation of an inflammatory exudate. With spread to the interstitium around the alveoli, consolidation and a degree of impaired gas exchange occur. Infection can also extend to the pleural space, causing **pleurisy** (pain on inspiration). The exudative response of the pleura to pneumonia is termed a **parapneumonic effusion**, which itself can become infected and develop into frank pus **(empyema)**.

Etiology

Despite technologic advances in diagnosis, the specific agents associated with community-acquired pneumonia cannot be identified in up to 50% of cases. Even in cases where a microbiologic diagnosis is made, there is usually a delay of several days before the pathogen can be identified and antibiotic susceptibility determined. Therefore, knowledge of the most common etiologic organisms is crucial in determining rational empiric antibiotic regimens. Patients with community-acquired pneumonia are subclassified into four groups by comorbid disease and severity of pulmonary infection to reflect the different bacterial organisms responsible for disease in these populations (Table 4-9).

Several organisms require special consideration because of differences in host susceptibility, therapy, severity, or public health importance. Table 4-10 classifies by patient risk factor the most common infectious agents associated with pneumonia and the postulated primary mechanism of infection. Symptoms, though helpful, are often nonspecific. Understanding and identifying patient risk factors (smoking, HIV infection, etc) and host defense mechanisms (cough reflex, cell-mediated immunity) focuses attention on the most likely etiologic agents, guides empiric therapy, and suggests possible contributing mechanisms that can be altered to decrease further risk. For example, hospital patients who have suffered a stroke and thus are at higher risk of aspirating oropharyngeal secretions are often colonized with nosocomial gram-negative bacteria. Aspiration precautions such as elevation of the head of the bed may decrease the risk of future lung infections. Likewise, a patient with AIDS is at high risk for pneumocystis pneumonia and should be given prophylactic antibiotics.

Pathogenesis

Although pneumonia is a relatively common disease, it occurs infrequently in immunocompetent individuals. This can be attributed to the effectiveness of host defenses, including anatomic barriers and cleansing mechanisms in the nasopharynx and upper airways and local humoral and cellular factors in the alveoli. Normal lungs are sterile below the first major bronchial divisions.

Pulmonary pathogens reach the lungs by one of four routes: (1) direct inhalation of respiratory droplets, (2) aspiration of upper airway contents, (3) spread along the mucosal membrane surface, and (4) hematogenous spread. The pulmonary antimicrobial defense mechanisms are shown in Table 4-11 and Figure 4-6. Incoming air with suspended particulate matter is subjected to turbulence in the nasal passages and then to abrupt changes in direction as the airstream is diverted through the pharynx and along the branches of the tracheobronchial tree. Particles

Table 4-9. Common etiologic agents of community-acquired pneumonia as determined by host characteristics.

	Outpatient		Hospitalized	
			Moderate Infection	Severe Infection
Etiologic Agent	Age < 60, No Comorbid Disease	Age > 60, Comorbid Disease	(Not Requiring ICU Admission)	(Requiring ICU Admission)
S pneumoniae	X	X	X	X
H influenzae	X	X	X	O
M catarrhalis		O	O	
S aureus	O	X	X	O
Aerobic gram-negative bacilli	O	X	X	X
Polymicrobial, anaerobic			X	
M pneumoniae	X		O	X
C pneumoniae	X		X	
Legionella species	O	O	X	X

Key: X = major cause; O = minor cause.

Table 4–10. Common risk factors and causes of pneumonia in specific adult hosts.

Risk Factor	Etiologic Agents		Pathogenetic Mechanism and Comments
	Acute Symptoms	Subacute or Chronic Symptoms	
Immunocompromised 1. Acquired: a. HIV-infected	*Streptococcus pneumoniae* *Haemophilus influenzae* *Pneumocystis carinii*	*Nocardia* *Mycobacterium tuberculosis*	Cell-mediated immune dysfunction Impaired humoral response
b. Transplant recipient	Cytomegalovirus Aspergillus Legionella *Pneumocystis carinii*	*Nocardia*	Cell-mediated immune dysfunction Granulocytopenia
2. Inherited: Complement deficiency, etc	*Streptococcus pneumoniae* *Neisseria meningitidis*		Impaired opsonization and cell lysis
Chronic lung disease	*S pneumoniae* *H influenzae* *Moraxella catarrhalis*		Decreased mucociliary clearance
Alcoholism	*Klebsiella pneumoniae*	Mixed anaerobic infection	Aspiration
Injection drug abuse	*Staphylococcus aureus*		Hematogenous spread
Environmental or animal exposure	*Legionella pneumophila* *Chlamydia psittaci* *Coxiella burnetti* (Q fever) Hanta virus	*Coccidioides immitis*, *Histoplasma capsulatum* *Cryptococcus neoformans*	Inhalation
Institutional exposure (hospital, nursing home, etc)	Gram-negative bacilli (eg, *Pseudomonas aeruginosa, Enterobacter cloacae*) *Staphylococcus aureus*		Microaspirations Bypass of upper respiratory tract defense mechanisms (intubation) Hematogenous (intravenous catheters)
Postinfluenza	*S aureus*		Disruption of respiratory epithelium Ciliary dysfunction Inhibition of PMNs

larger than 10 μm are trapped in the nose or pharynx; those with diameters of 2–9 μm are deposited on the mucociliary blanket; only smaller particles reach the alveoli. *M tuberculosis* and *Legionella pneumophila* are examples of bacteria that are deposited directly in the lower airways. Bacteria trapped in the upper airways can colonize the oropharynx and then be aspirated into the lungs, either by "microaspiration" or by overt aspiration through an open epiglottis (eg, in alcoholic patients who "pass out"). Likewise, chronic cigarette smokers have decreased mucociliary clearance secondary to damage of cilia and are often unable to clear respiratory secretions adequately. Patients who develop chronic bronchitis rely more heavily on the cough reflex to clear pathogens. The cough reflex is an important mechanism by which aspirated material, excess secretions, and foreign bodies are removed from the airway.

The respiratory epithelium has special mechanisms for fighting off infection. Epithelial cells are covered with beating cilia blanketed by a layer of mucus. Each cell has about 200 cilia that beat up to 500 times a minute, serving to move the mucus layer upward toward the larynx. The mucus itself contains antimicrobial compounds such as lysozyme and secretory IgA antibodies. Bacteria that reach the terminal bronchioles, alveolar ducts, and alveoli are inactivated primarily by alveolar macrophages and neutrophils. Opsonization of the microorganism enhances phagocytosis by these cells.

Table 4–11. Pulmonary antimicrobial defense mechanisms.[1]

Aerodynamic filtration
Cough reflex
Mucociliary transport system
Phagocytic cells (alveolar macrophages and polymorphonuclear leukocytes)
Immune responses (humoral and cellular)
Pulmonary secretions (surfactant, lysozyme, iron-binding proteins)

[1]Modified and reproduced, with permission, from LaForce FM: Bacterial pneumonias. In: *Infectious Diseases*. Gorbach SL, Bartlett JG, Blacklow NR (editors). Saunders, 1992.

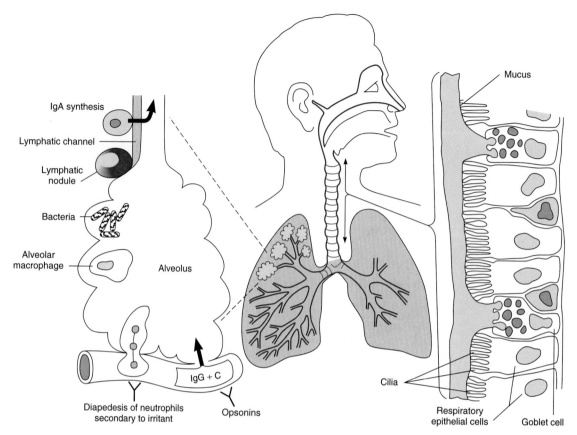

Figure 4–6. Pulmonary defense mechanisms. Abrupt changes in direction of air flow in the nasal passages can trap potential pathogens. The epiglottis and cough reflex prevent introduction of particulate matter in the lower airway. The ciliated respiratory epithelium propels the overlying mucus layer (right) upward toward the mouth. In the alveoli, cell-mediated immunity, humoral factors, and the inflammatory response defend against lower respiratory tract infections. (C, complement.) (Modified and reproduced, with permission, from Storch GA: Respiratory system. In: *Mechanisms of Microbial Disease,* 3rd ed. Schaechter M et al [editors]. Williams & Wilkins, 1998.)

Impairment at any level of host defenses increases the risk of developing pneumonia. Children with cystic fibrosis have defective ciliary activity and are prone to develop recurrent sinopulmonary infections, particularly with *S aureus* and *P aeruginosa*. Patients with granulocytopenia, whether acquired or congenital, are also susceptible to lung infections. Antigenic stimulation of T cells leads to the production of lymphokines which activate macrophages with enhanced bactericidal activity. HIV-infected patients have depleted CD4 T lymphocyte counts and are predisposed to a variety of bacterial, mycobacterial, and fungal infections.

Clinical Manifestations

Most patients with pneumonia have fever, cough, tachypnea, tachycardia, and an infiltrate on chest radiograph. Extrapulmonary manifestations that may provide clues to the etiologic agents involved in pneumonia include the presence of serum cold agglutinins *(Mycoplasma pneumoniae),* pharyngitis *(Chlamydia pneumoniae),* erythema nodosum rash (fungal and mycobacterial infections), hyponatremia (legionella), and diarrhea or abdominal pain (legionella).

The following questions should be answered to guide empiric therapy for a patient who presents with symptoms consistent with pneumonia:

Is this pneumonia community-acquired or institution-acquired (hospital, jail, nursing home, etc)?

Is this patient immunocompromised (HIV-infected, a transplant recipient)?

Is this patient an injection drug user?

Is this patient an alcoholic?

Has this patient had a recent loss of consciousness? (Suggestive of aspiration.)

Are the symptoms acute (days) or chronic (weeks to months)?

Has this patient lived in or traveled through geographic areas associated with specific endemic infections (histoplasmosis, coccidioidomycosis)?

Has the patient had recent zoonotic exposures associated with pulmonary infections (psittacosis, Q fever)?

Could this patient have a contagious infection of public health importance (tuberculosis)?

Could this patient's pulmonary infection be associated with a common source exposure (legionella outbreak)?

It is only by answering these epidemiologic questions that the practitioner can determine the probable causative organisms and begin efficacious empiric treatment.

> 17. How many cases of pneumonia occur in the U.S. annually?
> 18. What are the most likely pathogens for each of the four groups of patients with community-acquired pneumonia?
> 19. What host features influence the likelihood of particular causes of pneumonia?
> 20. What are the four mechanisms by which pathogens reach the lungs?
> 21. What are the defenses of the respiratory epithelium against infection?

INFECTIOUS DIARRHEA

Clinical Presentation

Each year throughout the world more than 5 million people—most of them children under 1 year of age—die of acute infectious diarrhea. (Infectious diarrhea is discussed in this chapter. Other forms of diarrhea are considered in Chapter 13.) The morbidity and mortality attributable to diarrhea are largely due to secretion of copious amounts of fluid into the intestinal lumen. All segments of the intestinal tract, from the proximal jejunum to the rectum, secrete water and electrolytes. For example, adults with cholera, if adequately hydrated, can sometimes excrete more than 1 L of fluid per hour. Contrast this with the normal volume of fluid lost daily in the stools (150 mL), and it is clear that massive fluid losses associated with infectious diarrhea can lead to dehydration, cardiovascular collapse, and death.

Gastrointestinal infections can present with primarily upper gastrointestinal symptoms (nausea, vomiting, crampy epigastric pain), small intestinal symptoms (profuse watery diarrhea), or large intestinal symptoms (tenesmus, fecal urgency, less profuse diarrhea). Sources of infection include person-to-person transmission (fecal-oral spread of shigella), water-borne transmission (cryptosporidium), food-borne transmission (salmonella or *S aureus* food poisoning), and overgrowth following antibiotic administration *(Clostridium difficile)*.

Etiology

A wide range of microorganisms infect the gastrointestinal tract. These agents include newly identified bacterial pathogens such as *Helicobacter pylori* and a growing number of viral causes of gastroenteritis. Rotavirus is thought to be the most common cause of severe diarrhea in infants and young children. Protozoal and fungal enteric pathogens can also produce diarrhea. In the United States, viral gastroenteritis causes about 35% of cases of infectious diarrhea; bacteria account for about 25% of cases; and in 40% the cause remains unknown. HIV-infected patients with very low CD4 lymphocyte counts (usually < 100/µL) can develop a severe, often unremitting watery diarrhea caused by the parasite cryptosporidium for which there is no effective antibiotic treatment.

Pathogenesis

A comprehensive approach to gastrointestinal infections starts with the classic host-agent-environment paradigm. A number of host factors influence gastrointestinal infections. Patients at extremes of age and with comorbid conditions (eg, HIV) are at higher risk for symptomatic infection. Use of medications that alter the gastrointestinal microenvironment or destroy normal bacterial flora also predispose patients to infection. Microbial agents responsible for gastrointestinal diarrheal illness can be categorized according to type of organism (bacterial, viral, parasitic), propensity to attach to different anatomic sites (stomach, small bowel, colon), and pathogenesis (enterotoxigenic, cytotoxigenic, enteroinvasive). Environmental factors can be divided into three broad categories based on mode of transmission: (1) water-borne, (2) food-borne, and (3) person-to-person transmission. Table 4–12 summarizes these relationships and provides a framework for assessing the pathogenesis of gastrointestinal infections.

Gastrointestinal infections range from those that involve primarily the stomach, causing nausea and vomiting, to those that affect the small and large bowel, with diarrhea as the predominant symptom. Gastroenteritis classically refers to infection of the stomach and proximal small bowel. Organisms causing this disorder include *Bacillus cereus, S aureus,* and a number of viruses (rotavirus, Norwalk-like agent). *Bacillus cereus* and *S aureus* produce a preformed **neurotoxin** that is responsible for symptomatic illness. Ingestion of the heat-stable neurotoxin, even in the absence of viable bacteria, is sufficient to cause disease, and these toxins represent major causes of food poisoning. While the exact mechanisms by which the neurotoxins exert their effects have not been well described, it is thought that they

Table 4–12. Approach to gastrointestinal infections.

Paradigm	Categories	Examples	Microbes
Environment	Water-borne	Water supply	*Vibrio cholerae*
	Food-borne	Contaminated food	*Staphylococcus aureus* *Bacillus cereus*
	Person-to-person	Child care centers	Shigella Rotavirus
Agent	Bacterial		Salmonella species
	Viral		Rotavirus
	Parasitic		*Entamoeba histolytica*
Host	Age	Children	Enterohemorrhagic *E coli* (EHEC)
	Comorbid conditions	HIV infection	Cryptosporidium Cytomegalovirus
	Gastric acidity	Antacid	Salmonella
	Gastrointestinal flora	Antibiotic use	*Clostridium difficile*

act locally, by activation of the sympathetic nervous system, with a resultant increase in peristaltic activity; and centrally, through activation of emetic centers in the brain.

The pathogenesis of diarrheogenic infections is typified by the diverse mechanisms by which *E coli* can cause diarrhea. Colonization of the human gastrointestinal tract by *E coli* is universal, typically occurring within hours after birth. However, when the host organism is exposed to pathogenic strains of *E coli* not normally present in the bowel flora, localized gastrointestinal disease or even systemic illness may occur. There are five major classes of diarrheogenic *E coli*: enterotoxigenic (ETEC), enteropathogenic (EPEC), enterohemorrhagic (EHEC), enteroaggregative (EAEC), and enteroinvasive (EIEC) (Table 4–13). Pathogenic *E coli* must fulfill the common criteria of evasion of host defenses, colonization of the intestinal mucosa, local multiplication, and host injury. This organism, like all gastrointestinal pathogens, must survive transit through the acidic gastric environment and be able to persist in the gastrointestinal tract despite the mechanical force of peristalsis and competition for scarce nutrients from existing

Table 4–13. *Escherichia coli* in diarrheal disease.

Class	Age at Higher Risk	Inoculum Size	Clinical Syndrome	Gastrointestinal Site	Enterotoxins or Cytotoxins	Site of Action of Toxin
Enteroaggregative *E coli* (EAggEC)	< 6 months	10^8–10^{10}	Watery diarrhea	Small bowel	Not well described	Not well described
Enteropathogenic *E coli* (EPEC)	< 1 year	10^8–10^{10}	Watery diarrhea	Small bowel	Not well described	Not well described
Enterotoxigenic *E coli* (ETEC)	> 1 year	10^8–10^{10}	Watery diarrhea	Small bowel	Heat-labile toxin (LT) (cholera-like) Heat-stable toxin (ST)	Adenylyl cyclase activation Guanylyl cyclase activation
Enteroinvasive *E coli* (EIEC)	> 2 years	10^8–10^{10}	Dysentery (bloody, inflammatory)	Small bowel, large bowel	Not well described	Not well described
Enterohemorrhagic *E coli* (EHEC)	2–10 years, elderly	< 10^3	Hemorrhagic colitis, hemolytic-uremic syndrome, (thrombotic thrombocytopenic purpura)	Small bowel, large bowel	Shiga toxin Stx1 Stx2	Binds to 60S ribosome and inhibits protein synthesis

Key: Stx = Shiga toxin.

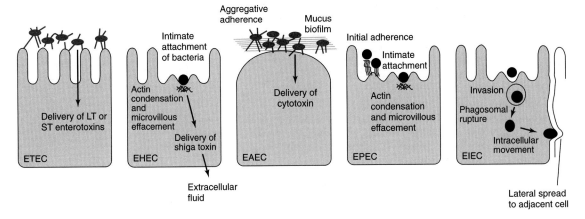

Figure 4–7. Attachment and interaction of the diarrheogenic *E coli* with intestinal epithelial cells. The five recognized categories of interaction are shown. (Modified and reproduced, with permission, from Nataro JP, Kaper JB: Diarrheogenic *Escherichia coli.* Clin Microbiol Rev 1998;11:142.)

bacterial flora. Adherence can be nonspecific (at any part of the intestinal tract) or, more commonly, specific, with attachment occurring at well-defined anatomic areas (Figure 4–7).

Once colonization and multiplication occur, the stage is set for host injury. Infectious diarrhea is clinically differentiated into secretory, inflammatory, and hemorrhagic types, with different pathophysiologic mechanisms accounting for these diverse presentations. **Secretory** (watery) diarrhea is caused by a number of bacteria (eg, *Vibrio cholerae,* ETEC, EPEC, EAEC), viruses (rotavirus, Norwalk agent),

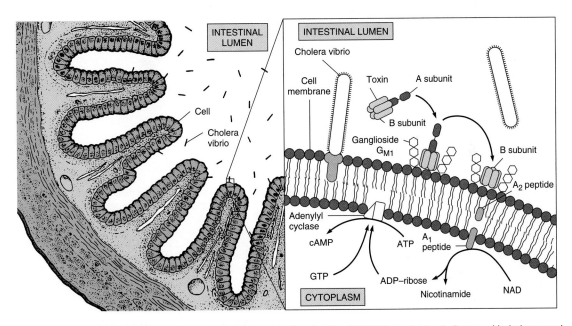

Figure 4–8. Pathogenesis of *Vibrio cholerae* and enterotoxigenic *E coli* (ETEC) in diarrheal disease. *V cholerae* and ETEC share similar pathogenetic mechanisms in causing diarrheal illness. The bacteria gain entry to the small intestinal lumen through ingestion of contaminated food **(left).** They elaborate an enterotoxin that is composed of one A subunit and five B subunits. The B subunits bind to the intestinal cell membrane and facilitate entry of part of the A subunit **(right).** Subsequently, this results in activation of adenylyl cyclase and formation of cAMP, which stimulates water and electrolyte secretion by intestinal endothelial cells. (Modified and reproduced, with permission, from Holmberg SD: Cholera and related illnesses caused by *Vibrio* species and *Aeromonas.* In: *Infectious Diseases.* Gorbach SL et al [editors]. Saunders, 1992.)

and parasites (giardia, cryptosporidium). These organisms attach superficially to enterocytes in the lumen of the small bowel. Stool examination is notable for the absence of fecal leukocytes, and in rare cases there is occult blood in the stools. Some of these pathogens elaborate **enterotoxins,** proteins that increase intestinal cAMP production, leading to net fluid secretion. The classic example is cholera. The bacterium *V cholerae* produces cholera toxin, which binds to epithelial adenylyl cyclase in the small bowel. This results in an increase in intestinal cAMP, with secretion of massive amounts of fluid and electrolytes into the intestinal lumen (Figure 4–8). Clinically, the patient presents with copious diarrhea ("rice-water stools"), progressing to dehydration and vascular collapse in the face of inadequate volume resuscitation. Enterotoxigenic *E coli* (ETEC), a common cause of acute diarrheal illness in young children, produces two enterotoxins. The heat-labile toxin (LT) activates adenylyl cyclase in a manner analogous to cholera toxin, while the heat-stable toxin (ST) activates guanylyl cyclase activity.

Inflammatory diarrhea is a result of bacterial invasion of the mucosal lumen, with resultant cell destruction and death. Patients with this syndrome are usually febrile, with complaints of crampy lower abdominal pain as well as diarrhea. The term **dysentery** is used when there are significant numbers of fecal leukocytes and gross blood. Pathogens associated with inflammatory diarrhea include enteroinvasive *E coli* (EIEC), shigella, salmonella, and *Entamoeba histolytica*. Shigella, the prototypical cause of bacillary dysentery, invades the enterocyte through formation of an endoplasmic vacuole which is lysed intracellularly (Figure 4–9). Bacteria then proliferate in the cytoplasm and invade adjacent epithelial cells. Production of a **cytotoxin,** the Shiga toxin, leads to local cell destruction and death. EIEC resembles shigella both clinically and with respect to the mechanism of invasion of the enterocyte wall; however, no specific cytotoxin has been identified (Figure 4–7).

Hemorrhagic diarrhea, a variant of inflammatory diarrhea, is primarily caused by enterohemorrhagic *E coli* (EHEC). Infection with *E coli* O157:H7 has been associated with a number of deaths secondary to the hemolytic-uremic syndrome, with several well-publicized outbreaks related to contaminated hamburger and apple juice consumption. EHEC causes a broad spectrum of clinical disease, with manifestations including (1) asymptomatic infection, (2) watery (nonbloody) diarrhea, (3) hemorrhagic colitis (bloody, noninflammatory diarrhea), (4) hemolytic-uremic syndrome (an acute illness, primarily of children, characterized by anemia and renal failure), and (5) thrombotic thrombocytopenic purpura (a variant of hemolytic-uremic syndrome seen in adults, associated with thrombocytopenia, fever, and altered mental status). EHEC does not invade enterocytes; however it

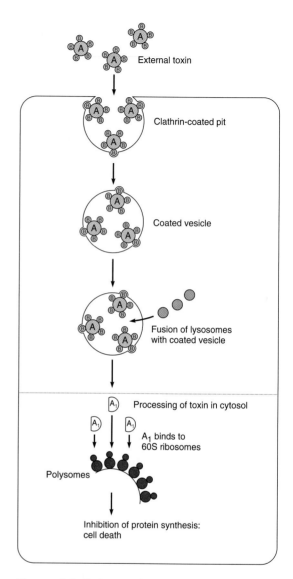

Figure 4–9. Pathogenesis of Shiga toxin. Shigella species and *E coli* O157:H7 probably cause diarrheal diseases by similar pathogenetic mechanisms. The A and B subunits enter the intestinal cells through receptor-mediated endocytosis. The active A_1 fragment binds to the 60S ribosome, leading to inhibition of protein synthesis and cell death. (Modified and reproduced, with permission, from O'Brien AD, Holmes RK: Shiga and Shiga-like toxins. Microbiol Rev 1987;51:206.)

does produce two Shiga toxins (Stx1 and Stx2) that closely resemble the Shiga toxin in structure and function. After binding of EHEC to the cell surface receptor, the A subunit of the Shiga toxin catalyzes the destructive cleavage of ribosomal RNA and halts protein synthesis, leading to cell death (Figure 4–9). Possible mechanisms whereby Shiga toxin causes systemic illness are shown in Figure 4–10.

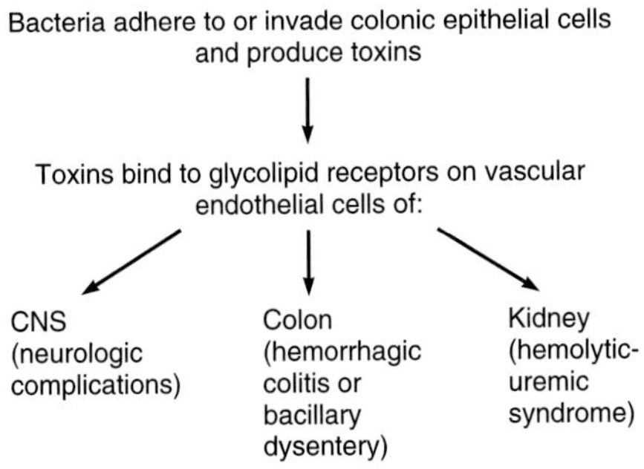

Figure 4–10. Possible mechanisms of complications of *E coli* O157:H7 and shigella species. Shigella species and *E coli* O157:H7 may share similar pathogenetic mechanisms in diarrheal illness and extraintestinal complications. A possible mechanism is that Shiga toxins damage vascular endothelial cells in various target organs. (Modified and reproduced, with permission, from Tesh VL, O'Brien AD: The pathogenic mechanisms of Shiga toxin and the Shiga-like toxins. Mol Microbiol 1991;5:1817.)

soning are profuse vomiting, nausea, and abdominal cramps, followed by diarrhea. Profuse watery (noninflammatory, nonbloody) diarrhea is associated with bacteria that have infected the small intestine and elaborated an enterotoxin (eg, *V cholerae*). In contrast, colitis-like symptoms (lower abdominal pain, tenesmus, fecal urgency) and an inflammatory or bloody diarrhea occur with bacteria that more commonly infect the large intestine. In this case, the incubation period is generally longer (days) and colonic mucosal invasion can occur, causing fever and systemic symptoms.

22. How many individuals in the world die yearly of infectious diarrhea?
23. What are different modes of spread of infectious diarrhea? Give an example of each.
24. What are the pathogenetic mechanisms by which infectious organisms cause diarrhea?

Clinical Manifestations

Table 4–14 summarizes infectious gastroenteritides and food poisoning syndromes. One organizational approach to gastrointestinal infections is to categorize the symptom complex associated with a known pathogenetic mechanism or anatomic site in the gastrointestinal tract. In staphylococcal food poisoning, symptoms develop several hours after ingestion of food contaminated with neurotoxin-producing *S aureus*. The symptoms of staphylococcal food poi-

SEPSIS & SEPTIC SHOCK

Clinical Presentation

Sepsis and septic shock is the leading cause of death in noncoronary intensive care units and the thirteenth leading cause of death in the United States. Approximately 400,000 cases of sepsis and 200,000 cases of septic shock occur annually, with an unadjusted mortality rate of 35%. The use of intravascular catheters, implantation of prosthetic material (eg, cardiac valves and artificial joints), and administra-

Table 4–14. Symptom-based approach to gastroenteritis and food poisoning syndromes.[1]

Symptoms	Syndrome	Anatomic Site	Incubation Period	Suspected Etiologin Agents
Nausea, vomiting	Gastroenteritis	Upper gastrointestinal tract	6 hours	*Staphylococcus aureus* *Bacillus cereus*
Watery noninflammatory diarrhea; passage of few voluminous stools, upper abdominal pain and cramps	Acute watery diarrhea	Small bowel	6–72 hours	Viral agents *B cereus* Enterotoxigenic *E coli* (ETEC) Enteroaggregative *E coli* (EAggEC) Enteropathogenic *E coli* (EPEC) *Vibrio cholerae* *Giardia lamblia*
Inflammatory ileocolitis; tenesmus, fecal urgency, dysentery; fever with invasion; passage of many small-volume stools	Colitis, dysentery	Large bowel origin; colitis; with or without mucosal invasion	16–72 hours	*Salmonella* *Shigella* *Campylobacter jejuni* Enterohemorrhagic *E coli* (EHEC)[2] Enteroinvasive *E coli* (EIEC) *Yersinia enterocolitica* *Vibrio parahaemolyticus*

[1]Modified and reproduced, with permission, from DuPont HL: Guidelines on acute infectious diarrhea in adults. Am J Gastroenterol 1997;92:1962.
[2]EHEC gastrointestinal infections are initially watery diarrhea followed by bloody diarrhea; inflammation occurs in only a small percentage of cases.

tion of immunosuppressive drugs and chemotherapeutic agents increase the risk of infection and subsequent sepsis among hospitalized patients.

The study of sepsis has been facilitated by the recent publication of a consensus definition (Table 4–15). The **systemic inflammatory response syndrome (SIRS)** is a nonspecific inflammatory state that may be seen with infection as well as with noninfectious states such as pancreatitis, pulmonary embolism, and myocardial infarction. Leukopenia and hypothermia, included in the SIRS case definition, are predictors of a poor prognosis when associated with sepsis. **Sepsis** is defined as the presence of SIRS in the setting of an identified infectious precipitant. A recent multicenter study found that only 56% of patients with SIRS fulfilled this definition of sepsis. **Severe sepsis** occurs when there is objective evidence of organ dysfunction (eg, renal failure, hepatic failure, altered mentation), usually associated with tissue hypoperfusion. The final stage of sepsis is **septic shock,** defined as hypotension (systolic blood pressure < 90 mm Hg or a 40 mm Hg decrease below the baseline systolic blood pressure) unresponsive to fluid resuscitation.

Etiology

While evidence of infection is a diagnostic criterion for sepsis, only 28% of patients with sepsis have bacteremia, and slightly more than 10% of these patients will have **primary bacteremia,** defined as positive blood cultures without an obvious source of bacterial seeding. Common sites of primary infection among patients with sepsis syndrome (in order of decreasing frequency) include the respiratory tract, the genitourinary tract, abdominal sources (gallbladder, colon), device-related infections, and wound or soft tissue infections.

The microbiology of sepsis has shifted in the last decade. Gram-negative organisms (Enterobacteriaceae and pseudomonas) account for approximately 40% of all documented infections, gram-positive organisms (*S aureus,* enterococcus, pneumococcus, etc) for 30%, polymicrobial infections for 16%, and fungi, particularly candida, for 6%. Significantly, gram-positive organisms, particularly the staphylococci, are the most common bacteria cultured from the bloodstream, presumably due to an increase in the prevalence of chronic indwelling venous access devices and implanted prosthetic material. *P aeruginosa,* candida, and polymicrobial infections are independent predictors of mortality.

Pathogenesis

The pathogenetic cascade of sepsis generally starts with a localized infection. Bacteria may then invade the bloodstream directly (leading to bacteremia and positive blood cultures) or may proliferate locally and release toxins into the bloodstream. These toxins can arise from a structural component of the bacteria (endotoxin, teichoic acid antigen, etc) or may be exotoxins, which are synthesized and released by the bacteria. **Endotoxin** is defined as the **lipopolysaccharide (LPS)** moiety contained in the outer membrane of gram-negative bacteria. Endotoxin is composed of an outer polysaccharide chain (the **O side chain**), which varies between species and is not toxic, and a highly conserved lipid portion **(lipid A),** which is embedded in the outer bacterial membrane (Figure 4–11). Injection of purified endotoxin or lipid A is highly toxic in animal models, causing a syndrome analogous to septic shock.

A variety of host mediators have been implicated in the pathogenesis of sepsis (Figure 4–12). Gram-negative bacterial endotoxin binds with either a soluble **LPS-binding protein (LPB)** or with a membrane-bound receptor in mononuclear cells, **CD14.** The net effect of these interactions is activation of monocytes, macrophages, and neutrophils to release inflammatory mediators such as **interleukin-1 (IL-1)** and **tumor necrosis factor (TNF),** accompanied by activation of the coagulation cascade, the complement system, and the kinin system. This inflammatory burst results in myocardial depression, changes in vasomotor tone, and organ dysfunction (kidney, liver, lung, and brain).

While much progress has been made in elucidating the pathogenesis of sepsis, current understanding of this complex process remains rudimentary, as evidenced by the failure of interventions aimed at blocking the host response. Multicenter clinical trials using immunotherapy to neutralize bacterial toxins (eg, monoclonal antibodies directed against endotoxin) and agents to ameliorate the host inflammatory response (blockade of IL-1 and TNF, bradykinin antagonists, inhibition of cyclooxygenase with ibuprofen, etc) have not shown a beneficial effect on survival. More concerning, one study actually showed an increase in mortality among patients receiving a pro-

Table 4–15. Definitions of the stages of sepsis.[1]

I. Systemic inflammatory response syndome (SIRS)
  Two or more of the following:
  (1) Temperature of > 38 °C or < 36 °C
  (2) Heart rate of > 90/min
  (3) Respiratory rate of > 20/min
  (4) WBC count of > 12×10^9/L or < 4×10^9/L or >10% immature forms (bands)
II. Sepsis
  SIRS plus a culture-documented infection
III. Severe sepsis
  Sepsis plus organ dysfunction, hypotension, or hypoperfusion (including but not limited to lactic acidosis, oliguria, or acute alteration in mental status)
IV. Septic shock
  Hypotension (despite fluid resuscitation) plus hypoperfusion abnormalities

[1]Reproduced, with permission, from Wenzel RP et al: Current understanding of sepsis. Clin Infect Dis 1996;22:407.

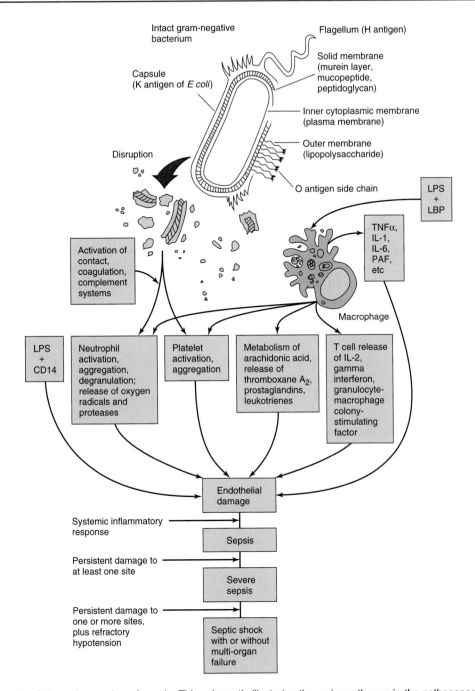

Figure 4–11. Schematic overview of sepsis. This schematic illustrates the major pathways in the pathogenesis of sepsis. See text for details. LPS, lipopolysaccharide; CD14, soluble CD14; LBP, LPS-binding protein. (Modified and reproduced, with permission, from Bone RC: The pathogenesis of sepsis. Ann Intern Med 1991;115:457.)

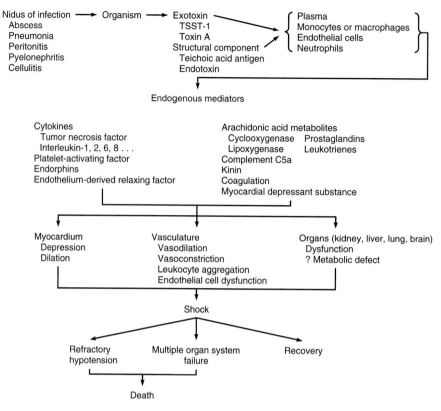

Figure 4–12. Pathogenetic sequence of the events in septic shock. TSST-1 denotes toxic shock syndrome toxin 1. Toxin A is *Pseudomonas aeruginosa* toxin A. (Reproduced, with permission, from Parrillo JE: Pathogenetic mechanisms of septic shock. N Engl J Med 1993;328:1471.)

tein that blocked TNF receptors. More study is needed to determine which components of the host response are responsible for organ damage and which ones are important for the control of infection.

A. Hemodynamic Alterations: All forms of shock result in inadequate tissue perfusion and subsequent cell dysfunction and death. In noninfectious forms (such as cardiogenic shock and hypovolemic shock), **systemic vascular resistance (SVR)** is elevated as a compensatory mechanism to maintain blood pressure. In the hypoperfused tissues, there is enhanced extraction of oxygen from circulating red blood cells leading to decreased pulmonary artery oxygenation. In contrast, early in septic shock there is hypovolemia from inappropriate arterial and venous dilation (low SVR) and leakage of plasma into the extravascular space. Even with correction of the hypovolemia, the SVR remains low despite a compensatory increase in **cardiac output.** Inefficient oxygen extraction and tissue hypoperfusion result in increased pulmonary artery oxygen content.

A hyperdynamic circulatory state, described as **distributive shock** to emphasize the maldistribution of blood flow to various tissues, is the common hemodynamic finding in sepsis. The release of vasoactive substances (including nitric oxide) results in loss of normal mechanisms of vascular autoregulation, producing regional and microcirculatory imbalances in blood flow with regional shunting and relative hypoperfusion of some organs. Animal studies have documented predictable changes in organ blood flow, with a marked reduction in blood flow to the stomach, duodenum, small bowel, and pancreas, a moderate reduction in blood flow to the myocardial and skeletal muscles, and normal perfusion of the kidneys and central nervous system.

Despite relative preservation of myocardial blood flow, myocardial depression is common in early septic shock. Initially, patients have low cardiac filling pressures and low cardiac output secondary to volume depletion and vasodilation. Following fluid replacement, cardiac output is normal or increased but ventricular function is abnormal. Twenty-four to 48 hours after the onset of sepsis, left and right ventricular ejection fractions are reduced and end-diastolic and end-systolic volumes are increased. This myocardial depression has been attributed to direct toxic effects of nitric oxide, TNF, and IL-1. Reduced ejection fraction and consequent myocardial depression are reversible in patients who survive septic shock. Failure of ventricular function to normalize despite inotropic agents is a poor prognostic feature

B. Vascular and Multiorgan Dysfunction: Most patients who die of septic shock have either refractory hypotension or multiple organ failure. Refractory hypotension can occur from two mechanisms. First, some patients cannot sustain high cardiac output in response to the septic state and develop progressive cardiac failure with hypodynamic shock. Second, circulatory failure may be associated with severe vasodilation and hypotension refractory to intravenous fluid resuscitation and vasopressor therapy.

The development of multiple organ failure represents the terminal phase of a hypermetabolic process that begins during the initial stages of shock. Organ failure results from microvascular injury induced by local and systemic inflammatory responses to infection. Maldistribution of blood flow is accentuated by impaired erythrocyte deformability, with microvascular obstruction. Aggregation of neutrophils and platelets may also reduce blood flow. Demargination of neutrophils from vascular endothelium results in release of mediators and subsequent migration of neutrophils into tissues. Components of the complement system are activated, attracting more neutrophils and releasing locally active substances such as prostaglandins and leukotrienes. These mediators cause local vasoconstriction and vasodilation and the accumulation of still more inflammatory cells. The net result of all of these changes is microvascular collapse and ultimately, organ failure.

The outcome of sepsis depends on the number of organs that fail: the mortality among patients with multi-organ failure (three or more organ systems) is 80–100%. Approximately 10% of patients with sepsis develop respiratory failure, most commonly **acute respiratory distress syndrome (ARDS),** which is characterized by severe refractory hypoxia, decreased lung compliance, noncardiogenic pulmonary edema, and pulmonary hypertension. ARDS is often fatal. Hepatic dysfunction is a sequela of sepsis in about 10% of cases. Initial manifestations are hyperbilirubinemia with modest elevations in serum aminotransferases and alkaline phosphatase. Renal failure develops later in the clinical course in about 4% of cases. Renal failure is usually a multifactorial process, with additive injury from intrarenal shunting, renal hypoperfusion, and administration of nephrotoxic agents (antibiotics and radiologic imaging dye). Other organs affected by sepsis include the central nervous system (altered mentation, coma) and the blood (disseminated intravascular coagulation).

Clinical Manifestations

The clinical manifestations of sepsis include those related to the systemic response to infections (tachycardia, tachypnea, alterations in temperature and leukocyte count) and those related to specific organ system dysfunction (cardiovascular, respiratory, renal, hepatic, and hematologic abnormalities). Sepsis sometimes begins with very subtle clues that can be easily confused with more common, less serious illnesses. Awareness of these early signs of sepsis can lead to early recognition and intervention. Nonspecific signs can include isolated tachypnea (without dyspnea), isolated tachycardia (with normal blood pressure), irritability or lethargy, and otherwise unexplained fever, rigors, or myalgias. Nonspecific laboratory abnormalities can include respiratory alkalosis, leukocytosis, and mild liver function abnormalities.

---

25. What is the incidence of sepsis and septic shock in the USA? What is the mortality rate?
26. What factors contribute to hospital-related sepsis?
27. Which organisms are most commonly associated with sepsis?
28. Which host mediators have been implicated in the pathogenesis of sepsis?
29. What activates these host mediators?
30. What are some distinctive hemodynamic features of septic shock versus other shock syndromes?

REFERENCES

General
Brooks GF et al: *Jawetz, Melnick, and Adelberg's Review of Medical Microbiology,* 21st ed. Appleton & Lange, 1998.
Mandell GL et al: *Mandell, Douglas and Bennett's Principles and Practices of Infectious Diseases,* 4th ed. Churchill Livingstone, 1995.
Schaechter M et al: *Mechanisms of Microbial Disease,* 2nd ed. Williams & Wilkins, 1993.

Infective Endocarditis
Bayer AD: Infective endocarditis. Clin Infect Dis 1993;17:313.
Brown M, Griffin GE: Immune responses in endocarditis. Heart 1998;79:1.

Meningitis
Quagliarello V, Scheld WM: Treatment of bacterial meningitis. N Engl J Med 1997;336:708.

Schuchat A et al: Bacterial meningitis in the United States in 1995. N Engl J Med 1997;337:970.

Van Furth AM et al: Roles of proinflammatory and anti-inflammatory cytokines in pathophysiology of bacterial meningitis and effect of adjunctive therapy. Infect Immunol 1996;64:4883.

Pneumonia

Bartlett JG et al: Community-acquired pneumonia in adults: Guidelines for management. Clin Infect Dis 1998;26:811.

Brown PD, Lerner SA: Community-acquired pneumonia. Lancet 1998;352:1295.

Infectious Diarrhea

Dupont HL: Guidelines on acute infectious diarrhea in adults. Am J Gastroenterol 1997;92:1962.

Nataro JP, Kaper JB: Diarrheogenic Escherichia coli. Clin Microbiol Rev 1998;11:142.

Sepsis, Sepsis Syndrome, and Septic Shock

Astiz ME, Rackow EC: Septic shock. Lancet 1998;351:1501.

Mark PE, Varon J: The hemodynamic derangements in sepsis. Chest 1998;119:854.

Natanson C (moderator): Selected treatment strategies for septic shock based on proposed mechanisms of pathogenesis. Ann Intern Med 1994;120:771.

Parrillo JE: Pathogenetic mechanisms of septic shock. N Engl J Med 1993;328:1471.

Sands KE et al: Epidemiology of sepsis syndrome in 8 academic medical centers. JAMA 1997;278:234.

Wenzel RP Current understanding of sepsis. Clin Infect Dis 1996;22:407.

Neoplasia 5

Debasish Tripathy, MD

Cell growth and maturation are normal events in organ development during embryogenesis, growth, and tissue repair and remodeling after injury. Disordered regulation of these processes can result in loss of control over cell growth, differentiation, and spatial confinement. Human neoplasia collectively represents a spectrum of diseases characterized by abnormal growth and invasion of cells. Although cancers are typically classified by their tissues of origin or anatomic location, many features are shared by all types. There is also considerable variation among patients with a given type of cancer in the nature of cellular alterations as well as the clinical presentation and course of disease. The recognition of overt malignancy by physical examination or imaging requires the presence in the body of about 1 billion malignant cells. A **preclinical phase** may sometimes be recognized. Preclinical signs may consist of (among others) polyps in the colon or dysplastic nevi on the skin—potential precursors of colon carcinoma and malignant melanoma, respectively. Such precursor lesions usually exhibit features of abnormal cell proliferation without the demonstration of invasiveness and may precede the development of an invasive malignancy by months to years—or may not progress to cancer within the individual's lifetime. More commonly, the preclinical phase goes undetected until invasive cancer, occasionally with regional or distant metastases, is already present. As is the case with other medical disorders, our understanding of the pathophysiology of neoplasia has been based on clinical and pathologic observations of large series of patients. More recently, cellular and molecular features of cancer cells have been described, and their relationships to certain neoplastic entities and clinical situations have extended our knowledge in this field.

1. What is the preclinical phase of cancer?
2. How many malignant cells must be present before overt signs of cancer are evident?

THE MOLECULAR & BIOCHEMICAL BASIS OF NEOPLASIA

The process of neoplasia is a result of stepwise alterations in cellular function. These phenotypic changes confer proliferative, invasive, and metastatic potential that are the hallmarks of cancer. It is generally believed—though not conclusively proved—that genetic alterations underlie all cellular and biochemical aberrations responsible for the malignant phenotype. An increasing number of genetic and cellular changes are being catalogued from the study of cancer cells—both in vivo, from primary tumors of patients, and in vitro, from established cancer cell lines grown in tissue culture. Some of these changes are specific to a certain tumor type or to a particular behavior, such as a high proliferative rate or metastatic potential. It can sometimes then be inferred—and subsequently proved experimentally—that a given genetic change directly or indirectly leads to a certain phenotype. Some genetic alterations can be observed across tumor types or at a high frequency. Others occur in combination with other aberrations, obscuring the exact role of these changes in producing the malignant phenotype.

3. What stepwise phenotypic changes are the hallmarks of cancer?

GENETIC CHANGES IN NEOPLASIA

Genetic changes in cancer can occur at random owing to the inherent genetic instability of malignant cells. Certain alterations, however, appear to produce or contribute to the malignant phenotype. These generally occur within the DNA base pair sequences that encode for a gene and can be broadly classified into two categories. Genes in which alterations result in a gain of function are referred to as **oncogenes,** whereas genes in which deletions or mutations result in loss of control functions are defined as **tumor suppressor genes.** Activation of oncogenes and loss of tumor suppressor genes can be shown to cause cancer by several laboratory methods, including in vitro cell culture and in vivo transgenic mouse models. Oncogene activation can occur as a result of a **point mutation, chromosomal translocation,** or **amplification** of genetic material. In some instances, an oncogene may be a transcribed unaltered gene that is normally silent or expressed only in regulated fashion during specific times, including embryogenesis and tissue repair. Alternatively, an oncogene can consist of a new **fusion gene** that is the result of a chromosomal translocation, and the corresponding **fusion protein** may exert a novel action that contributes to the malignant phenotype. Loss of tumor suppressor gene function can be the result of a **point mutation** or **frameshift mutation** or a **deletion,** either within the gene or over a large chromosomal segment that includes the tumor suppressor gene. In most instances, both tumor suppressor gene alleles must be inactivated, either by deletion or by mutation, to result in loss of function. There is increasing evidence that human neoplasia is the result of serial oncogene activation and tumor suppressor gene inactivation. For some tumor types, stereotypical oncogene and tumor suppressor gene alterations have been described, and the order in which the alterations occur.

Most genetic changes thus far described in human cancers are acquired somatic alterations seen only in the tumor cells of the affected individual. These changes can be produced by a variety of carcinogens or ionizing radiation. It is possible that some may arise without any inciting event, representing a net effect of DNA damage and natural repair processes. Populations of cells that normally exhibit a high growth fraction, such as hematopoietic and epithelial cells—or mesenchymal cells in growing children—may be particularly susceptible to genetic alterations introduced upon cellular division. In animals, many malignancies are the result of the activation or introduction of an oncogene by viral infection. In humans, however, few cancers are known to be directly caused by viral infection. One such virus, human T cell leukemia virus, is closely related to the human immunodeficiency virus and can cause a type of T cell leukemia due to proteins encoded by the viral genome which are able to activate latent human genes. Human papillomavirus has long been linked epidemiologically to cervical cancer, and the serotypes most often linked have recently been found to encode for proteins that can bind and inactivate host tumor suppressor gene products. In this situation, a causative gene is not necessarily introduced by the virus, but the viral genome is able to direct the inactivation of tumor suppressor gene products and thereby favor growth and proliferation as well as malignant potential. The ability of viruses to modulate the host cellular machinery—and in some cases retain altered mammalian genes that are oncogenic—is likely to have developed over the course of mammalian evolution, since an actively proliferating cell provides the optimal conditions for replication of virions and propagation of viral infections.

Inherited susceptibility to certain cancers has long been appreciated given the known increased risk of certain types of cancer if present in a family member. Certain tumors are passed on to progeny with high penetrance, suggesting that the genetic abnormality bears a strong causal relationship to the malignancy. Most of these rare familial malignancies are due to inherited allelic alterations of tumor suppressor genes, such that a somatic mutation or deletion in the remaining allele can then lead to expression of the malignant phenotype. Over recent years, tumor suppressor genes have been cloned and characterized through the study of families with malignancies such as retinoblastoma, neurofibromatosis (not itself a malignancy, but associated with a variety of tumors), and inherited colon or breast cancer. The same tumor suppressor genes can be involved in much more common nonheritable malignancies. In these cases, tumor suppression gene changes are somatic and are only seen in the primary tumor and not other host cells. Oncogenes, on the other hand, have not generally been found to be inherited. One exception is the familial syndrome of **multiple endocrine neoplasia type 2,** in which heterozygotes carrying an oncogene on chromosome 10 are at increased risk of developing two rare neural crest tumors: pheochromocytoma and medullary carcinoma of the thyroid.

ONCOGENES & TUMOR SUPPRESSOR GENES IN NORMAL PHYSIOLOGY & NEOPLASIA

The observation that cell-free tumor lysates could transform immortalized cells in tissue culture into cells with a more malignant phenotype has led to isolation of the responsible genetic elements. These proved to be genes that are homologous to normal human genes, termed **proto-oncogenes,** which encode for proteins responsible for a variety of physiologic cellular functions. In the altered form or in excessive amounts, however, proteins encoded by oncogenes possess deranged function that can confer proliferative or invasive properties on the cell. The functions of proteins encoded by known proto-oncogenes and their oncogene counterparts can be classified into surface membrane proteins, cytoplasmic proteins involved in signal transduction, and DNA-binding nuclear proteins that can modulate the expression of specific genes. By virtue of overexpression or activating mutation, surface membrane oncogene products can exhibit augmented or ligand-independent signal initiation compared with their physiologic counterparts. Cytoplasmic signaling modulator proteins can be similarly activated. Examples of this functional class are the ras family members, which are G proteins capable of being maintained in an active signal-transducing state when containing certain stereotypic mutations. Table 5–1 sets forth a partial list of oncogenes identified in human malignancies along with the tumor types in which they are commonly observed and the cellular function encoded by their proto-oncogene counterparts. Not surprisingly, these proteins are integral parts of the cellular machinery involved in growth, differentiation, and entry into the S phase of the cell cycle. Other cellular functions such as the inhibition of programmed cell death (apoptosis) have also been described. However, the disordered function of one or several of the individual components can be manifested as a malignant phenotype.

Tumor suppressor genes have been found to encode for proteins responsible for a variety of functions. These include regulatory proteins that regulate the cell cycle, adhesion proteins that govern cell-to-cell communication, and cytoplasmic proteins that modulate or attenuate signal transduction. Presumably, these functions are intended to keep the cell's proliferative and invasive potential in check. Since some cells need to proliferate, recruit vasculature, and invade tissue during embryogenesis, growth, and tissue repair, feedback mechanisms mediated by tumor suppressor gene products are presumably necessary physiologic controls. Table 5–2 presents a representative list of tumor suppressor genes, encoded functions, and tumor types in which somatic mutations or loss of function are common. Most of the tumor suppressor genes listed are also known to be involved in germline mutations that cause an inherited predisposition to one type or a spectrum of tumors. For example, the *p53* **gene** encodes for a nuclear phosphoprotein involved in the regulation of the cell cycle. Abnormalities in this gene are seen in a variety of tumor types and are thus among the most commonly observed genetic lesions in human malignancies. An inherited mutation in the *p53* gene can cause the rare Li-Fraumeni syndrome, characterized by the early development of soft tissue, bone, breast, and brain tumors.

A paradigm for sequential genetic alterations has been proposed as a necessary set of events leading to tumorigenesis. These include both gain of oncogenic function and loss of tumor suppressor function, occurring in series or in parallel. The largest body of evidence to support this theory has been generated from the molecular study of colon cancer and identifiable preneoplastic lesions, including adenomas and colonic polyps. In this model, the progressive development of neoplasia from premalignant to malignant to invasive lesions is associated with an increasing number of genetic abnormalities, including both oncogene activation and tumor suppressor gene inactivation. This theory is further supported by the identification of inherited abnormalities of several tumor suppressor genes, all associated with a strong familial tendency to develop colon cancer at a young age. Molecular techniques have been used to study many tumor types, and most abnormalities of oncogenes and tumor suppressor genes have been found in more than one tumor type, though certain aberrations tend to be common in certain tumor types as outlined in Table 5–1. In some cases, changes at the gene, messenger RNA, or protein level have also been found to correlate with certain clinical features, including clinical aggressiveness and survival. Given the pivotal

Table 5–1. Representative oncogenes identified in human neoplasia.[1]

Oncogene	Physiologic Function of Oncogene Product	Tumor Type
HER2/neu	Cell surface receptor	Breast, gastric, ovarian
PRAD1	Cyclin	Breast, esophageal, parathyroid adenoma
ras	G protein	Lung, colonic, pancreatic
myc	Transcription factor	Multiple tumor types
fos	Transcription factor	Multiple tumor types
int-2	Morphogen	Esophageal, gastric, head and neck
RET	Tyrosine kinase	Pheochromocytoma, medullary carcinoma of the thyroid (MEN type 2)
myb	Transcription factor	Leukemia
fes	Tyrosine kinase	Leukemia

[1]Oncogenic fusion genes are listed in Table 5–8.

Table 5–2. Representative tumor suppressor genes identified in human neoplasia.

Tumor Suppressor Gene	Chromosomal Location	Physiologic Function of Oncogene Product	Tumor Type
p53	17p13	Cell cycle regulator	Several
Retinoblastoma (Rb)	13q14	Cell cycle regulator	Retinoblastoma, small cell lung cancer, sarcoma
NF-1	17q11	GTPase activating protein	Sarcoma, glioma
NF-2	22q12	Membrane-cytoskeleton interface	Schwannoma
VHL	3p25	Surface receptor or cell adhesion	Hemangioblastoma, kidney, pheochromocytoma
WT-1	11p13	Transcription factor	Wilms' tumor
DCC	18q21	Cell adhesion	Colon
APC	5q21	Membrane/cell adhesion	Colon
MCC	5q21	Unknown, ? G protein	Colon
hMSH2	2p16	DNA repair	Colon
hMLH1	3p21	DNA repair	Colon
nm23	17q21	Nucleoside kinase	Colon, breast, others
BRCA1	17q21	DNA repair	Breast, ovarian
BRCA2	13q	Unknown	Breast (male and female)

role of oncogenes and tumor suppressor genes in human cancer, their targeting for diagnostic and therapeutic modalities is an area of active research.

HORMONES, GROWTH FACTORS, & GROWTH INHIBITORS

Specialized proteins are required for the normal growth, maturation, development, and function of cells and specialized tissue. The complexity of the human organism requires that these proteins be expressed at precisely coordinated points in space and time. An essential component of this regulation is the system of hormones, growth factors, and growth inhibitors, hereinafter referred to collectively as "factors." These proteins, upon binding to specific receptor proteins on the cell surface or in the cytoplasm, lead to a complex set of signals that can result in a variety of cellular effects, including mitogenesis, growth inhibition, changes in cell cycle regulation, apoptosis, differentiation, and the induction of a secondary set of genes. The actual end effects are not only dependent on the particular type of interacting factor and receptor but also on the cell type and milieu in which factor-receptor coupling occurs. This system allows for cell-to-cell interactions, whereby a factor secreted by one cell or tissue can enter the bloodstream and influence another set of distant cells (endocrine action) or act on adjacent cells (paracrine action). An autocrine action is also possible when a cell produces a factor that binds to a receptor on or in the same cell. Altered factor concentration as well as receptor mutations or overexpression can also change the signaling end effect, contributing to a malignant phenotype. Some growth factor receptors have actually been found to be the products of genes originally identified as transforming oncogenes. An example of this is the HER2/neu oncogene, which encodes for a receptor homologous to the epidermal growth factor receptor. It appears to be important in early neural and cardiac development. Artificial overexpression of this receptor can reproduce a malignant phenotype in laboratory models, including breast cancer in transgenic mice. The HER2/neu oncogene is amplified and overexpressed in human breast, ovarian, and gastric cancers, and in some of these cancer cell lines, inhibition of its function by specific antibodies can partially inhibit cell proliferation.

Other factor systems known to have physiologic effects can also be expressed aberrantly in some human malignancies. Insulin, for example, exerts well-known metabolic effects upon binding to the insulin receptor. Overexpression of the receptor can also lead to insulin-dependent malignant transformation in transfected cell lines, yet the overexpression of the insulin receptor seen in some breast cancers is of unclear significance. Therefore, gene amplification or other transcriptional regulatory mechanisms that allow for the overexpression or enhanced function of growth factor receptors can provide a growth advantage to cells. It is plausible that these changes are favored in the clonal evolution of a tumor. Some growth factor-mediated actions are not necessarily mitogenic—such as the fibroblast growth factor system, which can induce angiogenesis. This is another example of a controlled physiologic activity that can help support tumor growth when it is aberrantly controlled.

Naturally occurring growth inhibitors such as **transforming growth factor β (TGFβ)** may also be physiologic mediators of growth suppression in situations such as embryonic development and tissue repair. Although not directly implicated in tumorigenesis, it is possible that cell responsiveness to these inhibitors may be altered in cancer.

Steroid hormones and their cytoplasmic receptors constitute separate signaling pathways that mediate normal growth, development, and metabolism and are also known to interact with other factor systems. The expression of **estrogen receptors** on certain breast tumors can predict a greater likelihood of response to hormonal therapies, and the determination of their presence is therefore useful in clinical management.

Other functional membrane proteins not related to growth can also be present on tumors cells. The MDR-1 gene product belongs to a class of ATP-dependent channel transporter proteins and is present on some normal epithelial cells. Its physiologic role may be to pump toxic molecules out of the cell, but in some tumor cells its overexpression causes efflux of certain chemotherapeutic agents, leading to drug resistance. In some situations, its expression can be induced by long-term exposure to chemotherapy.

STROMAL, ADHESIVE, & PROTEOLYTIC PROTEINS

Several structural proteins such as actin, which is involved in scaffolding and movement, are known to be associated with signaling surface proteins. Adhesive proteins, most notably a class known as the **integrins,** are also felt to be involved in signaling to the nucleus. It is also likely that these interactions are altered in malignancy. Stromal proteins that constitute extracellular matrix, including basement membrane, are necessary for normal cell anchorage and separation of epithelial layers. Highly regulated proteolytic enzymes normally coordinate tissue remodeling at times of development, physical stress, or damage. In neoplasia, abnormal cell growth is also accompanied by cell invasion and the establishment of metastatic colonies. The invasive phenotype is therefore due in part to abnormalities of stromal proteins and disruption of the basement membrane. There is now evidence that these alterations can be directed by malignant tumor cells through elaboration of soluble factors that cause the synthesis and release of proteolytic enzymes by surrounding stroma. Likewise, tumor cells may be able to recruit other activities, such as angiogenesis, necessary to form a growing metastatic focus.

CELLULAR CHANGES IN NEOPLASIA

Functional and morphologic changes accompany molecular and biochemical changes in malignancy at both the cellular and tissue levels. These abnormalities may exist in a spectrum from normal to preinvasive to frankly malignant and invasive cells. Tissue architecture is also disrupted by the abnormal growth and invasive capacity of malignant cells. This disruption results in violation of the normal microanatomy at the site of origin of the tumor and at the sites of distant metastases. At both sites, the tumor cells not only possess the capacity to proliferate abnormally but also to break tissue boundaries such as the basement membrane in the case of epithelial malignancies.

Molecular and cellular changes in tumor cells are, in a sense, a modification of normal physiology that benefits their growth and spread. The initial alterations may be "preprogrammed" in rare inherited malignancies, or they may be acquired as a consequence of mutations brought about by environmental exposure or occurring by chance during normal cell division. In a process akin to evolution, albeit in a fast time frame, additional genetic changes occur that favor further growth, invasion, and spread. Evasion of the host's immune system, enhanced proliferative and invasive potential, and resistance to therapy are examples of early, middle, and late changes in the progression of neoplasia.

4. What is an oncogene?
5. What is a tumor suppressor gene?
6. What are the genetic mechanisms by which oncogenes can be activated or tumor suppressor genes inactivated?
7. Which is the more common mechanism of oncogene activation in humans, viral infection or somatic alteration?
8. What is a potential molecular explanation for the epidemiologic correlation of human papilloma virus infection with cervical cancer?
9. What is the molecular basis for most inherited susceptibilities to certain cancers?
10. Name some factors which support or inhibit tumor growth, although not directly implicated in tumorigenesis.
11. What is the role of proteolytic enzymes in metastasis?
12. Give some examples of early, middle, and late changes in the progression of neoplasia.

PATHOPHYSIOLOGY OF NEOPLASIA

The common property of all neoplasia is uncontrolled growth and invasion. From both the clinical and the pathophysiologic standpoints, the tissue type from which the malignant cells originate is also associated with certain unique characteristics. This uniqueness is due to underlying normal architecture and machinery possessed by the cells and tissue from which the tumor originates. Three general classifications of neoplasia have been chosen in this chapter to highlight the pathophysiology of all types of neoplasia: (1) epithelial neoplasia; (2) mesenchymal, neuroendocrine, and germ cell neoplasia; and (3) hematologic neoplasia. The malignant potential of these cells is related to the proliferative rate and perhaps to exposure to environmental, dietary, and endogenous hormonal or growth factor stimuli. In the growing infant and child, mesenchymal tumors from growing muscle, cartilage, and bone are common, whereas in adults tumors arising from epithelial elements in the colon, lung, breast, and prostate predominate.

EPITHELIAL NEOPLASIA

Epithelial cells are in constant turnover, arising from a basal layer that continually generates new cells. The mature and functional layer of cells performs specialized tissue or organ functions, and with senescence it is eventually sloughed off. Proliferating epithelial cells normally observe anatomic boundaries such as the basement membrane that underlies the basal layer of cells in the epithelium. The potential to divide, migrate, and differentiate is tightly controlled. The stimulus to divide may be autonomous or exogenous as a response to factors from adjacent or distant cells. Inhibitory signals and factors may also be present and serve to function as negative regulators to check uncontrolled growth. The neoplastic phenotype of epithelial cells can be seen as a spectrum from **hyperplastic** to **preinvasive** to frankly **invasive and metastatic** neoplasia as illustrated in Figure 5–1. By convention, malignancies of epithelial origin are termed **carcinomas.** Hyperplasia can be a normal physiologic response in some situations, such as that which occurs in the lining of the uterus in response to estrogens prior to the ovulatory phase of the menstrual cycle. It may also be a patho-

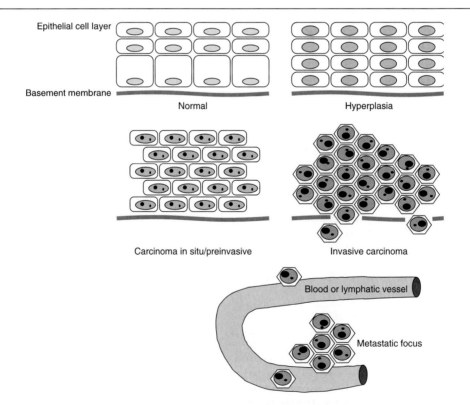

Figure 5–1. Schematic depiction of phenotypic transition of epithelial cells from hyperplasia to invasive carcinoma.

logic finding and associated with a predisposition to progress to invasive carcinoma. In such instances of hyperplasia, there are usually accompanying disorders of maturation that may be recognizable by microscopic examination. These changes are termed **dysplasia, atypical hyperplasia,** or **metaplasia** depending on the type of epithelium in which they are observed. More aggressive proliferation without the ability to invade though the basement membrane is termed **preinvasive carcinoma,** or **carcinoma in situ.** Technically, these cells do not have the capacity to metastasize, though they may progress to invasive carcinoma over time. The term **invasive carcinoma** implies that tissue boundaries, especially the basement membrane, have been breached. **Metastatic carcinoma** occurs via the lymphatic system to regional lymph nodes and via the bloodstream to distant organs and other tissues. This pattern of metastasis, however, is not unique to epithelial malignancies. Epithelial neoplasms in general have a variable propensity to spread to regional nodes and distant sites. It is assumed that the natural history of most tumors is to follow this pattern of spread over time. The specific genotypic and phenotypic changes necessary to accomplish this spread are not well understood; they may in some cases be shared across tumor types, and in other cases they are unique to a given neoplasia. Certain molecular characteristics have been linked to clinical characteristics, though the exact mode of action is not fully understood.

From a pathophysiologic standpoint, certain structural and functional characteristics must be acquired by malignant cells as outlined in Table 5–3. An increase in growth rate through several mechanisms has been described for different tumor types. It is known that the proliferative fraction (the percentage of cells in S phase, or actively synthesizing DNA) is elevated—and more so in histologically and clinically aggressive tumors. Changes in the tightly regulated cell cycle machinery have been observed, including abnormal levels of **cyclins** and other proteins that regulate cyclin-dependent kinases responsible for entry of the cell into S phase. Likewise, alterations of intermediate signaling proteins have been noted that couple external growth factor and hormonal stimuli to proliferation. The ability of cells to migrate and pass through cellular and extracellular matrix barriers can be enhanced in tumor cells. This can occur through the activation of proteolytic enzyme cascades from within the tumor cell or by the action of stromal cells that are directed to do so as a result of factors produced by nearby tumor cells. Through similar mechanisms, malignant cells can induce the formation of a microvasculature that is essential to support the continued growth of a tumor colony. Other functions necessary to breach the immune defenses and survive destruction by antitumor drugs can be mediated by the genetic program already possessed in latent form by tumor cells. Examples include modulation of antigens and alterations in drug metabolism or metabolic pathways that are targeted by certain drugs.

As described earlier, there is evidence that discrete phenotypic changes which arise from specific genetic alterations account for the progression from hyperplasia to metastatic neoplasia. Moreover, there is an interplay between these genetic changes and the inherent program of gene expression of a given epithelial type. This creates a specific spectrum of anatomic, pathophysiologic, and clinical entities for neoplasia of each epithelial type as listed in Table 5–4. Other highly regulated functions of epithelial cells include active or passive transport of ions or molecules as well as the synthesis and secretion of specific proteins. These functions may also be lost, altered, or even enhanced for specific tumor types and likewise can create specific pathophysiologic and clinical entities. Two epithelial neoplasms are discussed in further detail. Colon cancer is an example of an epithelial neoplasm for which precursor lesions have been well studied because we can seek out and biopsy such lesions by colonoscopy. Breast epithelial tissue is responsive to steroid hormones and growth factors that may play a role in the development and behavior of breast cancer.

Table 5–3. Phenotypic changes in the progression of neoplasia.

1. Enhanced proliferation
   Autonomous growth
   Abnormalities of cell cycle control
   Exaggerated response to hormonal or growth factor stimuli
   Lack of response to growth inhibitors or cell contact inhibition
2. Evasion of immune system
   Antigen modulation and masking
   Elaboration of immune response antagonistic molecules
3. Invasion of tissue and stroma
   Attachment to extracellular matrix
   Secretion of proteolytic enzymes
   Recruitment of stromal cells to produce proteolytic enzymes
   Loss of cell cohesion
4. Ability to gain access to and egress from lymphatics and bloodstream
   Enhanced cell motility
   Recognition of endothelial protein sequences
   Cytoskeletal modifications
5. Establishment of metastatic foci
   Cell adhesion and attachment
   Tissue-specific tropism
6. Ability to recruit vascularization to support growth of primary or metastatic tumor
7. Drug resistance
   Altered drug metabolism and drug inactivation
   Increased synthesis of targeted enzymes
   Enhanced drug efflux
   Enhanced DNA damage repair

13. What factors determine the malignant potential of epithelial vs mesenchymal tumors?
14. What is the term applied to malignancies of epithelial origin?
15. What is the spectrum of characteristics of the neoplastic phenotype in epithelial cells?

1. COLON CARCINOMA

The model of stepwise genetic alterations in cancer is best illustrated by observations made in colonic lesions representing different stages of progression to malignancy. Certain genetic alterations are found commonly in early-stage adenomas, whereas others tend to occur with significant frequency only after the development of invasive carcinoma. These changes are in keeping with the concept that serial phenotypic changes must occur in a cell for it to exhibit full malignant (invasive and metastatic) properties (Table 5–3). One early alteration seen in adenomas is a point mutation in the *ras* gene that results in enhanced cytoplasmic signaling. The end result of this mutation is not known, but it appears to be associated with a more rapid cell division rate. A later genetic abnormality is the loss of part or all of the *DCC* gene, which encodes for an adhesive protein. This may contribute to the loss of cell cohesion and the tendency to metastasize, an expected phenotypic change late in the neoplastic pathway.

Two principal lines of evidence support the model of stepwise genetic alterations in colon cancer:

Table 5–4. Epithelial neoplasia.

Epithelial Type	Hyperplasia or Dysplasia	Preinvasive	Invasive
Head and neck	Leukoplakia, erythroplakia (these lesions may contain dysplasia or carcinoma in situ)		Squamous cell carcinoma
Lung	Squamous metaplasia	Carcinoma in situ	Non-small cell carcinoma (squamous cell or adenocarcinoma)
Esophagus	Barrett's esophagus, chronic scarring	Carcinoma in situ	Squamous cell or adenocarcinoma
Stomach	Gastric ulcer, ?*Helicobacter pylori* infection	Carcinoma in situ	Adenocarcinoma
Colon	Adenomatous polyp	Carcinoma in situ (may be within polyp)	Adenocarcinoma
Liver and biliary tree	Hepatonodular liver regeneration, cirrhosis, biliary inflammation	Carcinoma in situ (biliary tree and gallbladder)	Adenocarcinoma
Exocrine pancreas	Chronic pancreatitis	Not seen clinically	Adenocarcinoma
Anus	Condyloma (anogenital warts)	Carcinoma in situ	Squamous cell or cuboidal (cloacogenic) carcinoma
Cervix	Dysplasia (cervical intraepithelial neoplasia grades I and II)	Carcinoma in situ (cervical intraepithelial neoplasia grade III)	Squamous carcinoma (rarely adenocarcinoma)
Uterus	Hyperplasia	Carcinoma in situ	Adenocarcinoma
Ovary	Preneoplastic ovary; epithelial lesions not seen clinically		Adenocarcinoma
Breast	Atypical hyperplasia	Ductal or lobular carcinoma in situ	Infiltrating ductal or lobular adenocarcinoma
Bladder and ureter	Hyperplasia, atypical hyperplasia and dysplasia	Carcinoma in situ	Squamous cell, transitional cell, or adenocarcinoma
Kidney	Papillary hyperplasia	Not seen clinically	Adenocarcinoma
Prostate	Prostatic hyperplasia	Not seen clinically	Adenocarcinoma
Skin	Many clinical entities, including actinic keratosis, acanthoma, cutaneous horn, and Bowen's disease	Carcinoma in situ	Basal cell and squamous cell carcinoma

(1) The rare familial syndromes associated with predisposition to colon cancer at an early age are now known to result from germline mutations. **Familial adenomatous polyposis** is the result of a mutation in the *APC* gene. In the tumors that subsequently develop, the remaining allele has been lost. Similarly, **hereditary nonpolyposis colorectal cancer** is associated with germline mutations in DNA repair genes such as *hMSH2* and *hMLH1*. These genes can also be affected in sporadic cancers.

(2) The carcinogenic effects of factors known to be linked to an increased risk of developing colon cancer constitute the second line of evidence for a genetic basis for colon cancer. Substances derived from bacterial colonic flora, ingested foods, or endogenous metabolites such as fecapentaenes, 3-ketosteroids, and benzo[α]pyrenes are mutagenic. Levels of these substances can be reduced by low-fat and high-fiber diets, and several epidemiologic studies confirm that such diets reduce the risk of colon cancer. Furthermore, since the risk of sporadic colon cancer in older individuals is mildly elevated in the presence of a positive family history, there may be other inherited genetic abnormalities that interact with environmental factors to cause colon cancer. The sequence of genetic changes may not need to be exact to lead to the development of an invasive cancer, though there is mounting evidence that some genetic lesions tend to develop early whereas others may develop late in the course of the natural disease. At present, all phenotypic changes cannot be explained by a known genetic abnormality, nor do all identified genetic alterations have a known phenotypic result.

The earliest change in the progression to colon cancer is the increase in cell number (hyperplasia) on the epithelial (luminal) surface. This produces an **adenoma,** which is characterized by gland-forming cells exhibiting increases in size and cell number but no invasion of surrounding structures (Figure 5–2). Presumably, these changes are due to enhanced proliferation and loss of cell cycle control but prior to acquisition of the capacity to invade extracellular matrix. Additional dysplastic changes such as loss of mucin production and altered cell polarity may be present to a variable degree. Some adenomas may progress to carcinoma in situ and ultimately to invasive carcinoma. An early feature associated with disrupted architecture even before invasion occurs is the development of fragile new vessels or destruction of existing vessels that can cause microscopic bleeding. This can be tested for clinically as a fecal occult blood determination used for screening and early diagnosis of preinvasive and invasive colon cancer. It is not known if all invasive colon cancers pass through a hyperplastic or preinvasive stage, nor is this information available for epithelial malignancies in general.

Further functional changes in the cell and surrounding tissue are also manifested in the preinvasive and invasive stage. Once the basement membrane is penetrated by invasive malignant cells, access can be gained to the regional lymphatics and spread to regional pericolic lymph nodes can occur. Entry of cells into the bloodstream can lead to distant spread in a pattern that reflects venous drainage. Therefore, hematogenous spread from primary colon tumors to the liver is common, whereas rectal tumors usually disseminate to liver, lung, and bone. In addition to anatomic considerations, there may exist specific tropism of malignant cells mediated by surface proteins that cause the cells to preferentially home in on certain organs or sites.

Colonic epithelium is specialized to secrete digestive enzymes and mucus proteins and to absorb specific nutrients (Chapter 9). The maintenance of a tight luminal barrier, intracellular charge differences, and the ability to exclude toxins are additional specialized functions. Some of these functions are maintained in the progression to neoplasia and may contribute to a specific phenotype of the malignant cell. One example is the expression of a transporter membrane protein, MDR-1, present on several types of epithelium including the colon. MDR-1 is known to cause efflux of several compounds out of the cells, presumably as a protective mechanism to exclude toxins. In advanced colon cancer, this protein may contribute to the relative resistance of this and other tumor types to a variety of chemotherapeutic agents

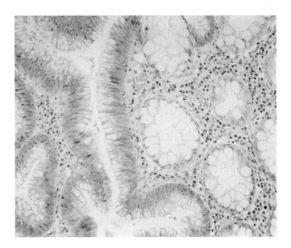

Figure 5–2. Edge of an adenomatous polyp, showing adenomatous change (left), compared with normal mucosal glands (right). Adenomatous change is characterized by increased size and stratification of nuclei and loss of cytoplasmic mucin. Note arrangement of nuclei of the adenoma perpendicular to the basement membrane (polarity). (Reproduced, with permission, from Chandrasoma P, Taylor CE: *Concise Pathology,* 3rd ed. Appleton & Lange, 1998.)

that are transported by MDR-1. In some cases, the activation of a latent gene encoding **carcinoembryonic antigen** (CEA) can result in measurable levels of the CEA protein in the serum of patients with localized or metastatic colon cancer as well as other adenocarcinomas.

> 16. What are the two principal lines of evidence in favor of the model of stepwise genetic alterations in colon cancer?
> 17. What is an explanation for the frequent appearance of occult blood in stools of patients with even early colon carcinoma?
> 18. What are two genes whose products contribute to the classic phenotype of colon carcinomas?

2. BREAST CARCINOMA

The female breast is a specialized gland that develops after puberty out of rudimentary ducts emanating from the nipples. Acinar cells and the terminal ductule they surround comprise the lobular unit from which most breast carcinomas arise. Breast tissue also responds to menstrual cycling of estrogen and progesterone, but both epithelial and stromal cells are also under the control of a variety of growth factors, including insulin-like growth factor-1 (IGF-1) and TGFβ. **Hypertrophy** of breast epithelial cells in response to the preovulatory estrogen surge and **hyperplasia** during pregnancy are examples of physiologic responses. Early stages of disordered growth through loss of cell cycle control or abnormalities in hormonal or growth factor response can result in benign proliferative changes such as adenosis or apocrine metaplasia. These changes by themselves are not necessarily associated with an increased risk of the subsequent development of breast cancer. Breast epithelial hyperplasia in the absence of pregnancy, however, is associated with an increased risk of carcinoma, especially if cell atypia is present.

Factors associated with an increased risk of breast cancer development may provide clues to early driving forces. Prolonged usage of high doses of exogenous estrogen is a risk factor that implicates some excessive mitogenic stimulus. Increased risk with a positive family history of breast cancer, as with other cancers, is evidence that inherited genes may on their own—or in concert with environmental factors—represent key steps toward breast neoplasia.

About 5–10% of breast cancer cases appear to be associated with an inherited predisposition. Familial clustering has long been noted in certain kindreds, and this led to the chromosomal localization of putative breast cancer susceptibility genes. This process is termed **linkage analysis,** whereby the characteristic of developing breast cancer can be shown to segregate with certain markers of known chromosomal location. The identification of two discrete genes, *BRCA1* and *BRCA2,* then followed through the use of **positional cloning,** a term that collectively describes a variety of strategies to pinpoint a gene over a large segment of the genome without knowledge of the gene's function but the presumption that mutations in this gene should be seen in susceptible individuals (eg, women with breast cancer in families with breast cancer clustering). Inherited mutations in the *BRCA1* and *BRCA2* genes appear to be associated with an up to 80% likelihood of developing breast cancer over a lifetime. *BRCA1* mutations also are associated with a predisposition for ovarian cancer, while *BRCA2* mutations lead to breast cancer in male carriers as well. Both of these genes probably function as tumor suppressor genes such that breast tumors contain both the inherited abnormality in one allele as well as a somatic loss of the remaining allele. While sporadic (nonfamilial) cases of breast cancer rarely contain *BRCA1* mutations, there may be abnormalities in other proteins that interact with BRCA1 to perform what appears to be a DNA repair function. It is likely that other inherited genetic abnormalities will be identified that confer an increased risk of breast cancer. Generally speaking, it will be more difficult to identify those that have only modest **penetrance** (ie, confer only a slight increase in breast cancer risk). The clinical usefulness of genetic testing for breast cancer risk remains undefined while information regarding the interventions and outcomes following such testing is being gathered.

The scheme depicted in Figure 5–1 applies to progressive changes toward invasive breast carcinoma, and this full spectrum may be seen in patients who undergo biopsy to evaluate breast masses or mammographic abnormalities. Carcinoma in situ of the breast represents a preinvasive lesion in which enhanced proliferation and malignant cell morphology are observed but no invasion of the basement membrane can be demonstrated. Therefore, lymph nodal or distant metastases cannot occur at this stage, presumably because the invasive phenotype has not yet been acquired. Certain molecular abnormalities can be seen at this stage, including *HER2/neu* oncogene overexpression and *p53* tumor suppressor gene mutations, though the mechanisms through which these abnormalities operate are not well understood.

The pathophysiology of breast cancer illustrates how stromal cells can be recruited to propagate tumor growth and invasion. A dense reaction of fibroblasts and extracellular matrix by breast tumors **(desmoplastic response)** can occasionally be seen. Soluble factors suspected of mediating this response include **TGFβ** and **platelet-derived growth factor (PGDF),** which are known to be secreted by breast tumors cells or nearby stromal cells in response to tumor cells. The desmoplastic response may be a mechanism to wall off the tumor or, conversely, may actually facilitate growth and cell migration. Stromal cell production of the metalloprotease **stromolysin 3** is elicited by uncharacterized soluble factors produced by breast tumor cells. Stromolysin 3 may be pivotal in allowing tumor cells to penetrate the basement membrane or blood and lymphatic vessels. Angiogenic factors such as fibroblast growth factor can also be produced by tumor or stromal cells and promote the formation of the new microvasculature that is necessary to support a growing tumor colony in the breast or at a site of metastasis.

The overexpression of HER2/neu, a growth factor receptor oncogene product, is associated with a higher growth rate and more aggressive clinical behavior. This suggests that in excessive amounts HER2/neu as a growth factor receptor turns on the cell division machinery in an exaggerated fashion. This may occur in response to its natural ligand or independently of any outside stimulus. Loss of expression of ***nm23,*** which encodes for a nucleoside kinase, has been linked to an increased likelihood of lymph node metastases as well as a lower survival rate. This putative tumor suppressor gene may therefore behave as an "antimetastasis gene" such that loss of its function could lead to increased potential for invasion and metastasis, though its mode of function remains unknown. The spread of tumor cells past the basement membrane to regional lymph nodes and to distant organs is therefore the result of several discrete changes in cellular function. The tendency for breast cancer to metastasize to certain organs such as bone, lung, and liver may be a result of cell surface recognition proteins on both tumor cells and target tissue cells. The **integrins** are a class of widely expressed adhesion and recognition proteins that may be altered in malignancy and may mediate invasion and distant metastases. Furthermore, the ability of a metastatic focus to continue to grow to a clinically significant size requires additional phenotypic changes, which may explain the clinical variability in the course of advanced cancer between tumor types and from patient to patient.

MESENCHYMAL, NEUROENDOCRINE, & GERM CELL NEOPLASIA

The pathophysiology of certain types of neoplasia can be described in terms of the embryonic tissue of origin. Table 5–5 is a representative list of mesenchymal, neuroendocrine, and germ cell tumors and the embryologic cell groups from which they arise. Owing to the extensive migration and convolution of embryonic cell layers during early development, these tumor types may not evolve in specific anatomic sites. Mesenchymal, neuroendocrine, and germ cell neoplasms account for a large proportion of the tumors of childhood and young adulthood, ostensibly because these cells are actively dividing and more

Table 5–5. Neoplasia of mesenchymal, neuroendocrine, and germ cells.

Neoplasia Type	Embryonic Derivation
Wilms' tumor	Metanephric blastema
Neuroblastoma Retinoblastoma Ganglioneuroma	Neuroblasts

Neuroendocrine tumors
  Small cell carcinoma
  Ewing's sarcoma
  Primitive neuroectodermal tumor
  Malignant melanoma
  Pheochromocytoma
  Carcinoid
  Gastrointestinal endocrine tumors
    Insulinoma
    Glucagonoma
    Somatostatinoma
    Gastrinoma
    VIPoma,
    GRFoma
  Pituitary tumors
	Neural crest

Intracranial brain tumors
  Glioblastoma/astrocytoma
  Ependymoma, oligodendroglioma, medulloblastoma
	Glial precursors

Germ cell tumors
  Teratoma (benign)
  Germinoma, dysgerminoma
  Testicular, extragonadal germ cell tumors
  Seminoma
  Choriocarcinoma
  Embryonal carcinoma
  Endodermal sinus, yolk sac tumors
  Ovarian germ cell tumors
	Germ cell

Sarcomas
  Rhabdomyosarcoma
  Leiomyosarcoma
  Liposarcoma
  Osteosarcoma
  Chondrosarcoma
  Malignant fibrous histiocytoma
  Synovial sarcoma
  Lymphangiosarcoma
  Hemangiosarcoma
  Kaposi's sarcoma
	Mesenchymal cell
	  Striated muscle
	  Smooth muscle
	  Adipocyte
	  Osteoblast
	  Chondrocyte
	  Fibroblast
	
	  Synovial cell
	  Lymphatic endothelium
	  Blood vessel endothelium
	  Endothelial cell + fibroblasts?

Hepatoblastoma	Mesenchymal cell + hepatocytes
Mesothelioma	Mesothelial cell
Schwannoma	Peripheral nerve sheath
Meningioma	Arachnoidal fibroblast

subject to mutational events. These tumor cells may produce specific proteins or appear morphologically similar to normal cells that derive from the same germ layer. Alternatively, they may exhibit no differentiated features at all or may maintain the ability to differentiate in an array of different directions.

1. CARCINOID TUMORS

Carcinoid tumors arise from neural crest tissue and, more specifically, from enterochromaffin cells, whose final resting place after embryonic migration is along the submucosal layer of the intestines and pulmonary bronchi. Reflecting this embryonic origin, carcinoid cells express the necessary enzymes to produce bioactive amines such as **5-hydroxytryptamine** and other vasoactive serotonin metabolites as well as a variety of small peptide hormones. Cytoplasmic granules typical of neuroendocrine cells are also commonly seen. These features may also be shared by other tumors of neural crest origin. In contrast to epithelial neoplasms, morphologic changes observed with the light microscope do not distinguish between malignant and benign cells. The anatomic distribution of primary carcinoid tumors is consistent with embryonic development patterns as listed in Table 5–6. Carcinoid tumors and other mesenchymal neoplasms have similar patterns of tissue invasion followed by local and distant spread to regional lymph nodes and distant organs. The characteristics of increased mitotic count (an indicator of rapid proliferation), nuclear pleomorphism, lymphatic and vascular invasion, and an undifferentiated growth pattern are associated with a higher rate of metastases and a less favorable clinical prognosis.

A frequent site of carcinoid metastasis is the liver. In this setting, especially with midgut carcinoid, there can be a constellation of symptoms (**carcinoid syndrome**) as a consequence of substances secreted into the blood (Table 5–7). These substances reflect the neuroendocrine origin of carcinoid and the latent machinery that can be activated inappropriately in the malignant state. Many of these peptides are vasoactive and can cause intermittent flushing as a result of vasodilation. Other symptoms often observed include secretory diarrhea, wheezing, and excessive salivation or lacrimation. Long-term tissue damage can also occur by exposure to these substances and their metabolites. Fibrosis of the pulmonary and tricuspid heart valves, mesenteric fibrosis, and hyperkeratosis of the skin have all been reported in patients with carcinoid syndrome. A urinary marker commonly used to aid in the diagnosis or to follow patients being treated is a metabolite of serotonin, **5-hydroxyindoleacetic acid (5-HIAA)**, since the production of serotonin is also characteristic of carcinoid and other neuroendocrine tumors that are able to take up and decarboxylate amine precursors.

Table 5–7. Peptides secreted by carcinoid cells.

Adrenocorticotropic hormone (ACTH)
Calcitonin
Gastrin
Glicentin
Glucagon
Growth hormone
Insulin
Melanocyte-stimulating hormone (β-MSH)
Motilin
Neuropeptide K
Neurotensin
Somatostatin
Pancreatic polypeptide
Substance K
Substance P
Vasoactive intestinal peptide

---

19. What are some of the hormones and growth factors to which breast tissue responds?
20. What are some factors associated with increased risk of breast cancer?
21. How do stromal cells contribute to the propagation of breast cancer growth?
22. To what tissues do breast cancers tend to metastasize and why?
23. What products produced by carcinoid tumors reflect their embryonic origin?
24. What are some common short-term symptoms and long-term complications precipitated by release of excessive amounts of these products?

2. TESTICULAR CANCER

Testicular cancer arises chiefly from germinal elements within the testes. Germ cells are the population of cells that give rise to spermatozoa through meiotic division and can therefore theoretically retain the ability to differentiate into any cell type. Some testicular neoplasms arise from remnant tissue outside the

Table 5–6. Carcinoid tumor location by site of embryonic origin.

Foregut	Midgut	Hindgut
Esophagus	Jejunum	Rectum
Stomach	Ileum	
Duodenum	Appendix	
Pancreas	Colon	
Gallbladder and bile duct	Liver	
Ampulla of Vater	Ovary	
Larynx	Testes	
Bronchus	Cervix	
Thymus		

testes owing to the midline migration of germline epithelium that occurs during early embryogenesis. This is followed by the formation of the urogenital ridge and eventually by the aggregation of germline cells in the ovary or testes. As predicted by this pattern of migration, extragonadal testicular neoplasms are found in the midline axis of the lower cranium, mediastinum, or retroperitoneum. The pluripotent ability of the germ cell—ie, the ability of one cell to give rise to an entire organism—is most evident in benign germ cell tumors such as **mature teratomas.** These tumors often contain differentiated elements from all three germ cell layers, including teeth and hair in lesions termed **dermoid cysts.** Malignant teratomas can also exist as a spectrum bridging other germ cell layer-derived neoplasms such as sarcomas and epithelium-derived carcinomas. Malignant testicular cancers may coexist with benign mature teratomas, and the benign component sometimes becomes apparent only after the malignancy has been eradicated with chemotherapy.

Proteins expressed during embryonic or trophoblastic development such as alpha-fetoprotein and human chorionic gonadotropin can be secreted and measured in the serum. Testicular carcinoma follows a lymphatic and hematogenous pattern of spread to regional retroperitoneal nodes and distant organs such as lung, liver, bone, and brain. The exquisite sensitivity of even advanced testicular cancers to radiation and chemotherapy may be a result of the foreign nature of malignant germ cells when present in a mature organism. This foreign nature may create more specific activity of cytotoxic insults and stimulate a more vigorous immune rejection of tumor.

> 25. From what cellular elements of the testes does testicular cancer generally arise?
> 26. What are some characteristic markers that may be followed in testicular tumor progression?

3. SARCOMAS

The sarcomas consist of a family of mesenchymal neoplasms whose morphologic appearance and anatomic distribution mirror the early mesenchymal elements from which they derive (Table 5–5). They arise in structures composed of the mesenchymal cell type or in locations where remnant cells eventually come to rest in the path of early tissue migration. Several of the less mature sarcomas that resemble more primitive cells are seen in children, since this compartment of cells is usually dividing more rapidly. These sarcomas include **rhabdomyosarcoma** and **osteosarcoma,** which are less common in adults. The morphologic appearance of sarcomas does not involve perceptible architectural changes, since cell polarity and gland formation do not occur in normal mature mesenchymal cells such as muscle or cartilage. Nuclear pleomorphism and mitotic rate determine the grade of a tumor, with higher grade correlating with a higher propensity to invade local and distant structures and a poorer survival. Sarcomas also have a tendency to retain the cell appearance and repertoire of expressed proteins of the cell of origin. Bone matrix of calcium and phosphorus can form within osteosarcomas, and calcification of these tumors can be observed on radiography. There is less of a propensity for direct tissue invasion by sarcomas than by epithelial malignancies. However, tissue destruction can result when a sarcoma compresses but does not invade adjacent tissue, leading to the formation of a **pseudocapsule.** Sarcomas exhibit metastatic dissemination to regional lymph nodes and distant organs, especially the lungs. High-grade histologic features and anatomic location are factors influencing the likelihood and timing of metastases.

Various genetic abnormalities have been detected in sarcomas. Mutations in the ***p53* tumor suppressor gene** are the most commonly detected lesion, though such changes are also seen in epithelial neoplasms. The ***NF-1* tumor suppressor gene** was originally identified through a germline mutation of this gene in patients with type 1 neurofibromatosis. This inherited syndrome is characterized by café au lait hyperpigmented skin spots and multiple benign **neurofibromas** (benign tumors of Schwann cells) under the skin and throughout the body. These can degenerate into malignant **neurofibrosarcomas (malignant schwannoma).** *NF-1* mutations have since been detected in sporadic sarcomas of different types. Defective or absent activity of the NF-1 protein is known to cause enhanced activation of the G protein-signaling pathways. Given the complex set of cellular activities governed by G protein-mediated pathways, the mechanisms by which NF-1 abnormalities contribute to the malignant phenotype is not fully understood.

> 27. From what two kinds of locations do sarcomas arise?
> 28. What kinds of sarcomas are more common in children?
> 29. Are sarcomas more or less likely to directly invade tissues compared with epithelial malignancies?
> 30. To what sites do sarcomas commonly metastasize?
> 31. What is the most common genetic lesion in sarcomas?
> 32. What are the characteristics of type 1 neurofibromatosis, and what is a likely molecular basis for the development of neoplasia in this syndrome?

HEMATOLOGIC NEOPLASMS

Hematologic neoplasms are malignancies of cells derived from hematopoietic precursors. The true hematopoietic stem cell has the capacity for self-renewal and the ability to give rise to precursors (**colony-forming units**) that proliferate and terminally differentiate toward one of any lineage, as shown in Figure 5–3. Distinct hematologic neoplasms can arise from each of the mature cell types. Many of these arise in the bone marrow, circulate in the blood stream, and can infiltrate certain organs and tissues. Others may form tumors in lymphoid tissue—particularly lymphomas, which arise from lymphoblasts.

The cellular ultrastructure and machinery of the malignant cell can somewhat resemble that of its cell of origin. A markedly enhanced proliferative rate and arrest of differentiation are the hallmarks of these neoplasms. Examination of the interphase nucleus of cells can sometimes reveal chromosomal abnormalities such as **deletions** (monosomy), **duplications** (trisomy), or **balanced translocations.** Certain types of hematologic neoplasms tend to have stereotypic chromosomal abnormalities. Given their clonal nature, these abnormalities will be evident on all malignant cells. In some cases of chromosomal translocation, a new fusion gene is formed and can result in production of a **fusion protein** possessing abnormal function compared with the original gene products (Table 5–8). This function usually involves loss of cell cycle control, abnormal signal transduction, or reprogrammed gene expression as a result of an aberrant **transcription factor.** In contrast to hematologic malignancies, solid tumors often contain multiple chromosomal abnormalities that are not as well characterized or as reproducible. Other genetic changes described in hematologic malignancies include mutations or deletions of the *p53*, retinoblastoma *(Rb)*, and Wilms tumor *(WT1)* suppressor genes and activating mutations in the N-*ras* oncogene. Additional genetic changes can be detected in the clonal evolution of leukemias as disease progresses to a more aggressive form in the patient's course. This finding lends further support to the theory that neoplasia is the result of stepwise genetic alterations that corre-

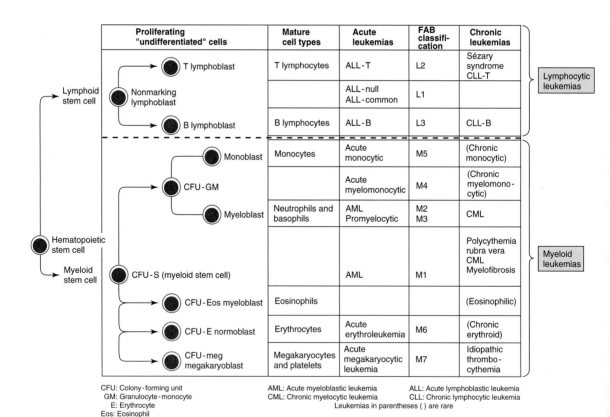

Figure 5–3. Classification of leukemias according to cell type and lineage. (Reproduced, with permission, from Chandrasoma P, Taylor CE: *Concise Pathology,* 3rd ed. Appleton & Lange, 1998.)

Table 5–8. Chromosomal translocations of hematologic neoplasms.

Neoplasm	Chromosomal Translocation	Fusion Gene Resulting From Translocation	Fusion Protein Function
Follicular lymphoma	t(14;18)	IgH-bcl-2	Inhibitor of apoptosis
Mantle cell lymphoma	t(11;14)	IgH-bcl-1	Cyclin
Follicular lymphoma	t(14;19)	IgH-bcl-3	Transcription inhibitor
Burkitt's lymphoma	t(8;14)	IgH-myc	Transcription factor
CML	t(9;22)	bcr-abl	Tyrosine kinase
AML M3	t(15;17)	PML-RAR	Transcription factor
AML	t(8;21)	AML1	Unknown
T cell ALL	t(1;14)	tal-1-TCR	Transcription factor

Key: IgH = immunoglobulin heavy chain enhancer; TCR = T cell receptor.

spond to the sequential acquisition of additional phenotypic changes that favor abnormal growth, invasion, and resistance to normal host defenses.

1. LYMPHOMA

The lymphomas comprise a set of entities characterized by the uncontrolled proliferation and potential dissemination of lymphocytes. Normal lymphocytes are able to proliferate under conditions of antigen stimulation and migrate to specific locations such as lymph nodes or lymphoid tissue surrounding the gastrointestinal tract and other mucosal surfaces. Following this tissue tropism, lymphomas typically arise in lymph nodes, though they may also develop in other tissues or organs where lymphoid elements normally reside. Normal lymphocytes also become committed upon maturation to respond to a given antigen by rearranging genes encoding immunoglobulins in the case of B cells and surface T cell receptors in the case of T cells. Analysis of these genes can prove that a given lymphoma population is clonal, or derived from a single cell, as would be expected in a dividing neoplasm. The association of lymphoma with AIDS has raised the possibility that chronic immune stimulation or modulation may be an early step in lymphomagenesis. This is further supported by the increased risk of developing lymphoma in patients with an assortment of autoimmune diseases. Iatrogenic immunosuppression in transplant patients can also increase the risk of B cell lymphoma, often seen with evidence of infection with the Epstein-Barr virus, though a causal relationship of the virus with lymphoma remains controversial. Many classification schemes for lymphomas have been devised, addressing different characteristics such as morphology, cell of origin, and cell surface antigen expression. The most recently adopted REAL (Revised European and American Lymphoma) classification is shown in Table 5–9 and incorporates clinical, biologic, and morphologic criteria. Staging is based on the extent of spread by clinical (physical examination plus radiographic studies) or surgical methods.

Lymphomas classified as well-differentiated or **low-grade** retain the morphology and patterns of gene expression of mature lymphocytes. Surface immunoglobulin in the case of B cell lymphomas and surface T cell receptor in the case of T cell lymphomas can usually be demonstrated. The appearance of individual malignant lymphocytes as well as the follicular architecture of the tumor reflect the preserved function of the cells. A slower growth rate and more favorable clinical course is also seen in low-grade lymphomas. Paradoxically, there is a tendency for patients with low-grade lymphomas to present at a more advanced stage than those with high-grade lymphoma. A common chromosomal translocation seen in low-grade follicular lymphomas juxtaposes the immunoglobulin heavy chain enhancer on chromosome 14 in front of the bcl-2 gene on chromosome 18, leading to enhanced expression of an inner mitochondrial protein encoded by bcl-2. This protein has been found to inhibit the natural process of programmed cell death, morphologically recognized as **apoptosis**. Apoptosis is required to expunge certain lymphoid clones whose function is not needed, and disordered regulation of this process may be a contributing feature in low-grade lymphomas.

Table 5–9. REAL (Revised European and American Lymphoma) classifications for lymphoma.

B cell
  Small lymphocytic
  Lymphoplasmacytic
  Follicular
  Marginal zone, MALT (mucosal-associated lymphocytic tumor)
  Marginal zone, nodal
  Mantle cell
  Diffuse large B cell
  Primary mediastinal large B cell
  Burkitt-like
T cell
  Peripheral T cell
  Anaplastic large T/null cell
  Lymphoblastic

High-grade lymphomas, on the other hand, express immature antigens and may fail to express differentiation markers such as immunoglobulin or T cell receptors. The nucleus is larger, with less organized chromatin and the presence of nucleoli, suggesting a higher growth rate and a greater loss of regulation of cell cycle. Effacement of the lymph node with an absence of follicular architecture and a tendency to exist in extranodal tissue such as the gastrointestinal tract and the central nervous system are other indications of a greater degree of genetic and cellular changes compared with low-grade lymphomas. In some cases, these changes can evolve in the clinical course of a patient with low-grade lymphoma and result in the emergence of high-grade lymphoma with a correspondingly aggressive clinical course. In these cases, additional chromosomal aberrations such as trisomy of chromosomes 7 or 3 may be seen.

Lymphomas cause a mass effect in lymph nodes or extranodal tissues and can occasionally invade and destroy adjacent tissue. Infiltration of the lungs, liver, and marrow can occur as a primary site or late in the course of the disease. Constitutional signs such as fever and weight loss, known as B symptoms, can also be seen, and these may be mediated through a variety of cytokines produced by lymphoma cells or as a reaction by normal immune cells. These cytokines include IL-1 and TNFα. In some cases of B cell lymphomas, the immunoglobulins produced by malignant cells are autoantibodies that can cause various syndromes. Among these are hemolytic anemia and thrombocytopenia, caused by autoantibodies to red cell and platelet surface proteins, respectively.

2. ACUTE MYELOGENOUS LEUKEMIA

Acute myelogenous leukemia (AML), also termed acute nonlymphocytic leukemia (ANLL), is a rapidly progressive neoplasm derived from hematopoietic precursors, or myeloid stem cells, that give rise to granulocytes, monocytes, erythrocytes, and platelets. There is increasing evidence that genetic events occurring early in stem cell maturation can lead to leukemia. First, there is a lag time of 5–10 years to the development of leukemia after exposure to known causative agents such as chemotherapy, radiation, and certain solvents. Second, many cases of secondary leukemia evolve out of a prolonged "preleukemic phase" manifested as a **myelodysplastic syndrome** of hypoproduction with abnormal maturation without actual malignant behavior. Finally, examination of precursor cells at a stage earlier than the malignant expanded clone in a given type of leukemia can reveal genetic abnormalities such as monosomy or trisomy of different chromosomes. In keeping with the general molecular theme of neoplasia, additional genetic changes are seen in the malignant clone compared with the morphologically normal stem cell that developmentally precedes it.

Table 5–10. Classification of acute myelogenous leukemias (AML).

M1	Myeloblasts without differentiation
M2	Myeloblasts with some degree of differentiation
M3	Acute promyelocytic leukemia
M4	Acute myelomonocytic leukemia
M5	Acute monocytic leukemia
M6	Erythroleukemia
M7	Megakaryoblastic leukemia

Acute myelocytic leukemias are classified by morphology and cytochemical staining, as shown in Table 5–10. **Auer rods** are crystalline cytoplasmic inclusion bodies characteristic of—though not uniformly seen in—all myeloid leukemias. In contrast to mature myeloid cells, leukemic cells have large immature nuclei with open chromatin and prominent nucleoli. The appearance of the individual types of AML mirrors the cell type from which they derive. M1 leukemias originate from early myeloid precursors with no apparent maturation toward any terminal myeloid cell type. This is apparent in the lack of granules or other features that mark more mature myeloid cells. M3 leukemias are a neoplasm of promyelocytes, precursors of granulocytes, and M3 cells exhibit abundant azurophilic granules that are typical of normal promyelocytes. M4 leukemias arise from myeloid precursors that can differentiate into granulocytes or monocytes, while M5 leukemias derive from precursors already committed to the monocyte lineage. Therefore, M4 and M5 cells both contain the characteristic folded nucleus and gray cytoplasm of monocytes, while M4 cells contain also granules of a granulocytic cytochemical staining pattern. M6 and M7 leukemias cannot be readily identified on morphologic grounds, but immunostaining for erythrocytic proteins is positive in M6 cells, and staining for platelet glycoproteins is apparent in M7 cells.

Chromosomal **deletions, duplications,** and **balanced translocations** had been noted on the leukemic cells of some patients prior to the introduction of molecular genetic techniques. Cloning of the regions where balanced translocations occur has in some cases revealed a preserved translocation site that reproducibly fuses one gene with another, resulting in the production of a new fusion protein. M3 leukemias show a very high frequency of the t(15;17) translocation that juxtaposes the *PML* gene with the *RARα* gene. *RARα* encodes for a retinoic acid steroid hormone receptor, and *PML* encodes for a transcription factor whose target genes are unknown. The fusion protein possesses novel biologic activity that presumably results in enhanced proliferation and a block of differentiation. Interestingly, retinoic acid can induce a temporary remission of M3 leukemia, supporting the importance of the RARα-PML fusion protein. Monosomy of chromosome 7 can be seen in leukemias arising out of the preleukemic syndrome of **myelodysplasia** or in de novo leukemias, and in both cases this finding is associated with a worse clinical prognosis. This monosomy as well as other serial cytogenetic changes can also be seen after relapse of treated leukemia, a situation characterized by a more aggressive course and resistance to therapy.

As hematopoietic neoplasms, acute leukemias involve the bone marrow and usually manifest abnormal circulating leukemic (blast) cells. Occasionally, extramedullary leukemic infiltrates known as **chloromas** can be seen in other organs and mucosal surfaces. A marked increase in the number of circulating blasts can sometimes cause vascular obstruction accompanied by hemorrhage and infarction in the cerebral and pulmonary vascular beds. This **leukostasis** results in symptoms such as strokes, retinal vein occlusion, and pulmonary infarction. In most cases of AML and other leukemias, peripheral blood counts of mature granulocytes, erythrocytes, and platelets are decreased. This is probably due to crowding of the bone marrow by blast cells as well as the elaboration of inhibitory substances by leukemic cells or alteration of the bone marrow stromal microenvironment and cytokine milieu necessary for normal hematopoiesis. Susceptibility to infections due to depressed granulocyte number and function and abnormal bleeding as a result of low platelet counts are common problems in patients initially presenting with leukemia.

Table 5–11. Direct systemic effects of neoplasms.

Effect	Clinical Syndrome
Vessel compression	Edema, superior vena cava syndrome
Vessel invasion and erosion	Bleeding
Lymphatic invasion	Lymphedema
Nerve invasion	Pain, numbness, dysesthesia
Brain metastases	Weakness, numbness, headache, coordination and gait abnormalities, visual changes
Spinal cord compression	Pain, paralysis, incontinence
Bone invasion and destruction	Pain, fracture
Bowel obstruction and perforation	Nausea, vomiting, pain, ileus
Airway obstruction	Dyspnea, pneumonia, lung volume loss
Ureteral obstruction	Renal failure, urinary infection
Liver invasion and metastases	Hepatic insufficiency
Lung and pleural metastases	Dyspnea, chest pain
Bone marrow infiltration	Pancytopenia, infection, bleeding

SYSTEMIC EFFECTS OF NEOPLASIA

Many effects of malignancies are mediated not by the tumor cells themselves but by direct and indirect effects as outlined in Tables 5–11 and 5–12. Direct effects (Table 5–11) include compression or invasion of vital structures such as blood and lymphatic vessels, nerves, spinal cord or brain, bone, airways, gastrointestinal tract, or urinary tract. These may cause a typical pain pattern as well as dysfunction of the involved organ and obstruction of a conduit. On occasion, an inflammatory or desmoplastic host response rather than the tumor itself can result in the same effect.

Indirect effects (Table 5–12) are heterogeneous and poorly understood. Likewise, the onset and clinical course are unpredictable. When affecting distant targets uninvolved by tumor they are collectively termed **paraneoplastic syndromes.** Some of these effects are stereotypic syndromes due to the elaboration of peptide hormones or cytokines with specific biologic activity, as shown in Table 5–12. The peptides secreted by a given neoplasm may reflect the tissue of origin or may be the result of activation of latent genes not normally expressed. In some malignancies such as carcinoid, several active peptides may act in concert to produce a constellation of symptoms and tissue effects. Cytokines such as the interleukins and tumor necrosis factor may be responsible for tumor-related fevers and weight loss. Some paraneoplastic syndromes are associated with the development of autoantibodies as a result of an immune response to tumor-associated antigens or an inappropriate production of antibody, as can be seen in lymphoid neoplasms. Finally, the nucleic acid, cytoplasmic, and membrane products of cell breakdown can result in electrolyte and other metabolic abnormalities as well as coagulopathic disorders, resulting in clotting or bleeding.

---

33. What are the hallmarks of hematologic malignancies?
34. What are some characteristics of low-grade lymphomas?
35. What are some characteristics of high-grade lymphomas?
36. What are "B symptoms," and what are they caused by?

Table 5–12. Indirect systemic effects of neoplasms.

Tumor Type	Cause of Indirect Effect	Clinical Syndrome
EFFECTS OF HORMONE OR PEPTIDE SECRETION		
Lung	ACTH	Cushing's syndrome
Lung, breast, kidney, others	PTH or PTH-related protein	Hypercalcemia
Lung	ADH, ANP	SIADH, hyponatremia
Germ cell, trophoblastic, hepatoblastoma	Gonadotropins (FSH, LH, βhCG)	Gynecomastia, precocious puberty
Lung, gastric	Growth hormone	Acromegaly
Carcinoid, neuroendocrine	Various vasoactive peptides	Flushing, wheezing, diarrhea
Sarcoma, mesothelioma, insulinoma	Insulin, insulin-like growth factor	Hypoglycemia
CUTANEOUS EFFECTS		
Gastrointestinal	Unknown	Acanthosis nigricans (hyperkeratosis and hyperpigmentation in skin folds)
Gastrointestinal, lymphoma	Unknown	Leser-Trelat (large seborrheic) keratoses
Lymphoma, hepatoma, melanoma	Melanin deposits	Melanosis (skin darkening)
Lymphoma	Autoantibodies to subepidermal proteins	Skin bullae (blisters)
Myeloid leukemia	Neutrophilic skin infiltrates	Sweet's syndrome
NEUROLOGIC EFFECTS		
Lung, prostate, colorectal, ovarian, cervical, others	Unknown	Subacute cerebellar degeneration
Lung, testicular, Hodgkin's disease	Unknown	Limbic encephalitis
Lung	Unknown	Dementia
Lung, others	Unknown	Amyotrophic lateral sclerosis
Lung, others	Unknown	Peripheral sensory or sensorimotor neuropathy
Lymphoma	Unknown, ?autoantibodies	Ascending radiculopathy (Guillain-Barré syndrome)
Lung, gastrointestinal	Autoantibodies to voltage-gated Ca^{2+} channels	Eaton-Lambert (myasthenia-like) syndrome
HEMATOLOGIC AND COAGULOPATHIC EFFECTS		
Several	Unknown	Anemia
Adenocarcinomas (especially gastric)	Unknown	Microangiopathic hemolytic anemia
Several	Interleukin-1, -3 and hematopoietic growth factors	Granulocytosis
Hodgkin's, others	Eosinophilic hematopoietic growth factors	Eosinophilia
Several	Unknown	Thrombocytosis
Adenocarcinomas (especially pancreatic), others	Unknown, ?exposed phospholipids from cell membranes	Thrombosis
Adenocarcinoma (especially prostate)	Urokinase, other mediators of fibrinolysis	Disseminated intravascular coagulation
METABOLIC EFFECTS		
Various	Interleukin-1, tumor necrosis factor α	Cachexia, anorexia
Lymphoma, others	Interleukins-1, -6	Fever
Hematologic neoplasms	Hypermetabolism/cell breakdown products	Hyperuricemia, hyperkalemia, hyperphosphatemia
Lymphoma, others	Tumor hypoxia	Lactic acidosis

Key: ACTH = adrenocorticotropic hormone; ADH = antidiuretic hormone (arginine vasopressin); ANP = atrial natriuretic protein; FSH = follicle-stimulating hormone; βhCG = human chorionic gonadotropin; LH = luteinizing hormone; PTH = parathyroid hormone; SIADH = syndrome of inappropriate secretion of antidiuretic hormone.

REFERENCES

General
DeVita VT, Hellman S, Rosenberg SA: *Cancer: Principles and Practice of Oncology,* 5th ed. Lippincott-Raven, 1997.

Lynch HT, Fusaro RM, Lynch JF: Cancer genetics in the new era of molecular biology. Ann N Y Acad Sci 1997;833:1.

Rowley J, Aster J, Sklar J: The clinical applications of new DNA diagnostic technology on the management of cancer patients. JAMA 1993;270:2331.

Colon Cancer
Marra G, Boland CR: Hereditary nonpolyposis colon cancer: The syndrome, the genes, and historical perspective. J Natl Cancer Inst 1995;87:1114.

Powell S et al: Molecular diagnosis of familial adenomatous polyposis. N Engl J Med 1993;329:1982.

Breast Cancer
Harris JR et al: Breast cancer. (Three parts.) N Engl J Med 1992;327:319, 390, 473.

Shattuck-Eidens D et al: *BRCA1* sequence analysis in women at high risk for susceptibility mutations. Risk factor analysis and implications for genetic testing. JAMA 1995;273:535.

Tripathy D, Benz CC: Activated oncogenes and putative tumor suppressor genes involved in human breast cancers. In: *Oncogenes and Tumor Suppressor Genes in Human Malignancies.* Benz CC, Liu E (editors). Kluwer, 1993.

Carcinoid
Caplin ME et al: Carcinoid tumor. Lancet 1998;352:799.

Kvols LK, Reubi JC: Metastatic carcinoid tumors and the malignant carcinoid syndrome. Acta Oncol 1993; 32:197.

Testicular Cancer
Bosl GJ, Motzer RJ: Testicular germ-cell cancer. N Engl J Med 1997;337:242.

Boyle P, Zaridze DG: Risk factors for prostate and testicular cancer. Eur J Cancer 1993;29:1048.

Oliver T, Mead G: Testicular cancer. Curr Opin Oncol 1993;5:559.

Sarcomas
Diller L: Rhabdomyosarcoma and other soft tissue sarcomas of childhood. Curr Opin Oncol 1992;4:689.

Shipley J, Crew J, Gusterson B: The molecular biology of soft tissue sarcomas. Eur J Cancer 1993;29:2054.

Lymphoma
Foon K et al: Genetic relatedness of lymphoid malignancies. Ann Intern Med 1993;119:63.

Ghia P, Nadler LM: Recent advances in lymphoma biology. Curr Opin Oncol 1997;9:403.

Harris NL et al: A revised European-American classification of lymphoid neoplasms: A proposal from the International Lymphoma Study Group. Blood 1994; 84:1361.

Paraneoplastic Syndromes
Pierce ST: Paraendocrine syndromes. Curr Opin Oncol 1993;5:639.

Posner JB: Paraneoplastic syndromes. Neurol Clin 1991;9:919.

Richardson GE, Johnson BE: Paraneoplastic syndromes in lung cancer. Curr Opin Oncol 1992;4:323.

6

Blood Disorders

J. Ben Davoren, MD, PhD

NORMAL STRUCTURE & FUNCTION

Blood is an extremely complex fluid, composed of both formed elements (red cells, white cells, platelets) and plasma. Red blood cells (**erythrocytes**) are the most common formed elements, carrying oxygen to the cells of the body via their main component, **hemoglobin.** White blood cells are generally present at about 1/700th the number of erythrocytes and function as mediators of immune responses to infection or other stimuli of inflammation. Platelets are the formed elements that participate in coagulation. Plasma is largely water, electrolytes, and plasma proteins, which are themselves very complex. The plasma proteins most important in blood clotting are the coagulation factors. Because blood circulates throughout the body, alterations in normal blood physiology—either formed elements or plasma proteins—may have widespread adverse consequences.

FORMED ELEMENTS OF BLOOD

Anatomy
A. The Bone Marrow and Hematopoiesis: Although the mature formed elements of blood are quite different from each other in both structure and function, all of these cells develop from a common progenitor cell, or **stem cell,** population, which resides in the bone marrow. The developmental process is called **hematopoiesis** and represents an enormous metabolic task for the body. More than 100 billion cells are produced every day. This makes the bone marrow one of the most active organs in the body, and—despite the fact that it is not localized to one part of the body—it (like the skin) should be considered an organ just as are the liver and kidneys. In the adult, most of the active marrow resides in the vertebrae, sternum, and ribs, with less activity in the long bones, where the marrow is more active in children.

The process of differentiation from stem cell to mature erythrocyte, granulocyte, lymphocyte, monocyte, or platelet is shown in Figure 6–1. It is not clear exactly what early events lead dividing stem cells down a particular path of development, but many different peptide hormones, called **cytokines,** are clearly involved (Table 6–1). Perhaps because mature white blood cells have a much shorter half-life in the circulation, white blood cell precursors usually outnumber red blood cell precursors by a ratio of 3:1 in the bone marrow.

The major hormone that stimulates the production of **erythrocytes** (ie, **erythropoiesis**) is **erythropoietin.** This peptide is produced by the kidney and regulates red blood cell production by a feedback system: When blood hemoglobin levels fall (**anemia**), oxygen delivery to the kidney falls, and the kidney produces more erythropoietin, which causes the marrow to produce more red cells. When hemoglobin levels rise, the kidney produces less erythropoietin and the marrow fewer red cells.

For white blood cells, the situation is more complex. The most common cells are the **granulocytes,** so named because their cytoplasms are filled with granules. Of these, the neutrophils are the most prevalent and the most important cells in producing inflammation. Granulocyte production (**myelopoiesis**) can be affected by many cytokines at different stages of development. Figure 6–1 shows that interleukin-3 (IL-3), granulocyte colony-stimulating factor (G-CSF), and granulocyte-macrophage colony-stimulating factor (GM-CSF) are the most important. All three proteins have been purified, sequenced, and cloned. The latter two proteins are now produced commercially for therapeutic use. Unlike G-CSF, GM-CSF also stimulates the maturation of a different white blood cell line, the **monocyte-macrophage line.** These cells are part of the immune system as well (ingesting foreign bacteria, for example) and can reside in skin and other tissues, not just blood. Their function, along with that of the B and T lymphocyte populations, is discussed more fully in Chapter 3.

Platelets are not cells but fragments of larger multinucleated cells in the marrow called **megakary-**

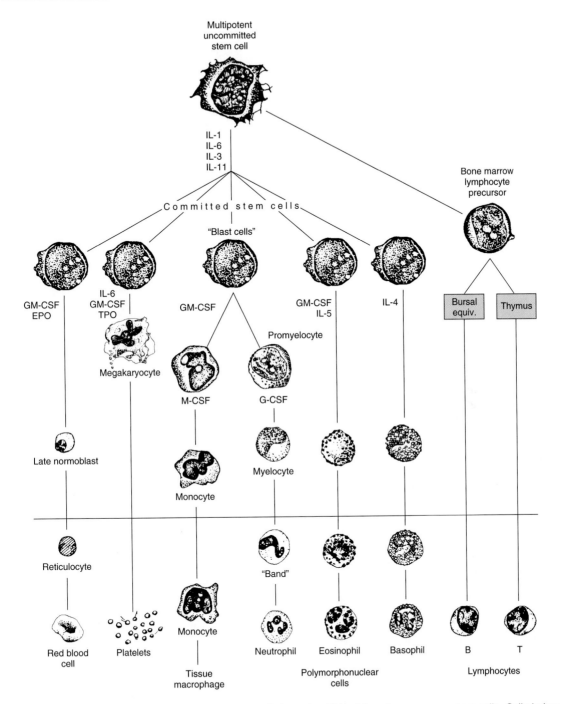

Figure 6–1. Hematopoiesis: development of the formed elements of blood from bone marrow stem cells. Cells below the horizontal line are found in normal peripheral blood. The principal cytokines that stimulate each cell lineage to differentiate are shown. (EPO, erythropoietin; TPO, thrombopoietin; CSF, colony-stimulating factors; G, granulocyte; M, macrophage; IL, interleukin.) See Table 6–1 for details. (Modified and reproduced, with permission, from Ganong WF: *Review of Medical Physiology,* 19th ed. Appleton & Lange, 1999.)

Table 6–1. Cytokines that regulate hematopoiesis.

Cytokine	Cell Lines Stimulated	Cytokine Source
IL-1	Erythrocyte Granulocyte Megakaryocyte Monocyte	Multiple cell types
IL-3	Erythrocyte Granulocyte Megakaryocyte Monocyte	T lymphocytes
IL-4	Basophil	T lymphocytes
IL-5	Eosinophil	T lymphocytes
IL-6	Erythrocyte Granulocyte Megakaryocyte Monocyte	Endothelial cells Fibroblasts Macrophages
IL-11	Erythrocyte Granulocyte Megakaryocyte	Fibroblasts Osteoblasts
Erythropoietin	Erythrocyte	Kidney Kupffer cells of liver
G-CSF	Granulocyte	Endothelial cells Fibroblasts Monocytes
GM-CSF	Erythrocyte Granulocyte Megakaryocyte	Endothelial cells Fibroblasts Monocytes T lymphocytes
M-CSF	Monocyte	Endothelial cells Fibroblasts Monocytes
Thrombopoietin	Megakaryocyte	Liver, kidney

Key: IL = interleukin; CSF = colony stimulating factor; G = granulocyte; M = macrophage.

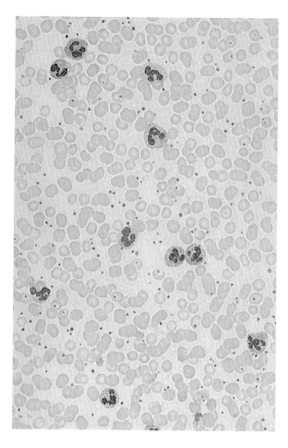

Figure 6–2. Normal thin blood smear, seen at low power (40×) with Wright's stain. Erythrocytes predominate and can be seen to be thin disks with central pallor (see text). Platelets are the numerous small, dark bodies. Larger cells with lobulated nuclei are mature neutrophils. Lymphocytes and monocytes are not present on this smear.

ocytes. Platelets are crucial to normal blood clotting. Platelet production is stimulated by multiple cytokines but is dependent mainly on the action of interleukins 6 and 11 (IL-6, IL-11) and a recently discovered peptide called **thrombopoietin.** This peptide is produced by the liver and kidney, probably at a constant rate, but the amount of this hormone free to interact with platelet precursors rises and falls, probably due to metabolism by the existing platelets in the blood, such that a low platelet count stimulates **thrombopoiesis.**

For all its complexity and metabolic activity, there is tremendous regulation of the marrow through the interaction of various cytokines. Normally, only the most mature elements in each cell lineage are released into the general circulation, demonstrating this exquisite control over development.

Examination of the appropriateness of blood cell development is best undertaken with the microscope, using the **thin blood smear** (Figure 6–2). Modern technical equipment, which can optically sort cells by size and various optical reflective parameters, gives important information, especially about whether cell numbers are out of the normal ranges (Table 6–2). Microscopic examination of the blood smear, usually using Wright's stain, gives additional information once an abnormality is detected, however, and should always be done when a blood disorder is suspected on clinical grounds.

Physiology

A. Erythrocytes: Mature red blood cells are biconcave disk-shaped cells filled with hemoglobin, which function as the oxygen-carrying component of the blood. In contrast to most other cells, they do not have nuclei at maturity; nuclei are extruded during the final phase of erythrocyte development, and the presence of erythrocytes with nuclei as seen on the

Table 6–2. Normal values obtained on automated blood count—formed elements of blood.

	Male Adult	Female Adult
Hemoglobin	14–18 g/dL	12–16 g/dL
Hematocrit (percentage of blood which is erythrocytes)	42–50%	37–47%
Red cell count	4.6–6 × 10^6/μL	4.2–5.4 × 10^6/μL
Mean corpuscular volume (MCV)	80–100 fL	80–100 fL
White blood cell (total) count	4,000–11,000/μL	4,000–11,000/μL
Neutrophils	2,500–7,500/μL	2,500–7,500/μL
Lymphocytes	1,500–3,500/μL	1,500–3,500/μL
Monocytes	200–800/μL	200–800/μL
Eosinophils	60–600/μL	60–600/μL
Basophils	<100/μL	<100/μL
Platelets	150,000–400,000/μL	150,000–400,000/μL

peripheral smear suggests an underlying disease state. Normal red cells are about 8 μm in diameter, a size that is larger than the smallest capillaries; however, their biconcave shape gives them enough flexibility so they can slip through small capillaries to deliver oxygen to the tissues. Once extruded from the bone marrow, individual erythrocytes function for about 120 days before they are removed from the circulation by the spleen.

On a typical blood smear (stained with Wright's stain), erythrocytes dominate the microscopic field, and their biconcave disk shape resembles a doughnut. There is a thicker outer rim that appears red owing to the hemoglobin present and an area of central pallor where the disk is thinnest. Young erythrocytes (reticulocytes) appear bluer (basophilic) because they still contain some ribosomes and mitochondria for a few days after the nuclei are extruded.

As noted, hemoglobin is the most important substance in the erythrocyte. This protein is actually a tetramer, made of two α-protein subunits and two β-protein subunits (in normal adult hemoglobin—called hemoglobin A), and each α- or β-subunit contains the actual oxygen-binding portion of the complex, **heme.** Heme is a compound whose centrally important atom is iron; it is this atom that actually binds oxygen in the lungs and subsequently releases it in the tissues of the body. A low level of hemoglobin in the blood, from a variety of causes (see below), is **anemia,** the most common general blood disorder.

B. Granulocytes—Neutrophils, Eosinophils, and Basophils: The granulocytes are the most common white blood cells; of these, neutrophils are most abundant, followed by eosinophils and basophils (Table 6–2). Developmentally, all three types are similar: As they mature, their nuclei become more convoluted and multilobed, and each develops a cytoplasm filled with granules. These granules contain a variety of enzymes, prostaglandins, and mediators of inflammation, with specific factors dependent on the cell type. Early progenitor cells for each type of granulocyte ("blasts") are indistinguishable on microscopic examination of the bone marrow, but under the influence of different cytokines they become morphologically distinct cell types.

Basophils contain very dark blue or purple granules (when stained with either Giemsa's stain or Wright's stain). Basophil granules are large and usually obscure the nucleus because of their density. Normally, basophils function in hypersensitivity reactions (as described in Chapter 3), but their numbers can be increased in diseases not associated with hypersensitivity, such as chronic myelogenous leukemia.

Eosinophils contain large, strikingly "eosinophilic" granules (staining red with Wright's or Giemsa's stain). Eosinophil nuclei are usually bilobed. Normally, eosinophils function as part of the inflammatory response to parasites too large to be engulfed by individual immune cells. They are also involved in some allergic reactions.

Neutrophils contain granules that are "neutrophilic," ie, neither eosinophilic nor basophilic. Although they predominate in the blood, their major function is actually in the tissues; they must leave the blood by inserting themselves between the endothelial cells of the vasculature to reach sites of injury or infection. Their granules contain highly active enzymes such as **myeloperoxidase,** which, along with the free radical oxygen ions produced by membrane enzymes such as **NADPH oxidase,** lead to the killing of bacteria which neutrophils ingest via endocytosis or phagocytosis. They are the "first line of defense" against bacterial pathogens, and low numbers of them lead directly to a high incidence of significant bacterial infections (see below). Of all the cells produced by the bone marrow, these comprise the greatest fraction because their life span in blood is much shorter than that of any other cell type—only about 6–8 hours. Demonstration of their importance and their short survival is commonly seen, because examination of the blood smear under the microscope in a patient with an active infection may show not only increased numbers of mature, multilobed neutrophils (neutrophilia) but also increased numbers of less mature cells. These less mature cells, released from a large storage pool in the bone marrow, are called **bands** and have a characteristic horseshoe-shaped nucleus which is not yet fully lobulated. The phenomenon of finding these cells in the peripheral blood is called a **left shift** of the granulocyte lineage.

C. Other White Blood Cells—Monocytes and Lymphocytes: Both monocytes and lymphocytes arise from the common stem cell. It is the widespread **pluripotential** ability of stem cells to differentiate into these cells in addition to the granulocytes, erythrocytes, and platelets that makes bone marrow transplantation a therapeutic option for immune system disorders and malignancies. Monocytes have a very long life span, probably several months, but spend only about 3 days in the circulation. They mostly reside in tissues and act there as immune cells that engulf (**phagocytose**) bacteria and subsequently can "present" components of these bacteria to lymphocytes in a way that further amplifies and refines the immune response (Chapter 3). On blood smear evaluation, monocytes are the largest cells seen, with irregular but not multilobed nuclei and pale blue cytoplasm, often with prominent vacuoles.

Lymphocyte precursors leave the marrow early and require extramedullary (outside of the marrow) maturation to become normally functioning immune cells in either the blood or the lymphatic system (Figure 6–3). Their crucial roles in recognizing "self versus nonself" and in modulating virtually all aspects of the immune response in infection are described in Chapter 3. On microscopic examination of the blood smear, lymphocytes are small cells, slightly larger than an erythrocyte, with dark nuclei essentially filling the entire cell; only a thin rim of light blue cytoplasm is normally seen. Granules are sparse or absent.

D. Platelets: Platelets are the smallest formed elements in the blood and have a half-life of about 4 days. They are fragments of larger, multinucleated cells which are the largest discrete constituents of the bone marrow (**megakaryocytes**), but platelets have no nuclei of their own. Most platelets remain in the circulation, but a substantial minority are trapped in the spleen; this phenomenon becomes important in a variety of immune-mediated decreases in platelet counts (**thrombocytopenia;** see below).

Platelets are integral components of the coagulation system. Their membranes provide an important source of phospholipids which are required for the function of the coagulation system proteins (Figure 6–4) and contain important receptors that allow attachment to endothelial cells (**platelet adhesion**) so that a **platelet plug** can be formed in response to blood vessel injury. This prevents further blood loss after trauma and contains the coagulation response at the site of injury rather than letting coagulation proceed inappropriately.

The cytoplasm is also important for platelet function, particularly the intracellular **dense granules** and **alpha granules.** The phenomenon of platelet activation is also called "degranulation" and can be initi-

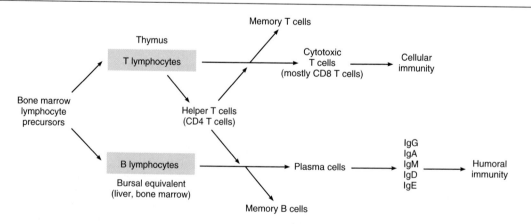

Figure 6–3. Development of the immune system from the common bone marrow stem cell. (Reproduced, with permission, from Ganong WF: *Review of Medical Physiology,* 19th ed. Appleton & Lange, 1999.)

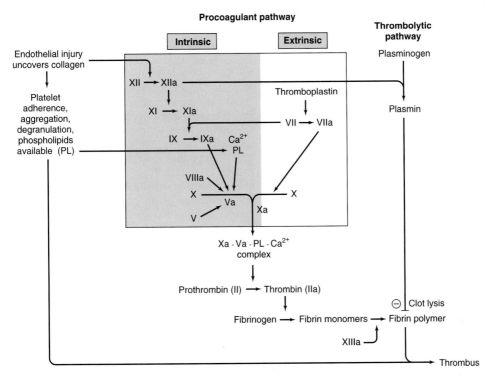

Figure 6–4. Coagulation and thrombolytic systems, showing balanced activity between them. (Modified and reproduced, with permission, from Chandrasoma P, Taylor CR: *Concise Pathology,* 3rd ed. Appleton & Lange, 1998.)

ated by exposure of platelets to the activated blood coagulation factor **thrombin,** adenosine 5′-diphosphate (ADP), or collagen. This last reaction is probably the most important, occurring when collagen, normally in the basement membrane below the endothelial cells, is exposed to the blood after injury. Platelet activation can also be induced by exposure to **platelet-activating factor (PAF),** a neutrophil-derived phospholipid cytokine.

During platelet activation, the dense and alpha granules release further activators of platelet activity, such as ADP, and several proteins, such as platelet factor 4, which is important in both activation and, possibly, binding to endothelial cells. It is also important because it binds to the most commonly used therapeutic anticoagulant, heparin (see below). The last step in platelet activity is platelet aggregation, where platelets stick to each other, firming up the platelet plug. On examination of the blood smear, platelets are small, irregularly shaped blue or purple granular bodies. In conditions where platelet numbers are rising as a result of increased marrow activity, more immature platelets can be identified by their size; they are much larger than normal platelets, and in some cases larger than erythrocytes (giant platelets).

1. What is the ratio of red blood cells to white blood cells in the bloodstream?
2. What is the number of cells produced daily by the bone marrow?
3. What are the different formed elements of blood and how can they and their subtypes be distinguished?

COAGULATION FACTORS & THE COAGULATION CASCADE

Anatomy

The coagulation system is remarkably complex in both structure and function. Many proteins are involved, produced by different cell types of the body, frequently with both inactive and active forms regulated in a fine balance. The coagulation system provides for immediate activation when there is blood loss that needs to be stemmed but usually confines its activity to the site of blood loss. Otherwise, coagulation might occur throughout the entire circulatory system, which would be incompatible with life.

There are two major components of the coagulation system: platelets (discussed in the previous section) and the coagulation factors, which are plasma proteins. The end result of coagulation factor activity is quite simple: the formation of a complex of cross-linked **fibrin** molecules and platelets that terminate hemorrhage after injury. However, the sophisticated **coagulation cascade** provides several points of control over this event (Figure 6–4).

The coagulation factors do not generally circulate in active forms. Most of them are enzymes (serine proteases) and remain "dormant" until they are needed. This is accomplished by having other enzymes (the other proteases in the cascade) available that can cleave the inactive factors into active ones. Presumably, the many steps in the cascade allow a small change in a very early enzyme, factor XII, to be amplified. This results in a timely change in the availability of thrombin, which cleaves fibrinogen, leaving fibrin to form the clot. All of the factors have roman numerals, and the inactive forms are written without annotation (eg, factor II, also known as prothrombin). The activated forms of the factors are signified by the letter "a" (eg, factor IIa, also known as thrombin).

Most of the coagulation factors are made by the liver, but factor XIII derives from platelets and factor VIII is made by endothelial cells. Factors II, VII, IX, and X are particularly important factors (Table 6–3) because they are all dependent on the liver enzyme γ-carboxylase. Gamma-carboxylase is dependent on vitamin K, and the oral anticoagulant **warfarin** acts by interfering with vitamin K activity. Two of the anticoagulant proteins, protein S and protein C (see below), are also vitamin K-dependent.

Physiology

The coagulation cascade, diagrammed in Figure 6–4, has two general procoagulant pathways, which converge at the step of activation of factor X to factor Xa. Factor Xa forms a complex with factor Va and calcium, and it is here also that the phospholipids (PLs) from platelet membranes come into play, helping to ensure that coagulation is proceeding in the appropriate place in the circulation where a clot is necessary, namely, at the platelet plug. This Xa-Va-Ca^{2+}-PL complex converts prothrombin to thrombin and can convert multiple molecules per complex. It is not the result of simple binding but rather of proteolytic cleavage of prothrombin, and the complex is free to act on other prothrombin molecules nearby. This mechanism provides more amplification of a system built on multiple levels of amplification.

Thrombin is also a serine protease. It cleaves the ubiquitous plasma protein fibrinogen into fibrin monomers, which are small insoluble proteins and which polymerize with each other to form the complex **fibrin.** This conglomerate can subsequently be solidified by chemical cross-links catalyzed by factor XIIIa, which is formed from factor XIII by the proteolytic activity of thrombin.

The two pathways that converge at the activation of factor X are called the **intrinsic** and **extrinsic systems.** The intrinsic system is so named because all the factors in it are intrinsic to the blood. The initial stimulus in this cascade is the activation of factor XII by high-molecular-weight kininogen (the precursor of the vasoactive peptide bradykinin) and kallikrein (an enzyme) in the presence of collagen. Exposed collagen usually becomes "available" for this reaction as a result of vascular injury and also leads to platelet adhesion and aggregation (see above).

Factor XIIa is a protease. It converts factor XI to XIa, which converts IX to IXa. At this point, factor VIII, which is normally complexed to the protein that allows platelets to adhere to endothelial cells, **von Willebrand factor (vWF),** is activated by its release from vWF. Factors VIIIa and IXa, in the presence of phospholipids (again, usually from platelets) and calcium, activate factor X. The complex of factor Xa with factor Va, phospholipid, and calcium can then become fully active as described above.

The extrinsic system is so named because the initial stimulus in this cascade is tissue-based (extrinsic to the blood). "Tissue factor," also called **thromboplastin,** is a lipid-rich protein material released upon tissue injury. It directly activates factor VII, and factor VIIa subsequently activates factor IX and factor X, with subsequent activity identical to that of the intrinsic system.

All of the factors described so far are **procoagulants,** ie, they accelerate the process of coagulation; but there are also two complex anticoagulant systems that help control the cascade. The first is the **throm-**

Table 6–3. Coagulation factors of plasma.

Name	Production Source
Procoagulant factors	
Factor I (fibrinogen)	Liver
Factor II (prothrombin)	Liver
Factor III (tissue thromboplastin)	Tissue
Factor IV (calcium)	. . .
Factor V (proaccelerin)	Liver
Factor VI (obsolete = factor Va)	. . .
Factor VII (proconvertin)	Liver
Factor VIII (antihemophilic factor)	Endothelial cells
Factor IX (Christmas factor)	Liver
Factor X (Stuart-Prower factor)	Liver
Factor XI (plasma thromboplastin antecedent)	Liver
Factor XII (Hageman factor)	Liver
Factor XIII (fibrin-stabilizing factor)	Platelets
Anticoagulant factors	
Antithrombin III	Liver
Protein C	Liver
Protein S	Liver
Plasminogen	Liver

bolytic system, which is principally involved in dissolving clots that have already formed. In this system, **plasmin,** a serum protease, cleaves fibrin, resulting in breakup of the clot and creating fibrin degradation products that inhibit thrombin. Completing this feedback loop, plasmin itself is formed from its own inactive precursor protein, **plasminogen,** by the enzymatic activity of thrombin. Plasminogen can also be cleaved by **tissue plasminogen activator (t-PA)** to form plasmin; t-PA and related proteins are now used clinically, injected intravenously or intraarterially, to break up clots that form in coronary arteries, causing heart attacks, and cerebral arteries, causing strokes.

The second anticoagulant system is characterized by a group of inhibitors of the coagulation factors. They are composed of antithrombin III, protein S, and protein C (see below). Antithrombin III is a protease inhibitor and physically blocks the action of the serine proteases in the cascade. Protein C, activated by thrombin, cleaves factor V into an inactive form so that the factor Xa-Va-Ca^{2+}-PL complex cannot cleave prothrombin into thrombin. It requires protein S as a cofactor. This complex also inactivates factor VIII.

---

4. Name the vitamin K-dependent clotting factors and the organ in which they are synthesized.
5. The extrinsic and intrinsic coagulation pathways converge with the activation of which clotting factor?
6. Describe the two anticoagulant systems that participate in clotting homeostasis.

OVERVIEW OF BLOOD DISORDERS

RED CELL DISORDERS

There are many red cell abnormalities, but the principal ones are a variety of anemias. **Anemia** is defined as an abnormally low hemoglobin concentration in the blood. There are several methods of classification, but the prevailing systems are based on red cell size and shape.

In normal persons, erythrocytes are of uniform size and shape, and the automated blood count shows a mean corpuscular volume (MCV) near 90 fL, which is the estimated volume of a single cell. Automated systems usually report abnormalities of red cells as changes in hemoglobin concentration, red cell number, and MCV. Small cells (with low MCVs) are termed **microcytic,** and cells larger than normal are termed **macrocytic.** The relative nonuniformity of cell shapes **(poikilocytosis)** or sizes **(anisocytosis)** can further aid in subclassifying erythrocyte disorders.

The morphologic classification of anemias is set forth in Table 6–4 and Figure 6–5. In general, the microcytic anemias are due to abnormalities in hemoglobin production, either in number of hemoglobin molecules per cell or in type of hemoglobin molecules **(hemoglobinopathies).** **Sickle cell anemia, iron deficiency anemia** due to chronic blood loss, and the **thalassemias** are examples of microcytic anemia.

The macrocytic anemias reflect either abnormal nuclear maturation or a higher fraction of young, large red cells (reticulocytes). When the nuclei of maturing red cells appear too young and large for the amount of hemoglobin in the cytoplasm, the macrocytic anemia is termed **megaloblastic.** These anemias are most often due either to vitamin deficiencies (vitamin B_{12} or folic acid) or drugs that interfere with DNA synthesis.

The normocytic anemias can be due to multiple causes: decreased numbers of red cell precursors in the marrow **(aplastic anemia,** or replacement of marrow elements with cancer), low levels of erythropoietin (due to chronic renal failure), or chronic inflammatory diseases that affect the availability of iron in the marrow and may have other effects as well. Other normocytic anemias can be secondary to a decreased life span of the cells that are produced. Examples of this phenomenon are acute blood loss; **autoimmune hemolytic anemias,** in which antibodies or complement bind to red cells and cause their destruction; and **hereditary spherocytosis** or **hereditary elliptocytosis,** in which defects in the erythro-

Table 6–4. Morphologic classification and common causes of anemia.

Type	MCV	Common Causes
Macrocytic	Increased	Folic acid deficiency Vitamin B_{12} deficiency Liver disease Alcohol Hypothyroidism Drugs (sulfonamides, zidovudine, antineoplastic agents)
Microcytic	Decreased	Iron deficiency Thalassemias
Normocytic	Normal	Aplastic anemia Anemia of chronic disease Chronic renal failure Hemolytic anemia Spherocytosis

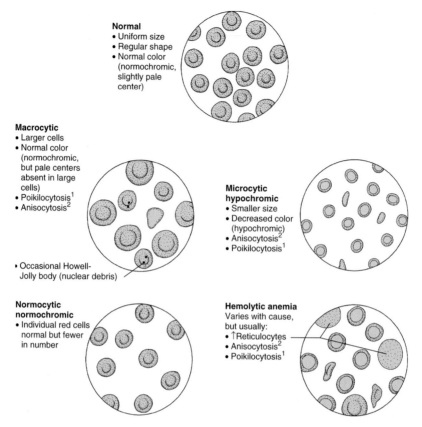

Figure 6–5. Thin blood smear appearance of erythrocytes in the different morphologic types of anemias. (1, Poikilocytosis [variation in shape]; 2, anisocytosis [variation in size].) (Modified and reproduced, with permission, from Chandrasoma P, Taylor CR: *Concise Pathology,* 3rd ed. Appleton & Lange, 1998.)

cyte membrane affect their ability to squeeze through the capillary microcirculation.

Anemias are very common. In contrast, an elevated hemoglobin concentration, termed **polycythemia,** is uncommon. Elevations in hemoglobin concentration can occur as a secondary phenomenon due to increased erythropoietin levels, such as that found in smokers or dwellers at high altitudes (whose low blood oxygen levels stimulate erythropoietin production). Some tumors, especially renal tumors, can also make the hormone. Primary polycythemia is an abnormality of the bone marrow itself—a **myeloproliferative disorder**—which leads to an increased red cell mass and consequent low erythropoietin levels by the negative feedback mechanism discussed previously.

WHITE BLOOD CELL DISORDERS

Abnormalities in white cell numbers occur commonly (Table 6–5), whereas abnormalities of *function* are rare. Neoplastic transformation in the form of leukemia (granulocytes and monocytes) or lymphoma (lymphocytes) is fairly common. The leukemias are discussed in Chapter 5.

Changes in neutrophil count are the most frequent white cell abnormality detected on the automated blood count. Increased numbers of neutrophils (**leukocytosis**) suggest acute or chronic infection or inflammation but can be a sign of many conditions, including stress, since adrenal corticosteroids cause **demargination** of neutrophils from blood vessel walls.

Decreased numbers of neutrophils (**neutropenia**) can be seen in overwhelming infection and benign diseases such as **cyclic neutropenia** (see below) but can also be seen when the bone marrow is infiltrated with tumor. Many drugs can also directly suppress marrow production, and since neutrophils have the shortest half-life in the blood of any cell produced by the marrow, their numbers fall quickly when this occurs.

Lymphocyte numbers can vary substantially (Table 6–6). Lymphocyte counts are classically elevated in viral infections, such as infectious mononucleosis, but persistent elevations are always worrisome for malig-

Table 6–5. Causes of abnormal neutrophil counts.

Neutrophilia
- *Increased marrow activity*
  - Bacterial infections
  - Acute inflammation
  - Leukemia and myeloproliferative disorders
- *Release from marrow pool*
  - Stress (catecholamines)
  - Corticosteroids
  - Endotoxin exposure
- *Demargination into blood*
  - Bacterial infections
  - Hypoxemia
  - Stress (catecholamines)
  - Corticosteroids
  - Exercise

Neutropenia
- *Decreased marrow activity*
  - Drugs (antineoplastic agents, antibiotics, gold, certain diuretics, antithyroid agents, antihistamines, antipsychotics)
  - Radiation exposure
  - Megaloblastic anemia
  - Cyclic neutropenia
  - Kostmann's (infantile) neutropenia
  - Aplastic anemias
  - Myelodysplastic syndromes
  - Marrow replacement by tumor
- *Decreased neutrophil survival*
  - Sepsis
  - Viral or rickettsial infection
  - Immune destruction associated with drugs
  - Immune destruction associated with autoantibodies (systemic lupus erythematosus, Felty's syndrome)
  - Hypersplenism

---

nancies, particularly **chronic lymphocytic leukemia**, which may not cause any symptoms and be incidentally discovered on a routine blood count.

Decreased lymphocyte counts (**lymphopenia**) are a common complication of corticosteroid therapy but

Table 6–6. Causes of abnormal lymphocyte counts.

Lymphocytosis
- Medium to large, atypical lymphocytes predominant
  - Viral infections (mononucleosis, mumps, measles, hepatitis, rubella)
  - Active immune responses, particularly in children
  - Toxoplasmosis
  - Lymphoma with circulating cells
  - Chronic lymphocytic leukemia
- Small, mature lymphocytes predominant
  - Chronic infections (tuberculosis)
  - Autoimmune diseases (myasthenia gravis)
  - Metabolic diseases (Addison's disease)
  - Lymphoma with circulating cells
  - Chronic lymphocytic leukemia
- Immature cells predominant
  - Acute lymphocytic leukemia
  - Lymphoblastic lymphoma

Lymphopenia
- Immunodeficiency states (AIDS)
- Corticosteroid therapy
- Toxic drugs
- Cushing's syndrome

---

are most worrisome for immunodeficiency states; the human immunodeficiency virus (HIV) directly infects lymphocytes, and the likelihood of opportunistic infections increases as lymphocyte counts fall, resulting in AIDS.

PLATELET DISORDERS

Abnormalities in platelet number are fairly common, particularly low counts (**thrombocytopenia**). Causes are listed in Table 6–7. Decreased production occurs when the marrow is affected by a variety of diseases or when thrombopoietin production by the liver is impaired, as in cirrhosis. Increased destruction is much more prevalent. There are three general mechanisms. Because a significant percentage of platelets normally resides in the spleen, any increase in spleen size or activity (**hypersplenism**) will lead to lower platelet counts. Platelet consumption because of ongoing clotting will also lower counts. Most commonly, however, there is immune-mediated consumption, due either to drugs or to autoantibodies, which are usually directed against a particular platelet membrane antigen called gpIIIa.

Table 6–7. Causes of platelet abnormalities.

Thrombocytosis
- Myeloproliferative disorders, especially essential thrombocythemia
- Postsplenectomy
- Reactive (postsurgical, posthemorrhage, anemias)
- Inflammatory disorders
- Malignancies

Thrombocytopenia
- *Decreased production*
  - Aplastic anemia
  - Marrow infiltration
  - Vitamin B_{12} and folate deficiencies
  - Radiation
  - Hereditary
  - Cirrhosis (low thrombopoietin levels)
- *Decreased survival*
  - Immune-mediated (idiopathic, systemic lupus erythematosus, drug-induced, neonatal from maternal IgG)
  - Hypersplenism
  - Disseminated intravascular coagulation
  - Thrombotic thrombocytopenic purpura, hemolytic uremic syndrome
  - Prosthetic valves

Qualitative platelet disorders
- *Inherited*
  - Bernard-Soulier syndrome (adhesion defect)
  - Glanzmann thrombasthenia (aggregation defect)
  - Storage pool disease (granule defect)
  - Von Willebrand's disease
  - Wiskott-Aldrich syndrome
- *Acquired*
  - Uremia
  - Dysproteinemias
  - Chronic liver disease
  - Drug-induced (especially aspirin)

Functional platelet disorders are not rare, especially the acquired disorders due to uremia (renal failure) or aspirin, which inhibits the platelet enzyme cyclooxygenase and decreases platelet aggregability. Inherited abnormalities are unusual, however, with the exception of **von Willebrand's disease,** which results from lack of the carrier protein for factor VIII, von Willebrand factor. This factor also acts as a bridge between platelets and the endothelium and thus is crucial for formation of the platelet plug in the coagulation cascade.

Elevations in the platelet count above the normal range (**thrombocytosis**) are not unusual and are especially apt to occur in association with iron deficiency anemia as the marrow attempts to compensate. In the myeloproliferative disorders, such as polycythemia discussed above, platelet counts are often high. In **essential thrombocythemia,** platelet counts may be over 1,000,000/μL.

COAGULATION FACTOR DISORDERS

The most important coagulation factor disorders are quantitative rather than qualitative and usually hereditary rather than acquired (Table 6–8). Exceptions to this rule are **acquired factor inhibitors,** which are antibodies that bind to one of the coagulation factors, most often factor VIII, which may or may not cause clinical bleeding problems, and a few qualitatively abnormal proteins, such as factor V or fibrinogen, discussed below.

The quantitative disorders that most commonly cause bleeding are **hemophilia A** (deficiency of factor VIII) and **hemophilia B** (deficiency of factor IX). Both are X chromosome-linked recessive traits, such that affected males have very low levels of factor VIII or IX. (It is not clear why all affected males do not have complete absence of factor VIII or IX activity, which would be predicted by this model.) Hemophilia A is most common, with a prevalence of 1:10,000 males worldwide. Both disorders lead to both spontaneous and excessive posttraumatic bleeding, particularly into joints and muscles. Females who carry the trait have 50% of the normal amount of either factor and tend not to have any bleeding problems; in general, one needs only half of the normal quantities of many of the coagulation factors to have normal coagulation.

Quantitative, inherited abnormalities of the anticoagulation systems also occur. Protein S deficiency, protein C deficiency, and antithrombin III deficiency all occur and lead to abnormal clotting problems as discussed in the next section.

Finally, the condition of **consumption coagulopathy** or **disseminated intravascular coagulation (DIC)** needs to be included. This condition is generally due to overwhelming infection, specific leukemias or lymphomas, or massive hemorrhage. In DIC, the coagulation factors become depleted. Often there is simultaneous activation of the fibrinolytic system as well, and uncontrolled bleeding may occur throughout the entire circulatory system.

---

7. Define anemia and suggest three causes each for macrocytic and microcytic anemia.
8. What are some categories of explanations for a white blood cell number that is substantially increased or decreased compared with the normal range?
9. What are the three general mechanisms of thrombocytopenia?
10. What is the nature of the defects in hemophilia A and B?

Table 6–8. Coagulation factor deficiencies.

Factor	Disease	Inheritance Pattern	Frequency	Disease Severity
Fibrinogen	Afibrinogenemia Dysfibrinogenemia	Autosomal recessive Autosomal dominant	Rare Rare	Variable Variable
Factor V	Parahemophilia	Autosomal recessive	Very rare	Moderate to severe
Factor VII		Autosomal recessive	Very rare	Moderate to severe
Factor VIII	Hemophilia A	X-linked recessive	Common	Mild to severe
vWF	Von Willebrand's disease	Autosomal dominant	Common	Mild to moderate
Factor IX	Hemophilia B	X-linked recessive	Uncommon	Mild to severe
Factor X		Autosomal recessive	Rare	Variable
Factor XI	Rosenthal's syndrome	Autosomal recessive	Uncommon	Mild
Factor XII	Hageman trait	Autosomal recessive or dominant	Rare	Asymptomatic
Factor XIII		Autosomal recessive	Rare	Severe

PATHOPHYSIOLOGY OF SELECTED BLOOD DISORDERS

RED CELL DISORDERS

1. IRON DEFICIENCY ANEMIA

Etiology

Iron deficiency anemia is the most common form of anemia. Although in many developing countries dietary deficiency of iron can occur, in developed nations the main cause is loss of iron, almost always through blood loss from the gastrointestinal or genitourinary tracts.

Because of recurrent menstrual blood loss, premenopausal women represent the population with the highest incidence of iron deficiency. The incidence in this group is even higher because of iron losses during pregnancy, since the developing fetus efficiently extracts maternal iron for use in its own hematopoiesis. In men or in postmenopausal women with iron deficiency, gastrointestinal bleeding is usually the cause. Blood loss in this case may be due to relatively benign disorders, such as peptic ulcer, arteriovenous malformations, or angiodysplasia (small vascular abnormalities along the intestinal walls). More serious causes are inflammatory bowel disease or malignancy. Investigation to exclude malignancy is mandatory in such cases.

There are other less frequent causes of iron deficiency, but almost all are related to blood loss: bleeding disorders, hemoptysis, and hemoglobinuria are the chief possibilities.

Pathogenesis

Body iron stores are generally sufficient to last several years, but there is a constant loss of iron in completely healthy persons, such that iron balance depends on adequate intake and absorption. Iron is found predominantly in hemoglobin and is stored in most body cells as **ferritin,** a combination of iron and the protein apoferritin. It is also stored as **hemosiderin,** which is ferritin partly stripped of the apoferritin protein shell. Iron is present also in **myoglobin,** the oxygen-storing protein of skeletal muscle. Lastly, iron is transported in blood bound to its carrier protein **transferrin.** Because of the complex interactions between these molecules, a simple measurement of serum iron rarely reflects body iron stores (see below).

The main role for iron is as the ion in the center of the body's oxygen-carrying molecule, **heme.** Iron, held stably in the ferrous form by the other atoms in heme, reversibly binds oxygen. Each protein subunit of hemoglobin contains one heme molecule; since hemoglobin exists as a tetramer, four iron molecules are needed in each hemoglobin unit. When there is iron deficiency, the final step in heme synthesis is interrupted (Figure 6–6). In this step, ferrous iron is inserted into protoporphyrin IX by the enzyme ferrochelatase; when heme synthesis is interrupted, there is inadequate heme production. Hemoglobin peptide synthesis is closely coupled to heme production, and hemoglobin biosynthesis is therefore inhibited in iron deficiency. This directly causes anemia, a decrease in the hemoglobin concentration of the blood.

As noted above, heme is also required as the oxygen acceptor in myoglobin; therefore, iron deficiency will also lead to decreased myoglobin production. Other proteins also are dependent on iron (Table 6–9), and most of these are enzymes. Many use iron in the heme molecule, but some use elemental iron. Although the exact implications of iron deficiency on their activity is not known, these enzymes are crucial to metabolism, energy production, DNA synthesis, and even brain function.

Pathology

As iron stores are depleted, the peripheral blood smear pattern evolves. In early iron deficiency, the hemoglobin level of the blood falls but individual erythrocytes appear normal. In response to a falling oxygen level, erythropoietin levels rise and stimulate the marrow, though the hemoglobin level cannot rise in response because of the iron deficiency. Other hormones are presumably also stimulated, however, and the resulting "revved-up" marrow usually causes an elevated blood platelet count. An elevated white cell count is less common. Reticulocytes are notably absent.

Eventually, the hemoglobin concentration of individual cells falls, leading to the classic picture of microcytic, hypochromic erythrocytes (Figure 6–4). This is most commonly found as an abnormally low MCV of red cells on the automated hemogram. There is also substantial anisocytosis and poikilocytosis, seen on the peripheral smear, and **target cells** may be seen as well. The target shape occurs because there is a relative excess of red cell membrane compared with the amount of hemoglobin within the cell, so that the membrane "bunches up" in the center.

Laboratory results are often confusing. A low serum ferritin level is diagnostic of iron deficiency, but even in obvious cases levels can be normal. This is because ferritin levels can rise in acute or chronic inflammation or significant illnesses, which can themselves be the cause of iron (blood) loss. Serum iron levels fall in many illnesses, and levels of its serum carrier, transferrin, fluctuate as well; neither is a consistent indicator of iron deficiency. Typically, however, the serum iron falls while the **total iron-binding capacity (TIBC)** of serum rises. The TIBC is mostly transferrin. The ratio of iron to TIBC is less

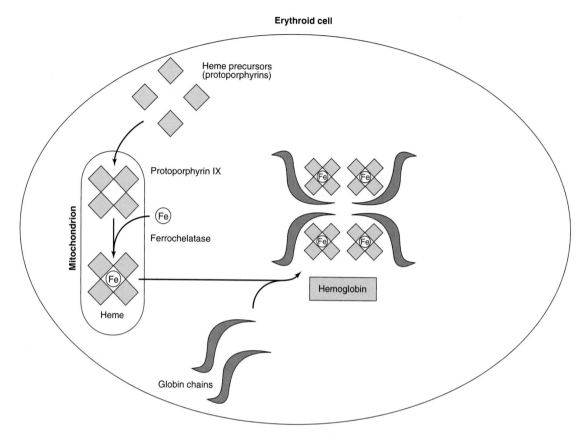

Figure 6–6. Heme synthesis, emphasizing the role of iron and the insertion of heme into individual globin chains to make hemoglobin.

than 20% in uncomplicated iron deficiency; it is higher in normal individuals and in those with other types of anemia. The blood test which is least often obtained but nonetheless suggestive of iron deficiency is the serum free erythrocyte protoporphyrin. Because of the lack of iron in the mitochondrion, the immediate precursor to heme, protoporphyrin IX, accumulates and can be measured in serum.

Other than observing a hematologic response to empiric iron supplementation, bone marrow biopsy is the only way to confirm a diagnosis of iron deficiency. Iron is normally found (as ferritin) in the macrophages of the marrow, where it supplies the erythrocyte precursors and is easily visualized with Prussian blue stain. These macrophages do not stain at all if there is iron deficiency.

Clinical Manifestations

All anemias lead to classic symptoms of decreased oxygen-carrying capacity, ie, fatigue, weakness, and shortness of breath—particularly dyspnea on exertion—and iron deficiency is no exception. Decreased oxygen-carrying capacity leads to decreased oxygen delivery to metabolically active tissues, which nonetheless must have oxygen; this leads directly to fatigue. The compensatory mechanisms of the body lead to additional symptoms and signs of anemia. Some patients appear pale not only because there is less hemoglobin per unit of blood (oxygenated hemo-

Table 6–9. Iron-associated proteins.

Protein	Function
Hemoglobin	Oxygen transport
Myoglobin	Oxygen storage and transport
Ferritin	Iron storage
Transferrin	Iron transport
Hemosiderin	Iron storage
Cytochromes of mitochondria	ATP production (electron transport)
Cytochrome P450	Drug and poison detoxification
Glucose-6-phosphate dehydrogenase	Anaerobic glycolysis
Ribonucleotide reductase	DNA nucleotide synthesis
Catalase	Peroxide metabolism
Monoamine oxidase	Catecholamine metabolism

globin is red and gives color to the skin) but also because superficial skin blood vessels constrict, diverting blood to more vital structures. Patients may also respond to the anemia with tachycardia. This increased cardiac output is appropriate since one way to increase oxygen delivery to the tissues is to increase the number of times each hemoglobin molecule is oxygenated in the lungs every hour. This tachycardia may cause benign cardiac murmurs due to the increased blood flow.

Abnormalities of the gastrointestinal tract occur because iron is also needed for proliferating cells. **Glossitis,** where the normal tongue papillae are absent, can occur, as can gastric atrophy with **achlorhydria** (absence of stomach acid). The achlorhydria may compound the iron deficiency, since iron is best absorbed in an acidic environment, but this complication is quite unusual.

In children, there may be significant developmental problems, both physical and mental. Iron-deficient children, mostly in developing regions, perform poorly on tests of behavior and cognition compared with iron-replete children. Iron therapy can reverse these findings if started early enough in childhood. The exact mechanism of cognitive loss in iron deficiency is not known. Another unexplained but often observed phenomenon in severe iron deficiency is **pica,** a craving for nonnutritive substances such as clay or dirt.

Many patients have no specific symptoms or findings at all, and their iron deficiency is discovered because of anemia noted on a blood count obtained for another purpose. It is of interest that mild anemias (hemoglobins of 11–12 g/dL) may be tolerated very well, since they develop slowly. In addition to the physiologic compensatory mechanisms discussed above (increased cardiac output, diversion of blood flow from less metabolically active areas), there is a biochemical adaptation as well. The ability to transfer oxygen from hemoglobin to cells is partly dependent on a small molecule in erythrocytes called **2,3-diphosphoglycerate (2,3-DPG).** In high concentrations, the ability to "unload" oxygen in the tissues is increased. Chronic anemia leads to elevated 2,3-DPG concentrations in erythrocytes.

Despite the frequency of anemia in iron deficiency, however, many patients do not present with symptoms directly related to the anemia; they present instead with symptoms or signs related directly to blood loss. Since the most common site of unexpected (nonmenstrual) blood loss is the gastrointestinal tract, patients often have visible changes in the stool. There may be gross blood (**hematochezia,** which is more common with bleeding sites near the rectum; or black, tarry, metabolized blood (**melena**) from more proximal sites. Significant blood loss from the urinary tract is very uncommon.

11. What is the most common form of anemia and its most likely cause in a premenopausal woman? In a man?
12. Why is the serum ferritin level often not a good indicator of whether anemia is due to iron deficiency?
13. What are some disorders associated with iron deficiency anemia?
14. What are the physiologic adaptations to slowly developing iron deficiency anemia?

2. PERNICIOUS ANEMIA

Etiology

Pernicious anemia is a megaloblastic anemia in which there is abnormal erythrocyte nuclear maturation. In contrast to many other anemias such as that due to iron deficiency, hemoglobin synthesis is normal. Pernicious anemia is the end result of a cascade of events which are autoimmune in origin. The ultimate effect is a loss of adequate stores of vitamin B_{12} (cobalamin), which is a cofactor involved in DNA synthesis. Rapidly proliferating cells are those most often affected, predominantly bone marrow cells and those of the gastrointestinal epithelium. The nervous system is also affected, demonstrating that this is a systemic disease. Anemia is merely the most common manifestation.

Besides pernicious anemia, cobalamin deficiency can also be due to bacterial overgrowth in the intestine (because bacteria compete with the host for cobalamin), intestinal malabsorption of vitamin B_{12} involving the terminal ileum (such as in Crohn's disease), surgical removal of the antrum of the stomach (gastrectomy), and, rarely, dietary deficiency, which occurs only in strict vegetarians. In the diet, cobalamin is found only in animal products.

Pernicious anemia is most common in older patients of Scandinavian descent but is found in a wide variety of ethnic groups. In the USA, black females are one of the most common groups. Pernicious anemia accounts for only a few percent of patients with anemia, however.

Pathogenesis

The initial events in the pathogenetic cascade begin in the stomach (Figure 6–7). The gastric parietal cells are initially affected by an autoimmune phenomenon that leads to two discrete effects: loss of gastric acid (**achlorhydria**) and loss of **intrinsic factor.** Pernicious anemia interferes with both the initial availability and the absorption of vitamin B_{12}: stomach acid is required for the release of cobalamin from foodstuffs, and intrinsic factor is a glycoprotein that binds cobalamin and is required for the effective absorption of cobalamin in the terminal ileum. Both

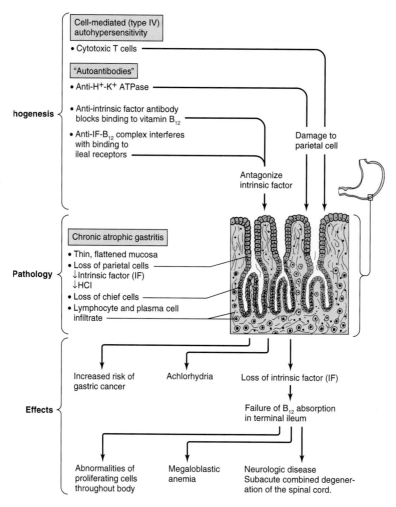

Figure 6–7. Pathogenesis and effects of pernicious anemia (autoimmune atrophic gastritis). (Modified and reproduced, with permission, from Chandrasoma P, Taylor CR: *Concise Pathology,* 3rd ed. Appleton & Lange, 1998.)

stomach acid and intrinsic factor are made exclusively by parietal cells.

Evidence for the autoimmune destruction of parietal cells is strong: Patients with pernicious anemia have atrophy of the gastric mucosa, and pathologic specimens show infiltrating lymphocytes, which are predominantly antibody-producing B cells (see below). In addition, 90% or more of patients have antibodies in their serum directed against parietal cell membrane proteins. The major protein antigen appears to be H^+-K^+ ATPase, or the **proton pump,** which is responsible for the production of stomach acid. More than half of patients also have antibodies to intrinsic factor itself or the intrinsic factor-cobalamin complex. Furthermore, patients with pernicious anemia have a higher incidence of other autoimmune diseases, such as Graves' disease. Lastly, corticosteroid therapy, used as first-line therapy for many autoimmune disorders, may reverse the pathologic findings in pernicious anemia. Despite this evidence, the exact mechanism of the initial inciting event remains unknown.

Complete vitamin B_{12} deficiency develops slowly, even after total achlorhydria and loss of intrinsic factor occur. Liver stores of vitamin B_{12} are adequate for several years. However, the lack of this vitamin eventually leads to alterations in DNA synthesis and, in the nervous system, altered myelin synthesis.

In DNA synthesis, cobalamin, along with folic acid, is crucial as a cofactor in the synthesis of deoxythymidine from deoxyuridine (Figure 6–8). Cobalamin accepts a methyl group from methyltetrahydrofolate, which leads to the formation of two important intracellular compounds. The first is methylcobalamin, which is required for the production of the amino acid methionine from homocys-

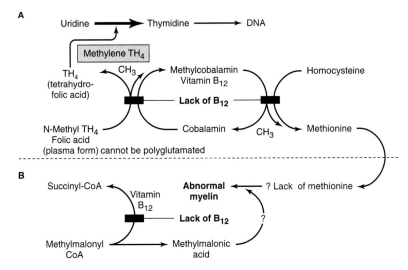

Figure 6–8. Role of cobalamin (vitamin B_{12}) and folic acid in nucleic acid and myelin metabolism. Lack of either cobalamin or folic acid retards DNA synthesis **(A)** and lack of cobalamin leads to loss of folic acid, which cannot be held intracellularly unless polyglutamated. Lack of cobalamin also leads to abnormal myelin synthesis, probably via a deficiency in methionine production **(B)**. (Modified and reproduced, with permission, from Chandrasoma P, Taylor CR: *Concise Pathology,* 3rd ed. Appleton & Lange, 1998.)

teine. The second is reduced tetrahydrofolate, which is required as the single-carbon donor in purine synthesis. Thus, cobalamin deficiency depletes stores of reduced tetrahydrofolate and impairs DNA synthesis because of lowered purine production. In cobalamin deficiency, other reduced folates may substitute for tetrahydrofolate (and may explain why pharmacologic doses of folic acid can partially reverse the megaloblastic blood cell changes—but not the neurologic changes—seen in pernicious anemia). However, methyltetrahydrofolate, normally the methyl donor to cobalamin, accumulates. This folate cannot be retained intracellularly since it cannot be **polyglutamated** (the addition of multiple glutamate residues leads to a charged compound that does not freely diffuse out of the cell). Therefore, there is relative folate deficiency in pernicious anemia as well. In addition, methionine may serve as a principal donor of methyl groups to these other "substituting" reduced folates; since methionine cannot be produced in cobalamin deficiency, this compounds the problems in purine synthesis.

The lack of methionine is also partly responsible for the neurologic effects (see below) of pernicious anemia. The exact mechanism of its role in **demyelination** (loss of the myelin sheaths around nerves) is not known, but the association seems clear, since hereditary defects in methionine synthesis or inactivation of methionine synthase by nitric oxide poisoning both lead to neuropathy.

The production of succinyl-CoA is also dependent on the presence of cobalamin. It is not clear whether a decrease in the production of succinyl-CoA, which may affect fatty acid synthesis, is also involved in the demyelinating disease.

Pathology

The gastric disorders associated with pernicious anemia are dominated by the picture of **chronic atrophic gastritis** (Figure 6–7). The normally tall columnar epithelium is replaced by a very thin mucosa, and there is obvious infiltration of plasma cells and lymphocytes. Pernicious anemia also increases the risk for gastric adenocarcinoma. Thus, pathologic examination may also reveal cancer.

The peripheral blood smear picture (Figure 6–5) varies, depending on the length of time the patient has been cobalamin-deficient. In early stages, patients may have mild macrocytic anemia, and large ovoid erythrocytes **(macro-ovalocytes)** are commonly seen. In full-blown megaloblastic anemia, however, there are abnormalities in all cell lines. The classic picture reveals significant anisocytosis and poikilocytosis of the red cell line, and there are hypersegmented neutrophils, revealing the nuclear dysgenesis from abnormal DNA synthesis (Figure 6–9). In severe cases of pernicious anemia, the red and white cell series are easily mistaken for acute leukemia because the cells look so atypical.

The bone marrow, however, is less suggestive of acute leukemia, and megaloblastic changes—nuclei that are too large and immature in cells with mature, hemoglobin-filled cytoplasm—are seen at each stage of erythrocyte development. These cells are not seen

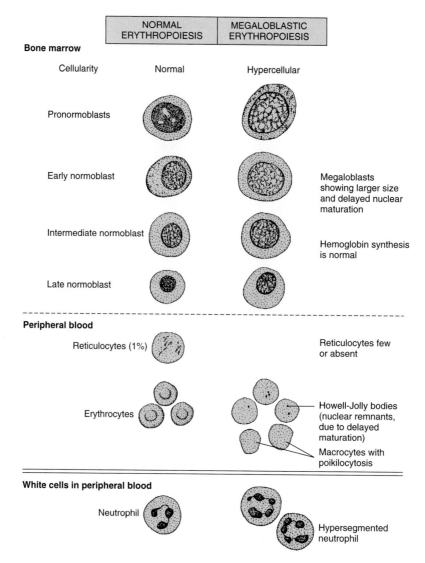

Figure 6–9. Megaloblastic hematopoiesis: morphologic changes visible with microscopic examination of bone marrow or peripheral blood. (Reproduced, with permission, from Chandrasoma P, Taylor CR: *Concise Pathology,* 3rd ed. Appleton & Lange, 1998.)

in the peripheral blood because the abnormal erythrocytes generally are destroyed in the marrow (**intramedullary hemolysis**) by unexplained processes. This compounds the anemia. Megaloblastic changes can be seen in the marrow even in the absence of obvious changes on the peripheral blood smear.

Spinal cord abnormalities—generally not visualized during life, of course—consist of demyelination of the posterolateral spinal columns, called **subacute combined degeneration.** Peripheral nerves may also show demyelination. Demyelination eventually results in neuronal cell death, which is also obvious on pathologic examination. Since neurons do not divide, new neurons cannot replace the dead ones.

Laboratory findings include elevated lactate dehydrogenase (LDH) and, sometimes, indirect bilirubin fraction consistent with the hemolysis occurring in the bone marrow. LDH is directly released from lysed red cells, and free hemoglobin is metabolized to bilirubin. Serum vitamin B_{12} levels are abnormally low, revealing the deficient state. The Schilling test, which assesses the oral absorption of radioactively labeled vitamin B_{12} with and without added intrinsic factor, must be done after cobalamin stores are repleted. This directly evaluates the mechanism of the vitamin B_{12} deficiency.

Clinical Manifestations

The clinical presentation consists of one or more symptoms related to the underlying deficiency. Anemia is the most commonly encountered abnormality and is often very severe; hemoglobin levels of 4 g/dL (less than a third of normal) can be seen. This degree of anemia is rare with other causes, such as iron deficiency. Typical symptoms are fatigue, dyspnea, or dizziness, since a decreased red cell mass equals decreased oxygen-carrying capacity of the blood. "High-output" congestive heart failure is relatively common, with tachycardia and signs of left ventricular failure (Chapter 10). Since oxygen demands are constant (or rise with exercise) and oxygen-carrying capacity is falling, the only way to maintain tissue oxygenation in anemia is to increase cardiac output, ie, the number of times per minute each red cell is fully oxygenated by the lungs. Eventually, however, the left ventricle cannot pump the amount of blood being returned to it from the body—this is heart failure.

However, symptoms may be mild, since the anemia occurs slowly due to the extensive liver storage of vitamin B_{12}. Patients with anemia usually adapt over time to slow changes in oxygen-carrying capacity. The same changes in 2,3-DPG that encourage oxygen delivery to the tissues from the hemoglobin in red cells in other anemias occur in vitamin B_{12} deficiency as well.

Gastrointestinal symptoms are less prevalent and include malabsorption, muscle wasting (unusual), diarrhea (more common) due to megaloblastic changes in the gut epithelium, and **glossitis** (most common). In glossitis, the normal tongue papillae are absent, no matter whether the tongue is painful, red and "beefy," or pale and smooth.

Neurologic symptoms are least likely to improve with cobalamin replacement therapy. Like other neuropathies involving loss of myelin from large peripheral sensory nerves, numbness and tingling (**paresthesias**) occur frequently and are the most common symptoms. Demyelination and neuronal cell death in the posterolateral "long tracts" of the spinal cord interfere with delivery of positional information to the brainstem, cerebellum, and sensory cortex. Patients therefore complain of loss of balance and coordination. Examination reveals impaired **proprioception** (position sense) and vibration sense. True dementia may also occur when demyelination involves the brain. Importantly but somewhat unexpectedly, neurologic symptoms may occur in the absence of any changes in the peripheral blood smear suggestive of pernicious anemia.

15. Name two crucial cofactors in DNA synthesis whose deficiency results in pernicious anemia. In what specific biochemical pathways do they participate?
16. Why are neurologic defects observed in prolonged pernicious anemia?
17. Why are symptoms of pernicious anemia usually relatively mild?
18. Are changes in the peripheral blood smear necessary for neurologic effects of vitamin B_{12} deficiency?

WHITE CELL DISORDERS

1. MALIGNANT DISORDERS

The most important leukocyte abnormalities are the malignant disorders leukemia and lymphoma. They are discussed in Chapter 5.

2. CYCLIC NEUTROPENIA

Neutropenia, characterized by neutrophil counts under 1500–2000/μL (> 2 SD below the mean in normals) is a commonly encountered problem in medicine and can be due to a large number of disease entities (Table 6–5).

Etiology

Cyclic neutropenia, however, is quite rare. It is of interest because it provides insight into normal neutrophil production and function. It is characterized by a lifetime history of neutrophil counts that decrease to zero or near zero for 3–5 days at a time every 3 weeks, then rebound.

The exact cause of cyclic neutropenia is unknown, and barely more than 100 cases have been reported in the literature. There does not seem to be a racial predilection or gender bias in incidence, but the disorder is usually diagnosed in children or adolescents. There is no specific genetic predisposition, but up to one-third of patients have affected first-degree relatives.

Pathogenesis

The neutrophil count in blood is stable in normal individuals, reflecting the fact that there is a large storage pool of these granulocytes in the marrow. This large pool is necessary because it takes nearly 2 weeks for the full development of a neutrophil from an early stem cell within the bone marrow, yet the average life span of a mature neutrophil in blood is less than 12 hours.

In cyclic neutropenia, the storage pool is not adequate. Daily measurements of neutrophil counts in

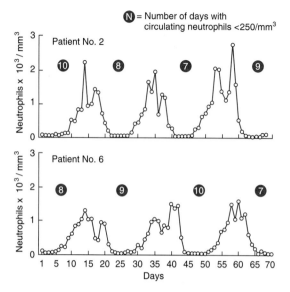

Figure 6–10. Daily blood neutrophil counts in two patients with cyclic neutropenia. All samples were obtained between 7 AM and 8 AM each day. (Reproduced, with permission, from Wright DG et al: Human cyclic neutropenia. Medicine 1981;60:1.)

the blood reveal striking variations in their number (Figure 6–10). Studies of neutrophil kinetics in affected patients reveal that the defect is in the abnormal production—rather than abnormal disposition—of neutrophils. Neutrophil production occurs in discrete waves, with trough production inadequate to maintain the normal reserve. However, the neutrophils appear to have a normal life span once they are extruded from the marrow.

The exact cause of the cyclic waves of maturation is not known, but the waves are remarkably constant in their periodicity. Almost every patient has a cycle between 19 and 22 days, and each patient's cycle length is constant during their lifetime. Neutrophils are not the only marrow elements that cycle, however, despite the name of the disorder. Platelet and reticulocyte counts also cycle with the same cycle length as the neutrophils; in contrast to the blood neutrophil count, however, clinically significant decreases are not observed. This is presumably because the blood life spans of these elements are so much longer than the life span of neutrophils.

Because multiple cell lines are seen to cycle, it is felt that there is either a defect in an early progenitor cell type or a defect in some cytokine or cytokines required for adequate marrow development. A defect in early cell progenitors is favored, because when stem cells were used in a bone marrow transplant from an affected individual to her sister with leukemia, the recipient developed cyclic neutropenia after marrow engraftment. The exact abnormality is still unknown, but there is a decreased responsiveness to the colony-stimulating factors G-CSF and GM-CSF when bone marrow cells from these individuals are placed in culture, while responsiveness to another important cytokine, interleukin-3, is maintained. This suggests that the underlying cause of cyclic neutropenia is a defect in either growth factor receptor binding or receptor activity.

Clinical support for this model comes from observations that administration of pharmacologic doses of G-CSF (filgrastim) to affected individuals had three interesting effects which partially overcame the problem. The first was that although cycling continued, mean neutrophil counts increased at each point in the cycle, such that patients were rarely neutropenic. The second was that the cycling periodicity decreased immediately from 21 days to 14 days. The third was that the other cell line fluctuations changed in parallel; their cycle periodicity also decreased to 14 days, suggesting that an early progenitor cell is indeed at the center of this illness. However, the fact that the cycling did not disappear demonstrates that there are other abnormalities yet to be discovered. It also suggests that there may be an inherent cycling of all stem cells in normal individuals which is modulated by multiple cytokines in the marrow.

Pathology

The pathologic features of cyclic neutropenia are seen mostly in the laboratory. The peripheral blood smear appears normal except for the paucity of neutrophils—mature or immature—during the nadirs of each cycle. Individual neutrophils appear normal. The bone marrow, however, shows striking differences depending on the day of the cycle on which it is examined. During the nadir of each cycle, there are increased numbers of early myeloid precursors such as promyelocytes and myelocytes, and mature neutrophils are rare. This picture is similar to that seen in acute leukemia, but 10 days later, as circulating neutrophil counts are rising, an entirely normal-appearing marrow is typical.

Clinical Manifestations

In general, neutropenia from any cause places patients at risk for severe bacterial infections, generally from enteric organisms, due to the alteration in host defenses in the gastrointestinal tract. Neutrophils, with their ability to engulf bacteria and deliver toxic enzymes and oxidizing free radicals to sites of infection, normally serve as the first line of host defenses against the bacteria that inhabit the gut. Such patients are also at risk for fungal infections if the neutropenia lasts more than several days—this is because it takes longer for fungi to reproduce and invade the bloodstream. Untreated infections of either type can be rapidly fatal, particularly if the neutrophil count is less than about 250/μL.

In cyclic neutropenia, then, recurrent infections

are to be expected, and deaths due to infections with intestinal organisms have been reported. Each cycle is characterized by malaise and fever coincident with the time neutrophil counts are falling. Cervical lymphadenopathy is almost always present, as well as oral ulcers. These symptoms usually last for about 5 days, then subside until the next cycle.

When infections occur, the site is usually predictable. Skin infections—specifically, small superficial pyogenic abscesses (**furunculosis**) or bacterial invasion of the dermis or epidermis (**cellulitis**)—are the most common and respond to antibiotic therapy with few sequelae. The next most common infection site is usually the gums, and chronic gingivitis is evident in about half of patients. It is also the most noticeably improved problem when patients receive therapy with filgrastim. Other infections are unusual, but, as noted above, any neutropenic patient is at risk for infection from organisms that reside in the gastrointestinal system. In the few patients who have required abdominal surgery during their neutropenia, ulcers similar to those seen in the mouth have been noted; this destruction of the normal mucosal barrier presumably eases entry of intestinal bacteria into the bloodstream. Because the period of greatest susceptibility to infection is only a few days in each cycle, most patients grow and develop normally.

> 19. How long does it take for a neutrophil to develop from a stem cell in the bone marrow? Once fully mature, what is its life span?
> 20. At what level of neutropenia does the incidence of infection dramatically increase?
> 21. What are the most common sites and types of infections observed in neutropenic patients?
> 22. What is the probable underlying abnormality in cyclic neutropenia?

PLATELET DISORDERS

1. DRUG-ASSOCIATED IMMUNE THROMBOCYTOPENIA

Etiology

Thrombocytopenia, defined as the occurrence of platelet levels below the normal laboratory range, is a commonly encountered blood count abnormality. Although there are many causes (Table 6–7), the possibility of a drug-induced immune thrombocytopenia needs to be considered in nearly every case.

Many drugs have been associated with this phenomenon, and the most common ones are listed in Table 6–10. There are no shared specific properties. In practice, the association between a given drug and thrombocytopenia is usually made clinically rather

Table 6–10. Common drugs that may cause thrombocytopenia.

Acetaminophen	Interferon-alpha
Acetazolamide	Iodinated contrast agents
Allopurinal	Methyldopa
Amiodarone	Nonsteroidal antiinflammatory drugs
Aspirin	Penicillins
Captopril	Phenothiazines
Carbamazepine	Phenytoin
Chlorothiazide	Procainamide
Chlorthalidone	Quinidine
Cimetidine	Quinine
Danazol	Ranitidine
Digoxin	Rifampin
Fluconazole	Sulfonamides (antibiotics and hypoglycemics)
Furosemide	
Gold salts	Valproic Acid
Heparin	Vancomycin
Hydrochlorothiazide	

than with specific tests; a suspect drug is stopped, and platelet counts rebound within a few days. Rechallenge with the drug, which is rarely done, almost always reproduces the thrombocytopenia.

Because of its frequent use in hospitalized patients and because its use requires frequent blood count monitoring, heparin is the most important cause of thrombocytopenia. The pathophysiology of heparin-induced thrombocytopenia is thus also the most completely described. Between 1% and 5% of patients treated with heparin will develop thrombocytopenia, though fewer have clinically significant complications.

Pathogenesis

Although the phenomenon of drug-induced thrombocytopenia has been known for decades to be immune in nature, the specific mechanisms have long been controversial. Antibodies are clearly involved, and the association of antibodies with platelets leads to their destruction usually because the platelets are recognized as being abnormal in the spleen because of shape changes due to antibody being bound to them. The spleen acts as the major "blood filter" and removes abnormal platelets as well as erythrocytes.

In the laboratory, the antibodies require the presence of the drug to bind to the platelets, suggesting that the drug binds to some platelet component, making the new combination antigenic; the antibody would thus bind to this combination. However, some antibody binding to platelets cannot be "competitively inhibited" by excess amounts of free drug in the test tube. This suggests that some antibodies are formed which bind to platelets not by their antigen-specific Fab fragments but rather by their common Fc portions; Fc receptors are definitely present on platelets.

For heparin, there is clear evidence of binding to a platelet protein, platelet factor 4 (PF4), which resides in the alpha granules of platelets and is released when they are activated. It binds back onto the platelet surface through a specific PF4 receptor molecule, further increasing platelet activation. It also binds with high affinity to heparin and to heparin-like glycosaminoglycan molecules present on the vascular endothelium. It is now known that the combination of heparin with PF4 is the antigenic stimulus which provokes the production of IgG, directed against the combination.

These antibodies occur in nearly 5% of patients treated with heparin; in about half of these patients, the IgG is clinically relevant and leads to thrombocytopenia. In most of the thrombocytopenic patients, the IgG binds to the heparin-PF4 complex in the blood, with PF4 having been previously released either by heparin itself (a weak platelet-aggregating agent on its own) or by other stimuli. This new complex (IgG-heparin-PF4) can bind to platelets through either the platelet Fc receptor (which would bind the IgG end) or the PF4 receptor (Figure 6–11). This binding can lead to one of two phenomena: platelet destruction by the spleen or platelet activation and consumption.

The first of these two phenomena leads to thrombocytopenia alone, and platelet counts fall with few sequelae. The second phenomenon, however, has more interesting clinical implications. Since each end of this IgG-heparin-PF4 molecule can bind to a platelet, it is possible that platelets can become "cross-linked" by a single molecule. One platelet would be bound via the Fc receptor-IgG interaction,

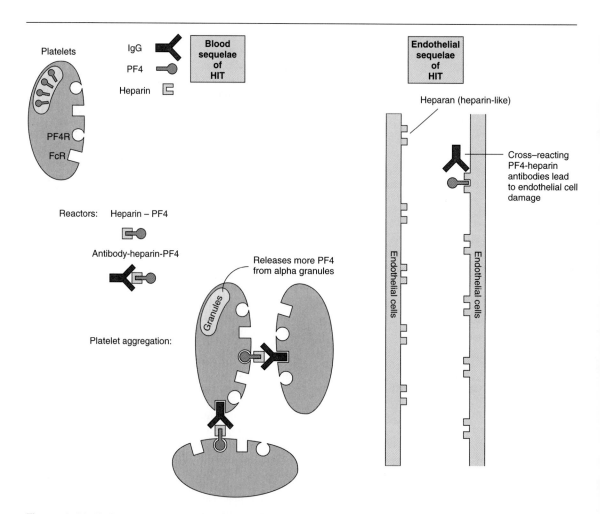

Figure 6–11. Pathogenesis of heparin-induced thrombocytopenia. IgG is the autoantibody against the heparin-PF4 complex. Platelets can bind to each other and become activated via either the IgG-Fc receptor interaction, or the PF4-PF4 receptor interaction, or both. Aggregation and thrombus formation may thus occur. Furthermore, IgG may bind to endothelial cell bound heparan-PF4 construct and cause vascular damage, which may also provoke thrombus formation.

another by the PF4-PF4 receptor interaction. Many platelets could actually interact in this fashion, leading to platelet aggregation and, as a result, platelet activation. Clinically, this decreases the numbers of circulating platelets causing thrombocytopenia, but it may also lead to creation of a thrombus at the site of activation. Thus, despite the fact that heparin is the most commonly used anticoagulant, in this case it may actually provoke coagulation. Furthermore, the activation of platelets via this mechanism leads to increased amounts of circulating PF4, which can bind to more heparin and continue the cycle. The excess PF4 can also bind to the endothelial surface via the heparin-like glycosaminoglycans described earlier. It is thus possible that the antibodies to the heparin-PF4 construct could bind to the endothelial cells as well, which may lead to endothelial cell injury, further increasing the risk of local thrombosis by generating tissue factor and ultimately thrombin. This syndrome is called **heparin-induced thrombocytopenia and thrombosis.**

Pathology

The peripheral blood smear is not strikingly abnormal unless platelet counts are under about 75,000/µL, and then it is usually only abnormal because relatively few platelets are seen. Platelet morphology, however, is usually normal, though large platelets can be seen. These large platelets are less mature and are a bone marrow compensation for a low peripheral platelet count, with platelet production from megakaryocytes being increased. Although drugs—heparin in particular—may cause platelet aggregation in vivo and in vitro, this is usually not apparent on review of the blood smear.

The bone marrow usually appears normal, though the megakaryocyte number may be relatively increased, presumably reflecting an attempt to increase the number of platelets (megakaryocyte fragments) in the circulation. In a few cases of immune-mediated thrombocytopenia, however, there may be decreased numbers of megakaryocytes. There are many hypotheses as to why this may occur, but it most likely means that the antigenic combination of drug-platelet protein is also occurring on megakaryocytes, so that they as well as the platelets in the peripheral circulation are being immunologically destroyed; this destruction would not involve the spleen, of course, but would require antibody-dependent cell killing instead.

In the patients who develop heparin-induced thrombocytopenia and thrombosis, thrombi are seen which are relatively rich in platelets when compared with "typical" thrombi seen in other situations. They are described as "white clots." In addition, the thrombi are more likely to be arterial, whereas most "typical" clots are in deep veins (see below).

Clinical Manifestations

Despite the fact that the platelet count in immune-mediated thrombocytopenia can be extremely low (< 10,000/µL, compared with a normal value of over 150,000/µL), significant bleeding is unusual. More often there is easy bruising with minimal trauma. With platelet counts under about 5000/µL, pinpoint hemorrhages (**petechiae**) may spontaneously occur in the skin or mucous membranes. These are self-limited because the plasma coagulation factors are still intact, and only a small number of aggregated platelets are needed to provide adequate phospholipid for the clotting cascade to proceed.

The relationship between the likelihood of bleeding and the platelet count is clearly not linear. The test used clinically to evaluate platelet function, the **bleeding time,** does not even begin to be prolonged (and thus become abnormal) until the platelet count is less than 90,000/µL. Spontaneous bleeding is unlikely until platelet counts are under 20,000/µL but is still uncommon until counts are under about 5000/µL. This assumes that patients do not have other abnormalities of hemostasis, which is not always true. For example, aspirin inhibits platelet aggregation and increases the likelihood of bleeding. When bleeding due to thrombocytopenia does occur, it is most often mucosal or superficial in the skin. This is most commonly seen as a nosebleed (epistaxis), but bleeding of the gums, gastrointestinal tract, or even from the bladder mucosa may be seen.

As mentioned above, however, when immune thrombocytopenia occurs due to heparin, a paradoxic clotting may occur instead of bleeding. This may cause a very confusing picture, since the heparin may have been given therapeutically for another thrombosis; it may be difficult to know if the new thrombosis is an extension of the initial clot or a new one referable to the heparin. However, the occurrence of the simultaneous thrombocytopenia provides a clue.

When heparin-induced thrombocytopenia and thrombosis does occur, the clinical manifestation of the new thrombosis will depend on the site of the thrombus. Most studies of this disorder suggest that when thrombosis occurs, it is at the site of previous vascular injury or abnormality. Thus, in patients with atherosclerotic vascular disease, arterial thromboses are much more common than in any other thrombotic disorder. Patients have the rapid onset of severe pain, usually in an extremity, with a cool, pale limb. Pulses are absent. This can be life-threatening or at least extremity-threatening, because oxygen flow to the affected area is cut off, and emergency clot removal or vascular bypass surgery may be necessary. Venous clots also occur in a manner similar to "typical" venous clots (see below).

23. What is the most common category of cause of thrombocytopenia?
24. Antibodies to which platelet protein are implicated in the pathogenesis of heparin-induced thrombocytopenia?
25. By what mechanism can heparin-induced thrombocytopenia actually increase clot formation?
26. Why is major bleeding unusual in drug-induced thrombocytopenia?

COAGULATION DISORDERS

1. THE INHERITED HYPERCOAGULABLE STATES

Etiology

The formation of blood clots in otherwise normal vessels is distinctly abnormal because the coagulation system in mammalian species is both positively and negatively balanced by so many factors. Nonetheless, there are a number of diseases that result in abnormal clotting (**thrombosis**). Abnormal clotting states may be either primary, in that the abnormalities are due to genetic predispositions involving the coagulation factors themselves, or secondary—ie, acquired, due to changes in coagulation factors, blood vessels, or blood flow.

As first noted by the pathologist Virchow over 150 years ago, there are three possible contributors to formation of an abnormal clot (thrombus): decreased blood flow, vessel injury or inflammation at the site, and changes in the intrinsic properties of the blood. Persistent physiologic changes in any of these three factors ("Virchow's triad") are referred to as the "hypercoagulable states."

The primary, or inherited, hypercoagulable states are all autosomal dominant genetic defects. This means that carriers (heterozygotes) are affected. Except for hyperprothrombinemia, all lead to only moderate (50%) decreases in the levels of these factors. Despite the relatively modest fall, affected individuals are predisposed to abnormal thrombosis. These disorders are relatively rare in the general population, but they do account for a significant percentage of young patients who come to medical attention with thromboses. The specific states to be discussed are activated protein C resistance (the most commonly encountered abnormality), protein C deficiency, protein S deficiency, antithrombin III deficiency, and the prothrombin 20210 AG abnormality.

Pathogenesis

In the coagulation cascade, activated factor V (Va) plays a pivotal role (Figure 6–12). It is required for significant activation of factor X (to Xa), which is

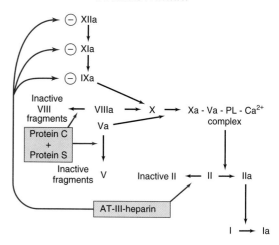

Figure 6–12. Central role of factor V in the control of the coagulation cascade, and action of each of the negative control factors (in brown) protein S, protein C, and antithrombin III.

the central factor involved in the entire cascade. Both the intrinsic and extrinsic pathways converge to activate this factor, which subsequently leads to thrombus formation. Factor Va thus makes an excellent negative control point, so that once clot formation has begun, it does not go on unchecked. Utterly unchecked coagulation throughout the circulatory system would be incompatible with life.

Protein C is the major inhibitor of factor Va. Although it is thus an anticoagulation factor, its production is contingent on vitamin K-dependent γ-carboxylation, just like the coagulation factors II, VII, IX, and X. Protein C, when activated by the presence of clotting that generates thrombin, cleaves factor Va into an inactive form, and activation of factor X is thus slowed. By itself, however, protein C only weakly influences factor Va; its negative effect on factor Va is enhanced by a protein cofactor, protein S.

Factor V does not provide the only negative control point, however. Protein C also inhibits activated factor VIII (VIIIa), and factors II, IX, X, XI, and XII (the serine proteases) are inhibited by a different molecule, antithrombin III (AT-III). AT-III's action itself is also regulated and is highly dependent on the binding of an accelerator, heparin, or similar molecules that are in present in abundance along the endothelial cells which line the vasculature.

The fact that deficiencies of protein S, C, and antithrombin III activity cause clinically significant thrombosis demonstrates an important concept: It is the lack of adequate *anticoagulant* activity rather than the overproduction of *procoagulant* activity that characterizes most of the hypercoagulable states.

A. Activated Protein C Resistance: Activated protein C resistance is the most common inherited hypercoagulable state, with as many as 2–5% of the general population heterozygous for the abnormality. It is due to a single DNA base pair mutation in the factor V gene, where guanine (G) is replaced by adenine (A). This single base change leads to substitution of the amino acid glutamine for arginine at position 506, and the altered factor V is referred to as "factor V Leiden," named for the town in the Netherlands where it was discovered. This amino acid change alters the three-dimensional conformation of the cleavage site within factor Va, where activated protein C normally binds to inactivate it. Thus, factor Va molecules can continue to enhance factor Xa's conversion of prothrombin to thrombin (factor IIa), and coagulation is not inhibited.

B. Protein C Deficiency: Protein C deficiency is probably very common, with up to 1:200 individuals in the population being heterozygotes. As noted above, protein C inactivates factors Va and VIIIa but requires protein S for its own action. Protein C is also dependent on the presence of platelet phospholipid and calcium. In protein C deficiency, both the intrinsic and the extrinsic coagulation cascades can activate factor X, and subsequently thrombin, leading to relatively unrestricted clot formation. Normally, some of the thrombin generated in the cascade binds to an endothelial cell protein, thrombomodulin, and this complex activates protein C in the first place. This "negative feedback loop" is thus lost in protein C deficiency.

Protein C deficiency is not all one disease, however, unlike the factor V Leiden abnormality discussed above. Both quantitative and qualitative abnormalities are found in different families.

C. Protein S Deficiency: Protein S deficiency is also an uncommon heterogeneous disorder. Abnormal quantities of a normal protein S are most frequently encountered, but abnormalities in protein S structure also exist. In the coagulation cascade, when factors Va and Xa are complexed together, the inactivation site on factor Va is "hidden" from protein C. Protein S, not a protease itself, exposes this site so that protein C can cleave Va. Since protein S is so crucial, deficiency of protein S also leads to the unregulated procoagulant action of factor Xa.

D. Antithrombin III Deficiency: Antithrombin III (AT-III) deficiency is less common than any of the above disorders, with a prevalence of one in several thousand. AT-III binds to and inhibits not just thrombin (whence its name) but also the activated forms of factors IX, X, XI, and XII. Unlike protein C's proteolytic cleavage of factor Va, AT-III binds to each factor, directly blocking their activity; it is not an enzyme. This action is accelerated—up to 2000 times—in a reversible manner by the anticoagulant molecule heparin. In AT-III deficiency, then, multiple coagulation steps are unbalanced, and the coagulation cascade may proceed unrestrained. As in protein S and protein C deficiencies, there may be either a quantitative or a qualitative defect in AT-III in a particular family, leading to the same clinical syndrome.

E. Hyperprothrombinemia: A mutation in the untranslated region of the prothrombin gene (a single base pair mutation, called 20210 AG) is associated with elevated plasma prothrombin levels and an increased risk of thrombosis. Presumably, this leads to excess thrombin generation when the Xa-Va-PL-Ca^{2+} complex is activated. This is probably the second-most common hereditary hypercoagulable state after factor V Leiden. It is the first hereditary thrombophilia associated with overproduction of procoagulant factors.

Pathology

The pathologic features of thrombi in hypercoagulable states are indistinguishable from those of genetically normal individuals on a gross anatomic or microscopic basis, except that there is a greater likelihood in hypercoagulable states of having clot in unusual sites. (See Clinical Manifestations, below.)

Most of the pathologic features of the hereditary hypercoagulable states consist of laboratory abnormalities, and findings depend on which laboratory tests are requested. In the evaluation of patients suspected of having a hereditary hypercoagulable state, there are two basic types of laboratory abnormalities. The first type is quantitative: Specific immunologic assays can define the relative amount of protein C, protein S, antithrombin III, or fibrinogen present in a given patient's serum, but they do not evaluate the function of any of these molecules. The second type is qualitative: The assays for protein C or protein S activity (rather than amount) measure the ability (or inability) of the patient's protein C or S to prolong a clotting time in vitro. Activated protein C resistance can be evaluated with a different clotting assay, but generally the presence of the specific mutation in factor V Leiden is assessed by the polymerase chain reaction, since the full sequence of the molecule is known. The polymerase chain reaction is also used for detecting the 20210 AG prothrombin abnormality. Prothrombin levels can also be measured and are consistently in the highest quartile of prothrombin levels found.

Clinical Manifestations

Most thromboembolic events encountered in clinical practice are secondary, not primary. Patients have blood clots usually in the deep veins of the legs for two reasons: (1) because of sluggish blood flow (in high-capacity, low-flow veins) compared with other sites, particularly when inactive (bedridden after surgery or due to illness); and (2) because the extremities are more likely to sustain injury than the trunk. Trauma causes blood vessel compression or injury; thus, two elements of Virchow's triad are more readily observed in the legs than elsewhere.

These venous clots in the legs (commonly referred to as deep venous thromboses, or DVTs) usually present with pain, swelling, and redness below the level of the thrombus, with normal arterial pulses and distal extremity perfusion. Because blood return to the central circulation is blocked in these high-capacity vessels, superficial collateral veins just under the skin may be prominent and engorged. The swelling is mechanical, since normal arterial blood flow continues to the extremity while venous return is compromised, leading to engorgement. Pain occurs primarily as a result of the swelling alone but can also occur from lactic acid buildup in the muscles of the legs. This happens when the pressure in the legs increases to the point that it compromises arterial blood flow and adequate oxygen delivery to those muscles.

Pulmonary emboli, the major source of morbidity and mortality after DVT of the lower extremity, typically present with acute-onset shortness of breath, hypoxemia, and a history suggesting an initial DVT that has now broken off and migrated through the right side of the heart to the pulmonary arterial system. The presence of the clot blocks blood flow from the heart to a portion of lung; thus, the blood returning from the lung to the heart is not fully oxygenated. The degree of hypoxemia depends on how much of the blood flow is blocked and whether the patient has any underlying lung disease.

The clinical presentations of all of the hypercoagulable states are similar, but there are some interesting differences. DVTs tend to occur (whether there is a hypercoagulable state or not) in patients with a history of trauma, pregnancy, oral contraceptive use, or immobility, but rarely in adolescents or young adults. The inherited hypercoagulable states are suspected in patients who present with a thromboembolic event, usually because they are young or have recurrent clots. Events that occur without any specific risks, of course, are particularly suspect. Because of the dominant pattern of inheritance, suspicion is aroused when other family members have had clotting problems, and this underscores the importance of taking a family history.

Despite the distinct coagulation abnormalities, most thromboses still occur in "usual" sites, ie, the deep veins of the legs with or without pulmonary embolism. Other unusual sites, however, are much more likely than in patients without underlying coagulation disorders, such as the sagittal sinus of the skull or the mesenteric veins in the abdomen. The propensity for clotting notwithstanding, arterial thromboses are extremely rare.

Interestingly, not all patients—probably not even a majority—with an inherited hypercoagulable state develop symptomatic thromboses; this is particularly true for heterozygotes. Each disorder is slightly different, presumably because of the redundancy of the factors in the coagulation cascade, and the penetrance of each state probably varies in individual patients because of other factors we do not yet understand. For this reason, many patients will come to medical attention with a clot in a "usual" spot with a "typical" risk factor: sustaining an injury, having an extremity immobilized, having surgery, or being pregnant.

Homozygous protein C or protein S deficiencies appear to have the highest likelihood of causing illness. Both of these conditions usually result in thrombosis which is often fatal in early life (neonatal purpura fulminans), though some patients may not present until their teens even with these profound defects. Heterozygotes for protein C deficiency are actually unlikely to develop a thrombosis over their lifetimes, though they are about six times more likely to do so than members of the general population. A similar propensity is true for the heterozygous protein S state.

Antithrombin III deficiency is the next most significant defect in terms of the likelihood of developing thrombosis; there is about an 85% lifetime risk of developing a clot with this abnormality even for heterozygotes.

The situation is also complex in the case of activated protein C resistance. Presumably, since proteins C and S can still cleave factor VIIIa and the factor V abnormality is a relative rather than absolute insensitivity to activated protein C, there is still negative control of the clotting cascade at the factor X step.

Heterozygotes for activated protein C resistance probably represent more than a third of all patients with familial thromboses. An individual's risk of developing a clot, however, is lower than with protein S or protein C deficiency. It is about five times higher than in an unaffected person.

Even homozygous factor V Leiden does not inevitably cause thrombosis. Families have been carefully described where homozygous females have had repeated pregnancies without difficulty. This is somewhat surprising since pregnancy, a hypercoagulable state itself, leads to decreases in protein S concentration, which would be expected to amplify the resistance to protein C. Nevertheless, case-control studies suggest at least a 30-fold increased risk of thrombosis versus the general population for homozygotes for factor V Leiden.

Persons with the prothrombin 20210 AG mutation are nearly all heterozygotes, with about a threefold higher risk of thrombosis than the general population.

---

27. What constitutes "Virchow's triad" of factors predisposing to formation of intravascular clots?
28. Deficiencies in what proteins can result in clinically significant thromboses?
29. What is the basis for activated protein C resistance?

REFERENCES

General Hematology
Beutler E, Williams W: *Williams Hematology*, 5th ed. McGraw-Hill, 1995.

Colman RW et al: *Hemostasis and Thrombosis: Basic Principles and Clinical Practice*, 3rd ed. Lippincott, 1993.

Hoffman R et al: *Hematology: Basic Principles and Practice*, 2nd ed. Churchill Livingstone, 1995.

Iron-Deficiency Anemia
Newton W: Laboratory diagnosis of iron deficiency anemia. J Fam Pract 1995;41:404.

Scrimshaw NS: Iron deficiency. Sci Am 1991;265:46.

Pernicious Anemia
Burman P et al: H^+,K^+-ATPase antibodies in autoimmune gastritis: Observations on the development of pernicious anemia. Scand J Gastroenterol 1991;26:207.

Healton EB et al: Neurologic aspects of cobalamin deficiency. Medicine 1991;70:229.

Pruthi RK, Tefferi A: Pernicious anemia revisited. Mayo Clinic Proc 1994;69:144.

Toh B-H et al: Pernicious anemia. N Engl J Med 1997;337:1441.

Welte K, Boxer LA: Severe chronic neutropenia: Pathophysiology and therapy. Semin Hematol 1997;34:267.

Cyclic Neutropenia
Hammond WP et al: Treatment of cyclic neutropenia with granulocyte colony-stimulating factor. N Engl J Med 1989;320:1306.

Hammond WP et al: Abnormal responsiveness of granulocyte-committed progenitor cells in cyclic neutropenia. Blood 1992;79:2536.

Welte K, Boxer LA: Severe chronic neutropenia: Pathophysiology and therapy. Semin Hematol 1997;34:267.

Wright DG et al: Human cyclic neutropenia: Clinical review and long-term follow-up of patients. Medicine 1981;60:1.

Drug-Induced Thrombocytopenia
Amiral J et al: Antibodies to macromolecular platelet factor 4. Heparin complexes in heparin-induced thrombocytopenia: A study of 44 cases. Thromb Haemost 1995;73:21.

Brieger DB: Heparin-induced thrombocytopenia. J Am Coll Cardiol 1998;31:1449.

Chong BH: Heparin-induced thrombocytopenia Br J Haematol 1995;89:431.

George JN et al: Drug-induced thrombocytopenia: A systematic review of published case reports. Ann Intern Med 1998;129:886.

Warkentin TE: Heparin-induced thrombocytopenia: Towards consensus. Thromb Haemost 1998;79:1.

Hypercoagulable States
Bertina RM et al: Mutation in blood coagulation factor V associated with resistance to activated protein C. Nature 1994;369:64.

Macik BG, Ortel TL: Clinical and laboratory evaluation of the hypercoagulable states. Clin Chest Med 1995; 16:375.

Poort SR: A common genetic variation in the 3'-untranslated region of the prothrombin gene is associated with elevated plasma prothrombin levels and an increase in venous thrombosis. Blood 1996;88:3698.

Rosendaal FR et al: High risk of thrombosis in patients homozygous for factor V Leiden (activated protein C resistance). Blood 1995;85:1504.

Schafer AI: Hypercoagulable states: Molecular genetics to clinical practice. Lancet 1994;344:1739.

7 Nervous System Disorders

Robert O. Messing, MD

The major functions of the nervous system are to detect, analyze, and transmit information. Information is gathered by sensory systems, integrated by the brain, and used to generate signals to motor and autonomic pathways for control of movement and of visceral and endocrine functions. These actions are controlled by neurons, which are interconnected to form signaling networks that comprise motor and sensory systems. In addition to neurons, the nervous system contains neuroglial cells that serve a variety of immunologic and support functions and modulate the activity of neurons. Understanding the pathophysiology of nervous system disease requires knowledge of neural and glial cell biology and the anatomy of neural networks. The first part of this chapter reviews several basic aspects of histology, cellular physiology, and anatomy of the nervous system.

Understanding the causes of neurologic diseases requires knowledge of molecular and biochemical mechanisms. For several neurologic diseases, the mechanisms are not known. However, recent discoveries in molecular biology and genetics have uncovered important information about the mechanisms of some disease states. Six neurologic disorders in which some of the molecular mechanisms of pathogenesis are known are discussed later in this chapter: motor neuron disease, Parkinson's disease, myasthenia gravis, epilepsy, Alzheimer's disease, and stroke.

NORMAL STRUCTURE & FUNCTION OF THE NERVOUS SYSTEM

HISTOLOGY & CELL BIOLOGY

Neurons

The major function of neurons is to receive, integrate, and transmit information to other cells. Neurons consist of three parts: **dendrites,** which are elongated processes that receive information from the environment or from other neurons; the **cell body,** which contains the nucleus; and the **axon,** which may be up to 1 m long and conducts impulses to muscles, glands, or other neurons (Figure 7–1). Most neurons are multipolar, containing one axon and several dendrites. Bipolar neurons have one dendrite and one axon and are found in the cochlear and vestibular ganglia, retina, and olfactory mucosa. Spinal sensory ganglia contain pseudounipolar neurons that have a single process emanating from the cell body which divides into branches extending to the spinal cord and to the periphery. Axons and dendrites usually branch extensively at their ends. Dendritic branching can be very complex, with the result that a single neuron may receive thousands of inputs. Axon branching allows several target cells to simultaneously receive a message from one neuron. Each branch of the axon terminates on the next cell at a **synapse,** a structure specialized for information transfer from the axon to muscle, to glands, or to another neuron. Synapses most often occur between axons and dendrites but may occur between an axon and a cell body, between two axons, or between two dendrites.

Signals are propagated electrically along axons. Like other cells, neurons maintain cell size and osmolarity primarily through the action of Na^+-K^+ ATPase, which actively pumps Na^+ out of cells in exchange for K^+. This results in formation of concentration gradients for Na^+ and K^+ across the cell membrane. The membrane is practically impermeable to Na^+, but the presence of K^+ leak channels permits the flow of K^+ out of cells. This produces a difference in electrical charge across the membrane that reaches a force which opposes further flow of K^+ from the cell. This maximal force is the **equilibrium potential** for K^+ (E_K) and is calculated by the Nernst equation:

$$E_K = 2.3 \frac{RT}{F} \log \frac{[K^+]_o}{[K^+]_i}$$

where

R = gas constant (2 kcal mol^{-1} °K^{-1})
T = absolute temperature (°K)

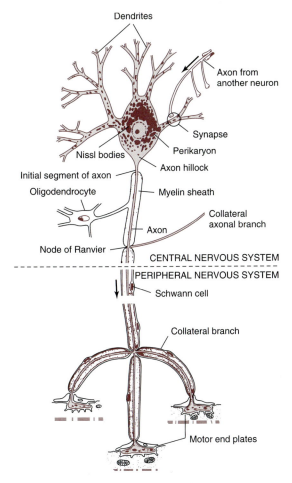

Figure 7–1. Schematic drawing of a Nissl-stained motor neuron. The myelin sheath is produced by oligodendrocytes in the central nervous system and by Schwann cells in the peripheral nervous system. Note the three motor end plates, which transmit the nerve impulse to striated skeletal muscle fibers. (Reproduced, with permission, from Junqueira LC, Carneiro J, Kelley RO: *Basic Histology,* 9th ed. Appleton & Lange, 1998.)

F = Faraday's constant (2.3×10^4 kcal V^{-1} mol^{-1})
$[K^+]_o$ = concentration of K$^+$ outside the cell
$[K^+]_i$ = concentration of K$^+$ inside the cell

In most neurons, the resting membrane potential (E_m) is 50–100 mV and lies close to E_K since the leak of K$^+$ is the major determinant of the charge difference across the membrane.

The membrane potential may be altered by increasing the permeability of the membrane to another ion, which drives the resting membrane potential toward the equilibrium potential for that ion. Neurons are highly specialized to use rapid changes in membrane potential to generate electrical signals. This is accomplished by **ligand-gated** and **voltage-gated** **ion channels** that allow the passage of Na$^+$, K$^+$, Ca^{2+}, or Cl$^-$ ions in response to electrical or chemical stimuli. These channels are composed of protein complexes embedded in the lipid membrane to form an aqueous pore to the inside of the cell. In general, channels are selective for a particular species of ion. An array of charged amino acids within voltage-dependent channels detects changes in voltage and induces a conformational change in the channel to alter ion permeability. Binding sites for **neurotransmitters** such as glutamate, γ-aminobutyric acid (GABA), glycine, and acetylcholine exist on ligand-gated channels and, when occupied, induce a conformational change to open the channel.

Electrical signals are propagated in neurons because a voltage change across the membrane in one part of a neuron is propagated to other parts. Passive spread of a voltage disturbance weakens with increasing distance from the source unless energy-dependent processes amplify the signal. Passive spread of electrical signals works well over short distances and is a major mechanism of signal propagation in dendrites. However, long-distance communication down axons to nerve terminals requires amplification. This is accomplished through the generation of self-propagating waves of excitation known as **action potentials.**

An action potential arises primarily from voltage-dependent changes in membrane permeability to Na$^+$ and K$^+$ (Figure 7–2). If a depolarizing stimulus raises the membrane potential to about –45 mV, voltage-gated Na$^+$ channels open, allowing influx of Na$^+$ and further depolarization toward E_{Na} (= +50 mV). Nearby areas of membrane are depolarized to the threshold for Na$^+$ channel activation, propagating a wave of depolarization from the initial site. The resting potential is restored quickly by a combination of events. First, Na$^+$ channels close rapidly and remain in an inactive state until the membrane potential returns to negative levels for several milliseconds. Voltage-dependent K$^+$ channels open as the membrane potential peaks, speeding the efflux of K$^+$ from cells and driving the membrane potential back to E_K. K$^+$ channels are also inactivated, but more slowly than Na$^+$ channels, and this may transiently hyperpolarize cells. Plasma membrane ion exchangers and ion pumps then counteract the ion fluxes and eventually restore the resting state.

Neurons transmit signals chemically to other cells at synapses (Figure 7–3). Presynaptic and postsynaptic cells are electrically isolated from each other and separated by a narrow synaptic cleft. Signaling across the cleft occurs through the release of neurotransmitters from the terminal of the presynaptic neuron. Most neurotransmitters are stored in membrane-bound synaptic vesicles and are released into the synaptic cleft by Ca^{2+}-dependent exocytosis. Depolarization of the nerve terminal opens voltage-gated Ca^{2+} channels, stimulating Ca^{2+} influx and neuro-

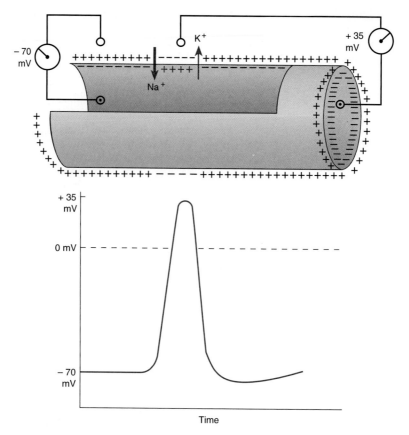

Figure 7–2. Conduction of the nerve impulse through an unmyelinated nerve fiber. In the resting axon, there is a difference of –70 mV between the interior of the axon and the outer surface of its membrane (resting potential). During the impulse passage, more Na$^+$ (thick arrow) passes into the axon interior than the amount of K$^+$ (thin arrow) that migrates in the opposite direction. In consequence, the membrane polarity changes (the membrane becomes relatively positive on its inner surface), and the resting potential is replaced by an action potential (+35 mV here). (Reproduced, with permission, from Junqueira LC, Carneiro J, Kelley RO: *Basic Histology*, 6th ed. Appleton & Lange, 1989.)

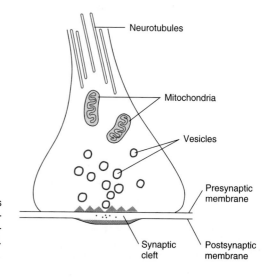

Figure 7–3. Schematic drawing of a synaptic terminal. Vesicles pass through the presynaptic membrane and release a transmitter substance into the synaptic cleft. (Reproduced, with permission, from Waxman SG: *Correlative Neuroanatomy*, 23rd ed. Appleton & Lange, 1997.)

transmitter release. Neurotransmitters diffuse across the cleft and bind to receptors on ligand-gated ion channels concentrated at the postsynaptic membrane. This produces local permeability changes, altering the membrane potential of the postsynaptic cell. If the response is depolarizing, an action potential may be generated if there are enough voltage-gated Na^+ channels nearby and the membrane potential has been raised to the threshold for their activation. Receptor-gated ion channels are highly selective for a particular neurotransmitter and for the type of ions they pass, which determines whether they generate excitatory or inhibitory responses. In general, **excitatory neurotransmitters** such as acetylcholine and glutamate open cation channels that allow influx of Na^+ or Ca^{2+} and generate a depolarizing **excitatory postsynaptic potential.** Inhibitory neurotransmitters such as GABA and glycine open Cl^- channels and generate an **inhibitory postsynaptic potential,** keeping the postsynaptic membrane near E_{Cl} (= –70 mV). Termination of the signal is achieved by removal of the neurotransmitter from the synaptic cleft. Acetylcholine is hydrolyzed by acetylcholinesterase at the postsynaptic membrane. Other neurotransmitters such as glutamate are removed by specific membrane transporters on nerve terminals or glial cells.

Not all neurotransmitter receptors are ion channels. Many receptors are coupled to cellular enzymes that regulate levels of **intracellular second messengers** to modulate the function of ion channels and many other cell proteins. A major mechanism by which messengers regulate ion channels is by promoting **phosphorylation** of channel subunits. For example, binding of the neurotransmitter norepinephrine to β-adrenergic receptors activates the enzyme **adenylyl cyclase** and stimulates the production of **cAMP.** Cyclic AMP in turn activates a cAMP-dependent protein kinase that can phosphorylate voltage-gated calcium channels. In many cases, this increases the duration of time the channel remains open once it is activated, resulting in increased Ca^{2+} influx through the channel. Other neurotransmitter receptors, such as α_1-adrenergic, muscarinic cholinergic, or metabotropic glutamate receptors, are coupled to the enzyme **phospholipase C,** which catalyzes the hydrolysis of the membrane lipid phosphatidylinositol-4,5-bisphosphate. Binding of neurotransmitter to the receptor activates phospholipase C to produce two second messengers, **1,2-diacylglycerol** and **inositol-1,4,5 trisphosphate.** Diacylglycerol activates several enzymes of the protein kinase C family, some of which phosphorylate ion channels and either enhance or suppress their function. Inositol 1,4,5-trisphosphate binds an intracellular receptor that is itself a calcium ionophore, allowing release of calcium from intracellular stores into the cytosol. This calcium signal activates several calcium-dependent enzymes, including phosphatases and kinases that can alter the phosphorylation state and function of several ion channels and all other cell proteins.

Astrocytes

Astrocytes serve a variety of metabolic, immunologic, structural, and nutritional support functions required for normal function of neurons. They possess numerous processes that radiate from the cell body, surrounding blood vessels and covering the surfaces of the brain and spinal cord (Figure 7–4). Astrocytes express voltage- and ligand-gated ion channels and regulate K^+ and Ca^{2+} concentrations within the inter-

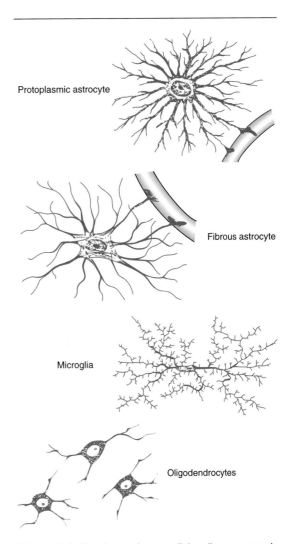

Figure 7–4. Drawings of neuroglial cells as seen in slides stained by metallic impregnation. Observe that only astrocytes exhibit vascular end-feet, which cover the walls of blood capillaries. (Reproduced, with permission, from Junqueira LC, Carneiro J, Kelley RO: *Basic Histology,* 9th ed. Appleton & Lange, 1998.)

stitial space. Many synapses are invested with astrocytic processes, and this may allow astrocytes to modulate neurotransmission by regulating extracellular concentrations of these cations. Astrocytes provide structural and trophic support for neurons through the production of extracellular matrix molecules such as laminin and through release of growth factors such as nerve growth factor, fibroblast growth factors, and brain-derived neurotrophic factor. Endfeet of astrocytic processes at blood vessels provide sites for release of cytokines and chemoattractants during central nervous system injury. Astrocytes respond to brain injury by increasing in size—and in some cases in number—through a process called **reactive astrocytosis.** This phenotypic change is characterized by an increase in expression of cells expressing glial-fibrillary acidic protein and by synthesis and release of cytokines that regulate inflammatory responses and entry of hematogenous cells into the central nervous system. Astrocytes play an important role also in terminating neuronal responses to glutamate, the most abundant excitatory neurotransmitter in the brain. In cell cultures, neurons die in the presence of high levels of glutamate unless astrocytes are present. Glutamate transporters present on astrocyte cell membranes remove glutamate from the synapse. Astrocytes also contain glutamine synthase, which converts glutamate to glutamine, detoxifying the central nervous system of both glutamate and ammonia.

Oligodendrocytes & Schwann Cells

Plasma membranes of oligodendrocytes in the central nervous system and Schwann cells in the peripheral nervous system envelop axons of neurons. For many axons, the membranes of these glial cells are wrapped layer upon layer around the axon, forming a myelin sheath (Figure 7–5). Gaps form between myelin sheaths from neighboring glia and produce **nodes of Ranvier** where a small portion of the axon is exposed to the interstitial space and where voltage-dependent Na$^+$ channels are clustered in the axonal membrane. Between the nodes, myelin insulates the axon from the extracellular space, allowing efficient spread of depolarization from one node to another. This allows action potentials to propagate rapidly by jumping from node to node in a process called **saltatory conduction,** resulting in much more rapid conduction down myelinated axons.

Microglia

Although peripheral blood lymphocytes and monocytes enter from the circulation and patrol the central nervous system, microglia cells, which reside in the central nervous system, function as the main immune effector cells. They appear to be derived from bone marrow precursors of macrophage-monocyte lineage and invade the central nervous system

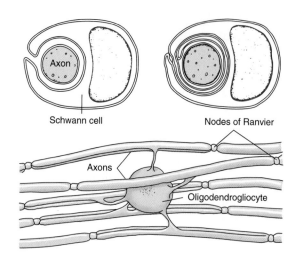

Figure 7–5. Myelination of axons. **Top left:** Unmyelinated axon. **Top right:** Myelinated axon. Note that the cell membrane of the Schwann cell has wrapped itself around the axon. **Bottom:** Myelination of several axons in the central nervous system by an oligodendrogliocyte. (Reproduced, with permission, from Ganong WF: *Review of Medical Physiology,* 19th ed. Appleton & Lange, 1999.)

during the perinatal period, where they differentiate into ramified cells in the central nervous system parenchyma. Microglia cells are activated by brain injury, infection, or neuronal degeneration. Activation is characterized by proliferation, migration into damaged tissue, increased or de novo expression of surface receptors, including CD45 (leukocyte common antigen), MHC class I and class II and immunoglobulin Fc receptors, and secretion of several cytokines, reactive oxygen intermediates, and proteinases. This response functions to remove dead tissue and destroy invading organisms but may contribute to central nervous system damage, particularly in certain central nervous system inflammatory and degenerative diseases.

1. What are the primary functions of neurons, astrocytes, and microglia?
2. What role does myelin play in axonal conduction?
3. What is responsible for the resting membrane potential and for the generation of action potentials?
4. What are some of the major neurotransmitters in the nervous system, and what effects do they produce when they bind to their receptors?

FUNCTIONAL NEUROANATOMY

To understand neuroanatomy, it is useful to study structures as parts of functional systems.

MOTOR SYSTEM

Large **alpha motor neurons** of the spinal cord ventral horns and brainstem motor nuclei (facial nucleus, trigeminal motor nucleus, nucleus ambiguus, hypoglossal nucleus) extend axons into spinal and cranial nerves to innervate skeletal muscles. Damage to these **lower motor neurons** results in loss of all voluntary and reflex movement, since they comprise the output of the motor system. Neurons in the precentral gyrus and neighboring cortical regions (**upper motor neurons**) send axons to synapse with lower motor neurons. Axons from these upper motor neurons comprise the **corticospinal** and **corticobulbar tracts**. The motor cortex and spinal cord are connected with other deep cerebral and brainstem motor nuclei, including the caudate nucleus, putamen, globus pallidus, red nuclei, subthalamic nuclei, substantia nigra, reticular nuclei, and neurons of the cerebellum. Neurons in these structures are distinct from cortical motor (**"pyramidal"**) neurons and are referred to as **"extrapyramidal"** neurons. Many parts of the cerebral cortex are connected by fiber tracts to the primary motor cortex. These connections are important for complex patterns of movement and for coordinating motor responses to sensory stimuli.

> 5. From where do lower motor neurons emanate, and to where do they send axons?
> 6. From where do upper motor neurons emanate, and with what do they synapse?

1. LOWER MOTOR NEURONS & SKELETAL MUSCLES

Anatomy

Each alpha motor neuron axon contacts up to about 200 muscle fibers, and together they constitute the **motor unit** (Figure 7–6). Axons of the motor neurons intermingle to form spinal ventral roots, plexuses, and peripheral nerves. Muscles are innervated from specific segments of the spinal cord, and each muscle is supplied by at least two roots. Motor fibers are rearranged in the plexuses so that most muscles are supplied by one peripheral nerve. Thus, the distribution of muscle weakness differs in spinal root and peripheral nerve lesions.

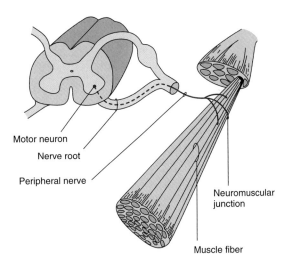

Figure 7–6. Anatomic components of the motor unit. (Reproduced, with permission, from Simon RP, Aminoff MJ, Greenberg DA: *Clinical Neurology*, 4th ed. Appleton & Lange, 1999.)

Physiology

The lower motor neurons are the final common pathway for all voluntary movement. Therefore, damage to lower motor neurons or their axons causes flaccid weakness of innervated muscles. In addition, muscle tone or resistance to passive movement is reduced, and deep tendon reflexes are impaired or lost. Tendon reflexes and muscle tone depend on the activity of alpha motor neurons, specialized sensory receptors known as muscle spindles, and smaller **gamma motor neurons** whose axons innervate the spindles (Figure 7–7). Some gamma motor neurons are active at rest, making the spindle fibers taut and sensitive to stretch. Tapping on the tendon stretches the spindles, which causes them to send impulses that activate alpha motor neurons. These in turn fire, producing the brief muscle contraction observed during the **myotactic stretch reflex**. Alpha motor neurons of antagonist muscles are simultaneously inhibited. Both alpha and gamma motor neurons are influenced by descending fiber systems, and their state of activity determines the level of tone and activity of the stretch reflex.

Each point of contact between nerve terminal and skeletal muscle forms a specialized synapse known as a **neuromuscular junction** composed of the presynaptic motor nerve terminal and a postsynaptic muscle membrane (Figure 7–8). Presynaptic terminals store synaptic vesicles that contain the neurotransmitter acetylcholine. The amount of neurotransmitter within a vesicle constitutes a quantum of neurotransmitter. Action potentials depolarize the motor nerve terminal, opening voltage-gated calcium

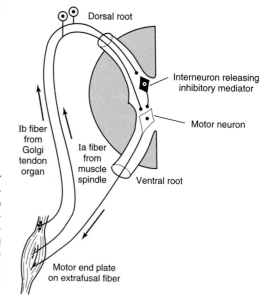

Figure 7–7. Diagram illustrating the pathways responsible for the stretch reflex and the inverse stretch reflex. Stretch stimulates the muscle spindle, and impulses pass up the Ia fiber to excite the motor neuron. It also stimulates the Golgi tendon organ, and impulses passing up the Ib fiber activate the interneuron to release the inhibitory mediator glycine. With strong stretch, the resulting hyperpolarization of the motor neuron is so great that it stops discharging. (Reproduced, with permission, from Ganong, WF: *Review of Medical Physiology,* 19th ed. Appleton & Lange, 1999.)

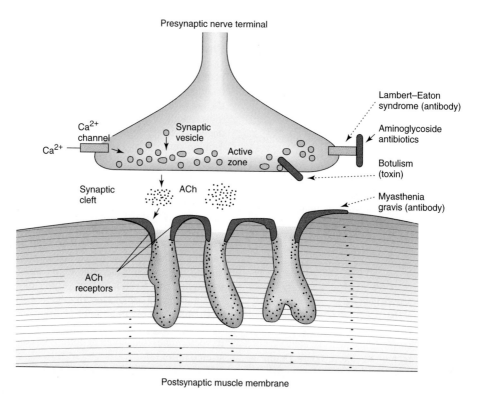

Figure 7–8. Sites of involvement in disorders of neuromuscular transmission. At left, normal transmission involves depolarization-induced influx of calcium (Ca^{2+}) through voltage-gated channels. This stimulates release of acetylcholine (ACh) from synaptic vesicles at the active zone and into the synaptic cleft. ACh binds to ACh receptors and depolarizes the postsynaptic muscle membrane. At right, disorders of neuromuscular transmission result from blockage of Ca^{2+} channels (Lambert-Eaton syndrome or aminoglycoside antibiotics), impairment of Ca^{2+}-mediated ACh release (botulinum toxin), or antibody-induced internalization and degradation of ACh receptors (myasthenia gravis). (Reproduced, with permission, from Simon RP, Aminoff MJ, Greenberg DA: *Clinical Neurology,* 4th ed. Appleton & Lange, 1999.)

channels and stimulating calcium-dependent release of neurotransmitter from the terminal. Released acetylcholine traverses the synaptic cleft to the postsynaptic (end plate) membrane, where it binds to nicotinic acetylcholine receptors. These receptors are ligand-gated cation channels, and, upon binding acetylcholine, they allow entry of extracellular sodium into the muscle fiber. This depolarizes the motor end plate and stimulates contraction of the muscle fiber. Following activation, acetylcholine receptors rapidly inactivate, reducing sodium entry. They remain inactive until acetylcholine dissociates from the receptor. This is facilitated by the enzyme acetylcholinesterase, which is present in the postsynaptic zone, degrades acetylcholine, and decreases the concentration of the neurotransmitter at the synapse.

Neuromuscular transmission may be disturbed in several ways (Figure 7–8). In the **Lambert-Eaton myasthenic syndrome,** antibodies to calcium channels inhibit calcium entry into the nerve terminal and reduce neurotransmitter release. In these cases, repetitive nerve stimulation facilitates accumulation of calcium in the nerve terminal and increases acetylcholine release. Clinically, limb muscles are weak, but if contraction is maintained, power increases. Electrophysiologically, there is an increase in the amplitude of the muscle response to repetitive nerve stimulation. **Aminoglycoside antibiotics** also impair calcium channel function and cause a similar syndrome. Proteolytic toxins produced by *Clostridium botulinum* cleave specific presynaptic proteins, preventing neurotransmitter release at both neuromuscular and parasympathetic cholinergic synapses. As a result, patients with **botulism** develop weakness, blurred vision, diplopia, ptosis, and large unreactive pupils. In **myasthenia gravis,** autoantibodies to the nicotinic acetylcholine receptor block neurotransmission by inhibiting receptor function and activating complement-mediated lysis of the postsynaptic membrane. Myasthenia gravis is discussed in greater detail later in this chapter.

Motor nerves exert trophic influences on the muscles they innervate. Denervated muscles undergo marked atrophy, losing more than half of their original bulk in 2–3 months. Nerve fibers are also required for organization of the muscle end plate and for the clustering of acetylcholine receptors to that region. Receptors in denervated fibers fail to cluster and become spread across the muscle membrane. Muscle fibers within a denervated motor unit may then discharge spontaneously, giving rise to a visible twitch (**fasciculation**) within a portion of a muscle. Individual fibers may also contract spontaneously, giving rise to **fibrillations,** which are not visible to the examiner but can be detected by electromyography. Fibrillations usually appear 7–21 days after damage to lower motor neurons or their axons.

> 7. What constitutes a motor unit?
> 8. Why does the distribution of weakness differ between spinal root and peripheral nerve lesions?
> 9. What are the features of lower motor neuron damage?
> 10. Describe the events in neuromuscular transmission.
> 11. What are some clinical syndromes in which neuromuscular transmission is disturbed?
> 12. What are some consequences of denervation on muscle structure and function?

2. UPPER MOTOR NEURONS

Anatomy

The motor cortex is the region from which movements can be elicited by electrical stimuli (Figure 7–9). This includes the primary motor area (Brodmann area 4), premotor cortex (area 6), supplementary motor cortex (medial portions of 6), and primary sensory cortex (areas 3, 1, and 2). In the motor cortex, groups of neurons are organized in vertical columns, and discrete groups control contraction of individual muscles. Planned movements and those guided by sensory, visual, or auditory stimuli are preceded by discharges from prefrontal, somatosensory, visual, or auditory cortices, which are then followed by motor cortex pyramidal cell discharges that occur several milliseconds before the onset of movement.

Cortical motor neurons contribute axons that converge in the corona radiata and descend in the posterior limb of the internal capsule, cerebral peduncles, ventral pons, and medulla. These fibers constitute the **corticospinal** and **corticobulbar tracts** and, together with fibers projecting from red nuclei, vestibular nuclei, midbrain tectal neurons, and the reticular formation, are known as upper motor neuron fibers (Figure 7–10). As they descend through the diencephalon and brainstem, fibers separate to innervate extrapyramidal and cranial nerve motor nuclei. The lower brainstem motor neurons receive input from crossed and uncrossed corticobulbar fibers, though neurons that innervate lower facial muscles receive primarily crossed fibers.

In the ventral medulla, the remaining corticospinal fibers course in a tract that on cross section is pyramidal in shape—thus the name **pyramidal tract.** At the lower end of the medulla, most fibers decussate, though the proportion of crossed and uncrossed fibers varies somewhat between individuals. The bulk of these fibers descend as the lateral corticospinal tract of the spinal cord.

Different groups of neurons in the cortex control muscle groups of the contralateral face, arm, and leg.

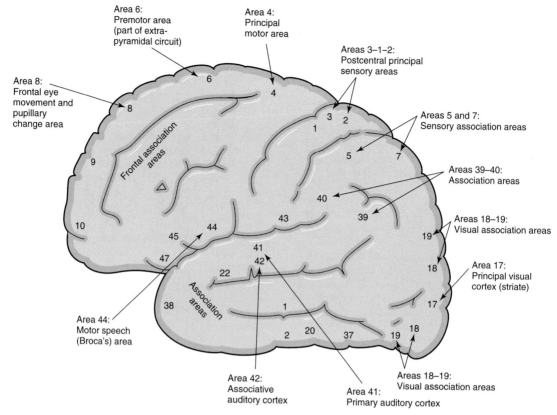

Figure 7–9. Lateral aspect of the cerebrum. The cortical areas are shown according to Brodmann, with functional localizations. (Reproduced, with permission, from Waxman SG: *Correlative Neuroanatomy,* 23rd ed. Appleton & Lange, 1997.)

Neurons near the ventral end of the central sulcus control muscles of the face, whereas neurons on the medial surface of the hemisphere control leg muscles (Figure 7–10). Because the movements of the face, tongue, and hand are complex in humans, a large share of motor cortex is devoted to their control. A somatotopic organization is also apparent in the lateral corticospinal tract of the cervical cord, where fibers to motor neurons that control leg muscles lie laterally and fibers to cervical motor neurons lie medially.

Physiology

Upper motor neurons control the planning, initiation, sequencing, and modulation of all voluntary movement. Much has been learned about the normal function of upper motor neurons through the study of animals and humans with focal brain lesions. Upper motor neuron pathways can be interrupted in the cortex, subcortical white matter, internal capsule, brainstem, or spinal cord. Unilateral upper motor neuron lesions spare muscles innervated by lower motor neurons that receive bilateral cortical input, such as muscles of the eyes, jaw, upper face, pharynx, larynx, neck, thorax, and abdomen. Unlike paralysis due to lower motor neuron lesions, paralysis from upper motor neuron lesions is rarely complete for a prolonged period of time. Acute lesions, particularly of the spinal cord, often cause flaccid paralysis and absence of spinal reflexes at all segments below the lesion. With spinal cord lesions, this state is known as **spinal shock.** After a few days to weeks, a state known as **spasticity** appears, characterized by increased tone and hyperactive stretch reflexes. A similar but less striking sequence of events can occur with acute cerebral lesions.

Upper motor neuron lesions cause a characteristic pattern of limb weakness and change in tone. Antigravity muscles of the limbs become more active relative to other muscles. The arms tend to assume a flexed, pronated posture, and the legs become extended. In contrast, muscles that move the limbs out of this posture (extensors of the arms and flexors of the legs) are preferentially weakened. Tone is increased in antigravity muscles (flexors of the arms and extensors of the legs), and if these muscles are

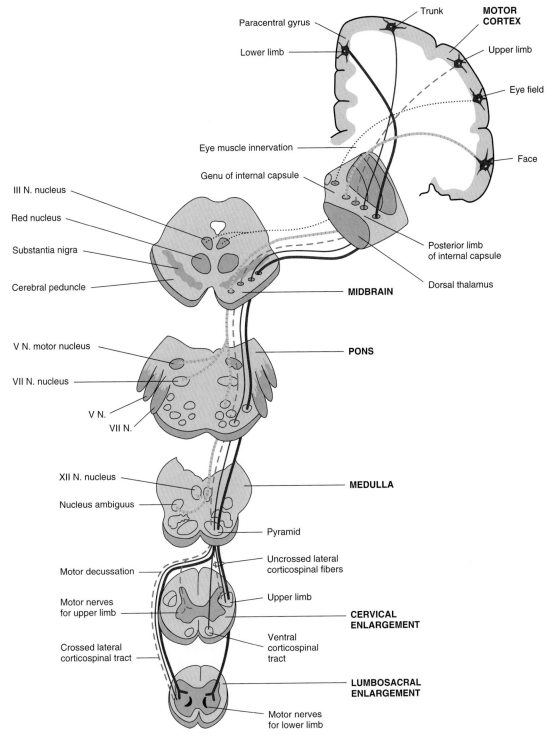

Figure 7–10. Schematic illustration of upper motor neuron pathways. (Reproduced, with permission, from Adams M, Victor RD: *Principles of Neurology,* 5th ed. McGraw-Hill, 1993.)

stretched rapidly, they respond with an abrupt catch, followed by a rapid increase and then a decline in resistance as passive movement continues. This sequence constitutes the **"clasp knife" phenomenon**. **Clonus**—a series of involuntary muscle contractions in response to passive stretch—may be present, especially with spinal cord lesions.

Pure pyramidal tract lesions in animals cause temporary weakness without spasticity. In humans, lesions of the cerebral peduncles also cause mild paralysis without spasticity. It appears that control of tone is mediated by other tracts, particularly corticorubrospinal and corticoreticulospinal pathways. This may explain why the degrees of weakness and spasticity often do not correspond in patients with upper motor neuron lesions.

The distribution of paralysis due to upper motor neuron lesions varies with the location of the lesion. Lesions above the pons impair movements of the contralateral lower face, arm, and leg. Lesions below the pons spare the face. Lesions of the internal capsule often impair movements of the contralateral face, arm, and leg equally, since motor fibers are packed closely together in this region. In contrast, lesions of the cortex or subcortical white matter tend to differentially affect the limbs and face, since the motor fibers are spread over a larger area of brain. Bilateral cerebral lesions cause weakness and spasticity of cranial and trunk muscles in addition to limb muscles and lead to dysarthria, dysphonia, dysphagia, bifacial paresis, and sometimes reflexive crying and laughing (**pseudobulbar paralysis**).

13. Define the motor cortex and describe its organization.
14. Fibers from which nuclei and in which tracts constitute upper motor neurons? What is their path?
15. Describe the somatotopic organization of motor neurons in the cortex.
16. What are the characteristics of weakness and tone in upper motor neuron lesions?
17. How is the distribution of paralysis and spasticity affected by the location of an upper motor neuron lesion?

3. CEREBELLUM

Anatomy

The cerebellar cortex can be divided into three anatomic regions (Figure 7–11B). The **flocculonodular lobe**, composed of the flocculus and the nodulus of the vermis, has connections to vestibular nuclei and is important for the control of posture and eye movement. The **anterior lobe** (Figure 7–11A) lies rostrad to the primary fissure and includes the re-

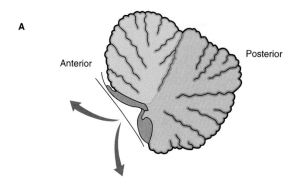

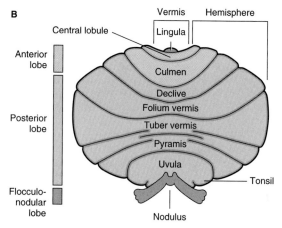

Figure 7–11. Anatomic divisions of the cerebellum in midsagittal view **(A)**; unfolded (arrows) and viewed from behind **(B)**. (Reproduced, with permission, from Simon RP, Aminoff MJ, Greenberg DA: *Clinical Neurology*, 4th ed. Appleton & Lange, 1999.)

mainder of the vermis. It receives proprioceptive input from muscles and tendons via the dorsal and ventral spinocerebellar tracts and influences posture, muscle tone, and gait. The **posterior lobe**, which comprises the remainder of the cerebellar hemispheres, receives major input from the cerebral cortex via the pontine nuclei and middle cerebellar peduncles and is important for the coordination and planning of voluntary skilled movements initiated from the cerebral cortex.

Efferent fibers from these lobes project to deep cerebellar nuclei, which in turn project to the cerebrum and brainstem through two main pathways (Figure 7–12). The fastigial nucleus receives input from the vermis and sends fibers to bilateral vestibular nuclei and reticular nuclei of the pons and medulla via the inferior cerebellar peduncles. Other regions of the cerebellar cortex send fibers to the **dentate, emboliform,** and **globose nuclei,** whose efferents form the superior cerebellar peduncles, enter the upper pons, decussate completely in the lower

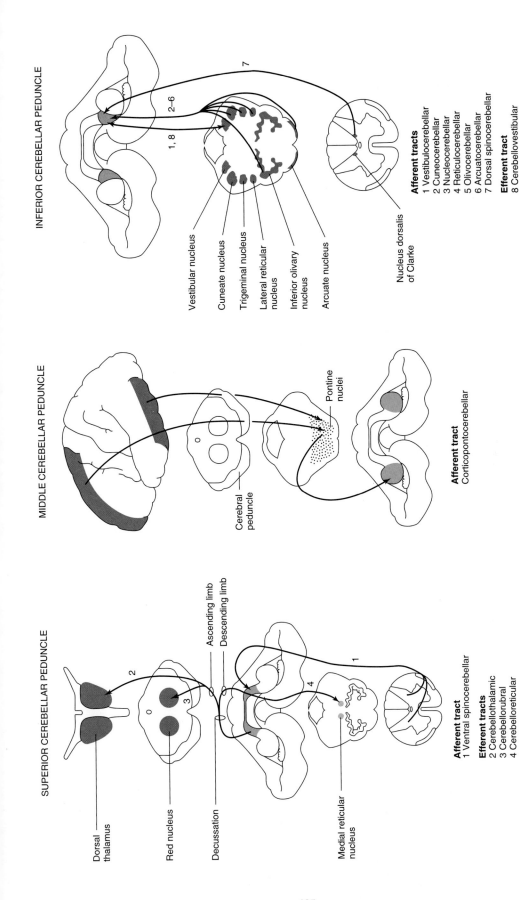

Figure 7–12. Cerebellar connections in the superior, middle, and inferior cerebellar peduncles. The peduncles are indicated by gray shading and the areas to and from which they project by brown shading. (Reproduced, with permission, from Simon RP, Aminoff MJ, Greenberg DA: *Clinical Neurology*, 4th ed. Appleton & Lange, 1999.)

midbrain, and travel to the contralateral red nucleus. At the red nucleus, some fibers terminate, whereas others ascend to the ventrolateral nucleus of the thalamus, whence thalamic neurons send ascending efferent fibers to the motor cortex of the same side. A smaller group of fibers descend after decussation in the midbrain and terminate in reticular nuclei of the lower brainstem. Thus, the cerebellum controls movement through connections with cerebral motor cortex and brainstem nuclei.

Physiology

The cerebellum is responsible for the coordination of muscle groups, control of stance and gait, and regulation of muscle tone. Rather than causing paralysis, damage to the cerebellum interferes with the performance of motor tasks. The major manifestation of cerebellar disease is **ataxia,** in which simple movements are delayed in onset and their rates of acceleration and deceleration are decreased, resulting in **intention tremor** and **dysmetria** ("overshooting"). Lesions of the cerebellar hemispheres affect the limbs, producing limb ataxia, whereas midline lesions affect axial muscles, causing truncal and gait ataxia and disorders of eye movement. Cerebellar lesions are often associated with **hypotonia** due to depression of activity of alpha and gamma motor neurons. If a lesion of the cerebellum or cerebellar peduncles is unilateral, the signs of limb ataxia appear on the same side as the lesion. However, if the lesion lies beyond the decussation of efferent cerebellar fibers in the midbrain, the clinical signs are on the side opposite the lesion.

18. What is the overall role of the cerebellum?
19. What are the anatomic regions of the cerebellum, what do they control, and through which other regions of the brain do they make connections?
20. What are the consequences of damage to the cerebellum, and what symptoms and signs are seen in patients with cerebellar lesions?
21. Below what point do unilateral cerebellar lesions manifest on the opposite side?

4. BASAL GANGLIA

Anatomy

Several subcortical, thalamic, and brainstem nuclei are critical for regulating voluntary movement and maintaining posture. These include the basal ganglia—caudate nucleus and putamen (corpus striatum), globus pallidus, claustrum, substantia nigra, and subthalamic nuclei—and the associated structures of the red nuclei and the mesencephalic reticular nuclei. The major pathways that involve these structures form three neuronal circuits (Figure 7–13). The first is the cortical-basal ganglionic-thalamic-cortical loop. Inputs mainly from premotor, primary motor, and primary sensory cortices (areas 1, 2, 3, 4, and 6) project to the corpus striatum, which sends fibers to the medial and lateral portions of the globus pallidus. Fibers from the globus pallidus form the ansa and fasciculus lenticularis, which sweep through the internal capsule and project onto ventral and intralaminar thalamic nuclei. Axons from these nuclei project to the premotor and primary motor cortices (areas 4 and 6), completing the loop. In the second loop, the substantia nigra sends dopaminergic fibers to the corpus striatum, which has reciprocal connections with the substantia nigra. The substantia nigra also projects to the ventromedial thalamus. The third loop is composed of reciprocal connections between the globus pallidus and the subthalamic nucleus. The subthalamic nucleus also sends efferents to the substantia nigra and corpus striatum.

Physiology

Basal ganglia circuits regulate the amplitude, speed, and initiation of movements. Diseases of the basal ganglia cause abnormalities of movement and are collectively known as **movement disorders.** They are characterized by motor deficits (bradykinesia, akinesia, loss of postural reflexes) or abnormal activation of the motor system, resulting in rigidity,

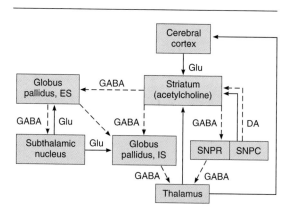

Figure 7–13. Diagrammatic representation of the principal connections of the basal ganglia. Solid lines indicate excitatory pathways, dashed lines inhibitory pathways. The transmitters are indicated in the pathways, where they are known. Glu, glutamate; DA, dopamine. Acetylcholine is the transmitter produced by interneurons in the striatum, ie, the putamen and the caudate nucleus, which have similar connections. SNPR, substantia nigra, pars reticulata; SNPC, substantia nigra, pars compacta; ES, external segment; IS, internal segment. The subthalamic nucleus also projects to the pars compacta of the substantia nigra; this pathway has been omitted for clarity. (Reproduced, with permission, from Ganong WF: *Review of Medical Physiology,* 19th ed. Appleton & Lange, 1999.)

tremor, and involuntary movements (chorea, athetosis, ballismus, and dystonia).

Several neurotransmitters are found within the basal ganglia, but their role in disease states is only partly understood. **Acetylcholine** is present in high concentrations within the corpus striatum, where it is synthesized and released by large Golgi type 2 neurons (Figure 7–14). Acetylcholine acts as an excitatory transmitter at medium-sized spiny striatal neurons that synthesize and release the inhibitory neurotransmitter **γ-aminobutyric acid (GABA)** and project to the globus pallidus. **Dopamine** is synthesized by neurons of the substantia nigra, whose axons form the nigrostriatal pathway that terminates in the corpus striatum. Dopamine released by these fibers inhibits striatal GABAergic neurons. In Parkinson's disease, degeneration of nigral neurons leads to loss of dopaminergic inhibition and a relative excess of cholinergic activity. This increases GABAergic output from the striatum and contributes to the paucity of movement that is a cardinal manifestation of the disease. Anticholinergics and dopamine agonists tend to restore the normal balance of striatal cholinergic and dopaminergic inputs and are effective in treatment. The pathogenesis of Parkinson's disease is discussed later in this chapter.

Huntington's disease is inherited as an autosomal dominant disorder. Patients develop involuntary, rapid, jerky movements **(chorea)** and slow writhing movements of the proximal limbs and trunk **(athetosis)**. The spiny GABAergic neurons of the striatum preferentially degenerate, resulting in a net decrease in GABAergic output from the striatum. This contributes to the development of chorea and athetosis. Dopamine antagonists, which block inhibition of remaining striatal neurons by dopaminergic striatal fibers, reduce the involuntary movements. The gene for the disease has been recently mapped to chromosome 4 and encodes for a protein, huntingtin, of unknown function. The gene is unique in that it contains a polymorphic trinucleotide (CAG) repeat of 11–34 copies that is expanded in patients with the disease. The expanded repeat encodes a polyglutamine domain that may alter the function or stability of huntingtin or of other proteins that interact with huntingtin within striatal neurons.

---

22. Which are the component nuclei of the basal ganglia, and what is their functional role?
23. What are the clinical consequences of lesions in the basal ganglia?
24. What are some of the neurotransmitters within the basal ganglia, and what is their role in disorders of basal ganglia function?

SOMATOSENSORY SYSTEM

Somatosensory pathways confer information about touch, pressure, temperature, pain, vibration, and the position and movement of body parts. This information is relayed to thalamic nuclei and integrated in the sensory cortex of the parietal lobes to provide conscious awareness of sensation. Information is also relayed to cortical motor neurons to adjust fine movements and maintain posture. Some ascending sensory fibers, particularly pain fibers, enter the midbrain and project to the amygdala and limbic cortex, where they contribute to emotional responses to pain. In the spinal cord, painful stimuli activate local pathways that induce the firing of lower motor neurons and cause a reflex withdrawal (Figure 7–7). Thus, somatosensory pathways provide tactile information, guide movement, and serve protective functions.

Anatomy

A variety of specialized end organs and free nerve endings transduce sensory stimuli into neural signals and initiate the firing of sensory nerve fibers. Fibers that mediate cutaneous sensation from the trunk and limbs travel in sensory or mixed sensorimotor nerves to the spinal cord (Figure 7–15). Cutaneous sensory nerves contain small myelinated Aδ fibers that transmit information about pain and temperature, larger myelinated fibers that mediate touch and pressure sensation, and more numerous unmyelinated pain and autonomic fibers. Myelinated proprioceptive

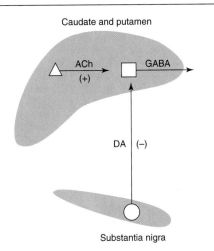

Figure 7–14. Simplified neurochemical anatomy of the basal ganglia. Dopamine (DA) neurons exert a net inhibitory effect and acetylcholine (ACh) neurons a net excitatory effect on the GABAergic output from the striatum. In Parkinson's disease, dopamine (DA) neurons degenerate. The net effect is to increase GABAergic output from the striatum. (Reproduced, with permission, from Simon RP, Aminoff MJ, Greenberg DA: *Clinical Neurology*, 4th ed. Appleton & Lange, 1999.)

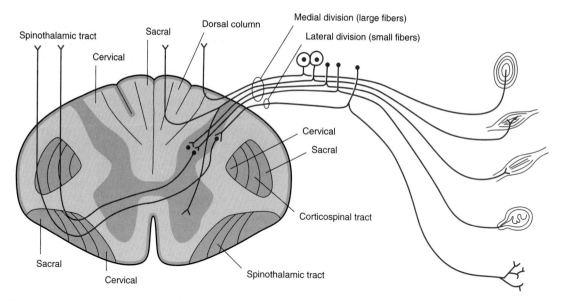

Figure 7–15. Schematic illustration of a spinal cord segment with its dorsal root, ganglion cells, and sensory organs. Sensory organs shown (from top to bottom) are the pacinian corpuscle, muscle spindle, tendon organ, encapsulated ending, and free nerve endings. The somatotopic arrangement of fibers in the dorsal columns, spinothalamic tract, and corticospinal tract is also shown. (Reproduced, with permission, from Waxman SG: *Correlative Neuroanatomy,* 23rd ed. Appleton & Lange, 1997.)

fibers and afferent and efferent muscle spindle fibers are carried in the larger sensorimotor nerves. The cell bodies of the sensory neurons are in the dorsal root ganglia, and their central projections enter the spinal cord via the dorsal spinal roots. Innervation of the skin, muscles, and surrounding connective tissue is segmental, and each root innervates a region of skin known as a **dermatome** (Figure 7–16). Cell bodies of the sensory neurons that innervate the face reside in the trigeminal ganglion and send their central projections in the trigeminal nerve to enter the brainstem. The trigeminal innervation of the face is subdivided into three regions, each innervated by one of the three divisions of the trigeminal nerve.

The dorsal roots enter the dorsal horn of the spinal cord (Figure 7–15). Large myelinated fibers divide into ascending and descending branches and either synapse with dorsal gray neurons within a few cord segments or travel in the **dorsal columns,** terminating in the gracile or cuneate nuclei of the lower medulla on the same side. Secondary neurons of the dorsal horn also send axons up the dorsal columns. Fibers in the dorsal columns are displaced medially as new fibers are added, so that in the cervical cord, leg fibers are located medially and arm fibers laterally (Figure 7–15). The gracile and cuneate nuclei send fibers that cross the midline in the medulla and ascend to the thalamus as the **medial lemniscus** (Figure 7–17). The dorsal column-lemniscal system car-

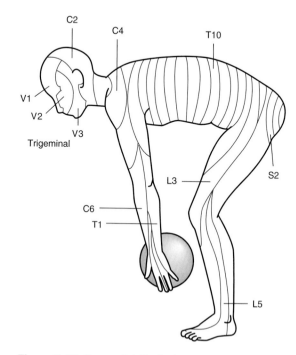

Figure 7–16. Segmental distribution of the body viewed in the approximate quadruped position, including sensory distribution of the trigeminal (V) cranial nerve. (Reproduced, with permission, from Waxman SG: *Correlative Neuroanatomy,* 23rd ed. Appleton & Lange, 1997.)

ture sensation terminate in the **nucleus of the spinal tract of cranial nerve V**, which is continuous with the dorsal horn of the cervical cord. Touch, pressure, and postural information are conveyed by fibers that terminate in the **main sensory** and **mesencephalic nuclei of the trigeminal nerve.** Axons arising from trigeminal nuclei cross the midline and ascend as the **trigeminal lemniscus** just medial to the spinothalamic tract. Fibers from the spinothalamic tract, medial lemniscus, and trigeminal lemniscus merge in the midbrain and terminate along with sensory fibers ascending from the spinal cord in the posterior thalamic nuclei, mainly in the nucleus ventralis posterolateralis. These thalamic nuclei project to the primary somatosensory cortex (Brodmann areas 3, 1, and 2) and to a second somatosensory area on the upper bank of the sylvian fissure (lateral cerebral sulcus). The primary somatosensory region is organized somatotopically like the primary motor cortex.

Physiology

A. Pain: Free nerve endings of unmyelinated C fibers and small-diameter myelinated A δ fibers in the skin convey sensory information in response to chemical, thermal, or mechanical stimuli. Intense stimulation of these nerve endings evokes the sensation of pain. In contrast to skin, most deep tissues are relatively insensitive to chemical or noxious stimuli. However, inflammatory conditions can sensitize sensory afferents from deep tissues to evoke pain upon mechanical stimulation. This sensitization appears to

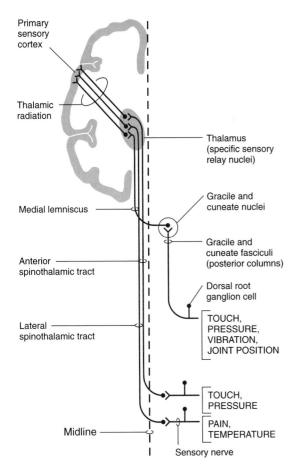

Figure 7–17. Sensory pathways conveying touch, pressure, vibration, joint position, pain, and temperature sensation. (Reproduced, with permission, from Simon RP, Aminoff MJ, Greenberg DA: *Clinical Neurology,* 4th ed. Appleton & Lange, 1999.)

ries information about pressure, limb position, vibration, direction of movement, recognition of texture and shape, and two-point discrimination.

Thinly myelinated and unmyelinated fibers enter the lateral portion of the dorsal horn and synapse with dorsal spinal neurons within one or two segments. The majority of secondary fibers from these cells cross in the anterior spinal commissure and ascend in the anterolateral spinal cord as the **lateral spinothalamic tracts.** Crossing fibers are added to the inner side of the tract, so that in the cervical cord the leg fibers are located superficially and arm fibers are deeper. These fibers carry information about pain, temperature, and touch sensation.

Sensation from the face is carried by trigeminal sensory fibers that enter the pons and descend to the medulla and upper cervical cord (Figure 7–18). Fibers carrying information about pain and tempera-

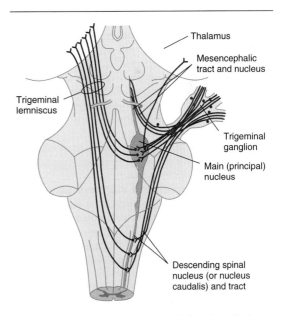

Figure 7–18. Schematic drawing of the trigeminal system. (Reproduced, with permission, from Waxman SG: *Correlative Neuroanatomy,* 23rd ed. Appleton & Lange, 1997.)

be mediated by bradykinin, prostaglandins, and leukotrienes released during the inflammatory response. Information from primary afferent fibers is relayed via sensory ganglia to the dorsal horn of the spinal cord and then to the contralateral spinothalamic tract, which connects to thalamic neurons that project to the somatosensory cortex.

Damage to these pathways produces a deficit in pain and temperature discrimination and may also produce abnormal painful sensations (**dysesthesias**) usually in the area of sensory loss. Such pain is termed **neuropathic pain** and often has a strange burning, tingling, or electric shock-like quality. It may arise from several mechanisms. Damaged peripheral nerve fibers become highly mechanosensitive and may fire spontaneously without stimulation. They also develop sensitivity to norepinephrine released from sympathetic postganglionic neurons. Electrical impulses may spread abnormally from one fiber to another (**ephaptic conduction**), enhancing the spontaneous firing of multiple fibers. Neuropeptides released by injured nerves may recruit an inflammatory reaction that stimulates pain. In the dorsal horn, denervated spinal neurons may become spontaneously active. In the brain and spinal cord, synaptic reorganization occurs in response to injury and may lower the threshold for pain. In addition, inhibition of pathways that modulate transmission of sensory information in the spinal cord and brainstem may promote neuropathic pain.

Pain-modulating circuits exert a major influence on the perceived intensity of pain. One such pathway (Figure 7–19) is composed of cells in the periaqueductal gray matter of the midbrain that receive afferents from frontal cortex and hypothalamus and project to rostroventral medullary neurons. These in turn project in the dorsolateral white matter of the spinal cord and terminate on dorsal horn neurons. Additional descending pathways arise from other brainstem nuclei (locus ceruleus, dorsal raphe nucleus, and nucleus reticularis gigantocellularis). Major neurotransmitters utilized by these systems include endorphins, serotonin, and norepinephrine, providing the rationale for the use of opioids, serotonin agonists, and serotonin and norepinephrine reuptake inhibitors in the treatment of pain.

B. Proprioception and Vibratory Sense: Receptors in the muscles, tendons, and joints provide information about deep pressure and the position and movement of body parts. This allows one to determine an object's size, weight, shape, and texture. Information is relayed to the spinal cord via large A α and A β myelinated fibers and to the thalamus by the dorsal column-lemniscal system. Detecting vibration requires sensing touch and rapid changes in deep pressure. This depends on multiple cutaneous and deep sensory fibers and is impaired by lesions of multiple peripheral nerves, the dorsal columns, medial lemniscus, or thalamus but rarely by lesions of

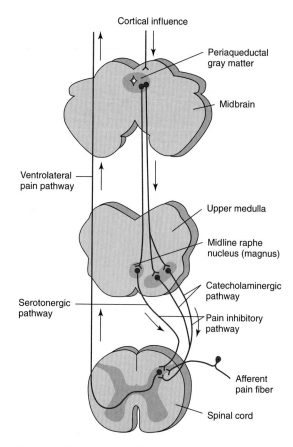

Figure 7–19. Schematic illustration of the pathways involved in pain control. (Courtesy of A Basbaum.) (Reproduced, with permission, from Waxman SG: *Correlative Neuroanatomy,* 23rd ed. Appleton & Lange, 1997.)

single nerves. Vibratory sense is usually impaired together with proprioception.

C. Discriminative Sensation: Primary sensory cortex provides awareness of somatosensory information and the ability to make sensory discriminations. Touch, pain, temperature, and vibration sense are considered the primary modalities of sensation and are relatively preserved in patients with damage to sensory cortex or its projections from the thalamus. In contrast, complex tasks that require integration of multiple somatosensory stimuli and of somatosensory stimuli with auditory or visual information are impaired. These include the ability to distinguish two points from one when touched on the skin (**two-point discrimination**), localize tactile stimuli, perceive the position of body parts in space, recognize letters or numbers drawn on the skin (**graphesthesia**), or identify objects by their shape, size, and texture (**stereognosis**).

D. Anatomy of Sensory Loss: The patterns of sensory loss often indicate the level of nervous system involvement. Symmetric distal sensory loss in the limbs, affecting the legs more than the arms, usually signifies a generalized disorder of multiple peripheral nerves (**polyneuropathy**). Sensory symptoms and deficits may be restricted to the distribution of a single peripheral nerve (**mononeuropathy**) or two or more peripheral nerves (**mononeuropathy multiplex**). Symptoms and signs limited to a dermatome indicate a spinal root lesion (**radiculopathy**).

In the spinal cord, segregation of fiber tracts and the somatotopic arrangement of fibers give rise to distinct patterns of sensory loss. Loss of pain and temperature sensation on one side of the body and of proprioception on the opposite side occurs with lesions that involve one-half of the cord on the side of the proprioceptive deficit (**Brown-Séquard's syndrome;** Figure 7–20). Compression of the upper

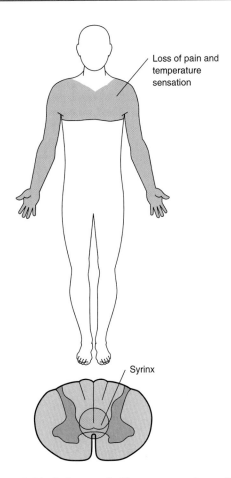

Figure 7–21. Syringomyelia (the presence of a cavity in the spinal cord due to breakdown of gliomatous new formations, presenting clinically with pain and paresthesias followed by muscular atrophy of the hands) involving the cervicothoracic portion of the cord. (Reproduced, with permission, from Waxman SG: *Correlative Neuroanatomy,* 23rd ed. Appleton & Lange, 1997.)

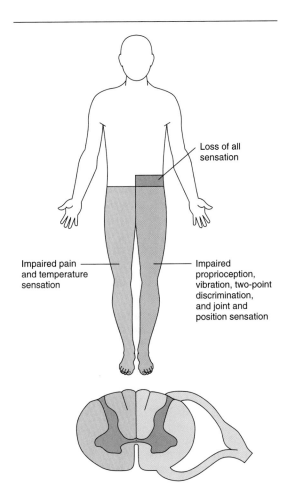

Figure 7–20. Brown-Séquard's syndrome with lesion at left tenth thoracic level (motor deficits not shown). (Reproduced, with permission, from Waxman SG: *Correlative Neuroanatomy,* 23rd ed. Appleton & Lange, 1997.)

spinal cord causes loss of pain, temperature, and touch sensation first in the legs, since the leg spinothalamic fibers are most superficial. More severe cord compression compromises fibers from the trunk. In patients with spinal cord compression, the lesion is often above the highest dermatome involved in the deficit. Thus, radiographic studies should be tailored to visualize the cord at and above the level of the sensory deficit detected on examination. Intrinsic cord lesions that involve the central portions of the cord often impair pain and temperature sensation at the level of the lesion since the fibers crossing the anterior commissure and entering the spinothalamic tracts are most centrally situated. Thus, enlargement of the central cervical canal in **syringomyelia** typically causes loss of pain and temperature sensation across the shoulders and upper arms (Figure 7–21).

Brainstem lesions involving the spinothalamic tract cause loss of pain and temperature sensation on the opposite side of the body. In the medulla, such lesions can involve the neighboring spinal trigeminal nucleus, resulting in a "crossed" sensory deficit involving the ipsilateral face and contralateral limbs. Above the medulla, the spinothalamic and trigeminothalamic tracts lie close together, and lesions there cause contralateral sensory loss of the face and limbs. In the midbrain and thalamus, medial lemniscal fibers run together with pain and temperature fibers, and lesions are more likely to impair all primary sensation contralateral to the lesion. Since sensory fibers converge at the thalamus, lesions there tend to cause fairly equal loss of pain, temperature, and proprioceptive sensation on the contralateral half of the face and body. Lesions of the parietal lobe impair discriminative sensation on the opposite side of the body, while detection of the primary modalities of sensation may remain relatively intact.

> 25. What fibers carry pain, and how are they segregated from fibers that carry proprioception information in the spinal cord?
> 26. What are the differences in characteristics of sensory loss at different levels of the nervous system?
> 27. What is the function of the primary sensory cortex, and what are the clinical features of damage to this region?

VISION & CONTROL OF EYE MOVEMENTS

The visual system provides our most important source of sensory information about the environment. The visual system and pathways for the control of eye movements are among the best-characterized pathways in the nervous system. Familiarity with these neuroanatomic features is often extremely valuable in localization of neurologic disease.

Anatomy

The cornea and lens of the eye refract and focus images on the photosensitive posterior portion of the retina. The posterior retina contains two classes of specialized photoreceptor cells, **rods** and **cones,** which transduce photons into electrical signals. At the retina, the image is reversed in the horizontal and vertical planes so that the inferior visual field falls upon the superior portions of the retina and the lateral field is detected by the nasal half of the retina.

Fibers from the nasal half of the retina traverse the medial portion of the optic nerve and cross to the other side at the **optic chiasm** (Figure 7–22). Each **optic tract** contains fibers from the same half of the visual field of both eyes. The optic tracts terminate in the **lateral geniculate nuclei** of the thalamus. Lateral geniculate neurons send fibers to the primary visual cortex in the occipital lobe (area 17, **calcarine cortex;** see Figure 7–9). These fibers form the **optic radiations,** which extend through the white matter of the temporal lobes and the inferior portion of the parietal lobes.

Eye movements are controlled by the extraocular muscles, which function in pairs to move the eyes along three axes (Figure 7–23). These muscles are innervated by the **oculomotor** (III), **trochlear** (IV), and **abducens** (VI) nerves. The oculomotor nerve innervates the ipsilateral **medial, superior,** and **inferior rectus muscles** and the **inferior oblique muscles.** It also supplies the ipsilateral levator palpebrae, which elevates the eyelid. The oculomotor nerve also carries parasympathetic fibers that mediate pupillary constriction (see below). Trochlear nerve fibers decussate before leaving the brainstem, and each trochlear nerve supplies the contralateral **superior oblique muscle.** The abducens nerve innervates the **lateral rectus muscle** of the same side.

Cortical and brainstem gaze centers innervate the extraocular motor nuclei and provide for supranuclear control of gaze. A **vertical gaze center** is located in the midbrain tegmentum, and **lateral gaze centers** are present in the pontine paramedian reticular formation. Each lateral gaze center sends fibers to the neighboring ipsilateral abducens nucleus and, via the **medial longitudinal fasciculus,** to the contralateral oculomotor nucleus. Therefore, activation of the right lateral gaze center stimulates conjugate deviation of the eyes to the right. Rapid **saccadic eye movements** are initiated by the **frontal eye fields** in the premotor cortex that stimulate conjugate movement of the eyes to the opposite side. Slower eye movements involved in pursuit of moving objects are controlled by parieto-occipital gaze centers, which stimulate conjugate gaze to the side of the gaze center. These cortical areas control eye movements through their connections with the brainstem gaze centers.

The size of the pupils is determined by the balance between parasympathetic and sympathetic discharge to the pupillary muscles. The parasympathetic oculomotor **nuclei of Edinger-Westphal** send fibers in the oculomotor nerves that synapse in the ciliary ganglia within the orbits and innervate the pupillary constrictor muscles.

The motor portion of pupillary dilation is controlled by a three-neuron system (Figure 7–24). It is composed of axons from neurons in the posterolateral hypothalamus that descend through the lateral brainstem tegmentum and the intermediolateral column of the cervical spinal cord to the level of T1. There they terminate on preganglionic sympathetic neurons within the lateral gray matter of the thoracic cord. These neurons send axons that synapse with postganglionic neurons in the superior cervical gan-

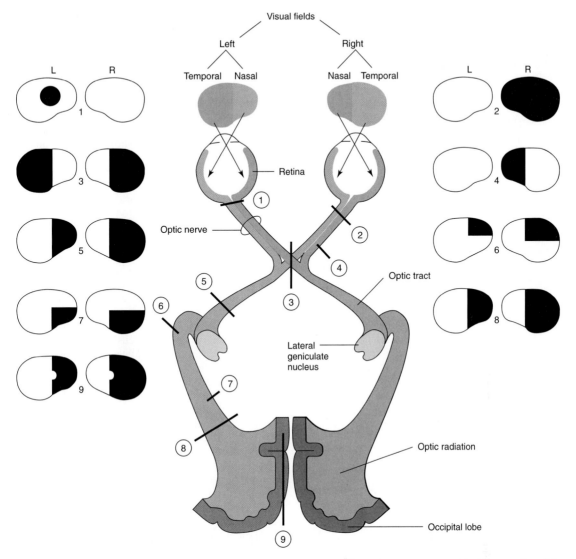

Figure 7–22. Common visual field defects and their anatomic bases. ① Central scotoma caused by inflammation of the left optic disk (optic neuritis) or optic nerve (retrobulbar neuritis). ② Total blindness of the right eye from a complete lesion of the right optic nerve. ③ Bitemporal hemianopia caused by pressure exerted on the optic chiasm by a pituitary tumor. ④ Right nasal hemianopia caused by a perichiasmal lesion (eg, calcified internal carotid artery). ⑤ Right homonymous hemianopia from a lesion of the left optic tract. ⑥ Right homonymous superior quadrantanopia caused by partial involvement of the optic radiation by a lesion in the left temporal lobe (Meyer's loop). ⑦ Right homonymous inferior quadrantanopia caused by partial involvement of the optic radiation by a lesion in the left parietal lobe. ⑧ Right homonymous hemianopia from a complete lesion of the left optic radiation. (A similar defect may also result from lesion 9.) ⑨ Right homonymous hemianopia (with macular sparing) resulting from posterior cerebral artery occlusion. (Reproduced, with permission, from Simon RP, Aminoff MJ, Greenberg DA: *Clinical Neurology,* 4th ed. Appleton & Lange, 1999.)

glion. Postganglionic neurons send fibers that travel with the internal carotid artery and the first division of the trigeminal nerve to innervate the iris. The fibers also innervate the tarsal muscles of the eyelids. Damage to these pathways causes **Horner's syndrome,** which consists of miosis, ptosis, and sometimes impaired sweating ipsilateral to the lesion.

Physiology

A. Vision: The rods are sensitive to low levels of light and are most numerous in the peripheral regions of the retina. In retinitis pigmentosa, there is degeneration of the retina that begins in the periphery. Poor twilight vision is thus an early symptom of this disorder. Cones are responsible for perception of

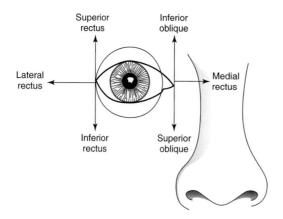

Figure 7–23. Extraocular muscles subserving the six cardinal positions of gaze. The eye is adducted by the medial rectus and abducted by the lateral rectus. The adducted eye is elevated by the inferior oblique and depressed by the superior oblique; the abducted eye is elevated by the superior rectus and depressed by the inferior rectus. (Reproduced, with permission, from Simon RP, Aminoff MJ, Greenberg DA: *Clinical Neurology,* 4th ed. Appleton & Lange, 1999.)

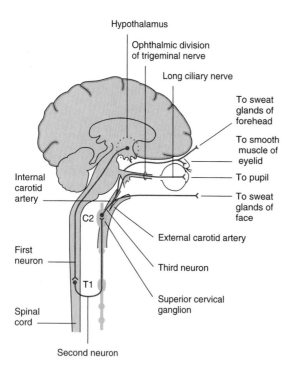

Figure 7–24. Oculosympathetic pathways. This three-neuron pathway projects from the hypothalamus to the intermediolateral column of the spinal cord, then to the superior cervical (sympathetic) ganglion, and finally to the pupil, the smooth muscle of the eyelids, and the sweat glands of the forehead and face. Interruption of these pathways results in Horner's syndrome. (Reproduced, with permission, from Simon RP, Aminoff MJ, Greenberg DA: *Clinical Neurology,* 4th ed. Appleton & Lange, 1999.)

stimuli in bright light and for discrimination of color. They are concentrated in the macular region, which is crucial for visual acuity. In disorders of the retina or optic nerve that impair acuity, diminished color discrimination is often an early sign.

Visual processing begins in the retina, where information gathered from rods and cones is modified by interactions between bipolar, amacrine, and horizontal cells. Amacrine and bipolar cells send their output to ganglion cells, whose axons comprise the optic nerve. Photoreceptors convey information about the absolute level of illumination. Retinal processing renders ganglion cells sensitive to simultaneous differences in contrast for detection of edges of objects.

Ganglion cell axons terminate in a highly ordered fashion in well-defined layers of the lateral geniculate nuclei. Because of the separation of fibers in the optic chiasm, the receptive fields of cells in the lateral geniculate lie in the contralateral visual field. Geniculate neurons are arranged in six layers, and ganglion cell axons from each eye terminate in separate layers. Cells in different layers are in register, so that the receptive fields of cells in the same part of each layer are in corresponding regions of the two retinas. A greater proportion of cells are devoted to the macular region of both retinas. This reflects use of the central retina for high acuity and color vision. Some visual processing occurs in the geniculate, particularly for contrast and edge perception and detection of movement.

In primary visual cortex, visual fields from the eyes are also represented in a topographic projection. Cortical neurons are functionally organized in columns perpendicular to the cortical surface. Geniculate fibers terminate within layer IV of the visual cortex, and cells within a column above and below layer IV show the same eye preference and similar receptive fields. Narrow alternating columns of cells supplied by one eye or the other lie next to each other **(ocular dominance columns).** A tremendous amount of visual processing occurs in primary visual cortex, including the synthesis of complex receptive fields and determination of axis orientation, position, and color. The retina is not simply represented as a map on the cortex—rather, each area of the retina is represented in multiple columns and analyzed with respect to position, color, and orientation of objects. As in the geniculate, a major portion of the primary visual cortex is devoted to analysis of information derived from the macular regions of both retinas. Cortical areas 18 and 19 provide higher levels of visual processing.

The anatomic organization of the visual system is useful for localizing neurologic disease (Figure 7–22). Lesions of the retina or optic nerves **(prechiasmal lesions)** impair vision from the ipsilateral eye. Lesions that compress the central portion of the chiasm, such as pituitary tumors, disrupt crossing fibers from the nasal halves of both retinas, causing **bitemporal hemianopia**. Lesions involving structures behind the chiasm (**retrochiasmal lesions**) cause visual loss in the contralateral field of both eyes. Lesions that completely destroy the optic tract, lateral geniculate nucleus, or optic radiations on one side produce a contralateral **homonymous hemianopia**. Selective destruction of temporal lobe optic radiations causes **superior quadrantanopia,** and lesions of the parietal optic radiations cause **inferior quadrantanopia.** The posterior portions of the optic radiations and the calcarine cortex are supplied mainly by the posterior cerebral artery, though the macular region of the visual cortex receives some collateral supply from the middle cerebral artery. Therefore, a lesion of primary visual cortex generally causes contralateral homonymous hemianopia, but if it is due to posterior cerebral artery occlusion it may spare macular vision.

B. Eye Movements: Conjugate eye movements are regulated by proprioceptive information from neck structures and information about head movement and position from the vestibular system. This information is used to maintain fixation on a stationary point when moving the head. In a comatose patient, the integrity of these oculovestibular and oculocephalic pathways can be assessed by the "doll's-eye" maneuver. This is elicited by briskly turning the head, which normally results in conjugate movement of the eyes in the opposite direction in a comatose patient. Irrigation of the ear with 10–20 mL of cold water reduces the activity of the labyrinth on that side and elicits jerk nystagmus, with the fast component away from the irrigated ear in a conscious individual. In coma, the fast saccadic component is lost, and the vestibular influence on eye movements dominates. Cold water irrigation then results in deviation of the eyes toward the irrigated ear. These caloric responses are lost with midbrain or pontine lesions, with damage to the labyrinths, or with drugs that inhibit vestibular function.

C. Pupillary Function: The size of the pupils is controlled by the amount of ambient light sensed by the retina (Figure 7–25). Fibers from each retina terminate within midbrain pretectal nuclei that send fibers to both Edinger-Westphal nuclei to activate pupillary constriction in bright light. In dim light, this reflex is inhibited and the influence of sympathetic fibers predominates, causing pupillary dilation. The pupillary constrictor fibers release acetylcholine, which activates muscarinic acetylcholine receptors and thus stimulates contraction of the pupillary sphincter muscle of the iris. Sympathetic pupillary fibers release norepinephrine, which activates α_1-adrenergic receptors, causing contraction of the radial muscle of the iris. Drugs that inhibit muscarinic receptors, such as atropine, or that stimulate α_1-adrenergic receptors, such as epinephrine, dilate the pupils, while drugs that stimulate muscarinic receptors or block α_1-adrenergic receptors cause pupillary constriction.

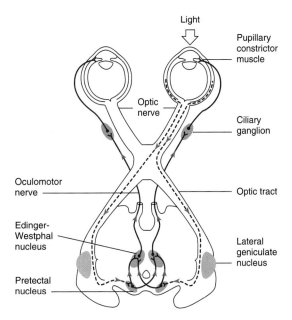

Figure 7–25. Anatomic basis of the pupillary light reflex. The afferent visual pathways from the retina to the pretectal nuclei of the midbrain are represented by dashed lines, the efferent pupilloconstrictor pathways from the midbrain to the retinas by solid lines. Note that illumination of one eye results in bilateral pupillary constriction. (Reproduced, with permission, from Simon RP, Aminoff MJ, Greenberg DA: *Clinical Neurology,* 4th ed. Appleton & Lange, 1999.)

---

28. What is the pathway of fibers from the retina to the visual cortex?
29. What is the innervation of the extraocular muscles?
30. Describe how lesions in various parts of the visual pathways produce characteristic visual field defects.

HEARING & BALANCE

Anatomy

Structures of the middle ear serve to amplify and transmit sounds to the cochlea, where specialized sensory cells (hair cells) are organized to detect ranges in amplitude and frequency of sound. The semicircular canals contain specialized hair cells that detect movement of endolymphatic fluid contained within the canals. Similar hair cells in the saccule and utricle detect movement of the otolithic membrane, which is composed of calcium carbonate crystals embedded in a matrix. The semicircular canal hair cells detect angular acceleration, while the hair cells of the utricle and saccule detect linear acceleration. Axons from auditory and vestibular neurons comprise the eighth cranial nerve, which traverses the petrous bone, is joined by the facial nerve, and enters the posterior fossa through the auditory canal. Auditory fibers terminate in the cochlear nuclei of the pons, and vestibular fibers terminate in the vestibular nuclear complex.

Cochlear neurons send fibers bilaterally to a network of auditory nuclei in the midbrain, and impulses are finally relayed through the medial geniculate thalamic nuclei to the auditory cortex in the superior temporal gyri. Vestibular nuclei have connections with the cerebellum, red nuclei, brainstem gaze centers, and brainstem reticular formation. The vestibular nuclei exert considerable control over posture through descending vestibulospinal, rubrospinal, and reticulospinal pathways.

Physiology

A. Hearing: There are three types of hearing loss: (1) **conductive deafness,** which is due to diseases of the external or middle ear that impair conduction and amplification of sound from the air to the cochlea; (2) **sensorineural deafness,** due to diseases of the cochlea or eighth cranial nerve; and (3) **central deafness,** due to diseases affecting the cochlear nuclei or auditory pathways in the central nervous system. Because of the redundancy of central pathways, almost all cases of hearing loss are due to conductive or sensorineural deafness. Besides hearing loss, auditory diseases may cause **tinnitus,** the subjective sensation of noise in the ear. Tinnitus due to disorders of the cochlea or eighth cranial nerve sounds like a constant nonmusical tone and may be described as ringing, whistling, hissing, humming, or roaring. Transient episodes of tinnitus occur in most individuals and are not associated with disease. When persistent, tinnitus is often associated with hearing loss.

Conductive and sensorineural deafness may be distinguished by examining hearing with a vibrating 512 Hz tuning fork. In the **Rinne test,** the tuning fork is held on the mastoid process behind the ear and then is placed at the auditory meatus. If the sound is louder at the meatus, the test is positive. Normally the test is positive, since sound transmitted through air is amplified by middle ear structures. In sensorineural deafness, although sound perception is reduced, the Rinne test is still positive since middle ear structures are intact. In conductive deafness, sounds are heard less well through air and the test is negative. In the **Weber test,** the tuning fork is applied to the forehead at the midline. In conductive deafness, the sound is heard best in the abnormal ear, whereas with sensorineural deafness the sound is heard best in the normal ear. **Audiometry** can distinguish types of hearing loss. In general, sensorineural deafness causes greater loss of high-pitched sounds, whereas conductive deafness causes more loss of low-pitched sounds.

B. Vestibular Function: In contrast to hearing, vestibular function is commonly disturbed by small brainstem lesions. The vestibular nuclei occupy a large portion of the lateral brainstem, extending from medulla to midbrain. Although there are extensive bilateral connections between vestibular nuclei and other motor pathways, these connections are not redundant but are highly lateralized and act in concert to control posture, balance, and conjugate eye movement.

Patients with diseases of the vestibular system complain of disequilibrium and dizziness. Cerebellar disease also causes disequilibrium, but this is often described as a problem with coordination rather than a feeling of dizziness in the head. Interpretation of the complaint of dizziness can often be difficult. Many patients use the term loosely to describe sensations of light-headedness, weakness, or malaise. Directed questioning is often required to establish whether there is truly an abnormal sensation of movement **(vertigo).**

Vertigo may be due to disease of the labyrinth or vestibular nerve (peripheral vertigo) or to dysfunction of brainstem and central nervous system pathways (central vertigo). In general, peripheral vertigo is more severe and associated with nausea and vomiting, especially if the onset is acute. Diseases of the semicircular canal neurons or their fibers frequently cause rotational vertigo, whereas diseases involving the utricle or saccule cause sensations of tilting or listing, as on a boat. Traumatic and ischemic lesions may cause associated hearing loss. Dysfunction of one labyrinth often causes horizontal and rotatory **jerk nystagmus.** The slow phase of the nystagmus is caused by the unopposed action of the normal labyrinth, which drives the eyes to the side of the lesion. The fast jerk phase is due to a rapid saccade, which maintains fixation.

Vertigo due to lesions of the central nervous system is usually less severe than peripheral vertigo and is often associated with other findings of brainstem dysfunction. In addition, nystagmus associated with central lesions may be present in vertical or multiple directions of gaze. Common causes of central vertigo include brainstem ischemia, brainstem tumors, and multiple sclerosis.

---

31. How does one distinguish between conductive and sensorineural hearing loss?
32. What are the major clinical features of unilateral vestibular dysfunction?

CONSCIOUSNESS, AROUSAL, & COGNITION

Anatomy

Consciousness is awareness of self and the environment. It has two aspects: **arousal,** which is the state of wakefulness; and **cognition,** which is the sum of mental activities. This distinction is useful, since neurologic disorders can affect arousal and cognition differently. Arousal is generated by activity of the ascending reticular activating system (Figure 7–26), which is composed of neurons within the central mesencephalic brainstem, the lateral hypothalamus, and the medial, intralaminar, and reticular nuclei of the thalamus. Widespread projections from these nuclei synapse on distal dendritic fields of large pyramidal neurons in the cerebral cortex and generate an arousal response. Cognition is the chief function of the cerebral cortex, particularly of prefrontal cortex and cortical association areas of the occipital, temporal, and parietal lobes. Some specialized mental functions are localized to specific cortical regions. Several subcortical nuclei in the basal ganglia and thalamus are intimately linked with cortical association areas, and damage to these nuclei or their interconnections with cortex may give rise to cognitive deficits similar to those observed with cortical lesions.

Physiology

A. Arousal: The reticular activating system is excited by a wide variety of stimuli, especially somatosensory stimuli. It is most compact in the midbrain and can be damaged by central midbrain lesions, resulting in failure of arousal, or **coma.** Higher nuclei and projections are less localized, and lesions rostrad to the midbrain must therefore be bilateral to cause coma.

Less severe dysfunction causes **confusional states** in which consciousness is clouded and the patient is sleepy, inattentive, and disoriented. Alertness is reduced, and the patient will appear drowsy or fall asleep easily without frequent stimulation. More awake patients perceive stimuli slowly but are distractible, assigning important and irrelevant stimuli equal value. Perceptions may be distorted, leading to **hallucinations,** and the patient may be unable to organize and interpret a complex set of stimuli. The inability to perceive properly interferes with learning and memory and with problem solving. Thoughts become disorganized and tangential, and the confused patient may maintain false beliefs in the face of evidence of their falsity (**delusions**). In some cases, the confusional state presents as **delirium,** which is characterized by heightened alertness, disordered perception, agitation, delusions, hallucinations, convulsions, and autonomic hyperactivity (sweating, tachycardia, hypertension).

Coma may result from structural or metabolic causes. Some structural lesions of the cerebral hemispheres, such as hemorrhages, large areas of ischemic infarction, abscesses, or tumors can expand over minutes or a few hours and cause brain tissue to herniate into the posterior fossa (Figure 7–27). If lateral within the temporal lobe, the expanding mass may drive the uncus of the temporal lobe into the ambient cistern surrounding the midbrain, compressing the ipsilateral third cranial nerve (**uncal herniation**). This causes pupillary dilation and impaired function of eye muscles innervated by that nerve. Continued pressure distorts the midbrain, and the patient lapses into coma with posturing of the limbs. With continued herniation, pontine function is impaired, causing loss of oculovestibular responses. Eventually, medullary function is lost, and breathing ceases. Hemispheric lesions closer to the midline compress thalamic reticular formation structures and can cause coma before eye findings develop (**central herniation**). With continued pressure, midbrain function is affected, causing the pupils to dilate and the limbs to posture. With progressive herniation, pontine vestibular and then medullary respiratory functions are lost.

Several nonstructural disorders that diffusely disturb brain function can produce a confusional state or, if severe, coma (Table 7–1). Most of these disorders are acute, and many—particularly those due to

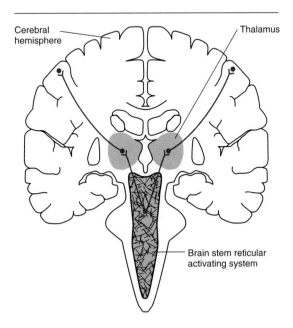

Figure 7–26. Brainstem reticular activating system and its ascending projections to the thalamus and cerebral hemispheres. (Reproduced, with permission, from Simon RP, Aminoff MJ, Greenberg DA: *Clinical Neurology,* 4th ed. Appleton & Lange, 1999.)

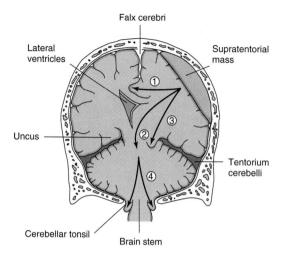

Figure 7–27. Anatomic basis of herniation syndromes. An expanding supratentorial mass lesion may cause brain tissue to be displaced into an adjacent intracranial compartment, resulting in (1) cingulate herniation under the falx cerebri, (2) downward transtentorial (central) herniation, (3) uncal herniation over the edge of the tentorium, or (4) cerebellar tonsillar herniation into the foramen magnum. Coma and ultimately death result when (2), (3), or (4) produces brainstem compression. (Reproduced, with permission, from Simon RP, Aminoff MJ, Greenberg DA: *Clinical Neurology,* 4th ed. Appleton & Lange, 1999.)

drugs and metabolic toxins—are reversible. Clues to the etiology of these "metabolic" encephalopathies are provided by the general physical examination, drug screens, and certain blood studies. When these disorders cause coma, pupillary light responses are usually preserved despite impaired oculovestibular or respiratory function. This finding is of great help in distinguishing metabolic from structural causes of coma.

Neurons in the dorsal midbrain and especially nuclei within the pontine reticular formation are impor-

Table 7–1. Nonstructural causes of confusional states and coma.

Drugs (sedative-hypnotics, ethanol, opioids)
Global cerebral ischemia
Hepatic encephalopathy
Hypercalcemia
Hyperosmolar states
Hyperthermia
Hypoglycemia
Hyponatremia
Hypoxia
Hypothyroidism
Meningitis and encephalitis
Seizure or prolonged postictal state
Subarachnoid hemorrhage
Thyrotoxicosis
Uremia
Wernicke's encephalopathy

---

tant for **sleep.** Thus, lesions involving the pons may preserve consciousness but disturb sleep. In contrast, diffuse lesions of the neocortex, such as those resulting from global cerebral ischemia, may preserve the reticular activating system and brainstem sleep centers, resulting in a patient with preserved sleep-wake cycles who cannot interact in any meaningful way with the environment (coma vigil or apallic state).

B. Cognition: Several disorders disturb cognition rather than the level of consciousness. Specific cortical regions generally mediate different cognitive functions, though there is considerable overlap and interconnection between cortical and subcortical structures in all mental tasks. When several of these abilities are impaired, the patient is said to suffer from **dementia.** Dementia is discussed in more detail later in this chapter.

The prefrontal cortex (Figure 7–9) generally refers to areas 9, 10, 11, 12, 45, 46, and 47 of Brodmann on the superior and lateral surfaces of the frontal lobes and the anterior cingulate, parolfactory, and orbitofrontal cortex inferiorly and mesially. These regions are essential for orderly planning and sequencing of complex behaviors, attending to several stimuli or ideas simultaneously, concentrating and flexibly altering the focus of concentration, grasping the context and meaning of information, and controlling impulses, emotions, and thought sequences. Damage to the frontal lobes or connections to the caudate and dorsal medial nuclei of the thalamus causes the **frontal lobe syndrome.** Patients may suffer dramatic alterations in personality and behavior, while most sensorimotor functions remain intact. Some patients become vulgar in speech, slovenly, grandiose, and irascible while others lose interest, spontaneity, curiosity, and initiative. The affect may become apathetic and blunted **(abulia).** Some patients lose the capacity for creativity and abstract reasoning and the ability to solve problems while becoming excessively concrete in their thinking. Often they are distractible and unable to focus attention when presented with multiple stimuli. The most dramatic manifestations are seen following bilateral frontal lobe damage; unilateral damage can lead to subtle alterations in behavior that may be difficult to detect. Involvement of premotor areas may lead to incontinence, the inability to perform learned motor tasks **(apraxia),** variable increases in muscle tone **(paratonia),** and the appearance of primitive grasp and oral reflexes (sucking, snouting, and rooting).

In about 90% of people, **language** is a function of the left hemisphere. While 99% of right-handed people are left hemisphere-dominant, about 40% of left-handed people are right hemisphere-dominant for language. In most left-handers hemispheric dominance for language is incomplete, and damage to the dominant hemisphere tends to disturb language less severely than in right-handed individuals. The cortical regions most critical for language include Broca's area (area 44), Wernicke's area (area 22), the primary auditory cortex (areas 41 and 42), and neighboring frontal and temporoparietal association areas (Figure 7–9). Injury to these areas or their connections to other cortical regions result in **aphasia.** Lesions in the frontal speech areas cause nonfluent, dysarthric, halting speech, whereas lesions of the temporal speech area cause fluent speech that contains many errors or may be totally devoid of understandable words. Patients with damage to temporal speech areas also lack comprehension of spoken words. Isolation of the temporal speech area from the occipital lobes causes an inability to read **(alexia).** Portions of the parietal lobe adjacent to the temporal lobe are important for retrieval of previously learned words, and damage here may result in **anomia.** The inferior parietal region is important for the translation of linguistic messages generated in the temporal language areas into visual symbols. Damage to this region may result in an inability to write **(agraphia).**

Memory requires that information be registered by the primary somatosensory, auditory, or visual cortex. Posterior cortical areas involved in comprehension of language are needed for immediate processing of spoken or written events and recalling them immediately. The hippocampi and their connections to the dorsal medial nuclei of the thalamus and the mamillary nuclei of the hypothalamus constitute a limbic system network crucial for learning and processing of events for long-term storage. When these areas are damaged, the patient is unable to learn new material or retrieve memories from the recent past. The most severe symptoms occur with bilateral lesions; unilateral disease causes more subtle learning deficits. Memories that remain with a person for years are considered remote memories and are stored in corresponding association cortex areas (eg, visual cortex for scenes). Remote memories remain intact in patients with damage to limbic structures required for learning. However, they may be lost by damage to cortical association areas. The mechanism by which recent memories are transferred from the limbic memory network to association cortex for long-term storage is not known.

The parietal association cortex is the region principally involved in visuomotor integration of constructional tasks. The visual cortex is required for observation, whereas the auditory cortex and the temporal language cortex are necessary for drawing objects on command. The inferior parietal cortex (areas 39 and 40) integrates visual and auditory information, and the output from this region is translated into motor patterns by motor cortex. Thus, lesions to the parietal lobes commonly cause constructional impairment. Damage to either hemisphere may result in constructional errors. Drawings may show rotation of objects, disorientation of objects on the background, fragmentation of design, inability to draw angles properly, or omission of parts of a figure presented for copying. It is often difficult to determine which side is damaged, though if language is preserved, a nondominant parietal deficit is more likely.

Calculation ability, abstract reasoning, problem solving, and several other aspects of intelligence are difficult to localize because they require integration of several cortical regions. They are frequently disturbed by diseases that cause widespread cortical dysfunction, such as those that cause dementia.

---

33. What is the network of neurons that maintain normal arousal and consciousness?
34. What are the symptoms and signs of cerebral herniation due to focal brain lesions?
35. Which cognitive functions are controlled by the frontal lobes and by the parietal association cortex?
36. What regions of the cortex are important for language and memory?

PATHOPHYSIOLOGY OF SELECTED NEUROLOGIC DISORDERS

Nervous system disease may be caused by a wide variety of degenerative, metabolic, structural, neoplastic, or inflammatory conditions that affect neurons, glia, or both. The resultant dysfunction is expressed either by neuronal hyperactivity, as seen during seizures, or by decreased activity of neurons, as observed following a stroke. The specific functional abnormalities observed depend on the network of neurons affected. For example, since amyotrophic lateral sclerosis is a disorder of upper and lower motor neurons, neurologic deficits are limited to the motor system. In Parkinson's disease, dopaminergic neurons of the substantia nigra degenerate, causing symptoms of extrapyramidal motor system dysfunction. In patients with ischemic stroke, the particular constellation of deficits is determined by the vascular territory affected. Therefore, an understanding of the pathophysiology of neurologic disease requires an analysis of events occurring at both the cellular level and the level of neural networks.

MOTOR NEURON DISEASE

Clinical Presentation

Motor neuron diseases predominantly affect the anterior horn cells of the spinal cord and are characterized by wasting and weakness of skeletal muscles. Spontaneous discharges of degenerating motor nerve fibers occur, giving rise to muscle twitches known as **fasciculations.** Electromyography characteristically shows features of denervation, including fibrillations in resting muscle and a reduction in the number of motor units detected during voluntary contraction. Sprouting of remaining healthy motor fibers may occur, leading to the appearance of large, polyphasic motor unit potentials.

The **spinal muscular atrophies** are genetic disorders that appear in childhood or early adolescence. Infantile spinal muscular atrophy **(Werdnig-Hoffman disease)** is an autosomal recessive disorder that manifests usually within the first 3 months of life. Infants with this condition have difficulty sucking, swallowing, and breathing. Atrophy and fasciculations are found in the tongue and limb muscles. The disorder is rapidly progressive, leading to death from respiratory complications usually by age 3. An intermediate form of the disease, also with an autosomal recessive mode of inheritance, begins in the latter half of the first year of life. It progresses more slowly than the infantile form, and patients may survive into adulthood. Both the infantile and the intermediate forms are due to deletions or mutations in the survival motor neuron *(SMN)* gene on chromosome 5. The SMN gene product appears to protect cells from programmed cell death **(apoptosis),** and absent or decreased anti-apoptotic activity of SMN appears to underlie the pathogenesis of SMA. **Kugelberg-Welander disease** is a mixed group of motor neuron diseases that develop in childhood or early adolescence. Patients develop weakness of proximal limb muscles with relative sparing of bulbar muscles. The course is gradually progressive, leading to disability in adulthood. In most cases, the mode of inheritance is autosomal recessive, but some are autosomal dominant or X-linked. The genetic basis for these disorders has not been determined. **Kennedy's disease** (progressive proximal spinal and bulbar muscular atrophy of late onset) is an X-linked recessive disorder that becomes manifest clinically in the fourth and fifth decades and is associated with an expanded CAG repeat in the androgen receptor gene. Androgen receptor function is normal in these patients, and the pathogenesis of neurodegeneration is not yet known.

In adults, motor neuron disease usually begins between the ages of 30 and 60 years and is commonly sporadic but may be familial in up to 10% of cases. Several varieties have been described, depending on relative involvement of upper or lower motor neurons and bulbar or spinal anterior horn cells. The most common form is **amyotrophic lateral sclerosis (ALS),** in which mixed upper and lower motor neuron deficits are found in limb and bulbar muscles. In 80% of patients, the initial symptoms are due to weakness of limb muscles. Complaints are often bilateral but asymmetric. Involvement of bulbar muscles causes difficulty with swallowing, chewing, speaking, breathing, and coughing. Neurologic examination reveals a mixture of upper and lower motor neuron signs. There is usually no involvement of extraocular muscles or sphincters. The disease is progressive and generally fatal within 3–5 years, with death resulting from pulmonary infection and respiratory failure.

Pathology & Pathogenesis

In ALS there is selective degeneration of motor neurons in the primary motor cortex and the anterolateral horns of the spinal cord. Many affected neurons show cytoskeletal disease with accumulations of neurofilaments in the cell body and in axons. There is only a subtle glial cell response and little evidence of inflammation. The cause is unknown, but recent biochemical and genetic studies have provided several clues.

A. Glutamate Transport: Glutamate (Figure 7–28) is the most abundant excitatory neurotransmitter in the central nervous system. Glutamate activates a large family of receptors that either open cation channels (ionotropic receptors) or activate phospholipase C (metabotropic receptors), which catalyzes the formation of the second messenger, inositol-1,4,5-trisphosphate (IP_3). Influx of Na^+ and Ca^{2+} through glutamate-gated cation channels depolarizes cells, while IP_3 stimulates release of Ca^{2+} from intracellular storage sites. The net effect of these events is to generate an excitatory postsynaptic potential and raise the concentration of free intracellular Ca^{2+} in the cytosol of the postsynaptic neuron. This Ca^{2+} signal activates calcium-sensitive enzymes and is quickly terminated by removal of glutamate from the synapse and by mechanisms for calcium sequestration and extrusion in the postsynaptic cell. Breakdown of normal mechanisms for terminating the excitatory signal leads to sustained elevations in intracellular Ca^{2+} that cause cell death.

Glutamate is removed from synapses by transport proteins on surrounding astrocytes and nerve terminals. In astrocytes, it is metabolized to glutamine and can be shuttled back to neurons for reconversion into glutamate. In 60% of patients with ALS, there is a large decrease in glutamate transport activity in the motor cortex and spinal cord but not in other regions of the central nervous system. This is associated with a loss of the astrocytic glutamate transporter protein EAAT2 due to a defect in splicing of its messenger RNA. In cultured spinal cord slices, pharmacologic inhibition of glutamate transport induces motor neuron degeneration. Thus, selective loss of a glutamate transporter may cause excitotoxicity in ALS by increasing extracellular levels of glutamate.

B. Free Radicals: In 1993 it was discovered that some familial forms of ALS are strongly linked to mutations in the **cytosolic copper-zinc superoxide dismutase (*SOD1*)** gene on the long arm of chromosome 21. *SOD1* catalyzes the formation of hydrogen peroxide from superoxide anion. Hydrogen

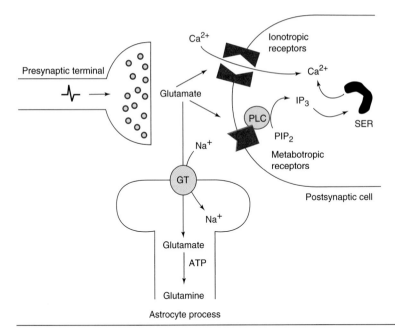

Figure 7–28. Glutamatergic neurotransmission. Depolarization stimulates release of glutamate from presynaptic terminals into the synaptic cleft, where it binds to ionotropic or metabotropic glutamate receptors, stimulating Ca^{2+} influx and activation of phospholipase C (PLC). PLC catalyzes hydrolysis of phosphatidyl-inositol-4,5-bisphosphate (PIP_2) to produce inositol-1,4,5-trisphosphate (IP_3), which causes release of Ca^{2+} from storage sites in smooth endoplasmic reticulum (SER). Synaptic actions of glutamate are terminated mainly by uptake through Na^+-dependent glutamate transporters (GT) on glia. In astrocytes, glutamate is converted into glutamine by glutamine synthetase.

peroxide is then detoxified by catalase or glutathione peroxidase to form water. Not all mutations reduce *SOD1* activity, and the disorder is inherited as an autosomal dominant trait, suggesting that mutations in familial ALS result in a gain rather than a loss of function. This is supported by the finding that transgenic mice expressing mutant *SOD1* develop motor neuron disease analogous to human familial ALS. Evidence indicates that the mutant enzyme has an altered substrate specificity and catalyzes the reduction of hydrogen peroxide to yield hydroxyl radicals. Support for involvement of free radicals in the pathogenesis of ALS comes from work demonstrating that the antioxidant vitamin E delays the onset of motor neuron disease in mice transgenic for mutant *SOD1*. In addition, brains of sporadic ALS patients have elevated levels of carbonyl proteins, suggesting oxidative damage.

C. Neurofilament Proteins: Motor neurons tend to be very large, with extremely long axons, and cytoskeletal proteins that maintain axonal structure may be critical targets for motor neuron injury. A role for neurofilament dysfunction in ALS is supported by the finding that neurofilamentous accumulations in cell bodies and proximal axons are an early feature of ALS pathology. In addition, mutations in the heavy chain neurofilament subunit have been detected in some patients with ALS. Moreover, transgenic mice overexpressing normal or mutant neurofilament proteins develop motor neuron disease. Increased or abnormal neurofilaments may interfere with axonal transport, resulting in failure to maintain axonal structure and transport of macromolecules such as neurotrophic factors required for motor neuron survival.

37. What are the clinical features of motor neuron disease?
38. What gene is responsible for some cases of familial ALS, and what is the postulated molecular mechanism by which the mutation causes disease?
39. What two other mechanisms may play a role in motor neuron degeneration?

PARKINSON'S DISEASE

Clinical Presentation

Parkinsonism is a clinical syndrome of rigidity, bradykinesia, tremor, and postural instability. Most cases are due to Parkinson's disease, an idiopathic disorder with a prevalence of about 1–2:1000. In the first half of this century, parkinsonism was a common sequela of von Economo's encephalitis, but since this infection no longer occurs, this type of parkinsonism is rare. Parkinsonism can also result from exposure to certain toxins such as manganese, carbon disulfide, or carbon monoxide. Several drugs, particularly butyrophenones, phenothiazines, metoclopramide, reserpine, and tetrabenazine, can cause reversible parkinsonism. Parkinsonism may also result from repeated head trauma or may be a feature of several basal ganglia diseases, including Wilson's disease, some cases of Huntington's disease, Shy-Drager syndrome, striatonigral degeneration, and progressive supranuclear palsy. In these disorders, other symptoms and signs are present along with parkinsonism.

Pathology & Pathogenesis

In Parkinson's disease, there is selective degeneration of monoamine-containing cell populations in the brainstem and basal ganglia, particularly of pigmented dopaminergic neurons of the substantia nigra. In addition, scattered neurons in basal ganglia, brainstem, spinal cord, and sympathetic ganglia contain eosinophilic inclusion bodies (**Lewy bodies**).

The mechanism by which dopaminergic neurons of the substantia nigra degenerate in Parkinson's disease is not understood. A mutation for the presynaptic protein α-synuclein on chromosome 4 has been found in a few families with autosomal dominant Parkinson's disease. In addition, mutations in the gene *parkin* on chromosome 6 have been identified in some cases of juvenile parkinsonism. The mechanisms by which these mutations cause disease and their relationship to sporadic Parkinson's disease are not known.

More has been learned about the pathogenesis of Parkinson's disease through study of the potent neurotoxin MPTP (1-methyl-4-phenyl-1,2,3,6-tetrahydropyridine). MPTP is a by-product of synthesis of a synthetic opioid derivative of meperidine. Illicit use of opioid preparations heavily contaminated with MPTP led to several cases of parkinsonism in the early 1980s. MPTP selectively injures dopaminergic neurons in the brain and produces a clinical syndrome very similar to Parkinson's disease.

MPTP enters the brain (Figure 7–29) and is converted by monoamine oxidase B present in glia and serotonergic nerve terminals to *N*-methyl-4-phenyldihydropyridine (MPDP$^+$), which diffuses across glial membranes and then undergoes nonenzymatic oxidation and reduction to the active metabolite *N*-methyl-4-phenylpyridinium (MPP$^+$). MPP$^+$ is taken up by plasma membrane transporters that normally act to terminate the action of monoamines by removing them from synapses. Internalized MPP$^+$ inhibits oxidative phosphorylation by interacting with complex I of the mitochondrial electron transport chain. This inhibits ATP production and reduces metabolism of molecular oxygen, allowing for increased formation of peroxide, hydroxyl radicals, and superoxide radicals that react with lipids, proteins, and nucleic acids to cause cell injury.

Despite clinical and pathologic similarities between MPTP toxicity and Parkinson's disease, no toxin has been identified in Parkinson's disease. However, exogenous dopamine is toxic to neurons in culture. Dopamine undergoes auto-oxidation to generate superoxide radicals or is metabolized by monoamine oxidase to generate hydrogen peroxide. Superoxide dismutase catalyzes the conversion of superoxide to H_2O_2, which is converted by glutathione peroxidase and catalase to water. However, H_2O_2 can also react with ferrous iron to form highly reactive hydroxyl radicals. In Parkinson's disease, conditions favor the formation of free radicals, since iron deposition in the substantia nigra is increased and levels of glutathione are reduced.

Treatment is directed toward restoring the balance of dopaminergic and cholinergic activity in the striatum and preventing further neural degeneration. This is accomplished by blocking the effect of acetylcholine with anticholinergic drugs or by increasing the effect of dopamine. For reasons that are not clear, anticholinergic drugs are more helpful in reducing tremor and rigidity than relieving bradykinesia, which is often the more disabling symptom. In contrast, dopaminergic drugs are quite effective in alleviating bradykinesia and rigidity. Levodopa, which is converted to dopamine, or ergot derivatives such as bromocriptine and pergolide that are dopamine agonists, can be given orally to relieve symptoms. Amantadine, an antiviral agent, also reduces manifestations of Parkinson's disease, probably by increasing the release of dopamine. Selegiline is an inhibitor of MAO-B that prevents experimental MPTP toxicity. Selegiline also inhibits metabolism of dopamine and therefore increases the antiparkinsonian effect of levodopa. Selegiline also delays the onset of disability in early Parkinson's disease, perhaps by inhibiting dopamine metabolism, which may reduce free radical formation and oxidative stress in surviving dopaminergic neurons.

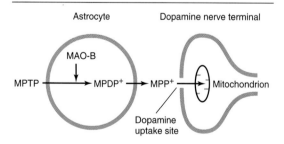

Figure 7–29. Proposed mechanism of MPTP-induced parkinsonism. MPTP enters brain astrocytes and is converted to MPDP$^+$ through the action of monoamine oxidase type B (MAO-B). MPDP$^+$ is then metabolized extracellularly to MPP$^+$, which is taken up through dopamine uptake sites on dopamine nerve terminals and concentrated in mitochondria. The resulting disturbance of mitochondrial function can lead to neuronal death. (Reproduced, with permission, from Simon RP, Aminoff MJ, Greenberg DA: *Clinical Neurology,* 4th ed. Appleton & Lange, 1999.)

40. What are the clinical features of parkinsonism?
41. What are some of the causes of this syndrome?
42. What is the pathophysiology of Parkinson's disease?

MYASTHENIA GRAVIS

Clinical Presentation

Myasthenia gravis is an autoimmune disorder of neuromuscular transmission. The major clinical features are fluctuating fatigue and weakness that improve after a period of rest and after administration of acetylcholinesterase inhibitors. Muscles with small motor units, such as ocular muscles, are most often affected. Oropharyngeal muscles, flexors and extensors of the neck, proximal limb muscles, and the erector spinae muscle are involved less often. In severe cases, all muscles are weak, including the diaphragm and intercostal muscles, and death may result from respiratory failure.

About 5% of patients have coexistent hyperthyroidism. Rheumatoid arthritis, systemic lupus erythematosus, and polymyositis are also more common in patients with myasthenia gravis than in the general population, and up to 30% of patients have a maternal relative with an autoimmune disorder. These associations suggest that patients with myasthenia gravis share a genetic predisposition to autoimmune disease.

Pathology & Pathogenesis

The major structural abnormality in myasthenia gravis is a simplification of the postsynaptic region of the neuromuscular synapse. The muscle end plate shows sparse, shallow, and abnormally wide or absent synaptic clefts. In contrast, the number and size of the presynaptic vesicles are normal. Scattered collections of lymphocytes, some within the vicinity of motor end plates, may be present. IgG and the C3 component of complement are present at the postsynaptic membrane.

Electrophysiologic studies indicate that the postsynaptic membrane has a decreased response to applied acetylcholine. Studies with ^{125}I-labeled α-bungarotoxin, which binds with high affinity to muscle nicotinic acetylcholine receptors, show a 70–90% decrease in the number of receptors per end plate in affected muscles. Circulating antibodies to the receptor are present in 70–90% of patients, and the disorder may be passively transferred to animals by administration of IgG from affected patients. Moreover, immunization with acetylcholine receptor protein from muscle can produce myasthenia in experimental animals. The antibodies block acetylcholine binding and receptor activation (Figure 7–30). In addition, the antibodies cross-link pairs of receptor molecules, increasing receptor internalization and degradation. Bound antibody also activates complement-mediated destruction of the postsynaptic region, resulting in simplification of the end plate.

During repetitive stimulation of a motor nerve, the number of quanta released from the nerve terminal declines with successive stimuli. Normally, this causes no clinical impairment because a sufficient number of acetylcholine receptor channels are opened by the reduced level of neurotransmitter. However, in myasthenia gravis, where there is a deficiency in the number of functional acetylcholine receptors, neuromuscular transmission fails at lower levels of quantal release. Electrophysiologically, this is measured as a decremental decline in the compound muscle action potential during repetitive stimulation of a motor nerve. Clinically, this is manifested by muscle fatigue with sustained or repeated activity.

Treatment has reduced the mortality rate from approximately 30% to 5% in generalized myasthenia gravis. The two basic strategies for treatment that stem from knowledge of the pathogenesis are to in-

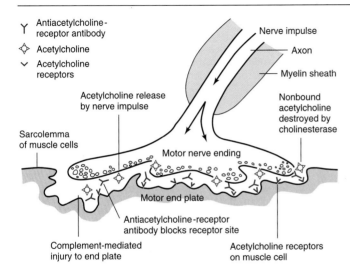

Figure 7–30. Pathogenesis of myasthenia gravis. Acetylcholine released at the nerve ending by the nerve impulse normally binds with acetylcholine receptors. This evokes the action potential in the muscle. In myasthenia gravis, antiacetylcholine receptor antibody binds to the acetylcholine receptor and inhibits the action of acetylcholine. Bound antibody evokes immune-mediated destruction of the end plate. (Reproduced, with permission, from Chandrasoma P, Taylor CE: *Concise Pathology*, 3rd ed. Appleton & Lange, 1998.)

crease the amount of acetylcholine at the neuromuscular junction and to inhibit immune-mediated destruction of acetylcholine receptors.

By preventing metabolism of acetylcholine, cholinesterase inhibitors can compensate for the normal decline in released neurotransmitter during repeated stimulation. The diagnosis of myasthenia gravis can also be confirmed by administration of the short-acting cholinesterase inhibitor edrophonium. A positive result consists of brief improvement in strength of affected muscles.

Therapy with cholinesterase inhibitors can cause a paradoxical increase in weakness known as a **cholinergic crisis.** This is due to an excess of acetylcholine. At the molecular level, binding of acetylcholine first opens nicotinic cation channels, but with continued exposure to the agonist, the channels desensitize and shut down again. The desensitized channels recover their sensitivity to acetylcholine only after the neurotransmitter is removed. Removal of acetylcholine is impaired when cholinesterase activity is inhibited. This can result in depolarization block of neurotransmission similar to the effect of the depolarizing paralytic agent succinylcholine or organophosphate insecticides and nerve gases that markedly inhibit acetylcholinesterase. Therefore, the dose of cholinesterase inhibitors must be carefully regulated to reduce myasthenia but avoid a cholinergic crisis.

Plasmapheresis, corticosteroids, and immunosuppressant drugs are effective in reducing levels of autoantibody to acetylcholine receptors and suppressing disease. The thymus is thought to play an important role in the pathogenesis of the disease by supplying helper T cells sensitized against thymic nicotinic receptors. In most patients with myasthenia gravis, the thymus is hyperplastic, and 10–15% have thymomas. Thymectomy is indicated if a thymoma is suspected. In patients with generalized myasthenia without thymoma, thymectomy induces remission in 35% and improves symptoms in another 45% of patients.

43. What is the clinical presentation of myasthenia gravis?
44. What causes this disorder?
45. What is the pathophysiology of symptoms in myasthenia gravis?

EPILEPSY

Clinical Presentation

Seizures are paroxysmal disturbances in cerebral function caused by an abnormal synchronous discharge of cortical neurons. The epilepsies are a group of disorders characterized by recurrent seizures. Approximately 0.6% of people in the United States suffer from recurrent seizures, and idiopathic epilepsy

Table 7–2. Simplified classification of seizures.

I. Partial (focal seizures)
   A. Simple partial seizures with motor, sensory, psychic, or autonomic symptoms
   B. Complex partial seizures
   C. Partial seizures with secondary generalization
II. Generalized seizures
   A. Absence seizures
   B. Tonic-clonic seizures
   C. Other (myoclonic, tonic, clonic, atonic)

accounts for more than 75% of all seizure disorders. In some forms of idiopathic epilepsy, a genetic basis is apparent. Other forms of epilepsy are secondary to brain injury from stroke, trauma, a mass lesion, or infection. About two-thirds of new cases arise in children, and most of these cases are idiopathic or due to trauma. In contrast, seizures or epilepsy with onset in adult life are more often due to underlying brain lesions or metabolic causes.

Seizures are classified by behavioral and electrophysiologic data (Table 7–2). **Generalized tonic-clonic seizures** are attacks characterized by sudden loss of consciousness followed rapidly by tonic contraction of muscles, causing limb extension and arching of the back. The tonic phase lasts 10–30 seconds and is followed by a clonic phase of limb jerking. The jerking builds in frequency to a peak after 15–30 seconds and then slows gradually over another 15–30 seconds. The patient then remains unconscious for several minutes. As consciousness is regained, there is a period of postictal confusion lasting several more minutes. In patients with recurrent seizures or an underlying structural or metabolic abnormality, confusion may persist for a few hours. Focal abnormalities may be present on neurologic examination during the postictal period. Such findings suggest a focal brain lesion requiring further laboratory and radiologic study.

Typical **absence seizures** begin in childhood and usually remit by adulthood. Seizures are characterized by brief lapses in consciousness lasting several seconds without loss of posture. These spells may be associated with eyelid blinking, slight head movement, or brief jerks of limb muscles. Immediately following the seizure, the patient is fully alert. The spells may occur several times through the day and impair school performance. The EEG shows characteristic runs of spikes and waves at a rate of three per second, particularly following hyperventilation (Figure 7–31). The disorder is transmitted as an autosomal dominant trait with incomplete penetrance.

Some forms of epilepsy cause seizures with only a tonic or clonic phase. In others, the seizure is manifested by sudden loss of muscle tone (atonic seizures). In myoclonic epilepsy, sudden, brief contractions of muscles occur. Myoclonic seizures are found in certain neurodegenerative diseases or fol-

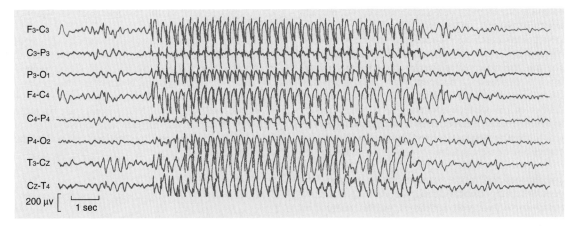

Figure 7–31. EEG of a patient with typical absence (petit mal) seizures, showing a burst of generalized 3-Hz spike-and-wave activity (center of record) that is bilaterally symmetric and bisynchronous. Odd-numbered leads indicate electrode placements over the left side of the head; even numbers, those over the right side. (Reproduced, with permission, from Simon RP, Aminoff MJ, Greenberg DA: *Clinical Neurology,* 4th ed. Appleton & Lange, 1999.)

lowing diffuse brain injury, as occurs during global cerebral ischemia.

Partial seizures are caused by focal brain disease. Therefore, in general, patients with simple or complex partial seizures should be investigated for underlying brain lesions. **Simple partial seizures** begin with motor, sensory, visual, psychic, or autonomic phenomena depending on the location of the seizure focus. Consciousness is preserved unless the seizure discharge spreads to other areas, producing a tonic-clonic seizure **(secondary generalization). Complex partial seizures** are characterized by the sudden onset of impaired consciousness with stereotyped, coordinated, involuntary movements **(automatisms).** Immediately prior to impairment of consciousness, there may be an aura consisting of unusual abdominal sensations, olfactory or sensory hallucinations, unexplained fear, or illusions of familiarity (déjà vu). Seizures usually last for 2–5 minutes and are followed by postictal confusion. Secondary generalization may occur. The seizure focus usually lies in the temporal or frontal lobe.

Pathogenesis

Normal neuronal activity occurs in a nonsynchronized manner, with groups of neurons inhibited and excited sequentially during the transfer of information between different brain areas. Seizures occur when neurons in a focal region or in the entire brain are activated synchronously. The kind of seizure depends on the location of the abnormal activity and the pattern of spread to different parts of the brain.

Interictal spike discharges are often observed on electroencephalographic recordings from epileptic patients. These are due to synchronous depolarization of a group of neurons in an abnormally excitable area of brain. Experimentally, this is known as the **paroxysmal depolarizing shift** and is followed by a hyperpolarizing afterpotential that is the cellular correlate of the slow wave that follows spike discharges on the EEG. The shift is produced by depolarizing currents generated at excitatory synapses and by subsequent influx of sodium or calcium through voltage-gated channels.

Normally, discharging excitatory neurons activate nearby inhibitory interneurons that suppress the activity of the discharging cell and its neighbors. Most inhibitory synapses utilize the neurotransmitter γ-aminobutyric acid (GABA). Voltage-gated and calcium-dependent potassium currents are also activated in the discharging neuron to suppress excitability. In addition, adenosine generated from ATP released during excitation further suppresses neuronal excitation by binding to adenosine receptors present on nearby neurons. Disruption of these inhibitory mechanisms by alterations in ion channels, or by injury to inhibitory neurons and synapses, may allow for the development of a seizure focus. In addition, groups of neurons may become synchronized if local excitatory circuits are enhanced by reorganization of neural networks after brain injury.

Spread of a local discharge occurs by a combination of mechanisms. During the paroxysmal depolarizing shift, extracellular potassium accumulates, depolarizing nearby neurons. Increased frequency of discharges enhances calcium influx into nerve terminals, increasing neurotransmitter release at excitatory synapses by a process known as **posttetanic potentiation.** This involves increased calcium influx through voltage-gated channels and through the N-methyl-D-aspartate (NMDA) subtype of glutamate receptor-gated ion channels. NMDA receptor-gated channels preferentially pass calcium ions but are relatively quiescent during normal synaptic transmission because they are blocked by magnesium ions. Magnesium block is relieved by depolarization. In contrast, the effect of inhibitory synaptic neurotransmission appears to decrease with high-frequency stimulation. This may be partly due to rapid desensitization of GABA receptors at high concentrations of released GABA. The net effect of these changes is to recruit neighboring neurons into a synchronous discharge and cause a seizure.

In secondary epilepsy, loss of inhibitory circuits and sprouting of fibers from excitatory neurons appear to be important for the generation of a seizure focus. In the idiopathic epilepsies, the biochemical or structural defects are generally not known. Studies in the lethargic mouse (lh/lh), however, reveal a possible mechanism for absence seizures. Absence seizures arise from synchronous thalamic discharges that are mediated by activation of low-threshold calcium currents (T or "transient" currents) in thalamic neurons. The anticonvulsant ethosuximide blocks T channels and suppresses absence seizures in humans. T channels are more likely to be activated following hyperpolarization of the cell membrane. Activation of $GABA_B$ receptors hyperpolarizes thalamic neurons and facilitates T channel activation. Lethargic mice demonstrate frequent absence spells accompanied by 5–6 Hz spike-wave discharges on the EEG and respond to drugs used in human absence epilepsy. A single mutation on chromosome 2 results in this autosomal recessive disorder. There is an increase in the number of $GABA_B$ receptors in the cerebral cortex in these mice, and the $GABA_B$ agonist baclofen worsens the seizures, whereas antagonists alleviate them. This suggests that abnormal regulation of $GABA_B$ receptor function or expression may be important in the pathogenesis of absence seizures.

The main targets for anticonvulsants are (1) voltage-gated ion channels that maintain the resting membrane potential and are involved in the generation of action potentials and neurotransmitter release, and (2) ligand-gated channels that modulate synaptic excitation and inhibition. Many agents act by more than one mechanism. Several anticonvulsants and some of their presumed mechanisms of action are listed in Table 7–3.

---

46. What is the clinical presentation of seizures?
47. What are some of the causes of seizure disorders?
48. What is the pathophysiology of seizures?

DEMENTIA & ALZHEIMER'S DISEASE

1. CLINICAL FEATURES OF DEMENTIA

Dementia is an acquired decline in intellectual function resulting in loss of social independence. There is impairment of memory and at least one other area of cortical function, such as language, calculation, spatial orientation, decision making, judgment, and abstract reasoning. In contrast to patients with confusional states, symptoms progress over months to years, and alertness is preserved until the very late stages of disease. Dementia affects 5–20% of persons over age 65, and, although not part of normal aging, its incidence increases with age. The most common causes listed in Table 7–4 account for almost 90% of cases. Treatable causes are important to

Table 7–3. Known mechanisms of action of some anticonvulsant drugs.

Drug	Main Indications	Mechanisms of Action
Phenytoin	Generalized tonic-clonic and partial seizures	Inhibition of voltage-gated sodium and calcium channels
Carbamazepine	Generalized tonic-clonic and partial seizures	Inhibition of voltage-gated sodium and calcium channels
Phenobarbital	Generalized tonic-clonic and partial seizures	Enhancement of $GABA_A$ receptor function
Valproate	Generalized tonic-clonic, absence, myoclonic, and partial seizures	Increases levels of GABA by inhibiting succinic semialdehyde dehydrogenase
Ethosuximide	Absence seizures	Inhibition of low-threshold (T-type) voltage-gated calcium channels
Felbamate	Generalized tonic-clonic and partial seizures	Antagonist of NMDA subtype of glutamate receptors; enhances action of GABA at $GABA_A$ receptors
Lamotrigine	Generalized tonic-clonic and partial seizures	Inhibition of voltage-gated sodium channels
Vigabatrin	Partial and secondarily generalized seizures	Increases GABA levels by inhibiting GABA transaminase
Tiagabine	Partial seizures	Increased GABA levels by inhibiting GABA reuptake

Table 7–4. Major causes of dementia.

Alzheimer's disease (>50% of cases)
Multiple cerebral infarcts
Dementia with Lewy bodies
Alcoholism
Normal pressure hydrocephalus
Primary or metastatic central nervous system neoplasms
Frontotemporal dementia
Parkinson's disease
Huntington's disease
Pick's disease
Prion diseases (eg, Creutzfeldt-Jakob disease)
Neurosyphilis
HIV infection
Hypothyroidism
Deficiency of vitamins B_{12}, B_6, B_1, or niacin
Chronic meningitis
Subdural hematoma

---

recognize and include hypothyroidism, vitamin B_{12} deficiency, neurosyphilis, brain tumor, normal pressure (communicating) hydrocephalus, and chronic subdural hematoma. In addition, although not curable, dementia associated with HIV infection may be slowed by antiretroviral treatment. About 10–15% of patients referred for evaluation of dementia suffer from depression **("pseudodementia")**, which may also respond to treatment.

Cerebrovascular disease is the second most common cause of dementia (after Alzheimer's disease). Dementia results from either multiple infarctions in the territory of major cerebral vessels **(multi-infarct dementia)** or from subcortical infarctions in the distributions of deep penetrating arterioles **(lacunar state, Binswanger's disease, subcortical arteriosclerotic encephalopathy)**. There is usually a history of stepwise progression of neurologic deficits, focal signs on neurologic examination, and multiple infarctions on brain imaging studies. Patients generally have a history of hypertension or other risk factors for atherosclerosis.

Chronic drug intoxication is often listed as a cause of dementia but actually produces a confusional state. The existence of alcohol-induced dementia is controversial. Although animal and cell culture studies provide evidence for a direct neurotoxic effect of alcohol, dementia in alcoholic patients also results from associated nutritional deficiency, from recurrent head trauma, and (rarely) from acquired hepatocerebral degeneration, a complication of chronic hepatic cirrhosis.

2. ALZHEIMER'S DISEASE

Clinical Features

Alzheimer's disease is the most common cause of dementia and accounts for over 50% of cases. It is a slowly progressive disorder that runs a course of 5–10 years and typically begins with impairment of learning and recent memory. Anomia, aphasia, and acalculia eventually develop, causing loss of employment and inability to manage finances. Spatial disorientation causes patients to become lost easily, and apraxias lead to difficulty with cooking, cleaning, and self-care. A frontal lobe gait disorder may appear, with short, shuffling steps, flexed posture, difficulty turning, and a tendency to fall backward **(retropulsion)** similar to that seen in Parkinson's disease. In later stages, social graces are lost, and psychiatric symptoms such as paranoia, hallucinations, and delusions may appear. Terminally, patients are bedridden, mute, and incontinent.

Pathology

The pathology of Alzheimer's disease is characterized by extracellular neuritic plaques in the cerebral cortex and in walls of meningeal and cerebral blood vessels (Figure 7–32). These plaques contain a dense core of amyloid material surrounded by dystrophic neurites (axons, dendrites), reactive astrocytes, and microglia. Other structural changes include the formation of intraneuronal neurofibrillary tangles, neuronal and synaptic loss, reactive astrocytosis, and microglial proliferation. Controversy exists as to which features are most related to the pathogenesis of the disease. Formation of neuritic plaques is particularly characteristic for Alzheimer's disease, but there is little evidence that the course or onset of disease correlates with plaque number. Neurofibrillary tangles are not specific for Alzheimer's disease and occur in several other neurodegenerative disorders. In general, all pathologic changes are most prominent in the hippocampus, entorhinal cortex, association cortex, and

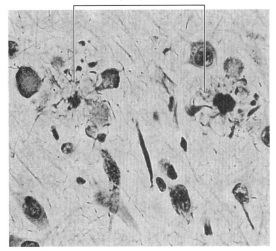

Figure 7–32. Amyloid plaques in cerebral cortex in Alzheimer's disease.

basal forebrain. This accounts for the early symptoms of memory loss and disturbance of higher cortical functions, with preservation of primary sensory and motor function until later in the course.

Pathophysiology

A. Amyloid β-Peptide: The major protein in neuritic plaques is **amyloid β-peptide (Aβ),** which is proteolytically derived from a membrane protein, the **β-amyloid precursor protein (APP)** encoded by a gene on chromosome 21. APP interacts with extracellular matrix and supports the growth of neurites in neuronal cultures. Genetic evidence implicates Aβ in the pathogenesis of Alzheimer's disease. Almost all patients with trisomy 21 (Down's syndrome) invariably develop pathologic changes indistinguishable from those seen in Alzheimer's disease, suggesting that having an increased copy of the *APP* gene increases the metabolism of APP to Aβ. About 10% of cases of Alzheimer's disease are familial, with early onset (< age 65) and autosomal dominant inheritance. In approximately 5% of these families, Alzheimer's disease is strongly linked to missense mutations within or immediately flanking the Aβ sequence in the *APP* gene, and at least one mutation has been associated with marked increases in Aβ production in cultured cells. Another *APP* mutation, with phenylalanine substituted for valine 717, has been expressed in transgenic mice. Animals heterozygous for this transgene develop Alzheimer-type neuropathology with numerous neuritic plaques, synaptic loss, reactive astrocytosis, and microglial infiltrates. Synthetic Aβ is toxic to cultured neurons and stimulates production of cytokines from microglial cells. This evidence links increased production of Aβ to Alzheimer's disease and suggests that Aβ causes the neurodegeneration.

B. Presenilins: The enzymatic pathways that regulate Aβ formation and the mechanisms of Aβ toxicity are critical areas of current research that may lead to new treatments. Some clues have come from analysis of additional families with Alzheimer's disease. Almost 70% of familial cases have been recently linked to the gene *S182* **(presenilin 1),** which encodes a seven-transmembrane protein on chromosome 14. Another 20% of cases have been linked to another gene, *STM2* **(presenilin 2),** on chromosome 1. The proteins encoded by these genes are 67% identical in amino acid sequence and therefore may have similar functions. Both are expressed in neurons and localize to the endoplasmic reticulum and Golgi apparatus. They are homologous to two proteins expressed in the nematode *Caenorhabditis elegans* that appear to be involved in processing and transport of proteins within cells. Recent evidence indicates that mutant variants of presenilins associated with familial Alzheimer's disease increase the production of the long, 42-amino-acid form of Aβ. This form fosters the development of amyloid plaques. This suggests a role for the presenilins in regulating *APP* metabolism.

C. Apolipoprotein E: The majority of patients with Alzheimer's disease are over age 60, and in about 50% of these patients the e4 isoform of **apolipoprotein E (apoE4)** has been identified as a risk factor. ApoE is a 34 kDa protein that mediates the binding of lipoproteins to the low-density lipoprotein (LDL) receptor and the LDL receptor-related protein (LRP). It is synthesized and secreted by astrocytes and macrophages and is thought to be important for mobilizing lipids during normal development of the nervous system and during regeneration of peripheral nerves after injury. There are three major isoforms (apoE2, apoE3, and apoE4), which arise from different alleles (e2, e3, and e4) of a single gene on chromosome 19. e3 is the most common, accounting for about 75% of all alleles, while e2 and e4 account for roughly 10% and 15%, respectively. The e4 allele is associated with increased risk and earlier onset of both familial and sporadic late-onset Alzheimer's disease. In contrast, inheritance of e2 is associated with decreased risk and later onset. It is important to note that Alzheimer's disease develops in the absence of e4 and also that many persons with e4 escape disease. Therefore, genotyping is not currently recommended as a useful genetic test.

The mechanism by which apoE alleles alter disease risk is not certain. In cultured neurons, apoE3 increases neurite outgrowth in the presence of very low density lipoproteins, whereas apoE4 inhibits outgrowth. Alzheimer patients who are homozygous for the e4 allele have larger and denser senile plaques than patients homozygous for the e3 allele. ApoE is found in neuritic plaques, and apoE4 binds Aβ more readily than does apoE3. Therefore, apoE4 may facilitate plaque formation. In addition, apoE enters neurons and binds the microtubule-associated protein tau, which is the major constituent of neurofibrillary tangles. ApoE3 binds tau much more avidly than apoE4. Binding of apoE3 to tau may prevent the formation of tangles and support normal microtubule assembly required for neurite outgrowth.

---

49. What are the treatable causes of dementia?
50. What are the clinical features of Alzheimer's disease?
51. In which proteins are there mutations associated with familial forms of Alzheimer's disease?
52. What is the association between apolipoprotein E and Alzheimer's disease?

STROKE

Clinical Presentation

Stroke is a clinical syndrome characterized by the sudden onset of a focal neurologic deficit that persists for at least 24 hours and is due to an abnormal-

NERVOUS SYSTEM DISORDERS / 159

Table 7–5. Classification of stroke.

Ischemic stroke
   Thrombotic occlusion
      Large vessels (major cerebral arteries)
      Small vessels (lacunar stroke)
      Venous occlusion
   Embolic
      Artery to artery
      Cardioembolic
Hemorrhage
   Intraparenchymal hemorrhage
   Subarachnoid hemorrhage
   Subdural hemorrhage
   Epidural hemorrhage
   Hemorrhagic ischemic infarction

Pathophysiology

A. Vascular Supply: The focal symptoms and signs that result from stroke correlate with the area of brain supplied by the affected blood vessel. Strokes may be classified into two major categories based on pathogenesis: ischemic stroke and hemorrhage (Table 7–5). In ischemic stroke, vascular occlusion interrupts blood flow to a specific brain region, producing a fairly characteristic pattern of neurologic deficits due to loss of functions controlled by that region. The pattern of deficits due to hemorrhage is less predictable, since it depends on the location of the bleed and also on factors that affect the function of brain regions distant from the hemorrhage. These factors include increased intracranial pressure, brain edema, compression of neighboring brain tissue, and rupture of blood into ventricles or subarachnoid space.

B. Ischemic Stroke: Ischemic strokes result from thrombotic or embolic occlusion of cerebral vessels. Neurologic deficits due to occlusion of large arteries (Figure 7–33) result from focal ischemia to the area of brain supplied by the affected vessel (Fig-

ity of the cerebral circulation. It is the third leading cause of death in the United States. The incidence of stroke increases with age and is higher in men than in women. Significant risk factors include hypertension, hypercholesterolemia, diabetes, smoking, heavy alcohol consumption, and oral contraceptive use.

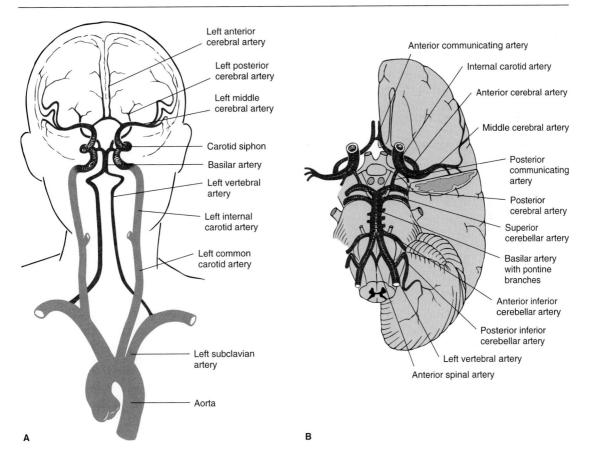

Figure 7–33. Major cerebral arteries. **A:** Anterior view. **B:** Inferior view showing the circle of Willis and principal arteries of the brainstem. (Reproduced, with permission, from Waxman SG: *Correlative Neuroanatomy,* 23rd ed. Appleton & Lange, 1997.)

ure 7–34) and produce recognizable clinical syndromes (Table 7–6). Not all signs are present in every patient, since the extent of the deficit depends on the presence of collateral blood flow, individual variations in vascular anatomy, blood pressure, and the exact location of the occlusion. Thrombosis usually involves the internal carotid, middle cerebral, or basilar arteries. Symptoms typically evolve over several minutes and may be preceded by brief episodes of reversible focal deficits known as **transient ischemic attacks.** Emboli from the heart, aortic arch, or carotid arteries usually occlude the middle cerebral artery, since it carries over 80% of blood flow to the cerebral hemisphere. Emboli that travel in the vertebral and basilar arteries commonly lodge at the apex of the basilar artery or in one or both posterior cerebral arteries.

Ischemic strokes involving occlusion of small arteries occur at select locations, where perfusion depends on small vessels that are end arteries. Most result from a degenerative change in the vessel, described pathologically as **lipohyalinosis,** that is caused by chronic hypertension and predisposes to occlusion. The most common vessels involved are the lenticulostriate arteries, which arise from the proximal middle cerebral artery and perfuse the basal ganglia and internal capsule. Also commonly affected are small branches of the basilar and posterior cerebral arteries that penetrate the brainstem and thalamus. Occlusion of these vessels causes small areas of tissue damage known as **lacunar infarctions.** These typically occur in the putamen, caudate, thalamus, pons, and internal capsule and less commonly in subcortical white matter and cerebellum. Lacunar infarctions produce several fairly stereotyped clinical syndromes. The two most common are pure motor stroke and pure sensory stroke. In pure motor stroke, the infarction is usually within the internal capsule or pons contralateral to the weak side. In pure sensory stroke, the infarction is usually in the contralateral thalamus.

Several vascular, cardiac, and hematologic disorders can cause focal cerebral ischemia (Table 7–7). The most common cause is **atherosclerosis** of the large arteries of the neck and base of the brain (Figure 7–35). Atherosclerosis is thought to arise from injury to vascular endothelial cells by mechanical, biochemical, or inflammatory insults (see Chapter 11). Endothelial injury stimulates attachment of circulating monocytes and lymphocytes that migrate into the vessel wall and stimulate proliferation of smooth muscle cells and fibroblasts. This leads to the formation of a fibrous plaque. Damaged endothelial cells also provide a nidus for aggregation and activa-

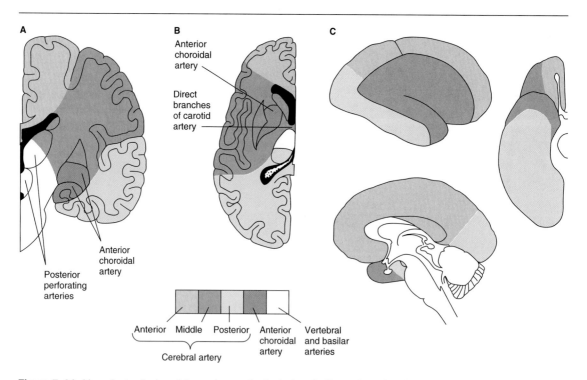

Figure 7–34. Vascular territories of the major cerebral arteries. **A:** Coronal section through the cerebrum. **B:** Horizontal section through the cerebrum. **C:** Vascular supply to the cerebral cortex. (Reproduced, with permission, from Chusid JG: *Correlative Neuroanatomy and Functional Neurology,* 19th ed. Lange, 1985.)

NERVOUS SYSTEM DISORDERS / 161

Table 7–6. Vascular territories and clinical features in ischemic stroke.

Artery	Territory	Symptoms and Signs
Anterior cerebral	Medial frontal and parietal cortex, anterior corpus callosum	Paresis and sensory loss of contralateral leg and foot
Middle cerebral	Lateral frontal, parietal, occipital, and temporal cortex and adjacent white matter, caudate, putamen, internal capsule	Aphasia (dominant hemisphere), neglect (nondominant hemisphere), contralateral hemisensory loss, homonymous hemianopia, hemiparesis
Vertebral (posterior inferior cerebellar)	Medulla, lower cerebellum	Ipsilateral cerebellar ataxia, Horner's syndrome, crossed sensory loss, nystagmus, vertigo, hiccup, dysarthria, dysphagia
Basilar (including anterior inferior cerebellar, superior cerebellar)	Lower midbrain, pons, upper and mid cerebellum	Nystagmus, vertigo, diplopia, skew deviation, gaze palsies, hemi- or crossed sensory loss, dysarthria, hemi- or quadraparesis, ipsilateral cerebellar ataxia, Horner's syndrome, coma
Posterior cerebral	Distal territory: Medial occipital and temporal cortex and underlying white matter, posterior corpus callosum	Contralateral homonymous hemianopia, dyslexia without agraphia, visual hallucinations and distortions, memory defect, cortical blindness (bilateral occlusion)
	Proximal territory: upper midbrain, thalamus	Sensory loss, ataxia, third nerve palsy, contralateral hemiparesis, vertical gaze palsy, skew deviation, hemiballismus, choreoathetosis, impaired consciousness

Table 7–7. Conditions associated with focal cerebral ischemia.[1]

Vascular disorders
  Atherosclerosis
  Fibromuscular dysplasia
  Inflammatory disorders
    Giant cell arteritis
    Systemic lupus erythematosus
    Polyarteritis nodosa
    Granulomatous angiitis
    Syphilitic arteritis
    AIDS
  Carotid or vertebral artery dissection
  Lacunar infarction
  Drug abuse
  Migraine
  Multiple progressive intracranial occlusions (moyamoya syndrome)
  Venous or sinus thrombosis
Cardiac disorders
  Mural thrombus
  Rheumatic heart disease
  Arrhythmias
  Endocarditis
  Mitral valve prolapse
  Paradoxic embolus
  Atrial myxoma
  Prosthetic heart valves
Hematologic disorders
  Thrombocytosis
  Polycythemia
  Sickle cell disease
  Leukocytosis
  Hypercoagulable states

[1]Reproduced, with permission, from Greenberg DA, Aminoff MJ, Simon RP: *Clinical Neurology*, 2nd ed. Appleton & Lange, 1993.

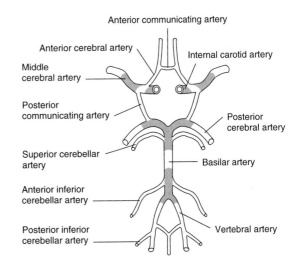

Figure 7–35. Sites of predilection (colored areas) for atherosclerosis in the intracranial arterial circulation. (Reproduced, with permission, from Simon RP, Aminoff MJ, Greenberg DA: *Clinical Neurology*, 4th ed. Appleton & Lange, 1999.)

tion of platelets. Activated platelets secrete growth factors that encourage further proliferation of smooth muscle and fibroblasts. The plaque may eventually enlarge to occlude the vessel or may rupture, releasing emboli.

C. Hemorrhage: Epidural and **subdural hematomas** typically occur as sequelae of head injury. Epidural hematomas arise from damage to an artery, typically the middle meningeal artery, which can be ruptured by a blow to the temporal bone. Blood dissects the dura from the skull and compresses the hemisphere lying below. Initial loss of consciousness from the injury is due to concussion and may be transient. Neurologic symptoms then return a few hours later as the hematoma exerts a mass effect that may be severe enough to cause brain herniation (Figure 7–27). Subdural hematomas usually arise from venous blood that leaks from torn cortical veins bridging the subdural space. These may be ruptured by relatively minor trauma, particularly in the elderly. The blood is under low pressure, and symptoms due to mass effect may not appear for several days.

Subarachnoid hemorrhage may occur from head trauma, from extension of blood from another compartment into the subarachnoid space, or from rupture of an arterial aneurysm. Cerebral dysfunction occurs because of increased intracranial pressure and from poorly understood toxic effects of subarachnoid blood on brain tissue and cerebral vessels. The most common cause of spontaneous (nontraumatic) subarachnoid hemorrhage is rupture of a **berry aneurysm**. Berry aneurysms are thought to arise from a congenital weakness in the walls of large vessels at the base of the brain. The aneurysms do not appear in childhood but become symptomatic usually after the third decade. Rupture of the aneurysm suddenly elevates intracranial pressure, which can interrupt cerebral blood flow and cause a generalized concussive injury. This results in loss of consciousness in about half of patients. In patients with very large hemorrhages, global cerebral ischemia can cause severe brain damage and prolonged coma. Focal ischemia may later result from vasospasm of arteries at or near the site of rupture. Recurrence of hemorrhage within the first few days is a common and often fatal complication.

Intraparenchymal hemorrhage may result from acute elevations in blood pressure or from a variety of disorders that weaken vessels. The resultant hematoma causes a focal neurologic deficit by compressing adjacent structures. In addition, metabolic effects of extravasated blood disturb the function of surrounding brain tissue, and nearby vessels are compressed, causing local ischemia. Chronic hypertension is the most common predisposing factor. In hypertensive patients, small **Charcot-Bouchard aneurysms** appear in the walls of small penetrating arteries and are thought to be the major sites of rupture. Most vulnerable are the small vessels that are also in-

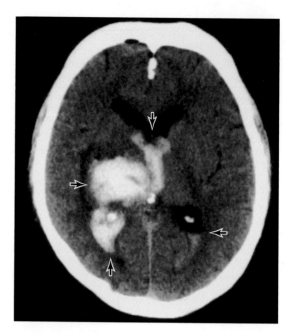

Figure 7–36. CT scan in hypertensive intracerebral hemorrhage. Blood is seen as a high-density signal at the site of hemorrhage in the thalamus (left arrow) and its extension into the third ventricle (top arrow) and the occipital horns of the ipsilateral (bottom arrow) and contralateral (right arrow) lateral ventricles. (Reproduced, with permission, from Simon RP, Aminoff MJ, Greenberg DA: *Clinical Neurology,* 4th ed. Appleton & Lange, 1999.)

volved in lacunar infarction. Hypertensive hemorrhages occur mainly in the basal ganglia, thalamus (Figure 7–36), pons, and cerebellum and less commonly in subcortical white matter. Other causes of intraparenchymal hemorrhage include **vascular malformations,** which contain abnormally fragile vessels susceptible to rupture at normal arterial pressures; and certain **brain tumors,** such as glioblastoma multiforme, which induce proliferation of fragile vessels within the tumor. Certain **platelet** and **coagulation disorders** may predispose to intracerebral hemorrhage by inhibiting coagulation. **Cocaine** and **amphetamines** cause rapid elevation of blood pressure and are common causes of intraparenchymal hemorrhage in young adults. Hemorrhage may be related to spontaneous bleeding from the acute elevation in blood pressure, rupture of an occult vascular abnormality, or drug-induced vasculitis. **Cerebral amyloid angiopathy** is an uncommon disorder that occurs mainly in the elderly and may be associated with Alzheimer's disease. Deposition of amyloid weakens the walls of small cortical vessels and causes lobar hemorrhage, often at several sites.

D. Excitotoxicity: Most efforts to intervene in stroke have focused on the vasculature. In ischemic stroke, these efforts include restoring circulation through surgical endarterectomy and reducing thrombosis with anticoagulant, antiplatelet, and thrombolytic drugs. More recently, a complementary approach has developed with the goal of reducing the vulnerability of brain tissue to ischemic damage. This is based on observations that central nervous system glutamate homeostasis is markedly altered during ischemia, leading to increased and toxic levels of extracellular glutamate.

Neurons deep within an ischemic focus die from energy deprivation. However, at the edge of the ischemic region, neurons appear to die because of excessive stimulation of glutamate receptors (Figure 7–37). As noted above, glutamate is released at excitatory synapses, and glutamate levels in the extracellular space are normally tightly regulated by sodium-dependent reuptake systems in neurons and glia. In glia, glutamate is further detoxified by conversion to glutamine via the ATP-dependent enzyme glutamine synthetase. Glutamine is then released by glia and taken up by neurons, where it is repackaged into synaptic vesicles for subsequent release. Ischemia deprives the brain of oxygen and glucose, and the resultant disruption in cellular metabolism depletes neurons and glia of energy reserves required to maintain normal transmembrane ion gradients. This leads to accumulation of intracellular Na^+ and collapse of the transmembrane Na^+ gradient, which in turn inhibits glutamate uptake. Declining energy reserves also reduce conversion of glutamate to glutamine in glia. Both events promote accumulation of extracellular glutamate, which stimulates glutamate receptors on surrounding neurons, causing entry of Ca^{2+} and Na^+. The influx of cations depolarizes these neurons, stimulating additional Ca^{2+} influx through voltage-gated channels.

Ischemia also disrupts K^+ homeostasis, leading to an increase in the concentration of extracellular K^+ ($[K^+]_o$). Neuronal activity can rapidly increase $[K^+]_o$, and one major function of glial cells is to keep $[K^+]_o$ at about 3 mmol/L to help neurons maintain their resting membrane potential. Two energy-dependent transporters are particularly important for removal of extracellular K^+ by glia: a Na^+-K^+ ATPase and an anion transporter that co-transports K^+ and Na^+ with Cl^-. In ischemia, these energy-dependent mechanisms fail, and K^+ released into the extracellular space can no longer be taken up by glia. This depolarizes neurons since the gradient of K^+ across neuronal membranes determines the level of the resting membrane potential. Depolarization activates release of neuro-

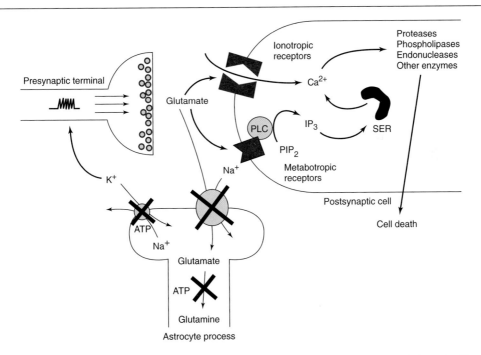

Figure 7–37. Excitotoxicity in neuronal ischemia. Depletion of energy supplies inhibits Na^+-K^+ ATPase, leading to accumulation of extracellular K^+ and a decline in extracellular Na^+. The rise in extracellular K^+ depolarizes nerve terminals, causing release of glutamate. The reduction in extracellular Na^+ reduces Na^+-dependent glutamate uptake, potentiating synaptic effects of released glutamate. This generates a sustained increase in intracellular Ca^{2+} in the postsynaptic cell, leading to cell death. Bold "X" denotes inhibition of Na^+-K^+ ATPase (left), glutamate transporters (right), and glutamine synthetase. Other abbreviations are defined in the legend to Figure 7–28.

transmitters, increasing accumulation of glutamate at excitatory synapses and in the extracellular space.

The net effect of these events is a tremendous influx of Na^+ and Ca^{2+} into neurons through glutamate- and voltage-gated ion channels. The resultant overload in intracellular Ca^{2+} appears to be especially toxic and may exceed the ability of the neuron to extrude or sequester the cation. This results in sustained activation of a variety of calcium-sensitive enzymes, including proteases, phospholipases, and endonucleases, leading to cell death. In support of an excitotoxic mechanism of cell death in stroke are animal studies that demonstrate a reduction in the size of ischemic lesions following treatment with glutamate receptor antagonists.

> 53. What is the clinical presentation of stroke?
> 54. What are some of the causes of stroke?
> 55. What role does glutamate play in neuronal injury during ischemia?

REFERENCES

General
Adams RD, Victor M, Popper AH: *Principles of Neurology*, 6th ed. McGraw-Hill, 1997.
Kandel ER, Schwartz JH, Tessel TM (editors): *Essentials of Neural Science and Behavior*. Appleton & Lange, 1995.
Rosenberg RN et al (editors): *The Molecular and Genetic Basis of Neurological Disease*, 2nd ed. Butterworth-Heinemann, 1997.

Histology & Cell Biology
Hille B: *Ionic Channels of Excitable Membranes*, 2nd ed. Sinauer, 1992.
McGeer PL et al: Microglia in degenerative neurological disease. Glia 1993;7:84.
Mucke L, Eddleston M: Astrocytes in infectious and immune-mediated diseases of the central nervous system. FASEB J 1993;7:1226.

Functional Neuroanatomy
Haerer A: *De Jong's The Neurologic Exam*, 5th ed. Lippincott, 1992.
Parent A: *Carpenter's Human Neuroanatomy*, 9th ed. Williams & Wilkins, 1996.
Simon RP, Aminoff MJ, Greenberg DA: *Clinical Neurology*, 4th ed. Appleton & Lange, 1999.
Wall PD, Melzack R (editors): *Textbook of Pain*, 3rd ed. Churchill-Livingstone, 1994.

Motor Neuron Disease
Brady ST: Motor neurons and neurofilaments in sickness and in health. Cell 1993;73:1.
Brown RH Jr: Amyotrophic lateral sclerosis: Recent insights from genetics and transgenic mice. Cell 1995; 80:687.
Iannacone ST: Spinal muscular atrophy. Semin Neurol 1998;18:19.
Lin C-LG et al: Aberrant RNA processing in a neurodegenerative disease: The cause for absent EAAT2, a glutamate transporter, in amyotrophic lateral sclerosis. Neuron 1998;20:589.

Parkinson's Disease
Edwards RH: Neural degeneration and the transport of neurotransmitters. Ann Neurol 1993;34:638.
Jenner P, Schapira AHV, Mardsen CD: New insights into the cause of Parkinson's disease. Neurology 1992;42:2241.
Kitada T et al: Mutations in the *parkin* gene cause autosomal recessive juvenile parkinsonism. Nature 1998; 392:605.
Olanov CW: An introduction to the free radical hypothesis in Parkinson's disease. Ann Neurol 1992;32(Suppl):52.
Polymeropoulos MH et al: Mutation in the α-synuclein gene identified in families with Parkinson's disease. Science 1997;276:2045.

Myasthenia Gravis
Drachman, DB: Myasthenia gravis. N Engl J Med 1994;330:1797.

Epilepsy
Engel J Jr: *Seizures and Epilepsy*. Vol 31 of *Contemporary Neurology Series*. Davis, 1989.
McNamara JO: Cellular and molecular basis of epilepsy. J Neurosci 1994;14:3413.
Schwartzkroin PA (editor): *Epilepsy: Models, Mechanisms, and Concepts*. Cambridge Univ Press, 1993.
Wyllie E (editor): *The Treatment of Epilepsy: Principles & Practice*, 2nd ed., William & Wilkins, 1997.

Dementia & Alzheimer's disease
Borchelt DR et al: Familial Alzheimer's disease-linked presenilin I variants elevate Aβ 1–42/1–40 ratio in vitro and in vivo. Neuron 1996;17:1005.
Corder EH et al: Gene dose of apolipoprotein E type 4 allele and the risk of Alzheimer's disease in late onset families. Science 1993;261:921.
Cummings JL, Benson DF: *Dementia: A Clinical Approach*, 2nd ed. Butterworth-Heinemann, 1992.
Levy-Lahad E et al: Candidate gene for the chromosome 1 familial Alzheimer's disease locus. Science 1995; 269:973.
Selkoe DJ: Normal and abnormal biology of the β-amyloid precursor protein. Ann Rev Neurosci 1994; 17:489.
Sherrington R et al: Cloning of a gene bearing missense mutations in early-onset familial Alzheimer's disease. Nature 1995;375:754.
Tomita T et al: The presenilin 2 mutation (N141I) linked to familial Alzheimer's disease (Volga German fami-

lies) increases the secretion of amyloid β protein ending at the 42nd (or 43rd) residue. Proc Nat Acad Sci U S A 1997;94:2025.

Stroke

Barnett HJM et al: *Stroke: Pathophysiology, Diagnosis and Management,* 2nd ed. Churchill Livingstone, 1992.

Caplan LR: *Stroke: A Clinical Approach,* 2nd ed. Butterworth-Heinemann, 1993.

Dugan LL, Choi DW: Excitotoxicity, free radicals and cell membrane changes. Ann Neurol 1994;35 (Suppl):S17.

Lipton SA, Rosenberg PA: Excitatory amino acids as a final common pathway for neurologic disorders. N Engl J Med 1994;330:613.

8 Diseases of the Skin

Timothy H. McCalmont, MD

NORMAL SKIN

The skin is the most accessible organ of the human body. Its most basic function is simply a protective one. As a barrier, the skin holds off desiccation and disease by keeping moisture in and pathogens out. Nevertheless, characterization of the skin as mere "plastic wrap" is a gross underestimation of the anatomic and physiologic complexity of this vital structure.

Unlike parenchymal organs, end organ dysfunction or failure is not a prerequisite for the diagnosis of a skin disease, since all skin diseases can be observed clinically irrespective of their functional effects. Among the spectacular array of neoplastic, inflammatory, infectious, and genetic cutaneous disorders, some elicit only trivial aberrations in skin structure or function, while others lead to profound and morbid consequences.

Anatomy

The integumentary system consists of a layer of tissue, 1–4 mm in thickness, that covers all exposed surfaces of the body. The skin merges uninterruptedly with the structurally similar envelope of the mucous membranes, but skin is distinct from mucosa in that it contains adnexal structures such as the eccrine units that exude sweat and the folliculosebaceous units that produce hairs and oils. There is considerable variation in skin thickness and composition, depending on the requirements of a particular body site. For example, the thinnest skin overlies the eyelids, where delicacy and mobility are essential. The thickest skin is present on the upper trunk, where sturdiness exceeds mobility in importance. The surfaces of the palms and soles are characterized by a high density of eccrine sweat units, reflecting the importance of this region in regulation of temperature; an absence of hairs, which would interfere with sensation; and accentuation of the cornified layer (see below), contributing to the tackiness needed to handle objects deftly. The size of the structures between sites can also vary greatly, best illustrated by the contrast between large terminal hair follicles found on the scalp, bearded areas, and genital skin and the small vellus hair follicles found at most other sites.

Histology

Using a light microscope, two important skin layers are easily identifiable: a stratified squamous epithelium, the **epidermis;** and a layer of connective tissue, the **dermis.** The underlying layer of adipose tissue is called the **subcutis.** The epidermis consists of keratinocytes arrayed in four distinct substrata: the basal, spinous, granular, and cornified layers (Figure 8–1). Basal keratinocytes comprise the proliferative

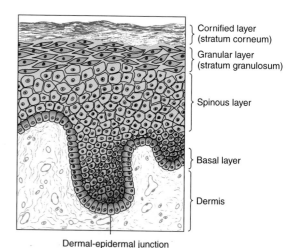

Figure 8–1. Although the epidermis biologically displays a gradient of differentiation, four distinct layers are recognized on the basis of microscopic appearance. Cuboidal germinative keratinocytes serve as a foundation in the basal layer; cells with ample cytoplasm and prominent desmosomes constitute the spinous layer; cells with cytoplasmic granularity due to an accumulation of keratin complexes and other structural proteins are found in the granular layer; and anucleate, flattened keratinocytes comprise the tough, membrane-like cornified layer. (Reproduced, with permission, from Orkin M, Maibach HI, Dahl MV [editors]. *Dermatology.* Appleton & Lange, 1991.)

pool of keratinocytes. These cells divide, giving rise to progeny that are displaced toward the skin surface. As the keratinocytes move outwardly, they progressively flatten and accumulate keratin filaments within their cytoplasm. Individual keratinocytes are

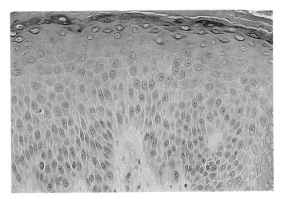

Figure 8–3. With conventional light microscopy, the numerous desmosomes of the spinous layer appear as delicate attachments ("spines") between individual keratinocytes.

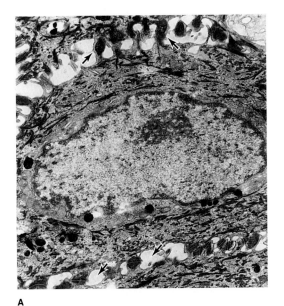

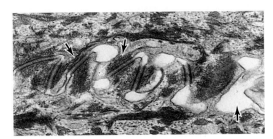

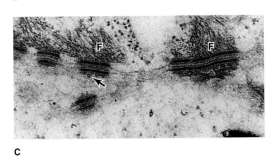

Figure 8–2. In an ultrastructural view of a human keratinocyte **(A)**, numerous desmosomes **(B)** appear as plaques that tightly bind two cell membranes together. With very high magnification **(C)**, the attachment of cytoplasmic keratin filaments **(F)** to the desmosomes can be appreciated. (Reproduced, with permission, from Junqueira LO, Carneiro J, Kelley R [editors]: *Basic Histology*, 9th ed. Appleton & Lange, 1998.)

tightly bound together by intracellular junctions called desmosomes (Figure 8–2). The desmosomal junctions appear as delicate "spines" between cells in conventional microscopic sections and are most conspicuous in the epidermal spinous layer (Figure 8–3). Keratin filaments are linked intracellularly and are also attached to the desmosomes, forming a network that is vital to structural integrity.

Melanocytes and Langerhans cells are dendritic cells that are intercalated among the keratinocytes of the epidermis. Melanocytes, which are positioned in the basal layer, synthesize a reddish brown biochrome, melanin, and dispense it to numerous adjacent keratinocytes through their dendrites (Figure 8–4). This distribution system permits melanin to provide a dispersed screen against the potentially harmful ultraviolet rays of the sun. Langerhans cells share a similar arborized morphology but are positioned in the midspinous layer. Langerhans cells are bone marrow-derived antigen-presenting cells (see also Chapter 3).

The epidermal-dermal junction, or basement membrane zone, is a structure that welds the epidermis to the dermis and contributes to the skin barrier. The juncture of the epidermis and dermis is arrayed in an undulating fashion to increase the surface area of binding between the two structures and to resist shearing forces. The downward projections of the epidermis are referred to as **rete ridges,** and the upward projections of the superficial dermis are called **dermal papillae** (Figure 8–5). Although the basement membrane comprises a thin eosinophilic (pink) band beneath the basal cells in conventional microscopic sections, it has a sophisticated multilayered structure that reaches from the hemidesmosomes of the basal keratinocytes to the collagen bundles of the superficial dermis (Figure 8–6). The lamina densa and lamina lucida are two of the layers of the base-

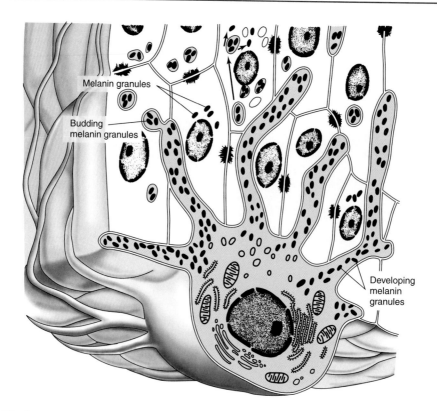

Figure 8–4. The human melanocyte displays a branching morphology, and the dendrites of the cell maintain contact with 35–40 adjacent keratinocytes in a multicellular structure termed the epidermal melanin unit. The function of the unit is the effective dispersion of melanin pigment, packaged in granules known as melanosomes, across a broad surface area. (Reproduced, with permission, from Junqueira LO, Carneiro J, Kelley R [editors]: *Basic Histology*, 9th ed. Appleton & Lange, 1998.)

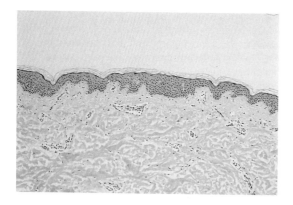

Figure 8–5. The undulating configuration of the epidermal-dermal junction consists of downward extensions of the epidermis, known as rete ridges, and upward extensions of the dermis, known as dermal papillae.

ment membrane zone and are so named because of their electron-dense and electron-lucid appearance when viewed ultrastructurally.

The dermis consists of a connective tissue gel composed largely of proteins and mucopolysaccharides (so-called ground substance). This matrix serves as the scaffolding that supports the complex neurovascular networks which course through the skin and also supports the eccrine (sweat gland) and follicular (hair) adnexal structures. The vast majority of the fibrous structural proteins of the dermis are composed of collagen types I and III, and a network of elastic microfibrils is also woven throughout the full dermal thickness. Fibrocytes, the synthetic units of the structural proteins, are ubiquitous, and there are also mast cells and dendritic immune cells arrayed throughout the dermis. The fine structure of the dermis—the dermal vascular and neural networks and the adnexal structures—is beyond the scope of this chapter.

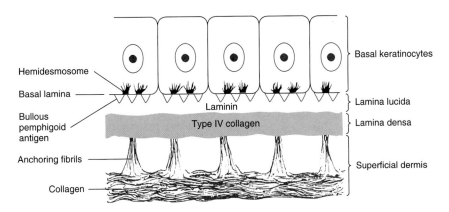

Figure 8–6. Schematic diagram of the basement membrane zone of human epidermis. (Reproduced, with permission, from Orkin M, Maibach HI, Dahl MV [editors]: *Dermatology.* Appleton & Lange, 1991.)

OVERVIEW OF SKIN DISEASES

In the broadest and simplest sense, there are two types of skin diseases: "growths" and "rashes." A skin growth is a cyst, a malformation, or a benign or malignant neoplasm. A rash is, with rare exception, a nonneoplastic skin disease; it is more precisely referred to as an inflammatory skin condition or a **dermatitis**. The pathophysiologic aspects of the huge number of described growths and rashes exceed the scope of this chapter, and our discussion will focus on five prototypical rashes.

Types of Skin Lesions

Physicians interested in the skin learned decades ago that the accurate diagnosis and classification of the many patterns of dermatitis were dependent upon a standardized nomenclature for the description and documentation of rashes. When used in association with a few well-chosen adjectives, the terms used to describe the prototypical types of inflammatory skin lesions (so-called primary lesions) permit vivid description of a rash. To illustrate the importance of terminology, imagine trying to describe a patient's condition over the phone to another physician. Talking about a "red raised rash" may truthfully describe the eruption in some sense, but the mental image evoked could be any one of dozens of skin diseases. The only way to accurately characterize an eruption is by the use of precisely defined terms.

The most important types of primary lesions include macules and patches, papules and plaques, vesicles and bullae, pustules, and nodules. The terms **macule** and **patch** denote flat areas of discoloration, without any discernible change in texture. Macules are 1 cm or less in diameter, while patches exceed 1 cm in size. **Papules** and **plaques** are elevated, palpable skin lesions, in which the breadth of the lesion exceeds its thickness. A papule is small, 1 cm or less in diameter, while a plaque exceeds 1 cm in size. **Vesicles** and **bullae** are fluid-filled spaces within the skin. Vesicles are less than 1 cm in diameter, while bullae exceed 1 cm in size. A vesicle or bulla containing purulent fluid is known as a **pustule**. A **nodule** is a solid, rounded skin lesion in which diameter and thickness are roughly equal.

Types of Inflammatory Skin Diseases

Different inflammatory processes involve different structures within the skin and display different microscopic patterns. Experience has shown that pattern analysis can serve as a useful means of diagnosis and classification. Pattern analysis is dependent upon accurate recognition of the distribution of inflammation within the skin as well as recognition of the specific structures affected by the inflammatory reaction. There are nine distinct patterns of dermatitis (Table 8–1; Figure 8–7). Four of these patterns and some of the diseases that produce them are discussed in detail in the paragraphs that follow.

---

1. What are the two most basic barrier functions of skin?
2. How is skin distinct from mucosa?
3. What are the histologic layers of the skin and how do they differ in structure and function?
4. What are the five categories of rashes that present as important primary lesions of skin, and what are their distinguishing characteristics?
5. What is the value of knowing the microscopic pattern of inflammation of a skin lesion? What additional information is needed for this information to be most useful?

Table 8–1. Patterns of inflammatory skin disease.

Pattern	Description	Prototypes
Perivascular dermatitis	Perivascular inflammatory infiltrate without significant involvement of the epidermis	Urticaria (hives)
Spongiotic dermatitis	Inflammatory infiltrate associated with intercellular epidermal edema (spongiosis)	Allergic contact dermatitis (poison oak dermatitis)
Psoriasiform dermatitis	Inflammatory infiltrate associated with epidermal thickening due to elongation of rete ridges	Psoriasis
Interface dermatitis	Cytotoxic inflammatory reaction with prominent changes in the lower epidermis, characterized by vacuolization of keratinocytes	Erythema multiforme Lichen planus
Vesiculobullous dermatitis	Inflammatory reaction associated with intraepidermal or subepidermal cleavage	Bullous pemphigoid
Vasculitis	Inflammatory reaction focused on the walls of cutaneous vessels	Leukocytoclastic vasculitis
Folliculitis	Inflammatory reaction directed against folliculosebaceous units	Acne folliculitis
Nodular dermatitis	Inflammatory reaction with a nodular or diffuse dermal infiltrate in the absence of significant epidermal changes	Cutaneous sarcoidosis
Panniculitis	Inflammatory reaction involving the subcutaneous fat	Erythema nodosum

PATHOPHYSIOLOGY OF SELECTED SKIN DISEASES

PSORIASIFORM DERMATITIS: PSORIASIS

Clinical Presentation

Psoriasis is a common chronic, persistent or relapsing, scaling skin condition. Individual lesions are distinctive in their classic form: sharply marginated and erythematous and surmounted by silvery scales (Figure 8–8). Most patients with psoriasis have a limited number of fixed plaques, but there is great variation in clinical presentation.

Epidemiology & Etiology

Psoriasis affects between 1% and 2% of individuals of both sexes in most ethnic groups. The most common age at onset is the third decade, but psoriasis can develop soon after birth, and psoriasis of new onset has been documented in a centenarian.

Several lines of evidence have established that genetic factors contribute to the development of psoriasis. There is a high rate of concordance for psoriasis in monozygotic twins and an increased incidence in relatives of affected individuals. The gene products of specific class I alleles of the major histocompatibility complex (MHC) are overexpressed in patients with psoriasis. Psoriasis is not merely a genetic disorder, however, since some susceptible individuals never develop characteristic lesions. In other predisposed individuals, a number of environmental factors, including infection and physical injury, can serve as triggers for the development of psoriasis (Table 8–2).

Histopathology & Pathogenesis

Psoriasis is the prototypical form of psoriasiform dermatitis, a pattern of inflammatory skin disease in which the epidermis is thickened as a result of elongation of rete ridges (Figures 8–7 and 8–9). In psoriatic lesions, epidermal thickening reflects excessive **epidermopoiesis** (epidermal proliferation). The increase in epidermopoiesis is reflected in shortening of the duration of the keratinocyte cell cycle and doubling of the proliferative cell population. Because of these alterations, lesional skin contains up to 30 times as many keratinocytes per unit area as normal skin. Evidence of excessive proliferation is also manifest microscopically as numerous intraepidermal mitotic figures.

During normal keratinocyte maturation, nuclei are eliminated as cells enter the cornified layer and condense to form a semipermeable envelope. In psoriasis, the truncation of the cell cycle leads to an accumulation of cells within the cornified layer with retained nuclei, a pattern known as **parakeratosis**. As parakeratotic cells accumulate, neutrophils migrate to the cornified layer. Histopathologically, the silvery scale of psoriatic plaques consists of a thick layer of parakeratotic keratinocytes with numerous intercalated neutrophils. At times, the number of neutrophils in the stratum corneum is so great that lesions assume a pustular appearance.

Psoriasis also induces endothelial cell hyperproliferation that yields pronounced dilation, tortuosity, and increased permeability of capillaries in the superficial dermis (Figure 8–10). The vascular alterations contribute to the bright erythema seen clinically. The

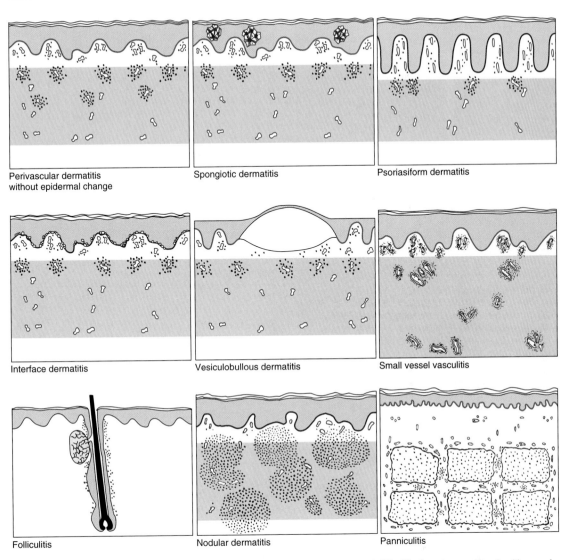

Figure 8–7. Nine patterns of inflammatory skin disease. (See also Table 8–1.) (Modified and reproduced, with permission, from Ackerman AB: *Histologic Diagnosis of Inflammatory Skin Diseases: A Method by Pattern Analysis.* Lea & Febiger, 1978.)

capillary changes are most pronounced at the advancing margins of psoriatic plaques.

After years of study, a large number of immunologic abnormalities have been documented in psoriatic skin, but a precise sequence of events that eventuates in epidermal hyperproliferation has not been established. The association between psoriasis and specific MHC class I molecules implicates CD8 lymphocytes because the complex of MHC class I protein and antigen is established as the ligand of the T cell receptor of CD8 cells (see also Chapter 3). Overexpression of a large number of cytokines has also been reported. Interleukin-2 (IL-2) overexpression is a common if not fundamental aberration, reflected in the observation that systemic IL-2 therapy for metastatic malignancy may precipitate severe exacerbations of psoriasis in predisposed individuals.

Clinical Manifestations

The cardinal features of the plaques of psoriasis include sharp margination, bright erythema, and nonconfluent whitish or silvery scales. Lesions can occur at any site, but the scalp, the extensor surfaces of the extremities, and the flexural surfaces are often in-

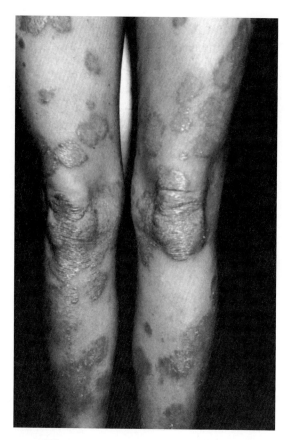

Figure 8–8. Classic plaque-type psoriasis (psoriasis vulgaris), consisting of sharply marginated scaling plaques accentuated over the extensor aspects of the extremities. (Reproduced, with permission, from Orkin M, Maibach HI, Dahl MV [editors]: *Dermatology.* Appleton & Lange, 1991.)

Table 8–2. Factors that induce or exacerbate psoriasis.

Physical factors
  Trauma (so-called Koebner phenomenon)
    Abrasions
    Contusions
    Lacerations
    Burns
    Sunburn[1]
    Bites
    Surgical incisions
  Cold weather
Infections
  Viral bronchitis
  Streptococcal pharyngitis
  Human immunodeficiency virus (HIV) infection
Medications or medication-related
  Antimalarial agents
  Lithium
  β-Adrenergic blocking agents
  Corticosteroid withdrawal

[1]Ultraviolet (UV) light in modest doses inhibits psoriasis and has been utilized as effective therapy for decades. UV light only exabcerbates psoriasis when presented in toxic doses (sunburn).

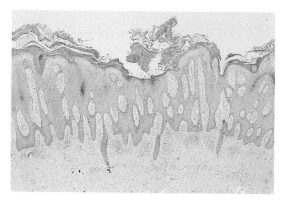

Figure 8–9. Histopathologic features of psoriasis at low magnification. The rete ridges are strikingly and evenly elongated, and the overlying cornified layer contains cells with retained nuclei (parakeratosis), a pattern that reflects the increased epidermal turnover.

volved. Psoriasis commonly affects the nail bed and matrix, yielding pitted or markedly thickened dystrophic nails. Mucosal surfaces are spared.

The only extracutaneous manifestation of psoriasis is psoriatic arthritis, a deforming, asymmetrical, oligoarticular arthritis that can involve small or large joints. The distal interphalangeal joints of the fingers and toes are characteristically involved. Psoriatic arthritis is classified as one of the seronegative spondyloarthropathies, distinguishable from rheumatoid arthritis by a lack of circulating autoantibodies (so-called rheumatoid factors) or circulating immune complexes and by linkage with specific MHC class I alleles, including HLA-B27.

There are many variants of psoriasis, all of which are histopathologically similar but which differ greatly in clinical distribution (Table 8–3).

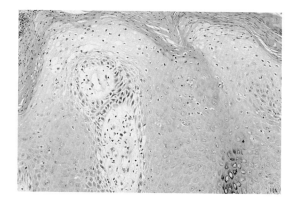

Figure 8–10. In a psoriatic plaque at high magnification, dilated capillaries are evident in an edematous portion of the superficial dermis.

DISEASES OF THE SKIN / 173

Table 8–3. Variants of psoriasis.

Variant	Cutaneous Findings and Distribution	Other Features
Plaque-type psoriasis (psoriasis vulgaris)	Large stationary plaques with prominent scales, commonly involving the scalp and the extensor surfaces of the extremities	
Guttate psoriasis	Scaling papules or small plaques, usually 0.5–1.5 cm in diameter, scattered on the trunk and proximal extremities	Lesions often induced or exacerbated by streptococcal pharyngitis
Erythrodermic psoriasis	Generalized erythematous plaques involving the face, trunk, and extremities, with only slight scaling	
Pustular psoriasis, generalized	Generalized eruption of sterile pustules involving erythematous skin of the trunk and extremities, often with sparing of the face	Associated with fever; may occur in pregnancy
Pustular psoriasis, localized	Scaling erythematous plaques, studded with pustules, involving the palms, soles, and nails	
Inverse psoriasis	Slightly scaling, erythematous plaques involving the axillary and inguinal regions, with sparing of areas usually involved in plaque-type disease	

6. What evidence supports genetic versus environmental causes of psoriasis?
7. Which cell types hyperproliferate in psoriasis?
8. What immunologic defects have been identified in psoriasis?

INTERFACE DERMATITIS: LICHEN PLANUS

Clinical Presentation

Lichen planus is a morphologically distinctive, itchy eruption that usually consists of numerous small papules. Individual lesions have angulate borders, flat tops, and a violaceous hue—attributes that form the basis of their alliterative description as pruritic polygonal purple papules (Figure 8–11). The individual papules of lichen planus sometimes coalesce to form larger plaques. White streaks, known as Wickham's striae, are characteristically found on the surfaces of lesions.

Epidemiology & Etiology

Lichen planus generally develops in adulthood and affects women slightly more commonly than men. Although the factors that trigger lichen planus remain obscure in many patients, it is clear that the rash represents a cell-mediated immune reaction that directly or indirectly damages basal keratinocytes of the epidermis. Observations that suggest a cell-mediated mechanism include the occurrence of lichen planus-like eruptions as a manifestation of graft-versus-host disease after bone marrow transplantation and the development of a lichen planus-like eruption in mice after injection of sensitized, autoreactive T cells. Although most lichen planus is idiopathic, drugs are one established cause of lichen planus or lichen planus-like reactions. Therapeutic gold and antimalarial agents are the medications most closely linked to the development of lichenoid eruptions, but a long list of other agents has accumulated (Table 8–4).

Histopathology & Pathogenesis

Lichen planus is a form of lichenoid interface dermatitis. It is a pattern of inflammatory skin disease in which a dense infiltrate of lymphocytes occupies the papillary dermis and the superficial dermis immediately subjacent to the epidermis, in association with vacuolization of the lower epidermis (Figure 8–12). The overwhelming majority of lymphocytes in the infiltrate are T cells. Some of the T cells are also found within the epidermis, where adjacent vacuolated, injured keratinocytes are found. Dense eosinophilic (pink) globules, known as **colloid bodies,** are

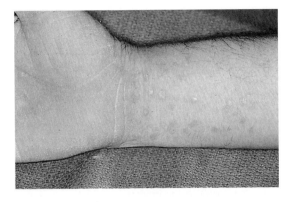

Figure 8–11. Pruritic polygonal flat-topped papules of lichen planus are present in a common location, the flexor surface of the wrist.

Table 8–4. Medications that induce lichenoid (lichen planus-like) reactions.

Therapeutic gold
Antimalarial agents
   Quinacrine
   Quinidine
   Quinine
   Chloroquine
Penicillamine
Thiazide diuretics
β-Blocking agents
Antibiotics
   Tetracycline
   Streptomycin
   Dapsone
   Isoniazid
Anticonvulsants
   Carbamazepine
   Phenytoin
Nonsteroidal anti-inflammatory drugs

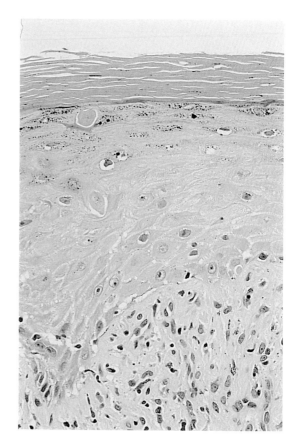

Figure 8–13. Necrotic keratinocytes (so-called colloid bodies) in a lesion of lichen planus appear as rounded globules along the epidermal-dermal junction. Necrotic cells are also evident in the upper epidermis.

also identifiable within the epidermis and the infiltrate (Figure 8–13). Colloid bodies represent condensed, anucleate keratinocytes that have succumbed to the inflammatory reaction. Although the keratinocytes bear the brunt of the lymphocyte attack, melanocytes are also destroyed in the reaction. Free melanin pigment is released as melanocytes are damaged, and the pigment is phagocytosed by dermal macrophages known as melanophages.

In incipient lesions of lichen planus, CD4 T helper lymphocytes predominate, and some of the cells have been found in proximity to macrophages and Langerhans cells (see also Chapter 3). In contrast, CD8 cytotoxic T cells comprise the bulk of the infiltrate in mature lesions. This shift in infiltrating T cell composition is thought to reflect the afferent and efferent aspects of lesional development. In the afferent phase, causative antigens are processed and presented to T helper cells, probably in the context of specific HLA determinants. The stimulated CD4 lymphocytes then elaborate specific cytokines that lead to the recruitment of cytotoxic lymphocytes. Cell-mediated cytotoxicity, cytokines, gamma interferon, and tumor necrosis factor are then thought to contribute to the vacuolization and necrosis of keratinocytes as a secondary event.

The clinical appearance of lichen planus lesions reflects several synchronous alterations in the skin. The dense array of lymphocytes in the superficial dermis yields the elevated, flat-topped appearance of each papule or plaque. The chronic inflammatory reaction induces accentuation of the cornified layer (hyperkeratosis) of the epidermis, which contributes to the superficial whitish coloration perceived as Wickham's striae. Although the many melanophages

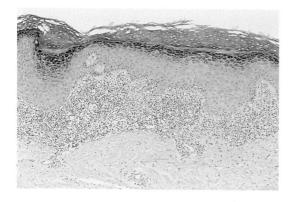

Figure 8–12. Histopathologic features of lichen planus at low magnification. There is a band-like infiltrate of lymphocytes that impinges upon the epidermal-dermal junction, and some keratinocytes adjacent to the infiltrate show cytoplasmic vacuolization.

that accumulate in the papillary dermis hold a brownish black pigment, the fact that the pigmented cells are embedded in a colloidal matrix such as the skin permits extensive scattering of light, an effect known as the Tyndall phenomenon. Thus, the human eye interprets a lesion of lichen planus as dusky or violaceous despite the fact that the pigment that serves as the basis for the coloration is melanin.

Clinical Manifestations

Lichen planus affects both skin and mucous membranes. Papules are generally distributed bilaterally and symmetrically. The sites most commonly involved include the flexor surfaces of the extremities, the genital skin, and the mucous membranes. Lesions are virtually never seen on the palms, soles, or face.

In general, lichen planus variants can be grouped into three categories:

A. Lichen Planus Papules Arrayed in an Unusual Configuration: In these variants, typical individual papules of lichen planus are grouped in a distinctive larger pattern. In annular lichen planus, small lichenoid papules are arrayed as a ring. Linear and zosteriform patterns of lichen planus have also been observed.

B. Lichen Planus Papules Arrayed at Distinctive Sites: Although most lichen planus is widespread, at times papules are restricted to a specific body site, such as the mouth (oral lichen planus) or genitalia. Nearly 25% of all lichen planus patients have disease limited to the mucous membranes.

C. Lichen Planus Papules With Unusual Clinical Appearances: Some examples of lichen planus defy clinical recognition because the appearance of the individual lesions is atypical. Erosive, vesiculobullous, atrophic, and hypertrophic lesions can be seen. In **erosive lichen planus,** the interface reaction that is directed against the epidermis is so profound that the entire epidermis becomes necrotic and ulceration ensues. The closely related entity **vesiculobullous lichen planus** is also characterized by an intense interface reaction that yields necrosis of the epidermal junctional zone across a broad front. As a result of basal layer necrosis, the epidermis becomes detached from its dermal attachments and a blister develops. In **atrophic lichen planus,** the rate of destruction of keratinocytes by the lichenoid interface reaction exceeds the rate of epidermal regeneration, and the epidermis becomes attenuated as a result. In contrast, in **hypertrophic lichen planus,** the rate of epidermal regeneration triggered by the interface reaction exceeds the rate of destruction, and thick, verrucous, hyperkeratotic lesions develop. All of these variants are histopathologically similar with the exception of the foci of ulceration seen in erosive lichen planus.

9. What skin cells are damaged by cell-mediated immune reactions in lichen planus?
10. Which drugs have been most commonly implicated in licheniform eruptions?
11. What synchronous alterations in the skin are reflected in the clinical appearance of lichen planus?

INTERFACE DERMATITIS: ERYTHEMA MULTIFORME

Clinical Presentation

Erythema multiforme is an acute cutaneous eruption that presents with a wide spectrum of clinical severity. The eruption is commonly brief and self-limited, but repetitive or generalized attacks can be disabling or even life-threatening. As the name implies, variation in lesional morphology can be seen, but most patients present with a monomorphous pattern in a given bout. The prototypical lesion is a red macule or thin papule that expands centrifugally and develops a dusky or necrotic center, creating a target-like pattern (Figure 8–14).

Epidemiology & Etiology

Erythema multiforme is an uncommon but distinctive skin disease that afflicts men and women in nearly equal numbers. The peak incidence is in the second to fourth decades of life, and onset during infancy or early childhood is a rarity. Like lichen planus, erythema multiforme represents a cell-mediated immune reaction that eventuates in necrosis of epidermal keratinocytes. Herpes simplex viral infection and reactions to medications have been established as the most common causes of erythema multiforme. Other cases are idiopathic.

Histopathology & Pathogenesis

Erythema multiforme is a prototypical form of vacuolar interface dermatitis. In contrast to lichen planus, which represents a pattern of lichenoid interface dermatitis characterized by dense inflammation within the superficial dermis, in erythema multiforme the inflammatory infiltrate is sparse. Thus, the vacuolated keratinocytes that are widely distributed within the epidermal basal layer are conspicuous in the face of a sparse infiltrate, and the damaged keratinocytes serve as the basis for the name of this pattern of inflammatory skin disease.

The dermal infiltrate in erythema multiforme is composed of a mixture of CD4 and CD8 T lymphocytes. CD8 cytotoxic cells are also found within the epidermis, in proximity to vacuolated and necrotic keratinocytes. Keratinocytes that are killed in the course of the inflammatory reaction become anucle-

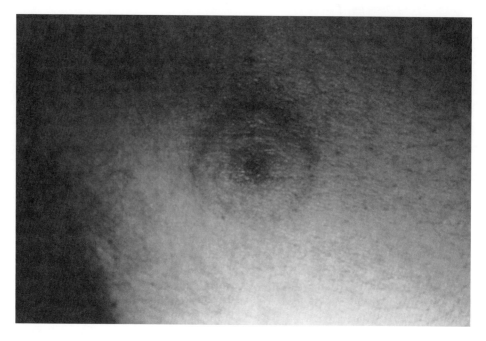

Figure 8–14. A target lesion—a characteristic pattern seen in erythema multiforme—consists of a papule or plaque with a central zone of epidermal necrosis surrounded by a rim of erythema. (Reproduced, with permission, from Jordon RE [editor]: *Immunologic Diseases of the Skin.* Appleton & Lange, 1991.)

ate and are manifest microscopically as round, dense, eosinophilic bodies similar to the colloid bodies of lichen planus (Figure 8–15).

Although lichen planus and erythema multiforme are clinically, microscopically, and etiologically distinct, both appear to share a common pathogenetic pathway in which specific inciting agents recruit effector lymphocytes into the epidermis and papillary dermis. After this recruitment, keratinocytes are injured and killed by the combined negative influences of cytotoxicity, cytokines, gamma interferon, and tumor necrosis factor.

Many cases of so-called erythema multiforme minor are triggered by herpes simplex viral infection. A relationship between erythema multiforme and herpetic infection had long been suspected, based upon the documentation of preceding herpes simplex lesions in patients with erythema multiforme. The relationship was strengthened after antiherpetic drug therapy, in the form of oral acyclovir, was shown to suppress the development of erythema multiforme lesions in some individuals. Recent molecular studies have substantiated the relationship by confirming the presence of herpes simplex DNA within skin from erythema multiforme lesions. Herpesvirus DNA is also demonstrable within peripheral blood lymphocytes and within lesional skin after resolution, but not within nonlesional skin. These findings suggest that viral DNA is disseminated from the primary infection in the peripheral blood and becomes integrated into the skin at specific target sites. The herpetic genomic fragments then contribute to the development of a cytotoxic effector response in their chosen target tissue, the skin.

The target-like clinical appearance of many erythema multiforme lesions reflects zonal differences in the intensity of the inflammatory reaction and its deleterious effects. At the periphery of an erythema multiforme lesion, only sparse inflammation, slight edema, and subtle vacuolization of the epidermis are apparent in the outer erythematous halo. In contrast, the dusky "bull's eye" often shows pronounced epidermal vacuolization, with areas of near-complete epidermal necrosis.

Clinical Manifestations

Erythema multiforme is generally limited to the skin and mucous membranes. The lesions develop rapidly in crops and are initially distributed on acral surfaces, though proximal spread to the trunk and face occurs not uncommonly. Mucosal erosions and ulcers are seen in roughly 25% of cases, and mucositis can be the sole presenting feature of the disease. Although erythema multiforme is an epithelial disorder, nonspecific constitutional symptoms such as malaise can also occur.

Although the spectrum of erythema multiforme exists as a continuum, a given patient is usually clas-

DISEASES OF THE SKIN / 177

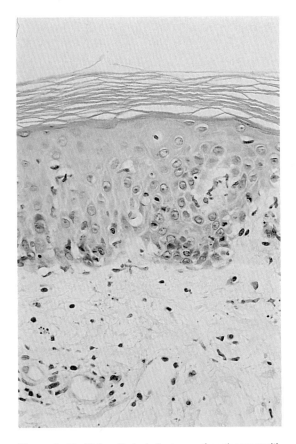

Figure 8–15. Histopathologic features of erythema multiforme, a type of vacuolar interface dermatitis. There is a modest infiltrate of lymphocytes in the vicinity of the epidermal-dermal junction where vacuolated and necrotic keratinocytes are conspicuous.

sified as having minor or major disease. The disorder is referred to as **erythema multiforme minor** when there are scattered lesions confined to the skin or when skin lesions are observed in association with limited mucosal involvement. A diagnosis of **erythema multiforme major** is based upon the presence of prominent involvement of at least one mucosal site, either oral, genital, or conjunctival. Many examples of erythema multiforme major also display severe, widespread cutaneous involvement. Erythema multiforme major encompasses **Stevens-Johnson syndrome,** a term that connotes profound mucosal involvement with or without cutaneous lesions, as well as **toxic epidermal necrolysis.** In the latter, which most commonly represents an idiosyncratic reaction to a medication, vast regions of the skin and mucosa undergo extensive necrosis (Figure 8–16). Pathologically, toxic epidermal necrolysis is similar to a severe burn in that the integrity of a patient's skin fails completely, with a resulting increased risk for infectious and metabolic sequelae.

12. What is the prototypical lesion in erythema multiforme?
13. In what ways is erythema multiforme similar to and in what ways different from lichen planus?
14. What are some complications of toxic epidermal necrolysis?

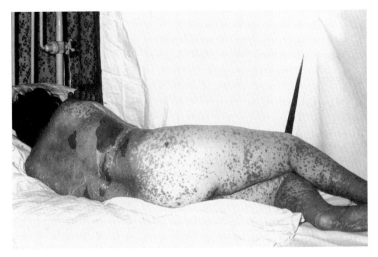

Figure 8–16. Toxic epidermal necrolysis is a form of erythema multiforme that usually represents an adverse reaction to a medication. Generalized maculopapular erythema of the trunk and extremities is followed by extensive desquamation, as illustrated on this patient's back, due to epidermal necrosis. Patients are often admitted to a burn unit for acute care. (Reproduced, with permission, from Orkin M, Maibach HI, Dahl MV [editors]: *Dermatology.* Appleton & Lange, 1991.)

VESICULOBULLOUS DERMATITIS: BULLOUS PEMPHIGOID

Clinical Presentation

Bullous pemphigoid is a blistering disease in which tense fluid-filled spaces develop within erythematous, inflamed skin. The blisters in bullous pemphigoid develop because of detachment of the epidermis from the dermis (subepidermal vesiculation) as the result of a specific inflammatory reaction. The term "pemphigoid" reflects the clinical similarity of bullous pemphigoid to pemphigus, another form of blistering skin disease that is characterized by intraepidermal rather than subepidermal vesiculation. The distinction between bullous pemphigoid and pemphigus is an important one, since bullous pemphigoid has a more favorable prognosis.

Epidemiology & Etiology

Bullous pemphigoid is a disorder of the elderly. There are rare reports of bullous pemphigoid in children and young adults, but the vast majority of patients are over 60 years of age. There is no sex predilection.

It has been known for years that immunoglobulins and complement are deposited along the epidermal-dermal junction in bullous pemphigoid. The deposited antibodies are specific for antigens within the basement membrane zone, and bullous pemphigoid thus represents a form of autoimmune skin disease. The specific factors that induce autoantibody production have not been identified.

Histopathology & Pathogenesis

Microscopically, biopsies from fully developed bullous pemphigoid lesions show a subepidermal cleft containing lymphocytes, eosinophils, neutrophils, and eosinophilic (pink) material, which represents extravasated proteins such as fibrin (Figure 8–17). An inflammatory infiltrate of eosinophils, neutrophils, and lymphocytes is also evident in the dermis beneath the cleft. These findings represent the aftermath of an inflammatory reaction centered on the basement membrane zone.

Insights into this reaction can be obtained from direct immunofluorescence microscopy, in which fluorochrome-labeled anti-IgG, anti-IgA, anti-IgM, and

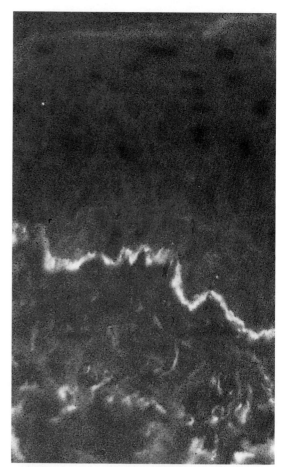

Figure 8–18. Direct immunofluorescence findings in lesional skin from a bullous pemphigoid patient. When fluorochrome-stained sections are viewed through an ultraviolet microscope, a bright linear band, signifying deposition of IgG, is evident along the epidermal-dermal junction. (Reproduced, with permission, from Jordon RE [editor]: *Immunologic Diseases of the Skin*. Appleton & Lange, 1991.)

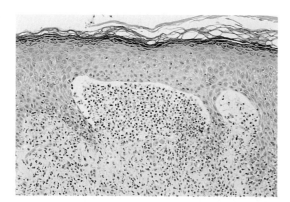

Figure 8–17. Histopathologic features of bullous pemphigoid. There is a subepidermal cleft that contains numerous eosinophils and lymphocytes, and a similar infiltrate is present in the superficial dermis. Ultrastructurally, the separation is within the lamina lucida of the basement membrane zone, at the level of the bullous pemphigoid antigen (see Figure 8–6).

anticomplement antibodies are incubated with lesional skin. Using an ultraviolet microscope to localize the fluorochrome, tagged antibodies that are specific for IgG and complement component C3 are found in a linear distribution along the epidermal-dermal junction (Figure 8–18). Circulating IgG that binds to the basement membrane zone of human epidermis is also identifiable in bullous pemphigoid patients. These antibodies are found to fix complement, and pathogenicity has been confirmed by injection into laboratory animals, in whom the antibodies bind to the junctional zone and induce blisters.

Characterization of the antigen bound by these autoantibodies has revealed a 230 kDa protein within the lamina lucida. The protein, known as the "bullous pemphigoid antigen," has been localized to the hemidesmosomal complex of the epidermal basal cell (Figure 8–6). Its exact structural or functional role has not been established.

Based upon these findings, blister formation is believed to begin with the binding of IgG to the bullous pemphigoid antigen with subsequent activation of the classic complement cascade (Chapter 3). Complement fragments induce mast cell degranulation and attract neutrophils. The presence of eosinophils in the infiltrate of bullous pemphigoid is probably a reflection of mast cell degranulation, since mast cell granules contain eosinophil chemotactic factors. Numerous enzymes are released by granulocytes and mast cells during the reaction, and enzymatic digestion is thought to be the primary mechanism behind the separation of the epidermis from the dermis. It is also possible that the bullous pemphigoid antigen plays a vital structural role that is compromised by autoantibody binding, leading to cleavage.

Clinical Manifestations

Patients with bullous pemphigoid present with large, tense blisters on an erythematous base (Figure 8–19). Lesions are most commonly distributed on the extremities and lower trunk, but blisters can develop at any site. Most patients experience considerable pruritus in association with their blisters. Mucous membrane lesions develop in up to one-third of patients and are usually clinically innocuous—in contrast to the variants of erythema multiforme.

Some patients with bullous pemphigoid present with itchy, erythematous plaques, with no blistering for an extended period of time, but blisters eventually develop in most patients. This pattern is known as "preeruptive" or "urticarial" bullous pemphigoid. Immunofluorescence and histopathologic examination of biopsies from such patients reveals junctional deposition of autoantibodies and complement in association with an eosinophil-rich infiltrate, implying that the inflammatory reaction is identical to that of conventional bullous pemphigoid. The explanation for the delayed blistering seen in these patients is not presently known.

Bullous pemphigoid is a disease of the skin only,

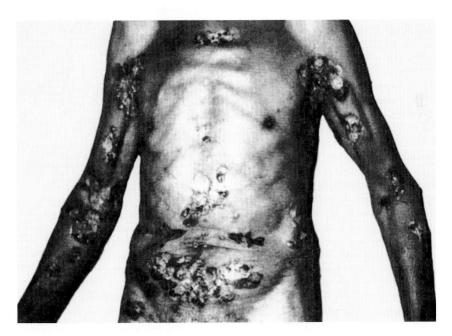

Figure 8–19. Large tense bullae on erythematous bases are distributed over the lower trunk and proximal extremities of this elderly man with bullous pemphigoid. (Reproduced, with permission, from Jordon RE [editor]: *Immunologic Diseases of the Skin.* Appleton & Lange, 1991.)

and systemic involvement has never been documented. Some patients with bullous pemphigoid have developed skin lesions synchronously with a diagnosis of malignancy, but careful studies with age-matched controls have not demonstrated an increased incidence of bullous pemphigoid in cancer patients.

> 15. How do pemphigus and pemphigoid differ and why is the distinction important?
> 16. How does Ig binding to the bullous pemphigoid antigen cause blistering in lesions of bullous pemphigoid?
> 17. Is there a connection between bullous pemphigoid and cancer?

VASCULITIS: LEUKOCYTOCLASTIC VASCULITIS

Clinical Presentation

Leukocytoclastic vasculitis is an inflammatory disorder affecting small blood vessels of the skin that typically presents as an eruption of reddish or violaceous papules, a pattern known as **palpable purpura** (Figure 8–20). The lesions develop in crops, and individual papules persist less than a month. Although each individual lesion is transient, the duration of the eruption can vary from weeks to months, and in exceptional cases crops can develop over a period of years.

Epidemiology & Etiology

Leukocytoclastic vasculitis can develop at any age, and the incidence is equal in both sexes. The most common precipitants include infections and medications. Bacterial, mycobacterial, and viral infections can all trigger bouts, but poststreptococcal and poststaphylococcal eruptions are most common.

A wide variety of drugs have been established as leukocytoclastic vasculitis elicitors, including antibiotics, thiazide diuretics, and nonsteroidal anti-inflammatory agents. Among antibiotics, penicillin derivatives are the foremost offenders.

Histopathology & Pathogenesis

The name of this disorder conveys its chief microscopic attributes—an inflammatory reaction involving blood vessels in association with an accumulation of necrotic nuclear (leukocytoclastic) debris. The key steps that contribute to this morphologic pattern include the accumulation of triggering molecules within the walls of small blood vessels, subsequent stimulation of the complement cascade with the elaboration of chemoattractants, and entry of neutrophils with oxidative enzyme release, eventuating in cellular destruction and nuclear fragmentation.

The molecules that trigger leukocytoclastic vasculitis are immune complexes, consisting of antibodies bound to exogenous antigens that are usually derived from microbial proteins or medications. Circulating immune complexes have been documented by laboratory assays of serum from patients with active leukocytoclastic vasculitis, and the presence of circulating complexes can also be deduced based upon the

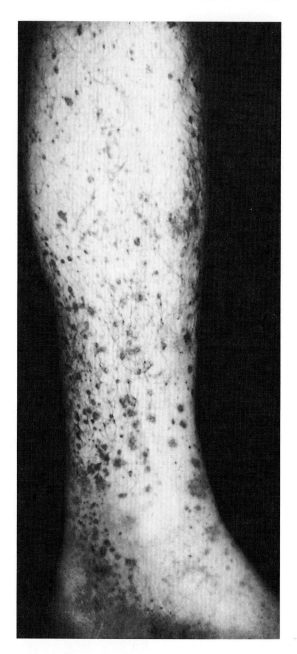

Figure 8–20. Purpuric papules are scattered on the lower extremity in leukocytoclastic vasculitis. (Reproduced, with permission, from Jordon RE [editor]: *Immunologic Diseases of the Skin*. Appleton & Lange, 1991.)

finding of low serum complement levels during exacerbations. The exact factors that lead to preferential deposition of immune complexes within small cutaneous vessels (venules) remain unknown, but the fact that venules exhibit relatively high permeability in the face of a relatively low flow rate is probably contributory. The deposited complexes are detectable within vessel walls by direct immunofluorescence testing (Figure 8–21).

After becoming trapped in tissue, immune complexes activate the complement cascade, and localized production of chemotactic fragments (such as C5a) and vasoactive molecules ensues (Chapter 3). Chemoattractants draw neutrophils out of vascular lumens and into vascular walls, where release of neutrophilic enzymes results in destruction of the immune complexes, the neutrophils, and the vessel. Microscopically, this stage is characterized by an infiltrate of neutrophils, neutrophilic nuclear dust, and protein (fibrin) in the vessel wall, a pattern that has historically been called "fibrinoid necrosis" (Figure 8–22). Throughout the inflammatory reaction, the integrity of the channel is progressively compromised.

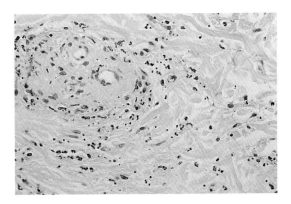

Figure 8–22. Histopathologic features of leukocytoclastic vasculitis, a form of small vessel vasculitis. Neutrophils, neutrophilic nuclear debris, and amorphous protein deposits are present within the expanded wall of a cutaneous venule.

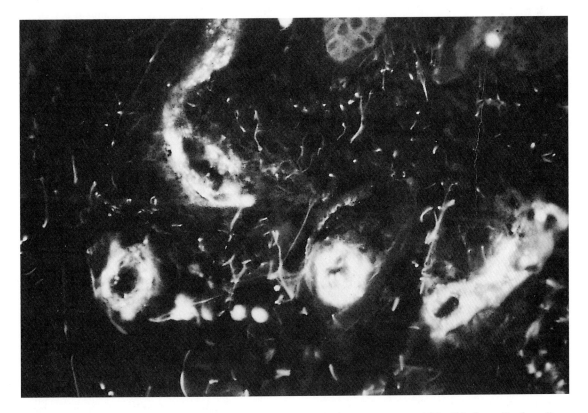

Figure 8–21. Direct immunofluorescence microscopy localizes complement component C3 within the walls of small cutaneous vessels. The complement fragments are present after activation of the complement cascade by immune complexes. Immunoglobulin deposition within vessel walls is detectable by the same method. (Reproduced, with permission, from Jordon RE [editor]: *Immunologic Diseases of the Skin.* Appleton & Lange, 1991.)

As cellular interstices widen, erythrocytes and fibrin exude through the vessel wall and enter the surrounding dermis.

Leukocytoclastic vasculitis lesions are papular because lesional skin is altered by an intense vasocentric inflammatory reaction containing numerous neutrophils. The erythematous or purpuric quality of leukocytoclastic vasculitis is attributable to the numerous extravasated erythrocytes that accumulate in the dermis of fully developed lesions. In patients with repetitive or persistent leukocytoclastic vasculitis, extravasated erythrocyte debris is metabolized into hemosiderin, which accumulates within macrophages (siderophages) within the deep dermis. The dermal hemosiderin can contribute to a dusky, violaceous clinical appearance, clinically similar to but pathologically distinct from the pigmentary changes seen in lichen planus. After resolution of the eruption, the hyperpigmentation resolves slowly over a period of weeks to months.

Clinical Manifestations

Lesions of leukocytoclastic vasculitis can develop at any site but are usually distributed on the lower extremities or in dependent areas. Although purpuric lesions comprise the most common clinical pattern, a variety of other morphologic patterns, including vesicopustules, necrotic papules, and ulcers, can develop. These patterns often reflect secondary ischemic changes that are superimposed upon the primary vasculitic papule. Vesicopustules develop after ischemic necrosis of the epidermis results in subepidermal separation or after massive dermal accumulation of neutrophils secondary to immune complex deposition. Necrotic papules, eschars, and ulcers are end stage lesions that develop after total necrosis of the epidermis and superficial dermis. In essence, these lesions represent vasculitic infarcts.

Leukocytoclastic vasculitis is not merely a dermatitis but often part of a systemic vasculitis involving small vessels. In such cases, the vascular eruption is accompanied by arthralgias, myalgias, and malaise. Arthralgias and myalgias are probably attributable to vasculitic changes in small vessels in joint capsules and soft tissue. Vasculitic involvement of the kidneys, liver, and gastrointestinal tract can also occur. Such involvement of abdominal organ systems often presents clinically as abdominal pain. Laboratory studies are important to evaluate possible renal or hepatic impairment.

---

18. Why are leukocytoclastic vasculitis lesions papular?
19. What are the most common precipitants of leukocytoclastic vasculitis?
20. When leukocytoclastic vasculitis is part of a systemic vasculitis, what additional symptoms are typically observed?

REFERENCES

General

Ackerman AB, Ragaz A: *The Lives of Lesions: Chronology in Dermatopathology.* Masson, 1984.

Arndt KA et al (editors): *Cutaneous Medicine and Surgery: An Integrated Program in Dermatology.* Saunders, 1996.

Fitzpatrick TB et al (editors): *Dermatology in General Medicine,* 4th ed. McGraw-Hill, 1993.

Orkin M, Maibach HI, Dahl MV (editors): *Dermatology.* Appleton & Lange, 1991.

Psoriasis

Barker JN: Psoriasis as a T cell-mediated autoimmune disease. Hosp Med 1998 Jul;59:530.

Bata-Csorgo Z et al: Fibronectin and alpha integrin regulate keratinocyte cell cycling: A mechanism for increased fibronectin potentiation of T cell lymphokine-driven keratinocyte hyperproliferation in psoriasis. J Clin Invest 1998;101:1509.

Bhalerao J, Bowcock AM: The genetics of psoriasis: A complex disorder of the skin and immune system. Hum Mol Genet 1998;7:1537.

Espinoza LR et al: Insights into the pathogenesis of psoriasis and psoriatic arthritis. Am J Med Sci 1998;316:271.

Guilhou J: Immunopathogenesis of psoriasis: News in an old concept. Dermatology 1998;197:310.

Roenighk HH, Jr, Maibach HI (editors): *Psoriasis,* 3rd ed. Marcel Dekker, 1998.

Zelickson BD, Muller SA: Generalized pustular psoriasis: A review of 63 cases. Arch Dermatol 1991;127:1339.

Lichen Planus

Eversole LR: Immunopathogenesis of oral lichen planus and recurrent aphthous stomatitis. Semin Cut Med Surg 1997;16:284.

Fox BJ, Odom RB: Papulosquamous diseases: A review. J Am Acad Dermatol 1985;12:597.

Porter SR et al: Immunologic aspects of dermal and oral lichen planus: A review. Oral Surg Oral Med Oral Pathol Oral Radiol Endod 1997;83:358.

Scully C et al: Update on oral lichen planus: Etiopathogenesis and management. Crit Rev Oral Biol Med 1998;9:86.

Erythema Multiforme

Aurelian L, Kokuba H, Burnett JW: Understanding the pathogenesis of HSV-associated erythema multiforme. Dermatology 1998;197:219.

Chrysomali E et al: Apoptosis in oral erythema multiforme. Oral Surg Oral Med Oral Pathol Oral Radiol Endod 1997;83:272.

Bullous Pemphigoid

Budinger L et al: Identification and characterization of autoreactive T cell responses to bullous pemphigoid antigen 2 in patients and healthy controls. J Clin Invest 1998;102:2082.

De Pita O et al: T-helper 2 involvement in the pathogenesis of bullous pemphigoid: Role of soluble CD30 (sCD30). Arch Dermatol Res 1997;289:667.

Gammon WR et al: Immunofluorescence on split skin for the detection and differentiation of basement membrane zone autoantibodies. J Am Acad Dermatol 1992;27:79.

Kitajima Y et al: Internalization of the 180 kDa bullous pemphigoid antigen as immune complexes in basal keratinocytes: An important early event in blister formation in bullous pemphigoid. Br J Dermatol 1998; 138:71.

Korman N et al: Bullous pemphigoid. J Am Acad Dermatol 1987;16 (5 Part 1):907.

Zhu XJ, Niimi Y, Bystryn JC: Molecular identification of major and minor bullous pemphigoid antigens. J Am Acad Dermatol 1990;23(5 Part 1):876.

Leukocytoclastic Vasculitis

Claudy A: Pathogenesis of leukocytoclastic vasculitis. Eur J Dermatol 1998;8:75.

Grunwald MH et al: Leukocytoclastic vasculitis—correlation between different histologic stages and direct immunofluorescence results. Int J Dermatol 1997; 36:349.

Sais G et al: Adhesion molecule expression and endothelial cell activation in cutaneous leukocytoclastic vasculitis: An immunohistologic and clinical study in 42 patients. Arch Dermatol 1997;133:443.

Sais G et al: Prognostic factors in leukocytoclastic vasculitis: a clinicopathologic study of 160 patients. Arch Dermatol 1998;134:309.

Hodge SJ, Callen JP, Ekenstam E: Cutaneous leukocytoclastic vasculitis: Correlation of histopathological changes with clinical severity and course. J Cutan Pathol 1987;14:279.

Sanchez NP, Van Hale HM, Su WP: Clinical and histopathologic spectrum of necrotizing vasculitis: Report of findings in 101 cases. Arch Dermatol 1985;121:220.

Smoller BR, McNutt NS, Contreras F: The natural history of vasculitis: What the histology tells us about pathogenesis. Arch Dermatol 1990; 126:84.

9　Pulmonary Disease

Thomas J. Prendergast, MD, & Stephen J. Ruoss, MD

ABBREVIATIONS AND SYMBOLS USED IN THIS CHAPTER

V	Volume of gas
V̇	Volume of gas per minute
Q̇	Flow of blood per minute
V̇/Q̇ ratio	Ratio of volume of gas per minute to blood flow per minute
V_D/V_T	Ratio of wasted ventilation (dead space) to tidal volume
P_{O_2}	Partial pressure of oxygen
P_{CO_2}	Partial pressure of carbon dioxide
Pa_{O_2}	Partial pressure of oxygen in arterial blood
Pa_{CO_2}	Partial pressure of carbon dioxide in arterial blood
F_{IO_2}	Fractional concentration of oxygen in inspired air
A–a ΔP_{O_2}	Difference between alveolar and arterial partial pressure of oxygen
D_{LCO}	Diffusing capacity of the lung for carbon monoxide
cm H_2O	Pressure measured in centimeters of water
mm Hg	Pressure measured in millimeters of mercury

When injury to components of the respiratory system occurs, the integrated function of the whole is disrupted. The consequences can be profound. Airway injury or dysfunction results in obstructive lung diseases, including bronchitis and asthma, while parenchymal lung injury can produce restrictive lung disease or pulmonary vascular disease. To understand the clinical presentations of lung disease, it is necessary first to understand the anatomic and functional organization of the lungs that determines normal function.

> 1. What are the two principal physiologic roles of the lungs?
> 2. What are the requirements for successful lung function?

NORMAL STRUCTURE & FUNCTION OF THE LUNGS

ANATOMY

The principal physiologic role of the lungs is to make oxygen available to tissues for metabolism and to remove the by-product of that metabolism, carbon dioxide. The lungs perform this function by placing inspired air in close proximity to the pulmonary capillary bed to permit gas exchange by simple diffusion. This is accomplished at a minimal work load, regulated efficiently over a wide range of metabolic demand, and takes place with close matching of ventilation to lung perfusion. The extensive surface area of the respiratory system must also be protected from a broad variety of infectious or noxious environmental insults.

Humans possess a complex and efficient respiratory system that satisfies these diverse requirements.

The mature respiratory system consists of visceral pleura-covered lungs contained by the chest wall and diaphragm, the latter serving under normal conditions as the principal bellows muscle for ventilation. The lungs are divided into lobes, each demarcated by intervening visceral pleura. Each lung possesses an upper and lower lobe; the middle lobe and lingula are the third lobes in the right and left lungs, respectively. At end-expiration, most of the volume of the lungs is air (Table 9–1), whereas almost half of the mass of the lungs is accounted for by blood volume. It is a testament to the delicate structure of the gas-exchanging region of the lungs that alveolar tissue has a total weight of only 250 g but a total surface area of 75 m².

LUNG VOLUMES, CAPACITIES, AND THE NORMAL SPIROGRAM

The volume of gas in the lungs is divided into volumes and capacities as shown in the bars to the left of the figure below. Lung volumes are primary: they do not overlap each other. Tidal volume (V_T) is the amount of gas inhaled and exhaled with each resting breath. A normal tidal volume in a 70-kg person is approximately 350–400 mL. Residual volume (RV) is the amount of gas remaining in the lungs at the end of a maximal exhalation. Lung capacities are composed of two or more lung volumes. The vital capacity (VC) is the total amount of gas that can be exhaled following a maximal inhalation. The vital capacity and the residual volume together constitute the total lung capacity (TLC), or the total amount of gas in the lungs at the end of a maximal inhalation. The functional residual capacity (FRC) is the amount of gas in the lungs at the end of a resting tidal breath. (IC, inspiratory capacity; IRV, inspiratory reserve volume; ERV, expiratory reserve volume.)

The spirogram at right in the figure is drawn in real time. The first tidal breath shown takes 5 seconds, indicating a respiratory rate of 12 breaths per minute. The forced vital capacity (FVC) maneuver begins with an inhalation from FRC to TLC (lasting about 1 second) followed by a forceful exhalation from TLC to RV (lasting about 5 seconds). The amount of gas exhaled during the first second of this maneuver is the forced expiratory volume in 1 second (FEV_1). Normal subjects expel approximately 80% of the FVC in the first second. The ratio of the FEV_1 to the FVC (referred to as the $FEV_1\%$) is diminished in patients with obstructive lung disease.

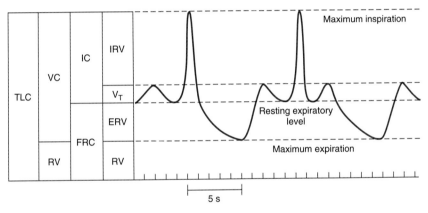

(Modified and reproduced, with permission, from Staub NC: *Basic Respiratory Physiology*. Churchill Livingstone, 1991.)

Two anatomic elements of support serve to maintain the anatomic integrity of this large and complex surface area: connective tissue fibers and surfactant. The connective tissue fibers are highly organized collagen and elastin structures. They radiate into the lungs, dividing segments, investing airways and vessels, and supporting alveolar walls with a very elastic and delicate fibrous network. The multidirectional elastic support provided by this network allows the lung, from alveoli to conducting airways, to support itself and retain airway patency despite large changes in volume.

Surfactant provides specific anatomic assistance in reducing the surface tension of alveoli. In the absence of a surface-active layer covering the alveolar surface, increasing surface tension associated with a reduction of alveolar volume during expiration would collapse alveoli. The distending pressure required to reexpand these alveoli would be greater than normal ventilatory effort could produce. Surfactant, a complex material produced by type II alveolar cells and composed of multiple phospholipids and specific associated proteins, produces a marked reduction of surface tension, allowing expansion of alveoli with a transpulmonary distending pressure of less than 5 cm H_2O.

Table 9–1. Components of normal human lung.[1]

Component	Volume (mL) or Mass (g)	Thickness (μm)
Gas (functional residual capacity)	2400	
Tissue	900	
Blood	400	
Lung	500	
Support structures	250	
Alveolar walls	250–300	
Epithelium	60–80	0.18
Endothelium	50–70	0.10
Interstitium	100–185	0.22

[1]Reproduced, with permission, from Murray JF, Nadel JA: *Textbook of Respiratory Medicine,* 2nd ed. Saunders, 1994.

Airway & Epithelial Anatomy

Further anatomic division of the lungs is based primarily on the separation of the tracheobronchial tree into **conducting airways,** which provide for movement of air from the external environment to areas of gas exchange, and **terminal respiratory units,** or **acini,** the airways and associated alveolar structures participating directly in gas exchange (Figure 9–1). The proximal conducting airways are lined by ciliated pseudostratified columnar epithelium, are supported by a cartilaginous skeleton in their walls, and contain secretory glands in the epithelial wall. The ciliated epithelium has a uniform orientation of cilia that beat in unison toward the pharynx. This ciliary action, together with the mucus layer produced by submucosal mucous secretory glands, provides a mechanism for the continuous transport of contaminating or excess material out of the lungs. Circumferential airway smooth muscle is also present but, as

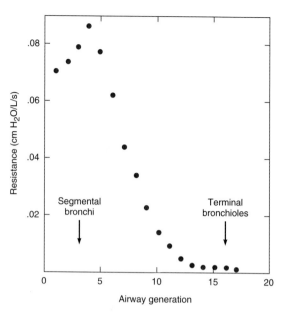

Figure 9–2. Location of the principal site of airflow resistance. The second- through fifth-generation airways include the segmental bronchi and larger bronchioles. They present the greatest resistance to airflow in normal subjects. The smaller airways contribute relatively little despite their smaller caliber because of the enormous number arranged in parallel. Compare with Figure 9–3. (Reproduced, with permission, from West JB: *Respiratory Physiology: The Essentials,* 4th ed. Williams & Wilkins, 1990.)

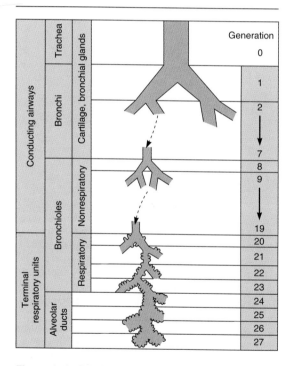

Figure 9–1. Subdivision of conducting airways and terminal respiratory units. This schematic illustration demonstrates the subdivisions of both the conducting airways and the respiratory airways. Successive branching produces increasing generations of airways, beginning with the trachea. Note that gas-exchanging segments of the lung are encountered only after extensive branching, with concomitant decrease in airway caliber and increase in total cross-sectional area (see Figures 9–2 and 9–3). (Modified and reproduced, with permission, from Weibel ER: *Morphometry of the Lung.* Springer, 1963.)

with secretory glands, is reduced and then lost as the airways branch farther into the lung and diminish in caliber. The smallest conducting airways are nonrespiratory **bronchioles.** They are characterized by a loss of smooth muscle and cartilage but retention of a cuboidal epithelium that may be ciliated and which is not a site of gas exchange. The lobes of the lung are divided into less distinct lobules, defined as collections of terminal respiratory units incompletely bounded by connective tissue septa. Terminal respiratory units are the final physiologic and anatomic unit of the lung, with walls of thin alveolar epithelial cells that provide gas exchange with the alveolar capillary bed.

The principal site of resistance to airflow in the lungs is in medium-sized bronchi (Figure 9–2). This at first seems counterintuitive, since one would expect airways of smaller caliber to be the major site of resistance. The small airways do not normally contribute significantly to airway resistance because of the profound increase in cross-sectional area in smaller airways as branching increases airway numbers (Figure 9–3). Under pathologic conditions such as asthma, where smaller bronchi and bronchioles

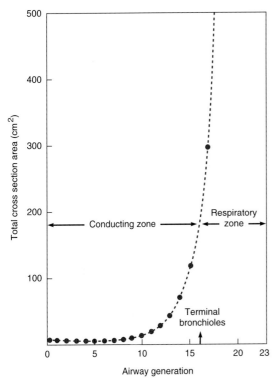

Figure 9–3. Airway generation and total airway cross-sectional area. Note the extremely rapid increase in total cross-sectional area in the respiratory zone (compare with Figure 9–1), and the fall in resistance as a consequence of the increase in cross-sectional area increase (compare with Figure 9–2). As a result, the forward velocity of gas during inspiration becomes very low at the level of the respiratory bronchioles, and gas diffusion becomes the chief mode of ventilation. (Reproduced, with permission, from West JB: *Respiratory Physiology: The Essentials,* 4th ed. Williams & Wilkins, 1990.)

become narrowed, airway resistance can increase dramatically.

As noted above, the pulmonary arterial system runs in close association with the branching bronchial tree throughout the lungs (Figure 9–4). By virtue of the ability to carefully regulate arterial and bronchial caliber, the anatomic arrangement provides the ideal setting for the continuous matching of ventilation and perfusion to lung segments.

Pulmonary Nervous System

The lungs are richly innervated with neural fibers from parasympathetic (vagal), sympathetic, and the so-called nonadrenergic, noncholinergic (NANC) systems. Efferent fibers include (1) parasympathetic fibers, with muscarinic cholinergic efferents that mediate bronchoconstriction, pulmonary vasodilation, and mucous gland secretion; (2) sympathetic fibers, whose stimulation produces bronchial smooth muscle relaxation, pulmonary vasoconstriction, and inhibition of secretory gland activity; and (3) the NANC system, with multiple transmitters implicated, including adenosine triphosphate (ATP), nitric oxide (NO), and peptide neurotransmitters such as substance P and vasoactive intestinal peptide (VIP). The NANC system participates in inhibitory events, including bronchodilation, and may function as the predominant reciprocal balance to the excitatory cholinergic system.

Pulmonary afferents consist principally of the vagal sensory fibers (Table 9–2). These include the following:

(1) Fibers from bronchopulmonary stretch receptors, located in the trachea and proximal bronchi. Stimulation of these fibers by lung inflation results in bronchodilation and an increased heart rate.

(2) Fibers from irritant receptors, which are also found in proximal airways. Stimulation of these fibers by diverse nonspecific stimuli elicits efferent responses including cough, bronchoconstriction, and mucus secretion.

(3) C fibers, or fibers from juxtacapillary (J) receptors, are unmyelinated fibers ending in lung parenchyma and bronchial walls and respond to mechanical and chemical stimuli. The reflex responses associated with stimulation of C fibers include a rapid shallow breathing pattern, mucus secretion, cough, and heart rate slowing with inspiration.

Vascular & Lymphatic Anatomy

The pulmonary vascular system has two main components: the pulmonary vessels and the bronchial vessels (Figure 9–4). Pulmonary arteries are smooth muscle-invested vessels running with the bronchial tree and providing perfusion to lung parenchyma. They are very sensitive to the alveolar P_{O_2}, with a prominent hypoxic vasoconstrictor response. This provides a sensitive mechanism for maintaining matching of alveolar perfusion with ventilation. Pulmonary veins in turn drain alveolar lung parenchyma, taking a course in the intralobular septa distinct from the pulmonary bronchovascular bundle. Bronchial vessels are systemic circulation vessels that supply blood to essentially all the intrapulmonary structures except the parenchyma, including the bronchial tree, pulmonary nervous system and lymphatics, and connective tissue septa (Figure 9–5). Bronchial arteries anastomose with capillaries of the pulmonary circulation but contribute little blood flow to the total pulmonary perfusion.

Pulmonary lymphatics develop along with the airway and vascular systems of the lung. Lymphatics are found in connective tissue spaces of the pleura, the peribronchovascular sheath, and interlobular septa. Lymphatics are found as far distally as the ter-

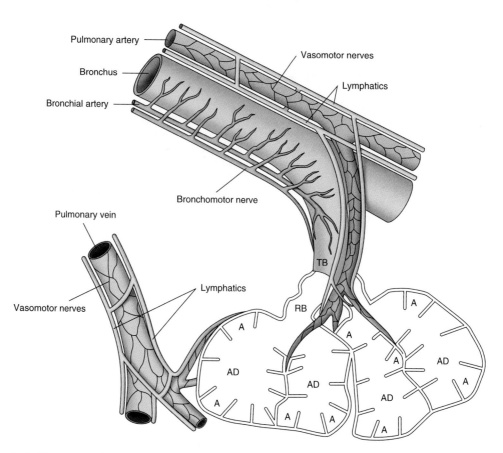

Figure 9–4. Airway, vascular, and lymphatic anatomy of the lung. This schematic diagram demonstrates the general anatomic relationships of the airways and terminal respiratory units with the vascular and lymphatic systems of the lung. Important points are as follows: (1) The pulmonary arterial system runs adjacent to the bronchial tree, while the draining pulmonary veins are found distant from the airways; (2) the bronchial wall blood supply is provided by bronchial arteries, branches of systemic arterial origin; (3) lymphatics are found adjacent to both the arterial and venous systems and are very abundant in the lung; and (4) lymphatics are found as far distally as the terminal respiratory bronchioles, but they do not penetrate to the alveolar wall. (A, alveolus; AD, alveolar duct; RB, respiratory bronchiole; TB, terminal bronchiole.) (Reproduced, with permission, from Staub NC: The physiology of pulmonary edema. Hum Pathol 1970;1:419.)

Table 9–2. Characteristics of the three pulmonary vagal sensory reflexes.[1]

Receptor	Location	Stimulus	Response
Pulmonary stretch, slowly adapting	Associated with smooth muscle of intrapulmonary airways	1. Lung inflation 2. Increased transpulmonary pressure	1. Hering-Breuer inflation reflex 2. Bronchodilation 3. Increased heart rate 4. Decreased peripheral vascular resistance
Irritant, rapidly adapting	Epithelium of (mainly) extrapulmonary airways	1. Irritants 2. Mechanical stimulation 3. Anaphylaxis 4. Lung inflation or deflation 5. Hyperpnea 6. Pulmonary congestion	1. Bronchoconstriction 2. Hyperpnea 3. Expiratory constriction of larynx 4. Cough 5. Mucous secretion

C fibers
  Pulmonary type (J)
  Bronchial
	Alveolar wall
	
	Airway and blood vessels
		1. Increased interstitial volume (congestion)
		2. Chemical injury
		3. Microembolism
			1. Rapid, shallow breathing
			2. Laryngeal and tracheobronchial constriction
			3. Bradycardia
			4. Spinal reflex inhibition
			5. Mucous secretion

[1]Modified and reproduced, with permission, from Murray JF: *The Normal Lung.* Saunders, 1986.

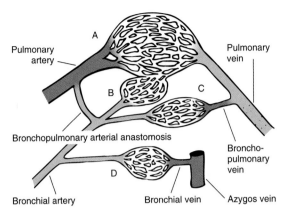

Figure 9–5. Relationship between bronchial and pulmonary circulations. The pulmonary artery supplies the pulmonary capillary network A. The bronchial artery supplies capillary networks B, C, and D. Network B represents the bronchial capillary supply to bronchioles that anastomose with pulmonary capillaries and drains through pulmonary veins. Network C represents the bronchial capillary supply to most bronchi; these vessels form bronchopulmonary veins that empty into pulmonary veins. Network D represents the bronchial capillary supply to lobar and segmental bronchi; these vessels form true bronchial veins that drain into the azygos, hemiazygos, or intercostal veins. Dark-colored areas represent blood of low O_2 content. (Reproduced, with permission, from Murray JF: *The Normal Lung*. Saunders, 1986.)

minal respiratory bronchioles but do not enter the connective tissue space of the alveolar walls (Figure 9–4). Thus, fluid that finds its way into the alveolar interstitium must move the short distance to the region of terminal bronchioles to gain access to draining lymphatics. Both visceral and parietal pleura contain associated lymphatics. These vessels—in particular the lymphatics associated with the parietal pleura—are responsible for the rapid clearance of fluid from the pleural space.

Immune Structure & Function

Of all the body's organs, the lungs are in a unique position with respect to exposure to hostile insults. Ventilatory requirements expose the lung to an enormous volume of environmental air daily—nonexertional ventilation in an adult totals about 6000 L of air per day, and the amount is increased substantially with activity. Ventilation in an open, nonsterile environment carries the continued risk of toxic or infectious insult. Furthermore, the pulmonary capillary bed is the only capillary bed in the body through which the entire circulating blood volume must flow in each cardiac cycle. As a consequence, the lung is an obligatory vascular sieve and functions as a principal site of defense against infection or other insult. Protection of the lungs from environmental and infectious injury involves a set of complex responses capable of providing a timely and successful defense against attack via the airways or the vascular bed. As outlined in Table 9–3, it is convenient for discussion to separate these responses into two major categories—nonspecific physical and chemical protections and specific immune structures and actions—all functioning in such a way as to prevent injury to or microbial invasion of the very large epithelial and vascular area of the lung (see Chapter 4 and Table 4–11).

Table 9–3. Lung defenses.[1]

I. Nonspecific defenses
  1. Clearance
    a. Cough
    b. Mucociliary escalator
  2. Secretions
    a. Tracheobronchial (mucus)
    b. Alveolar (surfactant)
    c. Cellular components (lysozyme, complement, surfactant proteins, defensins)
  3. Cellular defenses
    a. Nonphagocytic
      Conducting airway epithelium
      Terminal respiratory epithelium
    b. Phagocytic
      Blood phagocytes (monocytes)
      Tissue phagocytes (alveolar macrophages)
  4. Biochemical defenses
    a. Proteinase inhibitors (α_1-protease inhibitor, secretory leukoprotease inhibitor)
    b. Antioxidants (eg, transferrin, lactoferrin, glutathione, albumin)
II. Specific immunologic defenses
  1. Antibody-mediated (B lymphocyte-dependent immunologic responses)
    a. Secretory immunoglobulin (IgA)
    b. Serum immunoglobulins
  2. Antigen presentation to lymphocytes
    a. Macrophages and monocytes
    b. Dendritic cells
    c. Epithelial cells
  3. Cell-mediated (T lymphocyte-dependent) immunologic responses
    a. Cytokine-mediated
    b. Direct cellular cytotoxicity
  4. Nonlymphocyte cellular immune responses
    a. Mast cell dependent
    b. Eosinophil-dependent

[1]See also Table 4–11.

3. What are the roles of the connective tissue and surfactant systems in lung function?
4. What is the role of ciliary action of the respiratory epithelium?
5. Why is it that medium-sized bronchi rather than small airways are the major site of resistance to airflow in the lungs?
6. What are the physiologic functions of the efferent parasympathetic, sympathetic, and NANC neural systems of the lung?
7. What are the categories of afferent vagal sensory receptors?
8. What are the different roles of the pulmonary and bronchial arteries?
9. What sensitive mechanism do the pulmonary arteries have for matching alveolar perfusion with ventilation?
10. What are the components of the nonspecific defense system of the lungs?
11. What are the humoral and cellular components of the specific immune defense system of the lungs?

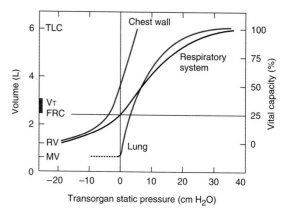

Figure 9–6. Interaction of the pressure-volume properties of the lungs and the chest wall. Resting lung volume (functional residual capacity [FRC]) represents the equilibrium point where the elastic recoil of the lung (tendency to collapse inward) and the chest wall (tendency to spring outward) are exactly balanced. Other lung volumes can also be defined by reference to this diagram. Total lung capacity (TLC) is the point where the inspiratory muscles cannot generate sufficient force to overcome the elastic recoil of the lungs and chest wall. Residual volume (RV) is the point where the expiratory muscles cannot generate sufficient force to overcome the elastic recoil of the chest wall. Compliance is calculated by taking the slope of these pressure-volume relationships at a specific volume. Note that the compliance of the lungs is greater at low lung volumes but falls considerably above two-thirds of vital capacity. (Reproduced, with permission, from Staub NC: *Basic Respiratory Physiology.* Churchill Livingstone, 1991.)

PHYSIOLOGY

At rest, the lungs take 4 L/min of air and 5 L/min of blood, direct them within 0.2 μm of each other, and then return both to their respective pools. With maximal exercise, flow may increase to 100 L/min of ventilation and 25 L/min of cardiac output. The lungs thereby perform their primary physiologic function of making oxygen available to the tissues for metabolism and removing the major by-product of that metabolism, carbon dioxide. The lungs perform this task largely free of conscious control, all the while maintaining $PaCO_2$ within 5% tolerance. It is a magnificent feat of evolutionary plumbing and neural control.

Static Properties: Compliance & Elastic Recoil

The lung maintains its extremely thin parenchyma over an enormous surface area by means of an intricate supporting architecture of collagen and elastin fibers. Anatomically—as well as physiologically and functionally—the lung is an elastic organ.

The lungs inflate and deflate in response to changes in volume of the semirigid thoracic cage in which they are suspended. An analogy would be to inflate a blacksmith's bellows by pulling the handles apart, thus increasing the volume of the bellows, lowering pressure, and causing inflow of air. Air enters the lungs when the pressure in the pleural space is reduced by the expansion of the chest wall. The volume of air entering the lungs depends on the change in pleural pressure and the **compliance** of the respiratory system. Compliance is an intrinsic elastic property that relates a change in volume to a change in pressure. The compliance of the chest wall and that of the lungs both contribute to the compliance of the respiratory system (Figure 9–6). The compliance of the chest wall does not change significantly with thoracic volume, at least within the physiologic range. The compliance of the lungs varies inversely with lung volume. At functional residual capacity (FRC), the lungs are normally very compliant, approximately 200 mL per cm H_2O. Thus, a reduction of 5 cm H_2O pressure in the pleural space will draw a breath of 1 L.

The tendency of a deformable body to return to its baseline shape is its **elastic recoil.** The elastic recoil of the chest wall is determined by the shape and structure of the thoracic cage. Two components contribute to lung elastic recoil. The first is tissue elasticity; the second is related to the forces needed to change the shape of the air-liquid interface of the alveolus (Figure 9–7). Expanding the lungs requires overcoming local surface forces that are directly proportionate to the local **surface tension.** Surface tension is a physical property that reflects the greater attraction between molecules of a liquid rather than between molecules of that liquid and adjacent gas. At

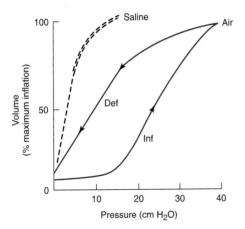

Figure 9–7. Effect of surface forces on lung compliance—a simple experiment demonstrating the effect of surface tension at the air-liquid interface of excised cat lungs. When inflated with saline, there are no surface forces to overcome and the lungs are both more compliant and show no difference (hysteresis) between the inflation and deflation curves. When inflated with air, the pressure required to distend the lung is greater at every volume. The difference between the two represents the contribution of surface forces. There is also a pronounced hysteresis that reflects surfactant recruited into the alveolar liquid during inflation (Inf), where it further reduces surface forces during deflation (Def). (Reproduced, with permission, from Morgan TE: Pulmonary surfactant. N Engl J Med 1971;284:1185.)

the air-liquid interface of the lung, molecules of water at the interface are more strongly attracted to each other than they are to the air above. This creates a net force drawing water molecules together in the plane of the interface. If the interface is stretched over a curved surface, that force acts to collapse the curve. The law of Laplace quantifies this force: The pressure needed to keep open the curve (in this case represented by a sphere) is directly proportionate to the surface tension at the interface and inversely proportionate to the radius of the sphere (Figure 9–8).

Surfactant is a mixture of phospholipid (predominantly dipalmitoylphosphatidylcholine [DPPC]) and proteins. These hydrophobic molecules displace water molecules from the air-liquid interface, thereby reducing surface tension. This reduction has three physiologic implications: First, it reduces the elastic recoil pressure of the lungs, thereby reducing the pressure needed to inflate them. This results in reduced work of breathing. Second, it allows surface forces to vary with alveolar surface area, thereby promoting alveolar stability and protecting against atelectasis (Figure 9–8). Third, it limits the reduction of hydrostatic pressure in the pericapillary interstitium caused by surface tension. This reduces the forces promoting transudation of fluid and the tendency to accumulate interstitial edema.

Pathologic states may result from changes in lung elastic recoil related to an increase in compliance (emphysema), a decrease in compliance (pulmonary fibrosis; Figure 9–9), or a disruption of surfactant with an increase in surface forces (infant respiratory distress syndrome [IRDS]).

Dynamic Properties: Flow & Resistance

Inflation of the lungs must overcome three opposing forces: elastic recoil, including surface forces; inertia of the respiratory system; and resistance to airflow. Since inertia is negligible, the work of breathing can be divided into work to overcome elastic forces and work to overcome flow resistance.

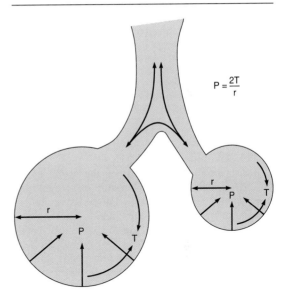

Figure 9–8. The importance of surface tension. If two connected alveoli have the same surface tension, then the smaller the radius, the greater the pressure tending to collapse the sphere. This could lead to alveolar instability, with smaller units emptying into larger ones. Alveoli typically do not have the same surface tension because surface forces vary according to surface area, due to the presence of surfactant. Since the relative concentration of surfactant in the surface layer of the sphere increases as the radius of the sphere falls, the effect of surfactant is increased at low lung volumes. This tends to counterbalance the increase in pressure needed to keep alveoli open at diminished lung volume and adds stability to alveoli which might otherwise tend to collapse into one another. Surfactant thus protects against regional collapse of lung units, a condition known as atelectasis, in addition to its other functions. (r, radius of alveolus; T, surface tension; P, gas pressure.)

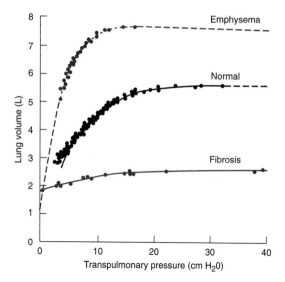

Figure 9–9. Static expiratory pressure-volume curves in normal subjects and patients with emphysema and pulmonary fibrosis. The underlying physiologic abnormality in emphysema is a dramatic increase in lung compliance. Such patients tend to breathe at very high lung volumes. Patients with pulmonary fibrosis have very noncompliant lungs and breathe at low lung volumes. (Modified and reproduced, with permission, from Pride NB, Mackem PT: Lung mechanics in disease. In: Vol III, Part 2, of *Handbook of Physiology.* Section 3. Respiratory System. Fishman AP [editor]. American Physiological Society, 1986.)

Resistance to flow depends on the nature of the flow. Under conditions of **laminar** or **streamlined flow,** resistance is described by Poiseuille's equation: Resistance is directly proportionate to the length of the airway and the viscosity of the gas and inversely proportionate to the fourth power of the radius. A reduction by one-half of airway radius leads to a 16-fold increase in airway resistance. Airway caliber is therefore the principal determinant of airway resistance under laminar flow conditions. Under conditions of **turbulent flow,** the driving pressure needed to achieve a given flow rate is proportionate to the square of the flow rate. Turbulent flow is also dependent on gas density and not on gas viscosity.

Most of the resistance to normal breathing arises in the medium-sized bronchi and not in the smaller bronchioles (Figure 9–2). There are two main reasons for this counterintuitive finding. First, airflow in the normal lung is not laminar but turbulent, at least from the mouth to the small peripheral airways. Thus, where flow is highest (in the segmental and subsegmental bronchi), resistance is dependent chiefly on flow rates. There is a transition to laminar flow approaching the terminal bronchioles as a consequence of increased cross-sectional area and decreased flow rates (Figure 9–3). In the respiratory bronchioles and alveoli, there is no bulk flow of gas, and gas movement occurs by diffusion. In small peripheral airways, airway caliber is the principal determinant of resistance. The caliber of peripheral airways is quite small, but repetitive branching creates a very large number of small airways arranged in parallel. Their resistance adds reciprocally, making their contribution to total airway resistance minor under normal conditions.

Airway resistance is determined by several factors. Many disease states affect bronchial smooth muscle tone and cause **bronchoconstriction,** producing an abnormal narrowing of the airways. Airways may also be narrowed by hypertrophy (chronic bronchitis) or infiltration (sarcoidosis) of the airway mucosa. Physiologically, the radial traction of the lung interstitium supports the airways and increases their caliber as lung volume increases. Conversely, as lung volume decreases, airway caliber also decreases and resistance to airflow increases. Patients with airflow obstruction often breathe at large lung volumes in an effort to maximize elastic lung recoil; this supports a larger airway caliber and thus minimizes resistance.

Analysis in terms of laminar and turbulent flow assumes that the airways are rigid tubes. In fact, they are highly compressible. The compressibility of the airways underlies the important phenomenon of **effort-independent flow.** It is an old clinical observation that airflow rates during expiration can be increased with effort only up to a certain point. Beyond that point, further increases in effort do not increase flow rates. The explanation for this phenomenon relies on the concept of an **equal pressure point.**

Pleural pressure is generally negative (subatmospheric) throughout quiet breathing. The peribronchiolar pressure that surrounds the conducting airways reflects pleural pressure. Hence, during quiet breathing, the airways are surrounded by negative pressure that helps to keep them open. Pleural and peribronchiolar pressure may become positive during forced expiration. In this case, the airways are surrounded by positive pressure. The equal pressure point occurs where the pressure inside the airway equals the surrounding peribronchiolar pressure, leading to instability and potential airway collapse (Figure 9–10).

The equal pressure point is not an anatomic site but a functional result that helps to clarify different mechanisms of airflow obstruction. Since the pressure driving expiratory airflow is lung elastic recoil pressure, a reduction in recoil pressure will lead to cessation of flow at higher lung volumes. Patients with emphysema lose lung elastic recoil and may have severely impaired expiratory flow even with airways of normal caliber. Conversely, an increase in recoil pressure will oppose dynamic compression. Patients with pulmonary fibrosis may have abnormally high flow rates despite severely reduced lung volumes. The presence of airway disease augments the drop in pressure along the airways and may generate an equal pressure point at high lung volumes.

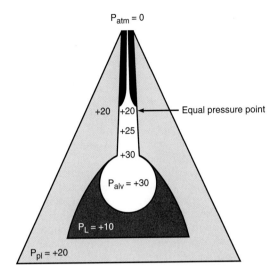

Figure 9–10. The concept of the equal pressure point. For air to flow through a tube, there must be a pressure difference between the two ends. In the case of forced expiration with an open glottis, this driving pressure is the difference between alveolar pressure (the sum of pleural pressure and lung elastic recoil pressure) and atmospheric pressure (assumed to be zero). Frictional resistance causes a fall in this driving pressure along the length of the conducting airways. At some point, the driving pressure may equal the surrounding peribronchial pressure; in this event, the net transmural pressure is zero. This defines the equal pressure point. Downstream (toward the mouth) from the equal pressure point, pressure outside the airway is greater than the driving pressure inside the airway. This net negative pressure tends to collapse the airway, resulting in dynamic compression. The more forcefully one expires, the more the pressure surrounding collapsible airways increases. Flow becomes effort-independent. (P_{pl}, pleural pressure; P_L, lung elastic recoil pressure; P_{alv}, alveolar pressure; P_{atm}, atmospheric pressure.)

The Work of Breathing

The amount of energy needed to maintain the respiratory muscles during quiet breathing is small, approximately 2% of basal oxygen consumption. Increasing ventilation in normal humans consumes relatively little oxygen until ventilation approaches 70 L/min. In patients with lung disease, the energy requirements are greater at rest and increase dramatically with exercise. Patients with emphysema may not be able to increase their ventilation by more than a factor of 2 because the oxygen cost of breathing exceeds the additional oxygen made available to the body.

A constant minute ventilation can be achieved through multiple combinations of respiratory rate and tidal volume. The two components of the work of breathing—elastic forces and resistance to airflow—are affected in opposite ways by changes in frequency and depth of breathing. Elastic resistance is minimized by rapid, shallow breathing; resistive forces are minimized by slow, large tidal volume breathing. Figure 9–11 shows how these two components can be summed to provide a total work of breathing for different frequencies at a constant minute ventilation. The set point for respiration is that point where the total work of breathing is minimized. In normal humans, this occurs at a frequency of approximately 15 breaths per minute. In different diseases, this pattern is altered to compensate for the underlying physiologic abnormality.

Distribution of Ventilation & Perfusion

Inhaled air is not distributed equally to all regions of the lung. In the healthy subject, this is due principally to the effects of gravity on pleural pressure. Pleural pressure varies from the top to the bottom of the lung by approximately 0.25 cm H_2O per centime-

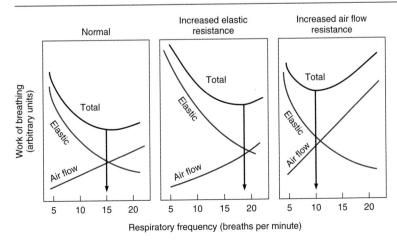

Figure 9–11. Minimizing the work of breathing. These diagrams divide the total work of breathing at the same minute ventilation into elastic and resistive components. In disease states that increase elastic forces (eg, pulmonary fibrosis), total work is minimized by rapid, shallow breathing; with increased airflow resistance (eg, chronic bronchitis), total work is minimized by slow deep breathing. (Reproduced, with permission, from Nunn JF: *Nunn's Respiratory Physiology,* 4th ed. Butterworth-Heinemann, 1993.)

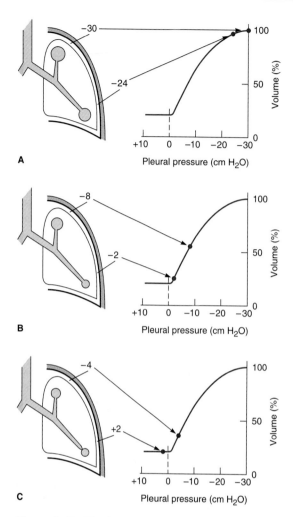

Figure 9–12. Distribution of ventilation at different lung volumes. The effect of gravity and the weight of the lung cause pleural pressure to become more negative toward the apex of the lung. The effect of this change in pressure is to increase the expansion of apical alveoli. **A:** Total lung capacity. At high lung volumes, the compliance curve of the lung is flat; alveoli are almost equally expanded because pressure differences cause small changes in lung volume. **B:** Functional residual capacity. During quiet breathing, the lower lobes are on the steep part of the pressure-volume curve. This increased compliance at lower volumes is why ventilation at FRC is preferentially distributed to the lower lobes. **C:** Residual volume. Below FRC, there may be dependent lung units that are exposed to positive pleural pressures. These units may collapse, leading to areas of lung that are perfused but not ventilated. (Modified and reproduced, with permission, from Murray JF: *The Normal Lung,* 2nd ed. Saunders, 1986.)

ter. It is more negative at the apex and more positive at the base. The effect is shifted to an anteroposterior distribution in the supine position and is greatly diminished (though not abolished) at zero gravity.

Regional ventilation is dependent on regional pleural pressure (Figure 9–12). More negative pleural pressure at the lung apex causes greater expansion of the apical alveoli. Given the shape of the lung's pressure-volume curve, lung compliance is greater at low lung volumes, and ventilation is preferentially distributed to the lower lobes at FRC.

Pulmonary blood flow is a low-pressure system that functions in a gravitational field across 30 vertical centimeters. The distribution of blood flow to the lungs is not uniform under resting conditions. In the upright position, there is a nearly linear increase in blood flow from the top to the bottom of the lung. The details of distribution are portrayed in Figure 9–13.

Multiple factors besides gravity regulate blood flow. The most important is **hypoxic pulmonary vasoconstriction.** The smooth muscle cells of the pulmonary arterioles are sensitive to alveolar PO_2 (much more so than to arterial PO_2). As alveolar PO_2 falls, there is arteriolar constriction, an increase in local resistance to flow, and redistribution of flow to regions of higher alveolar PO_2. This is an extremely effective mechanism when regionalized. It can greatly diminish local blood flow without a significant increase in mean pulmonary arterial pressure when it affects less than 20% of the pulmonary circulation. Global alveolar hypoxia results in pulmonary hypertension.

Matching of Ventilation to Perfusion

The functional role of the lungs is to place ambient air in close proximity to circulating blood to permit gas exchange by simple diffusion. To accomplish this, air and blood flow must be directed to the same place at the same time. In other words, ventilation and perfusion must be matched. A failure to match ventilation to perfusion, or **V̇/Q̇ mismatch,** lies behind most abnormalities in O_2 and CO_2 exchange.

In the normal subject, a typical resting minute ventilation is 6 L/min. Approximately one-third of this amount fills the conducting airways and constitutes dead space or wasted ventilation. Resting alveolar ventilation is therefore approximately 4 L/min, while pulmonary artery blood flow is 5 L/min. This yields an overall ratio of ventilation to perfusion of 0.8. As noted above, neither ventilation nor perfusion is homogeneously distributed. Both are preferentially distributed to dependent regions at rest, though the increase in gravity-dependent flow is more marked with perfusion than with ventilation. Hence, the ratio of ventilation to perfusion is highest at the apex and lowest at the base (Figure 9–14).

Alterations in the distribution of ventilation to per-

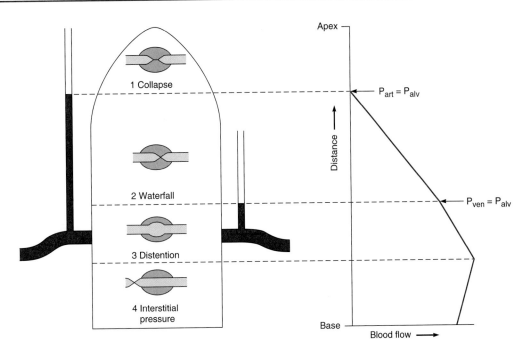

Figure 9–13. Effect of changing hydrostatic pressure on the distribution of pulmonary blood flow. Capillary blood flow in different regions of the lung is governed by three pressures: pulmonary arterial pressure, pulmonary venous pressure, and alveolar pressure. Pulmonary arterial pressure must be greater than pulmonary venous pressure to maintain forward perfusion; there are therefore three potential arrangements of these variables. **Zone 1:** $P_{alv} > P_{art} > P_{ven}$. There is no capillary perfusion in areas where alveolar pressure is greater than the capillary perfusion pressure. Since alveolar pressure is normally zero, this only occurs where mean pulmonary arterial pressure is less than the vertical distance from the pulmonary artery. **Zone 2:** $P_{art} > P_{alv} > P_{ven}$. Pulmonary arterial pressure exceeds alveolar pressure, but alveolar pressure exceeds pulmonary venous pressure. The driving pressure along the capillary is dissipated by resistance to flow until the transmural pressure is negative and compression occurs. This zone of collapse then regulates flow, which is intermittent and dependent on fluctuating pulmonary venous pressures. **Zone 3:** $P_{art} > P_{ven} > P_{alv}$. Flow is independent of alveolar pressure because the pulmonary venous pressure exceeds atmospheric pressure. **Zone 4:** Zone of extra-alveolar compression. In dependent lung regions, lung interstitial pressure may exceed pulmonary arterial pressure. In this event, capillary flow is determined by compression of extra-alveolar vessels.

The right side of the diagram shows a near-continuous distribution of blood flow from the top of the lung to the bottom, demonstrating that in the normal lung there are no discrete zones. The normal human lung at FRC spans 30 vertical centimeters, half of which distance is above the pulmonary artery and left atrium; and representative pulmonary arterial pressures are 33/11 cm H_2O with a mean of 19 cm H_2O. There is therefore no physiologic zone 1 in upright humans except perhaps in late diastole. Left atrial pressure averages 11 cm H_2O and is sufficient to create zone 3 conditions two-thirds of the distance from the heart to the apex. However, in patients undergoing positive-pressure mechanical ventilation, alveolar pressure is not atmospheric. Under conditions of positive end-expiratory pressure (PEEP), P_{alv} may be as high as 15–20 cm H_2O. This potentially shifts the entire distribution of pulmonary blood flow. (Reproduced, with permission, from Murray JF: *The Normal Lung*, 2nd ed. Saunders, 1986.)

---

fusion ratios are extremely important and underlie the functional impairment in many disease states. The distribution may favor **high V̇/Q̇ ratios,** with the limiting case being **alveolar dead space** (ventilation without perfusion, or V̇/Q̇ = ∞); or it may favor low V̇/Q̇ ratios, with the limiting case being a **shunt** (perfusion without ventilation, or V̇/Q̇ = 0). These two shifts affect respiratory function differently.

Approximately one-third of resting minute ventilation in normal subjects goes to fill the main conducting airways. This is the **anatomic dead space;** it represents ventilation to areas that do not participate in gas exchange. If gas-exchanging regions of the lung are ventilated but not perfused, as may occur in pulmonary embolism or various forms of pulmonary vascular disease, these regions also fail to function in gas exchange. They are referred to as **alveolar dead space,** or **wasted ventilation** (Figure 9–15, lower panel). Functionally, some percentage of the work of breathing then supports ventilation that does not participate in gas exchange, thus reducing the overall efficiency of ventilation. In the absence of respiratory

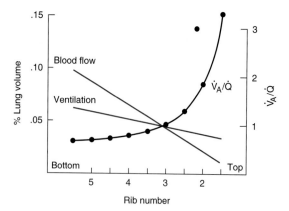

Figure 9–14. Changing distribution of ventilation and perfusion down the upright lung. The two straight lines reflect the progressive increases in ventilation and perfusion. The slope is steeper for perfusion. The ratio of ventilation to perfusion is therefore lowest at the base and highest at the apex. (Reproduced, with permission, from West JB: *Respiratory Physiology: The Essentials,* 4th ed. Williams & Wilkins, 1990.)

compensation, an increase in alveolar dead space will cause disturbances in both arterial PO_2 and arterial PCO_2: PaO_2 will fall and $PaCO_2$ will rise. However, since the respiratory control center is exquisitely sensitive to small changes in $PaCO_2$, the most common response to an increase in wasted ventilation is an increase in total minute ventilation that maintains $PaCO_2$ nearly constant. PaO_2 is normal or may be reduced if the fraction of wasted ventilation is large. The A–a ΔPO_2 is increased (see below).

A shunt occurs when ventilation is eliminated but perfusion continues, as might happen with atelectatic lung or in areas of lung consolidation (alveoli filled with fluid or infected debris) (Figure 9–15, mid panel). Such a right-to-left shunt permits mixed venous blood to pass to the systemic arterial circulation without coming in contact with alveolar gas. This typically causes a fall in *both* PO_2 and PCO_2. The reason can be seen in the diagram: The remaining respiratory unit is overventilated relative to its blood flow (large arrow).

The hyperventilation of some lung regions can compensate for a shunt through other regions but only for a possible rise in PCO_2 and not for the fall in PO_2. The reason is straightforward: The CO_2 content of blood is linearly related and inversely proportionate to alveolar ventilation. Increased ventilation to one respiratory unit can reduce the CO_2 content of blood leaving that unit. The CO_2 content of the mixture is the mean of the two units. Since the PCO_2 is directly proportionate to the CO_2 content, the reduced CO_2 content of the hyperventilated units compensates for lack of ventilation to the dead space.

The O_2 content of blood is not linearly related to

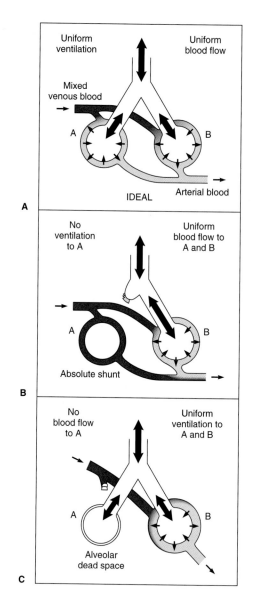

Figure 9–15. Three models of the relationship of ventilation to perfusion. In this schematic representation, the circles represent respiratory units, with tubes depicting the conducting airways. The colored channels represent the pulmonary blood flow, which enters the capillary bed as mixed venous blood (dark) and leaves it as arterialized blood (light). Large arrows show distribution of inspired gas; small arrows show diffusion of O_2 and CO_2. In the idealized case **(A)**, the PO_2 and PCO_2 leaving both units are identical. See text for details. (Reproduced, with permission, from Comroe J: *Physiology of Respiration,* 2nd ed. Year Book, 1974.)

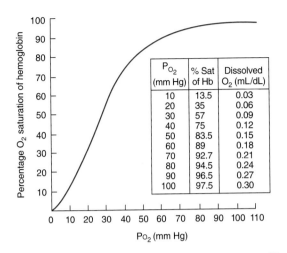

Figure 9–16. Oxygen-hemoglobin dissociation curve. pH 7.40, temperature 38 °C. (Reproduced, with permission, from Comroe JH Jr et al: *The Lung: Clinical Physiology and Pulmonary Function,* 2nd ed. Year Book, 1962.)

alveolar ventilation (Figure 9–16). The sigmoid shape of the hemoglobin-oxygen dissociation curve indicates that blood is nearly maximally saturated with oxygen at basal ventilation. Increasing ventilation to one respiratory unit does not significantly increase the O_2 content of blood leaving that unit. The O_2 content of blood leaving a low $\dot{V}/\dot{Q}$ area is the mean of normal blood oxygen content and desaturated, shunted blood. The reduced oxygen content of the mixture tends to lie on the steep portion of the hemoglobin-oxygen dissociation curve. The result is that modest falls in oxygen content lead to large falls in the P_{O_2}.

Ventilation/perfusion mismatching commonly occurs between the extremes of shunts and wasted ventilation. The effect on arterial blood gases of shifts in the distribution of $\dot{V}/\dot{Q}$ ratios can be predicted from the discussion of the limiting cases (Figure 9–17). At the top of Figure 9–17 is a respiratory unit where on one side (B) ventilation has been reduced but perfusion maintained. This defines an area of **low $\dot{V}/\dot{Q}$ ratio.** The effect on lung function can be understood by dividing it into an area with a normal $\dot{V}/\dot{Q}$ ratio (A) and an area of shunted blood (C). The physiologic effect of low $\dot{V}/\dot{Q}$ areas is similar to the effect of

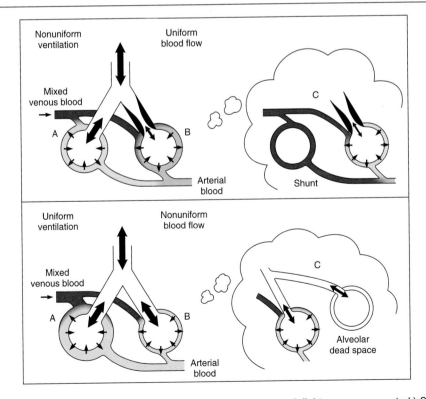

Figure 9–17. Ventilation-perfusion mismatching. (Dark areas, deoxygenated; light areas, oxygenated.) See text for details. (Reproduced, with permission, from Comroe J: *Physiology of Respiration,* 2nd ed. Year Book, 1974.)

shunts: hypoxemia without hypercapnia. The difference between them can also be seen in this schematic. Shunted blood comes into no contact with inspired air; therefore, no amount of additional oxygen supplied to the inspired air will reverse the fall in systemic arterial PO_2. A low $\dot{V}/\dot{Q}$ area does come in contact with inspired air and can be reversed with increased inspired oxygen. A true shunt is the limiting case of a low $\dot{V}/\dot{Q}$ area where the ratio is zero.

At the bottom of Figure 9–17 is a respiratory unit where on one side blood flow has been decreased (B) but ventilation maintained. This defines an area of **high $\dot{V}/\dot{Q}$ ratio.** The effect on lung function can be understood by dividing the unit into an area with a normal $\dot{V}/\dot{Q}$ ratio (A) and (this time) an area of wasted ventilation (C). As expected, the effect of high $\dot{V}/\dot{Q}$ ratios is to increase the amount of ventilation necessary to maintain a normal arterial PCO_2. Since the respiratory control system is very sensitive to small changes in $PaCO_2$ and since the lungs have enormous excess capacity, the physiologic effect of high $\dot{V}/\dot{Q}$ areas is to increase respiration to maintain $PaCO_2$. This may be done unconsciously. It becomes a clinical problem when the subject cannot maintain an increased minute ventilation.

Arterial blood gases detect major disturbances in respiratory function. One attempt to assess more subtle abnormalities of gas exchange is to calculate the difference between the alveolar and arterial PO_2. This is referred to as the A–a ΔPO_2 or **A–a DO_2.** The alveolar-capillary membrane permits full equilibration of alveolar and end capillary oxygen tension under normal $\dot{V}/\dot{Q}$ matching. There is nonetheless a small A–a ΔPO_2 in normal subjects as a result of right-to-left shunting through the bronchial veins and the thebesian veins of the left heart. This accounts for approximately 2% of resting cardiac output and leads to a normal A–a ΔPO_2 of 5–8 mm Hg. Increasing the fractional inspired concentration of oxygen (FIO_2) increases this value: A normal A–a ΔPO_2 breathing 100% oxygen is approximately 100 mm Hg. An increase in the A–a ΔPO_2 reflects areas of low $\dot{V}/\dot{Q}$ ratio, including shunting. It increases with age, presumably as a result of closure of dependent airways with a consequent shift toward low $\dot{V}/\dot{Q}$ ratios.

Control of Breathing

The lungs inflate and deflate passively in response to changes in pleural pressure. Therefore, control over respiration lies in control of the striated muscles—chiefly the diaphragm but also the intercostals and abdominal wall—that change pleural pressure.

These muscles are under both automatic and voluntary control. The rhythm of spontaneous breathing originates in the brainstem, specifically in several groups of interconnected neurons in the medulla. Research into the generation of the respiratory rhythm has identified neurons with at least half a dozen distinct electrical signatures. Respiratory neurons are either inspiratory or expiratory and may fire early, late, or in an accelerating fashion during the respiratory cycle. Their integrated output is an efferent signal via the phrenic nerve (diaphragm) and spinal nerves (intercostals and abdominal wall) to generate rhythmic contraction and relaxation of the respiratory musculature. The result is spontaneous breathing without conscious input. However, by attending to breathing, the reader may hold his or her breath. Eating, speaking, singing, swimming, and defecating all depend on voluntary control over automatic breathing.

A. Sensory Input: The frequency, depth, and timing of spontaneous breathing are modified by information provided to the respiratory center from both chemical and mechanical sensors (Figure 9–18).

There are chemoreceptors in the peripheral vasculature and in the brainstem. The peripheral chemoreceptors are the **carotid bodies,** located at the bifurcation of the common carotid arteries and the aortic bodies near the arch of the aorta. The carotid bodies are particularly important in humans. They function as sensors of arterial oxygenation. There is a graded increase in firing of the carotid body in response to a fall in the PaO_2. This response is most marked below 60 mm Hg. An increase in the $PaCO_2$ or a fall in arterial pH potentiates the response of the carotid body to decreases in the PaO_2.

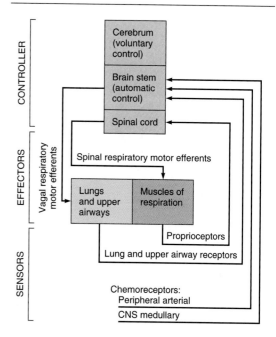

Figure 9–18. Schematic representation of the respiratory control system. The interrelationships among the central nervous system controller, effectors, and sensors are shown, as well as the connections among these components. (Reproduced, with permission, from Berger AJ et al: Regulation of respiration. [Three parts.] N Engl J Med 1977;297:92, 138, 194.)

In humans, the carotid bodies are solely responsible for the increased ventilation seen in response to hypoxia. Bilateral carotid body resection, which has been performed to treat disabling dyspnea and may happen as an unintended consequence of carotid thromboendarterectomy, results in a complete loss of this hypoxic ventilatory drive. The response to an increase in $PaCO_2$ remains intact. Central **chemoreceptors** mediate the response to changes in $PaCO_2$. There is growing evidence that these chemoreceptors are widely dispersed throughout the brainstem. They are separate from the neurons that generate the respiratory rhythm. The increased ventilatory response to elevation in $PaCO_2$ is mediated through changes in chemoreceptor pH. The blood-brain barrier permits free diffusion of CO_2 but not hydrogen ions. CO_2 is hydrated to carbonic acid, which ionizes and lowers brain pH. Central chemoreceptors probably respond to these changes in intracellular hydrogen ion concentration.

There are a variety of pulmonary **stretch receptors** located in airway smooth muscle and mucosa whose afferent fibers are carried in the vagus nerve. They discharge in response to lung distention. Increasing lung volume decreases the rate of respiration by increasing expiratory time. This is known as the Hering-Breuer reflex. There are unmyelinated C fibers located near the pulmonary capillaries (hence juxtacapillary [J] receptors). These fibers are quiet during normal breathing but can be directly stimulated by intravenous administration of irritant chemicals such as capsaicin. They appear to stimulate the increased respiratory drive in interstitial edema and pulmonary fibrosis. Skeletal movement transmitted by **proprioceptors** in joints, muscles, and tendons causes an increase in respiration and may have some role in the increased ventilation of exercise. Finally, there are muscle **spindle receptors** in the diaphragm and intercostals that provide feedback on muscle force. They may be involved in the sensation of dyspnea when the work of breathing is disproportionate to ventilation.

B. Integrated Responses: Under normal conditions in healthy people, the hydrogen ion concentration in the region of the central chemoreceptors determines the drive to breathe. Changes in chemoreceptor pH are largely determined by the $PaCO_2$. The PaO_2 is not an important part of the baseline respiratory drive under normal conditions.

Breathing is stimulated by a fall in the PaO_2, a rise in the $PaCO_2$, or an increase in the hydrogen ion concentration of arterial blood (fall in arterial pH).

Ventilation increases approximately 2–3 L/min for every 1 mm Hg rise in $PaCO_2$. This response (Figure 9–19) occurs first through sensitization of the carotid body receptor. The carotid body will increase its firing in response to an increased $PaCO_2$ even in the absence of changes in the PaO_2. This accounts for approximately 15% of the ventilatory response to hypercapnia. The majority of the response is mediated through pH changes in the region of the central chemoreceptors. Changes in arterial pH are additive to changes in $PaCO_2$. CO_2 response curves under conditions of metabolic acidosis have an identical slope but are shifted to the left. The ventilatory response to an increased $PaCO_2$ falls with age, sleep, and aerobic conditioning and with increased work of breathing.

The individual response to hypoxemia is extremely variable. Normally, there is little increase in ventilation until the PaO_2 falls below 50–60 mm Hg. At this point, there is a rapid increase in ventilation that reaches its maximum at approximately 32 mm Hg. Below this level, further decreases in PaO_2 lead to depression of ventilation. The response to hypoxia is affected by the $PaCO_2$. An increase in the alveolar PCO_2 will shift the isocapnic O_2 response curve upward and to the right (Figure 9–20).

A fall in arterial hydrogen ion concentration in-

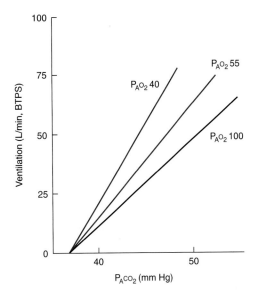

Figure 9–19. Ventilatory response to CO_2. The curves represent changes in minute ventilation plotted against changes in inspired PCO_2 at different values of alveolar PO_2. There is a linear increase in ventilation with increasing PCO_2. The rate of increase is greater at lower PO_2 values, but the curves begin from a common point where ventilation should cease in response to lowered PCO_2. In awake humans, arousal maintains ventilation even when the PCO_2 falls below this level; when lightly anesthetized, apnea does occur. In the case of metabolic acidosis, this x-intercept is shifted to the left but the slope of the lines remains virtually unchanged. This indicates that the effects of metabolic acidosis are separate from and additive to the effects of respiratory acidosis. (BTPS, body temperature and pressure, saturated with water vapor.) (Reproduced, with permission, from Ganong WF: *Review of Medical Physiology,* 19th ed. Appleton & Lange, 1999.)

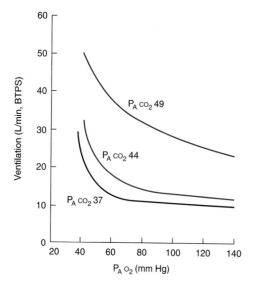

Figure 9–20. Isocapnic ventilatory response to hypoxia. These curves represent changes in minute ventilation plotted against changes in alveolar P_{O_2} when the alveolar P_{CO_2} is held constant at 37, 44, or 49 mm Hg. When the P_{CO_2} is in the normal range (37–44 mm Hg), there is little increase in ventilation until the P_{O_2} is reduced to between 50 and 60 mm Hg. This response is not linear, as is the response to an increased P_{CO_2}, but resembles a rectangular hyperbola asymptotic to infinite ventilation (at a P_{O_2} in the low 30s) and ventilation without tonic stimulation from the carotid bodies (which occurs above a P_{O_2} of 500 mm Hg). Not shown is the fall in minute ventilation that occurs with extreme hypoxia (P_{O_2} values below 30 mm Hg) due to depression of the respiratory center. (Reproduced, with permission, from Ganong WF: *Review of Medical Physiology,* 19th ed. Appleton & Lange, 1999.)

creases minute ventilation. This response results chiefly from stimulation of the carotid bodies and is independent of changes in $PaCO_2$. There is a response to severe metabolic acidosis in the absence of carotid bodies. It is assumed that this response is mediated by central chemoreceptors; it may represent breakdown of the blood-brain barrier.

C. Special Situations:

1. Chronic hypercapnia–In patients with chronic hypercapnia, brain pH is returned toward normal by compensatory changes in bicarbonate levels. This makes the central chemoreceptors less sensitive to further changes in arterial $PaCO_2$. In this instance, a patient's minute ventilation may depend on tonic stimuli from the carotid bodies. If such a patient were given high concentrations of inspired oxygen, it could reduce carotid body output and lead to a fall in minute ventilation. In rare cases, this can be extreme enough to cause a rapid rise in $PaCO_2$ and coma.

2. Chronic hypoxia–Long-term residence at high altitude—or sleep apnea with repeated episodes of severe oxygen desaturation—may blunt the hypoxic ventilatory response. In such patients, the development of lung disease and hypercapnia may remove any endogenous stimulus to breathing. This pattern is seen in patients with obesity-hypoventilation syndrome.

3. Exercise–Exercise may increase minute ventilation up to 25 times the resting level. Strenuous but submaximal exercise in a healthy subject typically causes no change or only a slight rise in PaO_2 due to increased pulmonary blood flow and better matching of ventilation and perfusion, with no change or a slight fall in $PaCO_2$. Changes in arterial oxygenation are therefore not a factor behind the increased ventilatory response to exercise. The reason for the increased ventilatory response is not known with certainty. Two contributing factors are the increased production of carbon dioxide and increased afferent discharge from joint and muscle proprioceptors.

12. What are the components of lung elastic recoil? What is the role of surfactant?
13. What three opposing forces must be overcome normally to inflate the lungs?
14. What are four factors affecting airway resistance?
15. What are the components of the work of breathing?
16. What factors regulate ventilation, and what factors regulate perfusion?
17. How are ventilation and perfusion normally matched?
18. What are the effects of changing CO_2 and O_2 levels on respiratory control?

PATHOPHYSIOLOGY OF SELECTED LUNG DISEASES

OBSTRUCTIVE LUNG DISEASES: ASTHMA & CHRONIC OBSTRUCTIVE PULMONARY DISEASE (COPD)

The fundamental physiologic problem in obstructive diseases is increased resistance to airflow as a result of caliber reduction of conducting airways. This increased resistance can be caused by processes (1) within the lumen, (2) in the airway wall, or (3) in the supporting structures surrounding the airway. Examples of luminal obstruction include the increased secretions seen in asthma and chronic bronchitis. Airway wall thickening and airway narrowing can result from the inflammation seen in both asthma and chronic bronchitis or from the bronchial smooth muscle contraction in asthma. Emphysema is the classic example of obstruction due to loss of surrounding supporting structure, with expiratory airway collapse resulting from the destruction of lung elastic tissue. Though the causes and clinical presentations of these diseases are distinct, the common elements of their physiology are instructive.

1. ASTHMA

Clinical Presentation

Asthma is a disease of airway inflammation and airflow obstruction characterized by the presence of intermittent symptoms, including wheezing, chest tightness, shortness of breath (dyspnea), and cough together with demonstrable bronchial hyperresponsiveness. Exposure to defined allergens or to various nonspecific stimuli initiates a cascade of cellular activation events in the airways, resulting in both acute and chronic inflammatory processes mediated by a complex and integrated assortment of locally released cytokines and other mediators. Release of mediators can alter airway smooth muscle tone and responsiveness, produce mucus hypersecretion, and damage airway epithelium. These pathologic events result in chronically abnormal airway architecture and function.

Inherent in the definition of asthma is the possibility of considerable variation in the magnitude and manifestations of the disease within and between individuals over time. For example, whereas many asthmatic patients have infrequent and mild symptoms, others may have persistent or prolonged symptoms of great severity. Similarly, initiating or exacerbating stimuli may be quite different between individual patients.

Etiology & Epidemiology

Asthma is the most common chronic pulmonary disease, affecting as much as 15–17% of some populations. The highest prevalence rates are reported in Australia and New Zealand; in the USA, the prevalence is 3–5%. Asthma is more common in children and occurs more frequently in boys than in girls. Data pertaining to deaths from asthma are incomplete and somewhat variable but suggest a trend toward an increased mortality rate in recent decades—this in spite of the greater availability of effective pharmacologic treatment. A number of explanations have been offered, including the deleterious side effects of medications and increasing exposure to industrial pollutants.

Atopy, or the production of IgE antibodies in response to exposure to allergens, is common in asthmatics and plays a role in evolution of the disease. Asthma has conventionally been divided into extrinsic and intrinsic asthma depending upon the presence or absence, respectively, of accompanying atopy. There are some characteristic differences between the two groups such as, in intrinsic asthma, the later age at onset, the lack of apparent allergic sensitization by testing, and the tendency toward greater disease severity. However, the two types share the pathologic features of airway inflammation, hyperresponsiveness, and obstruction, so the distinction has not proved useful clinically.

The fundamental abnormality in asthma is increased reactivity of airways to stimuli. As outlined in Table 9–4, there are many known provocative agents for asthma. These can be broadly categorized as (1) physiologic or pharmacologic mediators of asthmatic airway responses, (2) allergens that can induce airway inflammation and reactivity in sensitized individuals, and (3) exogenous physicochemical agents or stimuli that produce airway hyperreactivity. Some of these provocative agents will produce responses in asthmatics only (eg, exercise, adenosine), while others produce characteristically magnified responses in asthmatics that can be used to distinguish them from normals under controlled testing conditions (eg, histamine, methacholine; see below).

Asthmatics typically have early and late responses to provocative stimuli. In the early asthmatic response, there is an onset of airway narrowing within 10–15 minutes following exposure and improvement by 60 minutes. This can sometimes be followed by a late asthmatic response, which appears 4–8 hours following an initial stimulus. Although the mechanisms producing these two responses are different, they are part of a common process of airway inflammation.

Pathogenesis

There is no known single mechanism that serves to explain the occurrence of asthma in all individuals. There are, however, common events that characterize

Table 9–4. Asthma: Provocative factors.

I. Physiologic and pharmacologic mediators of normal smooth muscle contraction
Histamine
Methacholine
Adenosine triphosphate (ATP)
II. Physicochemical agents
Exercise; hyperventilation with cold, dry air
Air pollutants
Sulfur dioxide
Nitrogen dioxide
Viral respiratory infections (eg, influenza A)
Ingestants
Propranolol
Aspirin; NSAIDs
III. Allergens
Low-molecular-weight chemicals, eg, penicillin, isocyanates, anhydrides, chromate
Complex organic molecules, eg, animal danders, dust mites, enzymes, wood dusts

the pathologic processes which produce asthma. It is important to recognize the central role of airway inflammation in the evolution of asthma.

The earliest events in asthmatic airway responses are the activation of local inflammatory cells, principally mast cells and eosinophils. This can occur by specific IgE-dependent mechanisms or indirectly via other processes, eg, osmotic stimuli or chemical irritant exposure. Acute-acting mediators, including leukotrienes, prostaglandins, and histamine, rapidly induce smooth muscle contraction, mucus hypersecretion, and vasodilation with endothelial leakage and local edema formation. Epithelial cells appear also to be involved in this process, releasing leukotrienes and prostaglandins as well as inflammatory cytokines upon activation. Some of these preformed and rapidly acting mediators possess chemotactic activity, recruiting additional inflammatory cells such as eosinophils and neutrophils to airway mucosa.

A critical process that accompanies these acute events is the recruitment, multiplication, and activation of immune inflammatory cells through the actions of a network of locally released cytokines. These cytokines, including (among others) interleukins-2–6, -8, and -10, participate in a complex and prolonged series of events that result in perpetuation of the local airway inflammation and airway hyperresponsiveness (Table 9–5). These events include promoting growth of mast cells and eosinophils, the influx and proliferation of T lymphocytes, and the differentiation of B lymphocytes to IgE- and IgA-producing plasma cells. Thus, through their specific mediators, these cells in turn participate in the many proinflammatory processes that are active in the airways of asthmatics. Among these are injury to epithelial cells and denuding of the airway, greater exposure of afferent sensory nerves, and consequent neurally mediated smooth muscle hyperresponsiveness; the up-regulation of IgE-mediated mast cell and eosinophil activation and mediator release, including acute and long-acting mediators; and submucosal gland hypersecretion with increased mucus volume.

Pathology

The histopathologic features of asthma reflect the cellular processes at play. Airway mucosa is thickened, edematous, and infiltrated with inflammatory cells, principally lymphocytes, eosinophils, and mast cells. Hypertrophied and contracted airway smooth muscle is seen. Bronchial and bronchiolar epithelial cells are frequently damaged, in part by eosinophil products such as major basic protein and eosinophil chemotactic protein, which are cytotoxic for epithelium. Epithelial injury and death leave portions of the airway lumen denuded, exposing autonomic and probably noncholinergic, nonadrenergic afferents that can mediate airway hyperreactivity. Secretory gland hyperplasia and mucus hypersecretion are seen, with mucus plugging of airways a prominent finding in severe asthma. Even in mildly involved asthmatic airways, inflammatory cells are found in increased numbers in the mucosa and submucosa, and subepithelial myofibroblasts are noted to proliferate and produce increased interstitial collagen; this may explain the component of relatively fixed airway obstruction seen in some asthmatics. The pathologic findings seen in severe fatal asthma parallel the pathologic events described above but reflect the greater magnitude of the insult. More severe airway epithelial injury and loss is noted, often with severe and complete obstruction of the airway lumen by mucus plugs.

Pathophysiology

Local cellular events in the airways have important effects on lung function. As a consequence of the airway inflammation, smooth muscle hyperresponsiveness, and airway narrowing, airway resistance increases significantly. Thus, where under normal physiologic circumstances the small-caliber peripheral airways do not contribute significantly to airflow resistance, these airways now are the site of increased resistance. This will be worsened by the superimposed mucus hypersecretion and by any additional bronchoconstrictor stimuli. Bronchial neural function also appears to play a role in the evolution of asthma, though this is probably of secondary importance. Cough and reflex bronchoconstriction mediated by vagal efferents follows stimulation of bronchial irritant receptors. Peptide neurotransmitters may also play a role. The proinflammatory neuropeptide substance P can be released from unmyelinated afferent fibers in the airways and can induce smooth muscle contraction and mediator release from mast cells. Vasoactive intestinal peptide (VIP) is the pep-

Table 9–5. Asthma: Cellular inflammatory events.

I. Epithelial cell activation or injury
  Cytokine (IL-8) release with neutrophil chemotaxis or activation
  Antigen presentation to lymphocytes
  Secretory epithelial cell hyperplasia and hypersecretion
  Epithelial death; increased magnitude of airway sensory neural reflexes
II. Lymphocyte activation
  Antigen exposure with lymphocyte proliferation
  Increased cytokine expression; activation of additional effector cells (mast cells, eosinophils, macrophages)
  Activation of B cells; increased IgE synthesis
  Augmented lymphocyte activation by local cytokines
III. Mast cell and eosinophil activation
  Eosinophil release of cytotoxic and acute proinflammatory mediators
  IgE-mediated mast cell activation, with acute mediator release (eg, histamine, leukotrienes, platelet-activating factor)
  New expression of multiple cytokines by mast cells, with multiple effector cell activation, as with lymphocytes

tide neurotransmitter of some airway nonadrenergic, noncholinergic neurons and functions as a bronchodilator; interruption of its action by cleavage of VIP can promote bronchoconstriction.

Airway obstruction occurs diffusely, though not homogeneously, throughout the lungs. As a result, ventilation of respiratory units becomes nonuniform and the matching of ventilation to perfusion is altered. Areas of both abnormally low and abnormally high $\dot{V}/\dot{Q}$ ratios exist, with the low $\dot{V}/\dot{Q}$ ratio regions contributing to hypoxemia. Pure shunt is unusual in asthma even though mucus plugging is a common finding, particularly in severe, fatal asthma. Arterial CO_2 tension is usually normal to low, given the increased ventilation seen with asthma exacerbations. Hypercapnia is seen as a late and ominous sign, indicating progressive airway obstruction, muscle fatigue, and falling alveolar ventilation.

Clinical Manifestations

The manifestations of asthma are readily explained by the presence of airway inflammation and obstruction.

A. Symptoms and Signs: The variability of symptoms and signs is an indication of the tremendous range of disease severity, from mild and intermittent disease to chronic, severe, and sometimes fatal asthma.

1. Cough–Cough results from the combination of airway narrowing, mucus hypersecretion, and the neural afferent hyperresponsiveness seen with airway inflammation. It can also be a consequence of nonspecific inflammation following superimposed infections, particularly viral, in asthmatic patients. By virtue of the compressive narrowing and high velocity of airflow in central airways, cough provides sufficient shear and propulsive force to clear collected mucus and retained particles from narrowed airways.

2. Wheezing–Smooth muscle contraction, together with mucus hypersecretion and retention, results in airway caliber reduction and prolonged turbulent airflow, producing auscultatory and audible wheezing. The intensity of wheezing does not correlate well with the severity of airway narrowing; as an example, with extreme airway obstruction, airflow may be so reduced that wheezing is barely detectable if at all.

3. Dyspnea and chest tightness–The sensations of dyspnea and chest tightness are the result of a number of concerted physiologic changes. The greater muscular effort required to overcome increased airway resistance is detected by spindle stretch receptors, principally of intercostal muscles and the chest wall. Hyperinflation from airway obstruction results in thoracic distention. Lung compliance falls, and the work of breathing increases, also detected by chest wall sensory nerves and manifested as chest tightness and dyspnea. As obstruction worsens, increased $\dot{V}/\dot{Q}$ mismatching produces hypoxemia. Rising arterial CO_2 tension and, later, evolving arterial hypoxemia (each alone, or together as synergistic stimuli) will stimulate respiratory drive through the peripheral and central chemoreceptors. This stimulus in the setting of respiratory muscle fatigue produces progressive dyspnea.

4. Tachypnea and tachycardia–Tachypnea and tachycardia may be absent in mild disease but are virtually universal in acute exacerbations.

5. Pulsus paradoxus–Pulsus paradoxus is a fall of more than 10 mm Hg in systolic arterial pressure during inspiration. It appears to occur as a consequence of lung hyperinflation, with compromise of left ventricular filling, together with augmented venous return to the right ventricle during more vigorous inspiration in severe obstruction. With increased right ventricular end-diastolic volume during inspiration, the intraventricular septum is moved to the left, compromising left ventricular filling and output. The consequence of this decreased output is a decrease in systolic pressure during inspiration, or pulsus paradoxus.

6. Hypoxemia–The presence of increasing $\dot{V}/\dot{Q}$ mismatching with airway obstruction produces areas of low $\dot{V}/\dot{Q}$ ratios, resulting in hypoxemia. Shunt is unusual in asthma.

7. Hypercapnia and respiratory acidosis–In mild to moderate asthma, ventilation is normal or increased, and the arterial PCO_2 is either normal or decreased. In severe attacks, airway obstruction persists or increases and respiratory muscle fatigue supervenes, with the evolution of alveolar hypoventilation and increasing hypercapnia and respiratory acidosis. It is important to note that this can occur in the face of continued tachypnea, which is not equivalent to alveolar hyperventilation.

8. Obstructive defects by pulmonary function testing–Patients with mild asthma may have entirely normal pulmonary function between exacerbations. During active asthma attacks, all indices of expiratory airflow are reduced, including FEV_1, FEV_1/FVC ($FEV_1\%$); and peak expiratory flow rate (Figure 9–21). FVC is often also reduced as a result of premature airway closure before full expiration. Administration of a bronchodilator results in the improvement of airflow obstruction. As a consequence of the airflow obstruction, incomplete emptying of lung units at end-expiration results in acute and chronic hyperinflation; total lung capacity (TLC), functional residual capacity (FRC), and residual volume (RV) can be increased. Pulmonary diffusing capacity for carbon monoxide (DLCO) is often increased as a consequence of the increased lung (and lung capillary blood) volume.

9. Bronchial hyperresponsiveness–Bronchial provocation testing reveals hyperresponsiveness in all asthmatics, including those with mild disease and normal routine pulmonary function testing. Bronchial hyperresponsiveness is defined as either (1) a 20%

2. CHRONIC OBSTRUCTIVE PULMONARY DISEASE (COPD): CHRONIC BRONCHITIS & EMPHYSEMA

"Chronic obstructive pulmonary disease" is an intentionally imprecise term used to denote a process characterized by the presence of chronic bronchitis or emphysema that may lead to the development of airway obstruction. The obstruction may be partially reversible. Although chronic bronchitis and emphysema are often regarded as independent processes, they share some common etiologic factors and are frequently encountered together in the same patient. It is for the purpose of including both under the same broad category that the definition remains imprecise—it reflects what we currently know about the evolution of these diseases.

Clinical Presentation

A. Chronic Bronchitis: Chronic bronchitis is defined by a clinical history of productive cough for 3 months out of the year for 2 consecutive years. Dyspnea and airway obstruction, often with an element of reversibility, are intermittently to continuously present. Cigarette smoking is by far the leading cause, though other inhaled irritants may produce the same process. The predominant pathologic event is an inflammatory process in the airways, with mucosal thickening and mucus hypersecretion, resulting in diffuse obstruction.

B. Emphysema: Emphysema is properly a pathologic designation that in the lungs denotes a condition of abnormal permanent enlargement of the airspaces distal to the terminal bronchioles, accompanied by destruction of their walls without obvious fibrosis. In contrast to chronic bronchitis, the primary pathologic defect in emphysema is not in the airways but rather in the respiratory unit walls, where the loss of elastic tissue results in a loss of appropriate recoil tension to support airways during expiration. Progressive dyspnea and nonreversible obstruction accompany the airspace destruction without significant productive cough. Furthermore, the loss of alveolar surface area and the accompanying capillary bed for gas exchange contribute to the progressive hypoxia and dyspnea. Pathologic and etiologic distinctions can be made between various patterns of emphysema, but the clinical presentations of all are quite uniform.

Etiology & Epidemiology

Because of the overlap of these two diseases in individuals and the common causes encountered in both, epidemiologic data generally consider both diseases together under the rubric of COPD. COPD affects over 10 million persons in the United States, with chronic bronchitis the diagnosis in approximately 75% of cases and emphysema in the remainder. The incidence, prevalence, and mortality rates of

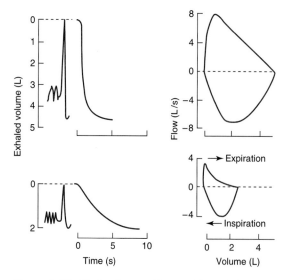

Figure 9–21. Obstructive ventilatory defect. Spirograms and flow-volume curves are shown for a normal patient (top panels) and a patient with an obstructive ventilatory defect (bottom panels). (Modified and reproduced, with permission, from Murray JF, Nadel JA: *Textbook of Respiratory Medicine*, 2nd ed. Saunders, 1994.)

decrease in FEV_1 in response to a provoking factor that, at the same intensity, causes less than a 5% change in a normal subject; or (2) a 20% increase in the FEV_1 in response to an inhaled bronchodilating drug. Methacholine and histamine are the agents for which standardized provocation testing has been established. Other agents have been used to establish specific exposure sensitivities; examples include sulfur dioxide and toluene diisocyanate.

---

19. What is the fundamental physiologic problem in obstructive lung disease? Give an example of each of its three principal sources.
20. What are the pathologic events that contribute to chronically abnormal airway architecture in asthma?
21. What are the three categories of provocative agents that can trigger asthma?
22. Which acute-acting mediators contribute to asthmatic airway responses?
23. What are some histopathologic features of asthma?
24. Name three reasons for increased airway resistance in asthma.
25. Why is arterial P_{CO_2} usually low in asthma exacerbations?
26. What are some of the common symptoms and signs of acute asthma?

COPD increase with age and are higher in men, whites, and persons of lower socioeconomic status. Cigarette smoking remains the principal cause of disease in up to 90% of patients with chronic bronchitis and emphysema. However, only 10–15% of smokers develop COPD. The reasons for differences in disease susceptibility are unknown but may include genetic factors. The most important identified single risk factor for the evolution of COPD—other than cigarette smoking—is deficiency of α_1-protease inhibitor. Its absence can lead to early onset of severe emphysema. **Alpha$_1$-protease inhibitor** is a circulating protein capable of inhibiting several types of proteases, including neutrophil elastase, which is implicated in the genesis of emphysema (see Pathophysiology, below). Autosomal dominant mutations, especially in northern Europeans, produce abnormally low serum and tissue levels of this inhibitor, altering the balance of connective tissue synthesis and proteolysis. A homozygous mutation (the ZZ genotype) results in inhibitor levels 10–15% of normal. The risk of emphysema, particularly in smokers who carry this mutation, is dramatically increased.

Population-based studies suggest that chronic dust (including silica and cotton) or chemical fume exposure can lead to COPD, but the contribution of these factors appears to be minor compared with tobacco use.

A. Chronic Bronchitis: A number of pathologic airway changes are seen in chronic bronchitis, though none are uniquely characteristic of this disease. The clinical features of chronic bronchitis can be attributed to chronic airway injury and narrowing. The principal pathologic features are inflammation of airways—particularly small airways—and hypertrophy of large airway mucous glands, with increased mucus secretion and accompanying mucus obstruction of airways (Figure 9–22). The airway mucosa is variably infiltrated with inflammatory cells, including polymorphonuclear leukocytes and lymphocytes. Mucosal inflammation can substantially narrow the bronchial lumen. As a consequence of the chronic inflammation, the normal ciliated pseudostratified columnar epithelium is frequently replaced by patchy squamous metaplasia. In the absence of normal ciliated bronchial epithelium, mucociliary clearance function is severely diminished or completely abolished. Hypertrophy and hyperplasia of submucosal glands is a prominent feature, with the glands often comprising over 50% of the bronchial wall thickness. Mucus hypersecretion accompanies mucous gland hyperplasia, contributing to luminal narrowing. Bronchial smooth muscle hypertrophy is common, and hyperresponsiveness to nonspecific bronchoconstrictor stimuli (including histamine and methacholine) can be seen. Bronchioles are often infiltrated with inflammatory cells and are distorted, with associated peribronchial fibrosis. Mucus impaction and

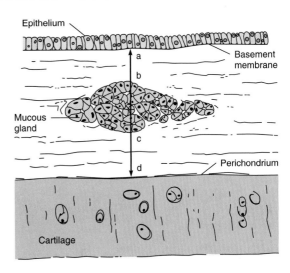

Figure 9–22. Bronchial wall anatomy. Structure of a normal bronchial wall. In chronic bronchitis, the thickness of the mucous glands increases and can be expressed as the ratio of (b–c)/(a–d); this is known as the Reid index. (Reproduced, with permission, from Thurlbeck WM: Chronic airflow obstruction in lung disease. In: *Major Problems in Pathology*. Bennington JL (editor). Saunders, 1976.)

luminal obstruction of smaller airways are often seen. In the absence of any superimposed process, such as pneumonia, the gas-exchanging lung parenchyma, composed of terminal respiratory units, is largely undamaged. The result of these combined changes is chronic airway obstruction and impaired clearance of airway secretions.

The nonuniform airway obstruction of chronic bronchitis has substantial effects on ventilation and gas exchange. Obstruction with prolonged expiratory time produces hyperinflation. Altered ventilation/perfusion relationships include areas of high and low $\dot{V}/\dot{Q}$ ratios. The latter is responsible in large part for the more significant resting hypoxemia seen in chronic bronchitis compared with emphysema. True shunt (perfusion with no ventilation) is unusual in chronic bronchitis.

B. Emphysema: The principal pathologic event in emphysema is thought to be a continuing destructive process due to an imbalance of local oxidant injury and proteolytic (particularly elastolytic) activity due to a deficiency of protease inhibitors (Figure 9–23). Oxidants, whether endogenous (superoxide anion) or exogenous (eg, cigarette smoke), can inhibit the normal protective function of protease inhibitors, allowing progressive tissue destruction.

In contrast to chronic bronchitis, emphysema is a disease not primarily of the airways but of the surrounding lung parenchyma. The physiologic consequences are the result of destruction of terminal res-

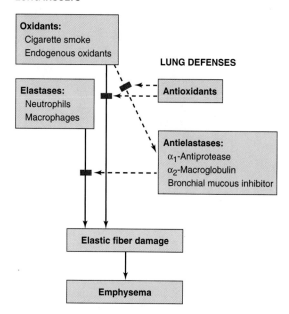

Figure 9–23. Schema of elastase-antielastase hypothesis of emphysema. Activation is represented by solid lines, inhibition by dashed lines. The lung is protected from elastolytic damage by α_1-protease inhibitor and α_2-macroglobulin. Bronchial mucus inhibitor protects the airways. Elastase is derived primarily from neutrophils, but macrophages secrete an elastase-like metalloprotease and may ingest and later release neutrophil elastase. Oxidants derived from neutrophils and macrophages or from cigarette smoke may inactivate α_1-protease inhibitor and may interfere with lung matrix repair. Endogenous antioxidants such as superoxide dismutase, glutathione, and catalase protect the lung against oxidant injury. (Modified and reproduced, with permission, from Snider GL: Experimental studies on emphysema and chronic bronchial injury. Eur J Respir Dis 1986;146[Suppl]:17.)

piratory units and loss of alveolar capillary bed and, very importantly, the supporting structures of the lung, including elastic connective tissue. The loss of elastic connective tissue produces a lung with diminished elastic recoil and increased compliance. In the absence of normal elastic recoil, the normal support of noncartilaginous airways is lost. Premature expiratory collapse of airways ensues, with characteristic obstructive symptoms and physiologic findings.

The pathologic picture of emphysema is one of progressive destruction of terminal respiratory units or lung parenchyma distal to terminal bronchioles. Airway inflammatory changes are minimal if present, though some mucous gland hyperplasia can be seen in large conducting airways. The interstitium of respiratory units harbors some inflammatory cells, but the chief finding is a loss of alveolar walls and enlargement of airspaces. Alveolar capillaries are also lost, which can result in decreased diffusing capacity and progressive hypoxemia, particularly with exercise.

Alveolar destruction is not uniform in all cases of emphysema. Anatomic variants have been described on the basis of the pattern of destruction of the terminal respiratory unit (or acinus, as it is also known). In **centriacinar emphysema,** destruction is focused in the center of the terminal respiratory unit, with the respiratory bronchioles and alveolar ducts relatively spared. This pattern is most frequently associated with prolonged smoking. **Panacinar emphysema** involves destruction of the terminal respiratory unit globally, with diffuse airspace distention. This pattern is typically—though not uniquely—seen in α_1-protease inhibitor deficiency. It is important to note that the distinction between these two patterns is largely pathologic—there is no significant difference in the clinical presentation. An additional emphysema pattern of clinical importance is **bullous emphysema.** Bullae are large confluent airspaces formed by greater local destruction or progressive distention of lung units. They are important because of the compressive effect they can have on surrounding lung and the large physiologic dead space associated with these structures.

Clinical Manifestations

A. Chronic Bronchitis: The clinical manifestations of chronic bronchitis are principally the result of the obstructive and inflammatory airway process.

1. Productive cough–Cough is productive of thick, often purulent sputum owing to the ongoing local inflammation and the high likelihood of bacterial colonization and infection. Sputum viscosity is increased, largely as a result of the presence of free DNA (of high molecular weight and highly viscous) from lysed cells. With increased inflammation and mucosal injury, hemoptysis can occur but is usually scant. The sputum usually does not have a putrid odor, as would be the case with anaerobic infection such as an abscess. Cough, which is very effective in clearing normal airways, is much less effective owing to the narrow airway caliber and the greater volume and viscosity of secretions.

2. Wheezing–Persistent airway narrowing and mucus obstruction can produce localized or more diffuse wheezing. This may be responsive to bronchodilators, representing a reversible component to the obstruction.

3. Inspiratory and expiratory coarse crackles–Increased mucus production, together with defective mucociliary escalator function, leaves excessive secretions in the airways, even with the increased coughing. These are heard prominently in larger airways during tidal breathing or with cough.

4. Cardiac examination–Tachycardia is common, especially with exacerbations of bronchitis or with hypoxemia. If hypoxemia is significant and chronic, pulmonary hypertension can result, with the cardiac examination revealing a prominent pulmonary valve closing sound (P_2) or elevated jugular venous pressure and peripheral edema because of right heart failure.

5. Imaging–Typical chest radiographic findings include increased lung volumes with relatively depressed diaphragms consistent with hyperinflation. Prominent parallel linear densities ("tram track lines") of thickened bronchial walls are common. Cardiac size may be increased, suggesting right heart volume overload. Prominent pulmonary arteries are common and are consistent with pulmonary hypertension.

6. Pulmonary function tests–Diffuse airway obstruction is demonstrated on pulmonary function testing as a global reduction in expiratory flows and volumes. FEV_1, FVC, and the FEV_1/FVC ($FEV_1\%$) ratio are all reduced. The expiratory flow-volume curve shows substantial limitation of flow (Figure 9–21). Some patients may respond to bronchodilators. Measurement of lung volumes reveals an increase in the RV and FRC, reflecting air trapped in the lung as a result of diffuse airway obstruction and early airway closure at higher lung volumes. DLCO is normal, reflecting a preserved alveolar capillary bed.

7. Arterial blood gases–Ventilation/perfusion mismatching is common in chronic bronchitis. The A–a ΔP_{O_2} is increased and hypoxemia is common, due mainly to significant areas of low $\dot{V}/\dot{Q}$ ratios (physiologic shunt); hypoxemia at rest tends to be more profound than in emphysema. With increasing obstruction, increasing P_{CO_2} (hypercapnia) and respiratory acidosis—with compensatory metabolic alkalosis—are seen.

8. Polycythemia–Chronic hypoxemia is associated with a variable erythropoietin-mediated increase in hematocrit. With more severe and prolonged hypoxia, the hematocrit may increase to well over 50%.

B. Emphysema: Emphysema presents as a noninflammatory disease manifested by dyspnea, progressive nonreversible airway obstruction, and abnormalities of gas exchange, particularly with exercise.

1. Breath sounds–Breath sounds in emphysema are typically decreased in intensity, reflecting decreased airflow, prolonged expiratory time, and prominent lung hyperinflation. Wheezes, when present, are of diminished intensity. Airway sounds, including crackles and rhonchi, are unusual in the absence of superimposed processes such as infection.

2. Cardiac examination–Tachycardia may be present as in chronic bronchitis, especially with exacerbations or hypoxemia. Pulmonary hypertension is a common consequence of pulmonary vascular obliteration and concomitant hypoxemia. Cardiac examination may reveal prominent pulmonary valve closure (increased P_2, pulmonary component of the second heart sound) or elevated jugular venous pressure and the peripheral edema due to right heart failure.

3. Imaging–Hyperinflation is common, with flattened hemidiaphragms and an increased anteroposterior chest diameter. Parenchymal destruction produces attenuated lung peripheral vascular markings, often with proximal pulmonary artery dilation due to secondary pulmonary hypertension. Cystic or bullous changes may also be seen.

4. Pulmonary function tests–Lung parenchymal destruction and the loss of lung elastic recoil are the fundamental causes of the observed abnormalities of pulmonary function. The loss of elastic recoil in lung tissue supporting the airways results in increased dynamic compression of airways (Figure 9–10), especially during forced expiration; all flow rates are reduced. With premature airway collapse, FEV_1, FVC, and the FEV_1/FVC ($FEV_1\%$ ratio) are all reduced. As with chronic bronchitis and asthma, the expiratory flow-volume curve shows substantial limitation in flow (Figure 9–21). Expiratory time prolongation, early airway closure due to loss of elastic recoil, and consequent air trapping produce increases in the RV and FRC. TLC is increased, though often a substantial amount of this increase comes from gas trapped in poorly or noncommunicating lung units, including bullae. The D_LCO is generally decreased in proportion to the extent of emphysema, reflecting the progressive loss of alveoli and their capillary beds. Incomplete hemoglobin saturation of pulmonary venous blood and arterial hypoxemia result from a combination of $\dot{V}/\dot{Q}$ mismatch, inability to increase minute ventilation with a fall in mixed venous P_{O_2}, and failure to oxygenate blood fully during capillary transit.

5. Arterial blood gases–Mild hypoxemia without hypercapnia is common in early emphysema. The A–a ΔP_{O_2} is increased; significant areas of abnormally low and high $\dot{V}/\dot{Q}$ ratios are found. With greater disease severity and greater decrease in DLCO, exercise-related (and, ultimately, even resting) arterial hemoglobin desaturation is seen. Hypercapnia, respiratory acidosis, and a compensatory metabolic alkalosis are common in severe disease.

6. Polycythemia–As in chronic bronchitis, chronic hypoxemia is frequently associated with an elevated hematocrit.

---

27. What is the leading cause of chronic bronchitis?
28. Describe the pathophysiologic changes in emphysema versus chronic bronchitis.
29. Mutations of which protein are strongly correlated with an increased risk of emphysema?
30. Name eight symptoms and signs of chronic bronchitis.
31. Name six symptoms and signs of emphysema.

RESTRICTIVE LUNG DISEASE: IDIOPATHIC PULMONARY FIBROSIS

The term "interstitial lung disease" is used to denote a broad collection of pulmonary processes, some of unknown cause, whose common feature is the infiltration or inflammation and scarring of lung parenchyma (Figure 9-24). The common consequence of these diverse pathologic processes is widespread lung fibrosis, producing increased lung elastic recoil and decreased lung compliance which we know as restrictive lung disease.

The modifier "interstitial" is an inadequate characterization of the process. Lung interstitium is considered to be the anatomic space bounded by the basement membranes of epithelium and endothelium and normally contains mesenchymal cells (eg, fibroblasts), extracellular matrix molecules (eg, collagen, elastin, and proteoglycans), and a few tissue leukocytes, including mast cells and lymphocytes. Interstitial lung diseases are not typically restricted to the anatomic interstitium but also involve inflammation of conducting airway mucosa and alveolar epithelium with an influx of recruited inflammatory cells. As a consequence, fibrosis is generally present throughout the lung parenchyma, with global effects on lung structure and function.

The pathologic events and physiologic consequences seen in idiopathic pulmonary fibrosis are shared by most of the other causes of interstitial lung disease. For that reason, idiopathic pulmonary fibrosis will be discussed as an example.

Clinical Presentation

Idiopathic pulmonary fibrosis, also known as interstitial pulmonary fibrosis or cryptogenic fibrosing alveolitis, is an uncommon disease of unknown cause marked by chronic inflammation of alveolar walls and resulting in diffuse and progressive severe fibrosis and destruction of normal lung architecture. This process produces not only a restrictive defect, with altered ventilation and increased work of breathing, but destructive and obliterative vascular injury that can severely impair normal pulmonary perfusion and gas exchange.

The usual presentation of idiopathic pulmonary fibrosis is with the insidious onset of progressive dyspnea, generally accompanied by a dry and persistent hacking cough. Fever and chest pain are generally absent. With disease progression, dyspnea often worsens and occurs even at rest. Digital cyanosis and clubbing are commonly seen. In the later stages of the disease, increasing pulmonary hypertension can lead to right heart failure and peripheral edema.

Etiology & Epidemiology

Idiopathic pulmonary fibrosis typically presents in the fifth to seventh decades of life, with a slight male predominance. There is no known causative agent. Many environmental exposures and specific systemic diseases can produce a clinical pattern similar if not identical to that seen in idiopathic pulmonary fibrosis. It is important to consider alternative causes when evaluating a patient with interstitial lung disease, as this may alter the evaluation or the treatment options. A familial form of interstitial pulmonary fibrosis has been described but is uncommon; typical cases do not appear to have a genetic basis.

Pathophysiology

The primary insult that leads to the fibrotic response is unknown. Even in interstitial diseases of known cause, such as hypersensitivity lung disease or asbestosis, the specific events in disease initiation

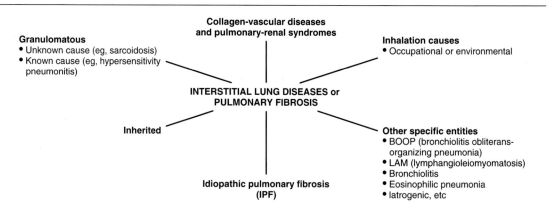

Figure 9–24. Categories of interstitial lung disease. In the absence of underlying malignancy or history of chemical or radiation therapy, interstitial lung disease can be broadly grouped into the clinical categories shown. Idiopathic pulmonary fibrosis occurs in a majority of these patients. (Reproduced, with permission, from Raghu G, Hert R: Interstitial lung diseases: Genetic predisposition and inherited interstitial lung diseases. Semin Respir Med 1993;14:323.)

Table 9–6. Cellular events involved in lung injury and fibrosis.

1. Tissue injury
2. Vascular endothelium activation and permeability changes, with thrombosis and thrombolysis
3. Epithelial injury and activation
4. Leukocyte influx, activation, and proliferation
5. Further tissue injury, remodeling, and fibrosis:
    Perpetuation of tissue inflammation
    Incomplete or delayed resolution of interstitial thrombosis
    Fibroblast proliferation and matrix molecule production or deposition
    Epithelial proliferation and repopulation

are not clearly established. There is, however, a common series of cellular events that mediate and regulate the inflammatory process and fibrotic response in idiopathic pulmonary fibrosis as well as in other interstitial lung diseases. This set of events, outlined in Table 9–6, includes (1) initial tissue injury; (2) vascular injury and activation, with increased permeability, exudation of plasma proteins into the extravascular space, and variable thrombosis and thrombolysis; (3) epithelial injury and activation, with loss of barrier integrity and release of proinflammatory mediators; (4) increased leukocyte adherence to activated endothelium, with transit of activated leukocytes into the interstitium; and (5) continued injury and repair processes characterized by alterations in cell populations and increased matrix production.

An extensive and complex array of effector and target cells and their specific products are thought to mediate the inflammatory and fibrotic events in idiopathic pulmonary fibrosis. A summary of the events is appropriate.

The initial pathophysiologic event in idiopathic pulmonary fibrosis is injury and activation of alveolar epithelium and endothelium. Type I epithelial cells are lost and replaced by proliferating type II cells. Airway epithelial cells participate in cytokine-mediated recruitment and activation of inflammatory cells, including neutrophils and lymphocytes. Recruitment and activation of both neutrophils and lymphocytes are also mediated by the injury and activation of vascular endothelium; this occurs through the coordinated action of multiple cytokines and the display of a specific repertoire of cellular adhesion molecules both on endothelial cells and on specific leukocytes. Fibroblasts are also activated by these local proinflammatory cytokines, with proliferation in the interstitium, submucosa, and alveolar lumen. Fibroblasts serve a dual role, magnifying local inflammatory events through their release of cytokines while producing the matrix molecules, including collagen, involved in tissue fibrosis. The perpetuation of this pattern of fibroblast activation and proliferation—and increased tissue matrix deposition—occurs under the influence of inflammatory cells. These include not only lymphocytes, alveolar macrophages, and neutrophils but also resident mast cells and eosinophils which are variably increased in number.

The histologic findings predict the physiologic abnormalities associated with interstitial lung disease. The process of lung injury and scarring is not uniform or synchronous. The disease is typically a nonhomogeneous process, with areas of intense injury and fibrosis often intermixed with relatively spared lung. In the early stages of disease, infiltration of alveolar structures by leukocytes accompanies patchy type II epithelial hyperplasia in alveoli. Destruction of normal alveolar epithelium also causes significant change in the production and turnover of surfactant, with an increase in the alveolar surface tension in affected lung units. This is followed by increasing tissue leukocytosis, fibroblast proliferation, and increasing scar formation. Lymphocytes—predominantly T cells—and mast cells are found in markedly increased numbers in alveolar interstitium and submucosal regions. Collagen and elastin deposition are markedly increased. Later in the course of the disease, progressive alveolar destruction is seen, with large areas of fibrosis and residual airspaces lined by cuboidal epithelium; this appears on radiographs as honeycombing. With this alveolar destruction, the accompanying vascular bed is obliterated, also in a patchy pattern.

This pattern of lung injury produces an altered physiology that includes increased elastic recoil and poor lung compliance, altered gas exchange, and pulmonary vascular abnormalities.

Clinical Manifestations
A. Symptoms and Signs:

1. Cough–With the bronchial and bronchiolar distortion that accompanies fibrotic damage to terminal respiratory units, chronic irritation of airways occurs, producing a chronic cough. Although epithelial cells may be injured, mucus hypersecretion and a productive cough are not seen.

2. Dyspnea and tachypnea–Multiple factors contribute to dyspnea in pulmonary fibrosis. With fibrosis of lung parenchyma as well as a decrease in normal surfactant effects, a greater distending pressure is required for inspiration. Increased stimuli from C fibers in fibrotic alveolar walls or stretch receptors in the chest wall may sense the increased force necessary to inflate the less compliant lungs. In severe disease, altered gas exchange with $\dot{V}/\dot{Q}$ mismatching can produce hypoxia even at rest. The diminished capillary bed and thickened alveolar-capillary membrane contribute to limitation of diffusion and increasing hypoxia with exercise. Tachypnea is the consequence of hypoxia and the apparent increased drive from lung sensory receptor stimuli. A rapid and shallow breathing pattern reduces ventilatory work in the face of increased lung elastic recoil.

3. Inspiratory crackles–Diffuse fine dry inspiratory crackles are common and reflect the successive opening on inspiration of respiratory units that are collapsed owing to the fibrosis and the loss of normal surfactant.

4. Digital clubbing–Clubbing of the fingers and toes is a common finding, but the cause is unknown. There is no established link with any specific physiologic variable, including hypoxemia.

5. Cardiac examination–As with hypoxemia from other causes, cardiac examination can reveal evidence of pulmonary hypertension with prominent pulmonary valve closure sound (P_2). This can be accompanied by right heart overload or decompensation, with elevated jugular venous pressure, the murmur of tricuspid regurgitation, or a right-sided third heart sound (S_3).

B. Imaging: The characteristic radiographic findings are of small lung volumes, with increased densities more prominent in the lung periphery. Fibrosis surrounding expanded small airspaces is seen as honeycombing. With pulmonary hypertension, central pulmonary arteries are enlarged, while the peripheral vascular destruction produces rapid attenuation of vessels out from the hilar regions.

C. Pulmonary Function Tests: Lung fibrosis typically produces a restrictive pattern, with reductions in TLC, FEV_1, and FVC, while maintaining a preserved or even increased ratio of FEV_1/FVC ($FEV_1\%$) (Figure 9–25). The increased elastic recoil produces normal to increased expiratory flow rates when adjusted for lung volume. With increased recoil pressure on airways, the traction maintains normal to increased airway caliber, with consequent decrease in resistance. The D_{LCO} in lung fibrosis is progressively reduced as a function of the fibrotic obliteration of lung capillaries.

D. Arterial Blood Gases: Hypoxemia is common in pulmonary fibrosis and results from an increased physiologic dead space and relatively fixed minute ventilation. This leads to an increase in both high and low $\dot{V}/\dot{Q}$ areas. Diffusion impairment worsens with the severity of fibrosis; this is a common and significant contributor to exercise-induced desaturation but less frequently causes resting hypoxia except in severe disease (Figure 9–26). The increased cardiac output during exercise reduces the transit time for blood through alveolar capillary beds, increasing the limitation in oxygen loading of hemoglobin. Arterial P_{CO_2} is also reduced as a consequence of increased ventilation under the stimuli of hypoxia and lung fibrosis. Only in the later stages of disease or during exercise, when the increased lung elastic recoil and work of breathing prevent appropriate ventilation, does the $PaCO_2$ rise above normal. Hypercapnia is a grave sign, implying an inability to maintain adequate alveolar ventilation due to elevated V_D/V_T or excess work of breathing.

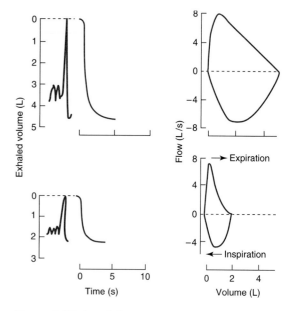

Figure 9–25. Restrictive ventilatory defect. Spirograms and flow-volume curves are shown for a normal patient (top panels) and a patient with a restrictive ventilatory defect (bottom panels). Compare with Figure 9–21. (Modified and reproduced, with permission, from Murray JF, Nadel JA: *Textbook of Respiratory Medicine,* 2nd ed. Saunders, 1994.)

---

32. How does interstitial lung disease affect lung function?
33. Name five events in the pathophysiology of idiopathic pulmonary fibrosis.
34. Name eight symptoms and signs of idiopathic pulmonary fibrosis.

PULMONARY EDEMA

Clinical Presentation

Pulmonary edema is the accumulation of excess fluid in the extravascular space of the lungs. This accumulation may occur slowly, as in a patient with occult renal failure, or with dramatic suddenness, as in a patient with left ventricular failure following an acute myocardial infarction. Pulmonary edema most commonly presents with dyspnea. Dyspnea is breathing perceived by a patient as both uncomfortable or anxiety-provoking and disproportionate to the preceding level of activity. The patient at first notices dyspnea only with exertion but may progress to ex-

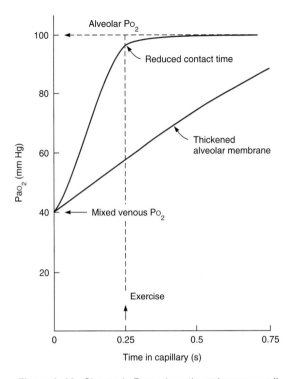

Figure 9–26. Change in PaO_2 along the pulmonary capillary. The typical transit time at rest for an erythrocyte through an alveolar capillary is 0.75 s. In the normal lung, the partial pressure difference and rate of diffusion of O_2 across the alveolar-capillary barrier assure complete saturation of hemoglobin in 0.25 s. Thus, even with the shorter capillary transit time of exercise, the normal lung allows for essentially complete saturation of hemoglobin in the alveolar capillary. If the alveolar-capillary barrier is thickened, as is the case in lung fibrosis, diffusion rates are diminished and alveolar-capillary blood may not be fully saturated with O_2 even at rest. Obviously, greater desaturation of arterial blood can occur with progressive exercise. (Reproduced, with permission, from West JB: *Pulmonary Pathophysiology: The Essentials.* Williams & Wilkins, 1992.)

perience dyspnea at rest. In severe cases, pulmonary edema may be accompanied by edema fluid in the sputum and cause acute respiratory failure.

Etiology

Pulmonary edema is a common problem associated with a variety of medical conditions (Table 9–7). In light of these multiple causes, it is helpful to think about pulmonary edema in terms of underlying physiologic principles.

Pathophysiology

All blood vessels leak. In the adult human, leakage from the pulmonary circulation represents less than 0.01% of pulmonary blood flow, or a baseline filtration of approximately 10–20 mL/h. Two-thirds of this flow occurs across the pulmonary capillary endothelium into the pericapillary interstitial space (Figure 9–27). This is one of two extravascular spaces in the lung—the interstitial space and the airspaces—which contain the alveoli and connecting airways. These two spaces are protected by different barriers. The pulmonary capillary endothelium limits extravasation into the interstitial space while the alveolar epithelium lines the airspaces and protects them against the free movement of fluid. Edema fluid does not readily enter the alveolar space because the alveolar epithelium is nearly impermeable to the passage of protein. This protein barrier creates a powerful osmotic gradient that favors accumulation of fluid in the interstitium.

The amount of fluid that crosses the pulmonary capillary endothelium is determined by the surface area of the capillary bed, the permeability of the vessel wall, and the net pressure driving it across that wall (transmural or driving pressure). The transmural pressure represents the balance between the net hydrostatic forces that tend to move fluid out of the

Table 9–7. Causes of pulmonary edema.

Increased pulmonary capillary transmural pressure
  Increased left atrial pressure
    Left ventricular failure, acute or chronic
    Mitral valve stenosis
  Pulmonary venous hypertension
    Pulmonary veno-occlusive disease
  Increased capillary blood volume
    Iatrogenic volume expansion
    Chronic renal failure
  Reduction of interstitial pressure
    Rapid reexpansion of collapsed lung
  Decreased plasma colloid osmotic pressure
    Hypoalbuminemia: nephrotic syndrome, hepatic failure
Increased pulmonary capillary endothelial permeability
  Circulating toxins: bacteremia, acute pancreatitis
  Infectious pneumonia
  Disseminated intravascular coagulation
  Nonthoracic trauma accompanied by hypotension ("shock lung")
  High-altitude pulmonary edema
  Following cardiopulmonary bypass
Increased alveolar epithelial permeability
  Inhaled toxins: oxygen, phosgene, chlorine, smoke
  Aspiration of acidic gastric contents
  Drowning and near-drowning
  Depletion of surfactant through high tidal volume positive-pressure mechanical ventilation
Reduced lymphatic clearance
  Lung resection (lobectomy) with regional lymph node sampling
  Lymphangitic spread of carcinoma
  Following lung transplant
Mechanism uncertain
  Neurogenic pulmonary edema
  Narcotic overdose
  Multiple transfusions

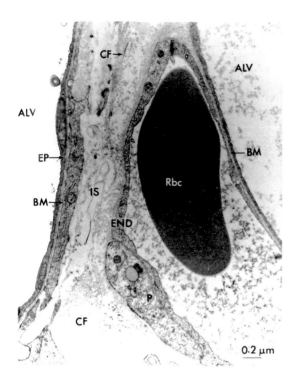

Figure 9–27. Interstitial pulmonary edema. Electron micrograph showing the alveolar septum and a pulmonary capillary in cross section. On the right, the basement membrane of the alveolar epithelium and the capillary endothelium are fused. This barrier is therefore thin (0.2 μm), which optimizes gas exchange and inhibits accumulation of edema fluid. On the other side, the interstitial space contains connective tissue that is in continuity with the loose connective tissue of the perivascular and peribronchial interstitium. Edema fluid first accumulates in this pericapillary space. The continuity of the interstitial spaces provides a pathway for movement of edema fluid centrally away from areas of gas exchange. (ALV, alveolus; EP, epithelial cell; BM, basement membrane; IS, interstitial space; Rbc, red blood cell; CF, pericapillary fluid; END, endothelial cell.) (Reproduced, with permission, from Fishman AP: Pulmonary edema. Circulation 1972; 46:390.)

capillary and the net colloid osmotic forces that tend to keep it in. An imbalance in one or more of these four factors—capillary endothelial permeability, alveolar epithelial permeability, hydrostatic pressure, and colloid osmotic pressure—lies behind nearly all clinical presentations of pulmonary edema.

In the shorthand of clinical practice, these four factors are grouped into two types of pulmonary edema: cardiogenic, referring to edema resulting from a net increase in transmural pressure (hydrostatic or osmotic); and noncardiogenic, referring to edema resulting from increased permeability. The former is primarily a mechanical process, the latter primarily an inflammatory one. However, these two types of pulmonary edema are not exclusive but closely linked: Pulmonary edema occurs when the transmural pressure is excessive for a given capillary permeability. For instance, in the presence of damaged capillary endothelium, small increases in otherwise normal transmural pressure may cause large increases in edema formation. Similarly, if the alveolar epithelial barrier is damaged, even the baseline filtration across an intact endothelium may cause alveolar flooding.

Several mechanisms aid in the clearance of ultrafiltrate and protect against its accumulation as pulmonary edema. Although there are no lymphatics in the alveolar septa, there are "juxta-alveolar" lymphatics in the pericapillary space that normally clear all the ultrafiltrate. The pericapillary interstitium is contiguous with the perivascular and peribronchial interstitium. The interstitial pressure there is negative relative to the pericapillary interstitium, so edema fluid tracks centrally, away from the airspaces. In effect, the perivascular and peribronchiolar interstitium acts as a sump for edema fluid. It can accommodate approximately 500 mL with only a small rise in interstitial hydrostatic pressure. Since this edema fluid is protein-depleted relative to blood, there is an osmotic balance that favors resorption from the interstitium into the bloodstream. This is the major source of resorption of fluid from these collection areas. The perivascular and peribronchiolar interstitium is also contiguous with the interlobular septa and the visceral pleura. In the event of pulmonary edema, there is increased interstitial flow into the pleural space where parietal pleural lymphatics are very efficient at clearance. Pleural effusions seen in patients with increased pulmonary venous pressure represent another reservoir for edema fluid, one that may compromise respiratory function less than would having the same fluid in the lung parenchyma. Finally, there is evidence that edema fluid may track along the interstitium into the mediastinum and be taken up by lymphatics there.

At some undefined critical level after the perivascular and peribronchiolar interstitium have been filled, increased interstitial hydrostatic pressure causes edema fluid to enter the alveolar space (Figure 9–28). The pathway into the alveolar space remains unknown.

In the case of cardiogenic pulmonary edema, increased transmural pressure may result from increased pulmonary venous pressure (causing increased capillary hydrostatic pressure), increased alveolar surface tension (thereby lowering interstitial hydrostatic pressure), or decreased capillary colloid osmotic pressure. When the rate of ultrafiltration rises beyond the capacity of the pericapillary lymphatics to remove it, interstitial fluid accumulates. If the rate of formation continues to exceed lymphatic clearance, alveolar flooding results. Since it is an ultrafiltrate of plasma,

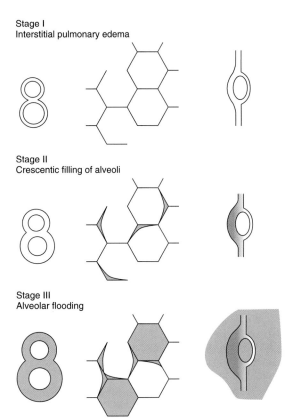

Figure 9–28. Stages in the accumulation of pulmonary edema fluid. The three columns represent three anatomic views of the progressive accumulation of pulmonary edema fluid. From left to right, the columns represent a cross section of the bronchovascular bundle showing the loose connective tissue surrounding the pulmonary artery and bronchial wall, a cross section of alveoli fixed in inflation, and the pulmonary capillary in cross section.

The first stage is eccentric accumulation of fluid in the pericapillary interstitial space. The limitation of edema fluid to one side of the pulmonary capillary maintains gas transfer better than symmetric accumulation. When formation of edema fluid exceeds lymphatic removal, it distends the peribronchovascular interstitium. At this stage, there is no alveolar flooding but there is some crescentic filling of alveoli. The third stage is alveolar flooding. Note that each individual alveolus is either totally flooded or has minimal crescentic filling. This pattern probably occurs because alveolar edema interferes with surfactant and, above some threshold, there is an increase in surface forces that greatly increases the transmural pressure and causes flooding. (Modified and reproduced, with permission, from Nunn JF: *Nunn's Applied Respiratory Physiology,* 4th ed. Butterworth-Heinemann, 1993.)

the edema fluid of cardiogenic pulmonary edema initially has a low protein content, generally less than 60% of the patient's plasma protein content.

Noncardiogenic (increased permeability) pulmonary edema is sometimes referred to clinically as acute (formerly "adult") respiratory distress syndrome (ARDS). Alveolar fluid accumulates as a result of loss of integrity of the alveolar epithelium, allowing solutes and large molecules such as albumin to enter the alveolar space. These changes may result from direct injury to the alveolar epithelium by inhaled toxins or pulmonary infection, or they may occur after primary injury to the capillary endothelium by circulating toxins. This is in contrast to cardiogenic pulmonary edema, in which both the alveolar epithelium and the capillary endothelium are usually intact. Owing to the disrupted epithelial barrier, edema fluid in increased permeability edema has a high protein content, generally more than 70% of the plasma protein content. The list of potential causes of injury is broad and associated with a diverse group of clinical entities (Table 9–7). The reason so many different problems are grouped together in this syndrome is that they share injury to the alveolar epithelium and damage to pulmonary surfactant, which results in characteristic changes in pulmonary mechanics and function.

With inhalation injury, like that produced by mustard gas during World War I, there is direct chemical injury to the alveolar epithelium that disrupts this normally tight cellular barrier. The presence of high-protein fluid in the alveolus—particularly the presence of fibrinogen and fibrin degradation products—inactivates pulmonary surfactant, causing large increases in surface tension. This results in a fall in pulmonary compliance and alveolar instability, leading to areas of atelectasis. Increased surface tension decreases the interstitial hydrostatic pressure and favors further fluid movement into the alveolus. A damaged surfactant monolayer may increase susceptibility to infection.

Circulating factors may act directly on the capillary endothelium or may affect it through various immunologic mediators. A common instance is gram-negative bacteremia. Bacterial endotoxin does not cause endothelial damage directly; it causes neutrophils and macrophages to adhere to endothelial surfaces and release a variety of inflammatory mediators such as leukotrienes, thromboxanes, and prostaglandins as well as oxygen radicals that cause oxidant injury. Both macrophages and neutrophils may release proteolytic enzymes that cause further damage. Alveolar macrophages may also be stimulated. Vasoactive substances may cause intense pulmonary vasoconstriction, leading to capillary failure.

The pathology of increased permeability pulmonary edema reflects these changes. The lungs appear grossly edematous and heavy. The surface appears violaceous, and hemorrhagic fluid exudes from the cut pleural surface. Microscopically, there is cellular infiltration of the interalveolar septa and the interstitium by inflammatory cells and erythrocytes. Type I pneumocytes are damaged, leaving a denuded alveolar barrier. Hyaline membranes form in the absence of alveolar epithelium. These are sheets of pink proteinaceous material composed of plasma proteins, fibrin, and coagulated cell debris. Fibrosis occurs in some cases. Complete recovery with regeneration from the type II pneumocytes of the alveolar epithelium may occur.

Clinical Manifestations

Cardiogenic and noncardiogenic pulmonary edema both result in increased extravascular lung water, and both may result in respiratory failure. Given the differences in pathophysiology, it is not surprising that the clinical manifestations are very different in the two syndromes.

A. Increased Transmural Pressure Pulmonary Edema (Cardiogenic Pulmonary Edema): Early increases in pulmonary venous pressure may be asymptomatic. The patient may notice only mild exertional dyspnea or a nonproductive cough stimulated by activation of irritant receptors coupled with C fibers. Orthopnea and paroxysmal nocturnal dyspnea both occur when recumbency causes redistribution of blood or edema fluid, respectively, pooled in the lower extremities, thereby increasing thoracic blood volume and pulmonary venous pressures.

Clinical signs begin with the accumulation of interstitial fluid. Physical examination may reveal a third heart sound, but there is a paucity of lung findings in purely interstitial edema. The earliest sign is frequently a chest radiograph showing an increase in the caliber of the upper lobe vessels ("pulmonary vascular redistribution") and fluid accumulating in the perivascular and peribronchial spaces ("cuffing"). It may also show Kerley B lines, which represent fluid in the interlobular septa. Pulmonary compliance falls, and the patient begins to breathe more rapidly and shallowly in order to minimize the increased elastic work of breathing. As alveolar flooding begins, there are further decreases in lung volume and pulmonary compliance. With some alveoli filled with fluid, there is an increase in the fraction of the lung that is perfused but poorly ventilated. This shift toward low $\dot{V}/\dot{Q}$ ratios causes an increase in A–a ΔP_{O_2}, if not frank hypoxemia. Supplemental oxygen corrects the hypoxemia. The Pa_{CO_2} is normal or low, reflecting the increased drive to breathe. The patient may become sweaty and cyanotic. The sputum may show edema fluid that is pink from capillary hemorrhage and frothy due to protein. Auscultation reveals inspiratory crackles—chiefly at the bases, where the hydrostatic pressure is greatest, but potentially throughout both lungs. Rhonchi and wheezing ("cardiac asthma") may occur. The radiograph shows areas of alveolar flooding.

B. Increased Permeability Pulmonary Edema (Noncardiogenic Pulmonary Edema): The most common form of increased-permeability pulmonary edema is the acute respiratory distress syndrome (ARDS). ARDS is generally a consequence of a separate serious medical condition. The range of clinical presentations includes all the diagnoses in the adult intensive care unit. Nevertheless, there are clinical observations that mirror the pathophysiology.

After the initial insult—eg, an episode of high-grade bacteremia—there is generally a period of stability, reflecting the time it takes for various immunologic mediators to wreak their havoc. Surfactant is inactivated, leading to a significant increase in surface forces and markedly reduced pulmonary compliance. For the first 24–48 hours after the insult, the patient may experience increased work of breathing, manifested by dyspnea and tachypnea but without abnormalities in the chest radiograph. At this early stage, the increased A–a ΔP_{O_2} reflects alveolar edema and $\dot{V}/\dot{Q}$ mismatching and is corrected by increased FI_{O_2} and increased minute ventilation. Pathologically, there is alveolar edema, hemorrhage, and atelectasis. The clinical picture may improve, or there may be a further fall in compliance and disruption of pulmonary capillaries leading to areas of true shunting and refractory hypoxemia. The combination of greatly increased work of breathing and severe hypoxemia generally mandates mechanical ventilation. However, the stiffness of the lungs increases nonhomogeneous ventilation, and there is a gross increase in ventilation of poorly perfused areas. The high pressures needed to ventilate these patients may overdistend normal alveoli and reduce blood flow to areas of adequate ventilation. Hypoxemia is profound, and hypercapnia may ensue. Radiographically, there is "whiteout" of the lungs that represents diffuse confluent alveolar filling. Pathologically, there is an increase in inflammatory cells and the formation of hyaline membranes. The mortality rate averages 40–50%. Most patients die from some complication of their presenting illness. Of those who survive, many will recover nearly normal lung function, but a significant number will develop new reactive airway disease or pulmonary fibrosis.

35. What four factors are involved in the production of pulmonary edema? How are they affected in cardiogenic versus noncardiogenic causes of pulmonary edema?
36. What are the common causes of noncardiogenic pulmonary edema?
37. Is lung damage from increased permeability pulmonary edema reversible? If so, how?
38. What are the two major reasons that mechanical ventilation is often required in severe pulmonary edema?

Table 9–8. Types of pulmonary emboli.

Material	Clinical Setting
Air	Cardiac surgery, neurosurgery, improper manipulation of central venous catheters
Amniotic fluid	Active labor
Fat	Long bone fracture, liposuction
Foreign body	Pieces of intravenous devices, talc
Oil	Lymphangiography
Parasite eggs	Schistosomiasis
Septic emboli	Endocarditis, thrombophlebitis
Thrombus	Deep venous thrombosis
Tumor	Renal cell carcinoma with invasion of vena cava

PULMONARY EMBOLISM

Clinical Presentation

The English word "embolus" derives from a Greek word meaning "plug" or "stopper." A pulmonary embolus consists of material that gains access to the venous system and then to the pulmonary circulation. Eventually, it reaches a vessel whose caliber is too small to permit free passage, and there it forms a plug, occluding the lumen and obstructing perfusion. There are many types of pulmonary embolization. The most common is pulmonary thromboembolism, which occurs when venous thrombi, chiefly from the lower extremities, migrate to the pulmonary circulation (Table 9–8).

It is a normal function of the pulmonary microcirculation to remove venous emboli. The lungs possess both excess functional capacity and a redundant vascular supply, making them a superb filter for preventing small thrombi and platelet aggregates from gaining access to the systemic circulation. However, large thromboemboli—or an accumulation of smaller ones—can cause substantial impairment of cardiac and respiratory function, and death.

Pulmonary thromboemboli are quite common and cause significant morbidity. They are found at autopsy in 25–50% of hospitalized patients and are considered a major contributing cause of death in a third of those. However, the diagnosis is made antemortem in only 10–20% of cases.

Etiology & Epidemiology

Thromboemboli almost never originate in the pulmonary circulation; they arrive there by a venous route. Pulmonary thromboembolism is therefore a secondary consequence of another disease, ie, venous thrombosis.

More than 95% of pulmonary thromboemboli arise from thrombi in the deep veins of the lower extremity: the popliteal, femoral, and iliac veins. Venous thrombosis below the popliteal veins or occurring in the superficial veins of the leg is clinically common but not a risk factor for pulmonary thromboembolism. Thrombi in these locations rarely migrate to the pulmonary circulation without first extending above the knee. Since fewer than 20% of calf thrombi will extend into the popliteal veins, isolated calf thrombi may be observed with serial tests to exclude extension into the deep system and do not necessarily require anticoagulation. Venous thromboses occasionally occur in the upper extremities or in the right side of the heart; this happens most commonly in the presence of intravenous catheters or cardiac pacing wires.

Risk factors for pulmonary thromboembolism are therefore the risk factors for the development of venous thrombosis in the deep veins of the legs (deep venous thrombosis) (Table 9–9). The German pathologist Rudolf Virchow stated these risk factors in 1856: venous stasis, injury to the vascular wall, and increased activation of the clotting system. His observations are still valid today.

The most prevalent risk factor in hospitalized patients is stasis from immobilization, especially in those undergoing surgical procedures. The incidence of calf vein thrombosis in patients who do not receive heparin prophylaxis following total knee replacement is reported to be as high as 84%; it is more than 50% following hip surgery or prostatectomy. The risk of fatal pulmonary thromboembolism in these patients may be as high as 5%. Physicians caring for these patients must therefore be aware of the magnitude of the risk and institute appropriate prophylactic therapy (Tables 9–9 and 9–10).

Malignancy and tissue damage at surgery are the two most common causes of increased activation of

Table 9–9. Risk factors for venous thrombosis.

Increased venous stasis
  Bed rest
  Immobilization, especially following orthopedic surgery
  Low cardiac output states
  Pregnancy
  Obesity
  Hyperviscosity
  Local vascular damage, especially prior thrombosis with incompetent valves
  Increasing age
Increased coagulability
  Tissue injury: surgery, trauma, myocardial infarction
  Malignancy
  Presence of a lupus anticoagulant
  Nephrotic syndrome
  Oral contraceptive use, especially estrogen administration
  Genetic coagulation disorders: Factor V Leiden; deficiency of antithrombin III; deficiency of protein C or its cofactor, protein S; deficiency of plasminogen; dysfunctional fibrinogen

Table 9–10. Risk of postoperative deep venous thrombosis or pulmonary embolus in patients who do not receive anticoagulant prophylaxis.[1]

Risk Category	Incidence of Calf Deep Venous Thrombosis	Incidence of Proximal Deep Venous Thrombosis	Incidence of Fatal Pulmonary Embolus

High risk
1. Age >40
2. Anesthesia >30 minutes
3. At least one of the following:
  a. Orthopedic surgery
  b. Pelvic or abdominal cancer surgery
  c. History of prior deep venous thrombosis or pulmonary embolus
  d. Hereditary coagulopathy
	40–80%	10–20%	1–5%

Moderate risk
1. Age >40
2. Anesthesia >30 minutes
3. At least one of the following secondary risk factors:
  a. Immobilization
  b. Obesity
  c. Malignancy
  d. Estrogen use
  e. Varicose veins
  f. Paralysis
	10–40%	2–10%	0.1–0.7%

Low risk 1. Any age 2. Anesthesia <30 minutes 3. No secondary risk factors	<10%	<1%	<0.01%

[1]Modified and reproduced, with permission, from Merli G: Update: Deep vein thrombosis and pulmonary embolism prophylaxis in orthopedic surgery. Med Clin North Am 1993;77:397.

the coagulation system. Genetic disorders are comparatively uncommon, representing 8% of diagnosed outpatients in one recent series. Abnormalities in the vessel wall contribute little to venous as opposed to arterial thrombosis. However, prior thrombosis can damage venous valves and lead to venous incompetence, which promotes stasis.

Pathophysiology

Venous thrombi are composed of a friable mass of fibrin, with many erythrocytes and a few leukocytes and platelets randomly enmeshed in the matrix. When a venous thrombus travels to the pulmonary circulation, it causes a broad array of pathophysiologic changes (Table 9–11).

Table 9–11. Pathophysiologic changes in pulmonary embolism.[1]

Basic Physiology	Effect of Thromboembolism	Mechanism
Altered hemodynamics	Increased pulmonary vascular resistance	Vascular obstruction Vasoconstriction by serotonin, thromboxane A_2
Impaired gas exchange	Increase in alveolar dead space	Vascular obstruction Increased perfusion of lung units with high $\dot{V}/\dot{Q}$ ratios
	Hypoxemia	Increased perfusion of lung units with low $\dot{V}/\dot{Q}$ ratios Right-to-left shunting Fall in cardiac output with fall in mixed venous P_{O_2}
Ventilatory control	Hyperventilation	Reflex stimulation of irritant receptors
Work of breathing	Increased airway resistance Decreased pulmonary compliance	Reflex bronchoconstriction Loss of surfactant with lung edema and hemorrhage

[1]Modified and reproduced, with permission, from Elliott CG: Pulmonary physiology during pulmonary embolism. Chest 1992;101(4 Suppl):163S.

A. Hemodynamic Changes: Every patient with a pulmonary embolus has some degree of mechanical obstruction. The effect of mechanical obstruction depends on the proportion of the pulmonary circulation obstructed and the presence or absence of preexisting cardiopulmonary disease. In patients without preexisting cardiopulmonary disease, pulmonary arterial pressure increases in proportion to the fraction of the pulmonary circulation occluded by emboli. If that fraction is greater than about one-third, pulmonary artery pressures will rise out of the normal range and cause right ventricular strain. The pulmonary circulation can adapt to increased flow, but this depends (1) on recruitment of underperfused capillaries, which may not be available because of obstruction; and (2) on relaxation of central vessels, which does not occur instantaneously. In patients with preexisting cardiopulmonary disease, increases in pulmonary artery pressures do not correlate with extent of embolization. In these studies, there were relatively few patients with both preexisting cardiopulmonary disease and extensive arterial occlusion. A correlation may be obscured by the possibility that massive emboli may either kill patients with preexisting cardiopulmonary disease or perhaps make them too unstable for angiography.

The most devastating and feared complication of acute pulmonary thromboembolism is sudden occlusion of the pulmonary outflow tract, reducing cardiac output to zero and causing immediate cardiovascular collapse and death. Large emboli that do not completely occlude vessels, particularly in patients with compromised cardiac function, may cause an acute increase in pulmonary vascular resistance. This leads to acute right ventricular strain and a fatal fall in cardiac output. Such dramatic presentations occur in less than 5% of cases and are essentially untreatable. They serve to highlight the importance of primary prevention of venous thrombosis.

B. Changes in Ventilation/Perfusion Relationships: Pulmonary thromboembolism reduces or eliminates perfusion distal to the site of the occlusion. The immediate effect is to increase the proportion of lung segments with high $\dot{V}/\dot{Q}$ ratios. If there is complete obstruction to flow, then the $\dot{V}/\dot{Q}$ ratio reaches infinity. This represents alveolar dead space. An increase in dead space ventilation impairs the excretion of carbon dioxide. This tendency is generally compensated by hyperventilation. After several hours, hypoperfusion interferes with production of surfactant by alveolar type II cells. Surfactant is depleted, resulting in alveolar edema, alveolar collapse, and areas of atelectasis. Edema and collapse may result in lung units with little or no ventilation. If there is perfusion to these segments, there will be an increase in lung units with low $\dot{V}/\dot{Q}$ ratios or areas of true shunting, both of which will contribute to arterial hypoxemia.

C. Hypoxemia: Mild to moderate hypoxemia

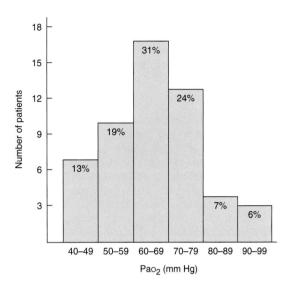

Figure 9–29. Arterial P_{O_2} in 54 patients with angiographically documented pulmonary embolism and no prior history of cardiopulmonary disease. (Reproduced, with permission, from Dantzker DR, Bower JS: Alterations in gas exchange following pulmonary thromboembolism. Chest 1982;81:495.)

with a low $PaCO_2$ is the most common finding in acute pulmonary thromboembolism. This finding may be obscured by the tendency to rely on oximetry alone, since two-thirds of patients will have oxygen saturations above 90% (Figure 9–29). A more sensitive indicator is to calculate the A–a ΔP_{O_2} in order to compensate for the presence of hypocapnia and to account for an increased inspired FIO_2. A widened A–a ΔP_{O_2} is a nearly universal finding in acute pulmonary thromboembolism.

There is no one mechanism that will fully account for hypoxemia. Two causes have been mentioned above. An increase in lung units with low $\dot{V}/\dot{Q}$ ratios impairs oxygen delivery. In patients whose underlying disease makes them unable to increase their minute ventilation, an increase in lung units with high $\dot{V}/\dot{Q}$ ratios can also result in hypoxemia. In some patients with preexisting impaired cardiac function or with large emboli that cause acute right ventricular strain, cardiac output may fall, with a resultant fall in the mixed venous oxygen concentration. This is an important cause of hypoxemia in seriously ill patients. Finally, there may be true right-to-left shunts. Such shunts have been described in a small percentage of patients with severe hypoxemia in the setting of an acute pulmonary thromboembolism. It is presumed that these represent pulmonary artery to pulmonary venous shunting—or perhaps opening of a foramen ovale—but their exact location is unknown.

Obstruction of small pulmonary arterial branches

that act as end arteries leads to pulmonary infarction in about 10% of cases. It is generally associated with some concomitant abnormality of the bronchial circulation such as is seen in patients with left ventricular failure and chronically elevated left atrial pressures.

Clinical Manifestations

A. Symptoms and Signs: The classic triad of a sudden onset of dyspnea, pleuritic chest pain, and hemoptysis occurs in only 20% of patients. Individually, these symptoms are present in 85%, 75%, and 30%, respectively, of diagnosed cases. Dyspnea probably results from reflex bronchoconstriction as well as increased pulmonary artery pressure, loss of pulmonary compliance, and stimulation of C fibers. In large emboli, there may be an element of acute right heart strain. Pleuritic chest pain is much more common than pulmonary infarction; one group has suggested that the pain is caused by areas of pulmonary hemorrhage. Hemoptysis is seen with pulmonary infarction but may also result from transmission of systemic arterial pressures to the microvasculature via bronchopulmonary anastomoses, with subsequent capillary disruption. It may reflect hemorrhagic pulmonary edema from surfactant depletion or neutrophil-associated capillary injury. Syncope may signal a massive embolus.

The most compelling physical finding is not in the chest but the leg: a swollen, tender, warm and reddened calf that provides evidence for deep venous thrombosis. The absence of such evidence does not exclude the diagnosis, since the clinical examination is insensitive, and the absence of signs may indicate that the entire thrombus has embolized. Auscultatory chest findings are common but nonspecific. Atelectasis may lead to inspiratory crackles; infarction may cause a focal pleural friction rub; and the release of mediators may cause wheezing. In large embolization, one may find signs of acute right ventricular strain such as a right ventricular lift and accentuation of the pulmonary component of the second heart sound.

B. Electrocardiography: Less than 25% of cardiograms are normal in the setting of acute pulmonary thromboembolism. However, the findings are usually nonspecific. The most common abnormalities are sinus tachycardia, T wave inversion in the precordial leads, and nonspecific ST and T wave changes. The classic finding of an acute right ventricular strain pattern on ECG—a deep S wave in lead I and both a Q wave and an inverted T wave in lead III ($S_1Q_3T_3$) was observed in 11% of patients in the Urokinase Pulmonary Embolism Trial.

C. Laboratory Findings: An increase in the A–a ΔP_{O_2} is seen in over 90% of cases, and hypoxemia is common in the setting of acute pulmonary thromboembolism. Measurement of the degradation product of cross-linked fibrin, D-dimers, is increasingly common in the diagnosis of venous thrombosis and pulmonary thromboembolism. Depending on the specific assay, the D-dimer has a high sensitivity (85–99%) and moderate specificity (40–70%) for pulmonary thromboembolism.

D. Imaging: The chest radiograph was normal in only 12% of patients with confirmed pulmonary thromboembolism in the Prospective Investigation of Pulmonary Embolism Diagnosis (PIOPED) study. The most frequent findings were atelectasis, parenchymal infiltrates, and pleural effusions. However, the prevalence of these findings was the same in hospitalized patients without suspected pulmonary thromboembolism. Local oligemia (Westermark's sign) or pleura based areas of increased opacity that represent intraparenchymal hemorrhage (Hampton's hump) are rare. The chest radiograph is necessary to exclude other common lung diseases and to permit interpretation of the ventilation/perfusion scan, but it does not itself establish the diagnosis. Paradoxically, it may be most helpful when normal in the setting of acute severe hypoxemia.

E. Ventilation/Perfusion Scanning: A perfusion scan is obtained by injecting microaggregated albumin with a particle size of 50–100 μm into the venous system and allowing the particles to embolize to the pulmonary capillary bed (approximate diameter 10 μm). The substance is labeled with a gamma-emitting isotope of technetium Tc 99m pertechnetate that permits imaging of the distribution of pulmonary blood flow. A ventilation scan is performed by having the patient breathe xenon 133 or a radioactive aerosol and doing sequential scans during inhalation and exhalation. A normal perfusion scan excludes clinically significant pulmonary thromboembolism. A segmental or larger perfusion defect in a radiographically normal area that shows normal ventilation is diagnostic. This is referred to as a "mismatched" defect and is highly specific (97%) for pulmonary thromboembolism.

A minority of ventilation/perfusion scans reveal clearly diagnostic findings. The PIOPED study demonstrated that nondiagnostic ventilation/perfusion scans can stratify a patient's risk of pulmonary thromboembolism. Furthermore, within the categories of high-, medium-, and low-probability studies, the clinician's pretest assessment of the probability of pulmonary thromboembolism can further stratify patients (Table 9–12).

F. Pulmonary Angiography: This is currently the definitive study for the diagnosis of pulmonary thromboembolism. Rapid sequence computed tomography scanning (spiral CT) appears to be both sensitive and specific in detecting thrombus in the central pulmonary arteries. It is effective up to the segmental level but not in smaller subsegmental branches.

G. Resolution: The variability among patients

Table 9–12. Pulmonary embolism (PE) status.[1,2]

V̇/Q̇ Scan Category[3]	Clinical Probability,[4] %							
	80–100		20–79		0–19		All Probabilities	
	PE+/No. of Pts	%	PE+/No. of Pts	%	PE+/No. of Pts	%	PE+/No. of Pts	%
High probability	28/29	96	70/80	88	5/9	56	103/118	87
Intermediate probability	27/41	66	66/236	28	11/68	16	104/345	30
Low probability	6/15	40	30/191	16	4/90	4	40/296	14
Near normal/normal	0/5	0	4/62	6	1/61	2	5/128	4
Total	61/90	68	170/569	30	21/228	9	252/887	28

[1]Reproduced, with permission, from The PIOPED Investigators: Value of the ventilation/perfusion scan in acute pulmonary embolism. JAMA 1990;263:2757.
[2]PE+ indicates angiogram reading that shows pulmonary embolism or determination of pulmonary embolism by the outcome classification committee on review. Pulmonary embolism status is based on angiogram interpretation for 713 patients, on angiogram interpretation and outcome classification committee reassignment for 4 patients, and on clinical information alone (without definitive angiography) for 170 patients.
[3]The division of V̇/Q̇ scan into normal, high, intermediate (or indeterminate), and low probability does stratify patients at risk for pulmonary embolus.
[4]The clinical evaluation of risk adds information to this assessment. For example, in a patient with a low-probability V̇/Q̇ scan, the risk of pulmonary embolus may be as high as 40% in those with a high clinical likelihood and as low as 4% in those with a low clinical likelihood. The V̇/Q̇ scan functions along with clinical judgment to weigh risks and benefits of pulmonary arteriography.

is so great that generalizations are hard to make. The largest number of patients followed serially with quantitative assessments was in the Urokinase Pulmonary Embolism Trial. In that study, serial perfusion scans showed substantial resolution in 9–14 days (Table 9–13). More modern studies, some involving quantitative angiography, have tended to support the time course of these findings.

In a few patients, pulmonary emboli do not resolve completely but become organized and incorporated into the pulmonary arterial wall as an epithelialized fibrous mass. Over time, this can lead to **chronic pulmonary thromboembolism.** This entity presents with stenosis of the central pulmonary arteries, pulmonary hypertension, and right ventricular failure (**cor pulmonale**). Treatment is surgical.

Table 9–13. Resolution of heparin-treated pulmonary thromboembolism assessed by serial perfusion scanning.[1]

Time After Event	Number of Patients	Resolution (% ± SD)
24 hours	70	7 ± 28
2 days	65	16 ± 30
3 days	65	21 ± 30
5 days	69	32 ± 31
7 days	67	42 ± 32
14 days	62	56 ± 30
3 months	60	75 ± 26
6 months	55	77 ± 25
12 months	50	77 ± 23

[1]From The Urokinase Pulmonary Embolism Trial: Circulation 1973;47(Suppl 2):1.

39. Where do 95% of pulmonary thromboemboli originate?
40. What are the risk factors for pulmonary thromboemboli?
41. What hemodynamic changes are brought about by significant pulmonary thromboemboli?
42. What changes in ventilation/perfusion relationships are brought about by significant pulmonary thromboemboli?
43. Suggest some possible explanations for hypoxemia in pulmonary thromboembolism.
44. What are the clinical manifestations of pulmonary thromboembolism?

REFERENCES

General
Crystal RG et al: *The Lung: Scientific Foundations*, 2nd ed. Lippincott-Raven, 1997.
Fishman AP et al: *Fishman's Pulmonary Diseases and Disorders*, 3rd ed. McGraw-Hill, 1998.
Levitzky MG: *Pulmonary Physiology*, 4th ed. McGraw-Hill, 1995.
Murray, JF: *The Normal Lung*, 2nd ed. Saunders, 1986.
Murray JF, Nadel JA: *Textbook of Respiratory Medicine*, 2nd ed. Saunders, 1994.
Nunn JF: *Applied Respiratory Physiology*, 4th ed. Butterworth-Heinemann, 1993.
West JB: *Respiratory Physiology: The Essentials*, 5th ed. Williams & Wilkins, 1994.

Normal Physiology
Berger AS et al: Regulation of respiration. (Three parts.) N Engl J Med 1977;297:92, 138, 194.
Gaston B et al: The biology of nitrogen oxides in the airways. Am J Respir Crit Care Med 1997;149:538.
Greene KE, Peters JI: Pathophysiology of acute respiratory failure. Clin Chest Med 1994;15:1.
Hillberg RE, Johnson DC: Noninvasive ventilation. N Engl J Med 1997;337:1746.
Krachman S, Criner GJ: Hypoventilation syndromes. Clin Chest Med 1998;19:139.
Meek PM et al: American Thoracic Society Consensus Statement. Dyspnea: Mechanisms, assessment and management: A consensus statement. Am J Respir Crit Care Med 1999;159:321.
Pasterkamp H et al: Respiratory sounds: Advances beyond the stethoscope. Am J Respir Crit Care Med 1997;156(3 Part 1):974.
Roussos C, Macklem PT: The respiratory muscles. N Engl J Med 1982;307:786.
Tobin MJ: Mechanical ventilation. N Engl J Med 1994;330:1056.
Wasserman K: Diagnosing cardiovascular and lung pathophysiology from exercise gas exchange. Chest 1997;112:1091.
West JB, Wagner PD: Pulmonary gas exchange. Am J Respir Crit Care Med 1998;157(4 Part 2):S82.

Obstructive Lung Disease
Celli BR: Pulmonary rehabilitation for patients with advanced lung disease. Clin Chest Med 1997;18:521.
Celli BR et al: American Thoracic Society Consensus Statement: Standards for the Diagnosis and Care of Patients with Chronic Obstructive Pulmonary Disease. Am J Respir Crit Care Med 1995;152(5 Part 2):S77.
Cherniak RM: Physiologic diagnosis and function in asthma. Clin Chest Med 1995;16:567.
MacNee W: Pathophysiology of cor pulmonale in chronic obstructive pulmonary disease. Am J Respir Crit Care Med. (Two parts.) 1994;150:833, 1158.
Owens GR et al: The diffusing capacity as a predictor of arterial oxygen desaturation during exercise in patients with chronic obstructive pulmonary disease. N Engl J Med 1984;310:1218.

Restrictive Lung Disease
Agostini C, Semenzato G: Immunology of idiopathic pulmonary fibrosis. Curr Opin Pulm Med 1996;2:364.
Cherniack RM et al: Correlation of structure and function in idiopathic pulmonary fibrosis. Am J Respir Crit Care Med 1995;151:1180.
Rochester CL, Elias JA: Cytokines and cytokine networks in the pathogenesis of interstitial and fibrotic lung disorders. Semin Respir Med 1993;14:389.

Pulmonary Edema
Hultgren HN: High altitude pulmonary edema: Hemodynamic aspects. Int J Sports Med 1997;18:20.
Ketai LH, Godwin JD: A new view of pulmonary edema and acute respiratory distress syndrome. J Thorac Imaging 1998;13:147.
Raijmakers PG et al: What is the cause of pulmonary oedema after acute myocardial infarction? A case study. Intens Care Med 1996;22:591.
Staub NC: Pathophysiology of pulmonary edema. In: *Edema*. Staub NC, Taylor AE (editors). Raven, 1984.

Acute Respiratory Distress Syndrome
Artigas A et al: The American-European Consensus Conference on ARDS. Part 2. Ventilatory, pharmacologic, supportive therapy, study design strategies, and issues related to recover and remodeling. Am J Respir Crit Care Med 1998;157(4 Part 1):1332.
Bersten AD et al: Respiratory mechanics and surfactant in the acute respiratory distress syndrome. Clin Exper Pharmacol Physiol 1998;25:955.
Connelly KG, Repine JE: Markers for predicting the development of acute respiratory distress syndrome. Annu Rev Med. 1997;48:429.
Dreyfuss D, Saumon G: Ventilator-induced lung injury: lessons from experimental studies. Am J Respir Crit Care Med 1998;157:294.
Gattinoni L et al: Lung structure and function in different stages of severe adult respiratory distress syndrome. JAMA 1994;271:1772.
Lesur O et al: Acute respiratory distress syndrome: 30 years later. Can Respir J 1999;6:71.
Luce JM: Acute lung injury and the acute respiratory distress syndrome. Crit Care Med 1998; 26:369.
Parsley E: Acute respiratory distress syndrome. Cellular biology and pathology. Respir Care Clin North Am 1998;4:583.
Pittet JF et al: Biological markers of acute lung injury: prognostic and pathogenetic significance. Am J Respir Crit Care Med 1997;155:1187.

Pulmonary Embolism
Clagett GP et al: Prevention of venous thromboembolism. Chest 1998;114(5 Suppl):531S.
Eliott CG: Pulmonary physiology during pulmonary embolism. Chest 1992;101(Suppl 4):163S.
Goldhaber SZ: Pulmonary embolism. N Engl J Med 1998;339:93.
Hyers TM: Venous thromboembolism. Am J Respir Crit Care Med 1999;159:1.
Jaeschke R et al: User's guide to the medical literature III: How to use an article about a diagnostic test. (Two parts.) JAMA 1994; 271:389, 703.

The PIOPED Investigators: Value of ventilation/perfusion scan in acute pulmonary embolism. JAMA 1990; 263:2753.

Pulmonary embolism: Epidemiology, pathophysiology, diagnosis, and management. Proceedings of an international symposium. Florence, Italy. Chest 1995; 107(1 Suppl):1S.

Santolicandro A et al: Mechanisms of hypoxemia and hypocapnia in pulmonary embolism. Am J Respir Crit Care Med 1995;152:336.

Tapson VF: Pulmonary embolism: New diagnostic approaches. N Engl J Med 1997; 336:1449.

10 Cardiovascular Disorders: Heart Disease

Fred Kusumoto, MD

Diseases of the cardiovascular system frequently confront the physician involved in the day-to-day care of patients. Knowledge of the underlying pathophysiologic processes associated with diseases of the heart and blood vessels provides a critical framework for patient management. This chapter deals with diseases of the heart and the next one with diseases of the blood vessels. Normal cardiac structure and function are summarized here, and pathophysiologic mechanisms for commonly encountered cardiac problems are then discussed, with emphasis on arrhythmias, congestive heart failure, valvular heart disease, coronary artery disease, and pericardial disease.

NORMAL STRUCTURE & FUNCTION OF THE HEART

ANATOMY

The heart is a complex organ whose primary function is to pump blood through the pulmonary and systemic circulations. It is composed of four muscular chambers: the main pumping chambers, the left and right ventricles, and the left and right atria that act as "priming pumps" responsible for the final 20–30% of ventricular filling (Figure 10–1A). Peripheral venous return from the inferior and superior venae cavae fill the right atrium and ventricle (through the open tricuspid valve) (Figure 10–1B). With atrial contraction, additional blood flows through the tricuspid valve and completes the filling of the right ventricle. Unoxygenated blood is then pumped to the pulmonary artery and lung by the right ventricle through the pulmonary valve (Figure 10–1C). Oxygenated blood returns from the lung to the left atrium via four pulmonary veins (Figure 10–1D). Sequential left atrial and ventricular contraction pumps blood back to the peripheral tissues. The mitral valve separates the left atrium and ventricle, and the aortic valve separates the left ventricle from the aorta (Figures 10–1D and 10–1E).

The heart lies free in the pericardial sac, attached to mediastinal structures only at the great vessels. During embryologic development, the heart invaginates into the pericardial sac like a fist pushing into a partially inflated balloon. The pericardial sac is composed of a serous inner layer (visceral pericardium) directly apposed to the myocardium and a fibrous outer layer called the parietal pericardium. Under normal conditions, approximately 40–50 mL of clear fluid, which probably is an ultrafiltrate of plasma, fills the space between the layers of the pericardial sac.

The left main and right coronary arteries arise from the root of the aorta and provide the principal blood supply to the heart (Figure 10–2). The large left main coronary artery usually branches into the left anterior descending artery and the circumflex coronary artery. The left anterior descending coronary artery gives off diagonal and septal branches that supply blood to the anterior wall and septum of the heart, respectively. The circumflex coronary artery continues around the heart in the left atrioventricular groove and gives off large obtuse marginal arteries that supply blood to the left ventricular free wall. The right coronary artery travels in the right atrioventricular groove and supplies blood to the right ventricle via acute marginal branches. The posterior descending artery, which supplies blood to the posterior and inferior walls of the left ventricle, arises from the right coronary artery in 80% of people (right-dominant circulation) and from the circumflex artery in the remainder (left-dominant circulation).

Contraction of the heart chambers is coordinated by several regions in the heart that are composed of myocytes with specialized automaticity (pacemaker) and conduction properties (Figure 10–3). Cells in the sinoatrial (SA) node and the atrioventricular (AV) node have fast pacemaker rates (SA node: 60–100 beats/min; AV node: 40–70 beats/min), and the His bundle and Purkinje fibers are characterized by rapid

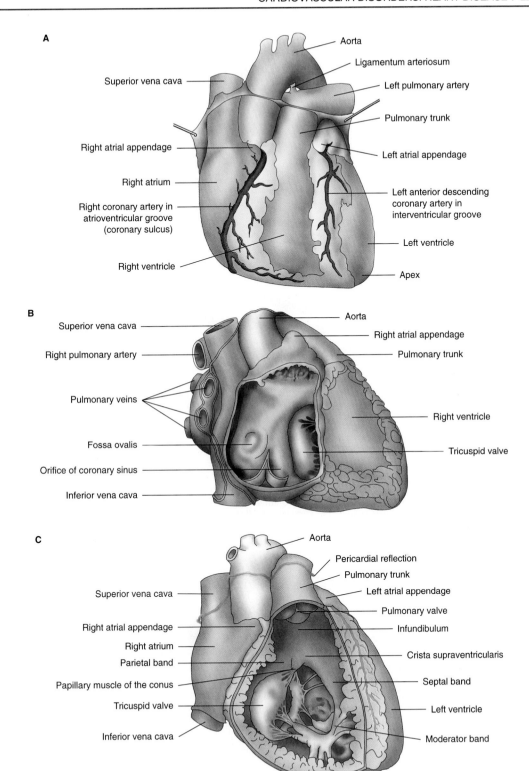

Figure 10–1. Anatomy of the heart. **A:** Anterior view of the heart. **B:** View of the right heart with the right atrial wall reflected to show the right atrium. **C:** Anterior view of the heart with the anterior wall removed to show the right ventricular cavity.

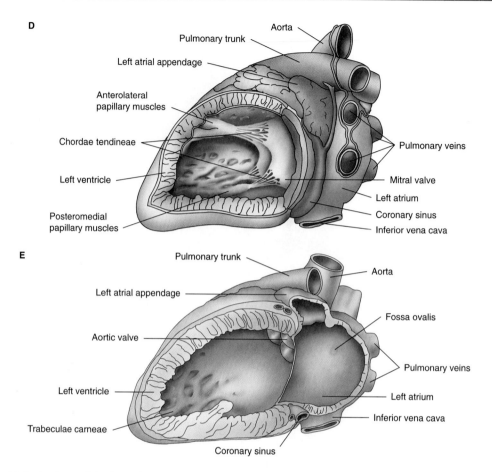

Figure 10–1. Anatomy of the heart. **D:** View of the left heart with the left ventricular wall turned back to show the mitral valve. **E:** View of the left heart from the left side with the left ventricular free wall and mitral valve cut away to reveal the aortic valve. (Reproduced, with permission, from Cheitlin MD, Sokolow M, McIlroy MB: *Clinical Cardiology,* 6th ed. Appleton & Lange, 1993.)

rates of conduction. Since it has the fastest intrinsic pacemaker rhythm, the SA node is usually the site of initiation of the cardiac electrical impulse during a normal cardiac beat. The impulse then rapidly depolarizes both the left and right atria as it travels to the AV node. Conduction velocity slows from 1 m/s in atrial tissue to 0.05 m/s in nodal tissue. After the delay in the AV node, the impulse moves rapidly down the His bundle (1 m/s) and Purkinje fibers (4 m/s) to simultaneously depolarize the right and left ventricles. The atria and ventricles are separated by a fibrous framework that is electrically inert, so that under normal conditions the AV node and the contiguous His bundle form the only electrical connection between the atria and ventricles. This arrangement allows the atria and ventricles to beat in a synchronized fashion and minimizes the chance of electrical feedback between the chambers.

The electrical activity of the heart can be measured from the body surface at standardized positions by electrocardiography. On the electrocardiogram (ECG), the P wave represents depolarization of atrial tissue; the QRS interval, ventricular depolarization; and the T wave, ventricular repolarization (Figure 10–3). Since normal ventricular depolarization occurs almost simultaneously in the right and left ventricle—usually within 60–100 ms—the QRS complex is narrow. While the electrical activity of the small specialized conduction tissues cannot be measured directly from the surface, the interval between the P wave and the start of the QRS complex (PR interval) represents primarily the conduction time of the AV node and His bundle.

HISTOLOGY

Ventricular myocytes are normally 50–100 μm long and 10–25 μm wide. Atrial and nodal myocytes are smaller, while myocytes of the Purkinje system

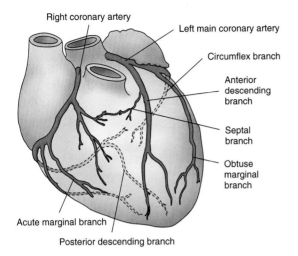

Figure 10–2. Coronary arteries and their principal branches in humans. (Modified and reproduced, with permission, from Ross G: The cardiovascular system. In: *Essentials of Human Physiology.* Ross G [editor]. Copyright © 1978 by Year Book Medical Publishers, Inc., Chicago.)

are larger in both dimensions. Myocytes are filled with hundreds of parallel striated bundles termed myofibrils. Myofibrils are composed of repeating units termed sarcomeres that form the major contractile unit of the myocyte (Figure 10–4). Sarcomeres are complex structures composed of the contractile proteins, myosin and actin; which are connected by cross-bridges; and a regulatory protein complex, tropomyosin. (See Cellular Physiology, below.)

PHYSIOLOGY

Physiology of the Whole Heart

Since the ventricles are the primary physiologic pumps of the heart, analysis has focused on the these chambers, particularly the left ventricle. Function of intact ventricles is traditionally studied by evaluating pressure-time and pressure-volume relationships.

In **pressure-time analysis** (Figure 10–5), pressures in the chambers of the heart and the great vessels are measured during the cardiac cycle and plotted as a function of time. At the beginning of the

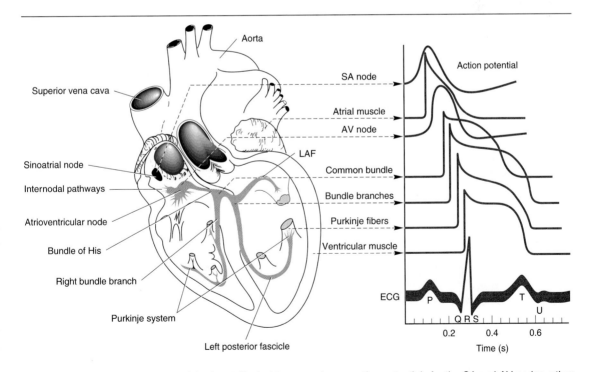

Figure 10–3. Conducting system of the heart. Typical transmembrane action potentials for the SA and AV nodes, other parts of the conduction system, and the atrial and ventricular muscles are shown along with the correlation to the extracellularly recorded electrical activity, ie, the electrocardiogram (ECG). The action potentials and ECG are plotted on the same time axis but with different zero points on the vertical scale. The PR interval is measured from the beginning of the P wave to the beginning of the QRS. (LAF, left anterior fascicle.) (Reproduced, with permission, from Ganong WF: *Review of Medical Physiology,* 19th ed. Appleton & Lange, 1999.)

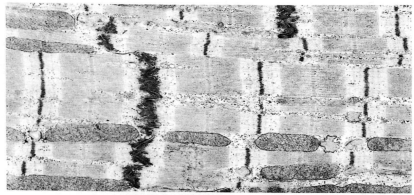
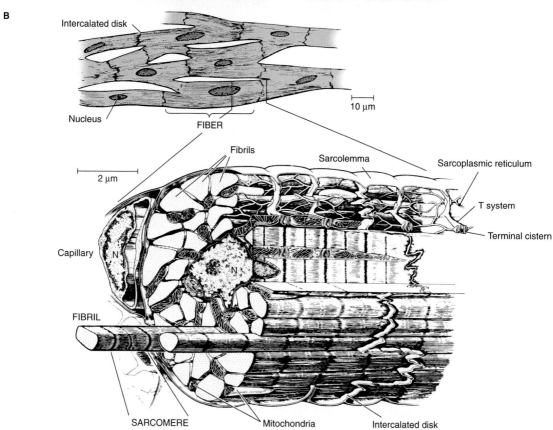
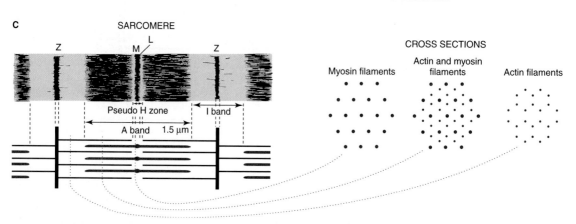

cardiac cycle, the left atrium contracts, forcing additional blood into the left ventricle and giving rise to an *a* wave on the left atrial pressure tracing. At end-diastole, the mitral valve closes, producing the first heart sound (S_1), and a brief period of isovolumic contraction follows during which both the aortic and the mitral valve are closed but the left ventricle is actively contracting. When intraventricular pressure rises to the level of aortic pressure, the aortic valve opens and blood flows into the aorta. After this point, the aorta and left ventricle form a contiguous chamber with equal pressures, but left ventricular volume decreases as blood is expelled. Left ventricular contraction stops and ventricular relaxation begins, and end-systole is reached when intraventricular pressure falls below aortic pressure. The aortic valve then closes, and the second heart sound (S_2) is heard. Throughout systole, blood has slowly accumulated in the left atrium (since the mitral valve is closed), giving rise to the *v* wave on the left atrial pressure tracing. During the first phase of diastole—isovolumic relaxation—no change in ventricular volume occurs, but continued relaxation of the ventricle leads to an exponential fall in left ventricular pressure. Left ventricular filling begins when left ventricular pressure falls below left atrial pressure and the mitral valve opens. Ventricular relaxation is a relatively long process that begins before the aortic valve closes and extends past mitral valve opening. The rate and extent of ventricular relaxation depend on multiple factors: heart rate, wall thickness, chamber volume and shape, aortic pressure, sympathetic tone, and the presence or absence of myocardial ischemia. Once the mitral valve opens, there is an initial period of rapid filling of the ventricle that contributes 70–80% of blood volume to the ventricle and occurs largely because of the atrioventricular pressure gradient. By mid diastole, flow into the left ventricle has slowed, and the cardiac cycle begins again with the next atrial contraction. Right ventricular pressure-time analysis would be similar, but with lower pressures since the impedance to flow in the pulmonary vascular system is much lower than in the systemic circulation.

In **pressure-volume analysis** (Figure 10–6A), pressure during the cardiac cycle is plotted as a function of volume rather than time. During diastole, as ventricular volume increases during both the initial rapid filling period and atrial contraction, ventricular pressure increases (curve **da**). The shape and position of this curve, the **diastolic pressure-volume relationship,** is dependent on relaxation properties of the ventricle, the elastic recoil of the ventricle, and the distensibility of the ventricle. The curve shifts to the left (higher pressure for a given volume) if relaxation of the ventricle is decreased, the ventricle loses elastic recoil, or the ventricle becomes stiffer. At the beginning of systole, active ventricular contraction begins and volume remains unchanged (isovolumic contraction period) (**ab**). When left ventricular pressure reaches aortic pressure, the aortic valve opens, and ventricular volume decreases as the ventricle expels its blood (curve **bc**). At end-systole (**c**), the aortic valve closes and isovolumic relaxation begins (**cd**). When the mitral valve opens, the ventricle begins filling for the next cardiac cycle, repeating the entire process. The area encompassed by this loop represents the amount of work done by the ventricle during a cardiac cycle. The position of point **c** is dependent on the **isovolumic systolic pressure-volume curve.** If the ventricle is filled with variable amounts of blood (preloads) and allowed to contract but the aortic valve is prevented from opening, a relatively linear relationship exists that is termed the isovolumic systolic pressure-volume curve (Figure 10–6B). The slope and position of this line describes the inherent contractile state of the ventricle. If contractility is increased by catecholamines or other positive inotropes, the line will be shifted to the left.

Pressure-volume relationships help illustrate the effects of different stresses on cardiac output. Cardiac output of the ventricle is the product of the **heart rate** and the volume of blood pumped with each beat **(stroke volume).** The width of the pressure-volume loop is the difference between end-diastolic volume and end-systolic volume, or the stroke volume (Figure 10–6). The stroke volume is dependent on three parameters: contractility, afterload, and preload (Figure 10–7). Changing the contractile state of the heart will change the width of the pressure-volume loop by changing the position of the isovolumic systolic pressure curve. The impedance against which the heart must work is termed **"afterload"**; increased afterload (aortic pressure for the left ventricle) will cause a decrease in stroke volume. **"Pre-**

Figure 10–4. A: Electron photomicrograph of cardiac muscle. The fuzzy thick lines are intercalated disks (× 12,000). (Reproduced, with permission, from Bloom W, Fawcett DW: *A Textbook of Histology,* 10th ed. Saunders, 1975). **B:** Diagram of cardiac muscle as seen under the light microscope **(top)** and the electron microscope **(bottom).** (N, nucleus.) (Reproduced, with permission, from Braunwald E, Ross J, Sonnenblick EH: Mechanisms of contraction of the normal and failing heart. N Engl J Med 1967;277:794.) **C:** An individual sarcomere from a myofibril. **At left,** a representation of the arrangement of myofilaments that make up the sarcomere; **at right,** cross sections of the sarcomere, showing the specific lattice arrangement of the myofilaments. (Reproduced, with permission, from Braunwald E, Ross J Jr, Sonnenblick EH: Mechanisms of contraction of the normal and failing heart. N Engl J Med 1967;277:794.)

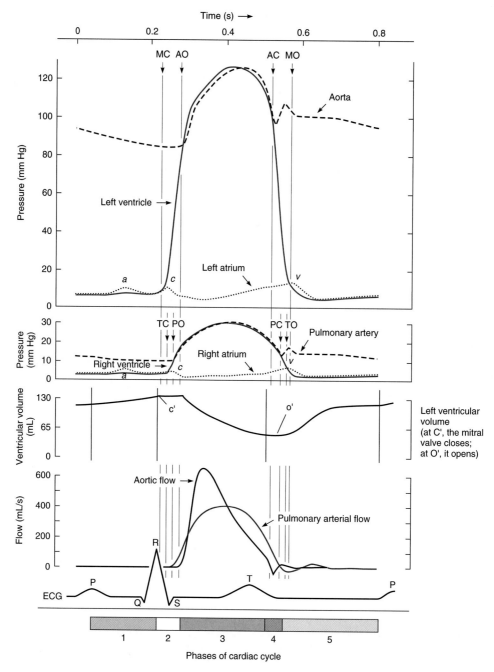

Figure 10–5. Diagram of events in the cardiac cycle. From top downward: pressure (mm Hg) in aorta, left ventricle, left atrium, pulmonary artery, right ventricle, right atrium; blood flow (mL/s) in ascending aorta and pulmonary artery; ECG. Abscissa, time in seconds. (Valvular opening and closing are indicated by AO and AC, respectively, for the aortic valve; MO and MC for the mitral valve; PO and PC for the pulmonary valve; TO and TC for the tricuspid valve.) Events of the cardiac cycle at a heart rate of 75 beats/min. The phases of the cardiac cycle identified by the numbers at the bottom are as follows: 1, atrial systole; 2, isovolumetric ventricular contraction; 3, ventricular ejection; 4, isovolumetric ventricular relaxation; 5, ventricular filling. Note that late in systole, aortic pressure actually exceeds left ventricular pressure. However, the momentum of the blood keeps it flowing out of the ventricle for a short period. The pressure relationships in the right ventricle and pulmonary artery are similar. (Modified and reproduced, with permission, from Milnor WR: The circulation. In: *Medical Physiology.* 2 vols. Mountcastle VB [editor]. Mosby, 1980; and from Ganong WF: *Review of Medical Physiology,* 19th ed. Appleton & Lange, 1999.)

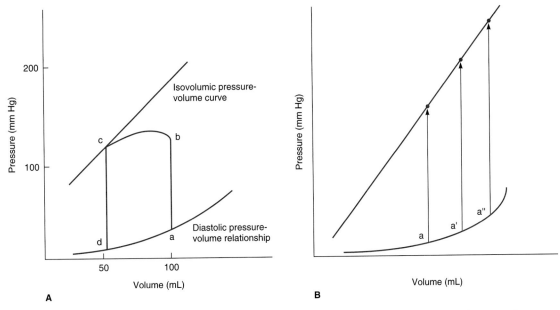

Figure 10–6. A: Pressure-volume loop for the left ventricle. During diastole the left ventricle fills and pressure increases along the diastolic pressure-volume curve from **d** to **a**. Line **ab** represents isometric contraction, and **bc** the ejection phase of systole. The aortic valve closes at point **c**, and pressure drops along **cd** (isovolumic relaxation), until the mitral valve opens at point **d** and the cycle repeats. The distance from **b** to **c** represents the stroke volume ejected by that beat. Point **a** represents end-diastole and point **c**, end-systole. **B:** If the left ventricle is filled by varying amounts **a, a′, a″**, and allowed to undergo isovolumic contraction, a relatively linear relationship, the isovolumic pressure-volume relation, can be defined.

load" is the amount of filling of the ventricle at end-diastole. Up to a point, the more a myocyte or ventricular chamber is stretched, the more it will contract (**Frank-Starling relationship**), so that increased preload will lead to an increase in stroke volume.

Pressure-time and pressure-volume relationships are critical for understanding the pathophysiologic mechanisms of diseases that affect the entire ventricular chamber function, such as heart failure and valvular abnormalities.

Cellular Physiology

A. Ventricular and Atrial Myocytes: The cellular mechanism of myocyte contraction after electrical stimulation is too complex to be fully addressed in this section, but excellent discussions of electromechanical coupling can be found. Briefly, when the myocyte is stimulated, sodium channels on the cell surface membrane (sarcolemma) open, and sodium ions (Na^+) flow down their electrochemical gradient into the cell. This sudden inward surge of ions is responsible for the sharp upstroke of the myocyte action potential (phase 0) (Figure 10–8). A plateau phase follows during which the cell membrane potential remains relatively unchanged owing to the inward flow of calcium ions (Ca^{2+}) and the outward flow of potassium ions (K^+) through several different specialized potassium channels. Repolarization occurs because of continued outward flow of K^+ after inward flux of Ca^{2+} has stopped.

Within the cell, the change in membrane potential from the sudden influx of Na^+ and the subsequent increase in intracellular Ca^{2+} causes the sarcoplasmic reticulum to release large numbers of calcium ions. The exact signaling mechanism is not known. Once in the cytoplasm, however, Ca^{2+} released from the sarcoplasmic reticulum binds with the regulatory proteins troponin and tropomyosin. Myosin and actin are then allowed to interact and the cross-bridges between them bend, giving rise to contraction (Figure 10–9). The process of relaxation is poorly understood also but appears to involve return of Ca^{2+} to the sarcoplasmic reticulum via two transmembrane sarcoplasmic reticulum-embedded proteins, Ca^{2+}-ATPase and phospholamban. Reuptake of Ca^{2+} is an active process that requires ATP.

B. Pacemaker Cells: The action potential of pacemaker cells is different from that described for ventricular and atrial myocytes (Figure 10–8). Fast sodium channels are absent, so that rapid phase 0 depolarization is not observed in SA nodal and AV nodal cells. In addition, these cells are characterized by increased automaticity from a relatively rapid spontaneous phase 4 depolarization. A combination

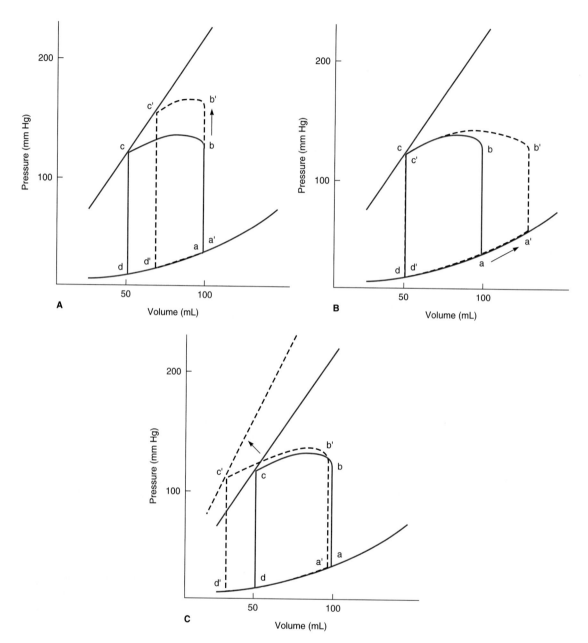

Figure 10–7. A: Increasing afterload from **b** to **b′** decreases stroke volume from **bc** to **b′c′**. **B:** Increasing preload from **a** to **a′** increases stroke volume from **bc** to **b′c′**, but at the expense of increased end-diastolic pressure. **C:** Increasing contractile state shifts the isovolumic pressure-volume relationship leftward, increasing stroke volume from **bc** to **b′c′**.

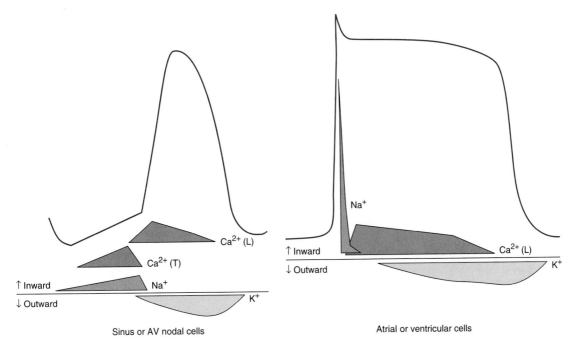

Figure 10–8. Changes in ionic conductances responsible for generating action potentials for ventricular or atrial tissue (right) and a sinus or AV node cell (left). In nodal cells rapid Na^+ channels are absent, so that the action potential upstroke is much slower. Diastolic depolarization observed in nodal cells is due to decreased K^+ efflux and slow Na^+ and Ca^{2+} influx Ca^{2+} (T): influx via Ca^{2+} (T) channels; Ca^{2+} (L): influx via Ca^{2+} (L) channels.

of reduced outward flow of K^+ and inward flow of Na^+ and Ca^{2+} via specialized channels appears to be responsible for this dynamic change in membrane potential. Myofibrils are sparse, though present, in the specialized pacemaker cells.

1. What are the differences in pacemaker and conduction properties in different regions of the heart, and why do these differences explain the observation that cardiac electrical impulses normally arise in the SA node?
2. Describe pressure-time analysis through the cardiac cycle.
3. Describe pressure-volume analysis through the cardiac cycle.
4. What are preload and afterload?
5. Briefly describe the molecular mechanism of electromechanical coupling in cardiac myocyte contraction.

PATHOPHYSIOLOGY OF SELECTED CARDIOVASCULAR DISORDERS

ARRHYTHMIAS

At rest, the heart is normally activated at a rate of 50–100 beats/min. Abnormal rhythms of the heart (arrhythmias) can be classified as either too slow (bradycardias) or too fast (tachycardias).

Bradycardia

Bradycardia can arise from two basic mechanisms. First, reduced automaticity of the sinus node can result in slow heart rates or pauses. As shown in Figure 10–10, if sinus node pacemaker activity ceases, the heart will usually be activated at a slower rate by other cardiac tissues with pacemaker activity. Re-

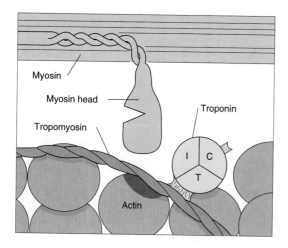 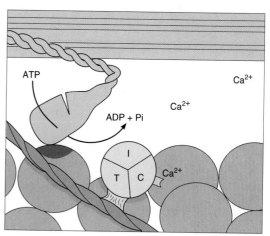

Figure 10–9. Initiation of muscle contraction by Ca^{2+}. When Ca^{2+} binds to troponin C, tropomyosin is displaced laterally, exposing the binding site for myosin on actin (dark area). Hydrolysis of ATP then changes the conformation of the myosin head and fosters its binding to the exposed site. For simplicity, only one of the two heads of the myosin-II molecule is shown. (Reproduced, with permission, from Ganong WF: *Review of Medical Physiology,* 19th ed. Appleton & Lange, 1999.)

duced sinus node automaticity can occur during periods of increased vagal tone (sleep, carotid sinus massage, "common faint"), with increasing age, and secondary to drugs (beta-blockers, calcium channel blockers).

Second, slow heart rates can occur if the cardiac impulse is prevented from activating the ventricles normally because of blocked conduction (Figure 10–11). Since the fibrous valvular annulus is electrically inert, normally the AV node and His bundle form the only electrically active connection between the atria and ventricles. While this arrangement is useful for preventing feedback between the two chambers, it also makes the AV node and His bundle vulnerable sites for blocked conduction between the atria and ventricles. While block can be observed in either the left or right bundle branches, bradycardia does not necessarily occur, since the ventricles can still be activated by the contralateral bundle. Atrioventricular block has been classified as first-degree when there is an abnormally long atrioventricular conduction time (PR interval > 0.22 s) but activation of the atria and ventricles still demonstrates 1:1 association. In second-degree atrioventricular block, some but not all atrial impulses are conducted to the ventricles. Finally, in third-degree block, there is no association between atrial and ventricular activity. Atrioventricular block can occur with increasing age, with increased vagal input, and as a side effect of certain drugs. Atrioventricular block can sometimes be observed also in congenital disorders such as muscular dystrophy, tuberous sclerosis, and maternal systemic lupus erythematosus and in acquired disorders such as sarcoidosis, gout, Lyme disease, systemic lupus erythematosus, ankylosing spondylitis, and coronary artery disease.

Bradycardia due to either decreased automaticity or blocked conduction calls for evaluation to detect reversible causes. However, implantation of a permanent pacemaker is often required.

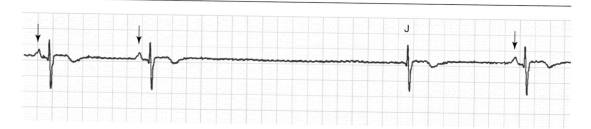

Figure 10–10. Rhythm strip showing bradycardia due to sinus node pause. Atrial activity **(arrows)** suddenly ceases, and after approximately 3 seconds a junctional escape beat is observed (J).

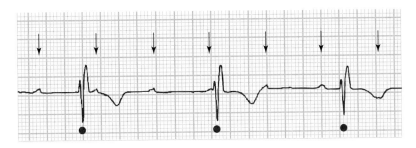

Figure 10–11. Rhythm strip demonstrating third-degree (complete) heart block with no association between atrial activity **(arrows)** and ventricular activity **(dots).**

Tachycardia

Tachycardias can arise from three basic cellular mechanisms (Figure 10–12). First, increased automaticity due to more rapid phase 4 depolarization can cause rapid heart rate. Second, if repolarization is delayed (longer plateau period), spontaneous depolarizations (due to reactivation of sodium or calcium channels) can sometimes occur in phase 3 or phase 4 of the action potential. These depolarizations are called triggered activity since they are dependent on the existence of a preceding action potential. If these depolarizations reach threshold, tachycardia can occur in certain pathologic conditions. Third—and most commonly—tachycardias can arise from a reentrant circuit. Any condition that gives rise to parallel but electrically separate regions with different conduction velocities (such as the border zone of a myocardial infarction or an accessory atrioventricular connection) can serve as the substrate for a reentrant circuit.

The best-studied example of reentrant tachyarrhythmias is the Wolff-Parkinson-White syndrome (Figure 10–13). As mentioned previously, the AV node normally forms the only electrical connection between the atria and ventricles. Perhaps because of incomplete formation of the annulus, an accessory atrioventricular connection is found in approximately one in 1000 persons. This accessory pathway is usually composed of normal atrial or ven-

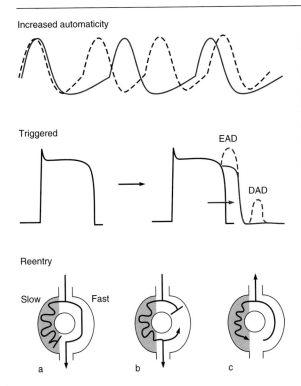

Figure 10–12. Tachyarrhythmias can arise from three different mechanisms. First, increased automaticity from more rapid phase 4 depolarization can cause arrhythmias. Second, in certain conditions, spontaneous depolarizations during phase 3 (early afterdepolarizations, EAD) or phase 4 (late afterdepolarizations, DAD) can repetitively reach threshold and cause tachycardia. This appears to be the mechanism of the polymorphic ventricular tachycardia (torsade de pointes) observed in some patients taking procainamide or quinidine and the arrhythmias associated with digoxin toxicity. Third, the most common mechanism for tachyarrhythmia is reentry. In reentry, two parallel pathways with different conduction properties exist (perhaps at the border zone of a myocardial infarction or a region of myocardial ischemia). The electrical impulse normally travels down the fast pathway and the slow pathway (shaded region), but at the point where the two pathways converge the impulse traveling down the slow pathway is blocked since the tissue is refractory from the recent depolarization via the fast pathway (a). However, when a premature beat reaches the circuit, block can occur in the fast pathway, and the impulse will travel down the slow pathway (shaded region) (b). After traveling through the slow pathway the impulse can then enter the fast pathway in retrograde fashion (which because of the delay has recovered excitability), and then reenter the slow pathway to start a continuous loop of activation, or reentrant circuit (c).

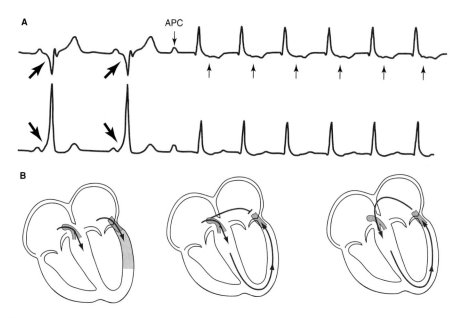

Figure 10–13. Reentrant tachyarrhythmia due to the Wolff-Parkinson-White syndrome. **A:** First two beats demonstrate sinus rhythm with preexcitation of the ventricles over an accessory pathway. The large arrows show the delta wave. An atrial premature contraction (APC) blocks in the accessory pathway, which leads to normalization of the QRS, and the atria are activated in retrograde fashion via the accessory pathway **(small arrows)** and supraventricular tachycardia ensues. **B:** The left panel schematically depicts the first two beats of the rhythm strip. The QRS is wide owing to activation of the ventricles over both the AV node and the accessory pathway. The middle panel depicts the atrial premature contraction, which is blocked in the accessory pathway but conducts over the AV node. In the right panel, the atria are activated in retrograde fashion over the accessory pathway, and a reentrant circuit is initiated.

tricular tissue. Since part of the ventricle is "preexcited" over the accessory pathway rather than via the AV node, the surface ECG shows a short PR interval and a relatively wide QRS with a slurred upstroke, termed a **delta wave.** Since the atria and ventricles are linked by two parallel connections, reentrant tachycardias are readily initiated. For example, a premature atrial contraction could be blocked in the accessory pathway but still conduct to the ventricles via the AV node. If enough time has elapsed so that the accessory pathway has recovered excitability, the cardiac impulse can travel in retrograde fashion to the atria over the accessory pathway and initiate a reentrant tachycardia.

Regardless of the mechanism, acute clinical management of tachycardias depends on whether the QRS complex is narrow or wide. If the QRS complex is narrow, depolarization of the ventricles must be occurring normally over the specialized conduction tissues of the heart, and the arrhythmia must be originating at or above the AV node (supraventricular) (Figure 10–14).

A wide QRS complex suggests that ventricular activation is not occurring normally over the specialized conduction tissues of the heart. The tachycardia is either arising from ventricular tissue or is a supraventricular tachycardia with aberrant conduction over the His-Purkinje system or an accessory pathway. Criteria have been developed for distinguishing between ventricular and supraventricular tachycardia with aberrance.

CONGESTIVE HEART FAILURE

Inadequate pump function of the heart, which leads to congestion resulting from fluid in the lungs and peripheral tissues, is a common end result of many disease processes. Congestive heart failure is present in approximately 3 million people in the United States, with more than 400,000 new cases reported annually. The clinical presentation is highly variable; for an individual patient, symptoms and signs depend on how quickly heart failure develops and whether it involves the left, right, or both ventricles.

1. LEFT VENTRICULAR FAILURE

Clinical Presentation

Patients with left ventricular failure most commonly present with a sensation of breathlessness

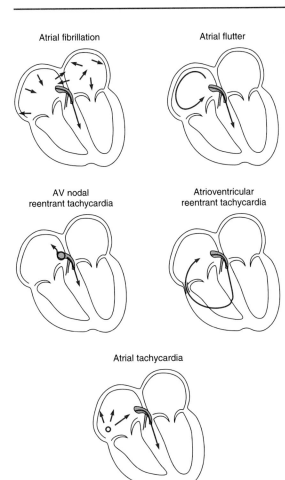

Figure 10–14. In supraventricular tachycardia, the QRS is narrow since the ventricles are depolarized over the normal specialized conduction tissues (colored region). There are five possible arrhythmias commonly encountered. First, in atrial fibrillation, multiple microreentrant circuits can lead to chaotic activation of the atrium. Since impulses are reaching the AV node at irregular intervals, ventricular depolarization is irregular. Second, in atrial flutter, a macroreentrant circuit, traveling up the interatrial septum and down the lateral walls can activate the atria in a regular fashion at approximately 300 beats/min. The AV node can conduct only every other or every third beat, so that the ventricles are depolarized at 150 or 100 beats/min. In AV nodal reentrant tachycardia, slow and fast pathways exist in the region of the AV node and a microreentrant circuit can be formed. Fourth, in atrioventricular reentry, an abnormal connection between the atrium and ventricle exists so that a macro reentrant circuit can be formed with the AV node forming the slow pathway, and the abnormal atrioventricular connection, the fast pathway. Finally, in atrial tachycardia an abnormal focus of atrial activity due to either reentry, triggered activity, or abnormal automaticity can activate the atria in a regular fashion.

(dyspnea), particularly when lying down (orthopnea) or at night (paroxysmal nocturnal dyspnea). In addition, the patient may complain of blood-tinged sputum (hemoptysis) and occasionally chest pain. Fatigue, nocturia, and confusion can also be caused by heart failure.

On physical examination, the patient usually has elevated respiratory and heart rates. The skin may be pale, cold, and sweaty. In severe heart failure, palpation of the peripheral pulse may reveal alternating strong and weak beats (pulsus alternans). Auscultation of the lungs reveals abnormal sounds called rales that have been described as "crackling leaves." In addition, the bases of the lung fields may be dull to percussion. On cardiac examination, the apical impulse is often displaced laterally and sustained. Third and fourth heart sounds can be heard on auscultation of the heart. Since many patients with left ventricular failure also have accompanying failure of the right ventricle, signs of right ventricular failure may also be present (see next section).

Etiology

Heart failure is a pathophysiologic complex associated with dysfunction of the heart and a common end point for many diseases of the cardiovascular system. As such, there are many possible causes of heart failure (Table 10–1), and the specific reason for heart failure in a given patient must always be sought. In general, heart failure can be caused by (1) inappropriate workloads placed on the heart, such as volume overload or pressure overload, (2) restricted filling of the heart, (3) myocyte loss, or (4) decreased myocyte contractility.

Pathophysiology

Pathophysiologically, heart failure can arise from worsening systolic or diastolic function or, more frequently, a combination of both. In **systolic dysfunc-**

Table 10–1. Causes of left ventricular failure.

Volume overload
Regurgitant valves (mitral or aortic)
High-output states: Anemia, hyperthyroidism
Pressure overload
Systemic hypertension
Outflow obstruction: Aortic stenosis, asymmetric septal hypertrophy
Loss of muscle
Myocardial infarction from coronary artery disease
Connective tissue disease: systemic lupus erythematosus
Loss of contractility
Poisons: Alcohol, cobalt, doxorubicin
Infections: Viral, bacterial
Restricted filling
Mitral stenosis
Pericardial disease: Constrictive pericarditis and pericardial tamponade
Infiltrative diseases: Amyloidosis

tion, the isovolumic systolic pressure curve of the pressure-volume relationship is shifted downward (Figure 10–15A). This reduces the stroke volume of the heart with a concomitant decrease in cardiac output. In order to maintain cardiac output, the heart can respond with three compensatory mechanisms: First, increased return of blood to the heart (preload) can lead to increased contraction of sarcomeres (Frank-Starling relationship). In the pressure-volume relationship, the heart operates at ***a'*** instead of ***a,*** and stroke volume increases—but at the cost of increased end-diastolic pressure (Figure 10–15D). Second, increased release of catecholamines can increase cardiac output both by increasing the heart rate and by

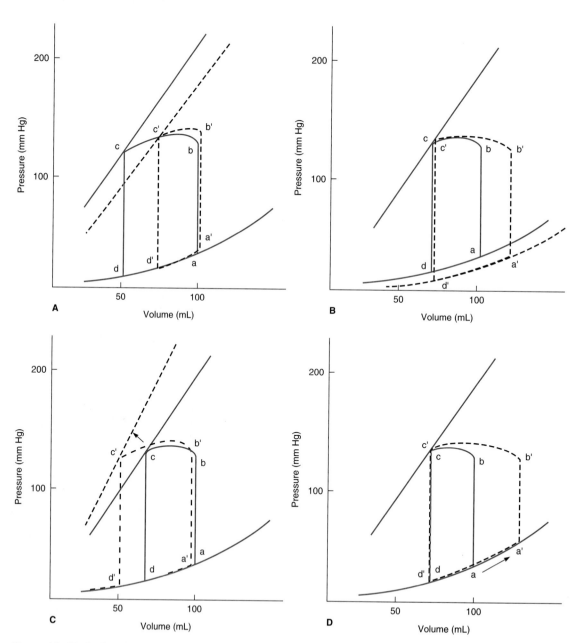

Figure 10–15. A: Systolic dysfunction is represented by shifting of the isovolumic pressure-volume curve to the right (dashed line), thus decreasing stroke volume. The ventricle can compensate by **(B)** shifting the diastolic pressure-volume relationship rightward (dashed line) by increasing left ventricular volume or elasticity, **(C)** increasing contractile state (dashed line) by activation of circulating catecholamines, and **(D)** increasing filling or preload (**a** to **a'**).

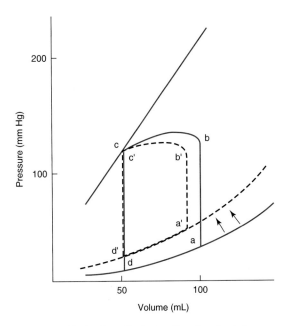

Figure 10–16. In diastolic dysfunction, the diastolic pressure-volume relation is shifted upward and to the left (dashed line), which leads to an elevated left ventricular end-diastolic pressure **a′** and reduced stroke volume.

shifting the systolic isovolumetric curve leftward (Figure 10–15C). Finally, cardiac muscle can hypertrophy and ventricular volume can increase, which shifts the diastolic curve rightward (Figure 10–15B). While each of these compensatory mechanisms can temporarily maintain cardiac output, each is of limited potential, and if the underlying reason for systolic dysfunction remains untreated, the heart ultimately fails.

In **diastolic dysfunction,** the position of the systolic isovolumic curve remains unchanged (contractility of the myocytes is preserved). However, the diastolic pressure-volume curve is shifted to the left, with an accompanying increase in left ventricular end-diastolic pressure and symptoms of congestive heart failure (Figure 10–16). Diastolic dysfunction can be present in any disease that causes decreased relaxation, decreased elastic recoil, or increased stiffness of the ventricle. Hypertension, which often leads to increases in left ventricular wall thickness, can cause diastolic dysfunction by changing all three parameters. Lack of sufficient blood to myocytes (ischemia) can also cause diastolic dysfunction by decreasing relaxation. If ischemia is severe, as in myocardial infarction, irreversible damage to the myocytes can occur, with replacement of contractile cells by fibrosis, which will lead to systolic dysfunction. In most patients, a combination of systolic and diastolic dysfunction is responsible for the symptoms of heart failure.

Clinical Manifestations

A. Symptoms:

1. Shortness of breath, orthopnea, paroxysmal nocturnal dyspnea–Although many details of the physiologic mechanisms for the sensation of breathlessness are unclear, the inciting event probably is a rise in pulmonary capillary pressures as a consequence of elevated left ventricular and atrial pressures. The rise in pulmonary capillary pressure relative to plasma oncotic pressure causes fluid to move into the interstitial spaces of the lung (pulmonary edema), which can be seen on chest x-ray (Figure 10–17). Interstitial edema probably stimulates juxtacapillary J receptors, which in turn causes reflex shallow and rapid breathing. Replacement of air in the lungs by blood or interstitial fluid can cause a reduction of vital capacity, restrictive physiology, and air trapping due to closure of small airways. The work of breathing increases as the patient tries to distend stiff lungs, which can lead to respiratory muscle fatigue and the sensation of dyspnea. Alterations in the distribution of ventilation and perfusion result in relative ventilation/perfusion $\dot{V}/\dot{Q}$ mismatch, with consequent widening of the alveolar-arterial O_2 gradient, hypoxemia, and increased dead space. Edema of the bronchial walls can lead to small airway obstruction and produce wheezing ("cardiac asthma"). Shortness of breath occurs in the recumbent position (orthopnea) because of reduced blood pooling in the extremities and abdomen—and, since the patient is operating on the steep portion of the diastolic pressure-volume curve, any increase in blood return leads to marked elevations in ventricular pressures. Patients usually learn to minimize orthopnea by sleep-

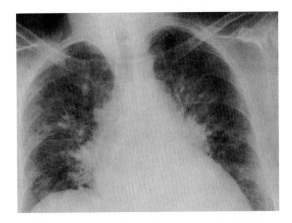

Figure 10–17. Posteroanterior chest x-ray in a man with acute pulmonary edema due to left ventricular failure. Note the bat's wing density, cardiac enlargement, increased size of upper lobe vessels, and pulmonary venous congestion. (Reproduced, with permission, from Cheitlin MD, Sokolow M, McIlroy MB: *Clinical Cardiology,* 6th ed. Appleton & Lange, 1993.)

ing with the upper body propped up by two or more pillows. Sudden onset of severe respiratory distress at night—paroxysmal nocturnal dyspnea—probably occurs because of the reduced adrenergic support of ventricular function that occurs with sleep, the increase in blood return as described above, and normal nocturnal depression of the respiratory center.

2. **Fatigue, confusion**–Fatigue probably arises because of inability of the heart to supply appropriate amounts of blood to skeletal muscles. Confusion may arise in advanced heart failure because of underperfusion of the cerebrum.

3. **Nocturia**–Heart failure can lead to reduced renal perfusion during the day while the patient is upright, which normalizes only at night while the patient is supine, with consequent diuresis.

4. **Chest pain**–If the cause of failure is coronary artery disease, patients may have chest pain secondary to ischemia (angina pectoris). In addition, even without ischemia, acute heart failure can cause chest pain from unknown mechanisms.

B. **Physical Examination:**

1. **Rales, pleural effusion**–Increased fluid in the alveolar spaces from the mechanisms described above can be heard as rales. Increased capillary pressures can also cause fluid accumulation in the pleural spaces.

2. **Displaced and sustained apical impulse**–In most people, contraction of the heart can be appreciated by careful palpation of the chest wall (apical impulse). The normal apical impulse is felt in the midclavicular line in the fourth or fifth intercostal space and is palpable only during the first part of systole. When the apical impulse can be felt during the latter part of systole, it is sustained. Sustained impulses suggest that increases in left ventricular volume or mass are present. In addition, when left ventricular volume is increased as a compensatory mechanism of heart failure, the apical impulse is displaced laterally.

3. **Third heart sound (S_3)**–The third heart sound is a low-pitched sound that is heard during rapid filling of the ventricle in early diastole (Figure 10–18A). The exact mechanism for the genesis of the third heart sound is not known, but the sound appears to result either from the sudden deceleration of blood as the elastic limits of the ventricular chamber are reached or from the actual impact of the ventricular wall against the chest wall. Although a third heart sound is normal in children and young adults, it is rarely heard in healthy adults over 40 years of age. In these individuals, the presence of a third heart sound is almost pathognomonic for ventricular failure. The increased end-systolic volumes and pressures characteristic of the failing heart are probably responsible for the prominent third heart sound. When it arises because of left ventricular failure, the third heart sound is usually heard best at the apex. It can be present in patients with either diastolic or systolic dysfunction.

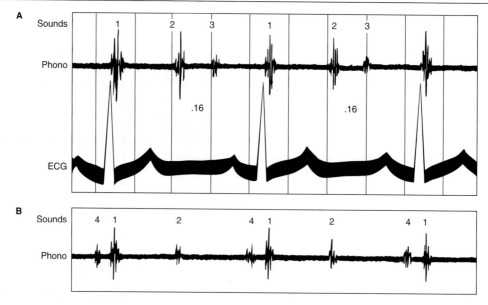

Figure 10–18. A: Phonocardiogram showing typical third heart sound (S_3). It follows the second sound (S_2) by 0.16 s. (Courtesy of Roche Laboratories Division of Hoffman-La Roche, Inc.) **B:** Phonocardiogram showing a fourth heart sound (S_4) and its relation to first sound (S_1).

4. **Fourth heart sound (S$_4$)**—Normally, sounds arising from atrial contraction are not heard. However, if there is increased stiffness of the ventricle, a low-pitched sound at end-diastole that occurs concomitantly with atrial contraction can sometimes be heard (Figure 10–18B). Like the third heart sound, the exact mechanism for the genesis of the fourth heart sound is not known. However, it probably arises from the sudden deceleration of blood in a noncompliant ventricle or from sudden impact of a stiff ventricle against the chest wall. It is best heard laterally at the apical impulse, particularly when the patient is rolled over onto the left side (left lateral decubitus position). The fourth heart sound is commonly heard in any patient with heart failure due to diastolic dysfunction.

5. **Pale, cold, and sweaty skin**—Patients with severe heart failure often have peripheral vasoconstriction, which maintains blood flow to the central organs and head. In some cases, the skin appears dusky because of reduced oxygen content in venous blood as a result of increased oxygen extraction from peripheral tissues that are receiving low blood flow. Sweating occurs because body heat cannot be dissipated through the constricted vascular bed of the skin.

2. RIGHT VENTRICULAR FAILURE

Clinical Presentation

Symptoms of right ventricular failure include shortness of breath, pedal edema, and abdominal pain.

The findings on physical examination are similar to those of left ventricular failure but in different positions, since the right ventricle is anatomically anterior and to the right of the left ventricle (Figure 10–1). Patients with right ventricular failure may have a third heart sound heard best at the sternal border or a sustained systolic heave of the sternum. Inspection of the neck reveals elevated jugular venous pressures. Since the most common cause of right ventricular failure is left ventricular failure, signs of left ventricular failure are often also present.

Etiology

Right ventricular failure can be due to several causes. As just mentioned, left ventricular failure can cause right ventricular failure because of the increased afterload placed on the right ventricle. Increased afterload can also be present from abnormalities of the pulmonary arteries or capillaries. For example, increased flow from a congenital shunt can cause reactive pulmonary artery constriction, increased right ventricular afterload, and, ultimately, right ventricular failure. Right ventricular failure can occur as a sequela of pulmonary disease (cor pulmonale) because of destruction of the pulmonary capillary bed or hypoxia-induced vasoconstriction of the pulmonary arterioles. Right ventricular failure

Table 10–2. Causes of right ventricular failure.

Left-sided failure
Precapillary obstruction
Congenital (shunts, obstruction)
Idiopathic pulmonary hypertension
Primary right ventricular failure
Right ventricular infarction
Cor pulmonale
Hypoxia-induced vasoconstriction
Pulmonary embolism
Chronic obstructive lung disease

can also be caused by right ventricular ischemia, usually in the setting of an inferior wall myocardial infarction (Table 10–2).

Pathophysiology

The pathophysiology of right ventricular failure is similar to that described for the left ventricle. Both systolic and diastolic abnormalities of the right ventricle can be present and usually occur because of inappropriate loads placed on the ventricle, or primary loss of myocyte contractility.

Patients with isolated right ventricular failure (pulmonary hypertension, cor pulmonale) can have a mechanical reason for left ventricular failure. The interventricular septum is usually bowed toward the thinner-walled and lower-pressure right ventricle. When right ventricular pressure increases relative to the left, the interventricular septum can bow to the left and prevent efficient filling of the left ventricle, which may lead to pulmonary congestion. Rarely, the bowing can be so severe that left ventricular outflow can be partially obstructed. This phenomenon is termed a "reversed Bernheim effect."

Clinical Manifestations

A. Shortness of Breath: If there is left ventricular failure, patients may be short of breath because of pulmonary edema as discussed above. In patients with right-sided failure due to pulmonary disease, shortness of breath may be a manifestation of the underlying disease (eg, pulmonary embolus, chronic obstructive pulmonary disease). In some patients with right ventricular failure, congestion of the hepatic veins with formation of ascites can impinge on normal diaphragmatic function and contribute to the sensation of dyspnea. In addition, reduced right-sided cardiac output alone can cause acidosis, hypoxia, and air hunger. If the cause of right-sided failure is a left-sided defect such as mitral stenosis, the onset of right heart failure can sometimes lessen the symptoms of pulmonary edema because of the decreased load placed on the left ventricle.

B. Elevated Jugular Venous Pressure: The position of venous pulsations of the internal jugular vein can be observed during examination of the neck (Figure 10–19A). The distance above the heart at

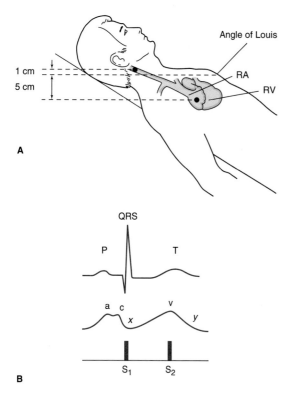

Figure 10–19. A: Examination of jugular venous pulse and estimation of venous pressure. (RA, right atrium; RV, right ventricle.) **B:** Jugular venous pressure waveforms in relation to the electrocardiogram (P wave, QRS, and T wave) and the first and second heart sounds (S_1 and S_2). The bottom of the x descent occurs coincident with the first heart sound (S_1). The v wave occurs just after the apical impulse is felt at the same time the second heart sound (S_2) is heard. See text for further explanation of jugular venous wave forms.

which venous pulsations are observed is an estimate of the right atrial or central venous pressure. Since the position of the right atrium cannot be precisely determined, the height of the jugular venous pulsation is measured relative to the angle of Louis on the sternum. Right atrial pressure can then be approximated by adding 5 cm to the height of the venous column (since the right atrium is approximately 5 cm inferior to the angle). Jugular venous pulsations are usually observed less than 7 cm above the right atrium. Elevated atrial pressures are present any time this distance is greater than 10 cm. Elevated atrial pressures indicate that the preload of the ventricle is adequate but ventricular function is decreased and fluid is accumulating in the venous system. Other causes of elevated jugular pressures besides heart failure include pericardial tamponade, constrictive pericarditis, and massive pulmonary embolus.

In addition to relative position, individual waveforms of the jugular venous pulse can be assessed.

Three positive waves (*a, c,* and *v*) and two negative waves (*x* and *y*) can be recognized (Figure 10–19B). The *a* wave is caused by transmitted right atrial pressure from atrial contraction. The *c* wave is usually not present on bedside examination; it is thought to arise from bulging of the tricuspid valve during isovolumic contraction of the right ventricle. The *x* descent is thought to be due to atrial relaxation and downward displacement of the tricuspid annulus during systole. The *v* wave arises from continued filling of the right atrium during the latter part of systole. Once the tricuspid valve opens, blood flows into the right ventricle and the *y* descent begins. Evaluation of the individual wave forms will become particularly important when pericardial disease is discussed.

C. Anasarca, Ascites, Pedal Edema, Hepatojugular Reflux, Abdominal Pain: Elevated right-sided pressure leads to accumulation of fluid in the systemic venous circulation. Venous congestion can be manifested by generalized edema (anasarca), ascites (collection of fluid in the peritoneal space), and dependent edema (swelling of the feet and legs). Pressing on the liver for approximately 5 seconds can lead to displacement of blood into the vena cava; when the right ventricle cannot accommodate this additional volume, an increase in jugular venous pressure ("hepatojugular reflux") can be observed. Expansion of the liver from fluid accumulation can cause distention of the liver capsule with accompanying right upper quadrant abdominal pain.

6. What are the clinical presentations of CHF? Of right ventricular failure?
7. What are the four general categories which account for almost all causes of CHF?
8. Explain the differences between the pathophysiology of CHF due to systolic vs diastolic dysfunction.
9. What are the major clinical manifestations and complications of left- vs right-sided heart failure?

VALVULAR HEART DISEASE

Dysfunctional cardiac valves can be classified as either narrow (stenosis) or leaky (regurgitation). While the tricuspid and pulmonary valves can become dysfunctional in patients with endocarditis, congenital lesions, or carcinoid syndrome, primary right-sided valvular abnormalities are relatively rare and will not be discussed further. In this section, the pathophysiologic mechanisms of stenotic and regurgitant aortic and mitral valves will be addressed.

A general classification of heart murmurs is presented in Figure 10–20. Any disease process that creates turbulent flow in the heart or great vessels can

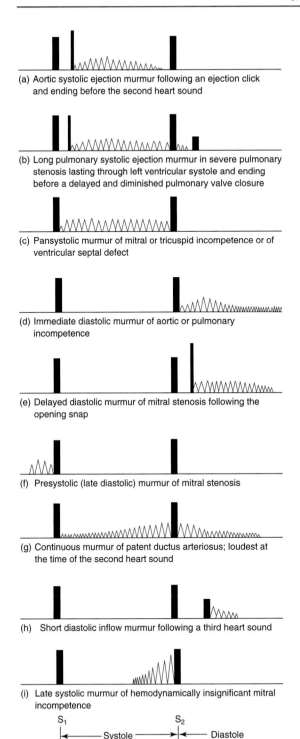

Figure 10–20. The timing of the principal cardiac murmurs. (Modified and reproduced, with permission, from Wood P: *Diseases of the Heart and Circulation,* 3rd ed. Lippincott, 1968.)

cause a murmur. For instance, ventricular septal defect is associated with a systolic murmur because of the abnormal interventricular connection and the pressure difference between the left and right ventricle; patent ductus arteriosus is associated with a continuous murmur because of a persistent connection between the pulmonary artery and the aorta. However, valvular lesions are the principal cause of heart murmurs. Thus, an understanding of heart murmurs gives insight into the underlying pathophysiologic processes of specific valvular lesions.

Heart murmurs can be either systolic or diastolic. During systole, while the left ventricle is contracting, the aortic valve is open and the mitral valve is closed. Turbulent flow can occur either because of an incompetent mitral valve, leading to regurgitation of blood back into the atrium, or from a narrowed aortic valve. In diastole, the situation is reversed, with filling of the left ventricle through an open mitral valve while the aortic valve is closed. Turbulent flow occurs when there is narrowing of the mitral valve or incompetence of the aortic valve. Stenosis of valves usually develops slowly over time; lesions that cause valvular regurgitation can be either chronic or acute.

1. AORTIC STENOSIS

Clinical Presentation

For all causes of aortic stenosis, there is usually a long latent period of slowly increasing obstruction before symptoms appear. In descending order of frequency, the three characteristic symptoms of aortic stenosis are chest pain (angina pectoris), syncope, and congestive heart failure (see above). Once symptoms occur, the prognosis is poor if the obstruction is untreated, with average life expectancies of 2, 3, and 5 years for angina pectoris, syncope, and heart failure, respectively.

On physical examination, palpation of the carotid upstroke reveals a pulsation (pulsus) that is both decreased (parvus) and late (tardus) relative to the apical impulse. Palpation of the chest reveals an apical impulse that is laterally displaced and sustained. On auscultation, a midsystolic murmur is heard, loudest at the base of the heart, and often with radiation to the sternal notch and the neck. Depending on the cause of the aortic stenosis, a crisp, relatively high-pitched aortic ejection sound can be heard just after the first heart sound. Finally, a fourth heart sound (S_4) is often present.

Etiology

Various causes of aortic stenosis are listed and described in Table 10–3.

Pathophysiology

The normal aortic valve area is approximately 3.5–4 cm^2. Critical aortic stenosis is usually present

Table 10–3. Causes of aortic stenosis.

Type	Pathology	Clinical Presentation
Congenital	The valve can be unicuspid, bicuspid, or tricuspid with partially fused leaflets. Abnormal flow can lead to fibrosis and calcification of the leaflets.	Patient usually develops symptoms before age 30.
Rheumatic	Tissue inflammation results in adhesion and fusing of the commissures. Fibrosis and calcification of the leaflet tips can occur because of continued turbulent flow.	Patient usually develops symptoms between ages 30 and 70. Often the valve will also be regurgitant. Accompanying mitral valve disease is frequently present.
Degenerative	Leaflets become inflexible because of calcium deposition at the bases. The leaflet tips remain relatively normal.	The most likely cause of aortic stenosis in patients over age 70. Particularly prevalent in patients with diabetes or hypercholesterolemia.

when the area is less than 0.8 cm². At this point, the systolic gradient between the left ventricle and the aorta can exceed 150 mm Hg, and most patients are symptomatic (Figure 10–21A). The fixed outflow obstruction places a large afterload on the ventricle. The compensatory mechanisms of the heart can be understood by examining Laplace's law for a sphere, where wall stress (T) is proportionate to the product of the transmural pressure (P) and cavitary radius (r) and inversely proportionate to wall thickness (w):

$$T \propto P \times \frac{r}{w}$$

In response to the pressure overload (increased P), left ventricular wall thickness markedly increases—while the cavitary radius remains relatively unchanged—by parallel replication of sarcomeres. These compensatory changes, termed "concentric hypertrophy," reduce the increase in wall tension observed in aortic stenosis (see Aortic Regurgitation). Analysis of pressure-volume loops reveals that in order to maintain stroke volume and because of decreases in ventricular compliance, left ventricular end-diastolic pressure increases significantly (Figure 10–21C). The thick ventricle leads to a prominent *a* wave on left atrial pressure tracings as the ventricle becomes more dependent on atrial contraction to fill the ventricle.

Clinical Manifestations
A. Symptoms:
1. Angina pectoris—Angina can occur because of several mechanisms. First, approximately half of all patients with aortic stenosis have significant concomitant coronary artery disease. Even without significant coronary artery disease, the combination of increased oxygen demands because of ventricular hypertrophy and decreased supply due to excessive compression of the vessels can lead to relative ischemia of the myocytes. Finally, coronary artery obstruction from calcium emboli arising from a calcified stenotic aortic valve has been reported, though it is an uncommon cause of angina.

2. Syncope—Syncope in aortic stenosis is usually due to decreased cerebral perfusion from the fixed obstruction, but it may also occur because of transient atrial arrhythmias with loss of effective atrial contribution to ventricular filling. In addition, arrhythmias arising from ventricular tissue are more common in patients with aortic stenosis and can cause syncope.

3. Congestive heart failure—(See Heart Failure, above.) The progressive increase in left ventricular end-diastolic pressure can cause elevated pulmonary venous pressure and pulmonary edema.

B. Physical Examination: Since there is a fixed obstruction to flow, the carotid upstroke is decreased and late. Left ventricular hypertrophy causes the apical impulse to be displaced laterally and to become sustained. The increased dependence on atrial contraction is responsible for the prominent S_4. Flow through the restricted orifice gives rise to a midsystolic murmur. The murmur is usually heard best at the base of the heart but often radiates to the neck and apex. The murmur is usually crescendo-decrescendo, and, in contrast to mitral regurgitation, the first and second heart sounds are usually easily heard. As aortic valve narrowing worsens, the murmur peaks later in systole. When calcified leaflets are present, the murmur tends to have a harsher quality. An aortic ejection sound, which is caused by the sudden checking of the leaflets as they open, is heard only when the leaflets remain fairly mobile, as in congenitally malformed valves.

While obstruction of blood flow from the left ventricle is usually due to valvular disease, obstruction can also occur above or below the valve and can present in somewhat the same way as valvular aortic stenosis. A membranous shelf that partially obstructs flow just above the valve in the aorta can sometimes be present from birth. In this condition, the systolic murmur is usually heard best at the first intercostal space at the right sternal border. Subvalvular stenosis

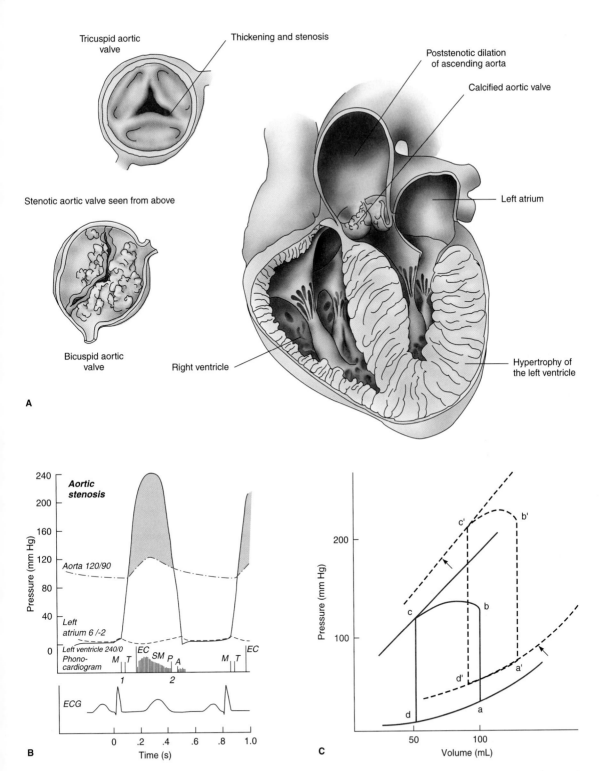

Figure 10–21. Aortic stenosis. **A:** Drawing of the left heart in left anterior oblique view showing anatomic features of aortic stenosis. Note structures enlarged: left ventricle (thickened); poststenotic dilation of the aorta. **B:** Drawing showing auscultatory and hemodynamic features of predominant aortic stenosis. Cardinal features include left ventricular hypertrophy; systolic ejection murmur. (EC, ejection click; SM, systolic murmur; P, pulmonary valve; A, aortic valve.) (Reproduced, with permission, from Cheitlin MD, Sokolow M, McIlroy MB: *Clinical Cardiology*, 6th ed. Appleton & Lange, 1993.) **C:** Pressure-volume loop in aortic stenosis. The left ventricle becomes thickened and less compliant, forcing the diastolic pressure-volume curve upward and to the right, which results in elevated left ventricular end-diastolic pressure **(a')**. Since the left ventricle must pump against a fixed gradient (increased afterload), **b** increases to **b'**. Finally, the hypertrophy of the ventricle results in increased inotropic force, which shifts the isovolumic pressure curve leftward.

Cardinal features:
Left ventricular (especially septal) hypertrophy, diastolic dysfunction; systolic outflow obstruction; systolic anterior motion of mitral valve; excessive left ventricular emptying.

Variable factors:
Severity; level of peripheral resistance; low resistance and low blood volume lead to obstruction.

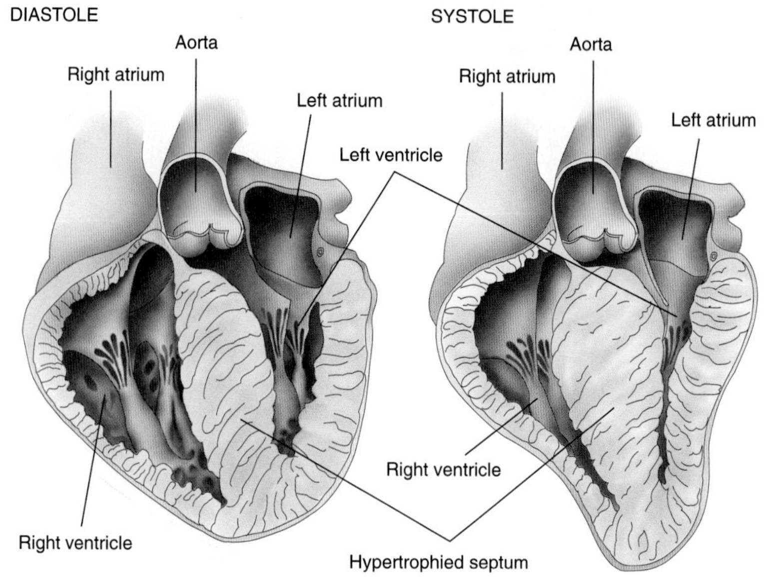

Figure 10–22. Hypertrophic cardiomyopathy (left lateral view). The cardinal features are displayed. (Reproduced, with permission, from Cheitlin MD, Sokolow M, McIlroy MB: *Clinical Cardiology,* 6th ed. Appleton & Lange, 1993.)

can occur in some patients who develop severe hypertrophy of the heart (Figure 10–22). This well-recognized clinical entity—hypertrophic cardiomyopathy—can also be manifested by a crescendo-decrescendo systolic murmur noted on physical examination. However, obstruction of the outflow tract in hypertrophic cardiomyopathy is dynamic, with greater obstruction when preload is decreased from decreased intraventricular volume. For this reason, having the patient stand or perform Valsalva's maneuver (forced expiration against a closed glottis), both of which decrease venous return, causes the murmur to increase. Both of these maneuvers cause a decrease in the murmur owing to valvular stenosis, since less absolute blood volume flows across the stenotic aortic valve.

2. AORTIC REGURGITATION

Clinical Presentation

Aortic regurgitation can be either chronic or acute. In chronic aortic regurgitation, there is a long latent period during which the patient remains asymptomatic as the heart responds to the volume load. When the compensatory mechanisms fail, symptoms of left-sided failure become manifest. In acute aortic regurgitation, there are no compensatory mechanisms, so shortness of breath, pulmonary edema, and hypotension, often with cardiovascular collapse, occur suddenly.

Physical examination of patients with chronic aortic regurgitation reveals hyperdynamic (pounding) pulses. The apical impulse is hyperdynamic and displaced laterally. On auscultation, three murmurs may be heard: a high-pitched early diastolic murmur, a diastolic rumble called the Austin Flint murmur, and a systolic murmur. A third heart sound is often present. However, in acute aortic regurgitation, the peripheral signs are often absent, and in many cases the left ventricular impulse is normal. On auscultation, the diastolic murmur is much softer, and the Austin Flint murmur, if present, is short. The first heart sound will be soft and sometimes absent.

Etiology

Acute and chronic aortic regurgitation can be due to either valvular or aortic root abnormalities (Table 10–4).

Pathophysiology

Aortic regurgitation places a volume load on the left ventricle, since during diastole blood enters the ventricle both from the left atrium and from the aorta. If the regurgitation develops slowly, the heart responds to the increased diastolic pressure by fiber elongation and replication of sarcomeres in series, which leads to increased ventricular volumes. Since systolic pressure remains relatively unchanged, increased wall stress—by Laplace's law—can be compensated for by an additional increase in wall thickness. This response, "eccentric hypertrophy" (so

Table 10–4. Causes of aortic regurgitation.

Site	Pathology	Causes	Time Course
Valvular	Cusp abnormalities	Endocarditis Rheumatic disease Ankylosing spondylitis Congenital	Acute or chronic Acute or chronic Usually chronic Chronic

Aortic	Dilation	Aortic aneurysm
		Heritable disorders of connective tissue
		  Marfan's syndrome
		  Ehlers-Danlos syndrome
		  Osteogenesis imperfecta
			Acute or chronic
			Usually chronic

	Inflammation	Aortitis (Takayasu)
		Syphilis
		Arthritic diseases
		  Ankylosing spondylitis
		  Reiter's syndrome
		  Rheumatoid arthritis
		  Systemic lupus erythematosus
		Cystic medial necrosis
			Usually chronic
			Usually chronic
			Usually chronic
			
			Acute or chronic

	Tears with loss of commissural support	Trauma Dissection, often from hypertension	Usually acute Usually acute

named because the ventricular cavity enlarges laterally in the chest and becomes eccentric to its normal position), explains the different ventricular geometry observed in patients with aortic regurgitation when compared with patients who have aortic stenosis (concentric hypertrophy due to the systolic pressure overload). Ultimately, chronic aortic regurgitation leads to huge ventricular volumes as demonstrated in the pressure-volume loops (Figure 10–23). The left ventricle operates as a low-compliance pump, handling large end-diastolic and stroke volumes, often with little increase in end-diastolic pressure. In addition, no truly isovolumic period of relaxation or contraction exists because of the persistent flow into the ventricle from the systemic circulation. Aortic pulse pressure is widened. Diastolic pressure decreases because of regurgitant flow back into the left ventricle and increased compliance of the large central vessels (in response to increased stroke volume); elevated stroke volume leads to increased systolic pressures (Figure 10–23C).

Clinical Manifestations

A. Shortness of Breath: Pulmonary edema can develop, particularly if the aortic regurgitation is acute and the ventricle does not have time to compensate for the sudden increase in volume. In chronic aortic regurgitation, compensatory mechanisms eventually fail and the heart begins to operate on the steeper portion of the diastolic pressure-volume relationship.

B. Physical Examination:

1. Hyperdynamic pulses–In chronic aortic regurgitation, a widened pulse pressure is responsible for several characteristic peripheral signs. Palpation of the peripheral pulse reveals a sudden rise and then drop in pressure (water-hammer or Corrigan's pulse). Head bobbing (DeMusset's sign), rhythmic pulsation of the uvula (Müller's sign), and arterial pulsation seen in the nail bed (Quincke's pulse) have been described in patients with chronic aortic regurgitation.

2. Murmurs–Three heart murmurs can be heard in patients with aortic regurgitation: First, flow from the regurgitant volume back into the left ventricle can be heard as a high-pitched, blowing, early diastolic murmur usually perceived best along the left sternal border. Second, the rumbling murmur described by Austin Flint can be heard at the apex during any part of diastole. The Austin Flint murmur is thought to result from regurgitant flow from the aortic valve impinging on the anterior leaflet of the mitral valve, producing functional mitral stenosis. Finally, a crescendo-decrescendo systolic murmur, which is thought to arise from the increased stroke volume flowing across the aortic valve, can be heard at the left sternal border.

In acute, severe aortic regurgitation, the early diastolic murmur may be softer owing to rapid diastolic equalization of ventricular and aortic pressures. The first heart sound is soft because of early mitral valve closure from aortic regurgitation and elevated ventricular pressures.

3. Third heart sound–A third heart sound can be heard because of concomitant heart failure or because of the exaggerated early diastolic filling of the left ventricle.

4. Apical impulse–The apical impulse is displaced laterally because of the increased volume of the left ventricle.

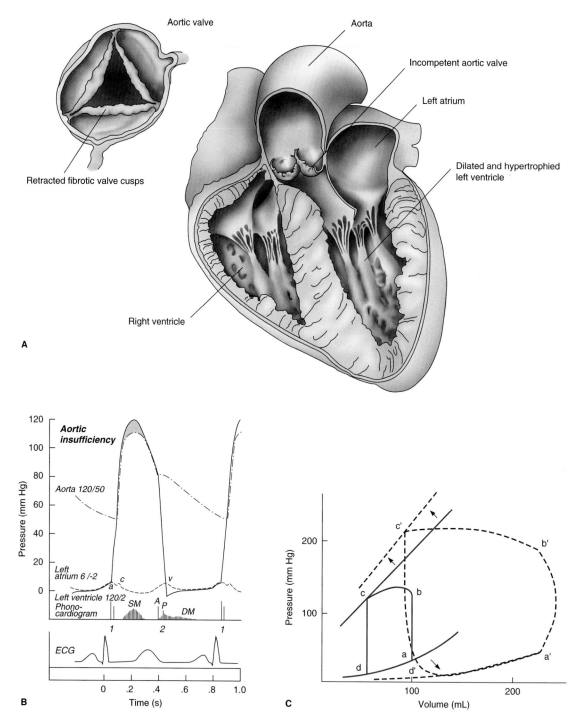

Figure 10–23. Aortic insufficiency (regurgitation). **A:** Drawing of the left heart in left anterior oblique view showing anatomic features of aortic insufficiency. Note structures enlarged: left ventricle, aorta. **B:** Drawing showing auscultatory and hemodynamic features of predominant aortic insufficiency. Cardinal features include large hypertrophied left ventricle; large aorta; increased stroke volume; wide pulse pressure; diastolic murmur. (SM, systolic murmur; A, aortic valve; P, pulmonary valve; DM, diastolic murmur.) (Reproduced, with permission, from Cheitlin MD, Sokolow M, McIlroy MB: *Clinical Cardiology,* 6th ed. Appleton & Lange, 1993.) **C:** Pressure-volume loop in chronic aortic insufficiency. Marked enlargement in left ventricular volume shifts the diastolic pressure-volume curve rightward. Hypertrophy of the ventricle shifts the isovolumic pressure-volume curve leftward. Stroke volume is enormous, although effective stroke volume may be minimally changed since much of the increase in stroke volume leaks back into the ventricle. Since the ventricle is constantly being filled from the mitral valve or the incompetent aortic valve, no isovolumic periods exist.

3. MITRAL STENOSIS

Clinical Presentation

The symptoms of mitral stenosis include dyspnea, fatigue, and hemoptysis. Occasionally, the patient complains of palpitations or a rapid heart beat. Finally, the patient with mitral stenosis may present with neurologic symptoms such as transient numbness or weakness of the extremities, sudden loss of vision, or difficulty with coordination.

The characteristic murmur of mitral stenosis is a late low-pitched diastolic rumble. In addition, an opening snap may be heard in the first portion of diastole (Figure 10–24). Auscultation of the lungs may reveal rales.

Etiology

Mitral stenosis is most commonly a sequela of rheumatic heart disease (Table 10–5). Infrequently, it may be caused by congenital lesions or calcium deposition. Atrial masses (myxomas) can cause intermittent obstruction of the mitral valve.

Pathophysiology

The mitral valve is normally bicuspid, with the anterior cusp approximately twice the area of the posterior cusp. The mitral valve area is usually 5–6 cm^2; clinically relevant mitral stenosis usually occurs when the valve area decreases to less than 1 cm^2. Since obstruction of flow protects the ventricle from pressure and volume loads, the left ventricular pressure-volume relationship shows relatively little abnormality other than decreased volumes. However, analysis of hemodynamic tracings shows the characteristic elevation in left atrial pressures (Figure 10–24B). For this reason, the main pathophysiologic abnormality in mitral stenosis is elevated pulmonary venous and right-sided (pulmonary artery, right ventricle, and right atrium) pressures. Dilation and reduced systolic function of the right ventricle are commonly observed in patients with advanced mitral stenosis.

Clinical Manifestations
A. Symptoms:
1. Shortness of breath, hemoptysis, and orthopnea–All of these symptoms occur because of elevated left atrial, pulmonary venous, and pulmonary capillary pressures (the actual mechanisms are described in the section on congestive heart failure).

2. Palpitations–Increased left atrial size predisposes patients with mitral stenosis to atrial arrhythmias. Chaotic atrial activity, or atrial fibrillation, is commonly observed. Since ventricular filling is particularly dependent on atrial contraction in patients with mitral stenosis, acute hemodynamic decompensation may occur when organized contraction of the atrium is lost.

3. Neurologic symptoms–Reduced outflow leads to dilation of the left atrium and stasis of blood flow. Thrombus in the left atrium is observed in approximately 20% of patients with mitral stenosis, and the prevalence increases with age, the presence of atrial fibrillation, the severity of stenosis, and any reduction in cardiac output. Embolic events that lead to neurologic symptoms occur in 8% of patients in sinus rhythm and 32% of patients with chronic or paroxysmal atrial fibrillation. In addition, left atrial enlargement can sometimes impinge on the recurrent laryngeal nerve and lead to hoarseness (Ortner's syndrome).

B. Physical Examination: On auscultation of the heart, the diastolic rumble occurs because of turbulent flow across the narrowed mitral valve orifice. An opening snap, analogous to the ejection click described for aortic stenosis, may be heard in early diastole. The opening snap is heard only when the patient has relatively mobile leaflets.

Rales occur because elevated pulmonary capillary pressures lead to accumulation of intra-alveolar fluid.

4. MITRAL REGURGITATION

Clinical Presentation

The presentation of mitral regurgitation depends on how quickly valvular incompetence develops. Patients with chronic mitral regurgitation develop symptoms gradually over time. Common complaints include dyspnea, easy fatigability, and palpitations. Patients with acute mitral regurgitation present with symptoms of left heart failure: shortness of breath, orthopnea, and shock. Chest pain may be present in patients whose mitral regurgitation is due to coronary artery disease.

On physical examination, patients have a pansystolic regurgitant murmur that is heard best at the apex and often radiates to the axilla. This murmur often obscures the first and second heart sounds. When mitral valve incompetence is severe, a third heart sound is often present. In chronic mitral regurgitation, the apical impulse is often hyperdynamic and displaced laterally.

Etiology

In the past, rheumatic heart disease accounted for most cases of mitral regurgitation. Mitral valve prolapse is now probably the most common cause, followed by coronary artery disease. The tips of the anterior and posterior mitral valve leaflets are held in place during ventricular contraction by the anterolateral and posteromedial papillary muscles. The valves are connected to the papillary muscles via thin fibrous structures called chordae tendineae. In patients with mitral valve prolapse, extra tissue present on the valvular apparatus can undergo myxomatous degeneration by the fifth or sixth decades. Mitral regurgita-

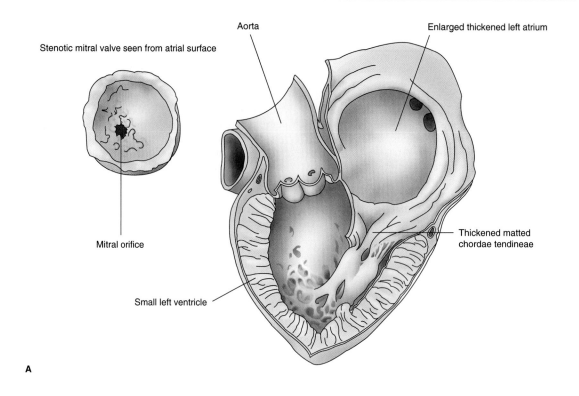
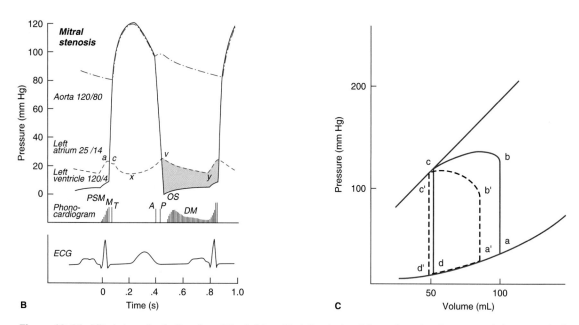

Figure 10–24. Mitral stenosis. **A:** Drawing of the left heart in left anterior oblique view showing anatomic features of mitral stenosis. Note enlarged left atrium, small left ventricle. **B:** Drawing showing auscultatory and hemodynamic features of mitral stenosis. Cardinal features include thickening and fusion of mitral valve cusps, elevated left atrial pressure, left atrial enlargement, opening snap, diastolic murmur. (PSM, presystolic murmur; OS, opening snap; M, mitral; T, tricuspid; A, aortic; P, pulmonary; DM, diastolic murmur). (Reproduced, with permission, from Cheitlin MD, Sokolow M, McIlroy MB: *Clinical Cardiology,* 6th ed. Appleton & Lange, 1993.) **C:** Pressure-volume loop in mitral stenosis. Filling of the left ventricle is restricted from **a** to **a′**, decreasing stroke volume to **b′c′**.

Table 10–5. Causes of mitral stenosis.

Type	Comments
Rheumatic	Most common. Narrowing results from fusion and thickening of the commissures, cusps, and chordae. Symptoms usually develop 20 years after acute rheumatic fever.
Calcific	Usually causes mitral regurgitation but can cause mitral stenosis in some cases.
Congenital	Usually presents during infancy or childhood.
Collagen-vascular disease	Systemic lupus erythematosus and rheumatoid arthritis (rare).

tion follows, either from poor coaptation of the valve leaflets or from sudden rupture of the chordae tendineae. In coronary artery disease, obstruction of the circumflex coronary artery can lead to ischemia or rupture of the papillary muscles (Table 10–6).

Pathophysiology

When the mitral valve fails to close properly, regurgitation of blood into the left atrium from the ventricle occurs during systole. In chronic mitral regurgitation, the compensatory mechanism to this volume load is similar to the changes seen in aortic regurgitation. The left ventricle and atrium dilate, and to normalize wall stress in the ventricle there is also concomitant hypertrophy of the ventricular wall (see discussion of Laplace's law). Diastolic filling of the ventricle increases since it is now the sum of right ventricular output and the regurgitant volume from the previous beat. In acute mitral regurgitation, the sudden volume load on the atrium and ventricle is not compensated for by chamber enlargement and hypertrophy. The sudden increase in atrial volume leads to prominent atrial v waves with transmission of this elevated pressure to the pulmonary capillaries and the development of pulmonary edema (Figure 10–25).

Table 10–6. Causes of mitral regurgitation.

Type	Causes
Acute	
Ruptured chordae	Infective endocarditis Trauma Acute rheumatic fever "Spontaneous"
Ruptured or dysfunctional papillary muscles	Ischemia Myocardial infarction Trauma Myocardial abscess
Perforated leaflet	Infective endocarditis Trauma
Chronic	
Inflammatory	Rheumatic heart disease Collagen vascular disease
Infection	Infective endocarditis
Degenerative	Myxomatous degeneration of the valve leaflets Calcification of the mitral annulus
Rupture or dysfunction of the chordae tendineae or papillary muscles	Infective endocarditis Trauma Acute rheumatic fever "Spontaneous" Ischemia Myocardial infarction Myocardial abscess
Congenital	Developmental anomalies

Clinical Manifestations

A. Symptoms:

1. Pulmonary edema–Rapid elevation of pulmonary capillary pressure in acute mitral regurgitation leads to the sudden onset of pulmonary edema, manifested by shortness of breath, orthopnea, and paroxysmal nocturnal dyspnea. In chronic mitral regurgitation, the symptoms develop gradually, but at some point the compensatory mechanisms fail and pulmonary edema develops, particularly with exercise.

2. Fatigue–Fatigue can develop because of decreased forward blood flow to the peripheral tissues.

3. Palpitations–Left atrial enlargement may lead to the development of atrial fibrillation and accompanying palpitations. Patients with atrial fibrillation and mitral regurgitation have a 20% incidence of cardioembolic events.

B. Physical Examination:

1. Holosystolic murmur–Regurgitant flow into the atrium produces a high-pitched murmur that is heard throughout systole. The murmur begins with the first heart sound and continues to the second heart sound and is of constant intensity throughout systole. It finally ends when left ventricular pressure drops to equal left atrial pressure during isovolumic relaxation. Unlike the murmur of aortic stenosis, there is little variation in the intensity of the murmur as the heart rate changes. In addition, the murmur does not change in intensity with respiration. It is usually heard best at the apex and often radiates to the axilla. If rupture of the anterior leaflet has occurred, the mitral regurgitation murmur will sometimes radiate to the back.

2. Third heart sound–A third heart sound is heard if heart failure is present. Because of increased and rapid filling of the ventricle during diastole, it may also be heard in the absence of overt failure in patients with severe mitral regurgitation.

3. Displaced and hyperdynamic apical impulse–The compensatory increase in left ventricular

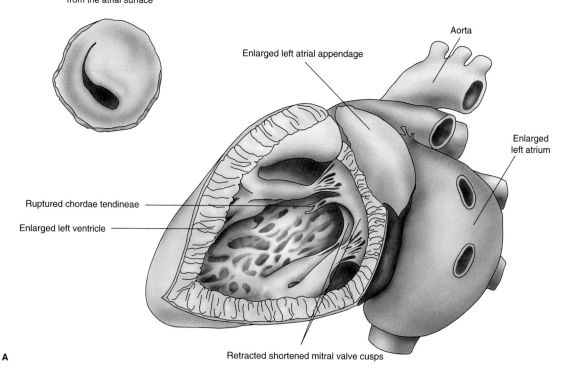
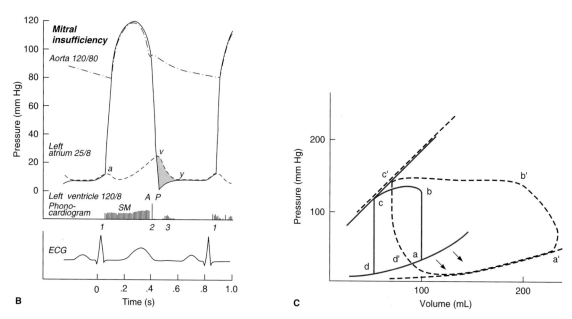

Figure 10–25. Mitral insufficiency (regurgitation). **A:** Drawing of the left heart in left lateral view showing anatomic features of mitral insufficiency. Note structures enlarged: left atrium, left ventricle. **B:** Drawing showing auscultatory and hemodynamic features of mitral insufficiency. Cardinal features include systolic backflow into left atrium, left atrial enlargement, left ventricular enlargement (hypertrophy in acute lesions), prominent v wave due to filling from both the pulmonary veins and the regurgitant jet, holosystolic murmur. (3, third heart sound; SM, systolic murmur; A, aortic; P, pulmonary.) (Reproduced, with permission, from Cheitlin MD, Sokolow M, McIlroy MB: *Clinical Cardiology,* 6th ed. Appleton & Lange, 1993.) **C:** Pressure-volume loop in mitral insufficiency. Increased ventricular volumes shift the diastolic pressure-volume curve rightward. Stroke volume is increased since the ventricle can now eject blood into the low-pressure left atrium.

volume and wall thickness in patients with chronic mitral regurgitation is manifested by a laterally displaced apical impulse. Since the ventricle now has a low pressure chamber (the left atrium) into which to eject blood, the apical impulse is often hyperdynamic. When mitral regurgitation develops suddenly, the apical impulse is not displaced or hyperdynamic, since the left ventricle has not had enough time for compensatory volume increases.

---

10. What are the clinical presentations of each of the four major categories of valvular heart disease?
11. What are the most common causes of each category of valvular heart disease?
12. What is the pathogenesis of each category of valvular heart disease?
13. What are the major clinical manifestations and complications of each category of valvular heart disease?

Table 10–7. Causes of coronary artery disease.

Type	Comments
Atherosclerosis	Most common cause. Risk factors include hypertension, hypercholesterolemia, diabetes mellitus, smoking, and a family history of atherosclerosis.
Spasm	Coronary artery vasospasm can occur in any population but is most prevalent in Japanese. Vasoconstriction appears to be mediated by histamine, serotonin, catecholamines, and endothelium-derived factors. Since spasm can occur at any time, the chest pain is often not exertion-related.
Emboli	Rare cause of coronary artery disease. Can occur from vegetations in patients with endocarditis.
Congenital	Congenital coronary artery abnormalities are present in 1–2% of the population. However, only a small fraction of these abnormalities cause symptomatic ischemia.

CORONARY ARTERY DISEASE

Clinical Presentation

Chest pain is the most common symptom associated with coronary artery disease. It is usually described as dull, and it can often radiate down the arm or to the jaw. It does not worsen with a deep breath and can be associated with shortness of breath, diaphoresis, nausea, or vomiting. This entire symptom complex has been termed **angina pectoris,** or "pain in the breast"; this phrase was first used by Heberden in 1772.

Clinically, angina is classified according to the precipitant and duration of symptoms. If the pain occurs only with exertion and has been stable over a long period of time, it is termed **stable angina.** If the pain occurs at rest, it is termed **unstable angina.** Finally, regardless of the precipitant, if the chest pain persists without interruption for prolonged periods and irreversible myocyte damage has occurred, it is termed **myocardial infarction.**

On physical examination, the patient with coronary artery disease may have a fourth heart sound or signs of congestive heart failure and shock. However, more than any other cardiovascular problem, the initial diagnosis relies on patient history.

Etiology

Atherosclerotic obstruction of the large epicardial vessels is by far the most common cause of coronary artery disease. Spasm of the coronary arteries from various mediators such as serotonin and histamine has been well described and is more common in Japanese. Rarely, congenital abnormalities can cause coronary artery diseases (Table 10–7).

Pathophysiology

Coronary blood flow brings oxygen to myocytes and removes waste products such as carbon dioxide, lactic acid, and hydrogen ions. The heart has a tremendously high metabolic requirement; although it accounts for only 0.3% of body weight, it is responsible for 7% of the body's resting oxygen consumption. Cellular ischemia occurs when there is either increased demand for oxygen relative to maximal arterial supply or when there is an absolute reduction in oxygen supply. While situations of increased demand, such as thyrotoxicosis and aortic stenosis, can cause myocardial ischemia, most clinical cases are due to decreased oxygen supply. Reduced oxygen supply can rarely arise from decreased oxygen content in blood, such as in carbon monoxide poisoning or anemia, but more commonly stems from coronary artery abnormalities (Table 10–7), particularly atherosclerotic disease. Myocardial ischemia may arise from a combination of increased demand and decreased supply; cocaine abuse increases oxygen demand (by inhibiting reuptake of norepinephrine at adrenergic nerve endings in the heart) and can reduce oxygen supply by causing vasospasm.

Atherosclerosis of large coronary arteries remains the predominant cause of angina and myocardial infarction. Raised fatty streaks, which appear as yellow spots or streaks in the vessel walls, are seen in coronary arteries in almost all members of any population by 20 years of age (see Chapter 11). They are found mainly in areas exposed to increased shear stresses such as bending points and bifurcations and are thought to arise from isolated macrophage foam cell migration into areas of minimal chronic intimal injury. In many people this process progresses, with additional migration of foam cells, smooth muscle cell proliferation, and extracellular fat and collagen deposition (Figure 10–26). The extent and incidence of these advanced lesions vary among persons in different geographic regions and ethnic groups.

The underlying pathophysiologic processes differ for each clinical presentation of coronary artery disease. In patients with **stable angina,** fixed narrowing of one or several coronary arteries is usually present. Since the large coronary arteries usually function as conduits and do not offer resistance to flow, the arterial lumen must be decreased by 90% to produce cellular ischemia when the patient is at rest. However, with exercise, a 50% reduction in lumen size can lead to symptoms. In patients with **unstable angina,** fissuring of the atherosclerotic plaque can lead to platelet accumulation and transient episodes of thrombotic occlusion, usually lasting 10–20 minutes. In addition, platelet release of vasoconstrictive factors such as thromboxane A_2 or serotonin and endothelial dysfunction may cause vasoconstriction and contribute to decreased flow. In **myocardial infarction,** deep arterial injury from plaque rupture may cause formation of a relatively fixed and persistent thrombus.

The heart receives its energy primarily from ATP generated by oxidative phosphorylation of free fatty acids, though glucose and other carbohydrates can be utilized. Within 60 seconds after coronary artery occlusion, myocardial oxygen tension in the affected cells falls essentially to zero. Cardiac stores of high-energy phosphates are rapidly depleted, and the cells shift rapidly to anaerobic metabolism with consequent lactic acid production. Dysfunction of myocardial relaxation and contraction occurs within seconds, even before depletion of high-energy phosphates occurs. The biochemical basis for this abnormality is not known. If perfusion is not restored within 40–60 minutes, an irreversible stage of injury characterized by diffuse mitochondrial swelling, damage to the cell membrane, and marked depletion of glycogen begins. The exact mechanism by which irreversible damage occurs is not clear, but severe ATP depletion, increased extracellular calcium concentrations, lactic acidosis, and free radicals have all been postulated as possible causes.

In experimental preparations, if ischemic myocardium is perfused within 5 minutes, systolic function returns promptly whereas diastolic abnormalities may take up to 40 minutes to normalize. With prolonged episodes of ischemia—up to 1 hour—it may take up to a month to restore ventricular function. When the heart demonstrates this prolonged period of decreased function despite normal perfusion, the myocardium is said to be "stunned." The biochemical basis for stunning is poorly understood. If reper-

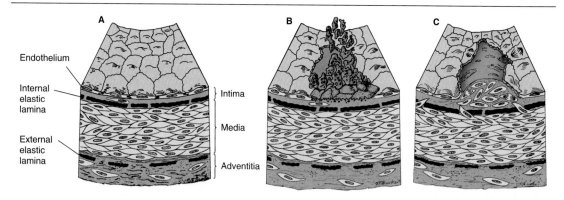

Figure 10–26. Mechanisms of production of atheroma. **A:** Structure of normal muscular artery. The adventitia, or outermost layer of the artery, consists principally of recognizable fibroblasts intermixed with smooth muscle cells loosely arranged between bundles of collagen and surrounded by proteoglycans. It is usually separated from the media by a discontinuous sheet of elastic tissue, the external elastic lamina. **B:** Platelet aggregates, or microthrombi, form as a result of adherence of the platelets to the exposed subendothelial connective tissue. Platelets that adhere to the connective tissue release granules whose constituents may gain entry into the arterial wall. Platelet factors thus interact with plasma constituents in the artery wall and may stimulate events shown in the next illustration. **C:** Smooth muscle cells migrate from the media into the intima through fenestrae in the internal elastic lamina and actively multiply within the intima. Endothelial cells regenerate in an attempt to re-cover the exposed intima, which thickens rapidly owing to smooth muscle proliferation and formation of new connective tissue. (Reproduced, with permission, from Ross R, Glomset JA: The pathogenesis of atherosclerosis. [Part 1.] N Engl J Med 1976;295:369.)

fusion occurs later or not at all, systolic function often will not return to the affected area.

Clinical Manifestations

A. Chest Pain: Chest pain in the past has traditionally been ascribed to ischemia. However, recent evidence suggests that in patients with coronary artery disease, 70–80% of episodes of ischemia are actually asymptomatic. When present, the chest pain is thought to be mediated by sympathetic afferent fibers that richly innervate the atrium and ventricle. From the heart, the fibers traverse the upper thoracic sympathetic ganglia and the five upper thoracic dorsal roots of the spinal cord. In the spinal cord, the impulses probably converge with impulses from other structures. This convergence is probably the mechanism for chest wall, back, and arm pain that can sometimes accompany angina pectoris. The importance of these fibers can be demonstrated in patients who have had a heart transplant. When these patients develop atherosclerosis, they remain completely asymptomatic, without development of angina.

Recent evidence suggests that the actual trigger for nerve stimulation is adenosine. Adenosine infusion into the coronary arteries can produce the characteristic symptoms of angina without evidence of ischemia. In addition, blocking the adenosine receptor (P_1) with aminophylline leads to reduced anginal symptoms despite similar degrees of ischemia.

The large proportion of asymptomatic episodes of ischemia probably has three causes: (1) Dysfunction of afferent nerves may cause silent ischemia. Patients with transplanted hearts do not sense cardiac pain despite significant atherosclerosis. Peripheral neuropathy in patients with diabetes may explain the increased episodes of silent ischemia described in this patient population. (2) Transient reduced perfusion may also be an important mechanism for silent ischemia. Within a few seconds after cessation of perfusion, systolic and diastolic abnormalities can be observed. Angina is a relatively late event, occurring after at least 30 seconds of ischemia. (3) Finally, differing pain thresholds between patients may explain the high prevalence of silent ischemia. The presence of angina is moderately correlated with a decreased pain tolerance. The mechanism for different pain thresholds is unknown but may be due to differences in plasma endorphins.

B. Fourth Heart Sound and Shortness of Breath: Both of these findings may occur because of diastolic and systolic dysfunction of the ischemic myocardium. (See the section on congestive heart failure, above.)

C. Shock: The site of coronary artery occlusion determines the clinical presentation of myocardial ischemia or infarction. As a general rule, the more myocardium that is supplied by the occluded vessel, the more significant and severe the symptoms. For example, obstruction of the left main coronary artery or the proximal left anterior descending coronary artery will usually present as severe cardiac failure, often with associated hypotension (shock). In addition, shock may be associated with coronary artery disease in several special situations. If necrosis of the septum occurs from left anterior descending artery occlusion, myocardial rupture with the formation of an interventricular septal defect can occur. Rupture of the anterior or lateral free walls from occlusion of the left anterior descending or circumflex coronary arteries, respectively, can lead to the formation of pericardial effusion and tamponade. Rupture of myocardial tissue usually occurs 4–7 days after the acute ischemic event, when the myocardial wall has thinned and is in the process of healing. Sudden hemodynamic decompensation during this period should arouse suspicion of these complications. Finally, circumflex artery occlusion may result in ischemia and dysfunction or overt rupture of the papillary muscles, which can produce severe mitral regurgitation and shock.

D. Bradycardia: Inferior wall myocardial infarctions usually arise from occlusion of the right coronary artery. Since the area of left ventricular tissue supplied by this artery is small, patients usually do not present with heart failure. However, the artery that provides blood supply to the AV node branches off the posterior descending artery, so that inferior wall myocardial infarctions are sometimes associated with slowed or absent conduction in the AV node. Besides ischemia, AV nodal conduction abnormalities can occur because of reflex activation of the vagus nerve, which richly innervates the AV node.

Dysfunction of the sinus node is rarely seen in coronary artery disease, since this area receives blood from both the right and the left coronary arteries.

E. Nausea and Vomiting: Nausea and vomiting may arise from activation of the vagus nerve in the setting of an inferior wall myocardial infarction.

F. Tachycardia: Levels of catecholamines are usually raised in patients with myocardial infarction. This helps to maintain stroke volume but leads to an increased heart rate.

---

14. What is the clinical presentation of coronary artery disease (CAD) along the continuum from stable angina to unstable angina to myocardial infarction?
15. What are the most common causes of CAD?
16. How are the pathophysiology of stable angina, unstable angina, and myocardial infarction different?
17. What are the major clinical manifestations and complications of CAD?

PERICARDIAL DISEASE

Pericardial disease may include inflammation of the pericardium (pericarditis) or abnormal amounts of fluid in the space between the visceral and parietal pericardium (pericardial effusion).

PERICARDITIS

Clinical Presentation

The patient presents with severe chest pain. Descriptions of the pain are variable, but the usual picture is of a sharp retrosternal onset with radiation to the back and worse with deep breathing or coughing. The pain is often position-dependent—worse when lying flat and improved while sitting up and leaning forward.

On physical examination, the pericardial rub is pathognomonic for pericarditis. It is a high-pitched squeaking sound, often with two or more components.

Occasionally, continual inflammation of the pericardium leads to fibrosis and the development of constrictive pericarditis (Figure 10–27). Examination of the jugular venous pulsation is critical in the patient who may have constrictive pericarditis. The jugular venous pressure is elevated, and the individual waveforms are often quite prominent. In addition, there can be an inappropriate increase in the jugular venous pulsation level with inspiration (Kussmaul's sign). Hepatomegaly and ascites may be noted on physical examination. On auscultation of the heart, a high-pitched sound called a pericardial knock can be heard just after the second heart sound, often mimicking a third heart sound.

Table 10–8. Causes of pericarditis.

Infections
Viral: Coxsackievirus
Bacterial
Tuberculosis
Purulent: Staphylococcal, pneumococcal
Protozoal: Amebiasis
Mycotic: Actinomycosis, coccidioidomycosis
Collagen-vascular disease
Systemic lupus erythematosus
Scleroderma
Rheumatoid arthritis
Neoplasm
Metabolic
Renal failure
Injury
Myocardial infarction
Postinfarction
Postthoracotomy
Trauma
Radiation
Idiopathic

Etiology

Table 10–8 lists the causes of acute pericarditis. Viruses, particularly the coxsackieviruses, are the most common cause of acute pericarditis. Viruses are also probably responsible for "idiopathic" pericarditis.

Pathophysiology

In pericarditis, microscopic examination of the pericardium shows signs of acute inflammation, with increased numbers of polymorphonuclear leukocytes, increased vascularity, and deposition of fibrin. If the inflammation is long-lived, the pericardium can become fibrotic and scarred, with deposition of calcium.

The heavily fibrotic pericardium can inhibit the filling of the ventricles. At this point, signs of constrictive pericarditis appear (see below).

Clinical Manifestations

A. Chest Pain: Chest pain is probably due to inflammation of the pericardium. Inflammation of adjacent pleura may account for the characteristic worsening of pain with deep breathing and coughing.

B. Physical Examination:

1. Friction rub—The pericardial friction rub is thought to arise from friction between the visceral and parietal pericardial surfaces. The rub is traditionally described as having three components, each as-

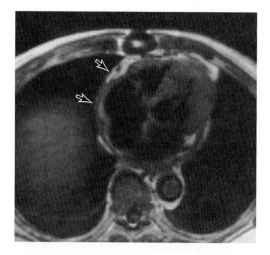

Figure 10–27. Magnetic resonance image of cross-section of thorax showing pericardial thickening (arrows) in a patient with constrictive pericarditis. (Courtesy of C Higgins. Reproduced, with permission, from Cheitlin MD, Sokolow M, McIlroy MB: *Clinical Cardiology,* 6th ed. Appleton & Lange, 1993.)

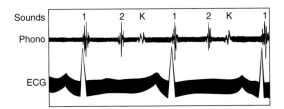

Figure 10–28. Phonocardiogram of typical sharp, early diastolic pericardial knock (K). (Courtesy of Roche Laboratories Division of Hoffman-La Roche, Inc.)

sociated with rapid movement of a cardiac chamber: The systolic component, which is probably related to ventricular contraction, is most common and most easily heard. During diastole, there are two components—one during early diastole, due to rapid filling of the ventricle; and another quieter component that occurs in late diastole, thought to be due to atrial contraction. The diastolic components often merge so that a two-component or "to-and-fro" rub is most commonly heard.

2. Signs of constriction—In the patient with constrictive pericarditis, early diastolic filling of the ventricle occurs normally but the filling is suddenly stopped by the nonelastic thickened pericardium. This cessation of filling can be observed on the pressure-time curve of the ventricle and is probably responsible for the diastolic knock (Figure 10–28). In addition, the rapid emptying of the atrium leads to a prominent y descent that makes the v wave more noticeable on the atrial pressure tracing (Figure 10–29). Systemic venous pressure is elevated, since flow entering the heart is limited. Usually with inspiration, the decrease in intrathoracic pressure is transmitted to the heart, and filling of the right side of the heart increases with an accompanying fall in systemic venous pressure. In patients with constrictive pericarditis, this normal response is prevented and the patient develops Kussmaul's sign (Figure 10–30). Elevated systemic venous pressure can lead to accumulation of fluid in the liver and intraperitoneal space, leading to hepatomegaly and ascites.

PERICARDIAL EFFUSION & TAMPONADE

Clinical Presentation

Pericardial effusion may occur in response to any cause of pericarditis, so the patient may develop chest pain or pericardial rub as described above. In addition, pericardial effusion may develop slowly and may be asymptomatic. However, sudden filling of the pericardial space with fluid can have catastrophic consequences by limiting ventricular filling (pericardial tamponade). Patients with pericardial tamponade often complain of shortness of breath, but the diagnosis is most commonly made by noting the characteristic physical examination findings associated with pericardial tamponade.

Pericardial tamponade is accompanied by characteristic physical signs that arise from the limited fill-

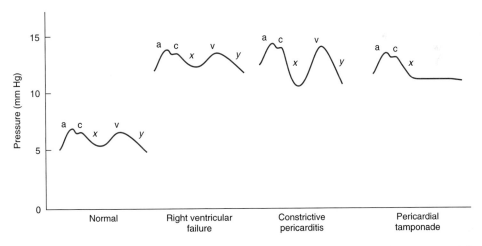

Figure 10–29. Jugular venous pressure waveforms in various kinds of heart disease. In right ventricular failure, mean jugular venous pressure is elevated, but the waveforms remain relatively unchanged. If right ventricular failure is accompanied by tricuspid regurgitation, the v wave may become more prominent (since the right atrium is receiving blood both from systemic venous return and the right ventricle). In constrictive pericarditis the y descent becomes prominent since the right ventricle rapidly fills in early diastole. In contrast, in pericardial tamponade, the right ventricle only fills during early systole, so that only an r descent is observed. In both constrictive pericarditis and pericardial tamponade, mean jugular venous pressure is elevated.

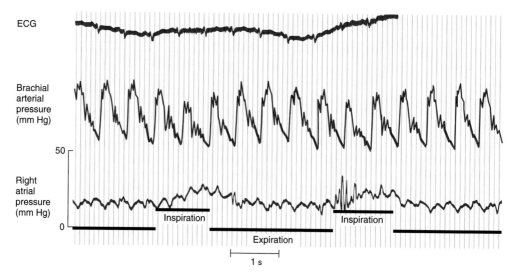

Figure 10–30. Brachial arterial and right atrial pressures showing pulsus paradoxus in a patient with constrictive pericarditis and an increase in right atrial pressure on inspiration (Kussmaul's sign). Both the systolic and diastolic atrial pressures rise with inspiration. (Reproduced, with permission, from Cheitlin MD, Sokolow M, McIlroy MB: *Clinical Cardiology*, 6th ed. Appleton & Lange, 1993.)

ing of the ventricle. The three classic signs of pericardial tamponade are called Beck's triad after the surgeon who described them in 1935: (1) hypotension, (2) elevated jugular venous pressure, and (3) muffled heart sounds. In addition, the patient may have a decrease in systemic pressure with inspiration ("paradoxic pulse").

Etiology

Almost any cause of pericarditis can cause pericardial effusion.

Pathophysiology

The pericardium is normally filled with a small amount of fluid (30–50 mL) with an intrapericardial pressure that is usually similar to the intrapleural pressure. With the sudden addition of fluid, the pericardial pressure can increase, at times to the level of the right atrial and right ventricular pressures. The transmural distending pressure of the ventricle decreases and the chamber collapses, preventing appropriate filling of the heart from systemic venous return. The four chambers of the heart occupy a relatively fixed volume in the pericardial sac, and evaluation of hemodynamics reveals equilibration of ventricular and pulmonary artery diastolic pressures with right atrial and left atrial pressures, all at approximately intrapericardial pressure.

Clinical Manifestations

Since the clinical manifestations of pericardial effusion without tamponade are similar to those of pericarditis, they will not be described here. Instead, the pathophysiologic mechanisms for the symptoms and signs of pericardial tamponade will be described.

A. Shortness of Breath: Dyspnea is the most common symptom of pericardial tamponade. The pathogenesis probably relates to a reduction in cardiac output and, in some patients, the presence of pulmonary edema.

B. Elevated Jugular Venous Pressure: Jugular venous pressure is elevated (Figure 10–29). In addition, cardiac tamponade alters the dynamics of atrial filling. Normally, atrial filling occurs first during ventricular ejection (*y* descent) and then later when the tricuspid valve opens (*x* descent). In cardiac tamponade, the atrium can fill during ventricular contraction, so that the *x* descent can still be seen. However, when the tricuspid valve opens, further filling of the right atrium is prevented because chamber size is limited by the surrounding pericardial fluid. For this reason, the *y* descent is not seen in the patient with pericardial tamponade. Loss of the *y* descent in the setting of elevated jugular venous pressures should always arouse suspicion of pericardial tamponade.

C. Hypotension: Hypotension occurs because of reduced cardiac output.

D. Paradoxic Pulse: Arterial systolic blood pressure normally drops 10–12 mm Hg with inspiration. Marked inspiratory drop in systolic blood pressure (> 20 mm Hg) is an important physical finding in the diagnosis of cardiac tamponade but can also be seen in severe pulmonary disease or, less commonly, in constrictive pericarditis (Figure 10–30). Marked inspiratory decline in left ventricular stroke volume occurs because of decreased left ventricular end-diastolic volume. With inspiration, increased blood return augments filling of the right ventricle which causes the interventricular septum to bow to the left and reduce left ventricular end-diastolic volume (reverse Bernheim effect). Also during inspiration, flow into the left atrium from the pulmonary veins is reduced, further reducing left ventricular preload.

E. Muffled Heart Sounds: Pericardial fluid can cause the heart sounds to become muffled or indistinct.

18. What are the clinical presentations of each form of pericardial disease discussed above?
19. What are the most common causes of pericarditis and pericardial effusion?
20. What are the major clinical manifestations and complications of pericarditis and pericardial effusion with tamponade?

REFERENCES

General
Kusumoto FM: *Cardiovascular Pathophysiology.* Fence Creek, 1998.
Schlant RC, Sonnenblick EC: Normal physiology of the cardiovascular system. In: *The Heart.* Schlant RC, Alexander RW (editors). McGraw-Hill, 1994.
Sperelakis N (editor): *Physiology and Pathophysiology of the Heart.* Kluwer, 1995.

Arrhythmias
Chakko S, Kessler KM: Recognition and management of cardiac arrhythmias. Curr Probl Cardiol 1995; 20:53.
The Sicilian Gambit: A new approach to the classification of antiarrhythmic drugs based on their actions on arrhythmogenic mechanisms. Circulation 1991;84:1831.
Zipes DP, Miles WM, Klein LS: Mechanisms of cardiac arrhythmias in patients. In: *Catheter Ablation of Arrhythmias.* Zipes DP (editor). Futura, 1994.

Congestive Heart Failure
Deedwania PC: Congestive heart failure. Cardiol Clin 1994;12:280.
Dell'Italia LJ, Freeman GL, Gaasch WH: Cardiac function and functional capacity: Implications for the failing heart. Curr Probl Cardiol 1993;18:705.
Shah PM, Pai RG: Diastolic heart failure. Curr Probl Cardiol 1992;17:781.

Young JB: Contemporary management of patients with heart failure. Med Clin North Am 1995;79:1171.

Valvular Heart Disease
Carabello B: Valvular heart disease. Cardiol Clin 1991;9:193.
Fenster MS, Feldman MD: Mitral regurgitation: An overview. Curr Probl Cardiol 1995;20:193.

Coronary Artery Disease
Califf RM: Acute ischemic syndromes. Med Clin North Am 1995;79:999.
Raines EW, Ross R: Smooth muscle cells and the pathogenesis of the lesions of atherosclerosis. Br Heart J 1993;69(1 Suppl):S30.
Ross R: Cell biology of atherosclerosis. Ann Rev Physiol 1994;57:791.
Theroux P, Lidon RM: Unstable angina: Pathogenesis, diagnosis, and treatment. Curr Probl Cardiol 1993; 18:157.

Pericardial Disease
Shabetai R: Diseases of the pericardium. Introduction. Cardiol Clin 1990;8:xiii.
Watkins MW, LeWinter MM: Physiologic role of the normal pericardium. Annu Rev Med 1993;44:171.

11

Cardiovascular Disorders: Vascular Disease

William F. Ganong, MD

This chapter reviews the normal structure and function of the vascular component of the cardiovascular system and then considers the pathophysiology of three common conditions frequently seen by practicing physicians: atherosclerosis, hypertension, and shock.

NORMAL STRUCTURE & FUNCTION

VASCULAR ANATOMY & HISTOLOGY

The blood vessels are a closed system of conduits that carry blood from the heart to the tissues and back to the heart. All of the blood flows through the lungs, but the systemic circulation is made up of many different circuits in parallel (Figure 11–1). This permits wide variation in regional systemic blood flow without changing the total systemic flow.

The characteristics of the various types of blood vessels in humans are summarized in Figure 11–2. Note that as the diameter of the vessels decreases, their number in the body increases so that the total cross-sectional area increases.

All the blood vessels are lined by endothelial cells. Collectively, the endothelial cells constitute a remarkable organ that secretes substances which affect the diameter of the vessels and provide for their growth, their repair when injured, and the formation of new vessels to carry blood to growing tissues.

Arterial Vessels

The aorta, the large arteries, and the arterioles are made up of an outer layer of connective tissue, the **adventitia;** a middle layer of smooth muscle, the **media;** and an inner layer, the **intima,** containing a layer of endothelial cells and some subendothelial connective tissue. The walls of the aorta and the large arteries contain abundant elastic tissue, much of it concentrated in the **internal elastic lamina,** a prominent band between the intima and the media; and another band, the **external elastic lamina,** between the media and the adventitia (Figure 11–3). The vessels are stretched by the force of cardiac ejection during systole, and the elastic tissue permits them to recoil during diastole. This maintains diastolic pressure and aids the forward motion of the blood. The walls of the arterioles contain less elastic tissue than the arteries but proportionately more smooth muscle (Figure 11–2). The muscle is extensively innervated by noradrenergic nerve fibers, which are constrictor in function. In some instances, there is a cholinergic innervation which is vasodilator in function. The arteries and the arterioles offer considerable resistance to the flow of blood and are known as the **resistance vessels.**

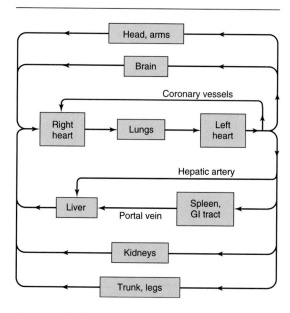

Figure 11–1. Diagram of the circulation in the adult. (Reproduced, with permission, from Ganong WF: *Review of Medical Physiology,* 19th ed. Appleton & Lange, 1999.)

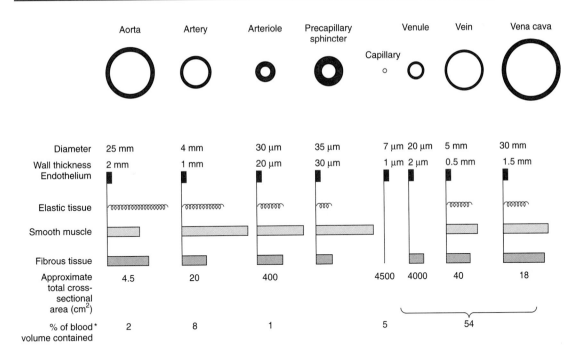

Figure 11–2. Characteristics of systemic blood vessels. Cross sections of the vessels are not drawn to scale because of the huge range in size from aorta and vena cava to capillaries. (Modified from Burton AC: Relation of structure to function of the tissues of the wall of blood vessels. Physiol Rev 1954;34:619.)

*In systemic vessels. There is an additional 12% in the heart and 18% in the pulmonary circulation.

Capillaries

The terminal portions of the arterioles, sometimes called metarterioles, drain into the **capillaries.** On the upstream side, the openings of the capillaries are surrounded by smooth muscle **precapillary sphincters.** There is debate about whether the metarterioles and sphincters are innervated. The capillaries themselves are made up of a single layer of endothelial cells. Outside these cells there are occasional pericytes, fibrous cells whose function is unknown (Figure 11–4). The capillaries anastomose extensively, and although each capillary is only 5–9 μm in diameter, they are so numerous that the total cross-sectional area of all the capillaries is about 4500 cm².

Some substances cross capillary walls by **vesicular transport,** a process that involves endocytosis of plasma, movement of the vesicles formed in this way across the endothelial cell cytoplasm, and exocytosis on the tissue side. However, relatively little material is moved in this fashion, and most fluid and solute exchange occurs at the junctions between endothelial cells. In the liver, there are large gaps between endothelial cells (Chapter 14). In endocrine tissues, the small intestine, and the kidneys, tissues in which there is bulk flow of material across capillary walls, the cytoplasm of the endothelial cells is attenuated to form gaps called **fenestrations.** These gaps appear to be closed by a discontinuous membrane which permits the passage of substances up to approximately 600 nm in diameter. In skeletal muscle, cardiac muscle, and many other tissues, there are no fenestrations, but the junctions between endothelial cells permit the passage of substances up to 10 nm in diameter. Finally, in brain capillaries, there are tight

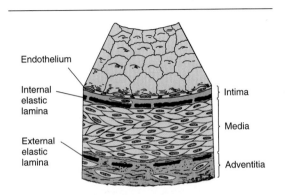

Figure 11–3. Structure of normal muscular artery. (Reproduced, with permission, from Ross R, Glomset JA: The pathogenesis of atherosclerosis [Part 1]. N Engl J Med 1976;295:369.)

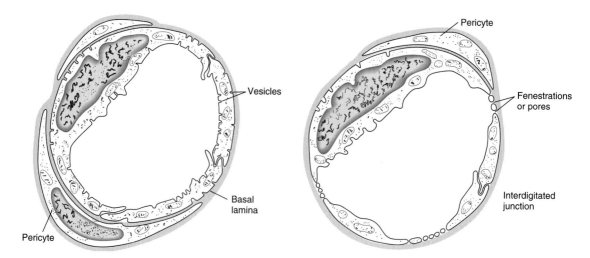

Figure 11–4. Cross sections of capillaries. **Left:** Continuous type of capillary found in skeletal muscle. **Right:** Fenestrated type of capillary. (Reproduced, with permission, from Fawcett DW: *Bloom and Fawcett, Textbook of Histology*, 11th ed. Saunders, 1986.)

junctions between the endothelial cells. These tight junctions permit very little passive transport and are a key component of the **blood-brain barrier.** Water and CO_2 enter the brain with ease, but movement of most other substances in and out of brain tissue is mainly via transport proteins in the endothelial cells.

Venules & Veins

The venules are very similar to capillaries; they are about 20 μm in diameter, and their approximate total cross-sectional area is 4000 cm². They drain into veins that have modest amounts of smooth muscle and elastic tissue in their relatively thin walls and average 5 mm in diameter. The veins drain into the superior and inferior vena cavas, which in turn drain into the right atrium of the heart. The walls of the veins, unlike those of the arteries and arterioles, are easily distended and can expand to hold more blood without much increase in intravascular pressure. Therefore, they are known as **capacitance vessels.** They are innervated, and their smooth muscle can contract in response to noradrenergic stimulation, pushing blood into the heart and the arterial side of the circulation. The intima of the limb veins is folded at intervals to form the venous valves that prevent retrograde flow.

Lymphatics

The smallest lymphatic vessels are made up of endothelial tubes. Fluid appears to enter them through loose junctions between the endothelial cells. They drain into larger endothelial tubes that have valves and contractile walls containing smooth muscle, so that the fluid they contain moves centrally. The central lymphatics drain into the right and left subclavian veins. Thus, the lymphatic system drains excess fluid in the tissues back into the vascular system.

1. How does the composition of the wall of an arteriole differ from that of an artery?
2. What are the modes of transport across the capillary wall? In what organ is transport greatest? In what organ is it most limited?
3. Why are veins termed capacitance vessels?

PHYSIOLOGY

Biophysical Considerations

In any system made up of a pump and a closed system of pipes such as the heart and the blood vessels, pressure is proportionate to the amount of fluid pumped into the pipes times the resistance to flow in the pipes.

Pressure = Flow × Resistance

In the cardiovascular system, this translates into:

Pressure = Cardiac output × Resistance

Thus, blood pressure increases when there is an increase in cardiac output or when the diameter of the blood vessels (principally the arterioles) is decreased.

Flow in blood vessels is laminar, ie, an infinitely thin layer of blood next to the vessel wall does not move, the next layer moves slowly, and the next layer moves more rapidly, with the fastest flow in the center. Usually the flow is smooth, and no sound is generated. However, if flow is accelerated, it becomes turbulent when a **critical velocity** is reached. Constriction of a blood vessel or a heart valve causes faster flow in the constricted region because the kinetic energy of flow is increased and the potential energy is decreased (**Bernoulli's principle**). Therefore, critical velocity is more often reached. The turbulence causes noise. The examining physician hears this noise through the stethoscope as a **bruit** or **murmur**. The two terms are often used interchangeably, though the term "murmur" is more commonly applied to noise heard over the heart "bruit" to that heard over blood vessels. The sounds of Korotkoff heard over an artery below a blood pressure cuff (see below) are another example.

The main factors that determine flow in a blood vessel are the pressure difference between its two ends, the radius of the vessel, and the viscosity of the blood. The relation can be expressed mathematically by the **Poiseuille-Hagen formula:**

$$F = (P_A - P_B) \times \left(\frac{\pi}{8}\right) \times \left(\frac{1}{\eta}\right) \times \left(\frac{r^4}{L}\right)$$

where

F = flow
$P_A - P_B$ = pressure difference between the two ends of the tube
η = viscosity
r = radius of tube
L = length of tube

Since flow is equal to pressure difference divided by resistance (R),

$$R = \frac{8\eta L}{\pi r^4}$$

Note that flow varies directly and pressure inversely with the fourth power of the radius of the vessel. This is why small changes in the diameter of the arterioles, the principal resistance vessels, cause large changes in pressure. For example, when the radius of a vessel is doubled, resistance is decreased to 6% of its previous value. Conversely, a small decrease in arterial diameter produces a relatively marked increase in blood pressure. Viscosity also has an effect, but except at very high or very low values, the effect is small. Viscosity is high in polycythemia and low in anemia.

The relation between distending pressure and wall tension is shown in Figure 11–5. This relation is called the **law of Laplace**. It states that the wall tension in a hollow viscus (T) is equal to the product of the **transmural pressure** (P) and the radius (r) divided by the thickness of the wall (w):

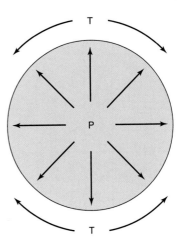

Figure 11–5. Law of Laplace. In a hollow object (viscus, blood vessel, etc), the distending pressure (P) equals the wall tension (T). (Reproduced, with permission, from Ganong WF: *Review of Medical Physiology,* 19th ed. Appleton & Lange, 1999.)

$$T = \frac{Pr}{w}$$

In thin-walled structures, w is negligible, but in structures such as arteries it becomes a significant factor. The transmural pressure is the pressure inside the viscus minus the pressure outside the viscus, but in the body the latter is negligible. Therefore, in a distensible hollow viscus, P at equilibrium is equal to T divided by the two principal radii of curvature of the object (r_1 and r_2):

$$P = T\left(\frac{1}{r_1} + \frac{1}{r_2}\right)$$

The operation of this law in the lungs is discussed in Chapter 9. In a cylinder such as a blood vessel, one radius is infinite, so:

$$P = \frac{T}{r}$$

Thus, the smaller the radius of a vessel, the lower the wall tension necessary to balance the distending pressure. For example, the wall tension in the aorta is about 170,000 dynes/cm, whereas in capillaries it is about 16 dynes/cm. This is why the thin-walled, delicate capillaries do not collapse. The law of Laplace also applies to the heart. When the heart is dilated, it must develop more wall tension to function. Consequently, its work is increased.

With these principles and Figure 11–2 in mind plus the fact that the major site of vascular resistance

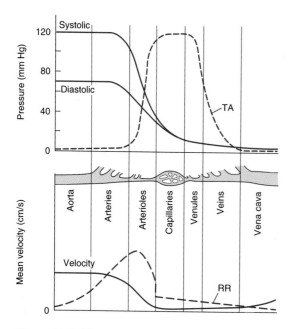

Figure 11–6. Diagram of the changes in pressure and velocity as blood flows through the systemic circulation. (TA, total cross-sectional area of the vessels, which increases from 4.5 cm^2 in the aorta to 4500 cm^2 in the capillaries [Figure 11–2]; RR, relative resistance, which is highest in the arterioles.) (Reproduced, with permission, from Ganong WF: *Review of Medical Physiology,* 19th ed. Appleton & Lange, 1999.)

is the arterioles, it is possible to understand the pressures in the various parts of the vascular system (Figure 11–6) and the velocity of flow in them. Systolic and diastolic pressures in the aorta and large arteries are stable, and there is a large pulse pressure. Normal pressure is about 120/80 mm Hg in healthy young adults. In the arterioles there is a sharp drop, so that pressure at the entrances to the capillaries is about 37 mm Hg and pulse pressure has disappeared. At the ends of the capillaries, it is about 17 mm Hg and falls steadily in the venous system to about 5 mm Hg at the entrance of the vena cavas into the right atrium. Velocity falls in the arterioles, is low in the capillaries because of the large total cross-sectional area, and increases again in the large veins.

The pressures mentioned above are of course those recorded with subjects in the supine position. Because of the weight of the blood, there is a pressure increase in the standing position in both arteries and veins of 0.77 mm Hg for each centimeter below the heart it is measured and a corresponding decrease of 0.77 mm Hg for each centimeter above the heart. Thus, when the mean arterial pressure at the level of the heart is 100 mm Hg, the mean arterial pressure in a large artery in the foot of a standing averaged-sized adult is about 180 mm Hg; and in the head, it is about 62 mm Hg.

Measurement of Arterial Pressure

Arterial pressure can be measured directly by inserting a needle into an artery. Alternatively (and usually), it can be measured by the auscultatory method. The familiar inflatable cuff attached to a manometer is placed around the upper arm at the level of the heart and a stethoscope is placed over the brachial artery below the cuff. The cuff is inflated to well above the suspected systolic pressure and then deflated slowly. At the systolic pressure, a faint tapping sound is heard as blood first begins to pass beyond the cuff. With further lowering of the pressure, the sound becomes louder, then dull and muffled before finally disappearing. These are the **sounds of Korotkoff,** which are produced by turbulent flow in the brachial artery. The change from staccato to muffled sound occurs when blood first passes under the cuff continuously, even though the artery is still partially constricted. Continuous flow has a different auditory quality than interrupted flow. Finally, at the diastolic pressure, the sound disappears. Although diastolic pressure measured directly with a catheter in the brachial artery correlates best with disappearance of sound in normal adults, in children and after exercise it correlates better with the change to a muffled sound.

Normal Arterial Pressure

Normal blood pressure in the brachial artery at heart level in healthy young adults is 120/80 mm Hg or less. It is affected by many factors, including emotion and anxiety, and in some individuals blood pressure is higher when taken by a physician in the clinic than it is during normal activities at home (**"white-coat hypertension"**). It is difficult to determine if blood pressure really increases with age because hypertension is common, and if all patients with an increase in blood pressure are thrown out of the sample being studied, there will obviously be no change with age. However, careful studies have now made it clear that there is a small rise with advancing age (Figure 11–7). Note in this figure the slightly lower blood pressure in women and the fall in blood pressure of approximately 20 mm Hg at night during sleep. This fall is normal, but it tends not to occur with the development of hypertension. In addition, at least in the population studied, there was not enough white-coat effect to produce a statistically significant difference between clinic blood pressures and pressures measured with a special recording device during normal daily activities.

Capillary Circulation

In the capillaries, the velocity of blood flow is decreased because although single vessel diameter is small, there is a large total cross-sectional area. It is

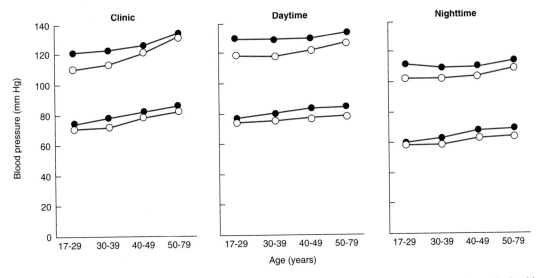

Figure 11–7. Blood pressure at various ages in men (solid circles) and women (open circles). The values obtained in a medical clinic are compared with average daytime and average nighttime values, measured with a constant recording device. Note that values in women are lower than in men but tend to catch up after the menopause. Note also the much lower values at right and the tendency for blood pressure to rise throughout life. (Data from O'Brien E et al: Twenty-four hour ambulatory blood pressure in men and women aged 17 to 80 years: The Allied Irish Bank Study. J Hypertens 1991;9:35.)

in the capillary bed that nutrients leave and wastes enter the circulation. The forces producing movement of solute and solvent across capillary walls are called **Starling forces** after the physiologist who first described them and analyzed their function. They are the hydrostatic pressure difference across the capillary wall (capillary pressure minus tissue pressure) and the osmotic pressure gradient across the capillary wall (capillary oncotic pressure minus tissue oncotic pressure). The pressure gradient is outward because tissue pressure is low, and the oncotic gradient is inward because large molecules in the blood do not cross the capillary wall. Obviously, most of the net movement of substances out of a typical capillary occurs at its arteriolar end where pressure is about 37 mm Hg (Figure 11–8). On the other hand, the inwardly directed oncotic pressure gradient is greater at the venular end because during flow through the capillaries, fluid enters the tissues and the osmotically active particles in the blood are more concentrated at the venular end. Thus, net flow is out of the capillary at the arteriolar end and into the capillary at the venular end. Any excess solute and solvent in the tissues is picked up by the lymph vessels and moved to the venous circulation by the main lymphatic ducts. Flow in the small lymphatics is passive, but in the larger lymphatic ducts, there are valves and the walls contract.

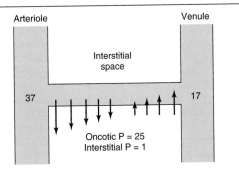

Figure 11–8. Schematic representation of pressure gradients across the wall of a muscle capillary. The numbers at the arteriolar and venular ends of the capillary are the hydrostatic pressures in millimeters of mercury at these locations. The arrows indicate the approximate magnitude and direction of fluid movement. In this example, the pressure differential at the arteriolar end of the capillary is 11 mm Hg ([37 − 1] − 25) outward; at the opposite end, it is 9 mm Hg (25 − [17 −1]) inward. (Reproduced, with permission, from Ganong WF: *Review of Medical Physiology*, 19th ed. Appleton & Lange, 1999.)

REGULATION OF THE CARDIOVASCULAR SYSTEM

Given the vital nature of the cardiovascular system in maintaining blood flow to vital organs and adjusting flow so that it is increased in active tissues and decreased in inactive tissues, it is not surprising that multiple cardiovascular regulatory mechanisms have evolved. Cardiovascular adjustments are effected by altering the output of the pump (the heart), changing the diameter of the resistance vessels (chiefly the arterioles), and altering the amount of blood pooled in the capacitance vessels (the veins).

Regulation of cardiac output is discussed in Chapter 10. The caliber of the arterioles is regulated by vasodilator metabolites produced in metabolically active tissues, by the process of autoregulation, by a variety of vasoregulatory substances produced by endothelial cells, by circulating vasoactive hormones, and by a system of vasomotor nerves to the blood vessels and the heart. Discharge in the vasomotor nerves is regulated in feedback fashion by carotid sinus and aortic arch baroreceptors that monitor pressure in the arteries (high-pressure baroreceptor system) and baroreceptors in the cardiac atria and great veins (low-pressure baroreceptor system).

Vasodilator Metabolites

Various metabolic changes occurring in active tissues produce substances that dilate vessels supplying the tissues. This helps ensure the increased blood flow necessary to support the increased tissue activity. One important vasodilator is CO_2. Another is K^+, and adenosine dilates blood vessels in some tissues. In addition, the rise in temperature and the fall in pH that occur in some metabolically active tissues has a vasodilator effect.

Autoregulation

Many tissues have the ability to maintain a relatively constant blood flow during changes in perfusion pressure; this is the process called **autoregulation**. The physiologic basis of autoregulation is unsettled. One factor is stretch of the smooth muscle in arterioles; as pressure inside a vessel rises, its smooth muscle is stretched, and its response is to contract. Smooth muscle contracts in the absence of extrinsic innervation. Another factor may be accumulation of vasodilator metabolites; when flow to a tissue is reduced, the metabolites are not washed away, and they accumulate even in the absence of increased activity.

Substances Secreted by the Endothelium

The blood vessels are lined by a continuous layer of endothelial cells, and these cells play a vital role in the regulation of vascular function. They respond to flow changes (shear stress), stretch, a variety of circulating substances, and inflammatory mediators. In response to these stimuli, they secrete growth regulators and vasoactive substances. The growth factors regulate vascular development and are important in a number of diseases. The vasoactive substances produced by the endothelium generally act in a paracrine fashion to regulate local vascular tone. They include prostaglandins such as prostacyclin and also thromboxanes, nitric oxide, and endothelins.

A. Prostaglandins and Thromboxanes: Prostacyclin is produced by endothelial cells and thromboxane A_2 by platelets from their common precursor, arachidonic acid. Thromboxane A_2 produces platelet aggregation and vasoconstriction, whereas prostacyclin promotes vasodilation. The balance between the two is one of the mechanisms favoring local vasoconstriction and clot formation at sites of vascular injury while keeping the clot from extending, thereby maintaining normal flow in neighboring uninjured areas. The balance between platelet thromboxane A_2 and endothelial prostacyclin can be shifted by administration of low doses of aspirin. Thromboxane A_2 and prostacyclin are both produced from arachidonic acid by the cyclooxygenase pathway. Aspirin produces irreversible inhibition of cyclooxygenase. However, endothelial cells make more cyclooxygenase within a few hours, whereas circulating platelets do not, and new platelet cyclooxygenase appears only as new platelets enter the circulation over a period of days. Therefore, chronic administration of small doses of aspirin reduces intravascular clotting for prolonged periods and is of value in the prevention of myocardial infarctions, unstable angina, transient ischemic attacks, and stroke.

B. Nitric Oxide: The production of a potent vasodilator by endothelial cells was first suspected when it was noted that removal of the endothelium from rings of arterial tissue converted the normal dilator response to acetylcholine into a pressor response. The responsible agent was first called **endothelium-derived relaxing factor (EDRF)**, but it is now known to be **nitric oxide (NO)**. NO is produced from arginine (Figure 11–9) in a reaction catalyzed by **nitric oxide synthase (NOS)**. Three forms of NOS have been cloned: NOS1, found in the nervous system; NOS2, found in macrophages and related immune cells; and NOS3, found in endothelial cells. NOS1 and NOS3 are activated by agents that increase intracellular Ca^{2+}, including the vasodilators acetylcholine and bradykinin, whereas NOS2 is activated by cytokines. The NO that is formed in endothelial cells diffuses to adjacent vascular smooth muscle cells, where it activates soluble guanylyl cyclase, producing cGMP (Figure 11–9). Cyclic GMP mediates relaxation of vascular smooth muscle.

The vasodilators that act by way of NO in vivo include not only acetylcholine and bradykinin but VIP, substance P, and some other polypeptides. In addition, various substances that produce vasoconstriction in vivo would have a much greater constrictor effect if they did not simultaneously release NO. Thus, NO is a major local regulator of blood flow. Its widespread role in regulation of the vascular system is indicated by the fact that infusion of amino acid analogs of arginine that inhibit NOS cause blood pressure to rise. Thus, it appears that NOS is acting in a chronic fashion to keep the vascular system dilated.

NO is responsible in large part for reactive hyperemia, the vasodilation and increased blood flow that

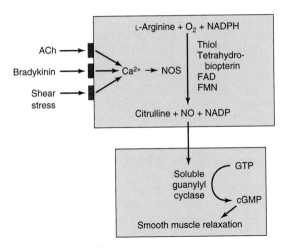

Figure 11–9. Synthesis of nitric oxide (NO) from arginine in endothelial cells and its action via stimulation of soluble guanylyl cyclase and generation of cGMP to produce relaxation in vascular smooth muscle cells. The endothelial form of nitric oxide synthase (NOS) is activated by increased intracellular Ca^{2+}, and an increase in Ca^{2+} is produced by acetylcholine (ACh), bradykinin, or shear stress acting on the cell membrane. Thiol, tetrahydrobiopterin, flavin adenine dinucleotide (FAD), and flavin mononucleotide (FMN) are requisite cofactors. (Reproduced, with permission, from Ganong WF: *Review of Medical Physiology,* 19th ed. Appleton & Lange, 1999.)

in the vicinity. Thus, ET-1 is primarily a local vasoconstrictor acting in a paracrine manner.

Circulating Hormones That Affect Vascular Smooth Muscle

Hormones in the circulation that have general effects on the vascular system include vasoconstrictors and vasodilators. The principal vasoconstrictors are norepinephrine and epinephrine (see Chapter 12), vasopressin (Chapter 19), and angiotensin II (Chapter 21). The principal vasodilators are vasoactive intestinal peptide (VIP; see Chapter 13), kinins, and natriuretic peptides.

A. Kinins: The kinins are two related vasodilator polypeptides called **bradykinin** and **lysylbradykinin** (Figure 11–11). The decapeptide lysylbradykinin can be converted to the nonapeptide bradykinin by aminopeptidase. Both are metabolized to inactive

occur in tissues and organs after a transient obstruction of their blood supply is removed. It can be seen in the forearm after occlusion of the blood supply above the elbow, and it can be quantitated by measuring the increase in forearm volume by plethysmography. NO-dependent vasodilation can also be measured clinically by determining the dilator response to graded doses of acetylcholine injected intra-arterially.

NO is present in many tissues in addition to the vascular system. Its function in some of these tissues is discussed in other chapters of this book.

C. Endothelins: Endothelial cells also produce endothelin-1 (ET-1), the most potent vasoconstrictor agent yet discovered. Three closely related endothelins have been identified in mammals: ET-1, endothelin-2 (ET-2), and endothelin-3 (ET-3). All are polypeptides related to the sarafotoxins, polypeptides found in snake venoms. They contain 21 amino acid residues and two disulfide bonds (Figure 11–10). All are apparently released from larger prohormones (big endothelins) by endothelin-converting enzymes. ET-2 and ET-3 are found in the intestine and the kidneys, and ET-3 is found also in the brain. Their functions in these organs are unsettled. In the endothelial cells, some of the ET-1 that is produced enters the circulation, but most of it diffuses to smooth muscle

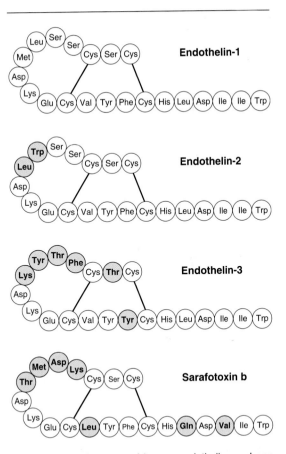

Figure 11–10. Structure of human endothelins and one of the snake venom sarafotoxins. The amino acid residues that differ from endothelin-1 are indicated in color. (Reproduced, with permission, from Ganong WF: *Review of Medical Physiology,* 19th ed. Appleton & Lange, 1999.)

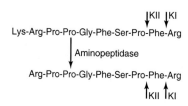

Figure 11–11. Kinins. Lysylbradykinin (top) can be converted to bradykinin (bottom) by aminopeptidase. The peptides are inactivated by kininase I (KI) or kininase II (KII) at the sites indicated by the short arrows. (Reproduced, with permission, from Ganong WF: *Review of Medical Physiology,* 19th ed. Appleton & Lange, 1999.)

fragments by the carboxypeptidase kininase I or the dipeptidylcarboxypeptidase kininase II. Kininase II and angiotensin-converting enzyme are the same enzyme, so inhibition of angiotensin-converting enzyme for the treatment of hypertension or heart failure increases plasma and tissue kinins.

Kinins are formed from two **kininogens:** high-molecular-weight (HMW) kininogen and low-molecular-weight (LMW) kininogen. These kinin precursor proteins are products of a single gene produced by alternative splicing. The proteases responsible for cleavage of kininogens are **kallikreins,** a family of enzymes encoded in humans by three genes situated on chromosome 19.

Lysylbradykinin and bradykinin are primarily tissue hormones produced, for example, by the kidneys and actively secreting glands, but small amounts are also found in the circulating blood. They act on two receptors, B_1 and B_2, both coupled to G proteins. Kinins increase blood flow to actively secreting glands by producing vasodilation, and when injected systemically they are relatively potent vasodilators.

B. Natriuretic Hormones: Atrial natriuretic peptide (ANP) is a polypeptide containing 28 amino acid residues that is secreted from the atria when atrial myocytes are stretched. **Brain natriuretic peptide (BNP)** and **CNP,** a third natriuretic polypeptide, are also found in humans. They cause natriuresis, probably by increasing the glomerular filtration rate, and this in turn causes excretion of salt and water, reducing blood volume and relieving the stretch on the atrial myocytes. They antagonize the pressor effects of angiotensin II and other pressor hormones. They act by increasing intracellular cGMP. All three have vasodilatory activity, but CNP differs in apparently having a greater effect on veins than arterioles. Their physiologic function is still unsettled. All three are found in various tissues other than the heart.

An additional natriuretic hormone that acts by inhibiting Na^+-K^+ ATPase is present in the circulation, but it raises rather than lowers blood pressure. There is substantial evidence that this hormone is actually ouabain and that it is secreted by the adrenal glands.

Neural Control Via the Sympathetic Vasomotor System

Factors affecting the caliber of the arterioles in the body and hence peripheral resistance and tissue blood flow are summarized in Table 11–1. This list includes the factors discussed above plus a few additional polypeptides that have minor or special effects. It also includes the control of blood pressure by noradrenergic and in some instances cholinergic sympathetic vasomotor nerves to the arterioles. In addition to the extensive nerve supply to these resistance vessels, there is a moderate innervation of the capacitance vessels.

Discharge of the noradrenergic vasomotor nerves causes constriction of the arterioles innervated by the nerves, and if the discharge is general rather than local, there is an increase in blood pressure. In addition, discharge of sympathetic noradrenergic nerves innervating the heart increases blood pressure by increasing the force and rate of cardiac contraction (inotropic and chronotropic effects), increasing stroke volume and cardiac output. Noradrenergic stimulation also inhibits the effect of vagal stimulation, which normally slows the heart and decreases cardiac output.

Table 11–1. Summary of factors affecting the caliber of the arterioles.

Constriction
Local factors
Decreased local temperature
Autoregulation
Locally released platelet serotonin
Endothelial cell products
Endothelin-1
Hormones
Norepinephrine
Epinephrine (except in skeletal muscle and liver)
Arginine vasopressin
Angiotensin II
Circulating Na^+-K^+ ATPase inhibitor
Neuropeptide Y
Neural control
Increased discharge of noradrenergic vasomotor nerves
Dilation
Local factors
Increased CO_2, K^+, adenosine, lactate
Decreased O_2
Decreased local pH
Increased local temperature
Endothelial cell products
Nitric oxide
Hormones
Vasoactive intestinal peptide
CGRPα (calcitonin gene-related peptide, the α form)
Substance P
Histamine
Kinins
Natriuretic peptides (ANP, BNP, CNP)
Epinephrine in skeletal muscle and liver
Neural control
Activation of cholinergic dilator fibers to skeletal muscle
Decreased discharge of noradrenergic vasomotor nerves

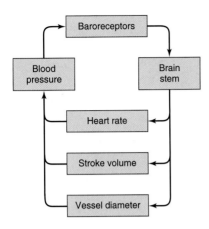

Figure 11–12. Feedback regulation of systemic blood pressure by baroreceptors. (Reproduced, with permission, from Ganong WF: *Review of Medical Physiology*, 19th ed. Appleton & Lange, 1999.)

The main control of vasomotor discharge is feedback regulation via the baroreceptors in the high-pressure and low-pressure portions of the circulatory system (Figure 11–12). The baroreceptors are stretch-sensitive nerve endings located in the carotid sinuses and aortic arch on the arterial side and in the walls of the great veins and the cardiac atria on the venous side. The nerve fibers relay impulses in cranial nerves IX and X to the medulla oblongata, where the fibers end in the nucleus tractus solitarius (Figure 11–13). From the nucleus, second-order neurons pass to the caudal portion of the ventrolateral medulla and environs. From there, third-order inhibitory neurons pass to the rostral ventrolateral medulla, the location of the cell bodies of the neurons that control blood pressure. The axons of these neurons descend into the spinal cord and innervate the cell bodies of the blood pressure-regulating preganglionic sympathetic neurons in the intermediolateral gray column of the spinal cord. The axons of the preganglionic neurons

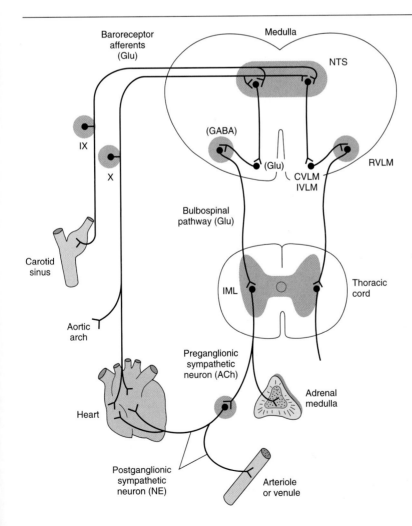

Figure 11–13. Basic pathways involved in the medullary control of blood pressure. The vagal efferent pathways to the heart are not shown. The probable neurotransmitters in the pathways are indicated in parentheses. (ACh, acetylcholine; GABA, γ-aminobutyric acid; Glu, glutamate; NE, norepinephrine; CVLM, IVLM, and RVLM, caudal, intermediate, and rostral ventrolateral medulla; IML, intermediolateral gray column; IX, glossopharyngeal nerve; NTS, nucleus tractus solitarius; X, vagus nerve.) (Modified from Reis DJ et al: Role of adrenaline neurons of the ventrolateral medulla [the C group] in the tonic and phasic control of arterial pressure. Clin Exp Hypertens [A] 1994;6:221.)

leave the spinal cord and synapse on the postganglionic neurons in the ganglionic chain and collateral ganglia as well as on the catecholamine-secreting cells in the adrenal medulla. The axons of the postganglionic noradrenergic neurons innervate the blood vessels and the heart. These pathways and the probable synaptic mediator at each synapse in the chain are shown in Figure 11–13. Note in particular that increased activity in the baroreceptor afferents produced by increases in blood pressure inhibits sympathetic vasomotor outflow, whereas decreased baroreceptor afferent discharge stimulates sympathetic vasomotor outflow. This is brought about by the inhibitory GABA-secreting neuron link between the caudal portion of the ventrolateral medulla and the rostral ventrolateral medulla. In addition, increased baroreceptor discharge stimulates afferents from the nucleus tractus solitarius to the dorsal motor nucleus of the vagus and the nucleus ambiguus. This increases vagal discharge to the heart, slowing the cardiac rate and decreasing cardiac output.

There are ancillary reciprocal circuits between the nucleus tractus solitarius and more dorsal portions of the brainstem and the hypothalamus which smooth and adjust the response of the baroreceptor pathway, but the primary neural regulation of blood pressure is mediated by the baroreceptor pathway in the medulla oblongata.

In addition to direct effects on vasomotor discharge, the baroreceptor pathway brings about changes in endocrine function that augment the homeostatic value of baroreceptor responses. Adrenal medullary secretion is increased by discharge of the sympathetic nervous system, though the contributions of circulating catecholamines to the increase in blood pressure are relatively small. Increased sympathetic discharge also increases renin secretion from the kidneys, and the resultant increase in circulating angiotensin II not only acts directly on vascular smooth muscle to cause constriction but increases aldosterone secretion. This in turn increases Na^+ and water retention, expanding extracellular fluid volume. Associated with increased vasomotor discharge there is also an increase in vasopressin secretion. This is mediated by a pathway from the medulla to the hypothalamus. The vasopressin expands total body water and in this way helps restore extracellular fluid volume, though its contribution is relatively small.

Baroreceptor function can be tested in experimental animals and judiciously in humans by infusing the pressor drug phenylephrine at different doses and at each dose measuring the slowing of the heart rate by determining the interval between the R waves (RR interval) of the ECG. An example of results of this type of testing is shown in Figure 11–14.

Sympathetic Vasodilator System

In addition to the sympathetic vasoconstrictor system, there appears to be a sympathetic vasodilator system consisting of anatomically sympathetic but cholinergic neurons innervating blood vessels in skeletal muscle. This system is activated by a pathway that passes from the cerebral cortex through the hypothalamus and medulla without interruption to the intermediolateral gray column of the spinal cord. The function of this system and its importance in cardiovascular control remain a matter of debate, but it may be responsible for the sharp fall in blood pressure and fainting that can occur in association with intense emotion.

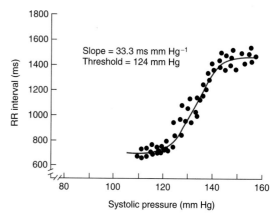

Figure 11–14. Baroreflex-mediated lowering of the heart rate during infusion of phenylephrine in a human subject. Note that the values for the RR interval of the ECG, which are plotted on the vertical axis, are inversely proportionate to the heart rate. (Reproduced, with permission, from Kotrly K et al: Effects of fentanyl-diazepam-nitrous oxide anaesthesia on arterial baroreflex control of heart rate in man. Br J Anaesth 1986;58:406.)

4. Why do small changes in the diameter of the arterioles have a relatively large effect on blood pressure?
5. Why does the velocity of blood flow decrease greatly in the capillaries and then increase in the veins?
6. What categories of factors are involved in regulating the diameter of arterioles?
7. By what mechanism does nitric oxide produced by endothelial cells act as a vasodilator?
8. What are the principal hormonal vasoconstrictors and vasodilators?
9. What is the role of baroreceptors in the feedback regulation of the high- and low-pressure portions of the circulatory system?

PATHOPHYSIOLOGY OF SELECTED VASCULAR DISORDERS

ATHEROSCLEROSIS

Prevalence & Significance

A condition that afflicts the large and medium-sized arteries of almost every human, at least in societies where cholesterol-rich foodstuffs are abundant and cheap, is **atherosclerosis**. This condition begins in childhood and, in the absence of accelerating factors, develops slowly until it is widespread in old age. It is characterized by localized fibrous thickenings of the arterial wall, associated with lipid-infiltrated plaques that may eventually calcify. Laymen call this "hardening of the arteries," though the term is not strictly correct. Atherosclerosis leads to vascular insufficiency in the limbs, abnormalities of the renal circulation, and dilations (aneurysms) and eventual rupture of the aorta and other large arteries. It also leads to common, severe, and life-threatening diseases of the heart and brain due to formation of intravascular clots at the site of the plaques. For example, in the United States and most developed countries, practically every patient with a myocardial infarction—and most with a stroke due to cerebral thrombosis—has atherosclerosis. The incidence of ischemic heart disease and strokes has been declining in the United States since 1963, but atherosclerosis is still the most common cause of death in individuals over age 45. Thus, atherosclerosis underlies and is fundamentally responsible for a large portion of the clinical problems seen by physicians whose patients are adults.

Etiology & Pathogenesis

Although there is still some debate on the matter, it appears that atherosclerosis starts early in life with localized injury to the endothelium. The endothelium is subject to **shear stress,** the tendency for it to be pulled along by the flowing blood or to be deformed. Injury occurs particularly at sites of high shear stress such as points where arteries branch. The endothelial injury causes the endothelial cells to express vascular cell adhesion molecules (VCAMs). Monocytes attach to the adhesion molecules and then enter the subendothelial region. Low-density lipoproteins (LDL; see below) also enter the vessel wall and are oxidized. The macrophages take up the oxidized LDL and become engorged with them, forming **foam cells** (Figure 11–15). The foam cells along the initial site of the endothelial injury form a **fatty streak.** These streaks are characteristic of developing atherosclerosis.

Oxidized LDL have a number of deleterious effects, including stimulation of release of cytokines and inhibition of NO production. Vascular smooth muscle cells in the vicinity of the initial injury are stimulated and move from the media to the intima, where they proliferate, lay down collagen and other matrix molecules, and contribute to the bulk of the lesion. In addition, smooth muscle cells also take up oxidized LDL and become foam cells. Eventually, the distorted, thickened wall of the artery takes up calcium, forming a brittle plaque.

T cells of the immune system also accumulate, and they secrete at least one of the factors responsible for conversion of monocytes to macrophages. Growth factors and cytokines involved in cell migration and proliferation are also produced by smooth muscle cells and endothelial cells, and there is evidence for shear stress response elements in the flanking DNA of relevant genes in the endothelial cells. Transforming a monocyte into a lipid-ingesting macrophage involves the appearance on its surface of a unique type of oxidized LDL receptor, the **scavenger receptor,** and monocytes are stimulated to produce these receptors by the action of **macrophage colony-stimulating factor** secreted by endothelial cells and vascular smooth muscle cells. When oxidized LDL-receptor complexes are formed, they are internalized and the receptors recycle to the membrane while the lipid is stored.

Obviously, accumulation of lipid in foam cells is a key event in the progression of atherosclerotic lesions, and it is well established that lowering plasma cholesterol slows the progress of atherosclerosis. The main pathways for the metabolism of ingested lipids are summarized in Figure 11–16. Since lipids are relatively insoluble, they are transported as special lipoprotein particles that increase their solubility. Dietary cholesterol and triglycerides are packaged in the protein-coated **chylomicrons** in intestinal epithelial cells. Under the influence of lipoprotein lipase, these particles release triglycerides to fat depots and muscles, and the resulting **chylomicron remnants** are taken up by the liver. The liver also synthesizes cholesterol and packages it with specific proteins to form **very low density lipoproteins (VLDL).** These lipoprotein particles enter the circulation and under the influence of lipoprotein lipase donate triglycerides to tissues. In this way, they become cholesterol-rich **intermediate-density lipoproteins (IDL) and low-density lipoproteins (LDL). High-density lipoproteins (HDL)** exchange cholesterol with VLDL, LDL, and tissues and transport it back to the liver, keeping plasma and tissue cholesterol low; this is why HDL cholesterol is called "good cholesterol." LDL provide cholesterol to all cells for production of cell membranes and other uses. LDL also provide most of the cholesterol that is the precursor for all steroid hormones. As noted above, oxidized LDL are taken up by macrophages and smooth muscle cells in atherosclerotic lesions. Low levels of plasma cholesterol and triglyceride limit the supply of oxidized

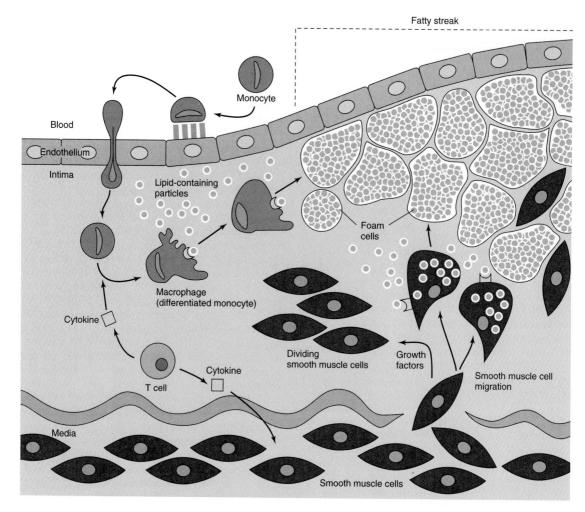

Figure 11–15. Formation of a fatty streak in an artery. Following vascular injury, monocytes bind to the endothelium, then cross it to the subendothelial space and become activated tissue microphages. The macrophages take up oxidized LDL, becoming foam cells. T cells release cytokines, which also activate macrophages. In addition, the cytokines cause smooth muscle cells to proliferate. Under the influence of growth factors, the smooth muscle cells then move to the subendothelial space where they produce collagen and take up LDL, adding to the population of foam cells. (Reproduced, with permission, from Hajjar DP, Nicholson AC: Atherosclerosis. Am Scientist 1995;83:460.)

LDL for deposition in atherosclerotic lesions and slow the progression of the lesions.

The similarity between atherosclerotic plaques and inflammatory processes deserves mention. Not only are they infiltrated with monocytes and T lymphocytes, but there are also multiple cytokines and chemokines in the lesions and there is connective tissue overgrowth. This has led some investigators to search for bacteria in plaques, and in a significant number *Chlamydia pneumoniae,* an organism usually associated with sexually transmitted disease, has been found. However, other organisms have also been found, and it is too early to say whether the chlamydiae are causative agents or merely coincidental tenants in the lesions.

A characteristic of atherosclerosis that is currently receiving considerable attention is its association with deficient release of NO and defective vasodilation. If acetylcholine is infused via catheter into normal coronary arteries, they dilate; but if it is infused when atherosclerosis is present, they constrict. This indicates that endothelial secretion of NO is defective. In the forearms of individuals with atherosclerosis, the NO-mediated vasodilator response to the termination of ischemia (reactive hyperemia) is reduced, indicating the presence of a defective endothelium in this vascular bed as well. This could be explained, of course, by the presence of atherosclerosis in the limb arteries as well as the coronary arteries. As noted above, oxidized LDL inhibit NO pro-

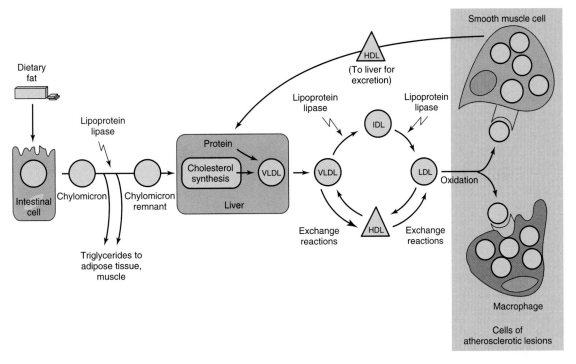

Figure 11–16. Lipid metabolism in relation to formation of atherosclerotic lesions. Fatty acids from dietary lipids are reesterified in intestinal cells and exported as protein-containing chylomicrons. Lipoprotein lipase from endothelial cells catalyzes the release of triglycerides from the chylomicrons, and the chylomicron remnants are taken up by the liver. In the liver, they take up cholesterol and are released into the blood stream as very low density lipoprotein (VLDL) particles. These engage in exchange reactions with high-density lipoproteins (HDL), and they form intermediate-density lipoproteins (IDL) and low-density lipoproteins (LDL). LDL are the major source of cholesterol for the tissues. When they enter the walls of arteries, they are oxidized, and oxidized LDL enter macrophages and smooth muscle cells, forming foam cells. In addition, HDL carry cholesterol from tissues to the liver for excretion in the bile, and LDL receptors in the liver (not shown) take up VLDL, IDL, and LDL, lowering circulating cholesterol. (Reproduced, with permission, from Hajjar DP, Nicholson AC: Atherosclerosis. Am Scientist 1995;83:460.)

duction. However, the endothelial NO response is also deficient in the limbs of individuals at risk for the development of atherosclerosis who have not as yet developed detectable disease. This has led to the hypothesis that in individuals who develop atherosclerosis, there is a diffuse defect in endothelial NO production which is either a primary cause or a predisposing factor in the development of the disease.

Clinical Manifestations

Since atherosclerosis is an abnormality of arterial blood vessels, it can affect almost any organ in the body. Clots tend to form at points where vessels are narrowed and distorted by atherosclerotic plaques. In addition, calcified plaques may ulcerate or rupture, and the resulting further arterial injury fosters clot formation. Bits of ruptured plaques can break off and form emboli.

Calcified atherosclerotic plaques are occasionally detected on x-ray, and angiographic visualization of deformed arterial walls is possible. In general, however, atherosclerosis is asymptomatic until one of its complications develops.

In coronary arteries, atherosclerotic narrowing that reduces the lumen of a coronary artery more than 75% causes **angina pectoris,** the chest pain that results when pain-producing substances accumulate in the myocardium. Typically, the pain comes on during exertion and disappears with rest, as the substances are washed out by the blood. When atherosclerotic lesions cause clotting and occlusion of a coronary artery, the myocardium supplied by the artery dies **(myocardial infarction).** Myocardial infarction is also discussed in Chapter 10.

In the cerebral circulation, arterial blockage at the site of atherosclerotic plaques causes **thrombotic strokes.** Strokes are discussed in Chapter 7. In the abdominal aorta, extensive atherosclerosis can lead to aneurysmal dilation and rupture of the vessel. In the renal vessels, localized constriction of one or both renal arteries causes **renovascular hypertension** (see below). In the circulation to the legs, vascular insufficiency causes **intermittent claudication** (fatigue and usually pain on walking that is relieved by rest). If the circulation of a limb is severely compromised, the skin can ulcerate, producing lesions that are slow to heal. Frank **gangrene** of the extremities may also occur. Less frequently, clot formation and obstruction may occur in vessels supplying the intestines or other parts of the body.

The development of atherosclerosis is accelerated in a number of conditions, ie, these conditions are risk factors for the disease. Estrogens increase cholesterol removal by the liver, and the progression of atherosclerosis is less rapid in premenopausal women than in men because of higher circulating estrogen during the female reproductive cycle. Other common conditions producing acceleration of atherosclerosis and the causes of the acceleration are summarized in Table 11–2. Understanding the processes involved in each of the conditions listed in the table is a good exercise in pathophysiologic reasoning.

The effect of increased plasma levels of homocysteine and related molecules such as homocystine and homocysteine thiolactone, a condition sometimes called hyperhomocyst(e)inemia, deserves emphasis. These increases are associated with accelerated atherosclerosis, and the magnitude of the plasma elevation is positively correlated with the severity of the atherosclerosis. Markedly elevated levels due to documented mutations of relevant genes are rare, but mild elevations occur in 7% of the general population. The mechanism responsible for the accelerated vascular damage is unsettled, but homocysteine is a significant source of H_2O_2 and other reactive forms of oxygen, and this may accelerate the oxidation of LDL.

Homocysteine is an intermediate in the synthesis of methionine. It is metabolized by enzymes that are dependent on vitamin B_6, vitamin B_{12}, and folic acid, and supplementation of the diet with these vitamins reduces plasma homocysteine, usually to normal. To determine whether such supplements also reduce the incidence of the accelerated atherosclerosis will require prolonged, careful clinical trials. The results of these trials are awaited with great interest.

Prevention

Treatment is outside the scope of this book, but it seems appropriate to mention prevention in the case of atherosclerosis, since the condition is so common and its complications affect so many people. For the most part, prevention involves avoiding risk factors or altering their effects. Obviously, little can be done about male sex and many of the genetic factors. However, it is possible to lower plasma cholesterol, LDL, and triglycerides and increase plasma HDL. Evidence is now overwhelming that lowering plasma cholesterol and triglyceride levels and increasing plasma HDL levels slows and in some cases reverses the atherosclerotic process. The desired decrease in lipids can sometimes be achieved with dietary restriction of cholesterol and saturated fat alone. When dietary treatment is not adequate, reducing conversion of mevalonate to cholesterol with drugs that inhibit HMG-CoA reductase, the enzyme which catalyzes this reaction, is beneficial. The currently available HMG-CoA reductase inhibitors include atorvastatin, cerivastatin, lovastatin, pravastatin, simvastatin, and fluvastatin. Administration to postmenopausal women of small doses of estrogen decreases the incidence of myocardial infarction and other ath-

Table 11–2. Conditions that accelerate the progression of atherosclerosis and the mechanisms responsible.

Condition	Mechanism
Male gender (and females after menopause)	Lack of LDL-lowering effect of estrogens; estrogens probably act by increasing the number of LDL receptors in the liver.
Family history of ischemic heart disease, stroke	Probably multiple genetic mechanisms.
Primary hyperlipidemia	Inherited disorders causing lipoprotein lipase deficiency (type I), defective LDL receptors (type IIa), abnormal apoprotein E (type III), deficiency of apoprotein C (type V), or unknown cause (types IIb and IV).
Secondary hyperlipidemia[1]	Increased circulating triglycerides produced by diuretics, β-adrenergic blocking drugs, excess alcohol intake.
Cigarette smoking	Probably carbon monoxide-induced hypoxic injury to endothelial cells.
Hypertension	Increased shear stress, with damage to endothelium.
Diabetes mellitus (both type 1 and type 2)	Decreased hepatic removal of LDL from the circulation; increased glycosylation of collagen, which increases LDL binding to blood vessel walls.
Obesity, particularly abdominal obesity	Unsettled, but obesity is associated with type 2 diabetes, hypertriglyceridemia, hypercholesterolemia, and hypertension, all of which are risk factors in their own right.
Nephrotic syndrome	Increased hepatic production of lipids and lipoprotein (a).
Hypothyroidism	Decreased formation of LDL receptors in the liver.
High lipoprotein (a)	Not known.
Elevated plasma homocysteine	Unsettled. Probably increased homocysteine provides more H_2O_2 and other reactive oxygen molecules that foster formation of oxidized LDL.

[1]Hypercholesterolemia and hypertriglyceridemia are both risk factors.

erosclerosis-induced vascular catastrophes. On the other hand, large oral doses of estrogen increase rather than decrease thromboembolic events. This is probably because the estrogens reach the liver in high concentration via the portal vein after absorption from the gastrointestinal tract and disrupt hepatic production of clotting factors. In cases in which there is severe hypercholesterolemia because of congenitally defective LDL receptors, gene therapy has been tried with promising preliminary results. Other approaches to slowing or preventing development of atherosclerosis by molecular biologic techniques are under development. Antioxidant treatment with agents such as α-tocopherol, vitamin E, and β-carotene has been used to inhibit oxidation of LDL, and this reduces the incidence of atherosclerotic changes in experimental animals. However, the results of antioxidant treatment in humans have generally been disappointing or negative.

Men who smoke a pack of cigarettes a day have a 70% increase in death rate from ischemic heart disease compared with nonsmokers, and there is also an increase in women. Smoking cessation lessens the risk of death and of myocardial infarction. The deleterious effects of smoking include endothelial damage due to carbon monoxide-induced hypoxia. Other factors may also be involved. Thus, stopping smoking is a major way to slow the progress of atherosclerosis.

Because of the increased shear stress imposed on the endothelium by an elevated blood pressure, hypertension is another important modifiable risk factor for atherosclerosis. Lowering blood pressure has its greatest effect in reducing the incidence of stroke, but there are beneficial effects on ischemic heart disease as well. With modern methods of treatment, blood pressure in hypertensives can generally be reduced to normal or near-normal values, and the decrease in strokes, myocardial infarctions, and renal failure produced by such treatment is clear testimony to the value of reducing or eliminating this risk factor. In diabetics, there are microvascular complications and macrovascular complications (see Table 18–9). The latter are primarily related to atherosclerosis. There is a twofold increase in the incidence of myocardial infarction compared with nondiabetics; severe circulatory deficiency in the legs with gangrene is relatively common; there are more thrombotic strokes, and renal failure is a serious problem (see Chapter 18). Tight control of diabetes decreases the incidence of retinopathy and nephropathy (microvascular complications), but it is not yet certain that tight control lowers the incidence of the macrovascular complications. The increased atherosclerosis seen in diabetes is related to insulin resistance, obesity, hypercholesterolemia, hypertriglyceridemia, and hypertension. Further studies of the interactions between these conditions should provide a clearer picture of why diabetes is a major risk factor for atherosclerosis.

The nephrotic syndrome and hypothyroidism also accelerate the progression of atherosclerosis and are treatable conditions.

---

10. What is the most common cause of death in the United States among individuals over the age of 45?
11. What is the hypothesized mechanism of atherosclerotic plaque formation?
12. What are some ways in which atherosclerotic plaques can cause cardiovascular disease?
13. Name five treatable risk factors for increased atherosclerosis.

HYPERTENSION

Hypertension is not a single disease but a syndrome with multiple causes. In most instances, the cause remains unknown, and the cases are lumped together under the term **essential hypertension** (Table 11–3). However, mechanisms are continuously being discovered that explain hypertension in new subsets of the formerly monolithic category of essential hypertension, and the percentage of cases in the essential category continues to decline. Essential hypertension is often called **primary hypertension** and hypertension in which the cause is known is called **secondary hypertension,** though this separation seems somewhat artificial. This chapter discusses the pathogenesis of hypertension and its complications in general terms and then discusses the specific causes of the presently defined subgroups and the unique features, if any, that each adds to the general findings in patients with high blood pressure.

Table 11–3. Estimated frequency of various forms of hypertension in the general hypertensive population.[1]

	Percentage of Population
Essential hypertension	93
Renal hypertension	
Renovascular	2
Parenchymal	3
Endocrine hypertension	
Primary aldosteronism	0.3
Cushing's syndrome	0.1
Pheochromocytoma	0.1
Other adrenal forms	0.2
Estrogen treatment ("pill hypertension")	1
Miscellaneous (Liddle's syndrome, coarctation of the aorta, etc.)	0.3

[1]Modified and reproduced, with permission, from Williams GH: Hypertensive vascular disease. In: *Harrison's Principles of Internal Medicine,* 14th ed. Fauci A et al (editors). McGraw-Hill, 1998.

Pathogenesis

Hypertension is generally defined as an arterial pressure over 140/90 mm Hg in adult humans on at least three consecutive visits to the doctor's office. The upper limits of normal pressure in children are somewhat lower, and in elderly individuals they are somewhat higher. In addition, isolated systolic hypertension, with systolic pressures over 140 mm Hg but diastolic pressures below 90 mm Hg, also occurs and is not as benign as once was thought. The most common cause of hypertension is increased peripheral vascular resistance. However, since blood pressure equals total peripheral resistance times cardiac output, prolonged increases in cardiac output can also cause hypertension. These are seen, for example, in hyperthyroidism and beriberi. In addition, increased blood volume causes hypertension, especially in individuals with mineralocorticoid excess or renal failure (see below); and increased blood viscosity, if it is marked, can increase arterial pressure.

Clinical Presentation

Hypertension by itself does not cause symptoms. Headaches, fatigue, and dizziness are sometimes ascribed to hypertension, but nonspecific symptoms such as these are no more common in hypertensives than they are in normotensive controls. Instead, the condition is picked up during routine screening or discovered when patients seek medical advice for its complications. These complications are serious and can be fatal. They include myocardial infarction, congestive heart failure, thrombotic and hemorrhagic strokes, hypertensive encephalopathy, and renal failure. This is why hypertension is called "the silent killer."

Physical findings are also absent in early hypertension, and observable changes are generally found only in advanced, severe cases. These may include **hypertensive retinopathy,** ie, narrowed arterioles seen on funduscopic examination, and, in more severe cases, retinal hemorrhages and exudates along with swelling of the optic nerve head (papilledema). Prolonged pumping against an elevated peripheral resistance causes left ventricular hypertrophy that can be detected by echocardiography and cardiac enlargement that can be detected on physical examination. It is important to listen with the stethoscope over the kidneys because in renal hypertension (see below), narrowing of the renal arteries may cause bruits. In addition, it has been recommended that the blood pressure response to rising from the sitting to the standing position be determined. A blood pressure rise on standing sometimes occurs in essential hypertension, presumably because of a hyperactive sympathetic response to the erect posture. This rise is usually absent in other forms of hypertension. Most individuals with essential hypertension (60%) have normal plasma renin activity, and 10% have high plasma renin activity. However, 30% have low plasma renin activity. There may be an as yet unidentified steroid causing salt retention in these patients, or their renin secretion may be reduced by an expanded blood volume from some other cause. However, the exact cause is unknown, and low-renin essential hypertension has not yet been separated from the rest of essential hypertension as a distinct entity.

In many patients with hypertension, the condition is benign and progresses slowly; in others, it progresses rapidly. Actuarial data indicate that on average, untreated hypertension reduces life expectancy by 10–20 years. Atherosclerosis is accelerated, and this in turn leads to ischemic heart disease with angina pectoris and myocardial infarctions (Chapter 10), thrombotic strokes and cerebral hemorrhages (Chapter 7), and renal failure (Chapter 16). Another complication of severe hypertension is **hypertensive encephalopathy,** in which there is confusion, disordered consciousness, and seizures. This condition, which requires vigorous treatment, is probably due to arteriolar spasm and cerebral edema.

In all forms of hypertension regardless of cause, the condition can suddenly accelerate and can enter the malignant phase. In **malignant hypertension,** there is widespread fibrinoid necrosis of the media with intimal fibrosis in arterioles, narrowing them and leading to progressive severe retinopathy, congestive heart failure, and renal failure. If untreated, malignant hypertension is usually fatal in 1 year.

Management

Treatment of disease is beyond the scope of this book. However, it should be noted that in all forms of hypertension, modern treatment with adrenergic blocking drugs, inhibitors of the renin-angiotensin system, vasodilators, and diuretics reduces blood pressure, usually to normal levels. In addition, these treatments delay or prevent complications and lengthen life expectancy. However, they are not curative and must be continued indefinitely. Thus, essential hypertension is like diabetes mellitus—it can be controlled but not cured. If a cause of hypertension can be identified, its treatment may result in a cure. Consequently, it is important to identify such cases.

Etiology

A. Coarctation of the Aorta: Congenital narrowing of the aorta usually occurs just distal to the origin of the left subclavian artery. Peripheral resistance is increased above the constriction. Therefore, blood pressure is elevated in the arms, head, and chest but lowered in the legs. However, since the constriction is proximal to the renal arteries, renin secretion is increased in most cases of coarctation as a result of the reduction in arterial pressure in the renal arteries. This tends to increase blood pressure throughout the body. Elimination of the constriction by resection of the narrowed segment of the aorta usually cures the condition.

Table 11–4. Salt sensitivity in humans.[1]

	Percentage of Individuals	
	Normal	Hypertensive
White		
Salt-sensitive[2]	30	55
Salt-resistant	70	45
Black		
Salt-sensitive[2]	32	73
Salt-resistant	68	27

[1]Courtesy of Weinberg MH. Data from Luft FC et al: Salt sensitivity and resistance of blood pressure. Hypertension 1991; 17(suppl I):I102.
[2]Mean blood pressure decrease >10 mm Hg with furosemide and low-salt diet.

B. Salt Sensitivity: Through selective inbreeding, Dahl was able to develop two strains of rats: salt-sensitive rats that showed an increase in blood pressure when fed a high-salt diet, and salt-resistant rats that did not. The genetic mechanisms responsible for these strain differences are currently under investigation. There may be a similar division of humans into salt-sensitive and salt-resistant, though obviously the lines between the groups are less distinct. As shown in Table 11–4, about 30% of whites with normal renal function and normal blood pressure are salt-sensitive. In whites with essential hypertension, the percentage is about 55. For unknown reasons, a larger percentage of black hypertensives are salt-sensitive. These figures have obvious significance in terms of recommendations about salt intake in hypertension.

It should be emphasized that the figures cited in the preceding paragraph refer to individuals with normal renal function and normal (or reduced) secretion of mineralocorticoid hormones. When renal function is reduced, mineralocorticoid secretion increased, or the effects of mineralocorticoids enhanced, there is abnormal retention of salt and water, and hypertension is produced on this basis (see below).

C. Renal Abnormalities: The observation by Goldblatt that **renal artery constriction** increased blood pressure in experimental animals was rapidly followed by the demonstration that the same thing occurred in humans. However, disappointment followed when it was found that **renal hypertension** due to constriction of one or both renal arteries accounted for only 2% of cases of clinical hypertension (Table 11–3). The narrowing can be due to atherosclerosis, to fibroelastic overgrowth of the wall of the renal artery, or to external pressure on the vessel. The initial constriction decreases renal arteriolar pressure, and this leads to increased renin secretion. The renin-angiotensin system is discussed in Chapters 16 and 21. However, in many cases, some other mechanism takes over chronically to maintain the hypertension. The nature of this other mechanism is unknown.

In rare instances, hypertension can be caused by tumors of the renin-secreting juxtaglomerular cells.

Ureteral obstruction can cause hypertension in animals and probably in humans by increasing renal interstitial pressure and thus decreasing the pressure gradient across the renin-secreting juxtaglomerular cells.

Acute and chronic glomerulonephritis and other forms of diffuse kidney disease can cause hypertension when loss of the ability to excrete salt is severe enough so that Na^+ and water are retained and blood volume is expanded.

In **Liddle's syndrome,** there is abnormal sodium retention by the kidneys with expanded extracellular fluid volume, producing hypertension but no increase in circulating mineralocorticoids. The sodium retention is due to constitutive activation of the epithelial sodium channel (ENaC). This channel, which is inhibited by amiloride, has three subunits, and activating mutations in the genes for the β or the γ subunit have been documented in patients with Liddle's syndrome.

An abnormality of the renin-angiotensin system that can cause significant hypertension is increased secretion of angiotensinogen from the liver. Secretion of this angiotensin precursor (Chapter 21) is under endocrine control and is stimulated by estrogens. Consequently, it is increased in women taking contraceptive pills containing large amounts of estrogens. When circulating angiotensinogen is increased, more angiotensin II is formed and blood pressure rises. The normal compensation for this response is decreased secretion of renin because angiotensin II feeds back directly on the juxtaglomerular cells to reduce renin secretion. However, in some women, the compensation is incomplete and the estrogens cause a significant increase in blood pressure. The incidence of this **pill hypertension** in the general hypertensive population is about 1% (Table 11–3). Some of the women with the condition have underlying essential hypertension which is triggered by the estrogens, but in others the hypertension is cured by stopping estrogen treatment. Mutations in the gene for angiotensinogen which produce slight increases in circulating angiotensinogen have been reported to be more common in patients with essential hypertension than in individuals with normal blood pressure.

D. Adrenal Gland Disorders: A remarkable number of adrenal abnormalities cause hypertension. These include mainly conditions in which mineralocorticoids are secreted in excess, but excess secretion of cortisol also causes hypertension, and so does excess secretion by tumors of the adrenal medulla.

1. Mineralocorticoid excess–The classic form of mineralocorticoid excess hypertension is primary hyperaldosteronism due to a tumor of the zona glomerulosa of the adrenal cortex (see Figure 21–17) that secretes large quantities of aldosterone (**Conn's syndrome**). The elevated circulating aldosterone level leads to Na⁺ retention with expansion of extracellular fluid volume and hypertension that is usually mild but can be severe. Because of the escape mechanism (see Chapter 21), edema does not occur, but there is chronic loss of K⁺ and H⁺. Consequently, the hallmark of Conn's syndrome is hypertension with the added feature of hypokalemia, and there may be alkalosis as well. The tumors are almost always benign and can be removed surgically.

Primary hyperaldosteronism can also be due to **bilateral hyperplasia** of the zona glomerulosa. This condition is less common than hyperaldosteronism due to an aldosterone-secreting tumor, and its cause is unknown.

Hypersecretion of deoxycorticosterone (DOC) can also cause mineralocorticoid-excess hypertension. DOC has less mineralocorticoid activity than aldosterone, but when present in increased amounts it can cause significant Na⁺ retention. DOC secretion, unlike aldosterone secretion, is increased by chronic hypersecretion of ACTH, so any condition that produces a chronic increase in ACTH secretion can also cause mineralocorticoid excess. This is the situation in **17α-hydroxylase deficiency;** the deficiency prevents the synthesis of cortisol, and ACTH secretion is consequently increased. However, the biosynthetic pathway leading to DOC is intact, and DOC secretion is increased. DOC is also the explanation of the hypertension found in the hypertensive form of **congenital adrenal hyperplasia.** This is due to 11β-hydroxylase deficiency, which prevents the conversion of DOC to corticosterone, causing circulating DOC to increase. In addition, the conversion of 11-deoxycortisol to cortisol is prevented, causing ACTH secretion to increase.

An interesting form of mineralocorticoid hypertension is **glucocorticoid-remediable aldosteronism (GRA).** In this autosomal dominant disorder, ACTH produces prolonged hypersecretion of aldosterone as well as glucocorticoids. The genes encoding aldosterone synthase and 11β-hydroxylase are 95% identical and located close together on chromosome 8. In GRA, there is unequal crossing over during development, and the regulatory 5′ portion of the 11β-hydroxylase gene is fused to the coding region of the aldosterone synthase gene, so that ACTH now causes induction of aldosterone synthase. The hypertension that results is variable in severity but is frequently more severe than the hypertension of primary hyperaldosteronism. Presumably this is because the tumors causing primary hyperaldosteronism develop later in life, whereas the congenital defect in GRA is present starting in early embryonic life. Strokes are common in GRA. GRA can be treated by administration of glucocorticoids in doses that suppress ACTH secretion. If the dose is chosen with care, inhibition of the secretion of ACTH can be achieved without producing the clinical features of Cushing's syndrome.

Another condition that mimics the effect of excess mineralocorticoid secretion is **apparent mineralocorticoid excess.** In vitro, mineralocorticoid receptors are as sensitive to glucocorticoids as they are to mineralocorticoids, but in vivo, mineralocorticoid effects are produced only by mineralocorticoid hormones. This is because of the presence in the vicinity of the receptor of 11β-hydroxysteroid dehydrogenase type 2, an enzyme that converts the glucocorticoids cortisol and corticosterone to their relatively inactive 11-oxo derivative (Figure 11–17). If this enzyme is congenitally absent or inhibited by substances such as licorice, which contains the enzyme inhibitor glycyrrhetinic acid, glucocorticoids have mineralocorticoid as well as glucocorticoid activity in vivo. Since glucocorticoids are normally present in much greater quantities than mineralocorticoids, their effect is relatively large.

2. Glucocorticoid excess–The incidence of hypertension is greater than normal in Cushing's syndrome, indicating that cortisol as well as mineralocorticoids can cause hypertension. The mechanism involved is unsettled, though there are a number of possibilities. First, glucocorticoids stimulate angiotensinogen secretion by the liver, and, as noted above, this increases circulating angiotensin II unless the feedback inhibition of renin secretion is able to compensate for the rise. Second, ACTH stimulates DOC secretion, and when present in increased amounts this steroid has appreciable mineralocorticoid activity. Third, there is evidence that glucocorticoids sensitize vascular smooth muscle to the contractile effect of catecholamines.

3. Excess secretion of catecholamines–Increases in adrenal medullary secretion of norepinephrine elevate systolic and diastolic pressure, and increases in epinephrine secretion may increase systolic pressure; but excess secretion from the normal adrenal medulla has not been reported to cause sustained hypertension. However, tumors of the adrenal medulla (**pheochromocytomas**) secrete enough catecholamines to cause hypertension. These tumors are discussed in Chapter 12. Norepinephrine-secreting pheochromocytomas may produce sustained hypertension as their only manifestation, though more commonly the hypertension is episodic or at least waxes and wanes in severity (Chapter 12). Epinephrine-secreting pheochromocytomas usually release epinephrine episodically, producing intermittent bouts of palpitation, headache, glycosuria, and systolic hypertension. Thus, the symptoms produced mirror the effects of injecting the two catecholamines. Pheochromocytomas can be diagnosed by measuring circulating or urinary catecholamines or their metabolites. If catecholamines are normal between episodic attacks, secretory responses can be provoked by injection of glucagon. However, this is not recommended because provoked attacks can be dangerous. Alternatively, one can administer clonidine, which blocks central α₂-adrenergic receptors

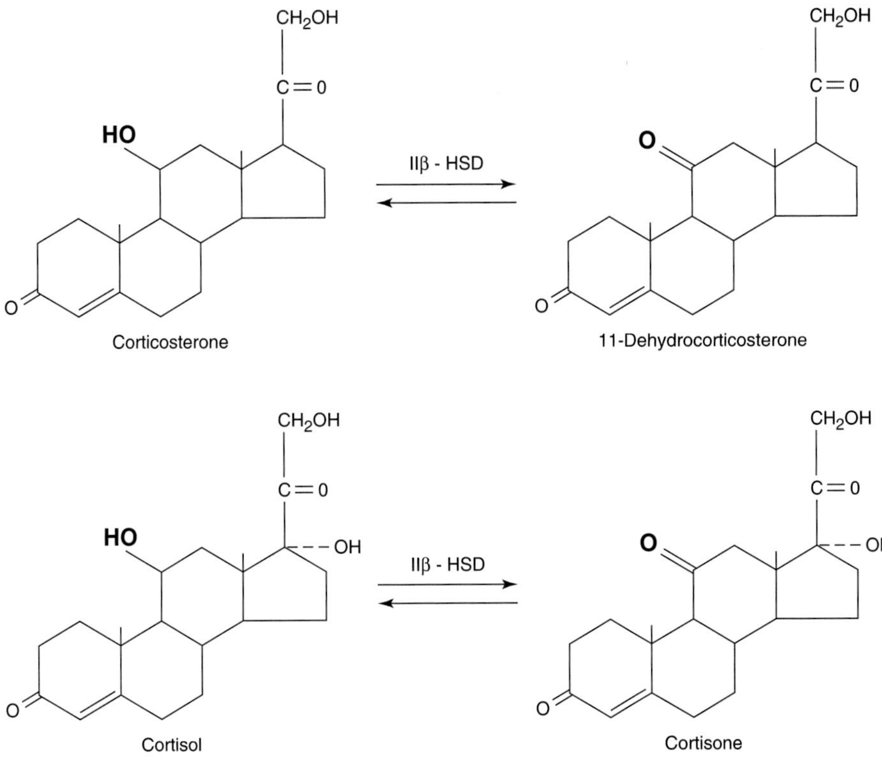

Figure 11–17. Formation of 11-keto derivatives of corticosterone and cortisol, catalyzed by 11β-hydroxysteroid dehydrogenase (11β-HSD). There are at least two isozymes of 11β-HSD. 11β-HSD type 1 is a reversible NADP(H)-dependent enzyme catalyzing both dehydrogenation and oxidation. 11β-HSD type 2 is an NAD-dependent enzyme that catalyzes dehydrogenation exclusively. It is this latter form that protects mineralocorticoid receptors from activation by glucocorticoids because 11-keto derivatives do not bind to mineralocorticoid receptors. (Modified from Seckl J: 11β-Hydroxysteroid dehydrogenase in the brain: A novel regulator of glucocorticoid action? Front Neuroendocrinol 1997;18:49.)

and lowers blood pressure in patients with essential hypertension but has little or no effect in patients with pheochromocytoma (see Chapter 12). Surgical removal of a pheochromocytoma effects a cure in many cases. However, pheochromocytomas can be multiple, can recur, and may be malignant, with metastases.

E. Natriuretic Hormones: In view of the fact that sodium retention due to mineralocorticoid excess causes hypertension, it may seem surprising that a natriuretic hormone is also a suspected cause of hypertension. Atrial natriuretic peptide (ANP) and other natriuretic peptides of cardiac origin cause sodium loss in the urine and generally lower blood pressure. However, there is in addition a digitalis-like natriuretic substance in the circulation. Its source seems to be the adrenals, though it has also been claimed that it is secreted by the hypothalamus. This substance, which may be naturally occurring ouabain, inhibits Na^+-K^+ ATPase. This results in loss of Na^+ in the urine, but Ca^{2+} accumulates in cells because of the decrease in Na^+ gradient across the cell membrane. The increase in intracellular Ca^{2+} causes vascular smooth muscle to contract. Consequently, blood pressure is increased. However, the physiologic and pathophysiologic significance of this natriuretic hormone remains unsettled, and hypersecretion of it cannot as yet be considered to be a proved cause of clinical hypertension.

F. Neurologic Disorders: The nervous system plays a key role in maintaining blood pressure in normal individuals (see above). Inhibition of central α_2 receptors by clonidine lowers blood pressure, and several of the most effective treatments for chronic hypertension act by decreasing the magnitude or effect of vasomotor sympathetic discharge to the blood vessels and heart. These and other observations suggest that clinical hypertension could be caused by central nervous system abnormalities. Interruption of the afferent input from the baroreceptors to the central nervous system in experimental animals causes increased blood pressure. However, emphasis has been placed recently on the variability of the blood pressure in such animals rather than any consistent elevation of mean arterial pressure. Furthermore, no comparable condition has been described in humans, and no definite syndrome due to a primary central nervous system abnormality has yet been identified as a cause of human hypertension.

G. Nitric Oxide: An intriguing recent observation in experimental animals is that administration of drugs that inhibit the production of nitric oxide (NO) increase blood pressure. Furthermore, there is a sustained elevation in blood pressure in knockout mice, in which the genetic expression of the endothelial form of nitric oxide synthase has been disrupted. These observations suggest that there is a chronic blood pressure-lowering effect of NO and raise the possibility that inhibition of the production or effects of NO could be a cause of hypertension in humans. As noted above, endothelium-dependent vasodilation is diffusely reduced in patients with atherosclerosis, and many of these are hypertensive.

H. Facilitation of Na^+-H^+ Exchange: In approximately 50% of patients with essential hypertension, the function of a ubiquitous pH-regulating Na^+-H^+ exchanger in cell membranes is enhanced. Recent evidence indicates that this is associated with a polymorphism in the gene for one of the β subunits of a G protein which facilitates the function of the G protein. However, the overall significance of this abnormality remains to be determined.

I. Relation to Insulin Resistance: There is a higher incidence of insulin resistance, hyperinsulinemia, hyperlipidemia, and obesity in patients with essential hypertension and in their normotensive relatives than there is in the general population or in patients with hypertension due to known causes. Hyperinsulinemia is present in about 45% of patients with essential hypertension compared with about 10% of the normotensive population. These observations have led some to speculate that in certain patients, insulin resistance increases insulin secretion, and the resulting hyperinsulinemia stimulates the sympathetic nervous system, causing the hypertension. However, patients with insulin-secreting pancreatic tumors (insulinomas) do not have an increased incidence of hypertension, and in dogs and normal humans, prolonged infusions of insulin have a slight vasodilator rather than a vasoconstricter effect. In addition, in a careful study of obese patients with essential hypertension, prolonged infusion of insulin caused a small decrease rather than an increase in blood pressure. Thus, although the cause of the insulin resistance, hyperinsulinemia, obesity, and hyperlipidemia in hypertension remains unknown, it seems unlikely that increased insulin resistance is a major cause of essential hypertension.

14. Describe five physical findings in long-standing or severe hypertension.
15. Name ten known causes of hypertension and a means by which each could be identified as the cause of hypertension in a patient.
16. What is the effect on blood pressure of disrupting the gene for the endothelial cell form of nitric oxide synthase in mice?

SHOCK

The term "shock" is used to denote various conditions. These include the response to passage of electric current through the body; the state that follows immediately after interruption of the spinal cord; and the stunned reaction to bad news. In the current context, it refers to an abnormality of the circulatory system in which there is inadequate tissue perfusion due to a relatively or absolutely inadequate cardiac output. The causes are divided into four groups: inadequate volume of blood to fill the vascular system (**hypovolemic shock**); increased size of the vascular system produced by vasodilation in the presence of a normal blood volume (**distributive, vasogenic, or low-resistance shock**); inadequate output of the heart as a result of myocardial abnormalities (**cardiogenic shock**); and inadequate cardiac output as a result of obstruction of blood flow in the lungs or heart (**obstructive shock**). Examples of the conditions or diseases that can cause each type are set forth in Table 11–5.

Table 11–5. Types of shock, with examples of conditions or diseases that can cause each type.

Hypovolemic shock (decreased blood volume)
Hemorrhage
Trauma
Surgery
Burns
Fluid loss associated with vomiting or diarrhea
Distributive shock (marked vasodilation; also called vasogenic or low-resistance shock)
Fainting (neurogenic shock)
Anaphylaxis
Sepsis (also causes hypovolemia due to increased capillary permeability with loss of fluid into tissues)
Cardiogenic shock (inadequate output by a diseased heart)
Myocardial infarction
Congestive heart failure
Arrhythmias
Obstructive shock (obstruction of blood flow)
Tension pneumothorax
Pulmonary embolism
Cardiac tumor
Pericardial tamponade

1. HYPOVOLEMIC SHOCK

Hypovolemic shock is characterized by hypotension; a rapid, thready pulse; a cold, pale, clammy skin; intense thirst; rapid respiration; and restlessness or, alternatively, torpor. Urine volume is markedly decreased. However, none of these findings are invariably present. Hypovolemic shock is commonly subdivided into categories on the basis of cause. The use of terms such as hemorrhagic shock, traumatic shock, surgical shock, and burn shock is of some benefit because although there are similarities between these various forms of shock, there are important features that are unique to each.

In hypovolemic and other forms of shock, inadequate perfusion of the tissues leads to increased anaerobic glycolysis, with production of large amounts of lactic acid. In severe cases, the blood lactate level rises from a normal value of about 1 mmol/L to 9 mmol/L or more. The resulting lactic acidosis depresses the myocardium, decreases peripheral vascular responsiveness to catecholamines, and may be severe enough to cause coma.

Multiple compensatory reactions come into play to defend extracellular fluid volume (Table 11–6). The large number of reactions that have evolved indicate the importance of maintaining blood volume for survival.

A decrease in pulse pressure or mean arterial pressure decreases the number of impulses ascending to the brain from the arterial baroreceptors, and the result is increased vasomotor discharge. The resulting vasoconstriction is generalized, sparing only the vessels of the brain and the heart. The coronary vessels are dilated because of the increased myocardial metabolism secondary to an increase in heart rate. Vasoconstriction in the skin accounts for the coolness and pallor, and vasoconstriction in the kidneys accounts for the shutdown in renal function.

The immediate cardiac response to hypovolemia is tachycardia. With more extensive loss of volume, tachycardia can be replaced by bradycardia, whereas with very severe hypovolemia, tachycardia reappears. Bradycardia may be due to unmasking of a vagally mediated depressor reflex, perhaps related to limiting blood loss.

Vasoconstriction in the kidney reduces glomerular filtration. This reduces water loss, but it reaches a point where nitrogenous products of metabolism accumulate in the blood (**prerenal azotemia**). If hypotension is prolonged, there may be severe renal tubular damage leading to acute renal failure.

The fall in blood pressure and the decreased O_2-carrying power of the blood due to loss of red cells results in stimulation of the carotid and aortic chemoreceptors. This not only stimulates respiration but increases vasoconstrictor discharge. In severe hypovolemia, the pressure is so low that there is no longer any discharge from the carotid and aortic baroreceptors. This occurs when the mean blood pressure is about 70 mm Hg. Under these circumstances, if the afferent discharge from the chemoreceptors via the carotid sinus and vagus nerves is stopped, there is a paradoxic further fall in blood pressure rather than a rise.

Hypovolemia causes a marked increase in the circulating levels of the pressor hormones angiotensin II, epinephrine, norepinephrine, and vasopressin. ACTH secretion is also increased, and angiotensin II and ACTH both cause an acute increase in aldosterone secretion. The resulting retention of Na^+ and water helps reexpand blood volume.

Refractory Shock

Depending largely on the severity of the shock, some patients die soon after the onset of hypovolemia, and others recover as compensatory mechanisms gradually restore the circulation to normal. In an intermediate group of patients, shock persists for hours and gradually progresses. It eventually reaches a state in which there is no longer any response to vasopressor drugs and in which—even if the blood volume is returned to normal—cardiac output remains depressed. This condition is known as **refractory shock.** The condition occurs in other forms of shock as well. It used to be called **irreversible shock,** and patients still die despite vigorous treatment. However, more and more patients are saved as understanding of the pathophysiologic mechanisms increases and treatment is improved. Therefore, "refractory shock" seems to be a more appropriate term.

Various factors appear to make shock refractory. Precapillary sphincters are constricted for several hours but then relax while postcapillary venules remain constricted. Therefore, blood flows into the capillaries and remains there. Various positive feedback mechanisms contribute to the refractory state. For example, cerebral ischemia depresses vasomotor

---

Table 11–6. Compensatory reactions activated by hypovolemia.

Vasoconstriction
Tachycardia
Venoconstriction
Tachypnea → Increased thoracic pumping
Restlessness → Increased skeletal muscle pumping (in some cases)
Increased movement of interstitial fluid into capillaries
Increased secretion of vasopressin
Increased secretion of glucocorticoids
Increased secretion of renin and aldosterone
Increased secretion of erythropoietin
Increased plasma protein synthesis

and cardiac discharge, causing blood pressure to fall and making the shock worse. This in turn causes a further reduction in cerebral blood flow. In addition, myocardial blood flow is reduced in severe shock. Myocardial failure makes the pumping action of the heart less effective and consequently makes the shock worse and further lowers myocardial blood flow.

A late complication of shock that has a very high mortality rate is pulmonary damage with production of acute respiratory distress syndrome (ARDS). This also occurs with severe injuries. The common feature appears to be capillary endothelial cell damage and damage to alveolar epithelial cells with the release of cytokines (see Chapter 9).

Forms of Hypovolemic Shock

Hemorrhagic shock is probably the most carefully studied form of shock because it is easily produced in experimental animals. With moderate hemorrhage (5–15 mL/kg body weight), pulse pressure is reduced but mean arterial pressure may remain normal. With more severe hemorrhage, blood pressure always falls.

After hemorrhage, the plasma protein lost in shed blood is gradually replaced by hepatic synthesis, and the concentration of plasma proteins returns to normal in 3–4 days. The increase in circulating erythropoietin increases red blood cell formation, but it takes 4–8 weeks to restore red cell counts to normal.

Traumatic shock develops when there is severe damage to muscle and bone. This is the type of shock seen in battle casualties and automobile accident victims. Bleeding into the injured areas is the principal cause of such shock. The amount of blood that can be lost into a site of injury that appears relatively minor is remarkable; the thigh muscles can accommodate 1 L of extravasated blood, for example, with an increase in the diameter of the thigh of only 1 cm.

Breakdown of skeletal muscle is a serious additional problem when shock is accompanied by extensive crushing of muscle **(crush syndrome)**. When pressure on tissues is relieved and they are once again perfused with blood, free radicals are generated, and these cause further tissue destruction **(reperfusion-induced injury)**. Increased Ca^{2+} in damaged cells can reach toxic levels. Large amounts of K^+ enter the circulation. Myoglobin and other products from reperfused tissue can accumulate in kidneys in which glomerular filtration is already reduced by hypotension, and the tubules can become clogged, causing anuria.

Surgical shock is due to combinations in various proportions of external hemorrhage, bleeding into injured tissues, and dehydration.

In **burn shock,** there is loss of plasma from burn surfaces and the hematocrit rises rather than falls, producing severe hemoconcentration. There are in addition complex metabolic changes. For these reasons plus the problems of easy infection of burned areas and kidney damage, the mortality rate when third-degree burns cover more than 75% of the body is close to 100%.

2. DISTRIBUTIVE SHOCK

In distributive shock, most of the symptoms and signs described above are present. However, vasodilation causes the skin to be warm rather than cold and clammy. **Anaphylactic shock** is a good example of distributive shock. In this condition, an accelerated allergic reaction causes release of large amounts of histamine, producing marked vasodilation. Blood pressure falls because the size of the vascular system exceeds the amount of blood in it even though blood volume is normal.

Another form of distributive shock is **septic shock.** This is now the most common cause of death in intensive care units in the United States. It is a complex condition that may include elements of hypovolemic shock due to loss of plasma into the tissues ("third spacing") and cardiogenic shock due to toxins that depress the myocardium. It is discussed in detail in Chapter 4.

A third type of distributive shock is **neurogenic shock,** in which a sudden burst of autonomic activity results in vasodilation and pooling of blood in the veins. The resulting decrease in venous return reduces cardiac output and frequently produces fainting, or **syncope,** a sudden transient loss of consciousness. A common form is **postural syncope,** which occurs on rising from a sitting or lying position. This is common in patients taking drugs that block sympathetic discharge or its effects on the blood vessels. Falling to the horizontal position restores blood flow to the brain, and consciousness is regained. Pressure on the carotid sinus produced, for example, by a tight collar can cause sufficient bradycardia and hypotension to cause fainting (carotid sinus syncope). Fainting brought on by a variety of activities has been given appropriate names such as micturition syncope, cough syncope, deglutition syncope, and effort syncope.

Syncope due to neurogenic shock is usually benign. However, it must be distinguished from syncope due to other causes and therefore merits investigation. About 25% of syncopal episodes are of cardiac origin and are due either to transient obstruction of blood flow through the heart or to sudden decreases in cardiac output caused by various cardiac arrhythmias. In addition, fainting is the presenting symptom in 7% of patients with myocardial infarctions.

3. CARDIOGENIC SHOCK

When the pumping function of the heart is impaired to the point that blood flow to tissues is no longer adequate to meet resting metabolic demands, the condition that results is called **cardiogenic shock.** This is most commonly due to extensive infarction of the left ventricle, but it can also be caused by other diseases that severely compromise ventricular function. The symptoms are those of hypovolemic shock plus congestion of the lungs and viscera due to failure of the heart to put out all the venous blood returned to it. Consequently, the condition is sometimes called "congested shock." The incidence of shock in patients with myocardial infarction is about 10%, and the mortality rate is 60–90%.

4. OBSTRUCTIVE SHOCK

The picture of congested shock is also seen in **obstructive shock.** Causes include massive pulmonary emboli, tension pneumothorax with kinking of the great veins, and bleeding into the pericardium with external pressure on the heart **(cardiac tamponade).** In the latter two conditions, prompt operation is required to prevent death. Pulsus paradoxus occurs in cardiac tamponade. Normally, blood pressure falls about 5 mm Hg during inspiration. In pulsus paradoxus, this response is exaggerated, and blood pressure falls 10 mm Hg or more as a result of increased pressure of the fluid in the pericardial sac on the external surface of the heart. However, pulsus paradoxus also occurs with labored respiration in severe asthma, emphysema, and upper airway obstruction.

---

17. What are the four major pathophysiologic forms of shock?
18. Name three pathophysiologic consequences of lactic acidosis in shock.
19. Name three factors that tend to make shock refractory.
20. Describe five specific forms of hypovolemic shock.
21. Name three specific forms of distributive shock and distinguish them from hypovolemic shock.

REFERENCES

General
Dampney RAL: Functional organization of central pathways regulating the cardiovascular system. Physiol Rev 1994;74:323.
Levin ER: Endothelins. N Engl J Med 1995;333:356.
Levin ER, Gardner DG, Samson WK: Natriuretic peptides. N Engl J Med 1998;339:321.
Margulius HS: Kallikreins and kinins. Hypertension 1995;26:221.
Resnick N, Gibrone MA Jr: Hemodynamic forces are complex regulators of endothelial gene expression. FASEB J 1995;9:874.
Rowell LB: *Human Cardiovascular Control.* Oxford Univ Press, 1993.

Atherosclerosis
Anderson TJ et al: Systemic nature of endothelial dysfunction in atherosclerosis. Am J Cardiol 1995;75:71B.
Hayden MR, Reidy M: Many roads lead to atheroma. Nat Med 1995;1:22.
Levine GN, Keaney JF Jr, Vita JF: Cholesterol reduction in cardiovascular disease: Clinical benefits and possible mechanisms. N Engl J Med 1995;332:512.
Myant NB: *Cholesterol Metabolism, LDL, and the LDL Receptor.* Academic Press, 1990.
Ross R: Atherosclerosis—an inflammatory disease. N Engl J Med 1999;340:116.
Walsh GN, Loscalzo J: Homocysteine and atherothrombosis. N Engl J Med 1998;338:1042.

Hypertension
Corvol P, Jeanmaitre X: Molecular genetics of human hypertension: Role of angiotensinogen. Endocr Rev 1998;18:662.
Kirkendall WM et al: Recommendations for human blood pressure determination by sphygmomanometers. Hypertension 1981;3:510A.
Reaven GM, Lithell H, Landsberg L: Hypertension and associated metabolic abnormalities: The role of insulin resistance and the sympathoadrenal system. N Engl J Med 1996;334:374.
Swales JD (editor): *Textbook of Hypertension.* Blackwell, 1994.

Shock
Califf RM, Bengston JR: Cardiogenic shock. N Engl J Med 1994;330:1724.
Odeh M: The role of reperfusion-induced injury in the pathogenesis of the crush syndrome. N Engl J Med 1991;324:1417.
Trunkey DD, Salber PR, Mills J: Shock. In: *Current Emergency Diagnosis & Treatment,* 4th ed. Saunders CE, Ho MT (editors). Appleton & Lange, 1992.

12 Disorders of the Adrenal Medulla

Stephen J. McPhee, MD

The **adrenal medulla** secretes catecholamines (epinephrine, norepinephrine, and dopamine). The catecholamines help prepare the individual to deal with emergency situations. The major disorder of the adrenal medulla is **pheochromocytoma,** a neoplasm characterized by excessive catecholamine secretion.

NORMAL STRUCTURE & FUNCTION OF THE ADRENAL MEDULLA

ANATOMY

The adrenal medulla is the reddish-brown central layer of the adrenal gland (Figure 21–2). Accessory medullary tissue is sometimes located in the retroperitoneum near the sympathetic ganglia or along the abdominal aorta (paraganglia) (Figure 12–1).

HISTOLOGY

The adrenal medulla is made up of polyhedral cells arranged in cords or clumps. Embryologically, the adrenal medullary cells derive from neural crest cells. Medullary cells are innervated by cholinergic preganglionic nerve fibers that reach the gland via the splanchnic nerves. Medullary parenchymal cells accumulate and store their hormone products in prominent, dense secretory granules, 150–350 nm in diameter. Histologically, these cells and granules have a high affinity for chromium salts **(chromaffin reaction)** and thus are called **chromaffin cells** and **chromaffin granules.** The granules contain the catecholamines epinephrine and norepinephrine. Morphologically, two types of medullary cells can be distinguished: epinephrine-secreting cells have larger, less dense granules, and norepinephrine-secreting cells have smaller, very dense granules. Separate dopamine-secreting cells have not been identified. Ninety percent of medullary cells are the epinephrine-secreting type and 10% the norepinephrine-secreting type.

PHYSIOLOGY

The catecholamines help to regulate metabolism, contractility of cardiac and smooth muscle, and neurotransmission.

Formation, Secretion, & Metabolism of Catecholamines

The adrenal medulla secretes three catecholamines: epinephrine, norepinephrine, and dopamine.

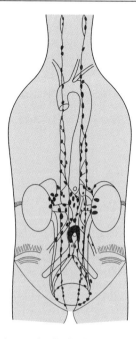

Figure 12–1. Anatomic distribution of extra-adrenal chromaffin tissue in the newborn. (Reproduced, with permission, from Coupland R: *The Natural History of the Chromaffin Cell.* Longman, Green, 1965.)

Secretion occurs following release of acetylcholine from the preganglionic neurons that innervate the medullary cells. The major biosynthetic pathways and hormonal intermediates for the catecholamines are shown in Figure 12–2. In humans, most (80%) of the catecholamine output of the adrenal medulla is epinephrine. Norepinephrine is principally found in nerve endings of the sympathetic nervous system and in the central nervous system, where it functions as a major neurotransmitter.

About 70% of the epinephrine and norepinephrine and 95% of the dopamine found in plasma are conjugated to sulfate and inactive. In the supine state, the normal plasma level of free epinephrine is about 30 pg/mL (0.16 nmol/L); there is a 50–100% increase upon standing. The normal plasma level of free norepinephrine is about 300 pg/mL (1.8 nmol/L), and the plasma free dopamine level is about 35 pg/mL (0.23 nmol/L).

In the circulation, the catecholamines have a short half-life of about 2 minutes. They are metabolized primarily by methoxylation to metanephrine and normetanephrine and by oxidation to 3-methoxy-4-hydroxymandelic acid (vanillylmandelic acid [VMA]) and excreted in the urine as free or conjugated metanephrine and normetanephrine (about 50%) and as VMA (about 35%). Normally, only very small quantities of free epinephrine (about 6 μg/d) and norepinephrine (about 30 μg/d) are excreted, but about 700 μg of VMA is excreted daily.

Regulation of Catecholamine Secretion

Physiologic stimuli affect medullary secretion through the nervous system. Medullary cells secrete catecholamines following release of acetylcholine from the preganglionic neurons that innervate them. Catecholamine secretion is low in the basal state and is reduced even further during sleep. In emergency situations, there is increased adrenal catecholamine secretion as part of a generalized sympathetic discharge that serves to prepare the individual for stress ("fight or flight" response). Hypoglycemia and certain drugs are also potent stimuli to catecholamine secretion.

Mechanism of Action of Catecholamines

The effects of epinephrine and norepinephrine are mediated by their actions on two classes of receptors: alpha- and beta-adrenergic receptors (Table 12–1). Alpha receptors are subdivided into α_1 and α_2 receptors and beta receptors into β_1, β_2, and β_3 receptors. Alpha$_1$ receptors mediate smooth muscle contraction in blood vessels and the genitourinary tract and increase glycogenolysis. Alpha$_2$ receptors mediate smooth muscle relaxation in the gastrointestinal tract and vasoconstriction of some blood vessels. Alpha$_2$ receptors also decrease insulin secretion. Beta$_1$ receptors mediate an increased rate and force of myocardial contraction and stimulate lipolysis and renin release. Beta$_2$ receptors mediate smooth muscle relaxation in the bronchi, blood vessels, genitourinary tract, and gastrointestinal tract and increase hepatic gluconeogenesis and glycogenolysis, muscle glycogenolysis, and release of insulin and glucagon.

The molecular mechanisms behind adrenergic receptor function are now at least partially understood. Stimulation of α_1-adrenergic receptors results in an increase in intracellular calcium concentrations. Several mechanisms are involved. First, there is activation of phospholipase C by the guanine nucleotide binding stimulatory protein, G_s. Phospholipase C hydrolyzes the membrane-bound phospholipid, phosphatidylinositol-4,5-bisphosphate, to generate two second messengers: diacylglycerol and inositol-1,4,5-trisphosphate. Diacylglycerol in turn activates protein kinase C, which phosphorylates various cel-

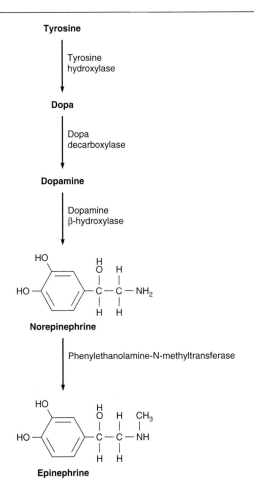

Figure 12–2. Biosynthesis of catecholamines. (Modified and reproduced, with permission, from Greenspan FS, Strewler GJ [editors]: *Basic and Clinical Endocrinology*, 5th ed. Appleton & Lange, 1997.)

Table 12–1. Physiologic effects of catecholamines on adrenergic receptors of selected tissues.[1]

Organ or Tissue	Adrenergic Receptor	Effect
Heart (myocardium)	β_1 α_1, β_1 β_1 β_1	Increased force of contraction (inotropic) Increased rate of contraction (chronotropic) Increased excitability (predisposes to arrhythmia) Increased AV nodal conduction velocity
Blood vessels (vascular smooth muscle)	α_1, α_2 β_2	Vasoconstriction, hypertension Vasodilation
Kidney (juxtaglomerular cells)	β_1	Increased renin release
Gut (intestinal smooth muscle)	α_1 β_2	Increased sphincter tone (hyperpolarization); decreased motility (relaxation) Decreased motility (relaxation)
Pancreas (B cells)	α_2 β_2	Decreased insulin release Decreased glucagon release Increased insulin release Increased glucagon release
Liver	α_1, β_2	Increased gluconeogenesis Increased glycogenolysis Release of potassium
Adipose tissue	α β_1, β_3	Decreased lipolysis Increased lipolysis
Skin (apocrine glands on hands, axillas, etc)	α_1	Increased sweating
Lung (bronchial smooth muscle)	β_2	Dilation of bronchi and bronchioles
Uterus (genitourinary smooth muscle)	α_1 β_2	Contraction Relaxation
Bladder (genitourinary smooth muscle)	α_1 β_2	Contraction Relaxation
Skeletal muscle	β_2	Vasodilation Increased glycogenolysis Increased release of lactic acid
Platelets	α_2	Aggregation
Central nervous system	α	Increased alertness, anxiety, fear
Peripheral nerves	α_2	Decreased norepinephrine release
Most tissues	β	Increased calorigenesis Increased metabolic rate

[1]Modified and reproduced, with permission, from Greenspan FS, Strewler GJ (editors): *Basic and Clinical Endocrinology,* 5th ed. Appleton & Lange, 1997.

lular substrates; and inositol-1,4,5-trisphosphate stimulates release of intracellular calcium, which then initiates various cellular responses.

Activation of α_2-adrenergic receptors results in a decrease in intracellular cAMP. The mechanism involves receptor interaction with an inhibitory G protein, G_i, leading to inhibition of adenylyl cyclase. The fall in cAMP level leads to a decrease in activity of the cAMP-dependent protein kinase A. The G_i protein also stimulates K^+ channels and inhibits voltage-sensitive calcium channels.

On the other hand, β-adrenergic receptors stimulate adenylyl cyclase through the mediation of G_s. Activation of β-adrenergic receptors thus leads to an increase in cAMP, activation of the cAMP-dependent protein kinase A, and consequent phosphorylation of various cellular proteins. The G_s protein can also directly activate voltage-sensitive calcium channels in the plasma membrane of cardiac and skeletal muscle.

The α_1- and β_1-adrenergic receptors are generally found in organs and tissues (eg, heart and gut) that are heavily innervated by—and situated so as to be readily activated by stimulation of—the sympathetic nerves. The α_1- and β_1-adrenergic receptors are preferentially stimulated by norepinephrine, especially that released by nerve endings. In contrast, the α_2- and β_2-adrenergic receptors are generally situated in postjunctional sites in organs and tissues (eg, uterine and bronchial skeletal muscle) remote from sites of norepinephrine release. The α_2- and β_2-adrenergic receptors are preferentially stimulated by circulating catecholamines, especially epinephrine.

Effects of Catecholamines

The catecholamines have been termed the hormones of "fight or flight" because their effects on the heart, blood vessels, smooth muscle, and metabolism assist the organism in responding to stress. The principal physiologic effects of the catecholamines are shown in Table 12-1.

In the peripheral circulation, norepinephrine produces vasoconstriction in most organs (via α_1 receptors). Epinephrine produces vasodilation via β_2 receptors in skeletal muscle and liver and vasoconstriction elsewhere. The former usually outweighs the latter, and for that reason epinephrine usually lowers total peripheral resistance.

Norepinephrine causes both systolic and diastolic blood pressures to rise. The rise in blood pressure stimulates the carotid and aortic baroreceptors, resulting in reflex bradycardia and a fall in cardiac output. Epinephrine causes a widening of pulse pressure but does not stimulate the baroreceptors to the same degree, so the pulse rises and cardiac output increases.

The effects of catecholamines on metabolism include effects on glycogenolysis, lipolysis, and insulin secretion, mediated by both alpha- and beta-adrenergic receptors. These metabolic effects result primarily from the action of epinephrine on four target tissues: liver, muscle, pancreas, and adipose tissue (see Table 12-1). The result is an increase in the levels of circulating glucose and free fatty acids. The increased supply of these two substances helps provide an adequate supply of metabolic fuel to the nervous system and muscle during physiologic stress.

The amount of circulating plasma epinephrine and norepinephrine needed to produce these various effects has been determined by infusing the catecholamines into resting subjects. For norepinephrine, the threshold for the cardiovascular and metabolic effects is about 1500 pg/mL, or about five times the basal level. In normal individuals, the plasma norepinephrine level rarely exceeds this threshold. However, for epinephrine, the threshold for tachycardia occurs at a plasma level of about 50 pg/mL, or about twice the basal level. The threshold for increasing systolic blood pressure and lipolysis is at about 75 pg/mL; for increasing glucose and lactate, about 150 pg/mL; and for increasing insulin secretion, about 40 pg/mL. In normal individuals, plasma epinephrine levels often exceed these thresholds.

The physiologic effect of circulating dopamine is unknown. Centrally, dopamine acts to inhibit prolactin secretion. Peripherally, in small doses, injected dopamine produces renal vasodilation, probably by binding to a specific dopaminergic receptor. In moderate doses, it also produces vasodilation of the mesenteric and coronary circulation and vasoconstriction peripherally. It has a positive inotropic effect on the heart, mediated by action on the β_1-adrenergic receptors. Moderate to large doses of dopamine increase the systolic blood pressure without affecting diastolic pressure.

---

1. What is the embryologic origin of the cells of the adrenal medulla?
2. What fibers innervate the adrenal medulla?
3. Which catecholamines are secreted by the human adrenal medulla? Of these, which is the major product?
4. What are the major physiologic stimuli of catecholamine secretion?
5. What are the subtypes and distribution of catecholamine receptors?
6. What physiologic processes do each subtype of catecholamine receptor control, and how do catecholamines affect the physiologic process?

OVERVIEW OF ADRENAL MEDULLARY DISORDERS

Pheochromocytoma is an uncommon tumor of adrenal medullary tissue that causes production of excessive amounts of catecholamines. Patients typically present with sustained or episodic hypertension or with a syndrome characterized by episodic palpitations, tachycardia, chest pain, headache, anxiety, blanching, excessive sweating, hyperglycemia, and glycosuria.

Two unusual catecholamine deficiency states have also been described. **Sympathetic neural failure** is caused by deficient production of norepinephrine, and **adrenomedullary failure** is caused by deficient production of epinephrine.

PATHOPHYSIOLOGY OF SELECTED DISORDERS OF THE ADRENAL MEDULLA

PHEOCHROMOCYTOMA

Pheochromocytomas are neoplasms of the chromaffin cells of the adrenal medulla or extramedullary sites. These tumors secrete excessive amounts of epinephrine, norepinephrine, or both. Most pheochromocytomas secrete norepinephrine and cause sustained or episodic hypertension. Pheochromocytomas that secrete epinephrine cause hypertension less often; more frequently, they produce episodic hyperglycemia, glucosuria, and other metabolic effects.

Table 12–2 summarizes the clinical features of pheochromocytomas. Pheochromocytomas are uncommon, probably found in less than 0.1% of all patients with hypertension and in approximately two individuals per million population. Pheochromocytomas occur in both sexes and in all age groups but are most often diagnosed in the fourth or fifth decades. The diagnosis is important because sudden release of catecholamines from these tumors during surgery or obstetric delivery may prove fatal. Pheochromocytoma is sometimes called "the 10% tumor" because 10% occur in extra-adrenal paraganglia, 10% are outside the abdomen, 10% are multiple, 10% are bilateral, about 10% are not associated with hypertension, 10% occur in children, 10% are malignant, and about 10% occur as part of a familial syndrome (Table 12–3).

Etiology

Pheochromocytomas usually occur sporadically but may also occur in familial distribution with an autosomal dominant pattern of inheritance (Table 12–3). Patients with type 1 neurofibromatosis (Recklinghausen's disease) have an increased incidence of pheochromocytoma. Pheochromocytoma is a frequent occurrence in families with von Hippel-Lindau disease, which is caused by mutations of the *VHL* tumor suppressor gene. More commonly, pheochromocytomas occur in association with other endocrine tumors. In the syndrome called multiple endocrine neoplasia (MEN) type 2a (Sipple's syndrome), pheochromocytomas occur in association with calcitonin-producing medullary carcinoma or C cell hyperplasia of the thyroid and parathyroid hormone-producing adenomas of the parathyroid. In MEN 2b, pheochromocytomas occur in association with medullary carcinoma of the thyroid and numerous oral mucosal neuromas. About 40% of patients with MEN 2a and 2b have bilateral pheochromocytomas.

The gene responsible for MEN types 2a and 2b has now been localized to chromosome 10q11.2. In 1993, more than two dozen different families with MEN 2a were found to have missense point mutations of the *RET* proto-oncogene, a tyrosine kinase receptor gene expressed at low levels in normal human thyroid tissue and at high levels in medullary thyroid carcinoma and pheochromocytoma tissue. Subsequently, it has been documented that the position of the *RET* mutation is related to disease phenotype. Any mutation of the *RET* proto-oncogene at one specific position (codon 634) is associated with pheochromocytoma as part of MEN type 2a and mutations at a different position (codon 918), with pheochromocytoma as part of MEN type 2b. These germline mutations of the *RET* proto-oncogene are the first examples of a dominantly acting oncogenic point mutation causing a heritable neoplasm in humans. These missense mutations can be detected by DNA analysis, allowing identification of MEN carri-

Table 12–2. Clinical features of pheochromocytoma.[1]

Epidemiology	Adults; both sexes; all ages, especially 30–50 years
Biologic behavior	90% benign; 10% malignant
Secretion	High levels of catecholamines; most secrete norepinephrine
Clinical presentation	Episodic or sustained hypertension, sweating, palpitations, hyperglycemia, glycosuria
Macroscopic features	Mass, often hemorrhagic; 10% bilateral; 10% extra-adrenal
Microscopic features	Nests of large cells, vascular stroma

[1]Modified from Chandrasoma P, Taylor CR (editors): *Concise Pathology,* 2nd ed. Appleton & Lange, 1994.

Table 12–3. Classification of pheochromocytoma.

A. Sporadic pheochromocytoma (90%)
B. Familial pheochromocytoma (10%)
  1. Recklinghausen's disease
      Pheochromocytoma (in 1% of familial cases) in association with neurofibromatosis
  2. Multiple endocrine neoplasia type 2a (Sipple's syndrome)
      Pheochromocytoma (in 40% of familial cases) in association with medullary carcinoma of thyroid or C cell hyperplasia, or with hyperparathyroidism
  3. Multiple endocrine neoplasia type 2b
      Pheochromocytoma (in 40% of familial cases) in association with medullary carcinoma of thyroid or C cell hyperplasia, mucosal neuromas, intestinal ganglioneuromas, and marfanoid habitus
  4. von Hippel-Lindau syndrome
      Pheochromocytoma (in 14% of familial cases) in association with CNS hemangioblastomas, retinal angiomas, renal cysts or carcinomas, pancreatic cysts, epididymal cystadenomas

ers. *RET* mutations have not been found in cases of sporadic pheochromocytoma.

Almost all pheochromocytomas (about 90%) occur in the abdomen, and most of these (85%) are in the adrenal medulla. Extra-adrenal pheochromocytomas (sometimes called gangliomas or paragangliomas) are found in the perirenal area, the organ of Zuckerkandl, the urinary bladder, the heart, the neck, and the posterior mediastinum (Figure 12–1). Extra-adrenal pheochromocytomas account for 10% of all pheochromocytomas in adults and 30–40% in children. They are usually larger than adrenal pheochromocytomas. About 10% of pheochromocytomas are multicentric, most commonly occurring in both adrenal glands and less commonly in the extra-adrenal paraganglia.

Grossly, pheochromocytomas are generally well-circumscribed but vary in size, with weights ranging from under 1 g to several kilograms (Figure 12–3). They are highly vascular tumors and frequently have cystic, necrotic, or hemorrhagic areas. Microscopically, the tumor consists of large pleomorphic cells arranged in sheets separated by a highly vascular stroma. In the cytoplasm, there are catecholamine-containing storage granules similar to those in normal adrenal medullary cells. Mitoses are rare, but tumor invasion of the adrenal capsule and blood vessels is common even in benign pheochromocytomas. About 10% of pheochromocytomas are malignant. Malignancy is established only when a metastasis is found in a site where chromaffin cells are not usually demonstrated (eg, liver, lung, bone, or brain). Unfavorable prognostic factors suggesting a malignant course include large tumor size, local extension, younger age, DNA aneuploid tumors, and the presence of familial pheochromocytoma.

Very rarely, a pathologic picture of diffuse adrenal medullary hyperplasia is found in the syndrome of multiple endocrine neoplasia.

Pathogenesis
(Table 12–4)

Most pheochromocytomas release predominantly norepinephrine, but most also release epinephrine. Rarely, a pheochromocytoma releases mostly or only epinephrine.

In about half of patients with pheochromocytoma, clinical manifestations vary in intensity and occur in an episodic or paroxysmal fashion. The paroxysms are related to sudden catecholamine discharge from the tumor. The sudden catecholamine excess causes hypertension, palpitations, tachycardia, chest pain, headache, anxiety, blanching, and excessive sweating. Such paroxysms usually occur several times a week but may occur only once every few months or up to 25 times daily. Paroxysms typically last for 15 minutes or less but may last for days. As time passes, the paroxysms usually become more frequent but generally do not change in character. A typical paroxysm may be produced by activities that compress the tumor (eg, bending, lifting, exercise, defecation, eating, or deep palpation of the abdomen) and by emotional distress or anxiety.

Other patients have persistently secreting tumors and more chronic symptoms, including sustained hypertension. However, such patients also usually experience paroxysms related to transient increases in catecholamine release. The long-term exposure to high levels of circulating catecholamines seems not to produce the classic hemodynamic responses observed after acute administration of catecholamines. This may be due in part to desensitization of the cardiovascular system to catecholamines and may explain why some patients with pheochromocytomas are entirely asymptomatic.

Clinical Manifestations

The clinical manifestations of pheochromocytoma are due to increased secretion of epinephrine and norepinephrine. Commonly reported manifestations are listed in Table 12–5.

The most common presenting feature of pheochromocytoma is hypertension. In about half of cases, hypertension is sustained but the blood pressure shows marked fluctuations, with peak pressures during symptomatic paroxysms. During a hypertensive episode, the systolic blood pressure can rise to as high as 300 mm Hg. In about one-third of cases, hypertension is truly intermittent. In some individuals with pheochromocytoma, hypertension is absent. The blood pressure elevation caused by the catecholamine excess results from two mechanisms: α-receptor-mediated vasoconstriction of arterioles, leading to an increase in peripheral resistance; and

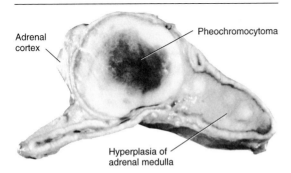

Figure 12–3. Cross section of adrenal, showing a pheochromocytoma associated with hyperplasia of the medulla in a patient with multiple endocrine neoplasia type 2a. He also had a medullary carcinoma of the thyroid and a large pheochromocytoma in the opposite adrenal. (Reproduced, with permission, from Chandrasoma P, Taylor CE: *Concise Pathology,* 3rd ed. Appleton & Lange, 1998.)

Table 12–4. Pathophysiologic and clinical manifestations of catecholamine excess.[1]

		Catecholamine Excess	
Target Tissue	Physiologic Effect	Pathophysiologic Manifestations	Clinical Manifestations
Heart	Increased heart rate	Tachycardia Tachyarrhythmia	Palpitations Angina pectoris
	Increased contractility	Increased myocardial O_2 consumption Myocarditis Cardiomyopathy	Angina pectoris Congestive heart failure
Blood vessels	Arteriolar constriction	Hypertension	Headache Congestive heart failure Angina pectoris
	Venoconstriction	Decreased plasma volume	Dizziness Orthostatic hypotension Circulatory collapse
Gut	Intestinal relaxation	Impaired intestinal motility	Ileus Obstipation
Pancreas (B cells)	Suppression of insulin release	Carbohydrate intolerance	Hyperglycemia Glucosuria
Liver	Increased glucose output	Carbohydrate intolerance	Hyperglycemia Glucosuria
Adipose	Lipolysis	Increased free fatty acids	Weight loss
Skin (apocrine glands)	Stimulation	Sweating	Diaphoresis
Bladder neck	Contraction	Elevated urethral pressures	Urinary retention
Most tissues	Increased basal metabolic rate	Increased heat production	Heat intolerance Sweating Weight loss

[1]Modified, with permission, from Werbel SS, Ober KP: Pheochromocytoma: Update on diagnosis, localization, and management. Med Clin North Am 1995;79:131.

β_1-receptor-mediated increases in cardiac output and in renin release, leading to increased circulating levels of angiotensin II. The increased total peripheral vascular resistance is probably primarily responsible for the maintenance of high arterial pressures.

Hypertensive crisis may be precipitated by a variety of drugs, including tricyclic antidepressants, antidopaminergic agents, metoclopramide, and naloxone. Administration of beta-blockers should always follow establishment of alpha blockade. Otherwise, blockade of β_2-adrenergic receptors, which promote vasodilation, will allow unopposed α-adrenergic receptor activation and produce marked vasoconstriction and hypertension.

Peripheral vasoconstriction, mediated by alpha receptors, causes both facial pallor and cool, moist hands and feet. Chronic vasoconstriction of the arterial and venous beds leads to a reduction in plasma volume and predisposes to postural hypotension. In others, orthostatic hypotension is associated with decreased cardiac stroke volume and an impaired response of total peripheral vascular resistance to changes in posture, perhaps indicative of diminished arteriolar and venous responsiveness. The reduced responsiveness of the vasculature to norepineprine in patients with pheochromocytoma is probably related to down-regulation of alpha-adrenergic receptors resulting from persistent elevations of norepinephrine levels.

Complications of pheochromocytoma are summarized in Table 12–6.

If unrecognized and untreated, pheochromocytoma may be complicated by hypertensive retinopathy (retinal hemorrhages or papilledema); nephropathy; myocardial infarction, due either to myocarditis or coronary artery vasospasm; pulmonary edema, secondary either to left-sided congestive heart failure or to noncardiogenic causes; and stroke from cerebral infarction, intracranial hemorrhage, or embolism. Cerebral infarction results from hypercoagulability, vasospasm, or both. Hemorrhage occurs secondary to severe arterial hypertension. Emboli can originate in mural thrombi in patients with dilated cardiomyopathy.

Table 12–5. Clinical findings in pheochromocytoma.[1]

	Frequency (%)
Symptoms	
Spells	67
Headache	59
Palpitations	50
Diaphoresis	50
Fainting episode	40
Bone pain	35
Weight loss	30
Anxiety	19
Nausea, vomiting	19
Dizziness	18
Flushing	14
Weakness, fatigue	14
Abdominal pain	14
Dyspnea	13
Paresthesias	13
Constipation	11
Chest pain	12
Flank pain	7
Visual symptoms	7
Diarrhea	6
Signs	
Hypertension	92
Sustained	48
Paroxysmal	44
Fever	28
Tachycardia	15
Orthostatic hypotension	12
Palpable mass	8
Shock	4
Laboratory findings	
Hyperglycemia	42
Hypercalcemia	4
Polycythemia	3

[1]Modified, with permission, from Werbel SS, Ober KP: Pheochromocytoma: Update on diagnosis, localization, and management. Med Clin North Am 1995;79:131.

Table 12–6. Complications of pheochromocytoma.

Cardiovascular
  Arrhythmias
    Ventricular tachycardia
    Torsades de pointes
    Wolff-Parkinson-White syndrome
    Ventricular fibrillation
  ECG changes
    ST segment elevations or depressions
    Inverted or flattened T waves
    Prolonged QT intervals
    High or peaked P waves
  Cardiomyopathy
    Dilated
    Hypertrophic
  Left ventricular hypertrophy
  Myocarditis
  Subendocardial, intramyocardial hemorrhages
  Acute myocardial infarction
Pulmonary
  Pulmonary edema (noncardiogenic)
Gastrointestinal
  Ileus
  Obstipation
  Acute abdominal pain
Renal
  Renal artery stenosis (from mass effect)
  Renal infarction
Endocrine and metabolic
  Hyperglycemia, glucose intolerance, diabetic ketoacidosis
  Hypoglycemia
  Thyrotoxicosis (transient)
  Reactivation of Graves' disease
  Hypercalcemia
  Lactic acidosis
  Fever
Skeletal
  Osseus microthrombi (from hemoconcentration)
  Brachydactyly
Skin
  Leukocytoclastic vasculitis
Crisis
  Obtundation, shock, disseminated intravascular coagulation, seizures, rhabdomyolysis, acute renal failure, death

Ileus and obstipation are typical. However, diarrhea may occur as a result of adrenal production of vasoactive intestinal peptide (VIP).

The metabolic effects of excessive circulating catecholamines increase both blood glucose and free fatty acid levels. Increased glycolysis and glycogenolysis, combined with an alpha receptor-mediated inhibition of insulin release, cause the increase in blood sugar levels. In addition, epinephrine stimulates glucose production by gluconeogenesis and decreases insulin-mediated glucose uptake by peripheral tissues such as skeletal muscle. In pheochromocytoma, impaired glucose homeostasis may also result from β-adrenergic receptor desensitization, which produces relative insulin resistance. Glucose intolerance is common, and diabetes mellitus may occur.

Epinephrine raises blood lactate concentrations by

stimulation of glycogenolysis and glycolysis. An increase in oxygen consumption from catecholamine stimulation of metabolism occurs in combination with a decrease in oxygen delivery to tissues from vasoconstriction, leading to lactate accumulation.

Hypercalcemia may occur, related to excessive production of PTHrP in cases of malignancy or of PTH itself in cases associated with hyperparathyroidism.

Occasionally, ectopic production of ACTH by pheochromocytoma may lead to severe hypokalemic metabolic alkalosis.

An increase in metabolic rate may cause weight loss (or, in children, lack of weight gain), and impaired heat loss from peripheral vasoconstriction may cause a mild elevation of basal body temperature, heat intolerance, flushing, or increased sweating.

During paroxysms, patients may experience marked anxiety, and when episodes are prolonged or severe there may be visual disturbances, paresthesias, or seizures. A feeling of fatigue or exhaustion usually follows these episodes. Some patients present with psychosis or confusion.

There may be abdominal discomfort due to a large adrenal mass. Remarkably, some patients with pheochromocytomas are entirely asymptomatic.

Somewhat different clinical manifestations occur with predominantly epinephrine-releasing pheochromocytomas. Symptoms and signs include hypotension, prominent tachycardia, widened pulse pressure, cardiac arrhythmias, and noncardiogenic pulmonary edema. Acute hemorrhagic necrosis of the tumor may present initially as acute abdominal pain with marked hypertension, followed by hypotension, shock, and sudden death as a consequence of sudden cessation of catecholamine production.

Patients with pure epinephrine-producing pheochromocytomas may be hypotensive because of epinephrine-induced peripheral vasodilation. Other patients with severe arterial vasoconstriction may appear to be in shock. In still others, the prolonged vasoconstriction of a hypertensive crisis may lead to shock.

Pheochromocytoma is diagnosed by demonstrating abnormally high concentrations of catecholamines or their breakdown products in the plasma or urine. Increases in plasma metanephrine concentrations are greater and more consistent than increases in plasma catecholamines or urinary metanephrines. A reliable assay showing increased plasma or urine levels of metanephrines is usually sufficient to establish the diagnosis. If the patient has paroxysmal symptoms, sampling of blood or timed urine collections during an episode may be needed to establish the diagnosis.

Elevated plasma levels of free metanephrines in patients with pheochromocytoma appear to be derived from catecholamines produced and metabolized within the tumors. Catechol-O-methyltransferase (COMT), the enzyme responsible for conversion of catecholamines to metanephrines, is present in pheochromocytomas. The consistent elevation of circulating free metanephrine levels in patients with pheochromocytoma is probably due mostly to metabolism before and not after release of the catecholamines into the circulation.

Administration of glucagon can precipitate a paroxysm, but this maneuver is not recommended. On the other hand, administration of the antihypertensive agent clonidine can be used to differentiate essential hypertension from hypertension due to pheochromocytoma. This potent α_2-agonist stimulates alpha receptors in the brain, reducing sympathetic outflow and blood pressure. A dose of 0.3 mg is given orally, and blood pressure and plasma catecholamine levels are determined periodically over the next 3 hours. Essential hypertension is dependent on centrally mediated catecholamine release. Administering clonidine normally suppresses sympathetic nervous system activity and substantially lowers plasma norepinephrine levels, reducing blood pressure. But in patients with pheochromocytoma, the drug has little or no effect on plasma catecholamine levels because these tumors, which are not thought to be innervated, behave autonomously. Thus, the blood pressure remains unchanged.

When a diagnosis of pheochromocytoma is made, the next step is to localize the neoplasm or neoplasms radiographically to permit surgical removal.

---

7. Why is pheochromocytoma called the "10% tumor"?
8. What are the symptoms and signs of pheochromocytoma?
9. What are some complications of untreated pheochromocytoma?
10. What are the metabolic and neurologic effects of pheochromocytoma?
11. How is the diagnosis of pheochromocytoma made?

ADRENAL MEDULLARY HYPOFUNCTION

Bilateral adrenalectomy obviously entails loss of the adrenal medulla. Yet individuals undergoing bilateral adrenalectomy suffer no clinically significant disability provided they receive glucocorticoid and mineralocorticoid replacement and have an otherwise intact sympathetic nervous system.

Patients with severe **primary autonomic failure (sympathetic neural failure)** have disabling orthostatic hypotension, abnormal autonomic function tests, and unresponsive plasma norepinephrine. Orthostatic hypotension is defined as a reduction of systolic blood pressure of at least 20 mm Hg or of diastolic blood pressure of at least 10 mm Hg within 3 minutes of standing. Some patients suffering from primary autonomic failure have isolated autonomic impairment (**pure autonomic failure**). Others have autonomic impairment plus central nervous system involvement, either with features of Parkinson's disease (**Parkinson's disease with autonomic failure**) or with parkinsonism and ataxia (**multiple system atrophy**). Multiple system atrophy is a sporadic, progressive adult-onset disorder, characterized by parkinsonism (bradykinesia with rigidity or tremor or both, usually with a poor or unsustained response to chronic levodopa therapy), cerebellar or corticospinal tract signs (ataxia or spasticity), and autonomic dysfunction (orthostatic hypotension, impotence, and urinary incontinence or retention). When autonomic dysfunction predominates, it is often called Shy-Drager syndrome. When parkinsonian features predominate, the condition is often called striatonigral degeneration. When cerebellar features predominate, multiple systematrophy is usually called sporadic olivopontocerebellar degeneration.

Adrenomedullary failure, caused by deficient production of epinephrine, usually causes little or no disability. However, in some patients with insulin-dependent diabetes mellitus, adrenomedullary failure is associated with glucagon deficiency (Table 12–7). This combined deficiency was originally described in patients with advanced **diabetic autonomic neuropathy.** More recently, the combined deficiency has been found in a subset of patients who do not develop hypoglycemia-related symptoms. In such patients, the central nervous system fails to recognize hypoglycemia and to mount defenses against it. The body's usual defense against hypoglycemia is to reduce the secretion of insulin, to increase the secretion of glucagon, and to increase the secretion of epinephrine. In addition to these physiologic endocrine defenses, warning symptoms of autonomic origin, such as anxiety, palpitations, hunger, sweating, irritability, and tremor, normally stimulate the patient to find and ingest food.

Patients who have combined deficiencies of their glucagon and epinephrine responses to hypoglycemia have a markedly increased risk for hypoglycemia during intensive insulin therapy of type 1 diabetes mellitus. They have the syndrome of **defective glucose counterregulation.** A related disorder, which also poses an increased risk for severe hypoglycemia, is the syndrome of **hypoglycemia unawareness** (loss of the warning symptoms of developing hypoglycemia). Awareness of hypoglycemia normally results from the perception of physiologic changes caused by the autonomic (both sympathetic neural and adrenomedullary) discharge triggered by falling glucose levels.

Failure of the central nervous system to recognize hypoglycemia results both from strict antecedent glucose control and from one or more recent hypoglycemic episodes (**hypoglycemia-associated autonomic failure**). Obviously, this failure predisposes to recurrent episodes of hypoglycemia in a vicious circle.

Episodes of iatrogenic hypoglycemia lead to reduced autonomic responses to subsequent hypoglycemia and thus predispose both to hypoglycemia unawareness and to defective glucose counterregulation. The specific mechanisms of the diminished autonomic responses induced by the antecedent hypoglycemia are unknown but are thought to involve increased blood-to-brain glucose transport. The increased uptake of glucose in the brain ultimately induces the unawareness of developing hypoglycemia.

Encouragingly, it has been established that the careful avoidance of hypoglycemia completely reverses the syndrome of hypoglycemia unawareness and at least partially corrects the reduced epinephrine response contributing to defective glucose counterregulation.

Table 12–7. Disorders associated with adrenal medullary hypofunction.[1]

Insulin-dependent diabetes mellitus
Familial dysautonomia
Shy-Drager syndrome
Parkinson's disease
Tabes dorsalis
Syringomyelia
Cerebrovascular disease
Idiopathic orthostatic hypotension
Sympathectomy
Drugs: antihypertensives, antidepressants

[1]Modified and reproduced, with permission, from Greenspan FS, Baxter JD (editors): *Basic and Clinical Endocrinology,* 4th ed. Appleton & Lange, 1994.

REFERENCES

General

Goldfien A: Adrenal medulla. In: *Basic and Clinical Endocrinology*, 5th ed. Greenspan FS, Strewler GJ (editors). Appleton & Lange, 1997.

Trendelenburg U, Weiner N (editors): Catecholamines. Vol 90 of *Handbook of Experimental Pharmacology.* Springer, 1988.

Pheochromocytoma

Bravo EL: Pheochromocytoma. Curr Ther Endocrinol Metabol 1997;6:195.

Bravo EL: Evolving concepts in the pathophysiology, diagnosis, and treatment of pheochromocytoma. Endocr Rev 1994;15:356.

Casanova S et al: Phaeochromocytoma in multiple endocrine neoplasia type 2A: Survey of 100 cases. Clin Endocrinol 1993;38:531.

Eng C et al: The relationship between specific RET proto-oncogene mutations and disease phenotype in multiple endocrine neoplasia type 2. International RET mutation consortium analysis. JAMA 1996;276:1575.

Miller JA, Norton JA: Multiple endocrine neoplasia. Cancer Treat Res 1997;90:213.

Neumann HPH et al: Pheochromocytomas, multiple endocrine neoplasia type 2, and von Hippel-Lindau disease. N Engl J Med 1993;329:1531.

Streeten DH, Anderson GH Jr: Mechanisms of orthostatic hypotension and tachycardia in patients with pheochromocytoma. Am J Hypertens 1996;9:760.

Werbel SS, Ober KP: Pheochromocytoma: Update on diagnosis, localization, and management. Med Clin North Am 1995;79:131.

Young WF Jr: Pheochromocytoma and primary aldosteronism: Diagnostic approaches. Endocrinol Metabol Clin North Am 1997;26:801.

Adrenal Medullary Hypofunction

Boyle PJ et al: Brain glucose uptake and unawareness of hypoglycemia in patients with insulin-dependent diabetes mellitus. N Engl J Med 1995;333:1726.

Consensus statement on the definition of orthostatic hypotension, pure autonomic failure, and multiple system atrophy. The Consensus Committee of the American Autonomic Society and the American Academy of Neurology. Neurology 1996;46:1470.

Cryer PE: Hypoglycemia-associated autonomic failure in insulin-dependent diabetes mellitus. Adv Pharmacol 1998;42:620.

Schatz IJ: Autonomic failure and orthostatic hypotension [editorial]. Hosp Pract (Off Ed) 1997 May;32:15.

Gastrointestinal Disease

13

Vishwanath R. Lingappa, MD, PhD

Gastrointestinal diseases most often present with one or more of four common classes of symptoms and signs: (1) abdominal or chest pain; (2) altered ingestion of food, eg, due to nausea, vomiting, **dysphagia** (difficulty swallowing), **odynophagia** (painful swallowing), or **anorexia** (lack of appetite); (3) altered bowel movements, ie, diarrhea or constipation; and (4) gastrointestinal bleeding, occurring either without warning or preceded by one or more of the foregoing (Table 13–1). However, not all cases of a particular gastrointestinal disease present in the same way. For example, peptic ulcer disease, while typically accompanied by abdominal pain, may be painless.

Gastrointestinal disease may be limited to the gastrointestinal tract (eg, reflux esophagitis, peptic ulcer, diverticular disease); may be a manifestation of a systemic disorder (eg, inflammatory bowel disease); or may present as a systemic disease resulting from a primary gastrointestinal pathologic process (eg, vitamin deficiencies due to malabsorption). Since different parts of the gastrointestinal tract are specialized for certain functions, the most prominent causes, consequences, and manifestations of disease differ from one anatomic site to another.

Acutely, gastrointestinal disease can be complicated by dehydration, sepsis, or bleeding or by their consequences, such as shock. **Dehydration** can occur as a consequence of even subtle alterations in fluid input or outflow because the volume of fluid traversing the gastrointestinal tract daily is enormous (see below). **Sepsis** can result from disruption of the barrier function against pathogens in the environment, including bacteria resident in the colon. The tendency to **bleeding** is a reflection of the tremendous vascularity of the gastrointestinal tract and the difficulty of applying pressure at the site of bleeding.

Chronically, gastrointestinal disease can be complicated by malnutrition and deficiency states. These occur because many primary gastrointestinal diseases result in **malabsorption** (failure to absorb one or more necessary nutrients in ingested food).

Gastrointestinal tract disease can present as partial or complete **obstruction** (blockage of movement of contents down the gastrointestinal tract) due to **adhesions** and **stenosis** resulting from proliferation of connective tissue in response to inflammation. The symptoms and signs of obstruction can range from mild nausea, abdominal pain, and anorexia to projectile vomiting, rebound tenderness with progression to perforation, infarction and bleeding, hypotension, shock, sepsis, and death. The severity of symptoms depends on the extent of obstruction, the degree to which the obstruction compromises blood flow to the affected region, and the stage in the natural history of the process at which the patient presents for medical attention.

1. What are the cardinal symptoms and signs of gastrointestinal disease?
2. What are some acute systemic complications of primary gastrointestinal disease?
3. What additional systemic manifestations can occur as a result of chronic gastrointestinal disease?

STRUCTURE & FUNCTION OF THE GASTROINTESTINAL TRACT

The gastrointestinal tract includes the continuous lumen from mouth to anus which is involved in separating ingested food into nutrients to be assimilated and wastes to be eliminated (Figure 13–1). The activities necessary to achieve these goals can be broadly categorized as motility, secretion, digestion, and absorption. **Motility** is achieved by muscular contractions of different segments of the gastrointestinal tract. **Secretion** involves two processes: (1) the transport of substances from the epithelial cells lining the gastrointestinal tract into the gut lumen via channels or transporters, and (2) release of proteins and other

Table 13–1. Common presentations of gastrointestinal disease.

Cardinal Gastrointestinal Symptom or Sign	Esophagus	Stomach	Intestines	Gallbladder
Pain	Achalasia, reflux	Gastric ulcer Gastric cancer	Duodenal ulcer Irritable bowel syndrome Diverticular disease	Cholelithiasis
Altered ingestion Dysphagia	Achalasia, reflux			
Nausea, vomiting	Achalasia, reflux Esophageal cancer	Gastroparesis	Acute gastroenteritis Obstruction	Cholelithiasis
Altered bowel movements Constipation			Diverticular disease Diabetic autonomic neuropathy	
Diarrhea (including steatorrhea)		Gastric surgery, dumping syndrome	Gastroenteritis Irritable bowel syndrome Inflammatory bowel disease Diabetic autonomic neuropathy	Cholelithiasis
Bleeding Hematemesis	Varices due to portal hypertension	Gastric ulcer Mucosal laceration (eg, after violent retching)	Duodenal ulcer	
Bloody stools (including melena, frank blood, and occult blood)	Varices	Gastric ulcer	Inflammatory bowel disease Duodenal ulcer Diverticular disease Colon cancer Gastroenteritis Infarction	

products either into the bloodstream or into the interstitial spaces between cells following the fusion of intracellular vesicles containing these products with the cellular plasma membrane of gastrointestinal endocrine cells. **Digestion** consists of the breakdown of substances within the gut lumen. **Absorption** refers to transport of the modified nutrients from the gut lumen across the lining epithelial cells and into the bloodstream. Different regions of the gastrointestinal tract are specialized for support of these processes, which are under complex neural and hormonal control.

Histologically, the wall of the gastrointestinal tract is composed of four major layers. From the lumen outward, these are the mucosa, submucosa, muscularis, and serosa (Figure 13–2). Each of these layers can be further subdivided into components with different structure and function. Thus, the mucosa consists not only of the epithelial cells that line the lumen of the gastrointestinal tract but also the immediately adjacent **lamina propria,** a layer of loose connective tissue rich in blood and lymph vessels and immune system cells, including both macrophages and lymphocytes active in secretion of IgA and IgM. In some regions of the gastrointestinal tract, glands and organized lymphoid tissue are also found in the lamina propria. Finally, the innermost aspect of the mucosa is demarcated by a thin layer of smooth muscle called the **muscularis mucosae.** It has both inner (circular) and outer (longitudinal) fibers. The muscularis mucosae is an important boundary in determining whether cancer of the gastrointestinal tract is still localized to its site of origin or is likely to have metastasized, ie, spread to distant regions of the body. In certain parts of the gastrointestinal tract, the mucosa is further organized into folds termed **villi** and **microvilli,** which serve to greatly increase the luminal surface area and which have important functional implications.

The **submucosa** is a layer of loose connective tissue directly beneath the mucosa containing not only larger blood and lymphatic vessels but also a nerve plexus of the intrinsic enteric nervous system termed the **submucosal nerve plexus (Meissner).** This nerve plexus is particularly important for control of secretion in the gastrointestinal tract. In some areas, the submucosa also contains glands and organized lymphoid tissue. The **muscularis externa** contains gut smooth muscle and is responsible for gastrointestinal tract motility. There are two layers of muscle fibers: an innermost circular layer, whose contraction decreases the diameter of the intestinal lumen; and an outer longitudinal layer, whose contraction shortens the tube. Between these muscle layers lies the **myen-

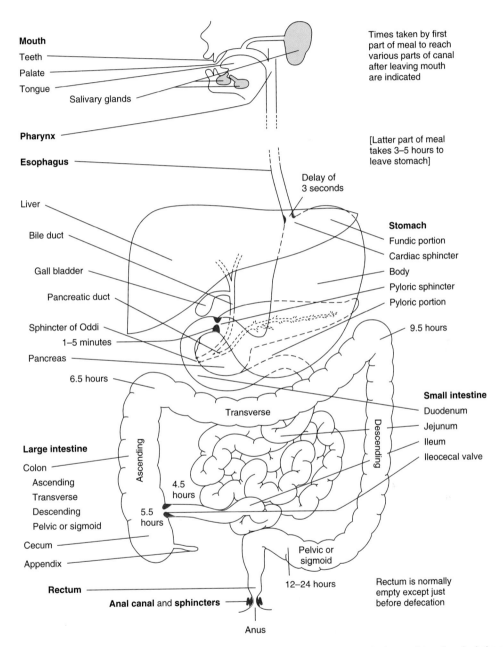

Figure 13–1. Progress of food along the alimentary canal. Food undergoes mechanical as well as chemical changes to render it suitable for absorption and assimilation. (Modified and reproduced, with permission, from Mackenna BR, Callander R: *Illustrated Physiology,* 5th ed. Churchill Livingstone, 1990.)

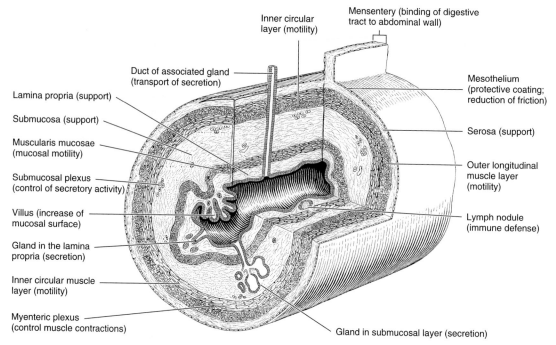

Figure 13–2. Schematic structure of a portion of the digestive tract with various possible components. (Redrawn and reproduced, with permission, from Bevelander G: *Outline of Histology,* 7th ed. Mosby, 1971.)

teric nerve plexus (**Auerbach**) of the enteric nervous system, involved primarily in control of motility. The **serosa** is the outermost layer, where larger nerves and blood vessels travel in a bed of connective and adipose tissue.

---

4. What are the broad classes of gastrointestinal tract functions?
5. Describe the key microscopic anatomic features of a cross-section of the gastrointestinal tract.
6. What features of gastrointestinal tract anatomy predispose to severe bleeding?

Functions of the Gastrointestinal Tract

A. Motility: The motility of the gastrointestinal tract is due to the contraction of smooth muscle. Smooth muscle cells have a resting membrane potential (small excess of negative charge) in their interior as a result of the activity of pumps in the plasma membrane. When a cell is depolarized, this potential difference is transiently abolished, generating a signal that (1) triggers events within that cell, leading to sliding of actin and myosin filaments; and (2) is propagated to neighboring cells, resulting in the coordinated response of muscle contraction. Depolarization of a cell can occur spontaneously or in response to a neural or hormonal stimulus depending on the specific characteristics of different cells. Gastrointestinal smooth muscle displays differences in contractile properties in different regions of the tract. "Slow wave" oscillating depolarizations occur in some areas and rapid "spike" depolarizations in other areas. Each type occurs with a characteristic intrinsic frequency, but each can also be triggered by specific stimuli such as stretch, neuronal input, or hormones. Short bursts of spikes cause phasic motor activity; longer bursts cause tonic muscle contraction. Tonic contraction occurs at **sphincters** ("gates" that allow further movement down the gastrointestinal tract only during relaxation). Phasic electrical activity occurs at the intervening regions of the gastrointestinal tract (between sphincters).

The degree of central nervous system control over gut motility varies from region to region: Striated muscle of the mouth, pharynx, and proximal esophagus is under direct central nervous system control; the small intestine is almost totally independent of the central nervous system, being controlled instead by a system of neurons localized entirely to the gastrointestinal tract and termed the **enteric nervous system;** the stomach, colon, and distal esophagus are each partially under control of the enteric and central nervous system control. Generally speaking, parasympathetic nerve stimulation causes muscle contraction and secretion while sympathetic nerve stimulation inhibits blood flow and motility. These effects of the autonomic nervous system can occur both directly and by interfacing with neurons of the enteric nervous system.

The myenteric plexus has two programmed responses, **segmental** and **peristaltic,** which characterize the motility of the gastrointestinal tract. The segmental program predominates in the postprandial period, the peristaltic pattern during fasting. Program selection is determined by hormonal, neural, and other factors and is manifested in different ways in different parts of the gastrointestinal tract.

B. Secretion: Certain epithelial cells lining the intestinal lumen (or glands that connect to the lumen) are specialized to secrete large volumes of fluid containing acid, digestive enzymes, or other products. The daily fluid load in the gastrointestinal tract is approximately 2 L of oral intake and 7 L of secretions (1.5 L saliva, 2.5 L gastric juice, 0.5 L bile, 1.5 L pancreatic juice, and 1 L intestinal secretions). From this total of 9 L, approximately 100 mL ends up in stool daily, with the balance recycled (Figure 13–3).

Several mechanisms can be used to transport substances in the gastrointestinal tract. Ions as well as small charged molecules such as amino acids, small peptides, and sugars are transported directly across the epithelial plasma membrane through channels via the processes of **diffusion** and **facilitated diffusion** or by transporters via the process of **active transport.** Active transport requires metabolic energy and can be of two sorts, either primary (where energy from ATP hydrolysis is used to transport a specific molecule directly across the membrane) or secondary (where transport of one substance is coupled to that of another). An example of primary active transport is the H^+-K^+ ATPase in the stomach. An example of secondary active transport is the coupling of monosaccharide and amino acid uptake to the Na^+ gradient established by Na^+-K^+ ATPase. For large molecules such as proteins, transport occurs by pinching-off from—and fusion of membrane vesicles with—the plasma membrane. These processes are termed **endocytosis** (uptake into epithelial cells) and **exocytosis** (export out of epithelial cells).

Structures in the proximal part of the gastrointestinal tract are predominantly involved in secretion. For example, saliva is secreted from the mouth, acid from the stomach, and mucus, bicarbonate, and digestive enzymes from the pancreas (Table 13–2). Conversely, structures in the distal part of the gastrointestinal tract (ie, intestine) are more involved in absorption. For example, the products of digestion are absorbed in the small intestine, while water is absorbed from the colon. Likewise, in the small intestine, epithelial cells of the villus tip are prominently involved in absorption while epithelial cells of the crypts are involved in secretion.

C. Digestion: The complex process of digestion actually starts in the mouth through the action of salivary amylase, lingual lipase, and the act of chewing. In the small intestine, the process involves hydrolysis both in the intestinal lumen and at the enterocyte brush border.

D. Absorption: This involves transport of nutrients into the enterocyte, processing of nutrients within the enterocyte, and export from the enterocyte into the portal or lymphatic circulation.

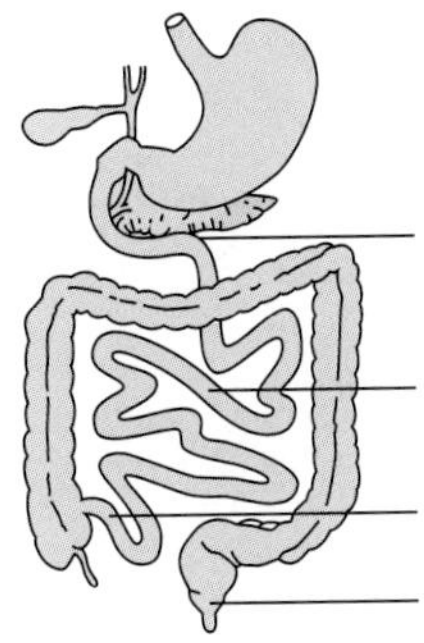

7. What kind of electrical activity occurs at sphincters, and what are its consequences?
8. Describe the range in extent of central nervous system control over gut motility in different parts of the gastrointestinal tract.
9. What are the programmed responses of the myenteric plexus of the enteric nervous system, and when do they occur?
10. What are the sources and approximate daily volumes of fluids entering the gastrointestinal tract?
11. By what mechanisms can substances be transported into or out of enterocytes?
12. What is the role of the villus tip versus crypts in absorption versus secretion?
13. List the key steps in carbohydrate, fat, and protein digestion.

	Flow rate mL/d	Ion concentrations meq/L				Osmolality mosm/kg
		Na^+	K^+	Cl^-	HCO_3^-	
	9000	60	15	60	15	Variable
	3000	140	6	100	30	Isotonic
	1000	140	8	60	70	Isotonic
	100	40	90	15	30	Isotonic

Colon absorption capacity (3–4 L/d)

Figure 13–3. Approximate flow rates per day and ionic constituents of fluid passing through different levels of the intestine. (Reproduced, with permission, from Fine KD, Krejs GJ, Fordtran JS: Diarrhea. In: *Gastrointestinal Disease,* 4th ed. Sleisenger MH, Fordtran JS [editors]. Saunders, 1989.)

Mechanisms of Control of Gastrointestinal Tract Functions

Neural and hormonal factors, separately and together, regulate the processes of motility, secretion, digestion, and absorption in the gastrointestinal tract (Figure 13–4).

Table 13–2. Secretory products of the gastrointestinal tract.[1]

Products	Physiologic Actions	Site of Release	Stimulus for Release	Disease Association
True hormones				
Gastrin	Stimulates acid secretion and growth of gastric oxyntic gland mucosa	Gastric antrum (and duodenum)	Peptides, amino acids, distention, vagal stimulation	Zollinger-Ellison syndrome, peptic ulcer disease
CCK	Stimulates gallbladder contraction, pancreatic enzyme and bicarbonate secretion, and growth of exocrine pancreas	Duodenum and jejunum	Peptides, amino acids, long chain fatty acids, (acid).	
Secretin	Stimulates pancreatic bicarbonate secretion, biliary bicarbonate secretion, growth of exocrine pancreas, pepsin secretion; inhibits gastric acid secretion, trophic effects of gastrin	Duodenum	Acid, (fat)	
GIP	Stimulates insulin release; (inhibits gastric acid secretion)	Duodenum, jejunum	Glucose, amino acids, fatty acids	
Candidate hormones				
Motilin	Stimulates gastric and duodenal motility	Duodenum and jejunum	Unknown	Irritable bowel syndrome; diabetic gastroparesis
Pancreatic polypeptide	Inhibits pancreatic bicarbonate and enzyme secretion	Pancreatic islets of Langerhans	Protein, (fat and glucose)	
Enteroglucagon	Elevates blood glucose?	Ileum	Glucose and fat	
Paracrines				
Somatostatin	Inhibits release of most other peptide hormones	Gastrointestinal tract mucosa, pancreatic islets of Langerhans	Acid stimulates, vagus inhibits release	Gallstones
Prostaglandins	Promote blood flow, increase mucus and bicarbonate secretion from gastric mucosa	Multiple	Various	NSAID-induced gastritis and ulcer disease
Histamine	Stimulates gastric acid secretion	Oxyntic gland mucosa	Unknown	
Neurocrines				
VIP	Relaxes sphincters and gut circular muscle; stimulates intestinal and pancreatic secretion	Mucosa and smooth muscle of gastrointestinal tract	Enteric nervous system	Secretory diarrhea
Bombesin	Stimulates gastrin release	Gastric mucosa	Enteric nervous system	
Enkephalins	Stimulates smooth muscle contraction; inhibit intestinal secretion	Mucosa and smooth muscle of gastrointestinal tract	Enteric nervous system	
Other products				
Intrinsic factor	Binds vitamin B_{12} to facilitate its absorption	Parietal cells of the stomach	Constitutive secretion	Autoimmune destruction resulting in pernicious anemia
Mucin	Lubrication and protection	Goblet cells along entire gastrointestinal tract mucosa	Gastrointestinal tract irritation	Viscid mucus in cystic fibrosis. Attenuation in some cases of peptic ulcer.
Acid	Prevents infection; initiates digestion	Parietal cells of the stomach	Gastrin, histamine, acetylcholine, NSAIDs (indirectly)	Acid-peptic disease

[1]Parentheses indicate minor components and effects.

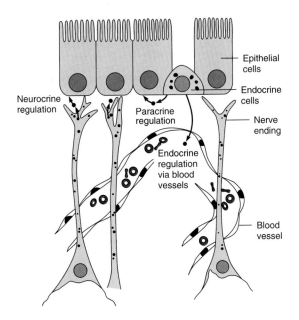

Figure 13–4. Neural and hormonal control of the intestine. (Reproduced, with permission, from Dharmsathaphorn K: Intestinal water and electrolyte transport. In: *Textbook of Internal Medicine*. Kelley WN [editor]. Lippincott, 1989.)

A. Neural Control: Gastrointestinal tract functions are controlled by both the central nervous system, working through autonomic components of the peripheral nervous system, and by the enteric nervous system. The size and complexity of the enteric nervous system are remarkable: It contains more neurons than the spinal cord and receives sensory input from neurons specialized to detect chemical, osmotic, thermal, and other changes in the lumen, or mechanical activity involving the gut wall. This information is integrated with and modified by input from the central nervous system via the sympathetic and parasympathetic neurons, which synapse with intramural neurons and provide the program for motor neurons. In this way, otherwise random and uncontrolled phasic motor and secretory activities of the gut become purposeful and coordinated, as manifested by characteristic gut programs such as peristalsis and sphincter control.

The enteric nervous system consists of two major networks of neurons and their processes—the myenteric plexus and the submucosal plexus—as well as several minor ones. The myenteric plexus is largely involved with muscular contraction while the submucosal plexus tonically suppresses fluid and electrolyte transport and limits the absorptive capacity of the intestine. These secretory effects are mediated by neurotransmitters released by the motor neurons that interact with receptors on intestinal epithelial cells to influence the function of ion channels.

Dependence of the enteric nervous system on central nervous system control varies with the embryologic origin of gut structures. The characteristic functions of structures derived from the embryonic foregut (proximal to the ampulla of Vater) are more dependent on central nervous system control (eg, esophageal peristalsis, relaxation of the lower esophageal sphincter, gastric accommodation and peristalsis, pyloric sphincter function). However, midgut- and hindgut-derived structures (ie, small and large intestine) function relatively well when their connections with the central nervous system are disrupted.

The clinical importance of the enteric nervous system itself is seen in clinical syndromes in which its function is lost, which can occur at several levels. In esophageal achalasia, for example, as a result of enteric nervous system defects, the body of the esophagus is quiet and the lower sphincter is tonically contracted, making ingestion of food difficult or impossible. Similarly, loss of enteric nervous system function in syndromes of pseudo-obstruction of the small bowel or Hirschsprung's disease in the colon have severe clinical consequences, including abdominal pain, distention, and a risk of catastrophic intestinal perforation.

B. Hormonal Control: Unlike the other endocrine glands, the gastrointestinal endocrine system is a diffuse aggregate of individual cells distributed throughout the mucosa of the tract. Armed with apical microvilli and crammed with basal secretory granules, they are ideally situated to respond to a change in the luminal environment by releasing their secretory products into the bloodstream.

Many peptides produced in the gastrointestinal tract function as neurotransmitters of the enteric nervous system rather than as true hormones. Other gastrointestinal peptides may be involved in **paracrine** rather than true endocrine actions (affecting neighboring cells rather than distant cells via the bloodstream). Some peptides play multiple roles in the gastrointestinal tract, and some do serve as true hormones. It is likely that each of these functional types of gastrointestinal peptides plays a role in the pathophysiology of gastrointestinal disease (Table 13–2).

Mechanisms of Defense of the Gastrointestinal Tract

The gastrointestinal tract is an interface between the external and internal environments where external products are broken down into nutrients and imported into the bloodstream. The gastrointestinal tract must be defended from pathogens that would use this route to enter the body as well as from corrosive products capable of digesting the gastrointestinal tract itself. Multiple lines of defense have evolved to deal with these diverse threats to gastrointestinal integrity and systemic homeostasis (Table 13–3; Figure 13–5).

Table 13–3. Mechanisms of defense of the gastrointestinal tract (and features of structure and function involved).

Forms of Defense	Structural Adaptations	Functional Adaptations	Mechanism of Defense
Defense from acid Mucus production	Large numbers of mucus-secreting goblet cells	Mucin gene expression	Prevents direct contact of acid with epithelium
Bicarbonate production (alkaline tide)			Neutralizes any acid that breaches epithelium
Prostaglandin production			Attenuates acid production
Tight junctions	Tight junction formation		Prevents breach of epithelium
Bicarbonate from pancreas	Pancreatic duct opening into duodenum	Response of secretin to gastric acid	Neutralizes acid leaving stomach
Defense from infection Secretory immune system		Machinery for transcytosis	Extends to gastrointestinal tract lumen the protective umbrella of blood-borne immunity
Rapid turnover of enterocytes	Villi with cell proliferation in crypts and cell release at tips		Limits the consequences of enterocyte infection
Normal colonic microflora			Impedes invasion or colonization by pathogenic organisms
Stomach acid	Gastric glands containing parietal cells	Multiple humoral controls on acid secretion (histamine, acetylcholine, and gastrin)	Kills pathogenic organisms upon ingestion

Recently, a family of proteins, termed **trefoil peptides,** have been identified as gastrointestinal luminal products secreted together with mucus. Among their many effects, they appear to promote healing of mucosal lesions. Further work is necessary to establish their position in the hierarchy of gastrointestinal defenses.

14. What are the roles of the myenteric and submucosal plexuses in control of the gastrointestinal tract?
15. What are some functions of each of the major families of gastrointestinal tract hormones?
16. Describe the defense mechanisms that serve to protect the gastrointestinal tract from acid and infection.

OROPHARYNX & ESOPHAGUS

Anatomy & Histology

The oropharynx provides entry to the gastrointestinal tract during swallowing and to the respiratory tract during breathing. It includes the vocal cords, which serve to separate the two tracts and provide the structural basis for speech. Much of the oropharynx is lined with a respiratory-type ciliated pseudocolumnar epithelium.

The esophagus is a hollow muscular tube, bounded by sphincters, that serves as a conduit from the pharynx to the stomach. Lined with stratified squamous epithelium, its muscular wall is notable for a transition from striated muscle (top third of its length, starting from the pharynx) to smooth muscle (bottom two-thirds). A key functional feature is the **lower esophageal (gastroesophageal) sphincter** at the transition from low pressure (intrathoracic) to high pressure (intra-abdominal) sections of the gastrointestinal tract. The lower esophageal sphincter remains closed as a result of tonic contractions, thereby keeping acidic stomach contents out of the esophagus. A specialized neural control mechanism governs relaxation of the lower esophageal sphincter to allow passage of food into the stomach during swallowing.

Physiology of Oropharyngeal & Esophageal Motility & Sphincter Tone

The major role of the oropharynx is to convey food into the esophagus without its ending up in the lungs or coming back out the nose. After mixing of food with saliva in the oropharynx (by the act of chewing), a bolus of food is directed posteriorly by the tongue and muscles of the mouth under voluntary control. Involuntary pharyngeal contraction then propels the bolus into the esophagus (swallowing) while the larynx is protected from food entry by involuntary forward and upward movement of the cricoid

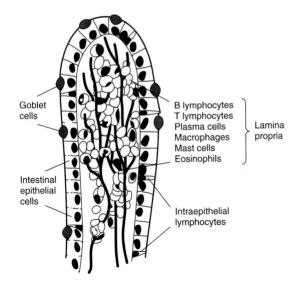

The key features of esophageal motility are primary and secondary peristalsis and lower esophageal sphincter tone. Various foods can increase (eg, protein) or decrease (eg, fat, ethanol, chocolate) lower esophageal sphincter pressure (Table 13–4). Disordered lower esophageal sphincter tone is a major cause of esophageal reflux, presenting as "heartburn."

> 17. What is the histologic difference between the proximal two-thirds and the distal one-third of the esophagus?
> 18. What foods affect lower esophageal sphincter pressure, and what are the potential pathologic consequences of these changes?

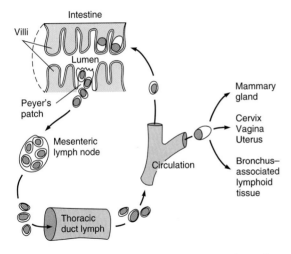

Figure 13–5. Systemic and local features of gut immunology. (Reproduced, with permission, from Kagnoff M: Immunology and disease of the gastrointestinal tract. In: *Gastrointestinal Disease,* 4th ed. Sleisenger MH, Fordtran JS [editors]. Saunders, 1989.)

Table 13–4. Factors influencing lower esophageal sphincter pressure.[1]

	Increase	Decrease
Hormones	Gastrin Motilin Substance P	Secretin Cholecystokinin Glucagon Somatostatin Gastric inhibitory peptide (GIP) Vasoactive intestinal peptide (VIP) Progesterone
Neural agents	Alpha-adrenergic agonists Beta-adrenergic antagonists Cholinergic agonists	Beta-adrenergic agonists Alpha-adrenergic antagonists Anticholinergic agents
Foods	Protein meals	Fat Chocolate Ethanol Peppermint
Other	Histamine Antacids Metoclopramide Domperidone Prostaglandin $F_{2\alpha}$ Migrating motor complex Raised intra-abdominal pressure	Theophylline Caffeine Gastric acidification Smoking Pregnancy Prostaglandins E_2, I_2 Serotonin Meperidine, morphine Dopamine Calcium channel-blocking agents Diazepam Barbiturates

[1]Reproduced with permission, from Diamant NE: Physiology of the esophagus. In: *Gastrointestinal Disease,* 4th ed. Sleisenger MH, Fordtran JS (editors). Saunders, 1989.

cartilage and approximation of the vocal cords (pharyngoesophageal sphincter).

The importance of oropharyngeal motility and its control through a complex combination of voluntary and involuntary muscle contraction is seen in patients who have had strokes or are demented: Inability to swallow properly often makes them unable to manage their own oral secretions, resulting in aspiration of oral contents into the lungs with development of pneumonia. This is a common cause of death in individuals with these kinds of central nervous system disorders.

STOMACH

Anatomy & Histology

In the stomach, ingested food is subjected to thorough mixing and initial breakdown by hydrochloric acid and the proteolytic enzyme pepsin. The mucosal surface of the stomach is a simple columnar epithelium of mucus-secreting cells interrupted occasionally by various types of glands in the form of surface invaginations (Figure 13–6). Within these glands, the surface epithelial cells are replaced by specialized exocrine or endocrine secretory cells. The endocrine cells secrete various substances from their apical surface (eg, acid from **parietal cells** and pepsin from **chief cells** of the oxyntic glands in the fundus and body of the stomach) into the gastrointestinal tract lumen. The exocrine cells secrete hormones from their basolateral surface (eg, gastrin from so-called **G cells** of the antral glands in the antral mucosa) into the adjacent capillary bloodstream.

Physiology of Stomach Motility

The proximal and distal stomach are functionally distinct. Both parts are involved in mixing ingested materials. Tonic contraction of the proximal stomach normally prevents reflux back into the esophagus, while the distal stomach promotes transit to the duodenum. Both of these functions involve **receptive relaxation,** which is the tendency of stretch of one part of the tract (eg, by food) to induce relaxation of muscle in the part of the tract immediately beyond it. This is followed by muscle contraction when the stretch is relieved, ie, when the food has passed beyond. As a result, material can be propelled from the esophagus through the stomach and into the intestine in an efficient, coordinated fashion. Furthermore, because the pyloric sphincter is triggered to start contracting at the same time as the distal stomach, most of the contents of the stomach impact against a closed pylorus and thus are churned within the stomach rather than being propelled forward into the duodenum. As a result of this churning action, large chunks of food are converted into fine suspensions of particles—in effect, put through a "strainer"—before leaving the stomach for the duodenum. Both the small particle size and the controlled release of small spurts of nutrient suspension from stomach to duodenum are critical for subsequent absorption. This process is under the control of fibers of the vagus nerve, but it responds also to a variety of luminal receptors. Thus, neutral, isotonic, noncaloric liquids leave the stomach most rapidly. The rate of gastric emptying slows with increasing acidity, fat, and amino acid content or caloric content of ingested food.

The importance of nervous system control over gastric motility is reflected in the high incidence of the so-called **dumping syndrome** (nausea, bloating, flushing, and explosive diarrhea) that occurs as a consequence of stomach dysmotility in some patients who have undergone surgical procedures such as partial gastrectomy or nonselective vagotomy.

Physiology of Stomach Secretion

A number of products are secreted from the stomach. Of these, hydrochloric acid is perhaps the most important from a pathophysiologic standpoint. Secretion of acid by the parietal cells of the gastric glands occurs in a basal diurnal pattern but can be stimulated by such diverse factors as the thought of food, distention of the stomach, and protein ingestion.

Acid secretion is controlled by a special mechanism that serves to deliver H^+-K^+ ATPase to the plasma membrane. Vesicle fusion causes H^+-K^+ ATPase to be localized to the plasma membrane, so that hydrogen ions pumped against a tremendous concentration gradient end up in the gastrointestinal lumen (Figure 13–7). A concentration of up to 100 mmol/L HCl (pH 1.0) can be achieved by this mechanism. Tight junctions keep H^+ in the lumen, with electroneutrality being maintained by export of K^+ and Cl^- through appropriate apical channels. Carbonic anhydrase generates bicarbonate, which is exported into the bloodstream in exchange for Cl^- via pumps on the basolateral side. Together with other pumps that export Na^+ in exchange for K^+ and H^+ in exchange for Na^+, electroneutrality and the ionic composition of the cytosol are maintained in the mucosal cells. Thus, HCl is secreted across the apical surface of the parietal cell while at the same time sodium bicarbonate is being exported across the basal surface of the parietal cell into the bloodstream. Perhaps this "alkaline tide" of bicarbonate-rich blood flowing through surface capillaries provides a last line of defense against acid-mediated mucosal injury.

At the cellular level, regulation of movement of the H^+-K^+ ATPase to the cell surface is a receptor-mediated process stimulated by histamine, gastrin, and acetylcholine working via both the cAMP and inositol phosphate pathways and inhibited by prostaglandins. The role of acetylcholine as a stimulant of acid secretion reflects yet another level of control of acid secretion. This allows higher centers in the central nervous system (eg, for satiety) to control acid production in anticipation of a meal via the autonomic nervous system.

The clinical importance of regulation of acid secretion is seen in the pathogenesis and therapy of acid-mediated injury to the gastrointestinal mucosa: Exacerbations are often traced to the use of drugs that inhibit prostaglandin synthesis (eg, aspirin, ibuprofen), thereby stimulating acid secretion (Figure 13–8). Clinical management of acid-mediated injury includes therapy with histamine H_2 receptor blocking agents (eg, cimetidine) and H^+-K^+ ATPase-blocking agents (eg, omeprazole) and avoiding stimulants of gastrin secretion (eg, protein-rich meals). In the pathophysiology of ulcer disease, chronic infection

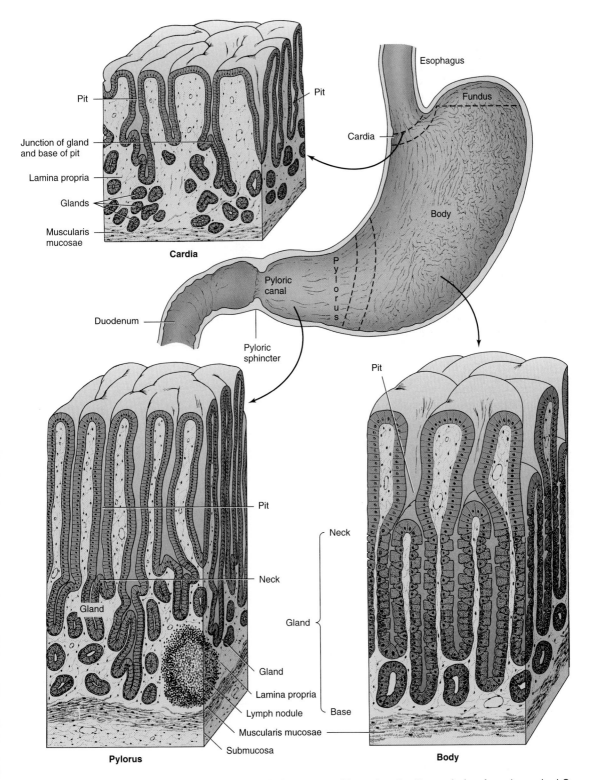

Figure 13–6. Regions of the stomach and their histologic structure. (Reproduced, with permission, from Junqueira LC, Carneiro J, Kelley RO: *Basic Histology,* 9th ed. Appleton & Lange, 1998.)

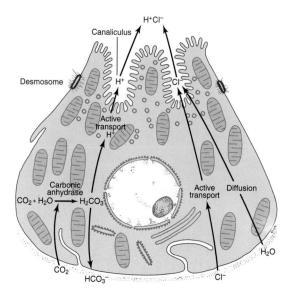

Figure 13–7. Diagram of parietal cell, showing the main steps in the synthesis of hydrochloric acid. Blood CO_2 under the action of carbonic anhydrase produces carbonic acid. This dissociates into a bicarbonate ion and a proton, H^+, which reacts with the chloride ion to produce hydrochloric acid. The tubulovesicles of the cell apex seem to be related to hydrochloric acid secretion, since they decrease in number after parietal cell stimulation. The bicarbonate ion returns to the blood and is responsible for a measurable increase in blood pH during digestion. (Reproduced, with permission, from Junqueira LC, Carneiro J, Kelley RO: *Basic Histology,* 9th ed. Appleton & Lange, 1998.)

by the bacterium *Helicobacter pylori* plays a key role in breaching the defenses against acid-mediated attack on the gastric and duodenal mucosa.

Other Stomach Products Secreted Into the Gut Lumen

Intrinsic factor is a vitamin B_{12}-binding protein required for the vitamin's uptake in the terminal ileum. It is secreted by a constitutive pathway from the same parietal cells that generate gastric acid. Thus, autoimmune destruction of parietal cells produces not only **achlorhydria** due to lack of acid secretion but also **pernicious anemia** from vitamin B_{12} deficiency.

---

19. What are the cell types that are found in the lining of the stomach?
20. What are the roles of the proximal and distal stomach?
21. Name two products secreted by the stomach into (1) the gut lumen and (2) the bloodstream, and describe their functions.

GALLBLADDER

Anatomy

The gallbladder is a muscular sac with a resting volume of about 50 mL that lies on the inferior surface of the liver (Figure 13–9). It is connected to the hepatic biliary system by the cystic duct, which leads

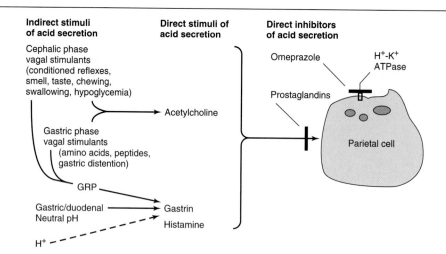

Figure 13–8. Regulation of gastric acid secretion. (GRP, gastric-releasing peptide.) Dashed arrow indicates inhibition.

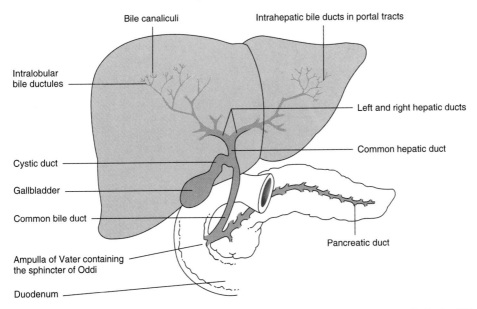

Figure 13–9. Anatomy of the biliary system. (Reproduced, with permission, from Chandrasoma P, Taylor CE: *Concise Pathology,* 3rd ed. Appleton & Lange, 1998.)

to the common bile duct whose opening into the proximal duodenum is controlled by the sphincter of Oddi. The common bile duct and the pancreatic duct usually join just proximal to this sphincter (Figure 13–9).

Physiology

Bile, which is produced by the liver, flows down the hepatic duct and into the gallbladder via the cystic duct. There it is stored until stimulation of gallbladder contraction expels the contents of the gallbladder back through the cystic duct into the common bile duct and, via the sphincter of Oddi, into the duodenum. Stimuli for gallbladder contraction and sphincter of Oddi relaxation necessary for proper bile flow include both hormones such as cholecystokinin (CCK), released in response to fat-rich meals, and neural inputs. Depending on how long it remains in the gallbladder, bile becomes concentrated. Bile composition is further modified by mucin production under the control of prostaglandins and by saturation of bile cholesterol controlled in part by estrogens.

The most prominent disorders of the gallbladder involve gallstone formation (see below).

SMALL INTESTINE

Anatomy & Histology

Three regions can be distinguished along the approximately 5-meter length of the small intestine. The pyloric sphincter marks the beginning of the **duodenum,** which is largely retroperitoneal and fixed in its location. Thanks to this sphincter, stomach contents normally enter the duodenum in small spurts containing tiny suspended particles. In the duodenum, gastric contents are mixed with the secretions of the common bile duct and pancreatic duct.

Beyond the duodenum, the small intestine is mobile and suspended in the peritoneal cavity by a mesentery. The proximal two-fifths is called the **jejunum.** The distal three-fifths is termed the **ileum,** which ends at the ileocecal valve at the start of the large intestine.

The most striking gross structural features of the small intestine are the numerous **villi** (projections of the mucosa approximately 1 mm in height) (Figure 13–10A). Each villus contains a single terminal branch of the arterial, venous, and lymphatic trees. These allow efficient transfer to the circulatory system of substances absorbed from the gut lumen by **enterocytes** (surface epithelial cells). By electron microscopy, each enterocyte displays numerous microvilli—plasma membrane evaginations that further increase the absorptive surface area (Figure 13–10B). The microvilli make up a brush border facing the intestinal lumen.

The crypts between villi are the site of cell proliferation. An as yet unidentified multipotential stem cell in the crypt serves as progenitor of the four mature cell types of the villus: enterocytes, goblet cells (which secrete mucus into the gastrointestinal lumen), enteroendocrine cells (which secrete hormones into the bloodstream), and Paneth cells (which produce antimicrobial peptides and growth factors).

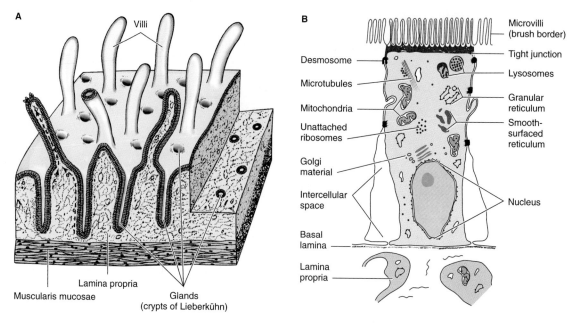

Figure 13–10. Structure of the small intestine. **A:** Schematic diagram illustrating the structure of the small intestine and the relationship of villi, epithelial cells, and the underlying lamina propria. (Redrawn and reproduced, with permission, from Ham AW: *Histology,* 6th ed. Lippincott, 1969.) **B:** Schematic diagram of an individual small intestine epithelial cell with microvilli. (Reproduced, with permission, from Sleisenger MH, Fordtran JS [editors]: *Gastrointestinal Disease,* 3rd ed. Saunders, 1986.)

While the other cell types migrate up the villus as they differentiate, with an average life span of 4–6 days, the Paneth cells stay in the crypt, which is where most fluid and electrolyte secretion by enterocytes into the gastrointestinal lumen occurs.

Physiology of Intestinal Motility

Two patterns of motility occur in the intestine: **fasting** and **feeding**. During fasting, the pattern is called the **migrating motor complex** and consists of a repetitive (every 80–100 minutes) three-phase cycle of activity that keeps the gastrointestinal tract clear of debris (bacteria, undigested material, desquamated cells, secretions) as one of the body's "housekeeping" duties. Phase I is quiescent, phase II is spontaneous irregular activity, and phase III is a burst of rhythmic propagated contraction. The migrating motor complex appears to be under the control of the gut hormone **motilin.** This pattern is interrupted upon feeding, with a new pattern of activity involving both segmental (to-and-fro) as well as propulsive contractions, and acts to promote optimal mixing and absorption.

Some common gastrointestinal tract disorders involve aberrant small intestine motility. Individuals with complaints of alternating constipation, diarrhea, and abdominal pain in whom no structural problem or underlying disease can be identified are said to have "irritable bowel syndrome." They probably have disordered small intestine motility. Similarly, disorders in which the migrating motor complex is disrupted or lacking can be a complication of diseases such as diabetes mellitus, familial pseudoobstruction, and scleroderma. Complications can include bezoar formation, intestinal bacterial overgrowth, excessively rapid small bowel transit time (diarrhea), nausea and vomiting, abdominal distention, and constipation.

Secretion in the Small Intestine

The intestinal mucosa is armed with an array of transporters that allow it to absorb a tremendous volume of fluids and electrolytes in the course of a normal day. Of the 9 L of fluid input, the small intestine typically absorbs 7–8 L, leaving 1–2 L to be dealt with by the colon. Absorption in the small intestine shares common features with fluid and electrolyte uptake by the proximal renal tubule. Absorption in the colon resembles that in the distal renal tubule in that both the colon and the distal renal tubule have aldosterone-sensitive sodium transporters.

However, absorption in the small intestine also has some distinctive features. In the crypts between villi, chloride can leave the enterocyte and enter the gastrointestinal lumen through a channel whose conductance is regulated by cAMP, with water following passively. The small intestine's capacity to resorb sodium and with it water is normally limited. Transport of sodium does occur, but such transport is normally used to take up precious small molecules such as glucose and amino acids. Enterocytes have sodium co-transporters, localized to the villi, that allow the energy expended by the Na^+-K^+ ATPase to be used for selective absorption against a concentration gradient. Activity of the Na^+-K^+ ATPase generates extracellular sodium, which is then used to drive these co-transporters. Under certain circumstances, this physiologic mechanism can be put to therapeutic use. In cholera, G protein modification by a toxin results in uncontrolled chloride channel activation in the crypts of the small intestinal villi. The resulting loss of huge amounts of chloride—and with it sodium and water—can rapidly cause dehydration and death. An inexpensive and effective treatment is oral rehydration with glucose-containing solutions. The glucose drives the sodium-glucose co-transporter to transport both molecules into enterocytes, and with them chloride and water, thereby offsetting the fluid efflux mediated by the bacterial toxin. Because these co-transporters are lacking in the colon, its maximum absorptive capacity (5 L/d) is considerably less than that of the small intestine (12 L/d).

Secretagogues (substances that stimulate secretion) can act from either the **apical** (gut lumen) or **basal** (blood) side of the enterocyte. Examples of **luminal secretagogues** are bacterial enterotoxins, bile salts, fatty acids, and some laxatives. **Humoral** (blood-borne) **secretagogues** include vasoactive intestinal peptide, calcitonin, prostaglandins, and serotonin.

Digestion & Absorption in the Small Intestine

The small intestine is the most important site of both digestion and absorption. The histologic specialization of villi and microvilli greatly expands the surface area on and across which digestion and absorption can take place. Similarly, the segmental motility program ensures even mixing and efficient extraction of substances in the lumen of the small intestine.

Most nutrients (eg, lipids, proteins, and carbohydrates) are digested and absorbed along the entire length of the small intestine. However, some specialized substances are absorbed only in particular regions. Thus, conjugated bile acids and vitamin B_{12} are absorbed in the terminal ileum, while absorption of iron occurs in the duodenum (free iron) and in the stomach (heme iron).

---

22. What are the programs of activity in the small intestine during fasting and feeding?
23. What are some consequences of disordered small intestinal motility?
24. What substances are absorbed in specialized regions of the small intestine?
25. Give an example of a luminal and of a humoral gastrointestinal tract secretagogue.

COLON

Anatomy & Histology

The adult colon is 1.5–1.8 meters in length. Its various segments (cecum; ascending, transverse, descending, and sigmoid colon; rectum and anal canal) are involved in absorption of water and electrolytes, secretion of mucus, and formation, propulsion, and storage of unabsorbed material (feces). The colon is also the home of the intestinal microbial flora.

The surface of the colon consists of a columnar epithelium with no villi and few folds except in the distal rectum. The epithelium has a few short, irregular microvilli. Numerous deep glands contain goblet cells, endocrine cells, and absorptive cells.

Physiology of Colonic Motility

Unlike the stomach and small intestine, the colon is rarely inactive, though its activity is less easily characterized than that of the stomach (which has the pattern known as receptive relaxation) or than that of the small intestine (which displays the pattern known as the migrating motor complex and segmental to-and-fro action). Some patterns are discernible, however, such as the **gastrocolic reflex** (colonic mass peristalsis following a meal). Disorders of colonic motility are common complications of autonomic neuropathy in patients with diabetes mellitus and can cause severe gastrointestinal complaints.

Secretion in the Colon

The major secretory product of the colon is mucin, a complex glycoprotein conjugate that serves lubricating and perhaps protective functions.

Digestion & Absorption in the Colon

Digestion in the colon occurs as a consequence of the action of the colonic microflora. Its physiologic significance is not well understood. However, some data suggest that short chain fatty acids released by microbial action on dietary fiber are an important source of energy for the colon. More importantly, short chain fatty acids promote survival of healthy colonic epithelium while inducing apoptosis (programmed cell death) in epithelial cells that are progressing toward malignant transformation.

Absorption of fluid and electrolytes has been well studied and is a major function of the colon. Up to 5 L of water can be absorbed per day across the colonic epithelium. Furthermore, the colonic epithelium can also take up sodium against a considerable concentration gradient. Aldosterone, a hormone involved in fluid and electrolyte homeostasis, increases colonic sodium conductance in response to volume depletion, thus playing an important role in maintaining fluid and electrolyte balance (see Chapter 21).

26. How does colonic motility differ from that in the small intestine?
27. What is the major secretory product of the colon?
28. What volume of water is the colon capable of absorbing per day?

OVERVIEW OF GASTROINTESTINAL DISORDERS

DISORDERS OF MOTILITY

Disorders of motility affect all major regions of the gastrointestinal tract. Because gastrointestinal tract motility is a complex result of smooth muscle contraction under neural and hormonal control, abnormal motility of the gastrointestinal tract can occur through damage to gastrointestinal smooth muscle or to the neural and hormonal mechanisms by which it is controlled—or to both. An example of muscle damage leading to abnormal motility is seen in esophageal stricture as a result of caustic ingestions or acid reflux. Abnormal neural control of motility is seen in esophageal achalasia. Esophageal motility disorders are typically characterized by dysphagia and odynophagia.

Motility disorders of the stomach include gastroparesis, a complication of diabetes mellitus; and dysmotility as a consequence of stomach surgery, either due to resection of part of the stomach or to **vagotomy.** Vagotomy entails surgical transection of the vagus nerve trunks, which prevents vagus-stimulated acid secretion and also cuts vagal fibers influencing motility via the enteric nervous system. Vagotomy is usually performed as treatment for Zollinger-Ellison syndrome, ie, acid hypersecretion and severe peptic ulcer disease due to a gastrin-secreting tumor.

The symptoms and signs of motility disorders in the stomach depend upon their cause. Because vagotomy cuts fibers influencing the enteric nervous system as well as the intended fibers that influence acid secretion, a classic complication of vagotomy is disordered gastric motility. This may present clinically as either partial outlet obstruction or as too rapid emptying of gastric contents into the duodenum, with resulting fluid shifts and vasomotor symptoms (**"dumping syndrome"**). Sometimes, however, patients may develop symptoms of stomach distention, nausea, early satiety, and vomiting suggestive of partial gastric outlet obstruction. To ameliorate the latter symptoms, **pyloroplasty** (severing the fibers of the pyloric sphincter) is done to render the sphincter less competent, so that food can pass more easily into the duodenum. Intrinsic neuropathy (eg, in diabetes mellitus) results in delayed gastric emptying, nausea, vomiting, and constipation rather than the classic dumping syndrome. The pathophysiologic basis for these differences is not known.

In the small intestine and colon, disordered motility is believed to be responsible for **irritable bowel syndrome,** characterized by recurrent episodes of abdominal pain, bloating, and diarrhea alternating with constipation. While the pathophysiology of this disorder is poorly understood, altered levels of gastrointestinal tract hormones such as motilin or CCK have been suggested as a cause, perhaps influenced by psychologic factors and stress-related release of inflammatory cytokines. Thus, a wide range of causes may result in abnormal motility, presumably as a consequence of interference with mechanisms of control of the gastrointestinal tract.

DISORDERS OF SECRETION

Clinically recognized disorders of secretion involve the production of acid, intrinsic factor, or mucus by the stomach, digestive enzymes and bicarbonate by the pancreas, bile by the liver, and water and electrolytes by the small intestine in response to secretagogues.

Either elevated gastric acid secretion or diminished mucosal defense can predispose to development of **peptic ulcers.** These are discrete regions of erosion through the mucosa which are surrounded by apparently normal tissue. Acid-induced damage may occur in the form of an ulcer either in the stomach (**gastric ulcer**) or in the first part of the small intestine (**duodenal ulcer**). Acid-induced injury may also occur in the form of more diffuse and less clearly demarcated inflammation anywhere along the gastrointestinal tract from the lower esophagus through the duodenum. It appears that elevated acid secretion is relatively more important in the development of duodenal ulcer, while diminished mucosal defense (eg, due to diminished mucus secretion in some cases) is a more crucial factor in development of gastric ulcer. Disorders of secretion involving the liver and pancreas are discussed in Chapters 14 and 15. Diarrhea, the major secretory disorder of the small intestine, is discussed below.

DISORDERS OF DIGESTION & ABSORPTION

Physiologically significant digestion and absorption can occur throughout the gastrointestinal tract. Indeed, the effectiveness of sublingual nitroglycerin therapy for patients with angina is a testimonial to the efficacy of sublingual absorption. Nevertheless, the clinically prominent disorders of digestion and absorption focus on the small intestine and colon and the accessory organs (pancreas and liver) whose secretions (digestive enzymes, bicarbonate, and bile) are necessary for digestion and absorption in the small intestine.

GASTROINTESTINAL MANIFESTATIONS OF SYSTEMIC DISEASE

A wide range of systemic conditions and diseases may produce symptoms and signs in the gastrointestinal tract. These include endocrine disorders that alter control of gastrointestinal tract functions or which predispose to pancreatitis or peptic ulcer disease; complications of diabetes mellitus, including autonomic neuropathy and ketoacidosis; pregnancy; deficiency disorders, including deficiency of zinc, niacin, and iron; and neoplastic, rheumatologic, and other syndromes (Table 13–5).

---

29. What are some common symptoms of esophageal dysmotility?
30. Why does vagotomy often create motor disorders in the stomach?
31. What are some suggested factors in the pathogenesis of the irritable bowel syndrome?

PATHOPHYSIOLOGY OF DISORDERS OF THE ESOPHAGUS

The major disorders of the esophagus are related to motor functions: Disordered peristalsis and increased lower esophageal sphincter tone are seen in esophageal achalasia, while inappropriate lower esophageal sphincter relaxation results in reflux esophagitis.

ESOPHAGEAL ACHALASIA

Clinical Presentation

Esophageal achalasia is a motor disorder in which the lower esophageal sphincter fails to relax properly. As a result, a **functional obstruction** (ie, obstruction due to abnormal function in the absence of a visible mass or lesion) is created that is manifested as dysphagia, regurgitation, and chest pain. It is a progressive disease in which severe radiographic distortion of the esophagus develops.

Etiology

The underlying cause of esophageal achalasia, which occurs with an incidence of 0.5–1:100,000 population per year, is unknown. It has been suggested that degenerative disease (due to any cause) of the myenteric plexus of the enteric nervous system of the lower two-thirds of the esophagus results in the clinical features of achalasia. Esophageal involvement in Chagas' disease, due to damage of the neural plexuses of the esophagus by the parasite *Trypanosoma cruzi*, bears a striking resemblance to esophageal achalasia. A number of other disorders, including malignancies, may present with manometric pressure characteristics or radiographic features similar to those observed in idiopathic esophageal achalasia (Table 13–6).

Pathology & Pathogenesis

While achalasia is manifested as a motor disorder of esophageal smooth muscle, it is actually due to defective innervation of smooth muscle in the esophageal body and lower esophageal sphincter. Lower esophageal sphincter tone is normally characterized by tonic contraction with intermittent relaxation due to a neural reflex arc (see above). In achalasia, it is even more tightly contracted and does not relax properly in response to swallowing, due to partial loss of neurons in the wall of the esophagus. Thus, achalasia can be thought of as a disorder due to defective inhibitory pathways of the esophageal enteric nervous system. Interestingly, injection of botulinum toxin into the lower esophageal sphincter diminishes the excitatory pathways and thereby ameliorates symptoms.

In addition to dysfunction of the lower esophageal sphincter, loss of normal peristalsis in the esophageal body is often seen in achalasia—consistent with the hypothesis of myenteric plexus degeneration. Variations of achalasia also exist in which normal peristalsis is replaced by simultaneous contractions of large or small amplitude.

Clinical Manifestations

Over months and years, lower esophageal sphincter dysfunction results in tremendous enlargement of the esophagus. Normally intended as a direct conduit to the stomach, the esophagus in advanced cases of achalasia can hold as much as 1 L of putrid, infected material, imposing a high risk of aspiration pneumonia. Without treatment, patients display progressive severe weight loss with worsening chest pain, mucosal ulceration, infection, and occasional esophageal rupture, culminating in death.

REFLUX ESOPHAGITIS

Clinical Presentation

The predominant presenting symptom of reflux is burning chest pain ("heartburn") due to recurrent mu-

Table 13–5. Gastrointestinal manifestations of systemic diseases and their pathophysiologic mechanisms.[1]

Disease or Condition	Commonly Associated Gastrointestinal Manifestations	Mechanism

Thyroid disease
  Autoimmune thyroiditis
  Hypothyroidism
 	
  Hyperthyroidism
	Achlorhydria and pernicious anemia
	Esophageal reflux
	Bezoars
	Constipation
	Malabsorption
	Diarrhea and weight loss
		Autoimmune destruction of parietal cells
		Lower esophageal sphincter dysfunction
		Gastric dysmotility
		Intestinal dysmotility
		Villous atrophy and pancreatic insufficiency
		Intestinal hypermotility with rapid transit and malabsorption

Adrenal disease Adrenal insufficiency	Abdominal pain Diarrhea	Unknown Malabsorption due to loss of trophic effect of corticosteroids on enterocyte brush border
Parathyroid disease Primary hyperparathyroidism	Nausea and vomiting Pancreatitis Acid-peptic disease	Hypercalcemia-induced alteration in signal transduction resulting in gastric atony and dysmotility Hypercalcemia-induced premature activation of pancreatic enzymes Hypercalcemia-induced increased acid secretion
Diabetes mellitus	Esophageal, gastric, small and large intestinal and rectal dysfunction Nausea, vomiting, abdominal pain	Autonomic neuropathy Ketoacidosis with gastric atony
Pregnancy	Esophageal reflux; nausea and vomiting; hematemesis; constipation and hemorrhoids	Pressure effects of gravid uterus on lower esophageal sphincter, gastric emptying, intestinal transit time, and venous return
Deficiency states Zinc, niacin	Malabsorption syndrome	Altered enterocyte brush border
Cancer	Pain, fever, bleeding, ascites, obstruction, perforation Paraneoplastic syndromes and hypercalcemia	Metastases (most commonly breast cancer, melanoma, bronchogenic carcinoma of lung) Tumor-produced peptides

Hematologic conditions
  Bleeding disorders
  Hypercoagulable states
  Dysproteinemias
	Intramural hematoma
	Bowel infarction
	Hemorrhage, obstruction, amyloidosis
		Hemorrhage
		Intestinal ischemia
		Infiltration

Rheumatologic disorders
  Scleroderma
  Systemic lupus erythematosus
  Rheumatoid arthritis
	Dysphagia, esophageal reflux, obstruction, bleeding, perforation, pseudo-obstruction, pancreatitis, malabsorption
	Nausea, vomiting, mucosal ulceration
	Gastric ulcers, gastritis
		Inflammation, vasculitis, vascular obliteration, villous atrophy
		Inflammation, vasculitis, vascular obstruction, villous atrophy
		Aspirin or NSAID use

Metabolic and infiltrative disorders (dyslipidemias; sarcoidosis, amyloidosis)	Malabsorption Infarction	Infiltration, muscle atrophy, dysmotility Infiltration, mucosal ischemia, infarction
Renal disorders (including chronic renal failure and transplantation)	Abdominal pain, gastrointestinal bleeding, intestinal perforation	Gastritis, duodenitis, pancreatitis
Neurologic disorders (including spinal cord injury, myotonic dystrophy, CNS disease)	Impaired gut motility with nausea, vomiting, chronic constipation	Disordered central and enteric nervous system communication

Pulmonary disorders
  Asthma
  Cystic fibrosis
	Esophageal reflux
	Diarrhea, malabsorption and weight loss
		Nocturnal aspiration
		Pancreatic exocrine insufficiency

[1]Reproduced, with permission, from Hunter TB, Bjeilard JC: Gastrointestinal complications of leukemia and its treatment. AJR Am J Roentgenol 1984;143:513; from Riley SA, Tumberg LA: Maldigestion and malabsorption. In: *Gastrointestinal Disease*, 4th ed. Sleisenger MH, Fordtran JS (editors). Saunders, 1989; and from Sack TL, Sleisenger MH: Effects of systemic and extraintestinal disease on the gut. In: *Gastrointestinal Disease*, 4th ed. Sleisenger MH, Fordtran JS (editors). Saunders, 1989.

Table 13–6. Disorders with manometric and radiologic features that mimic idiopathic achalasia.[1]

Malignancy
  Gastric adenocarcinoma
  Esophageal squamous cell carcinoma
  Lymphoma
  Lung carcinoma
  Pancreatic cancer
  Prostate cancer
  Hepatocellular cancer
  Anaplastic cancer
Chronic idiopathic intestinal pseudo-obstruction
Amyloidosis
Chagas' disease
Postvagotomy disturbance
Familial glucocorticoid deficiency syndrome
Multiple endocrine neoplasia type IIb
Juvenile Sjögren's syndrome with achalasia and gastric hypersecretion

[1]Reproduced, with permission, from Clouse RE: Motor disorders. In: *Gastrointestinal Disease,* 4th ed. Sleisenger MH, Fordtran JS (editors). Saunders, 1989.

cosal injury, often worse at night, when lying supine, or after consumption of foods or drugs that diminish lower esophageal sphincter tone.

Etiology

Common causes of reflux esophagitis are those conditions that result in persistent or repetitive acid exposure to the esophageal mucosa. These include disorders that increase the rate of spontaneous transient lower esophageal sphincter relaxations (Table 13–4) or impair reflexes that normally follow transient lower esophageal sphincter relaxations with a secondary wave of esophageal peristalsis. Conditions that increase gastric volume or pressure (eg, partial or complete gastric outlet obstruction and conditions that increase acid production) also contribute. (Figure 13–8). Occasionally, reflux esophagitis can be caused by alkaline injury, eg, pancreatic juice refluxing through both an incompetent pyloric sphincter and a relaxed lower esophageal sphincter.

Pathology & Pathogenesis

Normally, the tonically contracted state of the lower esophageal sphincter provides an effective barrier to reflux of acid from the stomach back into the esophagus. This is reinforced by secondary esophageal peristaltic waves in response to transient lower esophageal sphincter relaxation. Effectiveness of that barrier can be altered by loss of lower esophageal sphincter tone (ie, the opposite of achalasia), increased frequency of transient relaxations, loss of secondary peristalsis following a transient relaxation, increased stomach volume or pressure, or increased production of acid—all of which can make more likely reflux of acidic stomach contents sufficient to cause pain or erosion. Recurrent reflux can damage the mucosa, resulting in inflammation—hence the term "reflux esophagitis." Recurrent reflux itself predisposes to further reflux because the scarring that occurs with healing of the inflamed epithelium renders the lower esophageal sphincter progressively less competent as a barrier.

Although typically a consequence of acid reflux, esophagitis can also result from reflux of pepsin or bile. In most cases of esophageal reflux disease, a common pathophysiologic thread can be identified (Figure 13–11). Recurrent mucosal damage results in infiltration of granulocytes and eosinophils, hyperplasia of basal cells, and eventually the development of friable, bleeding ulcers and exudates over the mucosal surface. These pathologic changes set the stage for scar formation and sphincter incompetence, predisposing to recurrent cycles of inflammation.

Increased frequency of transient lower esophageal sphincter relaxations may be partly in response to increased gastric distention. Normally, transient lower esophageal sphincter relaxations are accompanied by increased esophageal peristalsis. Individuals with defects in excitatory pathways that promote peristalsis may therefore be at increased risk for the development of esophageal reflux.

Changes in the types of prostaglandins produced by the esophagus have been noted in reflux esophagitis, perhaps contributing to impairment of healing and predisposing to recurrences.

In contrast to other forms of acid-mediated injury, *H pylori* infection does not appear to contribute to the development of reflux or esophagitis.

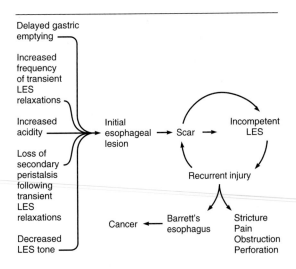

Figure 13–11. Pathophysiology of esophageal reflux disease. (LES, lower esophageal sphincter.)

Clinical Manifestations

Heartburn is the usual symptom of reflux esophagitis, typically worsening upon lying prone. With recurrent reflux, a range of complications may develop. The most common complication is the development of stricture in the distal esophagus. Progressive obstruction, initially to solid food and later to liquid, presents as dysphagia. Other complications of recurrent reflux include hemorrhage or perforation; hoarseness, coughing, wheezing; and pneumonia as a result of aspiration of gastric contents into the lungs, particularly during sleep. Epidemiologic studies suggest that cigarette smoking and alcohol abuse associated with recurrent reflux result in a change in the esophageal epithelium from squamous to columnar histology, termed **Barrett's esophagus.** In 2–5% of cases, Barrett's esophagus leads to the development of adenocarcinoma.

---

32. What are the roles of the lower esophageal sphincter structure in achalasia and in reflux esophagitis?
33. What is the relationship of esophageal reflux to Barrett's esophagus and cancer?

PATHOPHYSIOLOGY OF DISORDERS OF THE STOMACH

Common disorders involving the stomach reflect the importance of its role as a secretory organ, in particular of acid and intrinsic factor. Disorders of acid secretion result in acid-peptic disease, while loss of intrinsic factor secretion results in inability to absorb vitamin B_{12}, manifesting as **pernicious anemia.** The major motility disorder of the stomach is gastroparesis.

ACID-PEPTIC DISEASE

Clinical Presentation

Patients with acid-peptic disease typically present with chronic, mild, gnawing or burning abdominal or chest pain due to superficial or deep erosion of the gastrointestinal mucosa; with sudden complications such as gastrointestinal bleeding, resulting in hematemesis or melena; or with perforation and infection, resulting in severe abdominal pain and signs of acute abdomen (absence of bowel sounds, guarding, rebound tenderness). The latter presentation reflects the fact that in some cases acid-peptic disease can be painless in the early stages and can be detected only when it leads to an intra-abdominal catastrophe.

Classically, duodenal ulcer presents as gnawing or burning epigastric pain occurring 1–3 hours after meals, often waking the patient at night, with antacids or food producing relief. However, many patients later documented to have duodenal ulcer do not fit this symptom profile. Elderly patients in particular often present with a complication of duodenal ulcer but no history of pain.

Etiology

Various causes of absolute or relative increased acid production (Figure 13–8) or decreased mucosal defenses (Table 13–3) predispose to acid-peptic disease.

Pathology & Pathogenesis

Corrosive agents (acid and pepsin) secreted by the stomach play a key role in gastric ulcer, duodenal ulcer, and acute erosive gastritis. Each of these diseases has a distinctive but overlapping pathogenesis with the common themes of either excessive acid secretion or diminished mucosal defense. Exactly why one but not another form of acid-peptic disease should develop in a given individual remains unclear. A specific infectious agent, the bacterium *Helicobacter pylori,* has been implicated in predisposition to a number of forms of acid-peptic disease, including duodenal ulcer, gastric ulcer, and gastritis. *H pylori* can cause acid-peptic disease by multiple mechanisms, including altered signal transduction—resulting in inflammation, increased acid secretion, and diminished mucosal defenses. It may also affect apoptosis in the gastrointestinal tract.

H pylori is an extremely common pathogen, found in 50% of the world's population, with rates of infection even higher in the poorest countries where sanitation facilities and standards of personal hygiene are low. The most likely route of spread from person to person is fecal-oral. As many as 90% of infected individuals show signs of inflammation (gastritis or duodenitis) on endoscopy, though many of these individuals are clinically asymptomatic. Despite this high rate of association of inflammation with *H pylori* infection, the important role of other factors is indicated by the fact that only about 15% of infected individuals ever develop a clinically significant ulcer. These other factors (both genetic and environmental, such as cigarette smoking) must account for the individual variations and are pathophysiologically important. Nevertheless, the role of *H pylori* is of particular clinical importance because, of patients who do develop acid-peptic disease, almost all have *H pylori* infection. Furthermore, treatment that does not eradicate *H pylori* is associated with rapid recurrence of acid-peptic disease in most patients. Recent studies have also associated different strains of *H pylori* with different forms and degrees of acid-peptic disease and implicated *H pylori* infection in development of gastrointestinal tract cancers. These observations suggest the importance of altered local cytokine production by the host immune system in the pathophysiology of *H pylori*-induced disease. The details of these relationships remain to be clarified by further investigation.

1. GASTRIC ULCER

Gastric ulcer is distinguished from gastritis by the depth of the lesion, with gastric ulcers penetrating through the mucosa. The actual ulcer crater is often surrounded by an area of intact but inflamed mucosa, suggesting that gastritis is a predisposing lesion to development of gastric ulcer. Most gastric ulcers occur on the lesser curvature of the stomach. It is likely that gastric ulcer represents the outcome of a number of different abnormalities summarized below.

Some gastric ulcers are believed to be related to impaired mucosal defenses, since the acid and pepsin secretory capacity of some affected patients is normal or even below normal.

Motility defects have been proposed to contribute to development of gastric ulcer in at least three ways: (1) By a tendency of duodenal contents to reflux back through an incompetent pyloric sphincter. Bile acids in the duodenal reflux material act as an irritant and may be an important contributor to a diminished mucosal barrier against acid and pepsin. (2) By delayed emptying of gastric contents, including reflux material, into the duodenum. (3) By delayed gastric emptying and hence food retention, resulting in increased gastrin secretion and gastric acid production. It is not known whether these motility defects are a cause or a consequence of gastric ulcer formation.

Mucosal ischemia may play a role in the development of a gastric ulcer. Prostaglandins are known to increase mucosal blood flow as well as bicarbonate and mucus secretion and to stimulate mucosal cell repair and renewal. Thus, their deficiency—resulting from nonsteroidal anti-inflammatory drug (NSAID) ingestion or other insults—may predispose to gastritis and gastric ulcer, as might diminished bicarbonate or mucus secretion due to other causes. Subsets of gastric ulcer patients with each of these defects have been identified. Thus, the risk factors (NSAID ingestion, smoking, psychologic stress, *H pylori* infection) that have been associated with gastric ulcer probably act by diminishing one or more mucosal defense mechanisms.

Gastritis (inflammation of the gastric mucosa) as a result of aspirin and other NSAIDs, bile salts, alcohol, or other insults may predispose to ulcer formation (1) by attenuating the barrier created by the epithelial cells or the mucus and bicarbonate they secrete or (2) by reducing the quantity of prostaglandins the epithelial cells produce that might otherwise diminish acid secretion.

2. ACUTE EROSIVE GASTRITIS

Acute erosive gastritis includes inflammation due to superficial mucosal injury, mucosal erosion, or shallow ulcers due to a wide variety of insults, most notably alcohol, drugs, and stress. Ethanol ingestion predisposes to gastritis but not to development of gastric ulcer. Unlike gastric or duodenal ulcers, in erosive gastritis the submucosa and muscularis mucosae are not penetrated. Acid hypersecretion, gastric anoxia, altered natural defenses (especially diminished mucus secretion), epithelial renewal, tissue mediators (eg, prostaglandins), reduced intramucosal pH, and intramucosal energy deficits have been suggested as factors in the development of superficial gastric mucosal injury.

3. CHRONIC ATROPHIC GASTRITIS

This heterogeneous group of syndromes is characterized by inflammatory cell infiltration with gastric mucosal atrophy and loss of glands. In chronic disease—unlike acute erosive gastritis—endoscopic abnormalities may not be grossly apparent. The capacity to secrete gastric acid is progressively reduced, and the serum levels of gastrin are elevated. Autoantibodies to parietal cells, intrinsic factor, and gastrin are common findings. Chronic atrophic gastritis is associated with *H pylori* infection, development of pernicious anemia, gastric adenocarcinoma, and gastrointestinal endocrine hyperplasia with carcinoids (neuroendocrine tumors of the gastrointestinal tract producing serotonin metabolites and associated with dramatic symptoms of flushing and diarrhea).

4. DUODENAL ULCER

Like gastric ulcer, duodenal ulcer is believed to be a consequence of excessive acid and pepsin secretion relative to the level of mucosal defenses. Excessive acid secretion is believed to play the more important role, however, since duodenal ulcer rarely occurs in individuals who secrete less than 10 meq of acid per hour.

Since duodenal ulcer is an intermittent and recurrent disease, all of the predisposing factors may not be present in every patient at any given time (Figure 13–12). Patients found to have a duodenal ulcer are more likely to have (1) increased acid and peptic secretory capacity; (2) increased basal acid secretion; (3) an increased postprandial acid secretory response; (4) increased sensitivity of gastrin secretory cells to secretagogues and impaired acid inhibition of gastrin release; (5) impairment of other feedback mechanisms of gastric acid secretion; and (6) rapid gastric emptying. However, considerable overlap exists between patients who develop duodenal ulcer and those

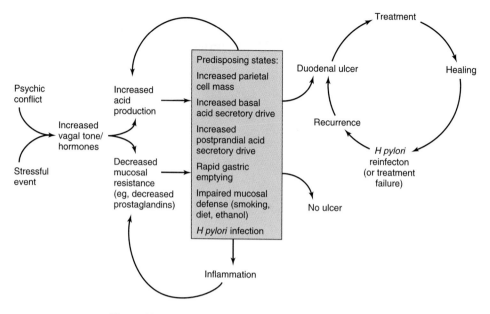

Figure 13–12. Pathophysiology of duodenal ulcer disease.

who do not, which may mean that important variables in pathogenesis are still unrecognized.

Various risk factors, including diet, smoking, *H pylori* infection, and excessive alcohol consumption, may influence the development of duodenal ulcers, though specific associations (eg, between coffee or spicy foods and the development of ulcers) have not been demonstrated. Genetic factors also play a role, with studies supporting the existence of a heritable component in duodenal ulcers distinct from that involved in gastric ulcer. Likewise, psychologic stress has been implicated in duodenal ulcer disease, perhaps by an autonomic-mediated influence on acid secretion (Figure 13–12).

Clinical Manifestations

Those forms of acid-peptic disease characterized by exclusively superficial mucosal lesions (eg, acute erosive gastritis) can result in either acute or chronic gastrointestinal bleeding, accompanied by a significant drop in hematocrit and related complications (eg, precipitating angina in a patient with coronary artery disease). Patients with acute massive bleeding present with hematemesis (vomiting of blood), rectal bleeding, or melena (tarry stools from the effect of acid on blood) depending on the site of origin, the rate of transit of blood through the gastrointestinal tract, and the extent of hemorrhage. Acute massive hemorrhage (> 10% of blood volume over minutes to hours) is manifested by hypotension, tachycardia, and orthostatic blood pressure and heart rate changes on standing, often with dizziness.

In addition to hemorrhage, complications of duodenal ulcer and gastric ulcer include life-threatening perforation and obstruction.

34. How does pernicious anemia result from a secretory disorder of the stomach?
35. What is the typical acid secretion status of patients with pernicious anemia?
36. In which acid-peptic disorder is diminished mucosal defenses more important than acid hypersecretion?
37. How might motility defects contribute to gastric ulcer?
38. What factors may predispose a patient to duodenal ulcer disease?
39. How do nonsteroidal anti-inflammatory agents contribute to acid-peptic disease?
40. What evidence indicates the importance of *H pylori* infection in acid-peptic disease?
41. What evidence suggests that other factors besides *H pylori* infection contribute to acid-peptic disease?

GASTROPARESIS

Clinical Presentation

A common complication of stomach disorders is delayed gastric emptying (Table 13–7). Known as gastroparesis, it is manifested by nausea, bloating, vomiting, and either constipation or diarrhea. The

Table 13–7. Conditions producing symptomatic gastric motor dysfunction.[1]

Acute Conditions	Chronic Conditions
Abdominal pain, trauma, inflammation	Mechanical
Postoperative state	Gastric ulcer
Acute infections, gastroenteritis	Duodenal ulcer
Acute metabolic disorders:	Idiopathic hypertrophic pyloric stenosis
Acidosis, hypokalemia, hypercalcemia or hypocalcemia, hepatic coma, myxedema	Superior mesenteric artery syndrome
	Acid-peptic disease
	Gastroesophageal reflux
Immobilization	Gastric ulcer disease, nonulcer dyspepsia
Hyperglycemia (glucose >200 mg/dL)	Gastritis
Phamaceutical agents and hormones	Atrophic gastritis with or without pernicious anemia
Opioids, including endorphins and narcotics (eg, morphine)	Viral gastroenteritis (acute, ?chronic gastritis)
	Metabolic and endocrine
Anticholinergics	Diabetic ketoacidosis (acute)
Tricyclic antidepressants	Diabetic gastroparesis (chronic)
Beta-adrenergic agonists	Addison's disease
Levodopa	Hypothyroidism
Aluminum hydroxide antacids	Pregnancy?
Gastrin	Uremia?
Cholecystokinin	Collagen-vascular diseases
Somatostatin	Scleroderma
	Dermatomyositis
	Polymyositis
	Systemic lupus erythematosus?
	Pseudo-obstruction
	Idiopathic, hollow visceral myopathy
	Secondary (eg, amyloidosis, Chagas' disease, muscular dystrophies, cancer-associated syndrome)
	Postgastric surgery
	Postvagotomy or postgastric resections
	Medications
	Anticholinergic, narcotic analgesics, levodopa, tricyclic antidepressants
	Hormones (pharmacologic studies)
	Gastrin, cholecystokinin, somatostatin
	Anorexia nervosa: bulimia
	Idiopathic
	Gastric dysrhythmias: tachygastria
	Gastroduodenal dyssynchrony
	Central nervous system: tabes dorsalis, depression

[1]Reproduced with permission, from McCallum RW: Motor function of the stomach in health and disease. In: *Gastrointestinal Disease,* 4th ed. Sleisenger MH, Fordtran JS (editors). Saunders, 1989.

condition can also occur silently, producing metabolic derangements (eg, of blood glucose in patients with diabetes mellitus) in the absence of somatic symptoms.

Etiology

Gastroparesis is a common complication of poorly controlled diabetes mellitus, with consequent autonomic neuropathy.

Pathology & Pathogenesis

Disorders of gastric motility result from alterations in a number of normal gastric functions. These include (1) serving as a reservoir for ingested solids and liquids (eg, alteration due to resection of the stomach); (2) mixing and homogenizing ingested food; and (3) functioning as a barrier that allows only small spurts of well-mixed chyme beyond the pyloric sphincter. The resulting disorders span the range from partial or complete gastric outlet obstruction to excessively rapid emptying and typically result from interference with the normal mechanisms by which these functions are controlled. These include the intrinsic contractility of gastric smooth muscle, the enteric nervous system, the autonomic nervous system's control over enteric nervous system function, and gut hormones.

Because the pyloric sphincter, like all sphincters, displays tonic contraction with intermittent transient relaxation, loss of vagal control results in excessive tonic contraction and symptoms of various degrees of gastric outlet obstruction. Disorders that affect the enteric nervous system such as the neuropathy of diabetes mellitus and surgical cutting of the stomach wall or vagal trunk typically cause delayed emptying. However, it is important to remember that in some cases, delayed emptying can result in symptoms expected from excessively rapid emptying. For example, an excessively contracted pylorus that can open completely but which does so infrequently can result in entry into the duodenum of too large a bolus of chyme from the excessively distended stomach. Such a bolus may not be efficiently handled by the small intestine, resulting in poor absorption and diarrheal symptoms characteristic of the dumping syndrome.

Hormones play an ill-defined but important role in regulation of gastrointestinal motility in health and disease. Erythromycin is of interest in this regard because, unrelated to its antibiotic properties, it recognizes the receptor for the gastrointestinal hormone motilin, causing increased gastrointestinal motility. Some patients with gastroparesis are observed to have substantial improvement with erythromycin analogs, especially when complaints related to partial gastric outlet obstruction, such as bloating, nausea, and constipation, are prominent.

Because different patients have different relative contributions of the intrinsic, enteric nervous system, autonomic nervous system, higher centers of the central nervous system, and hormones over control of their gastrointestinal tract motility, not all treatments for gastroparesis are effective for a majority of patients even with the same initial complaints.

Clinical Manifestations

Complications of gastroparesis include the development of bezoars from retained gastric contents, bacterial overgrowth, erratic blood glucose control, and, when nausea and vomiting are profound, weight loss. Elevated blood glucose can be either a cause or a consequence of delayed gastric emptying. Bacterial overgrowth itself can result in both malabsorption and diarrhea. For unknown reasons, the symptoms of gastroparesis are variable from patient to patient as well as over time in a given patient and often correlated poorly with delayed gastric emptying. In some cases, serotonin antagonists that decrease visceral perception may be more helpful than prokinetic agents in alleviating symptoms.

---

42. What are the symptoms of delayed versus rapid gastric emptying?
43. What are the complications of gastroparesis?
44. Why might erythromycin improve diabetic gastroparesis?

DISORDERS OF THE GALLBLADDER

Gallbladder disease is most commonly due to gallstones (cholelithiasis).

1. CHOLELITHIASIS

Clinical Presentation

Gallstones are most often asymptomatic, discovered incidentally at autopsy or during surgery for an unrelated condition. Of patients who do have symptoms referable to cholelithiasis, presentations range from mild nausea or abdominal discomfort after eating fatty or fried foods to severe right upper quadrant or midepigastric abdominal pain and jaundice. A history of chronic mild symptoms with dietary association typically predates an acute episode of abdominal pain. The typical patient with gallstones is female, has a history of high dietary fat intake, has had prior pregnancies—reflecting the role of estrogens in gallstone pathogenesis—and is in her forties, reflecting the time necessary for progression to symptomatic disease.

Etiology

Gallstones come in several varieties. Most are composed largely of cholesterol, with or without calcium deposits. Occasionally—especially in patients with a chronic hemolytic disease—bilirubin stones may form. Depending on the cause and the pathophysiologic mechanism involved, patients can have one or more of the following: a few large individual stones; many smaller stones; or "sludge"—a thickened viscous gel due to concentration of bile that is believed to be highly prone to formation of stones.

Pathology & Pathogenesis

Cholelithiasis is of multifactorial origin. However, the formation of cholesterol gallstones usually requires the formation of bile whose cholesterol concentration is greater than its percentage solubility. The normal processes that prevent gallstone formation probably include the fact that bile does not normally stay in the gallbladder long enough to become lithogenic (prone to stone formation). Thus, loss of gallbladder muscular wall motility (due either to intrinsic disease of the muscle wall, altered levels of hormones such as CCK, or altered neural control) and excessive sphincteric contraction, impairing emptying, are important predisposing factors. One consequence of decreased gallbladder emptying is excessive concentration of bile, leading to heightened lithogenicity. This can occur from excessive absorption of water or altered bile composition due to increased cholesterol content or saturation. Other factors can cause an increased tendency to form stones at any given degree of concentration and saturation, including the presence of nucleating versus antinu-

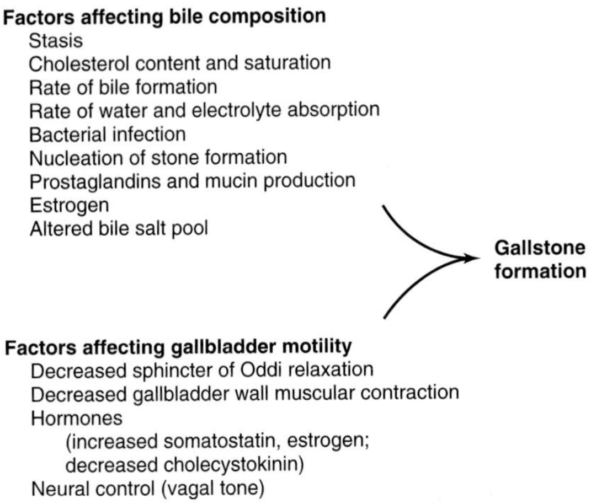

Factors affecting bile composition
  Stasis
  Cholesterol content and saturation
  Rate of bile formation
  Rate of water and electrolyte absorption
  Bacterial infection
  Nucleation of stone formation
  Prostaglandins and mucin production
  Estrogen
  Altered bile salt pool

→ Gallstone formation

Factors affecting gallbladder motility
  Decreased sphincter of Oddi relaxation
  Decreased gallbladder wall muscular contraction
  Hormones
    (increased somatostatin, estrogen;
    decreased cholecystokinin)
  Neural control (vagal tone)

Figure 13–13. Pathophysiology of cholelithiasis.

cleating factors in bile and the size and composition of the bile acid pool. Figure 13–13 summarizes the factors that predispose to gallstone formation, including estrogens, prostaglandins, increased mucus and glycoprotein production by the gallbladder epithelium, and chronic bacterial colonization or infection. Estrogens may play multiple roles, first affecting bile composition (increasing cholesterol and its saturation in bile) but also diminishing gallbladder motility (hence predisposing to stasis, sludge formation, and lithogenicity). Prostaglandins, which are protective in the stomach by increasing mucus production, actually may contribute to lithogenicity by the same mechanism. Thus, NSAIDs that block prostaglandin production are often beneficial for the prevention of gallstones in patients so predisposed, probably by decreasing mucus production.

Clinical Manifestations

The major clinical presentation of gallstones is inflammation of the gallbladder, or **cholecystitis**. Cholecystitis can be either acute or chronic—or acute against a background of chronic disease. An episode of acute cholecystitis can progress to acute pancreatitis if a stone travels down the common bile duct but fails to clear the sphincter of Oddi and thereby blocks the pancreatic duct. Likewise, an inflamed gallbladder can become infected or can undergo infarction and necrosis, setting the stage for systemic sepsis if the patient does not receive systemic broad-spectrum antibiotics and undergo emergency cholecystectomy (Figure 13–14).

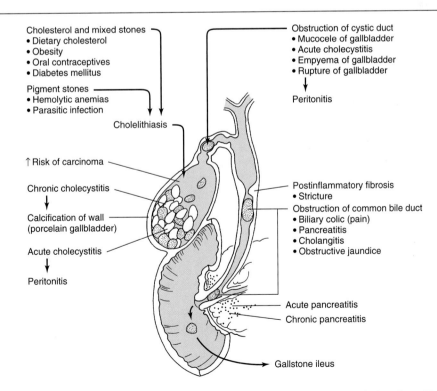

Figure 13–14. Clinical and pathologic effects of cholelithiasis. (Reproduced, with permission, from Chandrasoma P, Taylor CE: *Concise Pathology,* 3rd ed. Appleton & Lange, 1998.)

PATHOPHYSIOLOGY OF DISORDERS OF THE SMALL INTESTINE & COLON

Discussed below are diarrhea, inflammatory bowel disease, and diverticular disease. **Diarrhea** has many causes and diverse pathogenetic mechanisms, including altered motility, secretion, digestion, and absorption. While intestinal disorders are particularly prominent causes, disease of the stomach, pancreas, and biliary tract can also cause diarrhea. **Inflammatory bowel diseases** are poorly understood chronic autoimmune processes in the small intestine, colon, or both, with malabsorption as a prominent feature and with important systemic manifestations. **Diverticular disease** occurs most prominently in the colon, in part as a direct or indirect consequence of altered motor function.

DIARRHEA

Clinical Presentation

Diarrhea is defined as bowel movements which are excessive in volume, frequency, or liquidity. Any process that increases the frequency of defecation or volume of stool makes it more loose, since time-dependent absorption of water is responsible for the normal soft but formed consistency of stool.

Patients' subjective assessments of bowel movements are colored by their baseline bowel habits. An individual with chronic constipation, with bowel movements once every 3 days or so, may regard three soft stools in a day as "diarrhea." In contrast, an individual on a high-fiber diet may normally have bowel movements twice or even three times a day.

Diarrhea may be characterized as secretory, osmotic, or malabsorptive, depending on the physiologic basis for altered gut fluid homeostasis. **Osmotic diarrhea** is due to malabsorbed nutrients or poorly absorbed electrolytes that retain water in the lumen. **Secretory diarrhea** results when secretagogues maintain elevated rates of fluid transport out of epithelial cells into the gastrointestinal tract lumen. **Malabsorptive diarrhea** occurs when the ability to digest or absorb a particular nutrient is defective and can be due to disordered mixing (altered motility), to pancreatic insufficiency (altered digestion), or to damage to enterocytes or their surface transporters (altered absorption). These physiologic distinctions are useful in both diagnosis and therapy of diarrheal disorders. In transport capacity, the small intestine far exceeds the colon (owing to the enormous surface area of the brush border). Thus, infectious, toxic, or other causes of heightened secretion in the small intestine can overwhelm absorptive mechanisms in the colon, resulting in diarrhea.

Etiology

Flow in the gastrointestinal tract is a steady state involving massive fluid secretion into and absorption from the gastrointestinal lumen. Each process is controlled by both extrinsic and intrinsic factors. Subtle aberrations in input or output at any of several levels can result in diarrhea with or without nutrient malabsorption. Thus, an excessive osmotic load, increased secretion, or diminished fluid resorption may result in diarrhea (Table 13–8).

An excessive osmotic load in the gastrointestinal tract may come about in three different ways: By direct oral ingestion of excessive osmoles; by ingestion of a substrate that may be converted into excessive osmoles (eg, when bacterial action on the nondigestible carbohydrate lactulose generates a diarrhea-causing osmotic load in the colon); and as a manifestation of a genetic disease such as an enzyme deficiency in the setting of a particular diet (eg, milk consumption by a lactase-deficient individual).

Table 13–8. Mechanisms of diarrhea and major specific causes.[1]

Mechanisms of Diarrhea	Specific Causes
Osmotic	Disaccharidase deficiencies (eg, lactase deficiency) Glucose-galactose or fructose malabsorption Mannitol, sorbitol ingestion Lactulose therapy Some salts (eg, magnesium sulfate) Some antacids (eg, Maalox) Generalized malabsorption
Secretory	Enterotoxins Tumor products (eg, VIP, serotonin) Laxatives Bile acids Fatty acids Congenital defects
Malabsorption	Pancreatic enzyme deficiency Pancreatic enzyme inactivation (eg, by excess acid) Defective fat solubilization (disrupted enterohepatic circulation or defective bile formation) Ingestion of nutrient binding substances Bacterial overgrowth Loss of enterocytes (eg, radiation, infection, ischemia) Lymphatic obstruction (eg, lymphoma, tuberculosis)
Motility disorder	Diabetes mellitus Postsurgical
Inflammatory exudation	Inflammatory bowel disease Infection (eg, shigellosis)

[1]Reproduced, with permission, from Fine KD, Krejs GJ, Fordtran JS: Diarrhea. In: *Gastrointestinal Disease*, 4th ed. Sleisenger MH, Fordtran JS (editors). Saunders, 1989.

Secretion is increased by either blood-borne or intraluminal secretagogues. These include endogenous endocrine products (eg, overproduced by a tumor), exotoxins due to direct ingestion (eg, acute food poisoning) or infection (eg, cholera), or gastrointestinal luminal substances (eg, bile acids) that stimulate secretion.

Absorption of fluid, electrolytes, and nutrients can be diminished by many factors, including the toxic effects of alcohol and mucosal damage from infectious agents (Table 13–8) and from cytokines and prokinetic agents. Cytokines are released by immune and other cells, eg, in response to infection. Prokinetic agents speed up gastrointestinal motility, thereby diminishing the time available for absorption of any given nutrient, fluid, or electrolyte load. Finally, inflammatory and other disorders resulting in loss of mucus, blood, or protein from the gastrointestinal tract may be manifested as diarrhea. Symptoms and signs suggesting specific causes of diarrhea are listed in Table 13–9.

Pathology & Pathogenesis

Recognition of pathophysiologic subtypes of secretory, malabsorptive (Tables 13–10 and 13–11), and osmotic diarrheas provides a means of approaching diagnosis and therapy of diarrheal disorders. For example, nonbloody diarrhea that continues in the absence of oral intake must be due to a secretory mechanism, whereas diarrhea that diminishes as oral intake is curtailed (eg, in a patient receiving intravenous hydration) suggests an osmotic or malabsorptive cause. Likewise, the presence of white blood cells in the stool suggests an infectious or inflammatory origin of diarrhea, though their absence does not rule out such causes.

Of the many causes of diarrhea (Table 13–12), infectious agents are among the most important be-

Table 13–9. Clues to diagnosis of diarrhea from other symptoms and signs.[1]

Symptoms or Signs Associated With Diarrhea	Diagnoses to Be Considered
Arthritis	Ulcerative colitis, Crohn's disease, Whipple's disease, enteritis due to *Yersinia enterocolitica*, gonococcal proctitis
Liver disease	Ulcerative colitis, Crohn's disease, colon cancer with metastases to liver
Fever	Ulcerative colitis, Crohn's disease, amebiasis, lymphoma, tuberculosis, Whipple's disease, other enteric infections
Marked weight loss	Malabsorption, inflammatory bowel disease, colon cancer, thyrotoxicosis
Eosinophilia	Eosinophilic gastroenteritis, parasitic disease (particularly *Strongyloides*)
Lymphadenopathy	Lymphoma, Whipple's disease, AIDS
Neuropathy	Diabetic diarrhea, amyloidosis
Postural hypotension	Gastrointestinal bleeding, diabetic diarrhea, Addison's disease, idiopathic orthostatic hypotension
Flushing	Malignant carcinoid syndrome, pancreatic cholera syndrome
Erythema	Systemic mastocytosis, glucagonoma syndrome
Proteinuria	Amyloidosis
Collagen-vascular disease	Mesenteric vasculitis
Peptic ulcers	Zollinger-Ellison syndrome
Chronic lung disease	Cystic fibrosis
Systemic arteriosclerosis	Ischemic injury to gut
Frequent infections	Immunoglobulin deficiency
Hyperpigmentation	Whipple's disease, celiac disease, Addison's disease
Good response to corticosteroids	Ulcerative colitis, Crohn's disease, Whipple's disease, Addison's disease, eosinophilic gastroenteritis, celiac disease
Good response to antibiotics	Blind loop syndrome, tropical sprue, Whipple's disease

[1]Reproduced, with permission, from Fine KD, Krejs GJ, Fordtran JS: Diarrhea. In: *Gastrointestinal Disease,* 4th ed. Sleisenger MH, Fordtran JS (editors). Saunders, 1989.

Table 13–10. Histologic features of small intestinal diseases causing malabsorption.

Disease	Pathologic Features	Pattern of Distribution
Celiac (nontropical) sprue	Villus flattening, crypt hyperplasia, increased lymphocytes and plasma cells in lamina propria	Diffuse in proximal jejunum
Tropical sprue	Shortened villi, increased lymphocytes and plasma cells in lamina propria	Diffuse in proximal jejunum
Crohn's disease	Noncaseating granulomas with or without giant cells	Patchy lesions particularly affecting terminal ileum
Collagenous sprue	Subepithelial collagen deposits	Diffuse
Primary lymphoma	Malignant lymphocytes or histiocytes in lamina propria, variable villus flattening	Patchy
Whipple's disease	Lamina propria laden with PAS-staining foamy macrophages, bacilli in macrophages	Diffuse
Amyloidosis	Amyloid deposition in blood vessels, muscle layers	Diffuse in muscularis mucosae, mucosal sparing
Abetalipoproteinemia	Lipid-laden, vacuolated epithelial cells, normal villi	Diffuse
Radiation enteritis	Flattened villi, mucosal inflammation, fibrosis, ulceration	Patchy
Lymphangiectasia	Dilated lymphatics in lamina propria	Patchy
Eosinophilic gastroenteritis	Eosinophilic infiltrate in the intestinal wall	Patchy
Hypogammaglobulinemia	Villus flattening, *Giardia* trophozoites often present, few plasma cells	Patchy
Giardiasis	Trophozoites may be present, variable villus flattening	Patchy
Opportunistic infections	Organisms may be seen (*Isospora belli,* cryptosporidia, Microsporida), PAS-staining macrophages (*Mycobacterium avium* complex)	Patchy

cause they cause acute, sometimes life-threatening diseases whose pathogenesis is relatively well understood and because they are usually treatable. The symptoms of diarrhea due to infectious agents are due either to toxins that alter small bowel secretion and absorption or to direct mucosal invasion. The noninvasive toxin-producing bacteria are generally small bowel pathogens, while the invasive organisms are localized typically to the colon. Diarrheas due to infectious agents are discussed in Chapter 4.

Recent evidence suggests that infectious causes of diarrhea can interface more intimately with normal mechanisms of secretory control than had been previously realized. Thus, in addition to its direct affect on the G protein controlling chloride secretion in the crypts of the small intestinal epithelium, cholera activates the enteric nervous system to cause fluid and electrolyte secretion in the colon.

45. By what mechanisms do infectious agents cause diarrhea?
46. Name three ways in which an excessive osmotic load can occur in the gastrointestinal tract.

Clinical Manifestations

Dehydration, malnutrition, weight loss, and specific vitamin deficiency syndromes (eg, glossitis, cheilosis, and stomatitis) are common signs in diarrhea depending on its cause, severity, and chronicity (Tables 13–9 and 13–11).

In certain circumstances (eg, in young children), viral gastroenteritis is associated with a high mortality rate from dehydration when supportive measures (ie, oral or intravenous rehydration) are not promptly provided.

Some individuals with diarrhea due to parasitic infections remain relatively asymptomatic, while others may develop more severe symptoms and complications, including intestinal perforation.

INFLAMMATORY BOWEL DISEASE

Clinical Presentation

Noninfectious inflammatory bowel disease is distinguished from infectious entities by exclusion: recurrent episodes of mucopurulent (ie, containing mucus and white cells) bloody diarrhea characterized by lack of positive cultures for infectious organisms and

Table 13–11. Symptoms and signs of malabsorption.[1]

Clinical Features	Pathophysiology	Laboratory Findings
Diarrhea	Increased secretion and decreased absorption of water and electrolytes; unabsorbed fatty acids and bile salts	Increased fat excretion, decreased serum carotene, "osmotic gap" in stool electrolytes
Weight loss with hyperphagia	Decreased absorption of fat, protein, and carbohydrate	Increased fat excretion
Bulky, foul-smelling stools	Decreased fat absorption	Increased fat excretion
Muscle wasting, edema	Decreased protein absorption	Decreased serum albumin
Flatulence, borborygmi, abdominal distention	Fermentation of carbohydrates by intestinal bacteria	Increased fat excretion; Decreased D-xylose absorption
Abdominal pain	Small intestinal stricture, infiltration of the pancreas, intestinal ischemia	Increased fat excretion
Paresthesias, tetany	Decreased vitamin D and calcium absorption	Hypocalcemia, hypomagnesemia
Bone pain	Decreased calcium absorption	Hypocalcemia, increased alkaline phosphatase
Muscle cramps, weakness	Excess potassium loss	Hypokalemia, abnormal ECG
Easy bruisability, petechiae, hematuria	Decreased vitamin K absorption	Prolonged prothrombin time, increased fat excretion
Hyperkeratosis, night blindness	Decreased vitamin A absorption	Decreased serum carotene, increased fat excretion
Pallor	Decreased vitamin B_{12}, folate, or iron absorption	Macrocytic anemia, microcytic anemia
Glossitis, stomatitis, cheilosis	Decreased vitamin B_{12}, folate, or iron absorption	Decreased serum vitamin B_{12}, RBC folate, or serum iron
Acrodermatitis	Zinc deficiency	Decreased serum zinc

[1]Tables 13–10 and 13–11 reproduced, with permission, from Wright TL, Heyworth MF: Maldigestion and malabsorption. In: *Gastrointestinal Disease*, 4th ed. Sleisenger MH, Fordtran JS (editors). Saunders, 1989.

failure to respond to antibiotics alone. Because inflammatory bowel disease is characterized by exacerbations and remissions, favorable responses to therapy are difficult to distinguish from spontaneous remissions occurring as part of the natural history of the disease.

Etiology

The cause of noninfectious inflammatory bowel disease is unknown despite recent progress in understanding its pathogenesis.

Pathology & Pathogenesis

There are two forms of chronic noninfectious gastrointestinal inflammation—one superficial and limited to the colonic mucosa (**ulcerative colitis**), and the other transmural and granulomatous in character and occurring anywhere along the gastrointestinal tract (**Crohn's disease;** also called **regional enteritis**). Both have been proposed to result from aberrant host immune responses to normal gastrointestinal tract antigens. In mice, targeted disruption of the genes for the T cell receptor and the cytokine IL-2 results in gastrointestinal tract disease resembling ulcerative colitis, while similar disruption of the gene for the cytokine IL-10 results in a panenteritis resembling Crohn's disease. The onset and severity of disease in IL-2-deficient mice are significantly influenced by the background genetic strain, thus implicating other genes as well. These and other studies support the hypothesis that a delicate balance between helper and suppressor T cell effects on B cell function is disrupted in these diseases. The two forms of inflammatory bowel disease have characteristic differences and in many cases considerable overlap in manner of presentation (Table 13–13). The feature common to all forms of inflammatory bowel disease is mucosal ulceration and inflammation of the gastrointestinal tract—indistinguishable, in fact, from that which can occur acutely during invasive infectious diarrhea. Other factors besides the presence of key gene products, including infectious agents, altered host immune responses, immune-mediated intestinal damage, psychologic factors, and di-

Table 13–12. Most likely causes of diarrhea in seven different clinical categories.[1]

1. **Acute diarrhea (<2–3 weeks' duration)**
   Viral, bacterial, parasitic, and fungal infections
   Food poisoning
   Drugs[2] and food additives
   Fecal impaction
   Pelvic inflammation
   Heavy metal poisoning (acute or chronic)
2. **Traveler's diarrhea**
   Bacterial infections
   Mediated by enterotoxins produced by *E coli*
   Mediated mainly by invasion of mucosa and inflammation, eg, invasive *E coli*, *Shigella*
   Mediated by combinations of invasion and enterotoxins, eg, *Salmonella*
   Viral and parasitic infections
3. **Diarrhea in homosexual men without AIDS**
   Amebiasis
   Giardiasis
   Shigellosis
   Campylobacter
   Rectal syphilis
   Rectal spirochetosis other than syphilis
   Rectal gonorrhea
   Chlamydia trachomatis infection (lymphogranuloma venereum and non-LGV serotypes D–K)
   Herpes simplex
4. **Diarrhea in patients with AIDS**
   Cryptosporidium
   Amebiasis
   Giardiasis
   Isospora belli
   Herpes simplex, cytomegalovirus
   Mycobacterium avium-intracellulare complex
   Salmonella typhimurium
   Cryptococcus
   Candida
   AIDS enteropathy
5. **Chronic and recurrent diarrhea**
   Irritable bowel syndrome
   Inflammatory bowel disease
   Parasitic and fungal infections
   Malabsorption syndromes
   Drugs,[2] food additives, sorbitol
   Colon cancer
   Diverticulitis
   Fecal impaction
   Heavy metal poisoning (acute or chronic)
   Raw milk-related diarrhea
6. **Chronic diarrhea of unknown origin (previous workup failed to reveal diagnosis)**
   Surreptitious laxative abuse
   Defective anal sphincter competence masquerading as diarrhea
   Microscopic colitis syndrome
   Previously unrecognized malabsorption
   Pseudopancreatic cholera syndrome
   Idiopathic fluid malabsorption
   Hypermotility-induced diarrhea
   Neuroendocrine tumor
7. **Incontinence**
   Causes of sphincter dysfunction:
   Anal surgery for fissures, fistulas, or hemorrhoids
   Episiotomy or tear during childbirth
   Anal Crohn's disease
   Diabetic neuropathy
   Causes of diarrhea: same as under 5 and 6, above.

[1]Reproduced, with permission, from Fine KD, Krejs GJ, Fordtran JS: Diarrhea. In: *Gastrointestinal Disease,* 4th ed. Sleisenger MH, Fordtran JS (editors). Saunders, 1989.
[2]Digitalis, propranolol, quinidine, diuretics, colchicine, antibiotics, lactulose, antacids, laxatives, chemotherapeutic agents, bile acids, meclomen, and many others. (See drug compendiums for adverse effects of drugs the patient has been taking.)

etary and environmental factors, may contribute to a final common pathway of disordered immune response.

Clinical Manifestations

A. Crohn's Disease: Crohn's disease typically occurs in the distal ileum or the colon, though any region of the gastrointestinal tract from mouth to anus can be involved, generally in a discontinuous fashion. It is characterized by ulceration and inflammation involving the entire thickness of the bowel wall, with recurrence of disease in previously uninvolved regions of the intestine, and can even involve adjacent mesentery and lymph nodes. The combination of deep mucosal ulceration and submucosal thickening gives the involved mucosa a characteristic "cobblestone" appearance.

Perforation, fistula formation, abscess formation, and small intestinal obstruction are frequent complications of Crohn's disease, though an indolent course occurs in most patients. The full-thickness involvement of the bowel wall may predispose to these complications. Frank bleeding from the mucosal ulcerations can be either insidious or massive, as can **protein-losing enteropathy.** Another important complication is an increased incidence of intestinal cancer.

Patients with Crohn's disease often manifest symptoms outside of the gastrointestinal tract, including migratory arthritis. Inflammatory disorders of the skin, eye, and mucous membranes—particularly aphthous ulcers of the buccal mucosa, are also seen. Renal disorders, especially nephrolithiasis, are observed in a third of patients with Crohn's disease, probably related to increased oxalate absorption associated with steatorrhea. Amyloidosis is a serious complication of Crohn's disease, as is thromboembolic disease. Both of these complications are probably reflections of the systemic character of the inflammatory process. Patients are often malnourished and show evidence of deficiency states.

Table 13–13. Similarities and differences between ulcerative colitis and Crohn's disease.[1]

	Ulcerative Colitis	Crohn's Disease
Clinical features		
Rectal bleeding	>90%	<50%
Diarrhea	10–30%	>70%
Abdominal mass	<1%	30%
Perianal abscesses, sinuses, and fistulas	2%	30%
Bowel perforation (free)	2–3%	<1%
Toxic megacolon	5–10%	<5%
Cancer of colon	Definite increase (5%)	Questionable increase
Pyoderma gangrenosum	<5%	1%
Erythema nodosum	5%	15%
Renal stones	<5% (uric acid stones)	10% (oxalate stones)
Stomatitis	10%	10%
Cancer of colon	Definite increase (5%)	Questionable increase
Aphthous ulceration	4%	4%
Uveitis	45%	5–10%
Spondylitis	<5%	15–20%
Peripheral arthritis	10%	20%
Thromboembolism with increased platelets and increased coagulant activity	Occurs	Occurs
Radiologic, endoscopic, and pathologic findings		
Rectal involvement	Almost 100%	<50%
Ulcers	Superficial, multiple Irregular	Solitary ulcers in the rectum Linear, serpiginous, and aphthoid ulcers Collar-button ulcers
Crypt abscesses, pseudopolyps, diminished goblet cells	>70%	<40%
Lymphoid aggregates and noncaseating granulomas	<10%	60–70%
Extent of disease	Mucosal and continuous	Transmural and discontinuous with "skip lesions"
Ileal involvement	Nonspecific with mild inflammation and dilation (backwash ileitis)	Ulcers, fissures, and stenosis
Fatty liver	39–40%	30–40%
Pericholangitis	30%	20%
Sclerosing cholangitis	30%	20–30%
Cirrhosis	Rare	<1%
Gallstones	Rare	10–15%
Treatment		
General	Supportive and symptomatic	Supportive and symptomatic
Definitive (drugs)	Sulfasalazine, mesalamine, or olsalazine and corticosteroids	Sulfasalazine, corticosteroids, mercaptopurine

[1]Modified and reproduced, with permission, from Gopalswamy N: Inflammatory bowel disease. In: *Clinical Medicine: Selected Problems With Pathophysiologic Correlations.* Barnes HV et al (editors). Year Book, 1988.

B. Ulcerative Colitis: In contrast to Crohn's disease, inflammation in ulcerative colitis is restricted to the mucosa of the colon and rectum. At one time it was believed that ulcerative colitis and Crohn's disease were distinct entities. This view was based on the observation of characteristic necrotic lesions of the colonic crypts of Lieberkühn, termed crypt abscesses in patients with ulcerative colitis. However, it is now recognized that in 10% of patients, regions characteristic of both Crohn's disease and ulcerative colitis are present. The diseases are similar in presentation (eg, bloody diarrhea and malabsorption) and in at least some of the complications (eg, protein-losing enteropathy and malnutrition), reflecting widespread involvement of the mucosa in both entities. However, since ulcerative colitis generally is limited to the mucosa, obstruction, perforation, and fistula formation are not typical complications. Most patients have mild disease, and—as with Crohn's disease—some patients will have only one or two episodes during their lifetimes. For unknown reasons, the risk of development of carcinoma appears even higher in ulcerative colitis than in Crohn's disease. Toxic megacolon is the one complication of ulcerative colitis that carries a high risk of perforation. Its cause is unknown.

Both ulcerative colitis and Crohn's disease can go into remission after treatment with anti-inflammatory agents such as sulfasalazine and glucocorticoids. The natural history of both diseases is of periods of remission interrupted by active disease, with medical therapy during exacerbations directed toward supportive measures and attempts at inducing remission. Because these diseases can recur after resection of involved regions of the gastrointestinal tract, operative management is generally limited to relief of life-threatening intestinal obstruction or bleeding. Because of the variable response rate and the high risk of side effects, therapy with immunosuppressive agents such as mercaptopurine and azathioprine are limited to cases that have failed to respond to sulfasalazine and glucocorticoids.

---

47. How is inflammatory bowel disease distinguished from infectious diarrhea?
48. What are the differences between ulcerative colitis and Crohn's disease?
49. What are the complications of inflammatory bowel disease?

DIVERTICULAR DISEASE

Clinical Presentation

Nearly 80% of patients with diverticular disease are asymptomatic except for chronic constipation. Of those that develop other symptoms, the most common presentation is an intermittent and unpredictable gripping lower abdominal pain. Additional features of the presentation depend on which of the two major complications of diverticular disease the patient develops.

A patient who develops diverticulitis (see below) may present with fever and with symptoms and signs of peritoneal irritation (guarding, rebound tenderness, absence of bowel sounds). A patient who develops diverticular bleeding may present with either frankly bloody stools or stools that are positive for occult blood.

Etiology

Diverticular disease (diverticulosis) results from an acquired deformity of the colon in which the mucosa and submucosa herniate through the underlying muscularis (Figure 13–15). This is a disease of modern affluent life. A rarity at the turn of the century, today it afflicts 10% of the United States population. Its incidence increases with age, starting from about 40 years. Epidemiologic studies suggest that the consumption of highly refined foods and less fiber with resulting increased prevalence of chronic constipation are responsible for the increased prevalence of diverticular disease.

Pathology & Pathogenesis

A. Diverticulosis: Most acquired diverticula occur in the colon, with the sigmoid being involved in 95% of cases. Both structural and functional factors are believed to contribute to the development of diverticulosis. Abnormalities in colonic wall connective tissue are believed to be the structural basis of diminished resistance to mucosal and submucosal herniation (Figure 13–15). Thus, individuals with genetic diseases involving connective tissue, such as Ehlers-Danlos and Marfan's syndromes, are characterized by the appearance of diverticular disease at a much earlier age. The functional abnormality is believed to be related to the development of a transmural pressure gradient from colonic lumen to peritoneal space as a result of vigorous muscle contraction of the colonic wall. This functional abnormality is probably due to the change in dietary habits, with decreased dietary fiber making forward propulsion of feces at normal transmural pressures more difficult. This increased muscle contraction, which contributes to the development of diverticular disease, is also believed to cause the abdominal pain that is the cardinal symptom of uncomplicated diverticular disease. The pain may last hours to days, with sudden relief upon passing flatus or feces. Constipation or diarrhea and flatulence are common findings during such episodes, leading to the suggestion that there is a relationship between irritable bowel syndrome and the development of diverticulosis. Treatment of the pain of diverticular disease with opioids is contraindicated because they directly raise intraluminal pressure and hence may increase the risk of perforation.

B. Diverticular Bleeding: Branches of the colonic intramural arteries are closely associated with the diverticular sac, presumably leading to occasional rupture and bleeding. This is the most common cause of massive lower gastrointestinal bleeding in the elderly. Diverticular bleeding is typically painless and not believed to be associated with a focus of inflammation.

C. Diverticulitis: This most common complication of diverticulosis develops when a focal area of inflammation occurs in the wall of a diverticulum in response to irritation by fecal material. The patient develops symptoms of abdominal pain and fever with a risk of progression to abscess with or without perforation. The perforations usually are self-contained, but the potential for subsequent fistula formation and intestinal obstruction is high.

Clinical Manifestations

About one-fifth of all individuals with diverticular disease develop one of the two major complications—diverticular bleeding or diverticulitis—which must be distinguished from carcinoma, inflammatory bowel disease, and ischemic injury due to diffuse atherosclerosis.

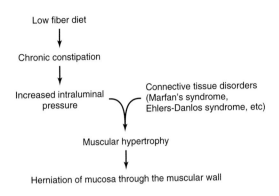
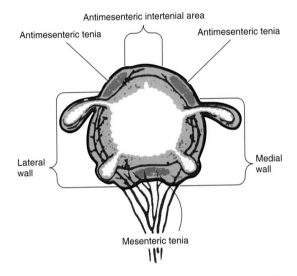

Figure 13–15. Top: Pathophysiology of diverticular disease. **Bottom:** Cross-sectional drawing of the colon, showing principal points of diverticula formation between mesenteric and antimesenteric teniae. (Reproduced, with permission, from Goligher JC: *Surgery of the Anus, Rectum and Colon,* 4th ed. Baillière Tyndall, 1980.

---

50. Where in the gastrointestinal tract do most diverticula occur?
51. What predisposing factors contribute to the development of diverticular disease?
52. What are the major complications of diverticular disease?

REFERENCES

General
Eberhart CE, Dubois RN: Eicosanoids and the gastrointestinal tract. Gastroenterology 1995;109:285.
Isselbacher K et al (editors): *Harrison's Principles of Internal Medicine,* 14th ed. McGraw-Hill, 1998.
Junqueira LC et al: *Basic Histology,* 8th ed. Appleton & Lange, 1995.
Sleisenger MH, Fordtran JS (editors): *Gastrointestinal Disease,* 5th ed. Saunders, 1993.
Toy LS, Mayer L: Basic and clinical overview of the mucosal immune system. Semin Gastrointest Dis 1996;7:2.
Yee LF, Mulvihill SJ: Neuroendocrine disorders of the gut. West J Med 1995;163:454.

Achalasia & Esophageal Reflux
Long JD, Orlando RC: Eicosanoids and the esophagus. Dig Dis 1997;15:145-154.
Mittal RK et al: Transient lower esophageal sphincter relaxation. Gastroenterology 1995;109:601.
Pasricha PJ et al: Intrasphincteric botulinum toxin for the treatment of achalasia. N Engl J Med 1995;332:774.
Spiess AE, Kahrilas PJ: Treating achalasia: From whalebone to laparoscope. JAMA, 1998;280:638.
Koshy SS, Nostrant TT: Pathophysiology and endoscopic/balloon treatment of esophageal motility disorders. Surg Clin North Am 1997;77:971.
van den Boogert J et al: Barrett's oesophagus: Patho-

physiology, diagnosis, and management. Scand J Gastroenterol 1998;33;:449.

Acid-Peptic Disease

Fisher RS, Parkman HP: Management of nonulcer dyspepsia. N Engl J Med 1998;339:1376.

Marchetti M et al: Development of a mouse model of *H pylori* infection that mimics human disease. Science 1995;267:1655.

McColl KE et al: The role of *Helicobacter pylori* in the pathophysiology of duodenal ulcer disease and gastric cancer. Semin Gastrointest Dis 1997;8:142.

Playford RJ: Trefoil peptides: What are they and what do they do? J R Coll Phys (Lond) 1997;31:37.

Shimoyama T, Crabtree JE: Bacterial factors and immune pathogenesis in *Helicobacter pylori* infection. Gut 1998;43(Suppl 1):S2.

Wallace JL, Granger DN: The cellular and molecular basis of gastric mucosal defense. FASEB J 1996;10:731.

Gastroparesis

Cullen JJ, Kelly KA: Gastric motor physiology and pathophysiology. Surg Clin North Am 1993;73:1145.

Enck P, Frieling T: Pathophysiology of diabetic gastroparesis. Diabetes 1997;46:S77.

Malagelada JR: Diabetic gastroparesis. Semin Gastrointest Dis 1995;6:181.

Morgan LM: The role of gastrointestinal hormones in carbohydrate and lipid metabolism and homeostasis: Effects of gastric inhibitory polypeptide and glucagon-like peptide-1. Biochem Soc Trans 1998;26:216.

Gallstone Disease

Moscati RM: Cholelithiasis, cholecystitis, and pancreatitis. Emerg Med Clin North Am 1996;14:719.

Diarrhea

Argenzio RA: Neuro-immune pathobiology of infectious enteric disease. Adv Exper Med Biol 1997;412:21.

Bueno L et al: Mediators and pharmacology of visceral sensitivity: from basic to clinical investigations. Gastroenterology 1997;112:1714.

Camilleri M, Ford MJ: Colonic sensorimotor physiology in health and its alteration in constipation and diarrheal disorders. Aliment Pharmacol Ther 1998;12:287.

Jodal M, Lundgren O: Nerves and cholera secretion. Gastroenterol 1995;108:287.

Lamberts SWJ et al: Octreotide. N Engl J Med 1996;334:246.

Maxwell PR, Mendall MA, Kumar D: Irritable bowel syndrome. Lancet 1997;350:1691.

Stenton GR, Vliagoftis H, Befus AD: Role of intestinal mast cells in modulating gastrointestinal pathophysiology. Ann Allergy Asthma Immunol 1998;81:1.

Wong MH, Stappenbeck TS, Gordon JI: Living and commuting in intestinal crypts. Gastroenterology 1999;116:208.

Inflammatory Bowel Disease

Binion DG et al: Acquired increase in leucocyte binding by intestinal microvascular endothelium in inflammatory bowel disease. Lancet 1998;352:1742.

Gusella JF: Inflammatory bowel disease: Is it in the genes? Gastroenterology 1998;115:1286.

Orchard T, Jewell DP: Review article: Pathophysiology of the intestinal mucosa in inflammatory bowel disease and arthritis: similarities and dissimilarities in clinical findings. Aliment Pharmacol Ther 1997;11 (Suppl 3):10.

Sartor RB: Current concepts of the etiology and pathogenesis of ulcerative colitis and Crohn's disease. Gastroenterol Clin North Am 1995;24:475.

Sleisenger MH, Law DH, Almy TP: The medical management of acute fulminant ulcerative colitis. Semin Gastrointest Dis 1998;9:31.

Diverticular Disease

Reynolds JC: Challenges in the treatment of colonic motility disorders. Am J Health Syst Pharm 1996;53:S17.

Uher EM, Swash M: Sacral reflexes: Physiology and clinical application. Dis Colon Rectum 1998;41:1165.

Liver Disease   14

Vishwanath R. Lingappa, MD, PhD

Although many different pathogenic agents and processes can affect the liver (Table 14–1), they are generally manifested in individual patients in a limited number of ways that can be assessed by evaluation of some key parameters. Liver disease can be acute or chronic; focal or diffuse; mild or severe; and reversible or irreversible. Most cases of **acute liver disease** (eg, due to viral hepatitis) are so mild that they never come to medical attention. Transient symptoms of fatigue, loss of appetite, and nausea are often ascribed to other causes (eg, "flu"), and minor biochemical abnormalities referable to the liver that would be identified in blood studies are not discovered. The patient recovers without any lasting medical consequences. In other cases of acute liver injury, symptoms and signs are severe enough to call for medical attention. The entire range of liver functions may be affected or only a few, as is the case with liver injury due to certain drugs that cause isolated impairment of the liver's role in bile formation **(cholestasis).** Occasionally, viral and other causes of acute liver injury occur in an overwhelming manner resulting in massive liver cell death. This syndrome of **fulminant hepatic failure** carries a high mortality rate, but if the patient survives, liver function returns to normal and there is no residual evidence of liver disease.

Liver injury may continue beyond the initial acute episode or may be recurrent **(chronic hepatitis).** In some cases of chronic hepatitis, liver function remains stable or the disease process ultimately resolves altogether. In other cases, there is progressive and irreversible deterioration of liver function.

Cirrhosis is ultimately the consequence of progressive liver injury. Cirrhosis can occur in a subset of cases of chronic hepatitis that do not resolve spontaneously or after repeated episodes of acute liver injury, as in the case of chronic alcoholism. In cirrhosis, the liver becomes hard, shrunken, and nodular and displays impaired function and diminished reserve due to a decreased amount of functioning liver tissue. More importantly, the physics of blood flow is altered such that the pressure in the hepatic portal vein is elevated. As a result, the blood is *diverted around* the liver rather than *being filtered through* the liver. This phenomenon, termed **portal-to-systemic shunting,** has profound effects on the function of various organ systems and sets the stage for certain devastating complications of liver disease that are described below.

While liver disease due to many different causes may present in common ways, the reverse is also true—ie, liver disease due to specific causes may have distinctly different presentations in different patients. For example, consider two patients with acute viral hepatitis: One may present with yellow eyes and skin—a manifestation of impaired liver function—complaining of nothing more than itching, fatigue, and loss of appetite, while the other may be brought to the emergency room moribund, with massive gastrointestinal bleeding and encephalopathy. Such variations in the severity of liver disease are probably due to genetic, immunologic, and environmental (including perhaps nutritional) factors that are at present poorly understood.

The consequences of liver disease can be either reversible or irreversible. Those arising directly from acute damage to the functional cells of the liver, most notably **hepatocytes,** without destruction of the liver's capacity for regeneration, are generally reversible. Like many organs of the body, the liver normally has both a huge reserve capacity for the various biochemical reactions it carries out and the ability to regenerate fully differentiated cells and thereby recover completely from injury. Thus, only in the most fulminant cases or in end-stage disease are there insufficient residual hepatocytes to maintain minimal essential liver functions. More commonly, patients display transient signs of liver cell necrosis and disordered function followed by full recovery. The symptoms and signs of this sort of acute liver injury can best be understood as an impairment of normal biochemical functions of the liver.

Other consequences of liver disease are irreversible, typically seen in the patient with cirrhosis. These are best understood as a result of portal-to-systemic shunting of blood flow. They include a heightened sensitivity to noxious substances absorbed from the gastrointestinal tract (encephalopathy), an increased risk of massive gastrointestinal bleeding (de-

Table 14–1. Categories of liver disease by presentation.[1]

Cholestasis
  Reactions to certain classes of drugs (including anabolic steroids, oral contraceptives, phenothiazines, erythromycins, oral hypoglycemic and antithyroid drugs)
  Direct causes (intrahepatic biliary atresia, cholangiocarcinoma, viral hepatitis, alcoholic hepatitis, primary biliary cirrhosis, pericholangitis)
  Secondary causes (postoperative, endotoxins, total parenteral nutrition, sickle cell crisis, hypophysectomy, some porphyrias)

Acute hepatitis
  Viral and bacterial, including hepatitis viruses A, B, C, D, and E, herpes simplex virus, cytomegalovirus, Epstein-Barr virus, yellow fever virus, *Brucella, Leptospira*
  Reactions to certain classes of drugs (anesthetics such as halothane, anticonvulsants such as phenytoin, antihypertensives such as methyldopa, chemotherapeutic agents such as isoniazid, and thiazide diuretics such as hydrochlorothiazide)
  Poisons (such as ethanol); reactions to drugs

Fulminant hepatic failure
  Infections (with hepatitis viruses A, B, and D, yellow fever virus, cytomegalovirus; herpes simplex virus, and *Coxiella burnetii*)
  Poisons and toxins, chemicals, and drugs (*Amanita phalloides* toxin, phosphorus, ethanol; solvents, including carbon tetrachloride and dimethylformamide; anesthetics, including halothane; analgesics, including acetaminophen; antimicrobials, including tetracycline and isoniazid; and other drugs, including methyldopa, monoamine oxidase inhibitors, and valproate)
  Ischemia and hypoxia (vascular occlusion, circulatory failure, heat stroke, gram-negative sepsis with shock, congestive heart failure, pericardial tamponade)
  Miscellaneous metabolic anomalies (acute fatty liver of pregnancy, Reye's syndrome, Wilson's disease, galactosemia)

Chronic hepatitis
  Viral hepatitis (types B, C, and D)
  Primary autoimmune disorders (idiopathic autoimmune chronic active hepatitis, primary biliary cirrhosis, and sclerosing cholangitis)
  Therapeutic drug-induced (methyldopa, nitrofurantoin, oxyphenisatin-containing laxatives)
  Genetic diseases (Wilson's disease, α_1-antiprotease deficiency)
  Infiltrative disorders (sarcoidosis, amyloidosis, hemochromatosis)

Cirrhosis
  Infectious (viral hepatitis types B, C, and D and toxoplasmosis)
  Genetic diseases (Wilson's disease, hemochromatosis, α_1-antiprotease deficiency, glycogen storage diseases, Fanconi's syndrome, cystic fibrosis)
  Drugs and poisons (eg, methotrexate, alcohol)
  Miscellaneous (sarcoidosis, graft-versus-host disease, inflammatory bowel disease, cystic fibrosis, jejunoileal bypass, diabetes mellitus)

Focal or extrinsic diseases with variable manifestations in the liver
  Vascular (hepatic vein thrombosis, occlusion by parasites such as *Echinococcus* or *Schistosoma*)
  Biliary (duct obstruction due to stones or tumor or bacterial infection)
  Infectious (systemic sepsis; bacterial, fungal, or parasitic abscesses)
  Granulomatous diseases (sarcoidosis, tuberculosis)
  Infiltrative diseases (hemochromatosis, amyloidosis, Gaucher's disease and other lysosomal storage diseases, lymphoma)

[1]Modified from Isslebacher KJ, Podolsky DK: Biological and clinical approach to liver disease. In: *Harrison's Principles of Internal Medicine,* 12th ed. Wilson JD et al (editors). McGraw-Hill, 1991.

velopment of varices and coagulopathy), and malabsorption of fat in the stool (due to decreased bile flow). In contrast to the consequences of acute hepatitis, those of cirrhosis are generally irreversible. Nevertheless, some of these consequences are treatable. Commonly, patients with cirrhosis present with superimposed acute liver injury (eg, due to an alcoholic binge or other drug exposure). Since they have a decreased hepatocyte mass and much less functional reserve, they are more sensitive to acute liver injury than is the patient with a normal liver.

1. What parameters must you consider in assessing a patient with liver disease?
2. What factors may determine the difference in severity of liver disease between two patients with acute hepatitis due to the same cause?
3. In what ways is the patient with underlying cirrhosis who presents with acute hepatitis likely to be different from the patient with a previously normal liver and acute hepatitis?

STRUCTURE & FUNCTION OF THE LIVER

ANATOMY, HISTOLOGY, & CELL BIOLOGY

The liver is located in the right upper quadrant of the abdomen in the peritoneal space just below the right side of the diaphragm and under the rib cage (Figure 14–1). It weighs approximately 1400 g in the adult and is covered by a fibrous capsule. It receives nearly 25% of the cardiac output, approximately 1500 mL of blood flow per minute, via two sources: venous flow from the **hepatic portal vein,** which is crucial to performance of the liver's roles in bodily functions; and arterial flow from the **hepatic artery,** which is important for liver oxygenation and which supplies the biliary system. These vessels converge within the liver, and the combined blood flow exits via the so-called **central veins** (also called terminal

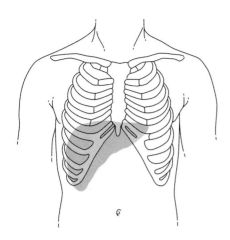

Figure 14–1. Location of the liver. (Reproduced, with permission, from Wolf DC: Evaluation of the size, shape and consistency of the liver. In: *Clinical Methods,* 3rd ed. Walker HK, Hall WD, Hurst JW [editors]. Butterworth, 1990.)

veins) that drain into the hepatic vein and ultimately the inferior vena cava.

The portal vein carries venous blood from the small intestine, rich in freshly absorbed nutrients—as well as drugs and poisons—directly to the liver. Also flowing into the portal vein prior to its entry into the liver is the pancreatic venous drainage, rich in pancreatic hormones (insulin, glucagon, somatostatin, and pancreatic polypeptide). The portal vein forms a specialized capillary bed that allows individual hepatocytes to be bathed directly in portal blood. In part because of this system of blood supply, the liver is a prime site for metastatic spread of cancer, especially from the gastrointestinal tract, breast, and lung.

Concepts of Liver Organization

The substance (**parenchyma**) of the liver is organized into plates of hepatocytes lying in a cage of supporting cells termed **reticuloendothelial cells** (Figure 14–2A). The plates of hepatocytes are generally only one cell thick, and individual plates are separated from each other by vascular spaces called **sinusoids**. It is in these sinusoids that blood from the hepatic artery is mixed with blood from the portal vein on the way to the central vein. The reticuloendothelial cell meshwork in which the hepatocytes reside includes diverse cell types, most importantly the **endothelial cells** that make up the walls of the sinusoids; specialized macrophages termed **Kupffer cells** are anchored in the sinusoidal space; and stellate cells or **lipocytes,** fat-storing cells involved in vitamin A metabolism, which lie between the hepatocytes and the endothelial cells. Approximately 30% of all cells in the liver are reticuloendothelial cells, and about one-third of these are Kupffer cells. Yet, because reticuloendothelial cells are smaller than hepatocytes, the reticuloendothelial system accounts for only 2–10% of the total protein in the liver. The reticuloendothelial cells are much more than just a cage for hepatocytes. They perform specific functions, including phagocytosis and secretion of cytokines, and communicate with each other as well as with hepatocytes. Their dysfunction contributes to both hepatocyte necrosis in acute liver disease and to hepatic fibrosis in chronic liver disease.

A. Lobules: Under the microscope at low-power magnification, liver architecture has been traditionally described in terms of the **lobule** (Figure 14–2B). Neat arrays of hepatocyte plates are organized around individual central veins to form hexagons with **portal triads** or **spaces** (sheath-like structures containing a portal venule, hepatic arteriole, and bile canaliculus) at their corners. The hepatocytes adjacent to the portal triad are termed the **limiting plate.** Disruption of the limiting plate is a significant diagnostic marker of some forms of immune-mediated liver disease. This may be seen in liver biopsies from patients with liver disease of unknown cause.

B. Functional Zonation: Physiologically, it is more useful to think of liver architecture in terms of the portal-to-central direction of blood flow: Blood entering the sinusoids from a terminal portal venule or hepatic arteriole flows past hepatocytes closest to those vessels first (termed zone 1 hepatocytes) and then percolates past zone 2 hepatocytes (so called because they are not the first hepatocytes reached by blood entering the hepatic parenchyma). The last hepatocytes reached by the blood before it enters the central vein are termed zone 3 hepatocytes. Thus, the microscopic organization of the liver can be viewed in terms of functional zones. A liver **acinus** is defined as the unit of liver tissue centered around the portal venule and hepatic arteriole whose hepatocytes can be imagined to form concentric rings of cells in the order in which they come into contact with portal blood, first to last (Figure 14–2C). Hepatocytes at either extreme of the acinus (zones 1 and 3) appear to differ in both enzymatic activity and physiologic functions. Zone 1 hepatocytes, exposed to the highest oxygen concentrations, are particularly active in gluconeogenesis and oxidative energy metabolism. They are also the major site of urea synthesis (since freely diffusible substances such as ammonia absorbed from protein breakdown in the gut will be largely extracted in zone 1). Conversely, zone 3 hepatocytes are more active in glycolysis and lipogenesis (processes requiring less oxygen). Zone 2 hepatocytes display attributes of both zone 1 and zone 3 cells.

C. Receptor-Mediated Uptake: Functional zonation applies only to processes driven by the presence of diffusible substances. The liver, however, is also involved in many pathways participating in receptor-mediated uptake and active transport of substances that are unable to diffuse freely into cells.

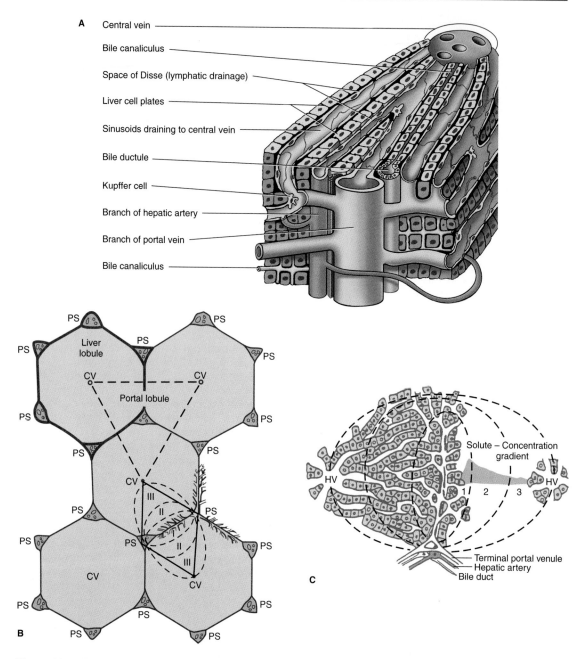

Figure 14–2. A: Detailed structure of the liver lobule. (Reproduced, with permission, from Chandrasoma P, Taylor CE: *Concise Pathology,* 3rd ed. Appleton & Lange, 1998.) **B:** Relationship of lobule to acinus. (Reproduced, with permission, from Junqueira LC, Carneiro J, Kelley RO: *Basic Histology,* 9th ed. Appleton & Lange, 1998.) **C:** Hepatic acinus. (CV, central vein; PS, portal space [or triad]; HV, hepatic venule; TPV, terminal portal venule.) (Reproduced, with permission, from Gumucio JJ: Hepatic transport. In: *Textbook of Medicine.* Kelley WN [editor]. Lippincott, 1989.)

These substances will enter whichever hepatocytes have the appropriate transporters, regardless of their zone. Similarly, substances that are tightly bound to carrier proteins for which the liver does *not* have receptors will be cleared equally poorly by hepatocytes in all three zones.

Hepatocytes: Polarized Cells With Segregation of Functions

All surfaces of a hepatocyte are not the same. One side, the **apical surface,** forms the wall of the bile canaliculus, while the **basolateral surface** is in contact with the bloodstream via the sinusoids. Very different activities go forward at these regions of the hepatocyte plasma membrane, with **tight junctions** between hepatocytes serving to maintain segregation of apical and basolateral plasma membrane domains. Processes related to bile transport and excretion act at the apical plasma membrane (Figure 14–3A). Uptake from and secretion into the bloodstream are activities that occur across the basolateral membrane (Figure 14–3B).

Effects of Hepatocyte Dysfunction

In view of this organization, it is perhaps not surprising that hepatocyte dysfunction can sometimes involve disruption of bile flow (cholestasis) with relative preservation of other functions. There is, however, no clear line between the consequences of disturbed apical and basolateral functions: Cholestasis, while initially a disorder of apical bile flow, is ultimately manifested at the basolateral surface. This is because it is at the basolateral surface that bilirubin and other substances to be excreted across the apical plasma membrane into the bile must first be taken up from the bloodstream. Similarly, disruption of energy metabolism or protein synthesis, while initially impinging on the secretory and metabolic processes of the hepatocyte, will ultimately affect the bile transport machinery in the apical plasma membrane as well.

Capacity for Regeneration

While the normal liver contains very few cells in mitosis, when hepatocytes are lost, poorly understood mechanisms stimulate proliferation of the remaining hepatocytes. This is why in most cases of fulminant hepatic failure with massive hepatocellular death, if the patient survives the acute period of hepatic dysfunction (usually with medical therapy in the hospital), recovery will be complete. Similarly, surgical resection of liver tissue is followed by proliferation of the remaining hepatocytes (**hyperplasia**). Numerous growth factors and cytokines are involved in positioning the liver on a continuum between cell proliferation and cell death.

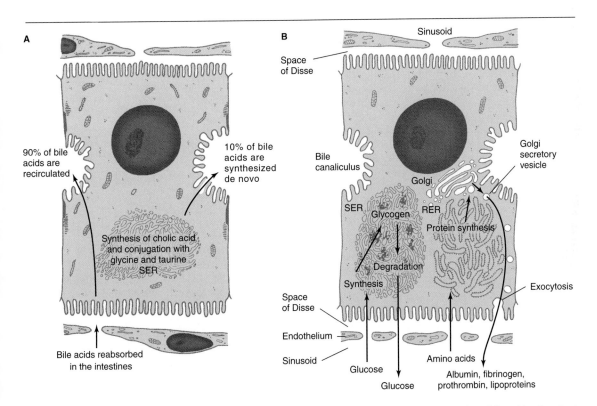

Figure 14–3. A: Mechanism of secretion of bile acids. About 90% of these compounds derive from bile acids absorbed in the intestinal epithelium and recirculated to the liver. The remainder are synthesized in the liver by conjugating cholic acid with the amino acids glycine and taurine. This process occurs in the smooth endoplasmic reticulum (SER). **B:** Protein synthesis and carbohydrate storage in the liver. Protein synthesis occurs in the rough endoplasmic reticulum, which explains why liver cell lesions or starvation lead to a decrease in the amounts of albumin, fibrinogen, and prothrombin in a patient's blood. In several diseases, glycogen degradation is depressed, with abnormal intracellular accumulation of this compound. (SER, smooth endoplastic reticulum; RER, rough endoplastic reticulum.) (Reproduced, with permission, from Junqueira LC, Carneiro J, Kelley RO: *Basic Histology,* 9th ed. Appleton & Lange, 1998.)

4. From which vascular beds do the hepatic central veins derive their blood flow?
5. Why is the liver a major site for metastasis of malignant neoplasms from other parts of the body?
6. What cell types make up the liver, and what are their distinguishing characteristics?
7. What is the difference between the lobule concept and the acinus concept of liver subarchitecture?
8. What are some physiologic consequences of functional zonation in the liver?
9. What activities are found in zone 1 hepatocytes? In zone 3 hepatocytes?
10. What structures normally maintain the separation of apical and basolateral plasma membrane domains of the hepatocyte?
11. What happens to the remaining hepatocytes when part of the liver is surgically resected?

Table 14–2. Functions of the normal liver.

Energy metabolism and substrate interconversion
  Glucose production through gluconeogenesis and glycogenolysis
  Glucose consumption by pathways of glycogen synthesis, fatty acid synthesis, glycolysis, and the tricarboxylic acid cycle
  Cholesterol synthesis from acetate, triglyceride synthesis from fatty acids, and secretion of both in VLDL particles
  Cholesterol and triglyceride uptake by endocytosis of HDL and LDL particles with excretion of cholesterol in bile, beta-oxidation of fatty acids, and conversion of excess acetyl-CoA to ketones
  Deamination of amino acids and conversion of ammonia to urea via the urea cycle
  Transamination and de novo synthesis of nonessential amino acids

Protein synthetic functions
  Synthesis of various plasma proteins, including albumin, clotting factors, binding proteins, apoliproproteins, angiotensinogen, and insulin-like growth factor I

Solubilization, transport, and storage functions
  Drug and poison detoxification through phase I and phase II biotransformation reactions and excretion in bile
  Solubilization of fats and fat-soluble vitamins in bile for uptake by enterocytes
  Synthesis and secretion of VLDL and pre-HDL lipoprotein particles and clearance of HDL, LDL, and chylomicron remnants
  Synthesis and secretion of various binding proteins, including transferrin, steroid hormone-binding globulin, thyroid hormone-binding globulin, ceruloplasmin, and metallothionein
  Uptake and storage of vitamins A, D, B_{12}, and folate

Protective and clearance functions
  Detoxification of ammonia through the urea cycle
  Detoxification of drugs through microsomal oxidases and conjugation systems
  Synthesis and export of glutathione
  Clearance of damaged cells and proteins, hormones, drugs, and activated clotting factors from the portal circulation
  Clearance of bacteria and antigens from the portal circulation

LIVER BLOOD FLOW & ITS CELLULAR BASIS

The portal blood flow, being venous in nature, is normally under low hydrostatic pressure (about 10 mm Hg). Accordingly, there must be little resistance to its flow within the liver, allowing the blood to percolate through the sinusoids and achieve maximal contact—for exchange of substances—with hepatocytes. Two unique features—fenestrations in the endothelial cells and lack of a typical basement membrane between endothelial cells and hepatocytes—aid in making the liver a low-pressure circuit for the flow of portal blood. These features are altered in cirrhosis, resulting in increased portal pressure and profound changes in liver blood flow, with devastating clinical consequences.

Fenestrations are spaces between the endothelial cells that make up the walls of the portal capillary system which allow plasma and its proteins—but not red blood cells—free and direct access to the surface of the hepatocytes. This feature is crucial to the liver's function of uptake from and secretion into the bloodstream. This feature also contributes to the efficiency of the liver as a filter of portal blood. Most of the capillary beds in the body lack such fenestrations.

PHYSIOLOGY

The diverse functions of the liver are listed as four broad categories in Table 14–2. While there is considerable overlap between them, systematic consideration of each category is a useful way of approaching the patient with liver disease.

Energy Generation & Substrate Interconversion

Much of the body's carbohydrate, lipid, and protein is synthesized, metabolized, and interconverted in the liver, with products removed from or released into the bloodstream in response to the energy and substrate needs of the body.

A. Carbohydrate Metabolism: After a meal, the liver achieves net glucose consumption (eg, for glycogen synthesis and generation of metabolic intermediates via glycolysis and the tricarboxylic acid cycle). This occurs as a result of a confluence of several effects. First, the levels of substrates such as glucose increase. Second, the levels of hormones that affect the amount and activity of metabolic enzymes change. Thus, when blood glucose increases, the ratio of insulin to glucagon in the bloodstream increases. The net effect is increased glucose utilization by the liver. In times of fasting (low blood glucose) or stress (when higher blood glucose is needed), hormone and substrate levels in the bloodstream drive metabolic pathways of the liver responsible for net glucose production (eg, the pathways of glycogenolysis and gluconeogenesis). As a result, blood glucose levels are raised to—or maintained in—the normal range in spite of wide and sudden changes in the rate of glucose input (eg, ingestion and absorption) and output (eg, utilization by tissues) from the bloodstream (Figure 14–4).

B. Protein Metabolism: Related to its important role in protein metabolism, the liver is a major site for processes of oxidative deamination and transamination (Figure 14–5). These reactions allow amino groups to be shuffled among molecules in order to generate substrates for both carbohydrate metabolism and amino acid synthesis. Likewise, the urea cycle allows nitrogen to be excreted in the form of urea, which is much less toxic than free amino groups in the form of ammonium ions. More will be said later about impairment of this function in liver disease.

C. Lipid Metabolism: Finally, the liver is the center of lipid metabolism. It manufactures nearly 80% of the cholesterol synthesized in the body from acetyl-CoA via a pathway that connects metabolism of carbohydrates with that of lipids (Figure 14–4). Moreover, the liver can synthesize, store, and export triglycerides (Figure 14–4). The liver is also the site of keto acid production via the pathway of fatty acid oxidation that connects lipid catabolism with activity of the tricarboxylic acid cycle.

In the process of controlling the body's level of cholesterol and triglycerides, the liver assembles, secretes, and takes up various lipoprotein particles (Figure 14–6). Some of these particles (**very low density lipoproteins [VLDL]**) serve to distribute lipid to adipose tissue for storage as fat or to other tissues for immediate use. In the course of these functions, the structure of VLDL particles is modified by loss of lipid and protein components. The resulting **low-density lipoprotein (LDL)** particles are then returned to the liver by virtue of their affinity for a specific receptor, the **LDL receptor,** found on the surface of various cells of the body, including he-

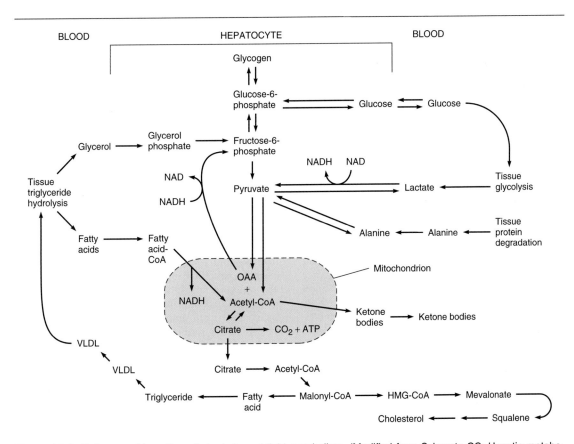

Figure 14–4. Pathways of hepatic carbohydrate and lipid metabolism. (Modified from Schwartz CC: Hepatic metabolism. In: *Textbook of Medicine.* Kelley WN [editor]. Lippincott, 1989.)

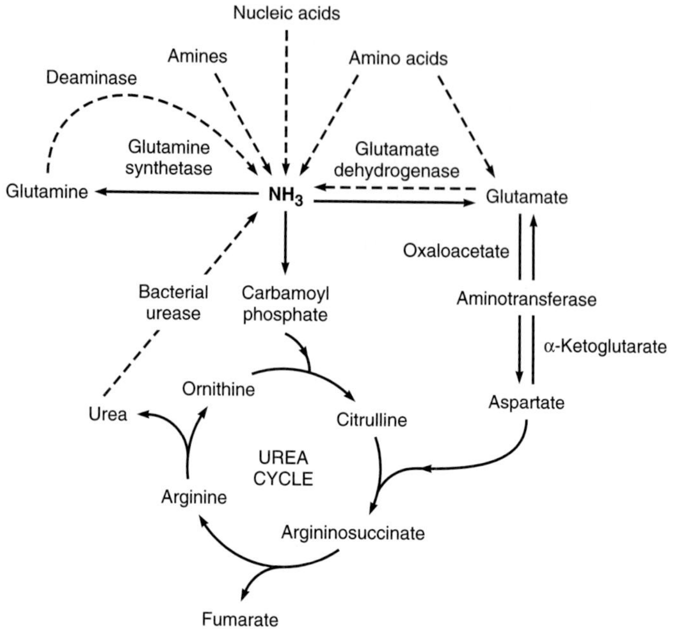

Figure 14–5. Urea cycle. Dashed lines signify pathways whose extent of involvement varies from patient to patient depending upon genetic, dietary, and other factors. (Reproduced, with permission, from Powers-Lee SG, Meister A: Urea synthesis and ammonia metabolism. In: *The Liver: Biology and Pathology,* 2nd ed. Arias IM et al [editors]. Raven Press, 1988.)

patocytes. Other lipoprotein particles (**high-density lipoproteins [HDL]**) are synthesized and secreted from the liver. They scavenge excess cholesterol and triglycerides from other tissues and from the bloodstream, returning them to the liver where they are excreted. Thus, secretion of HDL and removal of LDL are both mechanisms by which cholesterol in excess of that needed by various tissues is removed from the circulation (Figures 14–6B and 14–6C).

Synthesis & Secretion of Plasma Proteins

The liver manufactures and secretes many of the proteins found in plasma, including albumin, several of the clotting factors, a number of binding proteins, and even certain hormones and hormone precursors. By virtue of the actions of these proteins, the liver has important roles in maintaining plasma oncotic pressure (serum albumin), coagulation (clotting factor synthesis and modification), blood pressure (angiotensinogen), growth (insulin-like growth factor-1), and metabolism (steroid- and thyroid hormone-binding proteins). Table 14–3 lists some of the proteins synthesized by the liver and their physiologic functions.

Solubilizing, Transport, & Storage Functions

The liver plays an important role in solubilizing, transporting, and storing a variety of very different substances that would otherwise be difficult for the tissues to obtain or to move in and out of cells. Specific cells in the liver perform these functions by manufacturing specialized proteins that serve as receptors, binding proteins, or enzymes.

A. Enterohepatic Circulation of Bile Acids: Bile is a detergent-like substance synthesized by the liver that permits a variety of otherwise insoluble substances to be dissolved in an aqueous environment for transport into or out of the body. Bile acids are a major component of bile. Bile salts are recycled via the so-called **enterohepatic circulation** between the liver and the intestines. After synthesis and transport from hepatocyte cytoplasm into the bile canaliculus (across the apical plasma membrane of the hepatocyte), bile is collected in the biliary tract (and sometimes stored in the gallbladder) and excreted via the common bile duct into the duodenum. While still in the cytoplasm of the hepatocyte, many bile acids are conjugated to sugars, which increases their solubility. Once in the duodenum, bile acids serve to solubilize lipids, facilitating digestion and absorption of fats. In the terminal ileum, both conjugated and deconjugated bile salts are taken up and transported from enterocytes to portal blood flow. Portal blood returns them to the liver, where specialized bile acid transporters return them to the hepatocyte cytosol. There they are subject to reconjugation and secretion across the apical membrane along with other components (pigment, cholesterol, etc) to form new bile. Thereafter, they engage in another cycle of enterohepatic transport.

B. Drug Metabolism and Excretion: Most of the enzymes that catalyzes metabolic processes necessary for the detoxification and excretion of drugs and other substances are located in the endoplasmic

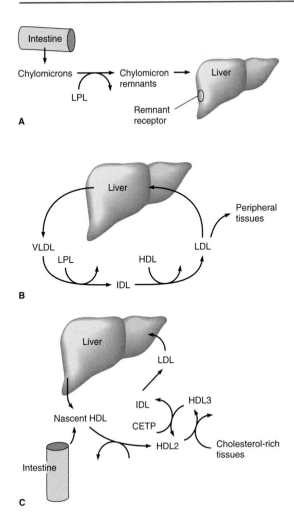

Figure 14–6. Lipoprotein metabolism in the liver. **A:** Exogenous fat transport pathway. **B:** Endogenous fat transport pathway. **C:** Pathway of reverse cholesterol transport. In each of these three pathways, lipoprotein particles are used to solubilize cholesteryl esters (and triglyceride), either for the purpose of import from the gastrointestinal tract **(A)**, distribution to various tissues **(B)**, or transport to the liver for excretion in bile **(C)**. During their circulation, specific lipoprotein particles are transformed by addition and removal of apoproteins and by the action of enzymes in plasma or in tissues (eg, LPL, lipoprotein lipase, CETP, cholesteryl ester transfer protein). Intermediate-density lipoproteins (IDL) are intermediates in the conversion of VLDL to LDL. (HDL, high-density lipoproteins; LDL, low-density lipoproteins.) (Modified from Breslow JL: Genetic basis of lipoprotein disorders. J Clin Invest 1989;84:373.)

reticulum of hepatocytes. These pathways are used not only for metabolism of exogenous drugs but also for many endogenous substances that would otherwise be difficult for cells to excrete (eg, bilirubin and cholesterol). In most cases, this metabolism involves the conversion of **lipophilic** (hydrophobic) substances (which are difficult to excrete from cells because they tend to partition into cellular membranes) into more **hydrophilic** substances. This process involves catalysis of covalent modifications to make the substance more charged, so that it will partition more readily into an aqueous medium or at least be solubilized sufficiently in bile. As a result of these processes, collectively termed biotransformations, some substances that would otherwise be retained in cellular membranes can be excreted directly in the urine or transported into the bile for excretion in feces.

C. Phases of Biotransformation: Biotransformation generally occurs in two phases. **Phase I reactions** involve oxidation-reductions in which an oxygen-containing functional group is added to the substance to be excreted. While oxidation itself does not necessarily have a major effect on water solubility, it usually introduces into the drug a reactive "handle" that makes possible other reactions which do render the modified substance water-soluble. These **phase II reactions** usually involve covalent attachment of the drug to a water-soluble carrier molecule such as the sugar glucuronic acid or the peptide glutathione. Unfortunately, by making substances more chemically reactive, phase I oxidation reactions often convert mildly toxic drugs into more toxic reactive intermediates. If conjugation by phase II enzymes is impaired for some other reason, the reactive intermediate can sometimes react with and damage other cellular structures. This feature of drug detoxification has important clinical implications.

D. Role of Apolipoprotein in Solubilization and Transport of Lipids: The detoxification and bile transport pathways allow hepatocytes to convert a wide range of hydrophobic low-molecular-weight substances (eg, drugs and bilirubin) into a more hydrophilic and hence water-soluble form in which they can be excreted (eg, in bile or by the kidney). However, these are not the only solubilization challenges facing the body. The body also needs a mechanism that makes lipids available to various tissues (eg, to synthesize membranes) and one that removes any excess lipid the tissues do not use. For these processes to occur, lipid must be solubilized in a dispersed form that can be carried through the bloodstream. Hepatocytes synthesize for this purpose a class of specialized **apolipoproteins.** Apolipoproteins assemble into a variety of lipoprotein particles that transport lipids to and from various tissues by receptor-mediated endocytosis (see Lipid Metabolism, above).

E. Role in Production of Binding Proteins: Various cells in the liver synthesize proteins that bind certain substances very tightly (eg, some vitamins, minerals, and hormones). In some cases, this allows their transport in the bloodstream, where they would otherwise not be soluble (eg, steroids bound to steroid-binding globulin, which is synthesized and

Table 14–3. Proteins synthesized by the liver: Physiologic functions and properties.[1]

Name	Principal Function	Binding Characteristics	Serum or Plasma Concentration
Albumin	Binding and carrier protein; osmotic regulator	Hormones, amino acids, steroids, vitamins, fatty acids	4500–5000 mg/dL
Orosomucoid	Uncertain; may have a role in inflammation		Trace; rises in inflammation
α_1-Antiprotease	Trypsin and general protease inhibitor	Proteases in serum and tissue secretions	1.3–1.4 mg/dL
α-Fetoprotein	Osmotic regulation; binding and carrier protein[2]	Hormones, amino acids	Found normally in fetal blood
α_2-Macroglobulin	Inhibitor of serum endoproteases	Proteases	150–420 mg/dL
Antithrombin-III	Protease inhibitor of intrinsic coagulation system	1 : 1 binding to proteases	17–30 mg/dL
Ceruloplasmin	Transport of copper	Six atoms copper/mol	15–60 mg/dL
C-reactive protein	Uncertain; has role in tissue inflammation	Complement C1q	<1 mg/dL; rises in inflammation
Fibrinogen	Precursor to fibrin in hemostasis		200–450 mg/dL
Haptoglobin	Binding, transport of cell-free hemoglobin	Hemoglobin 1 : 1 binding	40–180 mg/dL
Hemopexin	Binds to porphyrins, particularly heme for heme recycling	1 : 1 with heme	50–100 mg/dL
Transferrin	Transport of iron	Two atoms iron/mol	3.0–6.5 mg/dL
Apolipoprotein B	Assembly of lipoprotein particles	Lipid carrier	
Angiotensinogen	Precursor to pressor peptide angiotensin II		
Proteins, coagulation factors II, VII, IX, X	Blood clotting		20 mg/dL
Antithrombin III, protein C	Inhibition of blood clotting		
Insulin-like growth factor I	Mediator of anabolic effects of growth hormone	IGF-I receptor	
Steroid hormone-binding globulin	Carrier protein for steroids in bloodstream	Steroid hormones	3.3 mg/dL
Thyroxine-binding globulin	Carrier protein for thyroid hormone in bloodstream	Thyroid hormones	1.5 mg/dL
Transthyretin (thyroid-binding prealbumin)	Carrier protein for thyroid hormone in bloodstream	Thyroid hormones	25 mg/dL

[1]Adapted from Donohue TM et al: Synthesis and secretion of plasma proteins by the liver. In: *Hepatology: A Textbook of Liver Disease.* Zakim D, Boyer TD (editors). Saunders, 1990.
[2]The function of alpha-fetoprotein is uncertain, but because of its structural homology to albumin it is often assigned these functions.

secreted by hepatocytes). In other cases, binding proteins made by the liver (eg, thyroid hormone-binding globulin) allow transport of specific substances (eg, thyroxine) in a form not fully accessible to tissues. In this way, the effective concentration of the substance is limited to its free concentration at equilibrium, and the tightly bound fraction forms a reservoir of the substance that is made available slowly as the free fraction is metabolized, thereby prolonging its half-life.

In some cases, binding proteins allow the liver to accumulate specific substances in relatively high concentrations and store them in a nontoxic form. Consider iron, for example—an essential nutrient.

Free iron can be quite toxic to cells both directly as an oxidant and indirectly as an essential nutrient needed by infectious agents. The liver has the responsibility of making a variety of proteins crucial for the binding and metabolism of iron. Through the actions of these proteins, the body gets the iron it needs without allowing excess free iron to cause damage or support pathogens.

Transferrin is an iron-binding protein synthesized and secreted into the bloodstream by the liver. Upon binding of free iron at normal pH, transferrin undergoes a conformational change that gives it high affinity for a specific membrane receptor of the hepatocyte (**transferrin receptor**). Upon receptor binding, the transferrin–transferrin receptor complex is internalized into the endocytic pathway, a progressively more acidic environment. There, at low pH, iron no longer remains bound to transferrin. However, conformational changes that occur at low pH allow transferrin to maintain high-affinity binding to its receptor even in the absence of bound iron. Thus, when the receptor recycles back to the surface, it brings the "empty" transferrin with it. Upon presentation to the pH 7.4 environment of the bloodstream, transferrin lacking bound iron is released from the receptor, and the cycle can start over again. In this way, transferrin and its receptor keep the bloodstream free of iron. Meanwhile, the free iron released from transferrin in the acidic environment of the endosome is transported into the cytoplasm of the hepatocyte, where it binds to **ferritin,** a cytoplasmic iron storage protein. This provides a reservoir that can be mobilized in response to the body's needs but makes iron inaccessible to pathogens and keeps it from causing direct toxic effects. Similar dynamics of plasma binding proteins, receptors, or cytosolic storage proteins occur for many other substances, including fat-soluble vitamins and steroid hormones.

Whereas most solubilization functions are performed in hepatocytes, some of the binding and storage functions involve accessory cells. Thus, vitamin A storage occurs in fat droplets seen in the **lipocytes** of the reticuloendothelial system. Recently, lipocytes have been implicated in the pathogenesis of chronic liver injury and cirrhosis. It appears that they respond to certain cytokines by synthesizing collagen and other basement membrane components which contribute to the increased hydrostatic pressure in cirrhosis. These observations suggest that lipocytes have important roles other than vitamin A storage.

Protective & Clearance Functions

Many of the functions of the liver already discussed, such as drug detoxification and excretion of excess cholesterol by conversion to and solubilization in bile, can also be considered protective. Nevertheless, it is useful to conceptualize the protective function as a separate category because of its clinical importance in ameliorating the consequences of liver disease.

A. Phagocytic and Endocytic Functions of Kupffer Cells: The liver helps remove bacteria and antigens that breach the defenses of the gut to enter the portal blood and participates also in clearing the circulation of endogenously generated cellular debris. It appears that specialized receptors on the Kupffer cell surface bind to glycoproteins (via carbohydrate receptors), or to material coated with immunoglobulin (via the Fc receptor), or to complement (via the C3 receptor), thus allowing damaged plasma proteins, activated clotting factors, immune complexes, senescent blood cells, etc, to be recognized and removed.

B. Endocytic Functions of Hepatocytes: Hepatocytes have a number of specific receptors for damaged plasma proteins distinct from the receptors present on Kupffer cells (eg, the asialoglycoprotein receptor that specifically binds glycoproteins whose terminal sialic acid sugar residues have been removed). The precise physiologic significance of this metabolic action remains unclear.

C. Ammonia Metabolism: Ammonia generated from deamination of amino acids is metabolized within hepatocytes into the much less toxic substance urea. Loss of this function results in altered mental status, a common manifestation of severe or end-stage liver disease.

D. Hepatocyte Synthesis of Glutathione: Glutathione is the major intracellular (cytoplasmic) reducing reagent and thus is crucial for preventing oxidative damage to cellular proteins. This molecule is a nonribosomally synthesized tripeptide (γ-glutamyl-cistinyl-glycine) which is also a substrate for many phase II drug detoxification conjugation reactions. The liver may also export glutathione for use by other tissues.

Some additional indirect liver functions, such as its role in maintaining normal sodium and water balance, are inferred from the derangements observed in patients with liver disease, as will be discussed in the following section.

---

12. What are the roles of the liver in carbohydrate, protein, and lipid metabolism?
13. What are two physiologic mechanisms by which the body transports cholesterol?
14. Explain phase I and phase II reactions in drug detoxification.
15. Name and explain four clearance or protective functions of the liver.
16. What specializations allow the liver normally to be a low-pressure conduit for blood flow?

OVERVIEW OF LIVER DISEASE

TYPES OF LIVER DYSFUNCTION

Most of the clinical consequences of liver disease can be understood either as a failure of one of the liver's four broad functions (summarized in Table 14–2) or as a consequence of portal hypertension, the altered hepatic blood flow of cirrhosis.

Hepatocyte Dysfunction

One mechanism of liver disease—particularly in acute liver injury—is dysfunction of the individual hepatocytes that make up the liver parenchyma. The pathway and extent of hepatocellular dysfunction determine the specific manifestations of liver disease. The outcomes to be anticipated when normal hepatic functions fail are described below.

Portal Hypertension

Some consequences of liver disease—particularly of cirrhosis—are best understood in terms of what we know about hepatic blood flow. Of greatest clinical importance are the existence under normal circumstances of a low-pressure portal venous capillary bed throughout the liver parenchyma and the functional zonation of portal blood flow.

When pathologic processes (eg, fibrosis) result in elevation of the normally low intrahepatic venous pressure, blood "backs up" and a substantial fraction of it finds alternative routes back to the systemic circulation, bypassing the liver. Thus, blood from the gastrointestinal tract is, in effect, filtered less efficiently by the liver prior to entering the systemic circulation. The consequences of this portal-to-systemic shunting are loss of the protective and clearance functions of the liver; functional abnormalities in renal salt and water homeostasis; and a greatly increased risk of gastrointestinal hemorrhage from the development of engorged blood vessels carrying venous blood bypassing the liver (eg, **esophageal varices**).

Even in the absence of any intrinsic parenchymal liver disease, portal-to-systemic shunting of blood can produce or contribute to **encephalopathy** (altered mental status due to failure to clear poisons absorbed from the gastrointestinal tract); gastrointestinal bleeding (due to esophageal varices); and malabsorption of fats and fat-soluble vitamins (due to loss of enterohepatic recirculation of bile), with associated coagulopathy. In Table 14–4, the syndromes observed in liver disease are categorized as being a consequence of hepatocyte dysfunction, portal-to-systemic shunting, or both.

Table 14–4. Pathophysiology of syndromes of aberrant function in liver disease.

Syndromes of Aberrant Function in Liver Disease	Hepatocellular Dysfunction	Portal-to-Systemic Shunting
Energy metabolism and substrate conversion		
Alcoholic hypoglycemia	✔	
Alcoholic ketoacidosis	✔	
Hyperglycemia		✔
Familial hypercholesterolemia	✔	
Hepatic encephalopathy	✔	✔
Fatty liver	✔	
Solubilization, transport, and storage function		
Reactions to drugs	✔	
Drug sensitivity	✔	✔
Steatorrhea	✔	✔
Fat-soluble vitamin deficiency	✔	✔
Hemochromatosis	✔	✔
Coagulopathy	✔	✔
Protein synthetic function		
Edema due to hypoalbuminemia	✔	
Protective and clearance functions		
Hypergammaglobulinemia		✔
Hypogonadism and hyperestrogenism	✔	✔
Renal dysfunction		
Sodium retention		✔
Impaired water excretion		✔
Impaired renal concentrating ability		✔
Deranged potassium metabolism		✔
Prerenal azotemia		✔
Acute renal failure		✔
Glomerulopathies		✔
Impaired renal acidification		✔
Hepatorenal syndrome		✔

Pathophysiology of Functional Zonation

The fact that hepatocytes in the different zones of the acinus "see" blood in a particular sequence has great pathophysiologic significance. Since zone 1 hepatocytes see blood that has just left the portal venule or hepatic arteriole, they have access to the highest concentrations of various substances—both good (eg, oxygen and nutrients) and bad (eg, drugs and toxins absorbed from the gastrointestinal tract). Zone 2 hepatocytes receive blood containing less of these substances, and zone 3 hepatocytes are bathed in blood largely depleted of them. However, zone 3 hepatocytes see the highest concentrations of products (eg, drug metabolites) released into the bloodstream by hepatocytes of zones 1 and 2. Thus, direct poisons have their most severe impact on zone 1 hepatocytes, while poisons that are generated as a result of hepatic metabolism cause more damage to those of zone 3. Similarly, since sinusoidal blood around zone 3 has the lowest oxygen concentration, hepatocytes of this zone are at greatest risk of injury under conditions of hypoxia.

MANIFESTATIONS OF LIVER DYSFUNCTION

Whether due to hepatocyte dysfunction or portal-to-systemic shunting, prominent features of liver disease are manifestations of failure of normal functions. An understanding of these mechanisms offers insight into the probable causes of illness in a patient with acute or chronic liver disease.

Diminished Energy Generation & Substrate Interconversion

A first category of altered liver function involves the intermediary metabolism of carbohydrates, fats, and proteins.

A. Carbohydrate Metabolism: Severe liver disease can result in either hypo- or hyperglycemia. Hypoglycemia results largely from a decrease in functional hepatocyte mass, while hyperglycemia is a result of portal-to-systemic shunting, which decreases the efficiency of postprandial extraction of glucose from portal blood by hepatocytes, thus elevating systemic blood glucose concentration.

B. Lipid Metabolism: Disturbance of lipid metabolism in the liver can result in syndromes of fat accumulation within the liver early in the course of liver injury. Perhaps this is because the complex steps in assembly of lipoprotein particles for export of cholesterol and triglycerides from the liver are more sensitive to disruption than the pathways of lipid synthesis. Such disruption results in a buildup of fat that cannot be exported in the form of VLDL.

In certain chronic liver diseases such as primary biliary cirrhosis, bile flow decreases as a result of destruction of bile ducts. The decrease in bile flow results in decreased lipid clearance via bile, with consequent hyperlipidemia. These patients often develop subcutaneous accumulations of cholesterol termed **xanthomas.**

C. Protein Metabolism: Any disturbance of protein metabolism in the liver can result in a syndrome of altered mental status and confusion known as **hepatic encephalopathy.** As with carbohydrate metabolism, altered protein metabolism can result from either hepatocyte failure or portal-to-systemic shunting, with the net effect of elevation of blood concentrations of centrally acting toxins, including ammonia generated by amino acid metabolism.

Loss of Solubilization & Storage Functions

A. Disordered Bile Secretion: The clinical significance of bile synthesis can be seen in the prominence of cholestasis—failure to secrete bile—in many forms of liver disease. Cholestasis can occur as a result of extrahepatic obstruction (eg, from a gallstone in the common bile duct) or of selective dysfunction of the bile synthetic and secretory machinery within the hepatocytes themselves (eg, from a reaction to certain drugs). The mechanisms responsible for cholestatic drug reactions are not well understood. Regardless of the mechanism, however, the clinical consequences of severe cholestasis may be profound: A failure to secrete bile results in a failure to solubilize substances such as dietary lipids and fat-soluble vitamins, resulting in **malabsorption** and deficiency states, respectively.

The solubilization function of bile works both to excrete and to absorb substances. Thus, in cholestasis, endogenous substances that are normally excreted via the biliary tract can accumulate to high levels. One such substance is bilirubin, a product of heme degradation (Figure 14–7). The buildup of bilirubin results in **jaundice (icterus)**—yellow discoloration of the scleras and skin. In the adult, the most significant feature of jaundice is that it serves as a readily monitored index of cholestasis, which may occur alone or with other abnormalities in hepatocyte function (ie, as part of the presentation of acute hepatitis). In the neonate, however, elevated bilirubin concentrations can be toxic to the developing nervous system, producing a syndrome termed **kernicterus.**

Similarly, cholesterol is normally excreted either by conversion into bile salts or by forming complexes, termed micelles, with preexisting (recycled) bile salts. In cholestasis, the resultant buildup of bile salts can lead to their deposition in the skin. This is believed to cause intense itching, or **pruritus.** Recent data suggest that in at least some patients, cholestasis results in altered levels of endogenous opioids. Altered endogenous opioid-mediated neurotransmission may be responsible for pruritus instead of skin deposition of bile salts. Disorders of bile production are a basis for the formation of cholesterol gallstones. Nevertheless, as mentioned earlier, other hepatocyte functions are often relatively well preserved in the

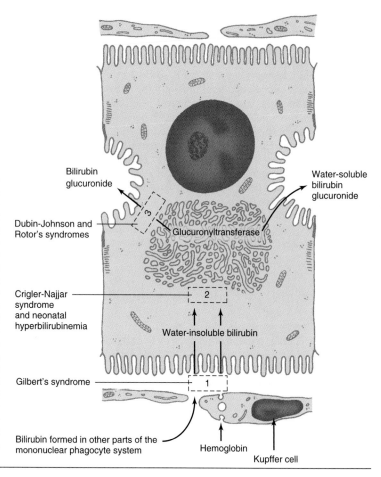

Figure 14–7. The secretion of bilirubin. This water-insoluble compound is derived from the metabolism of hemoglobin in macrophages of the mononuclear phagocyte system. Glucuronyl transferase activity in the hepatocytes causes bilirubin to be conjugated with glucuronide in the smooth endoplasmic reticulum, forming a water-soluble compound. Accumulation of bilirubin and bilirubin glucuronide in the tissues produces jaundice. Several defective processes in the hepatocytes can cause diseases that produce jaundice: a defect in the capacity of the cell to trap and absorb bilirubin (rectangle 1); the inability of the cell to conjugate bilirubin because of a deficiency in glucuronyl transferase (rectangle 2); or problems in the transfer and excretion of bilirubin glucuronide into the biliary canaliculi (rectangle 3). One of the most frequent causes of jaundice, however—unrelated to hepatocyte activity—is the obstruction of bile flow as a result of gallstones or tumors of the pancreas. This causes jaundice due primarily to accumulation of bilirubin glucuronide in the tissues. (Reproduced, with permission, from Junqueira LC, Carneiro J, Kelley RO: *Basic Histology,* 9th ed. Appleton & Lange, 1998.)

face of significant cholestasis. The syndromes that produce jaundice are summarized in Table 14–5.

Hemolysis causes an unconjugated hyperbilirubinemia because the hepatic capacity to take up and conjugate bilirubin is exceeded. Gilbert's syndrome reflects a genetic defect in bilirubin uptake. Thus, the findings in blood and urine are different from what is observed in hemolytic jaundice even though the pathway of bilirubin metabolism is "backed up" at a similar initial point. Extrahepatic biliary tract obstruction presents the other extreme, where the actual pathway of bile formation is entirely intact, at least initially. In obstruction, the bilirubin level in the urine is high because the backed-up metabolite is conjugated and hence much more water-soluble than unconjugated bilirubin, which accumulates in hemolysis. Most forms of jaundice that result from liver dysfunction due to hepatocellular damage reflect variable degrees of overlap between unconjugated and conjugated hyperbilirubinemia.

B. Impaired Drug Detoxification: Two features of the mechanisms of drug detoxification are of particular clinical importance. One is the phenomenon of **enzyme induction.** It is observed that the presence in the bloodstream of any of the large class of drugs inactivated by phase I enzymes increases the amount and activity of these enzymes in the liver. This property of enzyme induction makes physiologic sense (as a response to the body's need for increased biotransformation) but can have undesired effects as well: A patient who chronically consumes large amounts of a substance that is metabolized by phase I enzymes (eg, ethanol) will induce high levels of these enzymes and thus speed up the metabolism of other substances metabolized by the same detoxifying enzymes (eg, antiseizure or anticoagulant medications, resulting in subtherapeutic blood levels of the drugs).

A second clinically important phenomenon in drug metabolism has already been mentioned, namely, that phase I reactions often convert relatively benign compounds into more reactive and hence more toxic ones. Normally, this heightened reactivity of phase I reaction products serves to facilitate phase II reactions, making detoxification more efficient. However, under certain conditions when phase II reac-

Table 14–5. Laboratory findings in the differential diagnosis of jaundice.[1]

Type of Jaundice	Hct	Blood					Stool		Urine	
		Unconjugated Bilirubin (Indirect)	Conjugated Bilirubin (Direct)	Alkaline Phosphatase	Aminotransferases	Cholesterol	Color	Bilirubin		Urobilinogen
Hemolytic	↓	↑↑	N	N	N	N	N	NP		↑
Hepatocellular										
Gilbert's syndrome	N	↑	N	N	N	N	N	NP		N or ↓
Abnormal conjugation	N	↑	N	N	N	N	N	NP		N or ↓
Hepatocellular damage	N	↑	↑	N or ↑	↑↑	N	N	↑		↑
Obstructive										
Defective excretion	N	N	N	N	N	N	N	↑		N
Intrahepatic cholestasis	N	N	↑	N	N	N or ↑	Pale	↑		↓
Extrahepatic biliary obstruction	N	N	↑↑	↑↑	N or ↑	↑	Pale	↑		↓

[1]Modified and reproduced, with permission, from Chandrasoma P, Taylor CR: *Concise Pathology*, 2nd ed. Appleton & Lange, 1994.
Key: N = Normal; NP = Not present in significant amounts due to insolubility in water; ↑ = increased compared with normal; ↓ = decreased compared with normal.

tions are impaired (eg, during glutathione deficiency from inadequate nutrition), continued phase I enzyme activity can cause increased liver injury. This is because the products of many phase I reactions, in the absence of glutathione, react with and damage cellular components. Such damage rapidly kills the hepatocyte.

Thus, the combined effects of certain common conditions can make the individual abnormally sensitive to the toxic effects of drugs. For example, the combination of induced phase I activity (eg, due to alcoholism) with low phase II activity (eg, due to low glutathione levels from nutritional deprivation) can result in heightened generation of reactive intermediates with an inadequate capacity to conjugate and detoxify them. A classic example of this phenomenon is acetaminophen toxicity. As little as 2 g of acetaminophen can produce significant liver damage in such susceptible individuals. Table 14–6 lists common drugs and chemicals that cause morphologically distinctive changes in the liver.

C. Lipoprotein Dynamics and Dyslipidemias: The liver's role in lipid metabolism is illustrated by the genetic defect causing familial hypercholesterolemia. Lack of a functional LDL receptor in such cases renders the liver unable to clear LDL cholesterol from the bloodstream, resulting in markedly elevated serum cholesterol and accelerated atherosclerosis and coronary artery disease. Heterozygotes with one normal LDL receptor allele can be treated with drugs (eg, HMG-CoA reductase inhibitors) that inhibit endogenous cholesterol synthesis and thus upregulate LDL receptor levels. However, there is no effective drug therapy for homozygotes, since they have no normal LDL receptors. Hepatic transplantation is effective therapy for homozygous familial hypercholesterolemia because it provides a genetically different liver with normal LDL receptors.

In acquired liver diseases, the serum cholesterol is elevated in biliary tract obstruction due to blockage of cholesterol excretion in bile; and diminished in severe alcoholic cirrhosis, in which fat malabsorption prevents cholesterol intake.

D. Altered Hepatic Binding and Storage Functions: Liver disease influences the liver's ability to store various substances. As a result, patients with liver disease have a high risk of developing certain deficiency states such as folic acid and vitamin B_{12} deficiency. Since these vitamins are needed for DNA synthesis, their deficiency results in **macrocytic anemia** (low red blood cell count with large red cells reflecting abnormal nuclear maturation), a common finding in patients with liver disease.

Diminished Synthesis & Secretion of Plasma Proteins

The clinical significance of liver protein synthesis and secretion derives from the wide range of functions carried out by these proteins. For example, since albumin is the major contributor to plasma oncotic pressure, hypoalbuminemia as a consequence of liver disease or nutritional deficiency presents with marked edema formation. Other important proteins synthesized and secreted by the liver include clotting factors and hormone-binding proteins.

Loss of Protective & Clearance Functions

A crucial protective function of the liver is its role as a filter of blood from the gastrointestinal tract, by which various substances are removed from portal blood before it reenters the systemic circulation.

A. Clearance of Bacteria and Endotoxin: Clearance of bacteria by Kupffer cells of the liver is the final line of defense in keeping gut-derived bacteria out of the systemic circulation. Loss of this capacity in liver disease due to portal-to-systemic shunting may help to explain why, in patients with severe liver disease, infections can rapidly become systemic and result in sepsis.

B. Altered Ammonia Metabolism: Impairment of the liver's ability to detoxify ammonia to urea leads to hepatic encephalopathy, manifested as an altered mental status. This may be an early manifestation of acute fulminant hepatitis with massive hepatocellular dysfunction even before the development of maximal hepatocellular necrosis. It can be a final step in progressive chronic liver disease with diminished hepatocyte functional capacity. Most often it is a consequence of an increased ammonia load in a patient with marginal liver function or significant portal-to-systemic shunting. Thus, encephalopathy may occur as a first sign of renewed gastrointestinal bleeding (as a result of increased production of ammonia and other products due to breakdown of blood protein by gastrointestinal tract microbes) or may simply be due to increased protein intake (eg, a cheeseburger eaten by a patient with cirrhosis). Finally, the development of sepsis in these patients results in increased endogenous protein catabolism and therefore elevated ammonia production in the face of a decreased capacity for ammonia detoxification due to the liver disease. Thus, the development of encephalopathy in a patient with chronic liver disease calls for investigation of possible acute gastrointestinal bleeding as well as potentially catastrophic infection. Pending the outcome of diagnostic studies (eg, serial hematocrit measurements and cultures of blood, urine, and ascitic fluid), therapy is designed to improve mental status by diminishing the absorption of ammonia and other noxious substances from the gastrointestinal tract. When the patient is given the nonabsorbable carbohydrate **lactulose,** whose metabolism by microbes creates an acidic environment, ammonia is trapped as the charged NH_4^+ species in the gut lumen and excreted by the resultant osmotic diarrhea. Thus, this toxin is prevented from ever entering the portal circulation, and the patient's mental status gradually improves.

Table 14–6. Principal alterations of hepatic morphology produced by some commonly used drugs and chemicals.[1]

Principal Morphologic Change	Class of Agent	Example[2]
Cholestasis	Anabolic steroid	Methyltestosterone[3]
	Antithyroid	Methimazole
	Antibiotic	Erythromycin estolate
		Nitrofurantoin
	Oral contraceptive	Norethynodrel with mestranol
	Oral hypoglycemic	Chlorpropamide
	Tranquilizer	Chlorpromazine[3]
	Oncotherapeutic	Anabolic steroids
		Busulfan
		Tamoxifen
	Immunosuppressive	Cyclosporine
	Anticonvulsant	Carbamazepine
	Calcium channel blocker	Nifedipine
		Verapamil
Fatty liver	Antibiotic	Tetracycline
	Anticonvulsant	Sodium valproate
	Antiarrhythmic	Amiodarone
	Oncotherapeutic	Asparaginase
		Methotrexate
Hepatitis	Anesthetic	Halothane[4]
	Anticonvulsant	Phenytoin
		Carbamazepine
	Antihypertensive	Methyldopa[4]
		Captopril
		Enalapril
	Antibiotic	Isoniazid[4]
		Rifampin
		Nitrofurantoin
	Diuretic	Chlorothiazide
	Laxative	Oxyphenisatin[4]
	Antidepressant	Amitriptyline
		Imipramine
	Anti-inflammatory	Ibuprofen
		Indomethacin
	Antifungal	Ketoconazole
		Fluconazole
	Antiviral	Zidovudine
		Dideoxyinosine
	Calcium channel blocker	Nifedipine
		Verapamil
		Diltiazem
Mixed hepatitis and cholestasis	Immunosuppressive	Azathioprine
	Lipid-lowering	Nicotinic acid
		Lovastatin
Toxic (necrosis)	Hydrocarbon	Carbon tetrachloride
	Metal	Yellow phosphorus
	Mushroom	*Amanita phalloides*
	Analgesic	Acetaminophen
	Solvent	Dimethylformamide
Granulomas	Anti-inflammatory	Phenylbutazone
	Antibiotic	Sulfonamides
	Xanthine oxidase inhibitor	Allopurinol
	Antiarrhythmic	Quinidine
	Anticonvulsant	Carbamazepine

[1] Modified and reproduced, with permission, from Isselbacher K et al (editors): *Harrison's Principles of Internal Medicine,* 13th ed. McGraw-Hill, 1994.
[2] Several agents cause more than one type of liver lesion and appear under more than one category.
[3] Rarely associated with a primary biliary cirrhosis-like lesion.
[4] Occasionally associated with chronic active hepatitis or bridging hepatic necrosis or cirrhosis.

More recent studies suggest that altered ammonia metabolism exerts its effect on the brain by derangement of neuronal-astrocytic excitatory amino acid metabolism.

Furthermore, the resulting elevated blood ammonia and other nitrogen-containing compounds can up-regulate peripheral receptors for endogenous benzodiazepine-like products. These effects may contribute to altered systemic hemodynamics in liver disease.

C. Altered Hormone Clearance in Liver Disease: Normally, the liver removes from the bloodstream the fraction of steroid hormones not bound to steroid hormone-binding globulin. Upon uptake by hepatocytes, these steroids are oxidized, conjugated, and excreted into bile, where a fraction undergoes enterohepatic circulation. In liver disease accompanied by significant portal-to-systemic shunting, steroid hormone clearance is diminished; extraction of the enterohepatic circulated fraction is impaired; and enzymatic conversion of androgens to estrogens (termed peripheral aromatization) is increased. The net effect is an elevation of blood estrogens, which in turn alters hepatocyte protein synthesis and secretion and microsomal P450 activity. Synthesis of some hepatic proteins increases, while synthesis of others is diminished. P450 activity increases as the liver attempts to partially compensate for the higher blood estrogen levels by increased metabolism. Thus, male patients with liver disease display both gonadal and pituitary suppression as well as feminization.

Sodium & Water Balance

Patients with liver disease often display renal abnormalities and complications, most commonly sodium retention and difficulty in excreting water. An intrinsic renal lesion is apparently not involved, since the kidneys of patients with liver disease typically function normally when transplanted into patients with normal livers. Instead, renal abnormalities associated with liver disease are functional, occurring because liver disease induces altered intravascular pressures, and perhaps because of elevated nitric oxide levels or loss of as yet poorly understood factors secreted from the liver or the endothelium. By whatever homeostatic mechanisms, intravascular volume is perceived as being inadequate when it is really only maldistributed. Renal mechanisms of salt and water retention are then stimulated to correct what has been sensed as volume depletion. Some of the factors influencing renal sodium retention in liver disease are summarized in Table 14–7. Patients with severe liver disease are at risk of developing renal failure related to these hemodynamic alterations.

Table 14–7. Factors influencing renal sodium retention in liver disease.[1]

Hormonal
Elevated renal endothelin production
Hyperaldosteronism due to diminished clearance by the liver
Diminished angiotensinogen synthesis by the liver
Diminished renin and angiotensin II clearance by the liver
Altered kallikrein-kinin system
Loss of hepatic humoral natriuretic factors
Atrial natriuretic factor
Elevated blood estrogens
Prolactin
Vasoactive intestinal peptide
Elevated peripheral nitric acid production
Neural
Increased sympathetic nervous system activity
Hemodynamic
Alterations in intrarenal blood flow
Portal-to-systemic shunting
Hypoalbuminemia

[1]Modified and reproduced, with permission, from Epstein M: Functional renal abnormalities in cirrhosis: Pathophysiology and management. In: *Hepatology: A Textbook of Liver Disease,* 2nd ed. Zakim D, Boyer JD (editors). Saunders, 1990.

---

17. Under what circumstances is hypoglycemia seen in liver disease?
18. Name three clinical consequences of cholestasis.
19. Development of hepatic encephalopathy in a patient with chronic liver disease should lead you to investigate what possible precipitating factors?
20. By what mechanisms can coagulation defects be a consequence of liver disease?
21. What is an explanation for hypogonadism in male patients with liver disease?

PATHOPHYSIOLOGY OF SELECTED LIVER DISEASES

ACUTE HEPATITIS

Acute hepatitis is an inflammatory process causing liver cell death either by necrosis or by triggering apoptosis (programmed cell death). A wide range of clinical entities can cause global hepatocyte injury of sudden onset. Acute hepatitis is most commonly caused by infection with one of several types of viruses. Although these viral agents can be distinguished by serologic laboratory tests based on their antigenic properties, all produce clinically similar illnesses. Other less common infectious agents can result in liver injury (Table 14–1). Acute hepatitis is also sometimes caused by exposure to drugs (eg, isoniazid) or poisons (eg, ethanol).

Clinical Presentation

The severity of illness in acute hepatitis ranges from asymptomatic and clinically inapparent to fulminant and fatal. The presentation of acute hepatitis can be quite variable. Some patients are relatively asymptomatic, with abnormalities noted only by laboratory studies. Others may have a range of symptoms and signs, including anorexia, fatigue, weight loss, nausea, vomiting, right upper quadrant abdominal pain, jaundice, fever, splenomegaly, and ascites. The extent of hepatic dysfunction can also vary tremendously, correlating roughly with the severity of liver injury. The relative extent of cholestasis versus hepatocyte necrosis is also highly variable. The potential interrelationship of acute hepatitis, chronic hepatitis, and cirrhosis is illustrated in Figure 14–8.

Etiology

A. Viral Hepatitis: Acute hepatitis is commonly caused by one of five major viruses (Table 14–8): hepatitis A virus (HAV) (formerly: infectious or short-incubation hepatitis); hepatitis B virus (HBV) (formerly: serum or long-incubation hepatitis); hepatitis C virus (HCV) (one form of the illness formerly called non-A, non-B hepatitis, or posttransfusion hepatitis); hepatitis D virus (HDV) (also called HBV-associated delta agent); and hepatitis E virus (HEV) (another form of non-A, non-B hepatitis causing epidemic hepatitis in developing countries).

Table 14–8 summarizes important characteristics of these viral agents. Other viral agents that can cause acute hepatitis, though less commonly, include the Epstein-Barr virus (cause of infectious mononucleosis), cytomegalovirus (CMV), herpes simplex virus (HSV), rubella virus, and yellow fever virus.

Hepatitis A virus—a small RNA virus—causes liver disease both by direct killing of hepatocytes and by the host's immune response to infected hepatocytes. It is spread by the fecal-oral route from infected individuals. While most cases are mild, hepatitis A can occasionally present with fulminant liver failure and massive hepatocellular necrosis resulting in death. Regardless of the severity, patients who recover do so completely, show no evidence of residual liver disease, and have antibodies that protect them from reinfection.

Hepatitis B virus is a DNA virus that is transmitted by sexual contact or by contact with infected

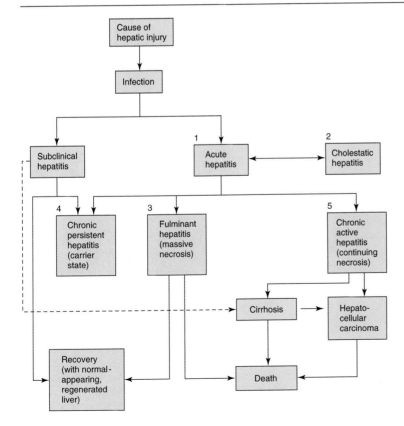

Figure 14–8. Clinical syndromes associated with hepatitis: Acute hepatitis **(1)**, which is sometimes associated with intrahepatic cholestasis **(2)**. Fulminant hepatitis **(3)** is associated with massive necrosis and is associated with a high mortality rate. Chronic viral hepatitis may be persistent **(4)** or active **(5)**. Chronic active hepatitis commonly progresses to cirrhosis of the liver, while chronic persistent hepatitis does not. (Reproduced, with permission, from Chandrasoma P, Taylor CE: *Concise Pathology,* 3rd ed. Appleton & Lange, 1998.)

Table 14–8. Characteristics of various types of viral hepatitis.[1]

	Hepatitis A	Hepatitis B	Hepatitis C	Hepatitis D	Hepatitis E
Clinical presentation					
Onset	Abrupt	Insidious	Insidious	Insidious	Abrupt
Incubation period					
Range (days)	15–20	28–160	14–160		
Mean (days)	30	8	50		40
Symptoms					
Arthralgia, rash	Uncommon	Common	Uncommon	Uncommon	Common
Fever	Common	Uncommon	Uncommon	Common	Common
Nausea, vomiting	Common	Common	Common	Common	Common
Jaundice	Uncommon in children	More common in hepatitis A	Uncommon	Common	Common
Laboratory data					
Duration of enzyme elevation	Short	Prolonged	Like hepatitis B	Like hepatitis B	
Virus type	RNA	DNA	RNA	RNA	RNA
	Picornavirus	Hepadnavirus	Flavivirus	Defective virus	Unclassified
Serologic tests					
Antigen	Yes	Yes	No	No	Yes
Antibody	Yes	Yes	Yes	Yes	Yes
Location of virus					
Blood	Transient	Prolonged	Prolonged	Prolonged	?Transient
Stool	Yes	No	No	No	Yes
Elsewhere	?	Yes	?	?	?
Outcome					
Severity of acute disease	Mild	Moderate	Mild	Moderate to severe	Severe
Mortality rate	Low (1%)	Low (1–3%)	Low (2%)	High (5%)	Moderate (+3%)
Chronic hepatitis	No	Yes	Yes	Yes	No
Chronic carrier	No	Yes	Yes	Yes	No
Associated with malignancy	No	Yes	Yes	Yes	No
Transmission					
Oral	+	±	?No	?No	+
Percutaneous	Rare	+	+	+	–
Sexual	+	+	–	+	?
Perinatal	–	+	±	–	?
Vaccine	Yes	Yes	No	No (vaccinate against HBV)	No

[1]Modified and reproduced, with permission, from Seeff LB: Diagnosis, therapy, and prognosis of viral hepatitis. In: *Hepatology: A Textbook of Liver Disease,* 2nd ed. Zakim D, Boyer JD (editors). Saunders, 1990.

blood. This virus does not kill the cells it infects. Rather, the infected hepatocytes die almost exclusively as a consequence of attack by the immune system after recognition of viral antigens on the hepatocyte surface. While most cases of hepatitis B infection are asymptomatic or produce only mild disease before clearance of the virus, an excessive immune response may produce fulminant hepatic failure. In even fewer patients—typically those with mild acute disease—the immune response is inadequate to clear the virus completely, and chronic hepatitis develops.

Hepatitis C virus, once known as non-A, non-B hepatitis virus, causes a form of hepatitis similar to HBV infection but with a greater proportion of cases progressing to chronic active hepatitis.

Hepatitis D virus, also known as delta agent, is a defective RNA virus that requires helper functions of HBV to cause infection. Thus, individuals who are chronically infected with HBV are at high risk for HDV infection, while individuals who have been vaccinated against HBV are at no risk. HDV infection causes a much more severe form of hepatitis, both in terms of the proportion of fulminant cases and in the percentage of cases that progress to chronic hepatitis.

B. Toxic Hepatitis: Some of the various drugs, poisons, and toxins known to cause acute hepatitis and fulminant hepatitis are listed in Table 14–9. Toxic acute hepatitis can be further subdivided into those for which hepatic toxicity is predictable and dose-dependent for most individuals and those which cause unpredictable (idiosyncratic) reactions without relationship to dose. Table 14–10 summarizes speculation on the mechanisms of dose-related drug-induced hepatic disease. In contrast, idiosyncratic reactions to drugs may be due to genetic predisposition in susceptible individuals to certain pathways of drug metabolism that generate toxic intermediates.

The time course of acute hepatitis is highly variable. In hepatitis A, jaundice is typically seen 4–8 weeks after exposure, while in hepatitis B, jaundice occurs usually from week 8 to week 20 after exposure (see Figure 14–9). Drug- and toxin-induced hepatitis typically occurs at any time during or shortly after exposure and resolves with discontinuance of the offending agent. This is usually the case for both idiosyncratic and dose-dependent reactions.

Table 14–9. Drugs implicated in idiosyncratic liver injury leading to acute liver failure.[1]

Infrequent Causes	Rare Causes	Synergistic Causes[2]
Isoniazid	Carbamazepine	Alcohol and acetaminophen
Valproate	Ofloxacin	Trimethoprim and sulfamethoxazole
Halothane	Ketoconazole	Rifampin and isoniazid
Phenytoin	Lisinopril	Acetaminophen and isoniazid
Sulfonamides	Niacin	Amoxicillin and clavulanic acid
Propylthiouracil	Labetalol	
Amiodarone	Etoposide (VP-16)	
Disulfiram	Imipramine	
Dapsone	Interferon alfa	
	Flutamide	

[1]Reproduced, with permission, from Lee WM: Acute liver failure. N Engl J Med 1993;329:1862.
[2]These are commonly used combinations of drugs with apparent systemic toxicity.

Table 14–10. Postulated mechanisms of drug-induced liver disease.[1]

Effect	Example
Alteration of the physical properties of membranes	Estrogens
Inhibition of membrane enzymes (eg, Na^+-K^+ ATPase)	Chlorpromazine metabolites
Interference with hepatic uptake processes	Rifampin
Impairment of cytoskeletal function	Chlorpromazine metabolites
Formation of insoluble complexes in bile	Chlorpromazine
Conversion to reactive intermediates Electrophils producing covalent modifications of tissue macromolecules	Acetaminophen
Free radicals producing lipid peroxidation	Carbon tetrachloride
Redox cycling with production of oxygen radicals	Nitrofurantoin

[1]Reproduced, with permission, from Bass NM, Ockner RK: Drug-induced liver disease. In: *Hepatology: A Textbook of Liver Disease*, 2nd ed. Zakim D, Boyer JD (editors). Saunders, 1990.

Acute hepatitis typically resolves in 3–6 months. Hepatic injury continuing for more than 6 months is arbitrarily defined as chronic hepatitis and suggests, in the absence of continued exposure to a noxious agent, that immune or other mechanisms are at work.

Pathogenesis

A. Viral Hepatitis: The viral agents responsible for acute hepatitis first infect the hepatocyte. During the incubation period, intense viral replication in the liver cell leads to the appearance of viral components (first antigens, later antibodies) in urine, stool, and body fluids. Liver cell death and an associated inflammatory response then ensue, followed by changes in laboratory tests of liver function and the appearance of various symptoms and signs of liver disease.

1. Liver damage—The host's immunologic response plays an important though incompletely understood role in the pathogenesis of liver damage. In hepatitis B, for example, the virus is probably not directly cytopathic. Indeed, there are asymptomatic HBV carriers who have normal liver function and histologic features. Instead, the host's cellular immune response has an important role in causing liver cell injury. Patients with defects in cell-mediated immunity are more likely to remain chronically infected with HBV than to clear the infection. Histologic

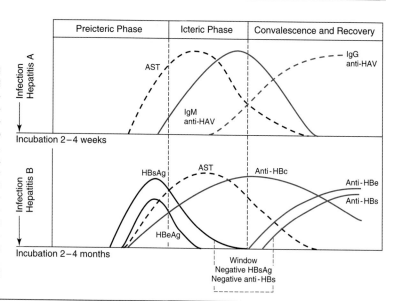

Figure 14–9. Serum antibody and antigen levels in hepatitis A and hepatitis B. (AST, aspartate aminotransferase, a marker for hepatocellular injury and necrosis; IgM anti-HAV, early antibody response to hepatitis A infection; IgG anti-HAV, late antibody response to hepatitis A infection; HBsAg, hepatitis B surface antigen, a marker of active viral gene expression; HBeAg, hepatitis B e antigen, a marker of infectivity.) Antibodies to the surface or e antigens (anti-HBs or anti-HBe) indicate immunity. (Reproduced, with permission, from Chandrasoma P, Taylor CE: *Concise Pathology,* 3rd ed. Appleton & Lange, 1998.)

specimens from patients with HBV-related liver injury demonstrate lymphocytes next to necrotic liver cells. It is thought that cytolytic T lymphocytes become sensitized to recognize hepatitis B viral antigens (eg, small quantities of HBsAg) and host antigens on the surfaces of HBV-infected liver cells.

2. Extrahepatic manifestations–Immune factors may also be important in the pathogenesis of the extrahepatic manifestations of acute viral hepatitis. For example, in hepatitis B, a serum sickness-like prodrome characterized by fever, urticarial rash and angioedema, and arthralgias and arthritis appears to be related to immune complex-mediated tissue damage. During the early prodrome, circulating immune complexes are composed of HBsAg in high titer in association with small quantities of anti-HBs. These circulating immune complexes are deposited in blood vessel walls, leading to activation of the complement cascade. In patients with arthritis, serum complement levels are depressed, and complement can be detected in circulating immune complexes containing HbsAg, anti-HBs, IgG, IgM, IgA, and fibrin.

Finally, immune factors are thought to be important in the pathogenesis of some clinical manifestations in patients who become chronic HBsAg carriers following acute hepatitis. For example, in patients developing glomerulonephritis with nephrotic syndrome, histopathologic investigation demonstrates deposition of HBsAg, immunoglobulin, and complement in the glomerular basement membrane. In patients developing polyarteritis nodosa, similar deposits have been demonstrated in affected small- and medium-sized arteries.

B. Alcoholic Hepatitis: Ethanol has both direct and indirect toxic effects on the liver as well as effects on many other organ systems of the body. Its direct effects may result from increasing the fluidity of biologic membranes and thereby disrupting cellular functions. Its indirect effects on the liver are in part a consequence of its metabolism. Ethanol is sequentially oxidized to acetaldehyde and then to acetate, with the generation of NADH and ATP. As a result of the high ratio of reduced to oxidized NAD that is generated, the pathways of fatty acid oxidation and gluconeogenesis are inhibited, while fatty acid synthesis is promoted. Ethanol can also quantitatively and qualitatively alter the pattern of gene expression in various tissues but especially in the liver, resulting in impaired homeostasis and greater sensitivity to other toxins. These and other biochemical mechanisms may contribute to the common observation of fat accumulation in the liver of alcoholics and the tendency to development of hypoglycemia in alcoholics whose liver glycogen has been depleted by fasting. Ethanol metabolism also affects the liver by generation of acetaldehyde, which reacts with primary amino groups to inactivate enzymes, resulting in direct toxicity to the hepatocyte in which it is generated. Furthermore, proteins so modified may activate the immune system against antigens that were previously tolerated as "self."

There is considerable variation among individuals in the amount of ethanol required to cause acute liver injury. Whether nutritional, genetic, or other factors are responsible for these differences has not been determined. The mechanisms thought to be responsible for ethanol-induced liver injury are listed in Table 14–11.

Pathology

In uncomplicated acute hepatitis, the typical histologic findings consist of (1) focal liver cell degenera-

Table 14–11. Mechanisms of hepatocyte injury by ethanol.[1]

Disorganizes the lipid portion of cell membranes, leading to adaptive changes in their composition:
  Increased fluidity and permeability of membranes
  Impaired assembly of glycoproteins into membranes
  Impaired secretion of glycoproteins
  Impaired binding and internalization of large ligands
  Formation of abnormal mitochondria
  Impairment of transport of small ligands
  Impairment of membrane-bound enzymes
  Adaptive changes in lipid composition, leading to increased lipid peroxidation
  Abnormal display of antigens on the plasma membrane

Alters the capacity of liver cells to cope with environmental toxins:
  Induces xenobiotic metabolizing enzymes
  Directly inhibits xenobiotic metabolizing enzymes
  Induces deficiency in mechanisms protecting against injury due to reactive metabolites
  Enhances the toxicity of O_2

Oxidation of ethanol produces acetaldehyde, a toxic and reactive intermediate:
  Inhibits export of proteins from the liver
  Modifies hepatic protein synthesis in fasted animals
  Alters the metabolism of cofactors essential for enzymatic activity—pyridoxine, folate, choline, zinc, vitamin E
  Alters the oxidation-reduction potential of the liver cell
  Induces malnutrition

[1]Reproduced, with permission, from Zakim D, Boyer TD, Montgomery C: Alcoholic liver disease. In: *Hepatology: A Textbook of Liver Disease*, 2nd ed. Zakim D, Boyer JD (editors). Saunders, 1990.

tion and necrosis, with cell drop-out, ballooning, and acidophilic degeneration (shrunken cells with eosinophilic cytoplasm and pyknotic nuclei); (2) inflammation of portal areas, with infiltration by mononuclear cells (small lymphocytes, plasma cells, eosinophils); (3) prominence of Kupffer cells and bile ducts; and (4) cholestasis (arrested bile flow) with bile plugs. Characteristically, although the regular pattern of the cords of hepatocytes is disrupted, the reticulin framework is preserved.

Recovery from acute hepatitis due to any cause is characterized histologically by regeneration of hepatocytes, with numerous mitotic figures and multinucleated cells, and by a largely complete restoration of normal lobular architecture.

Less commonly in acute hepatitis (1–5% of patients), there will be a more severe histologic lesion called **bridging hepatic necrosis** (also called subacute, submassive, or confluent necrosis). "Bridging" is said to occur between lobules because necrosis involves contiguous groups of hepatocytes, resulting in large areas of hepatic cell loss and collapse of the reticulin framework. Necrotic zones ("bridges") consisting of condensed reticulin, inflammatory debris, and degenerating liver cells link adjacent portal or central areas, or they may involve entire lobules.

Rarely, in massive hepatic necrosis or fulminant hepatitis (< 1% of patients), the liver becomes small, shrunken, and soft (acute yellow atrophy). Histologic examination reveals massive hepatocyte necrosis in most of the lobules, leading to extensive collapse and condensation of the reticulin framework and portal structures (bile ducts and vessels).

Clinical Manifestations

A. Viral Hepatitis: Acute viral hepatitis usually is manifested in three phases: the prodrome, the icteric phase, and the convalescent phase.

1. Prodrome–The prodrome is characterized by three sets of symptoms and signs: (1) nonspecific constitutional symptoms and signs: malaise, fatigue, and mild fever; (2) gastrointestinal symptoms and signs: anorexia, nausea, vomiting, altered senses of olfaction and taste (loss of taste for coffee or cigarettes), and right upper quadrant abdominal discomfort (reflecting the enlarged liver); and (3) extrahepatic symptoms and signs: headache, photophobia, cough, coryza, myalgias, urticarial skin rash, arthralgias or arthritis (10–15% of patients with HBV), and, rarely, hematuria and proteinuria.

2. Icteric phase–The constitutional symptoms usually improve, though mild weight loss may occur. Pruritus occurs if cholestasis is severe. Right upper quadrant abdominal pain as a result of the enlarged and tender liver, which was present in the prodromal phase, continues. Splenomegaly is noted in 10–20% of patients.

Jaundice may be observed as a yellowing of the scleras, skin, or mucous membranes. Jaundice is generally not appreciated on physical examination before the serum bilirubin rises above 2.5 mg/dL (41.75 μmol/L). **Direct hyperbilirubinemia** is elevation of the level of conjugated bilirubin in the bloodstream. Its occurrence indicates unimpaired ability of hepatocytes to conjugate bilirubin but a defect in the excretion of bilirubin into the bile as a result of intrahepatic cholestasis or posthepatic obstructive biliary tract disease, with overflow of conjugated bilirubin out of hepatocytes and into the bloodstream.

Changes in stool color (lightening) and urine color (darkening) often precede clinically evident jaundice. This reflects loss of bilirubin metabolites from the stool as a consequence of disrupted bile flow. Water-soluble (conjugated) bilirubin metabolites are excreted in the urine, while water-insoluble metabolites accumulate in tissues, giving rise to jaundice.

Ecchymoses suggest coagulopathy, which may be due to loss of vitamin K absorptive capacity from the intestine (caused by cholestasis) or decreased coagulation factor synthesis. Rarely, loss of clearance of activated clotting factors triggers disseminated intravascular coagulation. Coagulopathy in which the prothrombin time can be corrected by vitamin K injections but not by oral vitamin K suggests cholestatic disease, since vitamin K uptake from the gut is dependent on bile flow. If the prothrombin time cannot be corrected with either oral or parenteral vitamin

K, inability to synthesize clotting factor polypeptides (eg, due to massive hepatocellular dysfunction) should be suspected. Correction of prothrombin time with oral vitamin K alone suggests a nutritional deficiency rather than liver disease as the basis for the coagulopathy.

Tests for serum levels of various enzymes normally localized primarily within hepatocytes provide an indication of the extent of liver cell necrosis. Misnamed "liver function tests," these enzyme assays include aspartate aminotransferase (AST), alanine aminotransferase (ALT), and alkaline phosphatase. For unclear reasons, perhaps related to liver cell polarity, certain forms of liver disease typically result in disproportionate elevations in some parameters. Thus, in alcoholic hepatitis but not in viral hepatitis, AST is often disproportionately elevated relative to ALT (AST:ALT ratio > 2.0). Likewise, in cholestasis, alkaline phosphatase is commonly disproportionately elevated relative to AST or ALT.

Measurement of antigen and antibody titers is a convenient way to assess whether an episode of acute hepatitis is due to viral infection. Moreover, since IgM antibodies are produced early after exposure to antigens (ie, soon after onset of illness), the presence of IgM antibodies to either HAV or to core antigen of HBV (HBcAg) is strong evidence that an episode of acute hepatitis is due to the corresponding viral infection. Several months after onset of illness, IgM antibody titers wane and are replaced by antibodies of the IgG class, indicating immunity to recurrence of infection by the same virus. Moreover, since the presence of surface antigen of hepatitis B virus (HBsAg) correlates well with infectivity and infectivity correlates inversely with the titer of antibody to surface antigen, such serologic studies help determine whether a patient with acute hepatitis is infectious to others (Table 14–12).

Subtle or profound mental status changes are seen in fulminant hepatic necrosis. Encephalopathy is believed to be related in part to failure of detoxification of ammonia (which normally occurs through the urea cycle). Other products such as γ-aminobutyric acid (GABA) may not be metabolized. Although ammonia is a neurotoxin, it remains unclear whether it is the major agent of central nervous system dysfunction or whether elevated blood levels of GABA (or other compounds) may act synergistically to alter mental status because of its role as a major inhibitory neurotransmitter.

In addition to encephalopathic changes due to accumulation of toxins, acute hepatic failure is associated with encephalopathy due to cerebral edema caused by increased intracranial pressure, perhaps related to alterations in the blood-brain barrier.

Renal dysfunction may complicate fulminant hepatic failure. Affected patients may develop prerenal azotemia when the glomerular filtration rate falls secondary to intravascular volume depletion. A state of intravascular volume depletion can be induced by the combination of decreased oral intake, vomiting, and formation of ascites. If uncorrected, this process can lead to acute tubular necrosis and acute renal failure.

3. Convalescent phase–The convalescent phase is characterized by complete disappearance of constitutional symptoms but persistent abnormalities in liver function tests. Symptoms and signs gradually improve.

Table 14–12. Commonly encountered serologic patterns in hepatitis B infection.[1]

HBsAg	Anti-HBs	Anti-HBc	HBeAg	Anti-HBe	Interpretation
+	–	IgM	+	–	Acute HBV infection, high infectivity
+	–	IgG	+	–	Chronic HBV infection, high infectivity
+	–	IgG	–	+	Late acute or chronic HBV infection, low infectivity
+	+	+	+/–	+/–	1. HBsAg of one subtype and heterotypic anti-HBs (common) 2. Process of seroconversion from HBsAg to anti-HBs (rare)
–	–	IgM	+/–	+/–	1. Acute HBV infection 2. Anti-HBc window
–	–	IgG	–	+/–	1. Low-level HBsAg carrier 2. Remote past infection
–	+	IgG	–	+/–	Recovery from HBV infection
–	+	–	–	–	1. Immunization with HBsAg (after vaccination) 2. Remote past infection (?) 3. False-positive

[1]Reproduced, with permission, from Dienstag DL, Wards JR, Isselbacher KJ: Acute hepatitis. In: *Harrison's Principles of Internal Medicine*, 12th ed. Wilson JD et al (editors). McGraw-Hill, 1991.

22. Describe the range of clinical presentations of acute hepatitis.
23. Which viruses can cause hepatitis?
24. What are some extrahepatic manifestations of viral hepatitis?
25. What is the basis for the extrahepatic manifestations of viral hepatitis?

CHRONIC HEPATITIS

Chronic hepatitis is a category of disorders characterized by the combination of liver cell necrosis and inflammation of varying severity persisting for more than 6 months. It may be due to viral infection, drugs and toxins, genetic and metabolic factors, or unknown causes. The severity ranges from an asymptomatic stable illness characterized only by laboratory test abnormalities to a severe, gradually progressive illness culminating in cirrhosis, liver failure, and death. Based on clinical, laboratory, and biopsy findings, chronic hepatitis is often divided into two classes: chronic persistent and chronic active hepatitis. **Chronic persistent hepatitis** is seldom progressive despite persistent biochemical abnormalities reflecting ongoing liver cell necrosis. The clinical course is relatively benign, often characterized by spontaneous resolution (eg, clearance of persistent viral infection). **Chronic active (aggressive) hepatitis** is typically progressive, often resulting ultimately in cirrhosis and its complications or liver failure and death. The characteristics of the two types are summarized in Table 14–13.

Table 14–14. Autoimmune disorders and extrahepatic manifestations associated with chronic active hepatitis.[1]

Thyroiditis
Thyrotoxicosis (rare)
Hypothyroidism
Autoimmune hemolytic anemia
Polyarthritis
Capillaritis
Glomerulonephritis
Pulmonary disorders
    Fibrosing alveolitis
    Primary pulmonary hypertension
Amenorrhea and other menstrual abnormalities
Ulcerative colitis
Monoclonal gammopathy
Hyperviscosity syndrome
Lichen planus
Polymyositis
Uveitis

[1]Reproduced, with permission, from Maddrey WC: Chronic hepatitis. In: *Hepatology: A Textbook of Liver Disease*, 2nd ed. Zakim D, Boyer JD (editors). Saunders, 1990.

Clinical Presentation

Patients may present with fatigue, malaise, low-grade fever, anorexia, weight loss, mild intermittent jaundice, and mild hepatosplenomegaly. Others are initially asymptomatic and present late in the course of the disease with complications of cirrhosis, including variceal bleeding, coagulopathy, encephalopathy, jaundice, and ascites. In contrast to chronic persistent hepatitis, some patients with chronic active hepatitis—particularly those without serologic evidence of antecedent HBV infection—present with extrahepatic symptoms such as skin rash, diarrhea, arthritis, or various autoimmune disorders (Table 14–14).

Table 14–13. Chronic persistent and chronic active hepatitis.[1]

	Chronic Persistent Hepatitis	Chronic Active Hepatitis
Clinical features		
Onset like that of acute hepatitis	≈ 70%	≈ 30%
Recurrent acute episodes	Infrequent	Common
Extrahepatic involvement	Rare	Common
Prognosis	Good	Variable; typically poor
Liver histology		
Piecemeal necrosis	Inconstant	Typical
Site of inflammation	Portal	Portal, extending into lobule
Lobular architecture	Preserved	Distorted
Fibrosis	Slight	Common
Progression to cirrhosis	Rare	Common

[1]Reproduced, with permission, from Ward JR, Isselbacher KJ: Chronic hepatitis. In: *Harrison's Principles of Internal Medicine*, 12th ed. Wilson JD et al (editors). McGraw-Hill, 1991.

Etiology

Either type of chronic hepatitis can be caused by infection with several hepatitis viruses (eg, hepatitis B with or without hepatitis D superinfection and hepatitis C); a variety of drugs and poisons (eg, ethanol, isoniazid, acetaminophen), often in amounts insufficient to cause symptomatic acute hepatitis; genetic and metabolic disorders (eg, α_1-antiprotease [α_1-antitrypsin] deficiency, Wilson's disease, and hemochromatosis); or immune-mediated injury of unknown origin. Table 14–1 summarizes known causes of chronic hepatitis. A specific cause can be determined for only 10–20% of patients. Up to 10% of otherwise healthy individuals with acute hepatitis B remain chronically infected with HBV; of these patients, about two-thirds develop chronic persistent disease and one-third develop chronic active disease (see below). Superinfection with HDV of a patient with chronic HBV infection is associated with a much higher rate of development of chronic active hepatitis than is seen with isolated hepatitis B infection. Hepatitis D superinfection of patients with hepatitis B is also associated with a high incidence of fulminant hepatic failure. Finally, about 50% of individuals with acute posttransfusional or community-acquired hepatitis C develop chronic hepatitis.

Pathogenesis

Many cases of chronic hepatitis are thought to represent an immune-mediated attack on the liver occurring as a result of persistence of certain hepatitis viruses or after prolonged exposure to certain drugs or noxious substances (Table 14–15). In some, no mechanism has been recognized. Evidence that the disorder is immune-mediated is that liver biopsies reveal inflammation (infiltration of lymphocytes) in characteristic regions of the liver architecture (eg, portal versus lobular) (Table 14–13). Furthermore, a variety of autoimmune disorders occur with high frequency in patients with chronic hepatitis (Table 14–14).

A. Postviral Chronic Hepatitis: In approximately 2–10% of cases of HBV infection, the immune response is inadequate to clear the liver of virus, resulting in persistent infection. The individual becomes a chronic carrier, intermittently producing the virus and hence remaining infectious to others. Biochemically, these patients are often found to have viral DNA integrated into their genomes in a manner that results in abnormal expression of certain viral proteins with or without production of intact virus. Viral antigens expressed on the hepatocyte cell surface are associated with class I HLA determinants, thus eliciting lymphocyte cytotoxicity and resulting in hepatitis. The severity of chronic active hepatitis is largely dependent on the activity of viral replication and the response by the host's immune system.

Independently of the risk of progression to cirrhosis, chronic hepatitis B infection predisposes the patient to the development of hepatocellular carcinoma. It remains unclear whether hepatitis B infection is the initiator or simply a promoter in the process of tumorigenesis.

B. Alcoholic Chronic Hepatitis: Chronic liver disease in response to some poisons or toxins may represent triggering of an underlying genetic predisposition to immune attack on the liver. In alcoholic hepatitis, however, repeated episodes of acute injury ultimately cause necrosis, fibrosis, and regeneration, leading eventually to cirrhosis (Figure 14–10). As in other forms of liver disease, there is considerable variation in the extent of symptoms prior to development of cirrhosis.

C. Idiopathic Chronic Hepatitis: Some patients develop chronic active hepatitis in the absence of evidence of preceding viral hepatitis or exposure to noxious agents (Figure 14–11). These patients typically have serologic evidence of disordered immunoregulation, manifested as hyperglobulinemia and circulating autoantibodies. Nearly 75% of these patients are women, and many have other autoimmune disorders. A genetic predisposition is strongly suggested. Patients with idiopathic autoimmune chronic active hepatitis show histologic improvement in liver biopsies after treatment with systemic corticosteroids. The clinical response, however, can be variable.

Pathology

Both forms of chronic hepatitis share the common histopathologic features of (1) inflammatory infiltration of hepatic portal areas with mononuclear cells, especially lymphocytes and plasma cells; and (2) necrosis of hepatocytes within the parenchyma or immediately adjacent to portal areas (periportal hepatitis, or "piecemeal necrosis").

Table 14–15. Drugs implicated in the etiology of chronic hepatitis.[1]

Drug	Use
Acetaminophen	Analgesic
Amiodarone	Antiarrhythmic
Aspirin	Analgesic
Ethanol	Abuse
Isoniazid	Antituberculous therapy
Methyldopa	Antihypertensive
Nitrofurantoin	Antibiotic
Propylthiouracil	Antithyroid therapy
Sulfonamides	Antibiotic

[1]Modified and reproduced, with permission, from Bass NM, Ockner RK: Drug-induced liver disease. In: *Hepatology: A Textbook of Liver Disease*, 2nd ed. Zakim D, Boyer JD (editors). Saunders, 1990.

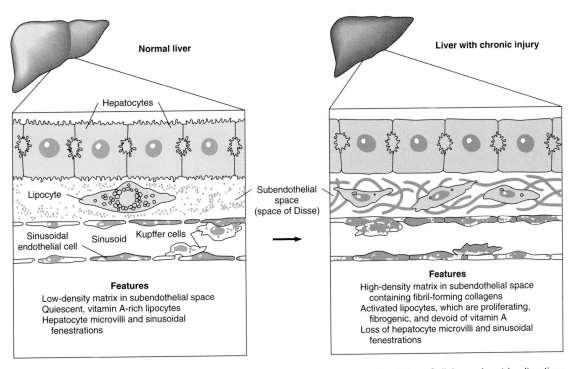

Figure 14–10. Changes in the hepatic subendothelial space during fibrosing liver injury. Cellular and matrix alterations in the space of Disse are critical events in the pathogenesis of hepatic fibrosis. The activation of lipocytes, characterized by proliferation and increased fibrogenesis, is associated with the replacement of the normal low-density matrix with a high-density matrix. These alterations are likely to underlie, at least in part, the loss of both endothelial fenestrations (pores) and hepatocytic microvilli typical of chronic liver injury. (Reproduced, with permission, from Friedman SL: The cellular basis of hepatic fibrosis. N Engl J Med 1993;328:1828.)

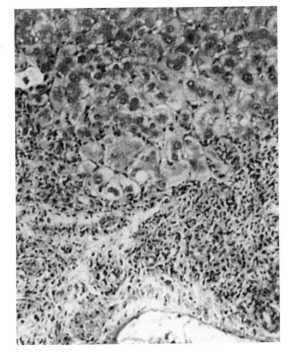

Figure 14–11. Chronic active hepatitis, showing marked lymphocytic infiltration and fibrosis of the portal areas. The lymphocytes extend into the peripheral part of the lobule through the limiting plate. There is ongoing necrosis of hepatocytes in the peripheral part of the lobule (piecemeal necrosis). (Reproduced, with permission, from Chandrasoma P, Taylor CE: *Concise Pathology,* 3rd ed. Appleton & Lange, 1998.)

In chronic persistent hepatitis, the overall architecture of the liver is preserved. Histologically, the liver reveals a characteristic lymphocyte and plasma cell infiltrate confined to the portal triad without disruption of the limiting plate and no evidence of active hepatocyte necrosis. There is little or no fibrosis, and what there is is generally restricted to the portal area; there is no sign of cirrhosis. A "cobblestone" appearance of liver cells is seen, indicating regeneration of hepatocytes.

In chronic active hepatitis, the portal areas are expanded and densely infiltrated by lymphocytes, histiocytes, and plasma cells. There is necrosis of hepatocytes at the periphery of the lobule, with erosion of the limiting plate surrounding the portal triads (piecemeal necrosis; Figure 14–11). More severe cases also show evidence of necrosis and fibrosis between portal triads. There is disruption of normal liver architecture by bands of scar tissue and inflammatory cells that link portal areas to one another and to central areas (bridging necrosis). These connective tissue bridges are evidence of remodeling of hepatic architecture, a crucial step in the development of cirrhosis. Fibrosis may extend from the portal areas into the lobules, isolating hepatocytes into clusters and enveloping bile ducts. Regeneration of hepatocytes is seen with mitotic figures, multinucleated cells, rosette formation, and regenerative pseudolobules. Progression to cirrhosis is signaled by extensive fibrosis and regenerating nodules.

Clinical Manifestations

Some patients with chronic persistent hepatitis are entirely asymptomatic and identified only in the course of routine blood testing; others have an insidious onset of nonspecific symptoms such as anorexia, malaise, and fatigue or hepatic symptoms such as right upper quadrant abdominal discomfort or pain. Fatigue in chronic hepatitis may be related to a change in the hypothalamic-adrenal neuroendocrine axis brought about by altered endogenous opioidergic neurotransmission. Jaundice, if present, is usually mild. There may be mild tender hepatomegaly and occasional splenomegaly. Palmar erythema and spider telangiectases are seen in severe cases. Other extrahepatic manifestations are unusual. By definition, signs of cirrhosis and portal hypertension (such as ascites, collateral circulation, and encephalopathy) are absent. Laboratory studies show mild to moderate increases in serum aminotransferase, bilirubin, and globulin levels. Serum albumin and the prothrombin time are normal until late in the progression of liver disease.

The clinical manifestations of chronic hepatitis probably reflect the role of a systemic genetically controlled immune disorder in the pathogenesis of chronic active hepatitis. Acne, hirsutism, and amenorrhea may occur as a reflection of the hormonal effects of chronic liver disease. Laboratory studies in patients with chronic active hepatitis are invariably abnormal to various degrees. Moreover, these abnormalities do not correlate with clinical severity. Thus, the serum bilirubin, alkaline phosphatase, and globulin levels may be normal and aminotransferase levels only mildly elevated at the same time that a liver biopsy reveals severe chronic active hepatitis. However, an elevated prothrombin time usually reflects severe liver disease.

The complications of chronic active hepatitis are those of progression to cirrhosis—variceal bleeding, encephalopathy, coagulopathy, hypersplenism, and ascites. These are largely due to portal-to-systemic shunting rather than diminished hepatocyte reserve (see below).

Patients with chronic liver disease can develop a poorly understood form of renal disease called **hepatorenal syndrome,** which has a dismal prognosis. This disorder is distinct from both prerenal azotemia and acute tubular necrosis. It is characterized by progressively rising serum creatinine and diminished urine volume. It occurs typically in patients with massive tense ascites and is often precipitated by overly aggressive attempts at diuresis in hospital. The urine produced is notable for an extremely low sodium content and an absence of casts, resembling the findings in prerenal azotemia. Yet when central venous pressures are measured the patient does not show intravascular volume depletion, and the disorder does not respond to hydration with normal saline. The renal abnormalities of the hepatorenal syndrome appear to be functional, since no pathologic changes are identifiable in the kidney, and when a kidney is transplanted from a patient dying of hepatorenal syndrome, it functions well in a recipient without liver disease. It remains to be determined whether this form of renal failure represents loss of an as yet unrecognized hormone produced by the liver that affects the kidneys or is the consequence of some combination of local hemodynamic effects resulting in diminished renal perfusion.

In recent years, the role of nitric oxide as an intracellular second messenger with vasodilatory effects on vascular beds and the role of endothelins, peptides synthesized by vascular endothelium which have vasoconstrictive properties, have been identified. A speculated role for nitric oxide-mediated peripheral arterial vasodilation combined with sympathetic nervous system and endothelin-mediated renal vasoconstriction has been proposed to explain the salt and water retention of cirrhosis. Those same mechanisms, in the extreme case, may give rise to the hepatorenal syndrome.

26. What are the categories of chronic hepatitis based on histologic findings on liver biopsy?
27. What are the causes of chronic hepatitis?
28. What are the consequences of chronic hepatitis?

CIRRHOSIS

Clinical Presentation

Cirrhosis is an irreversible distortion of normal liver architecture characterized by hepatic injury, fibrosis, and nodular regeneration. The clinical presentations of cirrhosis are a consequence of both progressive hepatocellular dysfunction and portal hypertension (Figure 14–12). As with other presentations of liver disease, not all patients with cirrhosis develop life-threatening complications. Indeed, in nearly 40% of cases of cirrhosis, it is diagnosed at autopsy in patients who did not manifest obvious signs of end-stage liver disease.

Etiology

The causes of cirrhosis are listed in Table 14–1. The initial injury can be due to a wide range of processes. A crucial feature is that the liver injury is not acute and self-limited but rather chronic and progressive. In the United States, alcohol abuse is the most common cause of cirrhosis. In other countries, infectious agents (particularly hepatitis B and hepatitis C viruses) are the most common causes. Other causes include chronic biliary obstruction, metabolic disorders, chronic congestive heart failure, and primary (autoimmune) biliary cirrhosis.

Pathogenesis

Increased or altered synthesis of collagen and other connective tissue or basement membrane components of the extracellular matrix is implicated in the development of hepatic fibrosis and thus in the pathogenesis of cirrhosis. The role of the extracellular matrix in cellular function is an important area of research, and recent studies suggest that it is involved in modulating the activities of the cells with which it

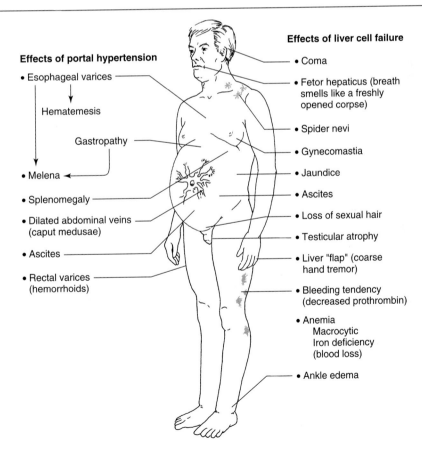

Figure 14–12. Clinical effects of cirrhosis of the liver. (Reproduced, with permission, from Chandrasoma P, Taylor CE: *Concise Pathology,* 3rd ed. Appleton & Lange, 1998.)

is in contact. Thus, fibrosis may affect not only the physics of blood flow through the liver but also the functions of the cells themselves.

Hepatic fibrosis appears to occur in three situations: (1) as an immune response, (2) as part of the process of wound healing, and (3) in response to agents that induce primary fibrogenesis. HBV and schistosoma species are good examples of agents producing fibrosis on an immunologic basis. Agents such as carbon tetrachloride or hepatitis A that attack and kill hepatocytes directly are examples of agents producing fibrosis as part of wound healing. In both immune responses and wound healing, the fibrosis is triggered indirectly by the effects of cytokines released from invading inflammatory cells. Finally, certain agents such as ethanol and iron may cause primary fibrogenesis by directly increasing collagen gene transcription and thus increasing also the amount of connective tissue secreted by cells.

The actual culprit in all of these mechanisms of increased fibrogenesis may be the fat-storing cells of the hepatic reticuloendothelial system. In response to cytokines, they differentiate from quiescent cells in which vitamin A is stored into myofibroblasts, which lose their vitamin A storage capacity and become actively engaged in extracellular matrix production. It appears that hepatic fibrosis occurs in two stages. The first stage is characterized by a change in extracellular matrix composition from non-cross-linked, non-fibril-forming collagen to collagen that is more dense and subject to cross-link formation. At this stage, liver injury is still reversible. The second stage involves formation of subendothelial collagen cross-links, proliferation of myoepithelial cells, and distortion of hepatic architecture with the appearance of regenerating nodules. This second stage is irreversible. Alterations in the composition of extracellular matrix can mediate changes in cellular functions of hepatocytes and other cells such as lipocytes (Figures 14–10 and 14–13). Thus, the change in collagen balance may play a crucial role in proceeding from reversible to irreversible forms of chronic liver injury by affecting hepatocyte function as well.

Regardless of the possible effects on hepatocyte function, the increased fibrosis markedly alters the nature of blood flow in the liver, resulting in important complications to be discussed below.

The manner in which alcohol causes chronic liver disease and cirrhosis is not well understood. However, chronic alcohol abuse is associated with impaired protein synthesis and secretion, mitochondrial injury, lipid peroxidation, formation of acetaldehyde and its interaction with cellular proteins and membrane lipids, cellular hypoxia, and both cell-mediated and antibody-mediated cytotoxicity. The relative importance of each of these factors in producing cell injury is unknown. Genetic, nutritional, and environmental factors (including simultaneous exposure to other hepatotoxins) also influence the development of liver disease in chronic alcoholics. Finally, acute

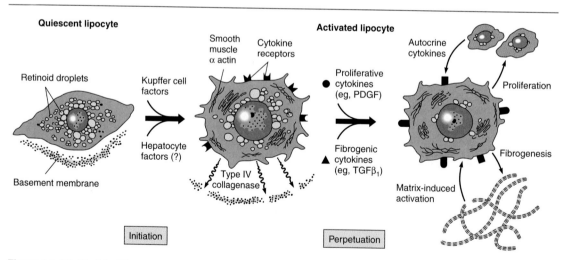

Figure 14–13. Model of lipocyte activation. Current evidence suggests that the process of lipocyte activation is a cascade occurring in at least two stages. Initiation is characterized by cellular enlargement, the expression of smooth muscle α actin, and the induction of cytokine receptors; initiating stimuli may include as yet uncharacterized paracrine factors from Kupffer cells, hepatocytes, or both. Initiation may also include the early disruption of the extracellular matrix through the secretion by lipocytes of type IV collagenase, leading to its eventual replacement with fibril-forming collagens. Perpetuation reflects the subsequent effects of proliferative and fibrogenic cytokines on the cells and the additional stimulation in response to the altered extracellular matrix. (PDGF, platelet-derived growth factor; TGFβ1, transforming growth factor β1.) (Reproduced, with permission, from Friedman SL: The cellular basis of hepatic fibrosis. N Engl J Med 1993;328:1828.)

liver injury (eg, from exposure to alcohol or other toxins) from which a person with a normal liver would fully recover may be sufficient to produce irreversible decompensation (eg, hepatorenal syndrome) in a patient with underlying hepatic cirrhosis.

Pathology

Grossly, the liver may be large or small, but it always has a firm consistency. Liver biopsy is the only method of definitively diagnosing cirrhosis.

Histologically, all forms of cirrhosis are characterized by three findings: (1) marked distortion of hepatic architecture, (2) scarring due to increased deposition of fibrous tissue and collagen, and (3) regenerative nodules surrounded by scar tissue. When the nodules are small (< 3 mm) and uniform in size, the process is termed **micronodular cirrhosis**. In **macronodular cirrhosis**, the nodules are over 3 mm and variable in size. Cirrhosis due to alcohol abuse is usually micronodular but can be macronodular or both micro- and macronodular. Scarring may be most severe in central regions, or dense bands of connective tissue may join portal and central areas.

More specific histopathologic findings may help to establish the cause of cirrhosis. For example, invasion and destruction of bile ducts by granulomas suggests primary (autoimmune) biliary cirrhosis; extensive iron deposition in hepatocytes and bile ducts suggests hemochromatosis; and alcoholic hyalin and infiltration with polymorphonuclear cells suggest alcoholic cirrhosis.

Clinical Manifestations

The clinical manifestations of progressive hepatocellular dysfunction in cirrhosis are similar to those of acute or chronic hepatitis and include constitutional symptoms and signs: fatigue, loss of vigor, and weight loss; gastrointestinal symptoms and signs: nausea, vomiting, jaundice, and tender hepatomegaly; and extrahepatic symptoms and signs: palmar erythema, spider angiomas, muscle wasting, parotid and lacrimal gland enlargement, gynecomastia and testicular atrophy in men, menstrual irregularities in women, and coagulopathy.

Clinical manifestations of portal hypertension include ascites, portosystemic shunting, encephalopathy, splenomegaly, and esophageal and gastric varices with intermittent hemorrhage (see Table 14–16).

A. Portal Hypertension: Portal hypertension is due to a rise in intrahepatic vascular resistance. The cirrhotic liver loses the physiologic characteristic of a low-pressure circuit for blood flow seen in the normal liver. The increased blood pressure within the sinusoids is transmitted back to the portal vein. Because the portal vein lacks valves, this elevated pressure is transmitted back to other vascular beds, resulting in splenomegaly, portal-to-systemic shunting, and many of the complications of cirrhosis discussed below.

Table 14–16. Complications of cirrhosis.

Due to portal hypertension with portal-to-systemic shunting
Ascites and increased risk of spontaneous bacterial peritonitis
Increased risk of sepsis
Increased risk of disseminated intravascular coagulation
Splenomegaly with thrombocytopenia
Encephalopathy
Varices
Drug sensitivity
Bile acid deficiency with malabsorption of fat and fat-soluble vitamins
Hyperestrogenemia
Hyperglycemia
Due to loss of hepatocytes
Hypoglycemia
Coagulopathy due to deficient clotting factor synthesis
Peripheral edema due to hypoalbuminemia
Hepatic coma
Other complications
Hepatorenal syndrome
Hepatocellular carcinoma

B. Ascites: Ascites is the presence of excess fluid in the peritoneal cavity. It can develop in patients with conditions other than liver disease, including protein-calorie malnutrition (due to hypoalbuminemia) and cancer (due to lymphatic obstruction). In patients with liver disease, ascites is due to portal hypertension.

Patients with ascites develop physical examination findings of increasing abdominal girth, a fluid wave, a ballotable liver, and shifting dullness. The mechanism by which portal hypertension results in accumulation of ascites in some patients with liver disease is complex and multifactorial (Figure 14–14). It is useful to first recognize that liver disease with ascites formation occurs in a wide clinical spectrum. At one end is fully compensated portal hypertension with no ascites present—because the volume of ascites generated is less than the approximately 800–1200 mL/d capacity of the peritoneal lymphatic drainage. At the other extreme is the typically fatal hepatorenal syndrome, in which patients with liver disease, usually with massive ascites, succumb to rapidly progressing acute renal failure. The hepatorenal syndrome seems to be precipitated by intense and inappropriate renal vasoconstriction and is characterized by extreme sodium retention typical of prerenal azotemia but in the absence of true volume depletion (see Chapter 16).

Over the years, various mechanisms have been proposed to explain ascites formation (Figure 14–14). Some hypotheses have proposed intravascular volume depletion, either real or "imagined" by the kidney, as a common theme in the pathophysiology of ascites. In this view, it is the underlying hemodynamic disorder that triggers reflex renal sodium retention. Thus, elevated hepatic sinusoidal pressure

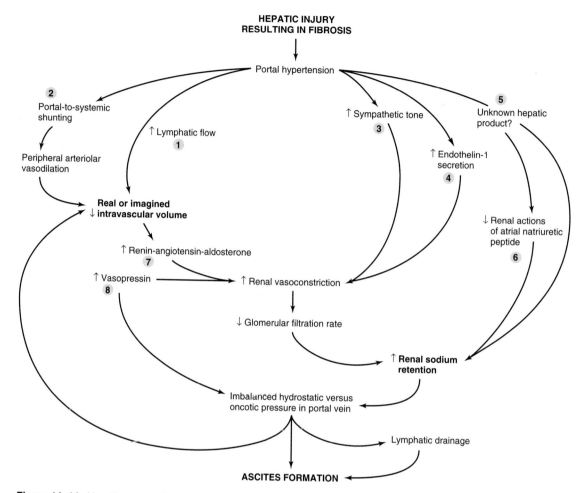

Figure 14–14. Hypotheses put forward to explain the pathophysiology of ascites formation in patients with liver disease. Hypotheses involving real or apparent intravascular volume depletion in triggering ascites formation: (1) "underfilling" hypothesis; (2) "peripheral vasodilation" hypothesis. Hypotheses involving inappropriate increased renal sodium retention: (3) increased sympathetic tone; (4) increased endothelin-1 secretion; unknown hepatic product working directly (5) or indirectly via antagonism of atrial natriuretic peptide, (6) or mechanisms (3) or (4) to trigger renal sodium retention. Regardless of the initiating mechanism, once ascites has formed, response to real or imagined intravascular volume depletion triggers (7) and (8).

results in "underfilling" of the central vein with diversion of intravascular volume to the hepatic lymphatics, which, like the central vein, drain the space of Disse. When this excess fluid exceeds the capacity of lymphatic drainage, hydrostatic pressure increases. The fluid can then be seen to visibly "weep" from the lymphatics and pool in the abdominal cavity as ascites. Another hemodynamic hypothesis involves portal-to-systemic shunting in liver disease. With shunting, vasodilatory products (eg, nitric oxide) that are normally cleared by the liver are instead delivered to the systemic circulation, where they cause peripheral arteriolar vasodilation, decreased renal arterial perfusion, and reflex renal arterial vasoconstriction and increased renal tubular sodium resorp-

tion. Retention of sodium expands the intravascular volume, which exacerbates portal venous hypertension. The imbalance between hydrostatic versus oncotic pressure in the portal vein results in ascites formation, as described above.

Others have proposed that inappropriate renal sodium retention is the inciting event in the development of ascites. In this view, ascites is the consequence of "overflow" from the intravascular volume-expanded portal system. But what triggers the inappropriate renal sodium retention? One possibility is that there may exist a hepatorenal reflex by which elevated sinusoidal pressure triggers increased sympathetic tone or endothelin-1 secretion. Either of these pathways could cause an inappropriate degree of renal vasoconstriction, fall in glomerular filtration rate, and, by tubuloglomerular feedback (see Chapter 16), sodium retention. Note that endothelin-1 is both a renal vasoconstrictor and a stimulant of epinephrine secretion, which in turn stimulates more endothelin-1 secretion. Alternatively, it is possible that an as yet unidentified product from the diseased liver interferes with atrial natriuretic peptide (ANP) action at the kidney or is in some other way responsible for an inappropriate increase in renal sodium retention. Regardless of the initial inciting event, once ascites formation has occurred, intravascular volume depletion will trigger activation of both the renin-angiotensin-aldosterone system and vasopressin (ADH) as mechanisms of compensation through sodium and water retention, respectively.

No single hypothesis of pathogenesis easily explains all findings, at all points in time, during the natural history of portal hypertension. Most likely, multiple mechanisms contribute to development of ascites and to its perpetuation, worsening, or improvement in diverse clinical situations. In any individual patient, depending on genetic, environmental, and other factors—including the patient's stage in the natural history of liver disease—one mechanism may dominate over others.

An important recent development has been the use of transhepatic intrajugular portal-to-systemic shunting (TIPS) as a means of decompressing the portal vein in patients with ascites. While encephalopathy can be a problem in some, most patients experience a remarkable lessening of ascites. As a result of the procedure, peripheral arteriolar vasodilation appears to increase (perhaps due to shunting of vasodilators such as nitric oxide that are normally cleared by the liver), yet ascites is generally dramatically improved. This finding suggests that arteriolar vasodilation is not the primary precipitant of ascites formation, though it may be a contributor. Other studies suggest a role for a sympathetic neural reflex as a trigger of renal sodium retention in response to elevated portal sinusoidal pressure, which would be relieved by TIPS. Regardless of the initial events, once fully established, many if not all of the mechanisms described in Figure 14–14 are likely to contribute to ascites formation.

C. Hypoalbuminemia and Peripheral Edema: Progressive worsening of hepatocellular function in cirrhosis can result in a fall in the concentration of albumin and other serum proteins synthesized by the liver. As the concentration of these plasma proteins goes down, the plasma oncotic pressure is lowered, thereby tilting the balance of hemodynamic forces toward the development of both peripheral edema and ascites.

These hemodynamic changes further contribute to an avid sodium-retaining state despite total body water and sodium overload seen by urinalysis in the cirrhotic patient. Serum sodium may be low as a result of superimposed water retention due to antidiuretic hormone release triggered by volume stimuli. A low serum potassium and metabolic alkalosis may be observed as a consequence of elevated aldosterone levels responding to renin release (and angiotensin II release) by the kidneys, which sense afferent intravascular depletion.

D. Spontaneous Bacterial Peritonitis: Spontaneous bacterial peritonitis is the development of infected ascites in the absence of a clear event (such as bowel perforation) that would account for the entry of pathogenic organisms into the peritoneal space. Symptoms and signs include fever, hypotension, abdominal pain or tenderness, decreased or absent bowel sounds, or abrupt onset of hepatic encephalopathy in a patient with ascites.

Patients with large-volume ascites or with very low ascitic fluid protein levels are at increased risk for this complication. Ascitic fluid is an excellent culture medium for a variety of pathogens, including Enterobacteriaceae (chiefly *E coli*), group D streptococci (enterococci), *Streptococcus pneumoniae,* and viridans streptococci. The greater risk in patients with low ascitic fluid protein levels may be due to a low level of opsonic activity in the fluid.

The exact pathogenesis of spontaneous bacterial peritonitis is unknown. Peritonitis may occur because of bacterial seeding of the ascitic fluid via the blood or lymph or by bacteria traversing the gut wall. Enteric organisms may enter the portal venous blood via the portosystemic collaterals, bypassing the reticuloendothelial system of the liver.

E. Gastroesophageal Varices and Bleeding: As blood flow through the liver is progressively impeded, hepatic portal venous pressure rises. In response to the elevated portal venous pressure, there is enlargement of blood vessels that anastomose with the portal vein, such as those on the surface of the bowel and lower esophagus. These enlarged vessels are termed **varices.** Physical examination may reveal enlargement of hemorrhoidal and periumbilical vessels. Gastroesophageal varices are of more significance clinically, however, because of their tendency to rupture. The resulting massive bleeding is often life-threatening, since varices in these sites are not easy to tamponade. Gastrointestinal bleeding from varices and other sources (eg, duodenal ulcer, gastritis) in patients with cirrhosis is often exacerbated by concomitant coagulopathy (see below).

F. Hepatic Encephalopathy: Hepatic encephalopathy is manifested by waxing and waning alterations in mental status that occur as a consequence of advanced decompensated liver disease or portal-to-systemic shunting (see Table 14–17 for a list of common precipitants). Abnormalities range from subtle alterations in mental status to profound obtundation. Cognitive changes include a full spectrum of mental abnormalities, ranging from mild confusion, apathy, agitation, euphoria, restlessness, and reversal of the

Table 14–17. Common precipitants of hepatic encephalopathy.[1]

Increased nitrogen load
  Gastrointestinal bleeding
  Excess dietary protein
  Azotemia
  Constipation
Electrolyte imbalance
  Hypokalemia
  Alkalosis
  Hypoxia
  Hypovolemia
Drugs
  Opioids, tranquilizers, sedatives
  Diuretics
Miscellaneous
  Infection
  Surgery
  Superimposed acute liver disease
  Progressive liver disease

[1]Reproduced, with permission, from Podolsky DK, Isselbacher KJ: Cirrhosis of the liver. In: *Harrison's Principles of Internal Medicine,* 12th ed. Wilson JD et al (editors). McGraw-Hill, 1991.

day-night sleep pattern to somnolence, marked confusion, and even coma. Motor changes range from fine tremor, slowed coordination, and asterixis to decerebrate posturing and flaccidity. **Asterixis** is a phenomenon of intermittent myoelectrical silence manifested by many muscle groups and enhanced by fatigue. It is best demonstrated by asking the patient to flex the wrists with fingers extended ("stop traffic") and then observing a flapping motion of the fingers. Cerebral edema, which is an important accompanying feature in patients with encephalopathy in acute liver disease, is not seen in cirrhotic patients with encephalopathy.

Common precipitants of encephalopathy are onset of gastrointestinal bleeding, increased dietary protein intake, and an increased catabolic rate due to infection (including spontaneous bacterial peritonitis). Similarly, because of compromised "first-pass" clearance of ingested drugs, affected patients are exquisitely sensitive to sedatives and other drugs normally metabolized in the liver.

The pathogenesis of hepatic encephalopathy is poorly understood. One proposed mechanism postulates that the encephalopathy is caused by toxins in the gut such as ammonia, derived from metabolic degradation of urea or protein; glutamine, derived from degradation of ammonia; or mercaptans, derived from degradation of sulfur-containing compounds. Because of anatomic or functional shunts, these toxins bypass the liver's detoxification processes and produce alterations in mental status. Increased levels of ammonia, glutamine, and mercaptans can be found in the blood and cerebrospinal fluid. However, blood ammonia and spinal fluid glutamine levels correlate poorly with the presence and severity of encephalopathy.

Alternatively, there may be impairment of the normal blood-brain barrier, rendering the central nervous system susceptible to various noxious agents. Increased levels of other substances, including metabolic products such as short-chain fatty acids and endogenous benzodiazepine-like metabolites, have also been found in the blood. Importantly, some patients show improvement in encephalopathy when treated with flumazenil, a benzodiazepine receptor antagonist.

A third proposed mechanism postulates a role for GABA, the principal inhibitory neurotransmitter of the brain. GABA is produced in the gut, and increased levels are found in the blood of patients with liver failure.

A fourth proposal postulates that there is an increased entry of aromatic amino acids into the central nervous system, resulting in increased synthesis of "false" neurotransmitters such as octopamine and decreased synthesis of normal neurotransmitters such as norepinephrine.

G. Coagulopathy: Factors contributing to coagulopathy in cirrhosis include loss of hepatic synthesis of clotting factors, some of which have a half-life of just a few hours. Under these circumstances, a minor or self-limited source of bleeding can become massive.

Hepatocytes are also functionally involved in maintenance of a normal coagulation cascade through the absorption of vitamin K (a fat-soluble vitamin whose absorption is dependent on bile flow), which is necessary for the activation of some clotting factors (II, VII, IX, X). An ominous sign of the severity of liver disease is the development of a coagulopathy that does not respond to parenteral vitamin K, suggesting deficient clotting factor synthesis rather than impaired absorption of vitamin K due to fat malabsorption. Finally, loss of the liver's capacity to remove activated clotting factors and fibrin degradation products may play a role in the increased susceptibility to **disseminated intravascular coagulation,** a syndrome of coagulation factor consumption that results in uncontrolled simultaneous clotting and bleeding.

H. Splenomegaly and Hypersplenism: Enlargement of the spleen is a consequence of elevated portal venous pressure and consequent engorgement of the organ. Thrombocytopenia and hemolytic anemia occur because of sequestering of formed elements of the blood in the spleen, from which they are normally cleared as they age and are damaged.

I. Hepatorenal Syndrome: This disorder is discussed in the section on clinical manifestations of chronic hepatitis.

J. Hepatocellular Carcinoma: Hepatocellular carcinoma occurs in up to 5% of cirrhotic patients. Several etiologic factors have been identified in the development of this tumor: (1) Malignant transformation is heightened in any form of chronic liver disease. (2) The risk of developing hepatocellular carcinoma is increased 100-fold in chronic HBV carriers. (3) Mycotoxins—metabolites of saprophytic fungi—are known hepatic carcinogens and have been proposed to act synergistically with cirrhosis and HBV infection in increasing the risk of liver cell cancer. (4) Hormonal factors have been implicated by experimental studies. The tumor is known to have a male predominance.

K. Miscellaneous Manifestations: Other findings on physical examination of patients with cirrhosis include **spider angiomas** (prominent blood vessels seen in the skin, particularly on the face and trunk), **Dupuytren's contractures** (fibrosis of the palmar fascia), testicular atrophy, **gynecomastia** (enlargement of breast tissue in men), palmar erythema, lacrimal and parotid gland enlargement, and diminished axillary and pubic hair (Figure 14–12). These findings are largely a consequence of estrogen excess due to decreased clearance of endogenous estrogens by the diseased liver combined with decreased hepatic synthesis of steroid hormone-binding globulin. Both of these mechanisms result in tissues receiving higher than normal concentrations of estrogens. In addition, a longer half-life of androgens may allow a greater degree of "peripheral aromatization" (conversion to estrogens by adipose tissue, hair follicles, etc), further increasing estrogen-like effects in patients with cirrhosis. Xanthomas of the eyelids and extensor surfaces of tendons of the wrists and ankles can occur with chronic cholestasis such as occurs in primary biliary cirrhosis. Finally, profound muscle wasting and cachexia in cirrhosis probably reflect diminution of the liver's synthesis of carbohydrate, lipid, and amino acids.

---

29. What are the defining features of cirrhosis?
30. What are the three categories of hepatic fibrosis? Name one agent causing each.
31. What are the two postulated stages in the development of cirrhosis?
32. What are some ways alcohol may injure the liver?
33. What are the major clinical manifestations of cirrhosis?
34. For each major clinical manifestation of cirrhosis, suggest a reasonable hypothesis to account for its pathogenesis.

REFERENCES

General

Achord JL: Alcohol and the liver. Scientific American Science and Medicine 1995 March/April:16.

Hill SA, McQueen MJ: Reverse cholesterol transport—a review of the process and its clinical implications. Clin Biochem 1997;30:517.

Jaeschke H: Cellular adhesion molecules: Regulation and functional significance in the pathogenesis of liver disease. Am J Physiol 1997;36:G602.

Kaplan LM: Leptin, obesity, and liver disease. Gastroenterology 1998;115:997.

Patel T et al: Dysregulation of apoptosis as a mechanism of liver disease: An overview. Semin Liver Dis 1998; 18:105.

Steer CJ: Liver regeneration. FASEB J 1995;9:1396.

Acute Liver Disease

Farrell GC: Drug-induced hepatic injury. J Gastroenterol Hepatol 1997;12:S242.

Koziel MJ: Immunology of viral hepatitis. Am J Med 1996;100:98.

Plevris JN, Schina M, Hayes PC: Review article: The management of acute liver failure. Aliment Pharmacol Ther 1998;12:405.

Chronic Liver Disease

Chung RT et al: Complications of chronic liver disease. Gastrointest Emerg 1995;11:431.

Bataller R et al: Hepatorenal syndrome: definition, pathophysiology, clinical features and management. Kidney International 1998;53(Suppl 66):S47.

Chang KM: The mechanisms of chronicity in hepatitis C virus infection. Gastroenterology 1998;115:1015.

Van Den Berg AP: Autoimmune hepatitis: pathogenesis, diagnosis and treatment. Scand J Gastroenterol 1998; 33(Suppl 225):66.

Cirrhosis

Williams EJ, Iredale JP: Liver cirrhosis. Postgrad Med J 1998;74:193.

15 | Disorders of the Exocrine Pancreas

Stephen J. McPhee, MD

The pancreas is a gland with both exocrine and endocrine functions. The exocrine pancreas contains **acini** that secrete pancreatic juice into the duodenum through the pancreatic ducts (Figure 15–1). Pancreatic juice contains a number of enzymes, some of which are initially made in an inactive form. Once activated, these enzymes help to digest food and prepare it for absorption in the intestine. Disorders interfering with normal pancreatic enzyme activity (pancreatic insufficiency) cause maldigestion of fat and steatorrhea (fatty stools). Dysfunction of the exocrine pancreas results from inflammation (acute pancreatitis, chronic pancreatitis), neoplasm (pancreatic carcinoma), or duct obstruction by stones or abnormally viscid mucus (cystic fibrosis).

The endocrine pancreas is composed of the **islets of Langerhans.** The islets are distributed throughout the pancreas and contain several different hormone-producing cells. The islet cells manufacture hormones such as insulin that are important in nutrient absorption, storage, and metabolism. Dysfunction of the endocrine pancreas causes diabetes mellitus (see Chapter 18).

Both exocrine and endocrine pancreatic dysfunction occur together in some patients.

NORMAL STRUCTURE & FUNCTION OF THE EXOCRINE PANCREAS

ANATOMY

The pancreas is a solid organ that lies transversely across the posterior abdominal wall deep within the epigastrium. It is firmly fixed in the retroperitoneum in front of the abdominal aorta and the first and second lumbar vertebrae. Thus, the pain of acute or chronic pancreatitis is situated deep in the epigastric region and frequently radiates to the back.

Normally, the pancreas measures about 15 cm long, though it weighs less than 110 g. The organ is covered by a thin capsule of connective tissue that sends septa into it, separating it into lobules.

The pancreas can be divided into four parts: a head—including the uncinate process—a neck, a body, and a tail. The head lies in the curved space between the first, second, and third portions of the duodenum. The uncinate process is that portion of the head which extends to the left behind the superior mesenteric vessels. The neck connects the head and body. The body is situated horizontally in the retroperitoneal space with the tail extending toward the hilum of the spleen.

The exocrine pancreas is drained by a major central duct called the **duct of Wirsung,** which runs the length of the gland. This duct is normally about 3–4 mm in diameter. In most individuals, the pancreatic duct enters the duodenum at the duodenal papilla alongside the common bile duct. The sphincter of Oddi surrounds both ducts. In about one-third of individuals, the duct of Wirsung and the common bile duct join to form a common channel before terminating at the **ampulla of Vater** (Figure 15–1).

Many individuals also have a separate accessory pancreatic duct called the **duct of Santorini** that runs from the head and body of the gland to enter the duodenum about 2 cm proximal to the duodenal papilla (Figure 15–1). Occasionally, the accessory duct joins with the major pancreatic duct.

HISTOLOGY

The exocrine pancreas consists of clusters of acini, or **lobules,** which are drained by ductules. The islets of Langerhans of the endocrine pancreas are clusters of a few hundred cells each located between the lobules.

Each pancreatic acinus is composed of several acinar cells surrounding a lumen (Figure 15–2). The acinar cells synthesize and secrete enzymes. On histologic examination, acinar cells are typical protein-

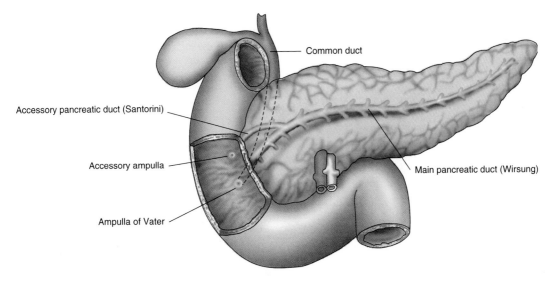

Figure 15–1. Anatomy of the pancreas. (Courtesy of W Silen.) (Reproduced, with permission, from Way LW [editor]: *Current Surgical Diagnosis & Treatment,* 10th ed. Appleton & Lange, 1994.)

secreting cells. They are pyramidal epithelial cells arranged in rows. Their apexes join to form the lumen of the acinus. **Zymogen granules** containing digestive enzymes are found in the acinar cells. These granules are discharged by exocytosis from the apexes of the cells into the lumen. The number of zymogen granules in the cells varies, with more being found during fasting and fewer after a meal.

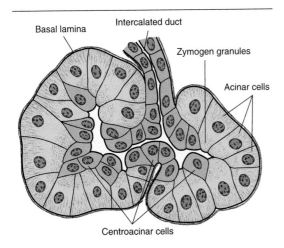

Figure 15–2. Schematic drawing of the pancreatic acini. Acinar cells are pyramidal in shape, with zymogen granules at their apexes. (Reproduced, with permission, from Junqueira LC, Carneiro J, Kelley RO: *Basic Histology,* 9th ed. Appleton & Lange, 1998.)

PHYSIOLOGY

Composition of Pancreatic Juice

About 1500 mL of pancreatic juice is secreted each day. Pancreatic juice contains water, ions, and a variety of proteins. The principal ions in pancreatic juice are HCO_3^-, Cl^-, Na^+, and K^+. Of these, HCO_3^- is particularly important. At maximum flow rates, the concentration of HCO_3^- in pancreatic juice may reach 150 meq/L (versus 24 meq/L in plasma), and the pH of the juice may reach 8.3. The alkaline nature of pancreatic juice plays a major role in neutralizing the gastric acid entering the duodenum with ingested food (chyme) from the stomach. The pH of the duodenal contents rises to 6.0–7.0, and by the time the chyme reaches the jejunum, its pH is nearly neutral.

Most of the proteins in pancreatic juice are enzymes and proenzymes (enzyme precursors that require some structural change to render them active). These enzymes aid in the intraluminal phase of digestion and absorption of fats, carbohydrates, and proteins. The rest of the proteins in pancreatic juice are plasma proteins, mucoproteins, and trypsin inhibitors (see below).

Some of the pancreatic enzymes (lipase, amylase, deoxyribonuclease, and ribonuclease) are secreted by the acinar cells in their active forms. The remaining enzymes are secreted as inactive proenzymes or **zymogens** (trypsinogen, chymotrypsinogen, proelastase, procarboxypeptidase, and phospholipase A_2) that are activated in the lumen of the proximal intestine. Activation of zymogens within the acinar cell might otherwise lead to acute pancreatitis and pancreatic autodigestion.

When the pancreatic juice enters the duodenum, trypsinogen is converted to the active form trypsin by an enzyme found in the intestinal brush border called enteropeptidase (or enterokinase). Trypsin then converts the remaining proenzymes into active enzymes, eg, chymotrypsinogen into chymotrypsin. Trypsin can also activate its own precursor, trypsinogen, producing the potential for an autocatalytic chain reaction. It is thus not surprising that pancreatic juice normally contains a trypsin inhibitor so that this autocatalytic reaction does not occur under normal circumstances.

Regulation of Secretion of Pancreatic Juice

Between and after meals, pancreatic secretion is regulated by hormonal and neural actions and by neurohumoral interactions.

Secretion of pancreatic juice is controlled primarily by two different hormones—**secretin** and **cholecystokinin (CCK)**—that are produced by specialized enteroendocrine cells of the duodenal mucosa.

Secretion of secretin is triggered by gastric acid and by the products of protein digestion in the duodenum. Secretin acts chiefly on the pancreatic duct cells to cause an outpouring of very alkaline pancreatic juice. In response to secretin, the pancreas produces a large volume of watery fluid rich in bicarbonate content but with little enzyme activity.

Secretion of CCK is triggered by the products of protein and fat digestion (peptides, amino acids, and fatty acids) when they enter the duodenum. The release of CCK from specific intestinal cells is thought to be regulated by a cholecystokinin-releasing peptide in the proximal small intestine that is trypsin-sensitive and active in the lumen. CCK acts chiefly on the acinar cells to cause release of enzymes from zymogen granules. Thus, in response to CCK, the pancreas secretes a small volume of juice low in bicarbonate but very high in enzyme content. In addition, CCK increases the secretion of enteropeptidase (enterokinase) from other endocrine cells of the duodenal mucosa. The integrated action of both secretin and CCK produces abundant secretion of enzyme-rich, alkaline pancreatic juice.

The secretion of pancreatic juice is also controlled in part by a reflex mechanism. Acetylcholine released by the vagus nerve acts like CCK on acinar cells to cause discharge of zymogen granules. Thus, stimulation of the vagus nerve causes production of a small volume of pancreatic juice rich in enzymes.

Digestive Functions of Pancreatic Juice

The secretion of pancreatic juice aids digestion in several ways. The large amount of bicarbonate in the juice helps to neutralize the acidic chyme from the stomach so that the pancreatic enzymes can function optimally in a neutral pH range.

Each of the enzymes also has an important digestive function. In digesting carbohydrates, pancreatic **amylase** splits straight-chain glucose polysaccharides (so-called amyloses in starch) into smaller α-limit dextrins, maltose and maltotriose. In digesting fat, pancreatic **lipase** splits triglycerides into fatty acids and monoglyceride. **Phospholipase A_2** splits a fatty acid off from lecithin to form lysolecithin. **Ribonuclease** and **deoxyribonuclease** attack the nucleic acids. The remaining enzymes help to digest proteins. **Trypsin, chymotrypsin,** and **elastase** are endopeptidases—ie, they cleave peptide bonds in the middle of polypeptide chains. **Carboxypeptidase** is an exopeptidase—ie, it splits peptide bonds adjacent to the carboxyl terminals of peptide chains. Together, these proteases break down proteins into oligopeptides and free amino acids.

---

1. What histologic features allow the pancreas to secrete digestive enzymes into the gastrointestinal tract?
2. What is the volume, composition, and function of pancreatic juice?
3. What are the neural and hormonal controls over exocrine pancreatic function?
4. Why does trypsinogen not self-activate before arriving in the duodenum?

PATHOPHYSIOLOGY OF SELECTED EXOCRINE PANCREATIC DISORDERS

ACUTE PANCREATITIS

Clinical Presentations

Acute pancreatitis is a clinical syndrome resulting from acute inflammation and destructive autodigestion of the pancreas and peripancreatic tissues. Clinically, acute pancreatitis is a common and important cause of acute upper abdominal pain, nausea, vomiting, and fever. Laboratory findings of marked elevations of serum amylase and lipase help to differentiate pancreatitis from other entities causing these symptoms. The severity of inflammation varies, and the prognosis ranges from mild, self-limited illness lasting 1–2 days to death from pancreatic necrosis, hemorrhage, or sepsis. Acute pancreatitis often recurs (relapsing acute pancreatitis). With repeated attacks, the gland may eventually be permanently damaged, resulting in chronic pancreatitis.

Etiology

Acute pancreatitis has many causes (Table 15-1), but in none of them is the exact mechanism of damage to the gland completely understood. However, in all there is escape of activated proteolytic enzymes from the ducts, leading to tissue injury, inflammation, necrosis, and in some cases infection.

The two most common conditions associated with acute pancreatitis are alcohol abuse and biliary tract disease.

Alcohol abuse is a common cause of acute pancreatitis in the USA, accounting for 65% of cases in some series. Acute pancreatitis usually occurs following an episode of heavy drinking. The exact mechanism by which alcohol damages the gland is not clear. Alcohol may have a direct toxic effect on pancreatic acinar cells, leading to intracellular trypsin activation by the lysosomal enzymes, or may cause inflammation of the sphincter of Oddi, leading to retention of hydrolytic enzymes in the pancreatic duct and acini. Alternatively, alcohol may cause decreased tone at the sphincter of Oddi, predisposing to reflux of bile or duodenal contents into the pancreatic duct and leading to parenchymal injury.

In patients who do not drink alcohol, about 50% of cases of acute pancreatitis are associated with biliary tract disease. In such cases, the hypothesized mechanism is obstruction of the common bile duct and the main pancreatic duct when a gallstone becomes lodged at the ampulla of Vater. Reflux of bile or duodenal contents into the pancreatic duct leads to parenchymal injury. Others have proposed that bacterial toxins or free bile acids travel via lymphatics from the gallbladder to the pancreas, giving rise to inflammation. In either case, acute pancreatitis associated with biliary tract disease is more common in women because gallstones are more common in women.

Acute pancreatitis may result from a variety of infectious agents, including viruses (mumps virus, coxsackievirus, hepatitis A virus, human immunodeficiency virus, or cytomegalovirus) and bacteria (*Salmonella typhi* or hemolytic streptococci). Patients with human immunodeficiency virus (HIV) infection can develop acute pancreatitis from the HIV

Table 15-1. Causes of acute pancreatitis.

Alcohol ingestion (acute or chronic alcoholism)	**Drugs**
Biliary tract disease	Definite association
Trauma	Immunosuppressives: azathioprine, mercaptopurine
Blunt abdominal trauma	Diuretics: thiazides, furosemide
Postoperative	Antimicrobials: sulfonamides, tetracyclines, pentamidine, didanosine, metronidazole, erythromycin
Post-endoscopic retrograde cannulation of pancreatic duct, injection of pancreatic duct	Steroids: estrogens, oral contraceptives, corticosteroids, ACTH
Post-electric shock	Miscellaneous: valproic acid, phenformin, intravenous lipid infusion
Infections	Probable association
Viral: Mumps, rubella, cocksackievirus B, echovirus, viral hepatitis A, B, adenovirus, cytomegalovirus, varicella, Epstein-Barr virus, human immunodeficiency virus	Immunosuppressives: asparaginase
	Diuretics: ethacrynic acid, chlorthalidone
	Miscellaneous: procainamide
Bacterial: *Mycoplasma pneumoniae, Salmonella typhi,* group A streptococci (scarlet fever), staphylococci, actinomycosis, *Mycobacterium tuberculosis, Mycobacterium avium* complex, *Legionella, Campylobacter jejuni, Leptospira icterohaemorrhagiae*	Possible association
	Antimicrobials: isoniazid, rifampin, nitrofurantoin
	Analgesics: acetaminophen, propoxyphene, salicylates, sulindac, other NSAIDs
	Miscellaneous: methyldopa
Parasitic: *Ascaris lumbricoides,* hydatid cyst, *Clonorchis sinensis*	**Vascular**
	Vasculitis: systemic lupus erythematosus, polyarteritis nodosa, malignant hypertension, thrombotic thrombocytopenic purpura
Metabolic	
Hyperlipidemia, apolipoprotein CII deficiency syndrome, hypertriglyceridemia	Shock, hypoperfusion, myocardial or mesenteric infarction
Hypercalcemia, eg, hyperparathyroidism	Atheromatous embolism
Uremia	**Mechanical**
Post-renal transplant	Pancreas divisum with accessory duct obstruction
Pregnancy, eclampsia	Ampulla of Vater stenosis, tumor, obstruction (regional enteritis, duodenal diverticulum, duodenal surgery, worms, foreign bodies)
Hemochromatosis, hemosiderosis	
Malnutrition: kwashiorkor, sprue, postgastrectomy, Whipple's disease	Choledochocele
Diabetic ketoacidosis	Penetrating duodenal ulcer
Hereditary	Pancreatic carcinoma
Familial pancreatitis	**Idiopathic**
Cystic fibrosis	
Poisons and toxins	
Venom: scorpion (*Tityus trinitatis*)	
Inorganic: zinc, cobalt, mercuric chloride, saccharated iron oxide	
Organic: Methanol, organophosphates	

infection itself, from related opportunistic infections, or from antiretroviral therapies. In HIV-infected patients, pancreatitis has been associated with intravenous drug abuse, pentamidine therapy, *Pneumocystis carinii* and *Mycobacterium avium-intracellulare* infections, and gallstones.

Blunt or penetrating trauma and other injuries may cause acute pancreatitis. Pancreatitis sometimes occurs following surgical procedures near the pancreas (duodenal stump syndrome; pancreatic tail syndrome following splenectomy). Infarction of the pancreas may result from occlusion of vessels supplying the gland. Shock and hypothermia may cause decreased perfusion, resulting in cellular degeneration and release of pancreatic enzymes. Radiation therapy of retroperitoneal malignant neoplasms can sometimes cause acute pancreatitis.

Marked hypercalcemia, such as that associated with hyperparathyroidism, sarcoidosis, hypervitaminosis D, or multiple myeloma, causes acute pancreatitis in about 10% of cases. Two mechanisms have been hypothesized. The high plasma calcium concentration may cause calcium to precipitate in the pancreatic duct, leading to ductal obstruction. Alternatively, hypercalcemia may stimulate activation of trypsinogen in the pancreatic duct.

Pancreatitis is also associated with hyperlipidemia, particularly those types characterized by increased plasma levels of chylomicrons (types I, IV, and V). In these cases, it is postulated that free fatty acids liberated by the action of pancreatic lipase cause gland inflammation and injury. Alcohol abuse or oral contraceptive use increases the risk of acute pancreatitis in patients with hyperlipidemia.

A variety of drugs have been associated with pancreatitis, including corticosteroids, thiazide diuretics, immunosuppressants, and cancer chemotherapeutic agents.

Rarely, acute pancreatitis may be familial, occurring with an autosomal dominant inheritance pattern. Hereditary recurrent acute pancreatitis has been associated with a mutation of the cationic trypsinogen gene. The point mutation—an arginine to histidine substitution at residue 117—makes trypsin resistant to cleavage at this site, which ordinarily leads to trypsin inactivation. Loss of this cleavage site thus permits active trypsin to autodigest the pancreas.

In about 25% of cases of acute pancreatitis, no etiologic factor can be identified. It is thought that idiopathic acute pancreatitis is often caused by occult biliary microlithiasis.

Whatever the cause of the acute pancreatitis, once the pathogenetic mechanisms have been brought into play the course and outcome of the disease are no longer influenced by the underlying etiologic factor.

Pathology & Pathogenesis

The symptoms, signs, laboratory findings, and complications of acute pancreatitis can all be explained on the basis of the pathologic damage to the ductules, acini, and islets of the pancreas. However, both the degree of damage and the clinical consequences are quite variable.

When the damage is limited in extent, the pathologic features consist of mild to marked swelling of the gland, especially the acini, and mild to marked infiltration with polymorphonuclear neutrophils. However, damage to tissue is usually only minimal to moderate, and there is no hemorrhage. In some cases, suppuration may be found along with edema, and this may result in tissue necrosis and abscess formation. In severe cases, massive necrosis and liquefaction of the pancreas occurs, predisposing to pancreatic abscess formation. Vascular necrosis and disruption may occur, resulting in hemorrhage. Hemorrhagic pancreatitis, which usually involves the entire gland, is the most serious form of pancreatitis.

In addition, a brownish serous fluid is often found in the peritoneal cavity ("pancreatic ascites"). This fluid contains blood, fat globules ("chicken broth"), and high levels of amylase and other pancreatic enzymes. Fat necrosis may occur in and around the pancreas, omentum, and mesentery, appearing as chalky white foci that may later calcify.

The mechanism by which enzymes and bioactive substances become activated within the pancreas is a major unanswered question in acute pancreatitis. The early initiating events probably occur at a membrane or intracellular level.

A recently proposed theory of the pathogenesis of alcoholic pancreatitis emphasizes disordered agonist-receptor interaction on the membrane of pancreatic acinar cells. According to this theory, alcohol induces alterations in the control of exocrine pancreatic secretion which in turn result in hyperstimulation of pancreatic acinar cells and their muscarinic receptors. This hyperstimulation mimics the mechanism of acute pancreatitis caused by scorpion stings, anti-acetylcholinesterase-containing insecticide poisoning, or administration of supramaximal doses of secretagogues such as acetylcholine and CCK.

Other recent studies suggest that lysosomal enzymes within the pancreatic acinar cell may play an important role. Morphologic studies during the first 24 hours after ligation of the pancreatic duct in animals indicate that the earliest lesions occur in acinar cells. Digestive enzyme zymogens and lysosomal hydrolases such as cathepsin B become localized together, suggesting that intra-acinar cell activation of the zymogens by lysosomal hydrolases may be an important initiating event. One speculation is that obstruction, bile reflux, and duodenal reflux disturb pancreatic acinar cell function, causing intracellular trypsin activation by the lysosomal enzymes. Other factors might also trigger this mechanism, including the toxic effects of alcohol and other drugs, hypercalcemia, ischemia, and the products of digestion of certain lipoproteins.

The pathologic changes all result from the action of activated pancreatic enzymes on the pancreas and surrounding tissues. In a manner still not understood, small amounts of trypsin escape from the duct system into the pancreatic parenchyma to initiate pancreatitis, perhaps through inhibition of the trypsin inhibitor. Once there, trypsin activates the proenzymes of chymotrypsin, elastase, and phospholipase A_2, and the activated enzymes cause damage in several ways (Figure 15–3). For example, chymotrypsin activation leads to edema and vascular damage. Similarly, elastase, once activated from proelastase, digests the elastin in blood vessel walls and causes vascular injury and hemorrhage; damage to peripancreatic blood vessels can lead to hemorrhagic pancreatitis. Phospholipase A_2 splits a fatty acid off lecithin, forming lysolecithin, which is cytotoxic to erythrocytes and damages cell membranes. Formation of lysolecithin from the lecithin in bile may contribute to disruption of the pancreas and necrosis of surrounding fat. Phospholipase A_2 also liberates arachidonic acid, which is then converted to prostaglandins, leukotrienes, and other mediators of inflammation, contributing to coagulation necrosis.

Pancreatic lipase, released directly as a result of pancreatic acinar cell damage, acts enzymatically on surrounding adipose tissue, causing fat necrosis (Figure 15–3).

Furthermore, trypsin and chymotrypsin activate kinins, complement, coagulation factors, and plasmin, leading to edema, inflammation, thrombosis, and hemorrhage within the gland. For example, trypsin activation of the kallikrein-kinin system leads to the release of bradykinin and kallidin, causing vasodilation, increased vascular permeability, edema, and inflammation (Figure 15–3).

The activated pancreatic enzymes also enter the bloodstream and may produce effects elsewhere in the body. Circulating phospholipases interfere with the normal function of pulmonary surfactant, contributing to the development of an adult respiratory distress syndrome in some patients with acute pancreatitis. Elevated serum lipase levels are sometimes associated with fat necrosis outside of the abdomen.

Finally, during acute pancreatitis, cytokines and other inflammatory mediators such as tumor necrosis factor-α (TNF-α), interleukins (especially IL-1, IL-6, and IL-8), and endotoxin are released rapidly and predictably from inflammatory cells. This release appears to be independent of the underlying etiology. Production of cytokine during clinical pancreatitis begins shortly after pain onset and peaks 36–48 hours later. These agents are now thought to be principal mediators in the transformation of acute pancreatitis from a local inflammatory process to a systemic illness (Figure 15–4). The degree of TNF-α-induced inflammation correlates with the severity of pancreatitis. Systemic complications of acute pancreatitis, such as respiratory failure, shock, or even multisystem organ failure, are accompanied by significant increases in monocyte secretion of TNF-α, IL-1, IL-6, and IL-8, and up-regulation of the number of receptors for these cytokines on target cells. This finding suggests that TNF-α, IL-1, IL-6, and IL-8 play a central role in the pathophysiology of these manifestations. Whether endotoxin is a marker for or a mediator of these systemic complications remains under investigation.

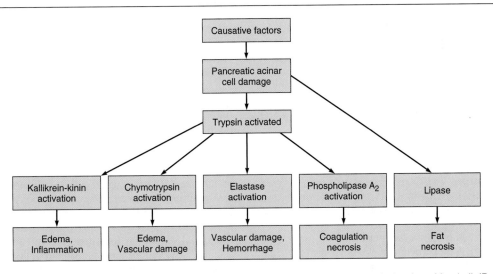

Figure 15–3. Hypothesized pathogenesis of acute pancreatitis. (Reproduced with permission from Marshall JB: Acute pancreatitis: A review with an emphasis on new developments. Arch Intern Med 1993;153:1185.)

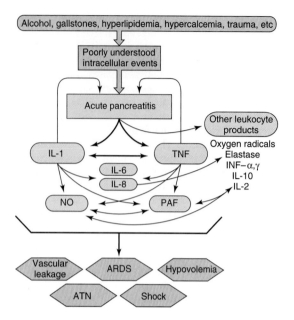

Figure 15–4. Inflammatory mediators of acute pancreatitis include interleukin-1B (IL-1) and tumor necrosis factor-α (TNF-α). As depicted, these two cytokines can induce other inflammatory mediators, such as interleukins (IL) 2, 6, 8, and 10; nitric oxide (NO); platelet activating factor (PAF); and interferon (INF) alpha and gamma, while at the same time producing a direct noxious effect on the pancreas itself. Each of the mediators shown plays a role in development of the systemic manifestations of acute pancreatitis. ARDS, acute respiratory distress syndrome; ATN, acute tubular necrosis. (Reproduced, with permission, from Norman J: The role of cytokines in the pathogenesis of acute pancreatitis. Am J Surg 1998;175:76.)

Table 15–2. Clinical manifestations and complications of acute pancreatitis.

Pancreas
 Edema, inflammation, local fat necrosis
 Necrosis, hemorrhage
 Phlegmon
 Pseudocyst: pain, rupture, hemorrhage, infection, obstruction of gastrointestinal tract (stomach, duodenum, colon)
 Abscess
Contiguous organs
 Extension of inflammation, fat necrosis, hemorrhage into peritoneum and retroperitoneum
 Thrombosis of adjacent blood vessels
 Ileus, bowel obstruction, perforation, infarction
 Pancreatic ascites: disruption of main pancreatic duct, leaking pseudocyst
 Obstructive jaundice
Systemic
 Cardiovascular: shock, hypovolemia, peripheral vasodilation, pericardial effusion, nonspecific ECG changes, sudden death
 Pulmonary: pleural effusion, pulmonary edema, adult respiratory distress syndrome, atelectasis, pneumonitis, mediastinal abscess
 Renal: renal failure, acute tubular necrosis, renal artery or vein thrombosis
 Hematologic: disseminated intravascular coagulation (DIC)
 Metabolic: hypocalcemia, hypoglycemia, hyperglycemia, hypertriglyceridemia
 Gastrointestinal: erosive gastritis, peptic ulcer, hemorrhage, bowel obstruction, portal vein thrombosis, variceal hemorrhage
 Nervous system: encephalopathy, retinopathy (sudden blindness), psychosis, fat emboli
 Distant fat necrosis (skin, bones, joints)

Clinical Manifestations

The major clinical consequences—symptoms, signs, and complications—of acute pancreatitis (Table 15–2) are readily explained by pathologic destruction of ductules, acini, and islets of the pancreas. The extent of damage is highly variable from patient to patient, as are the clinical manifestations, ranging from mild episodes of epigastric pain, nausea, and vomiting to severe (sometimes fatal) episodes of peritonitis, shock, and cyanosis.

The diagnosis of pancreatitis is primarily a clinical one. Distinguishing pancreatitis from other, potentially lethal causes of abdominal pain and identifying those patients with severe pancreatitis who may develop serious complications from the remote systemic effects of the disease are major diagnostic concerns.

Computed tomography is useful in diagnosis (Figure 15–5). It is particularly useful in distinguishing between edematous and necrotizing forms and providing prognostic information by detecting extrapancreatic involvement.

A. Pain: Patients with acute pancreatitis usually present with severe, constant, deep epigastric pain, often radiating to the back and flanks. The pain is thought to derive in part from stretching of the pancreatic capsule by distended ductules and parenchymal edema, inflammatory exudate, digested proteins and lipids, and hemorrhage. In addition, these materials may seep out of the parenchyma into the retroperitoneum and lesser sac, where they irritate retroperitoneal and peritoneal sensory nerve endings and produce intense back and flank pain. The clinical findings of generalized peritonitis may follow.

B. Nausea, Vomiting, and Ileus: Stretching of the pancreatic capsule may also produce nausea and vomiting. Increasing abdominal pain, peritoneal irritation, and electrolyte imbalance (especially hypokalemia) may cause a paralytic ileus with marked abdominal distention. If gastric motility is inhibited and the gastroesophageal sphincter is relaxed, there may be emesis. Both small and large bowel often dilate during an acute attack. Sometimes only a localized segment of bowel dilates. For example, there

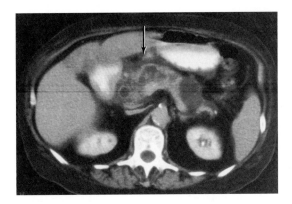

Figure 15–5. Acute pancreatitis on CT. Findings include enlargement and edema of the pancreas plus peripancreatic inflammatory change and fluid collections (arrow). (Courtesy of Henry I. Goldberg, MD, Department of Radiology, University of California, San Francisco.)

may be localized dilation of a segment of jejunum overlying the pancreas. In such cases, a plain x-ray of the abdomen shows thickening of the valvulae conniventes and air-fluid levels ("sentinel loop"). In other cases, there may be segmental dilation of a portion of the overlying transverse colon. The x-ray shows a sharply demarcated area of localized colonic dilation and edema ("colon cut-off sign").

C. Fever: Almost two-thirds of patients with acute pancreatitis develop fever. The pathophysiologic mechanism responsible for fever involves the extensive tissue injury, inflammation, and necrosis and the release of endogenous pyrogens, principally interleukin-1, from polymorphonuclear leukocytes into the circulation. In most cases of acute pancreatitis, fever does not indicate a bacterial infection. However, persistent fever beyond the fourth or fifth day of illness—or spiking temperatures to 40 °C or more—may signify development of infectious complications such as pancreatic abscess or ascending cholangitis.

D. Shock: Hypovolemia, hypotension, and shock may occur as a result of several interrelated factors. Hypovolemia results from massive exudation of plasma and hemorrhage into the retroperitoneal space and from accumulation of fluid in the gut due to ileus. Hypotension and shock may also result from release of kinins into the general circulation. For example, activation during acute inflammation of the proteolytic enzyme kallikrein results in peripheral vasodilation via liberation of the vasoactive peptides, bradykinin and kallidin. This vasodilation causes the pulse rate to rise and the blood pressure to fall. Cytokines like platelet-activating factor (PAF), a very potent vasodilator and leukocyte activator, have been implicated in the development of shock and other manifestations of the systemic inflammatory response syndrome. The contracted intravascular volume combined with the hypotension may lead to myocardial and cerebral ischemia, respiratory failure, and decreased urinary output or renal failure due to acute tubular necrosis.

E. Hyperamylasemia and Hyperlipasemia: The cardinal laboratory finding in acute pancreatitis is elevation of the serum amylase level, often up to 10–20 times normal. The elevation occurs almost immediately (within hours), but amylase concentration usually returns to normal within 48–72 hours even if symptoms continue. The sensitivity of the serum amylase in acute pancreatitis is estimated to be 70–95%, meaning that 5–30% of patients with acute pancreatitis have normal or minimally elevated serum amylase values. The specificity of the test is considerably lower. Serum amylase elevation can be present in a variety of other conditions.

The serum amylase concentration reflects the steady state between the rates of amylase entry into and removal from the blood. Hyperamylasemia can result from either an increased rate of entry or a decreased metabolic clearance of amylase from the circulation. The pancreas and salivary glands have much higher concentrations of amylase than any other organs and probably contribute almost all of the serum amylase activity in normal persons. Amylase of pancreatic origin can be now be distinguished from that of salivary origin by a variety of techniques. Pancreatic hyperamylasemia results from injuries to the pancreas, ranging from minor (cannulation of the pancreatic duct) to severe (pancreatitis). In addition, injuries to the bowel wall (infarction or perforation) cause pancreatic hyperamylasemia due to enhanced absorption of amylase from the intestinal lumen. Salivary hyperamylasemia is observed in salivary gland diseases such as mumps parotitis but also (inexplicably) in a host of unrelated conditions such as chronic alcoholism, postoperative states (particularly following coronary artery bypass graft surgery), lactic acidosis, anorexia nervosa or bulimia nervosa, and certain malignancies. Hyperamylasemia can also result from decreased metabolic clearance of amylase due to renal failure or macroamylasemia (a condition in which there is an abnormally high-molecular-weight amylase in the serum).

Patients with marked elevations of serum amylase (more than three times the upper limit of normal) usually have acute pancreatitis. Patients with lesser elevations of serum amylase often have other conditions.

Determination of serum lipase activity is often helpful diagnostically. In acute pancreatitis, the serum lipase level is elevated, usually about 72 hours after onset of symptoms. The serum lipase measurement may be a better diagnostic test than serum amylase because it is just as easy to perform, may be a more sensitive test than the serum amylase (85% versus 79%), is more specific for acute pancreatitis, and decreases to normal more slowly than the amylase level.

F. Coagulopathy: Tissue factor release and expression during proteolysis may cause activation of the plasma coagulation cascade and may lead to disseminated intravascular coagulation (DIC). In other cases, hypercoagulability of the blood is thought to be due to elevated concentrations of several coagulation factors, including factor VIII, fibrinogen, and perhaps factor V. Clinically affected patients may present with hemorrhagic discoloration (purpura) in the subcutaneous tissues around the umbilicus (Cullen's sign) or in the flanks (Grey Turner's sign).

G. Pleuropulmonary Complications: Pleuropulmonary complications of acute pancreatitis include pleural effusion, pulmonary edema, and respiratory failure (acute respiratory distress syndrome [ARDS]). Quite often, acute pancreatitis is accompanied by a small (usually left-sided) pleural effusion. The effusion may be secondary to a direct effect of the inflamed, swollen pancreas on the pleura abutting the diaphragm or to tracking of exudative fluid from the pancreatic bed retroperitoneally into the pleural cavity through defects in the diaphragm. Characteristically, the pleural fluid is an exudate with high levels of protein, LDH, and amylase. The effusion may contribute to segmental atelectasis of the lower lobes, leading to ventilation/perfusion mismatch and hypoxia. Pulmonary edema may occur and has been attributed to the effects of circulating activated proteolytic enzymes on the pulmonary capillaries, leading to transudation of fluid into the alveoli. The most dreaded pulmonary complication is the development of ARDS. This is most often seen 3–7 days after the onset of severe hemorrhagic pancreatitis and is thought to be related to hypotension ("shock lung") and damage to endothelial and epithelial cells and to production of IL-1 and TNF-α within the pulmonary parenchyma.

H. Jaundice: Jaundice (hyperbilirubinemia) and bilirubinuria occur in about one-fifth of patients with acute pancreatitis. Several factors undoubtedly contribute. A gallstone underlying the pancreatitis may cause transient common bile duct obstruction. Partial obstruction of the common bile duct may also result from swelling of the head of the pancreas. In other cases, more protracted and severe jaundice may result from compression of the common bile duct by inflammatory **pseudocysts,** non-epithelium-lined cavities that contain plasma, blood, pus, and pancreatic juice (see below).

I. Hypocalcemia: In severe cases of acute pancreatitis, the serum calcium level may fall precipitously, occasionally low enough to cause frank tetany. This is a state of neuromuscular irritability that is manifested clinically by positive Chvostek and Trousseau signs. Chvostek's sign is unilateral facial spasm elicited by a slight tap over the facial nerve; Trousseau's sign is unilateral carpal spasm elicited by compression of the upper arm by a tourniquet or blood pressure cuff (Figure 17–16). Most often, hypocalcemia occurs between the third and tenth days of illness. Several factors contribute to the decline in serum calcium. Lipolysis of the peripancreatic, retroperitoneal, and mesenteric fat releases free fatty acids that combine with ionized calcium to form soaps. With the ensuing rapid fall in serum calcium, the parathyroid glands are unable to respond quickly and adequately enough to compensate for the hypocalcemia. If there is associated hypomagnesemia, the hypocalcemia may prove to be both severe and refractory, since normal serum magnesium concentrations are required for normal parathyroid function. Severe hypocalcemia is clinically manifested by tetany, stupor, seizures, coma, and even death due to laryngospasm.

J. Acidosis: Metabolic acidosis occurs in many patients with severe acute pancreatitis. The acidosis is primarily a lactic acidosis resulting from hypotension and shock. However, in patients with extensive pancreatic necrosis and hemorrhage, there may be destruction or dysfunction of the pancreatic islets, causing deficient insulin production and acute diabetic ketoacidosis. Hyperglycemia is seen in about 25% of patients and transient glycosuria in about 10%.

K. Hyperkalemia and Hypokalemia: The initial phase of acute pancreatitis, marked by acute inflammation and tissue necrosis, often causes release of large amounts of potassium into the circulation. This release, combined with hypovolemia and acidosis, often results in hyperkalemia. Later, following fluid repletion and correction of acidosis, the serum potassium may fall to dangerously low levels.

L. Hyperlipidemia: Acute attacks of pancreatitis, particularly when caused by alcohol abuse, are often accompanied by marked hyperlipidemia. The mechanism is thought to relate to decreased release and activity of the endothelial and plasma enzyme lipoprotein lipase.

M. Hyperglycemia: Hyperglycemia is common and is thought to be related to a decreased release of insulin by pancreatic islet cells in combination with increased levels of circulating catecholamines and glucocorticoids from the adrenal gland.

N. Pancreatic Phlegmon, Pseudocysts, Ascites, or Abscess: See Table 15–2. A pancreatic **phlegmon** is a solid mass of inflamed pancreatic tissue, detectable by CT or MRI, that usually resolves spontaneously.

Infected pancreatic necrosis and **pancreatic abscess** occur when there is bacterial infection of necrotic tissue in and around the inflamed pancreas. An abscess is defined by the presence of one or more localized collections of pus. Infected necrosis occurs an average of 2 weeks and abscesses an average of 5 weeks after the onset of symptoms. These septic complications are serious—potentially life-threatening—complications of acute pancreatitis.

Inflammatory **pseudocysts** are so called because they are non-epithelium-lined cavities that contain plasma, blood, pus and pancreatic juice. They generally occur after recovery from the acute attack and are the result of both parenchymal destruction and ductal obstruction. Some acini continue to secrete pancreatic juice, but because the juice cannot drain normally, it collects in an area of necrotic tissue, forming the ill-defined pseudocyst (Figure 15–6). As more juice is secreted, the cyst may grow progressively larger and may cause compression of nearby structures such as the portal vein (producing portal hypertension), common bile duct (producing jaundice or cholangitis), or gut (producing gastric outlet or bowel obstruction). Less commonly, the pseudocyst will erode through the bowel wall and rupture into the gut, causing gastrointestinal hemorrhage.

Pancreatic ascites occurs when a direct connection develops between a pancreatic pseudocyst and the peritoneal cavity. Given its origin, it is not surprising that the ascitic fluid resembles pancreatic juice, characteristically an exudate with high protein and extremely high amylase levels.

Course & Prognosis

The severity of acute pancreatitis can be estimated by various methods: clinical assessment, biochemical tests, Ranson's prognostic criteria, peritoneal lavage, and computed tomography. Table 15–3 lists Ranson's criteria—adverse prognostic signs that correlate with morbidity and mortality in acute pancreatitis.

Most patients with acute pancreatitis recover completely with supportive medical management. The pancreas then regenerates and returns to normal except for some mild residual scarring. Diabetes mellitus almost never occurs after a single attack of pancreatitis. However, in some cases, one or more pancreatic pseudocysts form in the weeks to months following recovery.

The initial course of alcoholic pancreatitis is characterized by recurrent acute exacerbations and the later course by progressive pancreatic insufficiency. However, among individuals with recurrent acute alcoholic pancreatitis, two groups can be distinguished in terms of prognosis. About three-fourths of cases progress to advanced chronic pancreatitis, typically with pancreatic calcification and pancreatic insufficiency. The remainder do not progress and do not develop pancreatic duct dilation. The factors responsible for progression have not yet been elucidated.

A minority of patients (8–25% in various series) develop severe pancreatitis and may die as a consequence of hemorrhage, shock, DIC, ARDS, or septic pancreatic abscess.

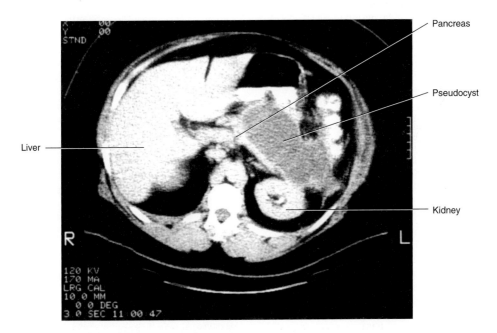

Figure 15–6. Pancreatic pseudocyst on CT. (Reproduced, with permission, from Way LW [editor]: *Current Surgical Diagnosis & Treatment,* 10th ed. Appleton & Lange, 1994.)

Table 15–3. Adverse prognostic signs in acute pancreatitis: Ranson's criteria of severity of acute pancreatitis.[1]

Criteria present at diagnosis or admission
Age over 55 years
White blood cell count > 16,000/μL
Blood glucose > 200 mg/dL
Serum LDH > 350 IU/L
AST > 250 IU/L
Criteria developing during first 48 hours
Hematocrit fall > 10%
BUN rise > 5 mg/dL
Serum calcium < 8 mg/dL
Arterial P_{O_2} < 60 mm Hg
Base deficit > 4 meq/L
Estimated fluid sequestration > 6 L

Mortality rates correlate with number of criteria present

Number of Criteria	Mortality Rate
0–2	1%
3–4	16%
5–6	40%
7–8	100%

[1]Modified from Way LW (editor): *Current Surgical Diagnosis & Treatment*, 10th ed. Appleton & Lange, 1994.

---

5. What are the presenting symptoms and signs of acute pancreatitis?
6. What are the most common causes of acute pancreatitis?
7. Which drugs are commonly associated with pancreatitis?
8. What is the pathophysiologic mechanism by which hemorrhagic pancreatitis occurs?
9. What are the complications of severe pancreatitis?
10. What are the pathophysiologic mechanisms by which each of the complications of severe pancreatitis occurs?

CHRONIC PANCREATITIS

Clinical Presentations

Chronic pancreatitis is a relapsing disorder causing severe abdominal pain, exocrine and endocrine pancreatic insufficiency, severe duct abnormalities, and pancreatic calcifications. The prevalence of the disorder is about 30 per 100,000 individuals, and the yearly incidence is less than 10 per 100,000. In chronic pancreatitis, there is chronic inflammation of the parenchyma, leading to progressive destruction of the acini, stenosis and dilation of the ductules, and fibrosis of the gland. Eventually, there is impairment of the gland's exocrine functions (see Pancreatic Insufficiency, below) and sometimes of its endocrine functions as well (Chapter 18).

Etiology

It was at one time believed that chronic pancreatitis simply resulted from recurrent attacks of acute pancreatitis. Indeed, long-term clinical and histopathologic studies do suggest that alcoholic chronic pancreatitis evolves from severe acute pancreatitis. However, there is some evidence that acute and chronic pancreatitis due to other causes are distinct pathogenetic entities. Patients developing acute pancreatitis are a mean 13 years older than individuals with onset of chronic calcified pancreatitis. Furthermore, the two diseases have been linked to different causes. Finally, in acute pancreatitis, the pancreas is normal before the attack and the pathologic changes are completely reversible if the patient survives, whereas in chronic pancreatitis the gland is abnormal before the attack, and the pathologic changes are not reversible.

The major cause of chronic pancreatitis is chronic alcoholism, which accounts for about 70–80% of cases. The remainder are due to diverse causes listed in Table 15–4. In 1788, Cawley first reported the association of alcoholism with chronic pancreatitis. He described a "free living young man" with diabetes and emaciation. At autopsy, his pancreas was "full of stones." Patients with chronic pancreatitis due to alcohol abuse usually have a long history (6–12 years) of heavy alcohol consumption (150–175 g/d) before the onset of the disease. In alcoholics, deficiencies of zinc and selenium may inhibit quenching of oxygen free radicals. Long term obstruction of the pancreatic duct can also cause chronic pancreatitis. The obstruction can be caused by a periampullary tumor, papillary stenosis, cyst, scarring or stricture, or trauma. Pancreas divisum, an anatomic variant in which the head and body of the pancreas are separate glands, can also cause a relative obstruction to the flow of pancreatic juice at the lesser papilla. Tropical pancreatitis is thought to be caused by protein or micronutrient deficiencies, which may cause impaired clearance of free radicals, or by ingestion of a toxic substance, such as cyanogens in cassava root. Cyanogens are known to inhibit a variety of antioxidant enzymes. Thus, ingestion of cassava may promote unrestrained generation of free radicals with

Table 15–4. Causes of chronic pancreatitis.

Alcohol abuse
Duct obstruction (eg, gallstones)
Pancreas divisum[1]
Tropical (malnutrition, toxin)
Hypercalcemia (eg, hyperparathyroidism)
Hyperlipidemia
Drugs
Trauma
Autoimmune
Hereditary
Cystic fibrosis (mucoviscidosis)
Idiopathic

[1]An anatomic variant in which the head and body of the pancreas are separate glands.

toxic effects. Chronic hypercalcemia may cause pancreatitis. For example, about 10–15% of patients with hyperparathyroidism develop pancreatitis. Intraductal precipitation of calcium and stimulation of pancreatic enzyme secretion are thought to be important in pathogenesis. In some cases of chronic pancreatitis with features of Sjögren's syndrome, an autoimmune mechanism may be involved. Chronic hereditary pancreatitis, characterized by recurrent episodes of abdominal pain beginning in childhood, accounts for about 1% of cases. It is transmitted as an autosomal dominant genetic disorder with incomplete penetrance. Hereditary chronic pancreatitis has also been associated with mutations in the cationic trypsinogen gene (discussed above). Some cases are due to cystic fibrosis (mucoviscidosis; see Chapter 2). In many cases, no cause can be identified. The incidence of chronic pancreatitis has been increasing recently for unknown reasons.

Pathology

As noted above, in acute pancreatitis, peripancreatic and intrapancreatic fat necrosis is the key pathologic finding. In resolving acute pancreatitis, there is organization of fat necrosis with early perilobular fibrosis or peripancreatic pseudocysts. However, if acute pancreatitis is severe, affecting the intrapancreatic fat deposits, it may perhaps evolve into chronic pancreatitis.

In the early stage of chronic pancreatitis, pseudocysts are present in half (52%), and there is a focally accentuated fibrosis of the perilobular and, to a lesser degree, intralobular type. While intralobular and perilobular fibrosis of the pancreas is a hallmark of alcoholic pancreatitis, it is also common among patients with alcohol dependence and abuse who have no history of pancreatitis. Marked fibrosis, ductal distortions, and the presence of intraductal calculi are the main features of advanced chronic pancreatitis. Pseudocysts are less frequent (36%). CD4 and CD8 T lymphocytes are the predominant T cell subsets in the inflammatory infiltrates in chronic pancreatitis.

Thus, pathologically, chronic pancreatitis is characterized by scarring and shrinkage of the pancreas due to fibrosis and atrophy of acini and by stenosis and dilation of ductules. Grossly, the process usually involves the whole gland, but in about one-third of cases it is localized, most often involving the head and body of the gland. The ductules and ducts are often filled with inspissated secretions or calculi. Between 36% and 87% of patients with chronic pancreatitis have ductal stones. The gland may be rock hard as a result of diffuse sclerosis and calcification, and biopsy may be required to differentiate chronic pancreatitis from pancreatic carcinoma (see Carcinoma of the Pancreas, below). Microscopically, there is loss of acini, dilation of ductules, marked fibrosis, and a lymphocytic infiltrate. The islets of Langerhans are usually well preserved.

Table 15–5. Pathogenetic classification of pancreatitis.[1]

Pathogenetic Class	Subclassification	Pathologic Features
Acute pancreatitis	Mild pancreatitis Severe (necrotizing) pancreatitis	Fat necrosis Coagulation necrosis Hemorrhagic necrosis
Chronic pancreatitis	Lithogenic pancreatitis Obstructive pancreatitis Inflammatory pancreatitis Pancreatic fibrosis	Protein plugs Calculi Obstruction of main pancreatic duct Mononuclear cell infiltration Acinar cell necrosis Diffuse perilobular fibrosis

[1]Modified, with permission, from Sarles H et al: Pathogenesis of chronic pancreatitis. Gut 1990;31:629; and Sidhu SS, Tandon RK: The pathogenesis of chronic pancreatitis. Postgrad Med J 1995;71:67.

Pathogenesis

Table 15–5 presents a classification of pancreatitis based on pathogenesis.

For chronic lithogenic pancreatitis, several different pathogenetic mechanisms have been postulated. One theory postulates **acinar protein (trypsinogen) hypersecretion** as an initial event (Figure 15–7A). Ultrastructural studies of exocrine pancreatic tissue from patients with chronic pancreatitis show signs of protein hypersecretion, including a larger diameter of cells, nuclei, and nucleoli; increased length of the endoplasmic reticulum; increased numbers of condensing vacuoles; and decreased numbers of zymogen granules. The hypersecretion of protein occurs without increased fluid or bicarbonate secretion by ductal cells. At the same time, there is an increase in the ratio of lysosomal hydrolases (cathepsin B) to digestive hydrolases (trypsinogen). Co-localization of lysosomes and zymogens (see Acute Pancreatitis, above) results in activation of trypsinogen. Precipitation of intraductal protein into plugs is then thought to occur in the following fashion: **Lithostathines** (formerly called pancreatic stone proteins, or **PSPs**) are peptides secreted into pancreatic juice that normally inhibit the formation of protein plugs and the aggregation of calcium carbonate crystals to form stones. Acinar cell secretion of lithostathine is impaired by alcohol. Furthermore, when hydrolyzed by trypsin and cathepsin B, lithostathine H2/PSP-S1 is created. This insoluble peptide polymerizes into fibrils that form the matrix of protein plugs. At the same time, there is hypersecretion of calcium into the pancreatic juice. The calcium hypersecretion is first triggered by neural (cholinergic, vagally mediated) or hormonal stimuli. Later, as the basal lamina of the pancreatic

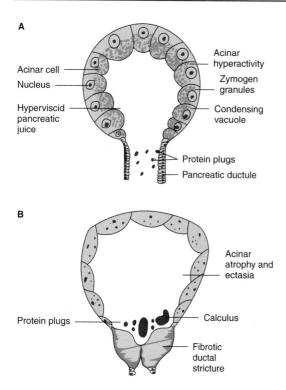

pancreatitis causes cellular anoxia, necrosis, chronic inflammation, and subsequent fibrosis. In particular, periacinar and periductal fat necrosis induces periductal fibrosis, which partially obstructs the interlobular ducts. Stasis within the ductules then leads

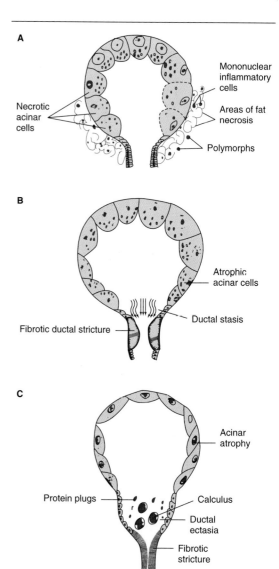

Figure 15–7. Proposed pathogenetic model of chronic pancreatitis emphasizing acinar protein hypersecretion. **A:** In early chronic pancreatitis, there is acinar cell hyperactivity and secretion of a hyperviscid pancreatic juice with an imbalance of pancreatic stone promoters and inhibitors, resulting in protein plug formation. **B:** In advanced chronic pancreatitis, there are acinar cell atrophy, ductal strictures and ectasia, and intraductal stones. (Reproduced, with permission, from Sidhu SS, Tandon RK: The pathogenesis of chronic pancreatitis. Postgrad Med J 1995;71:67.)

duct is eroded by contact with the protein plugs, there is transudation of serum protein and calcium into the pancreatic juice. The combination of protein plug formation in pancreatic juice that is thick, viscid, and protein-rich and supersaturated with calcium carbonate leads to formation of **calculi** (stones) (Figure 15–7B). Decreased levels of other nucleation-inhibitory factors, such as local trypsin inhibitor and citrate, in pancreatic juice further enhance formation of pancreatic plugs and stones. Eventually, the stones provoke formation of fibrotic ductal strictures and ductal ectasia, acinar cell atrophy, and parenchymal atrophy distal to obstructed ducts in the advanced stages of chronic pancreatitis.

Another theory postulates a **necrosis-fibrosis sequence**, in which focal necrosis during recurrent attacks of acute pancreatitis induces scarring and fibrosis, leading to chronic lithogenic pancreatitis (Figure 15–8A). In this scenario, vascular damage in acute

Figure 15–8. Proposed pathogenetic model of chronic pancreatitis emphasizing the sequence of acute pancreatitis followed by chronic pancreatitis. **A:** In acute pancreatitis, there is necrosis of acinar cells and fat and infiltration of inflammatory cells. **B:** Later, there is healing and fibrosis. **C:** Finally, changes of chronic pancreatitis appear, including acinar cell atrophy, formation of protein plugs and calculi, and ductal strictures and ectasia. (Reproduced, with permission, from Sidhu SS, Tandon RK: The pathogenesis of chronic pancreatitis. Postgrad Med J 1995;71:67.)

to protein plug and stone formation in the pancreatic juice (Figure 15–8B). Subsequently, total obstruction of ducts by calculi induces acinar cell necrosis, inflammation, and fibrosis (Figure 15–8C). Transforming growth factor-β (TGF-β) appears to be a mediator of collagen synthesis after pancreatic injury.

Oxidative stress may also be responsible for chronic pancreatitis. According to this theory, inappropriate activation of pancreatic cytochrome P450 enzymes (eg, by alcohol), results in lipid peroxidation by excess free radicals of oxygen. Resultant lipid deposition in the basal cytoplasm of acinar cells is thought to trigger the development of fibrosis. Oxidative stress and membrane lipid oxidation lead to an inflammatory process, perhaps mediated by chemokines attracting mononuclear cells.

In cases of chronic pancreatitis due to **obstruction of the pancreatic ducts,** the obstruction antedates the development of pancreatitis. The pathogenesis probably involves elevated pressures in the pancreatic duct, resulting in ischemia, necrosis, and inflammation of acinar cells. However, the ductal epithelium is preserved. Calcified protein plugs and stones are less often present. Many patients with idiopathic chronic pancreatitis also have ductal hypertension.

Finally, chronic inflammatory pancreatitis is thought to be produced by an **autoimmune** mechanism. Associated clinical features may include bilateral sialadenitis, intrahepatic cholestasis, and the nephrotic syndrome. Elevated levels of serum immune globulins are typical.

Pathophysiology

Studies of patients with chronic pancreatitis have found no differences from healthy individuals in basal plasma levels of CCK and pancreatic polypeptide, but there is impaired interdigestive cycling and postprandial release of CCK and PP. Chronic pancreatitis does not seem to have any effect on intestinal motility.

There is a direct correlation between severity of histologic findings and exocrine pancreatic dysfunction as estimated by the CCK-secretin test (see below).

Hepatic insulin resistance has been demonstrated in patients with chronic pancreatitis, perhaps related to a decrease in high-affinity insulin receptors on the hepatocyte cell membrane. In rats, insulin binding improves following administration of pancreatic polypeptide.

In chronic pancreatitis, fecal bile acid excretion has been found to be three times that of healthy individuals. Bile acid malabsorption is related to impairment of pancreatic bicarbonate secretion; it is generally not observed until bicarbonate output is markedly reduced (< 0.05 meq/kg/h). Such bile acid malabsorption may cause the hypocholesterolemia seen in patients with chronic pancreatitis.

Impairment of exocrine function in chronic pancreatitis may also lead to increased CCK-mediated stimulation of the pancreas.

Table 15–6. Clinical manifestations of chronic pancreatitis.

Abdominal pain
Nausea
Vomiting
Weight loss
Malabsorption
Hyperglycemia
Jaundice

Clinical Manifestations

The clinical manifestations of chronic pancreatitis are listed in Table 15–6. The major symptom of chronic pancreatitis is severe abdominal pain that can be either constant or intermittent. The abdominal pain often radiates to the mid back or scapula and increases after eating. It is sometimes relieved by sitting upright or leaning forward. The pain is thought to derive from dilation of the duct system, causing ductal and parenchymal hypertension, from inflammation of the parenchyma, causing pancreatic ischemia, or from local enzymatic activity and destruction of the perineural sheath, exposing axons to cytokines released by inflammatory cells and ultimately causing perineural fibrosis. Patients may have recurrent attacks of severe abdominal pain, vomiting, and elevation of serum amylase (chronic relapsing pancreatitis). Continued alcohol intake may increase the frequency of painful episodes, at least when there is still relatively preserved pancreatic function; in severe pancreatic insufficiency, alcohol intake appears to have less influence on the development of abdominal pain. Pancreatic parenchymal pressure measurements have not been found to correlate with pain.

Between 10% and 20% of patients have "painless pancreatitis," presenting with diabetes, jaundice, malabsorption, or steatorrhea. Anorexia and weight loss occur frequently, related both to poor nutrition and to malabsorption from pancreatic insufficiency.

Physical findings include epigastric or upper abdominal tenderness. A fever or a palpable mass suggests a complication such as an abscess or a pseudocyst.

The diagnosis of chronic pancreatitis is based mainly on symptoms and signs. The serum amylase and lipase levels are elevated in only a minority of cases. In the remaining cases, the amylase and lipase levels are normal or low, probably because there is little residual pancreatic tissue. A finding of pancreatic calcifications on abdominal x-ray often suggests the diagnosis. Such pancreatic calcifications are visible in about 30% of cases. The calcifications are actually the intraductal pancreatic calculi composed of calcium carbonate and lithostathines (PSPs). Ultrasonography typically reveals pancreatic enlargement and ductal dilation and may demonstrate pseudocysts in up to 10% of patients. Computed tomography may reveal calcifications and cystic areas not noted on plain abdominal x-rays or ultrasound.

About 5% of patients develop severe sclerosing pancreatitis involving the head of the pancreas, leading to obstruction of the common bile and pancreatic ducts. Obstruction may also be caused by a pseudocyst in the head of the pancreas. Common bile duct obstruction results in profound and persistent jaundice, resembling that produced by pancreatic carcinoma. The serum bilirubin and alkaline phosphatase are elevated.

Endoscopic retrograde cholangiopancreatography is the best imaging procedure for assessing the severity and extent of ductal changes. ERCP findings include dilated ducts, frequently with adjacent areas of stricture, yielding a "chain of lakes" or "string of pearls" appearance, or ducts of normal caliber, with adjacent small ducts lacking side branches, yielding a "tree in winter" appearance.

Exocrine pancreatic function is estimated by the CCK-secretin test. In this test, measurements are made of pancreatic juice volume, amylase output, and bicarbonate concentration in the basal state, then 30 minutes after intravenous injection of CCK, and then 60 minutes after intravenous administration of secretin.

Simpler, less invasive tests include the bentiromide test, the pancreolauryl test, and the cholesteryl-[^{14}C]octanoate breath test (see Pancreatic Insufficiency, below).

Failure to secrete pancreatic juice results in malabsorption of fat (steatorrhea) and fat-soluble vitamins and in weight loss. Endocrine dysfunction produces hyperglycemia, glycosuria, and frank diabetes mellitus in approximately 30–40% of cases of long-standing chronic pancreatitis. Impairment of exocrine function is manifested by pancreatic insufficiency (see below).

The major complications of chronic pancreatitis are pseudocyst formation and mechanical obstruction of the common bile duct and duodenum. Less common complications include pancreatic fistulas with pancreatic ascites, pleural effusion, or sometimes pericardial effusion; splenic vein thrombosis with portal hypertension; and formation of a pseudoaneurysm, with hemorrhage or pain due to expansion and pressure on adjacent structures. Fistulas result from disruption of the pancreatic duct. Splenic vein thrombosis occurs because the splenic vein, which courses along the posterior surface of the pancreas, may become involved in peripancreatic inflammation. Pseudoaneurysms may affect any of the arteries in proximity to the pancreas, most commonly the splenic, hepatic, gastroduodenal, and pancreaticoduodenal arteries.

In patients followed for more than 10 years, the mortality rate is 22%, with pancreatitis-induced complications accounting for 13% of the deaths. The major causes of death are alcoholic liver disease, postoperative complications, and cancer. Older age at diagnosis, cigarette smoking, and alcohol intake are major predictors of mortality among individuals with chronic pancreatitis. Pancreatic carcinoma occurs in 3% and extrapancreatic carcinoma in 4%.

PANCREATIC INSUFFICIENCY

Clinical Presentations

Pancreatic exocrine insufficiency is the syndrome of maldigestion resulting from disorders interfering with effective pancreatic enzyme activity. Because pancreatic lipase is essential for fat digestion, its absence leads to steatorrhea—the occurrence of greasy, bulky, light-colored stools. On the other hand, while pancreatic amylase and trypsin are important for carbohydrate and protein digestion, other enzymes in gastric and intestinal juice can usually compensate for their loss. Thus, patients with pancreatic insufficiency seldom present with maldigestion of carbohydrate and protein (nitrogen loss).

Etiology

Pancreatic insufficiency usually results from chronic pancreatitis in adults or cystic fibrosis (mucoviscidosis) in children (Table 15–7). In some cases it is a consequence of pancreatic resection or carcinoma of the pancreas. Pancreatic insufficiency occurs after bone marrow transplantation and appears to be related to prior acute or chronic graft-versus-host disease. Each of these conditions markedly re-

Table 15–7. Causes of pancreatic insufficiency.

Primary
  A. Acquired decreased enzyme secretion
    Chronic pancreatitis (alcohol abuse, trauma, hereditary, idiopathic)
    Pancreatic, ampullary and duodenal neoplasms
    Pancreatic resection
    Severe protein-calorie malnutrition, hypoalbuminemia
  B. Congenital decreased enzyme secretion
    Cystic fibrosis
    Hemochromatosis
    Shwachman's syndrome (pancreatic insufficiency with anemia, neutropenia, and bony abnormalities)
    Enzyme deficiencies (trypsinogen, enterokinase, amylase, lipase, proteases, α_1-antiprotease deficiency)

Secondary
  A. Intraluminal enzyme destruction: Gastrinoma (Zollinger-Ellison syndrome)
  B. Decreased pancreatic stimulation: Small intestinal mucosal disease (nontropical sprue)
  C. Mistiming of enzyme secretion: Gastric surgery
    1. Subtotal gastrectomy with Billroth I anastomosis
    2. Subtotal gastrectomy with Billroth II anastomosis
    3. Truncal vagotomy and pyloroplasty

duces the amount of pancreatic enzymes secreted, often to less than 5% of normal.

Less commonly, pancreatic insufficiency results from disease states that cause hypersecretion of gastric acid. For example, excessive gastrin secretion from a gastrinoma (an islet cell neoplasm composed of G cells) leads to continuous hypersecretion of gastric acid and a very low pH of gastric juice. In affected patients, the excess gastric acid overwhelms the normal pancreatic bicarbonate production and results in an abnormally acidic pH in the duodenum. This acid pH, in turn, causes decreased activity of otherwise adequate amounts of pancreatic enzymes.

Pathology & Pathogenesis

Normally, the activities of the various pancreatic enzymes decrease during their passage from the duodenum to the terminal ileum. However, the degradation rates of individual enzymes vary, with lipase activity lost rapidly and protease and amylase activity lost slowly. Lipase activity is usually destroyed by proteolysis, mainly by the action of residual chymotrypsin. This mechanism persists in patients with pancreatic insufficiency, helping to explain why fat malabsorption develops earlier than protein or starch malabsorption.

Normal fat digestion begins in the duodenum, where pancreatic lipase hydrolyzes triglycerides into free fatty acids and monoglycerides and bile salts permit micellar solubilization of the fatty acids and monoglycerides.

Patients with destruction of the exocrine pancreas develop impaired digestion and absorption of fat. Clinically, fat malabsorption is manifested as steatorrhea. While the steatorrhea is caused mostly by the deficiency of pancreatic lipase, the absence of pancreatic bicarbonate secretion also contributes to its occurrence. Without bicarbonate, acidic chyme from the stomach inhibits the activity of pancreatic lipase and causes precipitation of bile salts. Deficiency of bile salts in turn causes failure of micelle formation and interference with fat absorption.

Finally, chronic alcohol intake interferes with both of the major mechanisms regulating exocrine pancreatic secretion: the cholinergic and the CCK pathways.

Pathophysiology

Causes of maldigestion from exocrine pancreatic insufficiency include chronic pancreatitis, cystic fibrosis, pancreatic cancer, partial or total gastrectomy, and pancreatic resection. Each of these causes is associated with specific related changes in gastrointestinal physiology, including changes in intraluminal pH, bile acid metabolism, gastric emptying, and intestinal motility.

For example, during the course of chronic pancreatitis, there is a close relationship between gastric acidity, exocrine pancreatic insufficiency, and impaired digestion. Postprandial gastric acidification has been found to be significantly greater among patients with severe pancreatic insufficiency than among those with mild or no insufficiency. Inhibition of gastric acid secretion by H_2 blockers such as cimetidine or proton pump inhibitors such as omeprazole improves the response to pancreatic enzyme replacement and decreases fecal fat excretion. However, it does not lead to complete elimination of steatorrhea.

On the other hand, loss of the stomach can cause considerable change in function of the exocrine pancreas. After total gastrectomy, patients frequently develop severe primary exocrine pancreatic insufficiency with maldigestion and weight loss. Postoperatively, pancreatic juice volume, bicarbonate output, and enzyme (amylase, trypsin, and chymotrypsin) secretion are reduced significantly compared with preoperative levels. These reductions probably result from changes in gastrointestinal hormone secretion, altering regulation of pancreatic function. For example, following gastrectomy, most patients exhibit decreased baseline and postprandial gastrin and pancreatic polypeptide secretion and increased postprandial CCK secretion.

Clinical Manifestations

The symptoms and signs (Table 15–8) exhibited by patients with pancreatic insufficiency vary to some extent with the underlying disease. For example, patients with chronic pancreatitis often have persistent symptoms of abdominal pain, anorexia, nausea, and vomiting. In severe cases of chronic pancreatitis, calcification of the gland and loss of islet cells leading to diabetes mellitus may ensue (see Chronic Pancreatitis, above). In addition, the clinical manifestations of malabsorption depend both on what is being malabsorbed and on how long the process has been occurring.

A. Steatorrhea: Patients with steatorrhea usually describe their stools as voluminous or bulky, foul-smelling, greasy, frothy, pale yellow, and floating. However, significant steatorrhea may occur without any of these characteristics. It can be docu-

Table 15–8. Clinical manifestations of pancreatic insufficiency.[1]

Symptoms and Signs	Percentage
Weight loss	90%
Steatorrhea (stool fat > 6 g/d)	48%
Edema, ascites	12%
Weakness	7%
Hypoproteinemia	14%
Malabsorption of vitamin B_{12}	40%

[1]Modified from Evans WB, Wollaeger EE: Incidence and severity of nutritional deficiency states in chronic exocrine pancreatic insufficiency: Comparison with nontropical sprue. Am J Dig Dis 1966;11:594.

mented by placing the patient on a high-fat (50–150 g/d diet and collecting all stools for 3 days and determining the average daily fecal fat excretion. An abnormal fat excretion is more than 7 g of fat per day.

B. Diarrhea: In patients with fat malabsorption, diarrhea may result from the cathartic action of hydroxylated fatty acids. These fatty acids inhibit the absorption of sodium and water by the colon. Less commonly, watery diarrhea, abdominal cramping, and bloating are due to carbohydrate malabsorption. Indeed, because salivary amylase production remains undisturbed and because pancreatic amylase production must be markedly reduced before intraluminal starch digestion is slowed, symptomatic carbohydrate malabsorption is uncommon in pancreatic insufficiency.

C. Hypocalcemia: Hypocalcemia, hypophosphatemia, tetany, osteomalacia, osteopenia (low bone mineral density), and osteoporosis can occur both from deficiency of the fat-soluble vitamin D and from the binding of dietary calcium to unabsorbed fatty acids, forming insoluble calcium-fat complexes (soaps) in the gut.

D. Nephrolithiasis: The formation of insoluble calcium soaps in the gut also prevents the normal binding of dietary oxalate to calcium. Dietary oxalate remains in solution and is absorbed from the colon, causing hyperoxaluria and predisposing to nephrolithiasis.

E. Vitamin B_{12} Deficiency: About 40% of patients with pancreatic insufficiency demonstrate malabsorption of vitamin B_{12} (cobalamin), though clinical manifestations of vitamin B_{12} deficiency are rare (anemia, subacute combined degeneration of the spinal cord, and dementia). The malabsorption of vitamin B_{12} appears to result from reduced degradation by pancreatic proteases of the normal complexes of vitamin B_{12} and its binding protein (R protein), resulting in less free vitamin B_{12} to bind to intrinsic factor in the small intestine.

F. Weight Loss: Long-standing malabsorption leads to protein catabolism and consequent weight loss, muscle wasting, fatigue, and edema. At times weight loss occurs in patients with chronic pancreatitis because eating exacerbates their abdominal pain or because narcotics used to control pain cause anorexia. In patients who develop diabetes mellitus, weight loss may be due to glycosuria. Weight loss may also be due to patients' prolonged fasting during repeated hospitalizations.

Laboratory Tests & Evaluation

The diagnosis of pancreatic insufficiency is enhanced by several noninvasive tests of exocrine pancreatic function. These tests include the bentiromide test, the pancreolauryl test, and the cholesteryl-[^{14}C]octanoate breath test. In these tests, substrates for pancreatic digestive enzymes are administered orally and their products of digestion are measured.

In the bentiromide test, N-benzoyl-L-tyrosine-p-aminobenzoic acid is administered as a substrate for chymotrypsin. Enzymatic cleavage yields p-aminobenzoic acid, which is absorbed from the gut and measured in the urine. In the pancreolauryl test, fluorescein dilaurate is administered and pancreatic esterases release fluorescein, which is then absorbed and measured in the urine. The cholesteryl-[^{14}C]octanoate breath test measures $^{14}CO_2$ output in the breath at 120 minutes after ingestion, allowing rapid detection of pancreatic exocrine insufficiency. Patients with chronic pancreatitis have markedly diminished excretion of the p-aminobenzoic acid or fluorescein in the urine or output of $^{14}CO_2$ in the breath.

---

11. How is chronic pancreatitis different from acute pancreatitis in terms of symptoms and signs?
12. What are the symptoms and signs of pancreatic insufficiency?

CARCINOMA OF THE PANCREAS

Epidemiology & Etiology

Pancreatic carcinoma is increasing dramatically in incidence, and the reason is obscure. In 1998, there were approximately 29,000 new cases of pancreatic cancer in the United States. The disease accounts for approximately 5% of cancer deaths and is the fourth leading cause of cancer death in the USA. Pancreatic cancer usually occurs after age 50 and increases in incidence with age. It is somewhat more frequent in men than in women. A study from England estimated an age-standardized incidence of 8.4 cases per 100,000 among women and 10.1 cases per 100,000 among men. Autopsy series document that pancreatic cancer has been identified in up to 2% of individuals undergoing a postmortem examination. Pancreatic cancer is rarely curable; even with surgical resection, the 5-year survival rate is little more than 5%.

The cause is unknown. The disease is six times more common in diabetic than nondiabetic women (but not in diabetic men) and two and a half to five times more common in cigarette smokers. Cholelithiasis and chronic pancreatitis have also been found to be associated with pancreatic cancer. There appears to be a five- to sixfold increase in the risk of pancreatic adenocarcinoma in patients with long-standing alcohol-related chronic pancreatitis. The role of dietary factors (decaffeinated coffee, high fat intake, and alcohol use) is much debated. Diets containing fresh fruits and vegetables are thought to be protective. There is an increased incidence of pancreatic cancer among patients with hereditary pancreatitis, particularly among those who develop pancreatic calcifications. Rarely, pancreatic carcinoma is inherited in an autosomal dominant fashion in association with diabetes mellitus and exocrine pancreatic insufficiency. A genetic predisposition has also been identified in a number of familial cancer syndromes, the most common being hereditary nonpolyposis colorectal cancer syndrome.

Pathology

Carcinomas occur more often in the head (70%) and body (20%) than in the tail (10%) of the pancreas. Virtually all pancreatic carcinomas (99%) originate in ductular cells and only a few (1%) in acinar cells. Results of molecular analyses (eg, for mutations in the proto-oncogene K-*ras*) suggest a monoclonal cellular origin in at least 95% of cases.

Grossly, pancreatic cancer presents as an indurated infiltrating tumor that obstructs the pancreatic duct and thus often causes inflammation of the distal gland. Carcinomas of the head of the pancreas tend to obstruct the common bile duct early in their course, leading to jaundice and—if the tumor is a large one—to widening of the duodenal C loop on contrast x-ray or imaging studies. Tumors of the body and tail tend to present later in their course and thus to be very large when found. Pancreatic cancer frequently causes marked fibrosis in adjacent areas (desmoplastic reaction).

Microscopically, almost all pancreatic cancers (90%) are adenocarcinomas; the remainder are adenosquamous, anaplastic, and acinar cell carcinomas. Pancreatic cancer tends to spread into surrounding tissues, invading neighboring organs along the perineural fascia, causing severe pain, and via the lymphatics and bloodstream, causing metastases in regional lymph nodes, liver, and other more distant sites.

Pathogenesis

As with other malignancies, it appears that specific molecular genetic alterations occur during development of pancreatic cancer, including activation of oncogenes, inactivation of tumor suppressor genes, and mutations of DNA mismatch repair genes. For example, point mutations in the proto-oncogene K-*ras* at codon 12 have been identified in 70–95% of pancreatic cancers. These mutations can be identified from cytologic brushings or from pancreatic juice obtained at the time of endoscopic retrograde cannulation of the pancreatic duct. Mutation in the *p53* tumor suppressor gene has also been detected in adenocarcinoma of the pancreas. Concurrent loss of *p53* and K-*ras* function may contribute to the clinical aggressiveness of the cancer. Mutation of cell cycle regulators, such as the inhibitor of the *p16* tumor suppressor gene, or of cyclin-dependent kinases may occur as a new molecular event in pancreatic cancer.

Malignant transformation of human pancreatic duct cells frequently results in deregulation of expression of various growth factors and receptors. Specifically, in comparison to normal human pancreatic duct epithelium, pancreatic carcinoma cell lines commonly demonstrated in vitro overexpression of epidermal growth factor receptor, erbB2, transforming growth factor-α, Met/hepatocyte growth factor receptor, vascular endothelial growth factor, and keratinocyte growth factor. How these alterations relate to pathogenesis is still uncertain.

Clinical Manifestations

The clinical presentation of pancreatic cancer may sometimes be indistinguishable from that of chronic pancreatitis, in part because inflammatory changes commonly occur in association with carcinoma. The clinical manifestations (Table 15–9) of pancreatic cancer vary both with location and with histologic type of tumor.

Patients with carcinoma of the head of the pancreas usually present with painless, progressive jaundice due to common bile duct obstruction. Sometimes the obstruction caused by carcinoma in the head of the pancreas is signaled by the presence of both jaundice and a dilated gallbladder palpable in the right upper quadrant (**Courvoisier's law**). Courvoisier's law states that palpable enlargement of the gallbladder in a patient with jaundice is caused by carcinoma of the head of the pancreas and not by gallstones in the common bile duct, because with

Table 15–9. Clinical manifestations of pancreatic carcinoma.

	Percentage
Symptoms and signs[1]	
Abdominal pain	73–74%
Anorexia	70%
Weight loss	60–74%
Jaundice[2]	65–72%
Diarrhea	27%
Weakness	21%
Palpable gallbladder	9%
Constipation	8%
Hematemesis or melena	7%
Vomiting	6%
Abdominal mass	1–38%
Migratory thrombophlebitis	<1%
Abnormal laboratory tests[3]	
↑ Alkaline phosphatase	82%
↑ 5′-Nucleotidase	71%
↑ LDH	69%
↑ AST	64%
↑ Bilirubin	55%
↑ Amylase	17%
↑ α-Fetoprotein	6%
↑ Carcinoembryonic antigen (CEA)	57%
↓ Albumin	60%

[1]Modified from Anderson A, Bergdahl L: Carcinoma of the pancreas. Am Surg 1976;42:173; and from Hines LH, Burns RP: Ten years' experience treating pancreatic and periampullary cancer. Am Surg 1976;42:442.
[2]With carcinoma of the head of the pancreas.
[3]Modified from Fitzgerald PJ et al: The value of diagnostic aids in detecting pancreas cancer. Cancer 1978;41:868.

gallstones the gallbladder is usually scarred from inflammation and does not become distended.

Patients with carcinoma of the body or tail of the pancreas usually present with epigastric abdominal pain, profound weight loss, an abdominal mass, and anemia. These patients usually present at later stages and more often have distant metastases, particularly in the liver.

Adenocarcinomas of the pancreas are sometimes associated with superficial thrombophlebitis or disseminated intravascular coagulation, thought to be related to thromboplastins in the mucinous secretions of the adenocarcinoma. The uncommon acinar cell carcinomas sometimes secrete lipase into the circulation, causing fat necrosis in subcutaneous tissues (manifested as skin rashes) and bone marrow (manifested as lytic bone lesions) throughout the body.

A variety of tumor markers, such as carcinoembryonic antigen (CEA), alpha-fetoprotein, pancreatic oncofetal antigen, and galactosyl transferase II, can be found in the serum of patients with pancreatic cancer. However, none of these tumor markers have sufficient specificity or predictive value to be useful in screening for the disease. Measurements of serum amylase or lipase are not helpful in diagnosis.

In evaluating patients who are suspected of having pancreatic cancer, ultrasound is very useful both in detecting tumors and in evaluating their extent. If ultrasound fails to provide the information being sought, CT is performed. For patients with an equivocal or inconclusive ultrasound or CT examination, endoscopic retrograde cannulation of the pancreatic duct (ERCP) is recommended. With the newer imaging technique of positron emission tomography (PET), an increased uptake of the radiolabeled tracer, $2[^{18}F]$-fluoro-2-deoxy-D-glucose, is seen in about 95% of patients with pancreatic cancer. Such uptake is not seen in patients with chronic pancreatitis. Percutaneous fine-needle aspiration (FNA) biopsy is used to confirm the diagnosis, particularly in patients with cancer of the body or tail of the pancreas, and to evaluate patients with suspected metastases. Angiography is often performed preoperatively to delineate the regional vascular anatomy and to look for major vascular invasion by tumor, a sign of unresectability.

Clinical prognostic factors have been identified. These include tumor size, tumor site, clinical stage, lymph node metastasis, type of surgery, anemia requiring blood transfusion, performance status, and adjuvant radiation therapy. Prognosis is influenced also by histologic characteristics such as capsular invasion, blood vessel invasion, multicentricity of the tumor, epithelial atypia in the uninvolved areas of the pancreas, and a lymphocytic infiltrate at the tumor margin. Finally, DNA flow cytometry and nuclear morphometric analysis of the mitotic rate can differentiate patients prognostically. For example, in studies using DNA analysis of cytologic specimens obtained with fine-needle aspiration biopsy, about one-fourth of patients were found to have diploid tumors and the remainder tetraploid or aneuploid tumors. The corresponding patient survival times were 8, 5, and 4 months, respectively, and resectable tumors were more often DNA diploid than nonresectable ones. These findings suggest that DNA diploid tumors represent a somewhat less aggressive subset of pancreatic carcinomas. Other measurements reflecting the proliferative activity of the cancer cells, such as S-phase fraction and mitotic rate, have prognostic significance.

Unfortunately, only about 10% of pancreatic carcinomas are diagnosed at an early stage when cure by radical resection is possible. In a large retrospective review of 37,000 cases of pancreatic cancer, only 4100 patients had undergone resection and only 156 patients were long-term survivors—an overall survival rate of only 0.4%.

13. What are the risk factors for pancreatic cancer?
14. What are common symptoms and signs of pancreatic cancer?
15. How can you make the diagnosis of pancreatic cancer in a patient with suggestive symptoms and signs?

REFERENCES

General

Chandrasoma P, Taylor CR: *Concise Pathology*, 3rd ed. Appleton & Lange, 1997.

Chey WY: Regulation of pancreatic exocrine secretion. Int J Pancreatol 1991;9:7.

Acute Pancreatitis

De Beaux AC, Fearon KC: Circulating endotoxin, tumour necrosis factor-alpha, and their natural antagonists in the pathophysiology of acute pancreatitis. Scand J Gastroenterol 1996;219(Suppl):43.

Larvin M: Circulating mediators in acute pancreatitis as predictors of severity. Scand J Gastroenterol 1996; 219(Suppl):16.

Lerch MM, Hernandez CA, Adler G: Gallstones and acute pancreatitis—mechanisms and mechanics. Dig Dis 1994;12:242.

Marshall JB: Acute pancreatitis: A review with an emphasis on new developments. Arch Intern Med 1993;153:1185.

Norman J: The role of cytokines in the pathogenesis of acute pancreatitis. Am J Surg 1998;175:76.

Steinberg W, Tenner S: Acute pancreatitis. (Medical Progress.) N Engl J Med 1994;330:1198.

Chronic Pancreatitis

Adler G, Schmid R: Chronic pancreatitis: Still puzzling? (Editorial.) Gastroenterology 1997;112:1762.

Ammann RW, Heitz PU, Kloppel G: Course of alcoholic chronic pancreatitis: A prospective clinicomorphological long-term study. Gastroenterology 1996; 111:224.

Braganza JM: The pathogenesis of chronic pancreatitis. Q J Med 1996;89:243.

Hayakawa T et al: Relationship between pancreatic exocrine function and histological changes in chronic pancreatitis. Am J Gastroenterol 1992;87:1170.

Kloppel G, Maillet B: Chronic pancreatitis: Evolution of the disease. Hepatogastroenterology 1991;38:408.

Lankisch PG et al: Natural course in chronic pancreatitis: Pain, exocrine and endocrine pancreatic insufficiency and prognosis of the disease. Digestion 1993; 54:148.

Longnecker DS: Role of the necrosis-fibrosis sequence in the pathogenesis of alcoholic chronic pancreatitis. Gastroenterology 1996;111:258.

Mergener K, Baillie J: Chronic pancreatitis. Lancet 1997;350:1379.

Owyang C: Negative feedback control of exocrine pancreatic secretion: Role of cholecystokinin and cholinergic pathway. J Nutr 1994;124(Suppl):1321S.

Sidhu SS, Tandon RK: The pathogenesis of chronic pancreatitis. Postgrad Med J 1995;71:67.

Steer ML, Waxman I, Freedman S: Chronic pancreatitis. N Engl J Med 1995;332:1482.

Pancreatic Insufficiency

Bruno MJ et al: Simultaneous assessments of exocrine pancreatic function by cholesteryl-$[^{14}C]$octanoate breath test and measurement of plasma p-aminobenzoic acid. Clin Chem 1995;41:599.

Durie PR, Forstner GG: Pathophysiology of the exocrine pancreas in cystic fibrosis. J R Soc Med 1989;82 (Suppl 16):2.

Friess H et al: Maldigestion after total gastrectomy is associated with pancreatic insufficiency. Am J Gastroenterol 1996;91:341.

Moran CE et al: Bone mineral density in patients with pancreatic insufficiency and steatorrhea. Am J Gastroenterol 1997;92:867.

Pancreatic Carcinoma

Chu TM: Molecular diagnosis of pancreas carcinoma. J Clin Lab Anal 1997;11:225.

Evans JD, Morton DG, Neoptolemos JP: Chronic pancreatitis and pancreatic carcinoma. Postgrad Med J 1997;73:543.

Gudjonsson B: Cancer of the pancreas: 50 years of surgery. Cancer 1987;60:2284.

Liu N et al: Comparative phenotypic studies of duct epithelial cell lines derived from normal human pancreas and pancreatic carcinoma. Am J Pathol 1998;153:263.

Lowenrels AB et al: Pancreatitis and the risk of pancreatic cancer. N Engl J Med 1993;328:1433.

Warshaw AL, Fernandez-del Castillo C: Pancreatic carcinoma. N Engl J Med 1992;326:455.

16

Renal Disease

Vishwanath R. Lingappa, MD, PhD

Patients with renal disease who present early in the course of illness typically have abnormalities of urine volume or composition (eg, the presence of red blood cells or abnormal amounts of protein). Later, they manifest systemic symptoms and signs of lost renal function (eg, edema, fluid overload, electrolyte abnormalities, and anemia). Depending on the nature of the renal disease, they may progress—rapidly or slowly—to display a wide range of chronic complications due to inadequate residual renal function.

Because there are no pain receptors within the substance of the kidney, pain is a prominent presenting complaint only in those renal diseases (eg, nephrolithiasis) in which there is impingement on the ureter or the renal capsule.

Because of the crucial role of the kidney in filtering blood, a wide range of systemic diseases and disease of other organ systems may be manifested most prominently in the kidney. Thus, renal disease is a prominent presentation of long-standing diabetes mellitus, hypertension, and autoimmune disorders such as systemic lupus erythematosus.

Without treatment, renal disease may result in sufficient loss of kidney function to be incompatible with life. However, not all renal disease has an inexorable downhill course and dismal outcome. The consequences of renal disease depend on the extent and nature of the injury and its natural history and time course. Some forms of renal disease are transient. Even when severe, they may be self-limited and reversible and, if managed properly, may have no permanent ill consequences. Other forms progress eventually to renal failure, either rapidly or slowly, with a host of metabolic and hemodynamic consequences along the way. When renal disease progresses, there can be loss of aspects of renal filtration capacity (eg, disordered regulation of body electrolyte and volume status) as well as loss of nonexcretory renal functions such as the production of erythropoietin (resulting in anemia).

1. What are some important causes of renal disease?
2. What are some consequences of renal failure?

NORMAL STRUCTURE & FUNCTION OF THE KIDNEY

ANATOMY, HISTOLOGY, & CELL BIOLOGY

The kidneys are a pair of encapsulated organs located in the retroperitoneal area (Figure 16–1). A renal artery enters and a renal vein exits from each kidney at the hilum. Approximately 25% of cardiac output goes to the kidneys. Blood is filtered in the kidneys to remove wastes—in particular urea and nitrogen-containing compounds—and to regulate extracellular electrolytes and intravascular volume. Because renal blood flow is from cortex to medulla and because the medulla has a relatively low blood flow for a high rate of metabolic activity, the normal oxygen tension in the medulla is lower than in other parts of the kidney. This makes the medulla particularly susceptible to ischemic injury.

The anatomic unit of kidney function is the **nephron,** a structure consisting of a tuft of capillaries termed the **glomerulus,** the site at which blood is filtered, and a **renal tubule** from which water and salts in the filtrate are reclaimed (Figure 16–2). Each human kidney has approximately 1 million nephrons.

A glomerulus consists of an **afferent** and an **efferent arteriole** and an intervening tuft of capillaries lined by endothelial cells and covered by epithelial cells that form a continuous layer with those of **Bowman's capsule** and the renal tubule. The space between capillaries in the glomerulus is called the **mesangium.** Material comprising a basement mem-

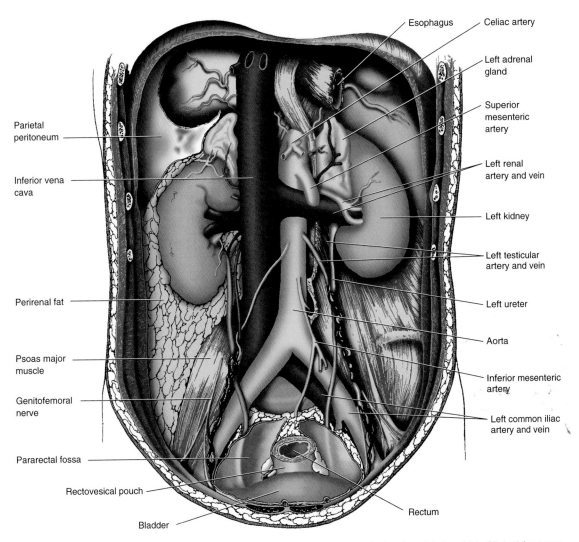

Figure 16–1. Vessels and organs of the peritoneum. (Reproduced, with permission, from Lindner HH: *Clinical Anatomy.* Appleton & Lange, 1989.)

brane is located between the capillary and the epithelial cells (Figure 16–2).

Closer examination of glomerular histology and cell biology reveals features not found in most peripheral capillaries (Figure 16–2). First, the glomerular capillary endothelium is fenestrated. However, because the endothelial cells have a coat of negatively charged glycoproteins and glycosaminoglycans, they normally exclude plasma proteins such as albumin. On the other side of the glomerular basement membrane are the epithelial cells. Termed "podocytes" because of their numerous extensions or foot processes, these cells are connected to one another by modified desmosomes.

The mesangium is an extension of the glomerular basement membrane but is less dense and contains two distinct cell types, intrinsic glomerular cells and tissue macrophages. Both cell types contribute to the development of immune-mediated glomerular disease by their production of—and response to—cytokines such as TGFβ.

The complex organization of the glomerulus is crucial not only for renal function but also for explaining the differences observed in glomerular disease. Thus, in some conditions immune complexes may accumulate under the epithelial cells, whereas in others they accumulate under the endothelial cells. Likewise, because immune cells are not able to cross

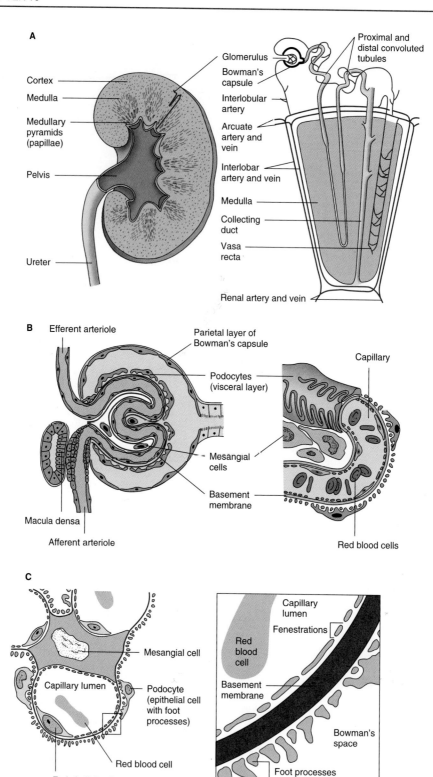

Figure 16–2. Structures of the kidney. **A:** Landmarks of the normal kidney. **B:** Glomerulus and glomerular capillary. **C:** Detailed structure of the glomerulus and the glomerular filtration membrane composed of endothelial cell, basement membrane, and podocyte. (Reproduced, with permission, from Chandrasoma P, Taylor CE: *Concise Pathology,* 3rd ed. Appleton & Lange, 1998.)

the glomerular basement membrane, immune complex deposition under the epithelial cells is generally not accompanied by a cellular inflammatory reaction (see below).

The renal tubule itself has a number of different structural regions: the **proximal convoluted tubule,** from which approximately 80% of the electrolytes and water are reclaimed; the **loop of Henle;** and a **distal convoluted tubule** and **collecting duct,** where the urine is concentrated and additional electrolyte and water changes are made in response to hormonal control (Figure 16–3).

PHYSIOLOGY

Glomerular Filtration & Tubular Resorption

Approximately 120 mL/min of glomerular filtrate are generated in a normal person with two fully functional kidneys. The approximate size cutoff of substances for filtration is 70 kDa. However, substances smaller than this are often retained, either due to charge effects (eg, albumin) or because they are tightly bound to other proteins to give them a larger effective size (eg, various growth factors and nonprotein hormones).

After filtration at the glomerulus, most of the Na^+—and, under normal conditions, almost all of the K^+ and glucose—are actively resorbed from the tubular fluid in the proximal tubule. Water is resorbed osmotically. In addition to absorption, a number of substances are secreted into the tubular fluid through the action of transporters along the renal tubule. Examples of substances that are secreted include organic anions and cations such as creatinine, histamine, and many drugs and toxins.

Normally, about 30 mL/min of isotonic filtrate is delivered to the loops of Henle, where a countercurrent multiplier mechanism achieves concentration of the urine. The loop of Henle passes down into the medulla of the kidney, where active secretion of Na^+ from the cells in the thick ascending limb establishes a hypertonic concentration gradient to resabsorb water from the tubular fluid across the cells of the descending limb.

Under normal circumstances, no more than about 5–10 mL/min of glomerular filtrate is delivered to the collecting tubules. Water absorption in the collecting tubule occurs directly through water channels controlled by **vasopressin** (also known as **antidiuretic hormone [ADH]**). Under the control of aldosterone, Na^+ resorption from tubular fluid and K^+ and H^+ transport into tubular fluid occur in different types of cells in the renal collecting tubule. Phosphoric and sulfuric acid and other acids are not volatile and therefore cannot be excreted by the lungs. Instead, they must be excreted as salts by the kidney and are thus termed "fixed acids." Urinary excretion of fixed acids also occurs in the collecting tubule. Even though it deals with less than one-tenth of the total glomerular filtrate, the collecting tubule is the site of regulation of urine volume and the site at which water, Na^+, acid-base, and K^+ balance are achieved. The crucial role of the collecting tubule in regulation of kidney function depends on two features: First, the collecting tubule is under hormonal control—in contrast to the proximal tubule, whose actions are generally a simple function of volume and composition of tubular fluid and constitutively active transporters. Second, the collecting tubule is the last region of the renal tubule traversed before the remaining 1–2 mL/min of the original glomerular filtrate exits into the ureters as urine. Insight into the functional roles of the proximal and distal renal tubules can be seen in the clinical features of the various forms of renal tubular acidosis (Table 16–1).

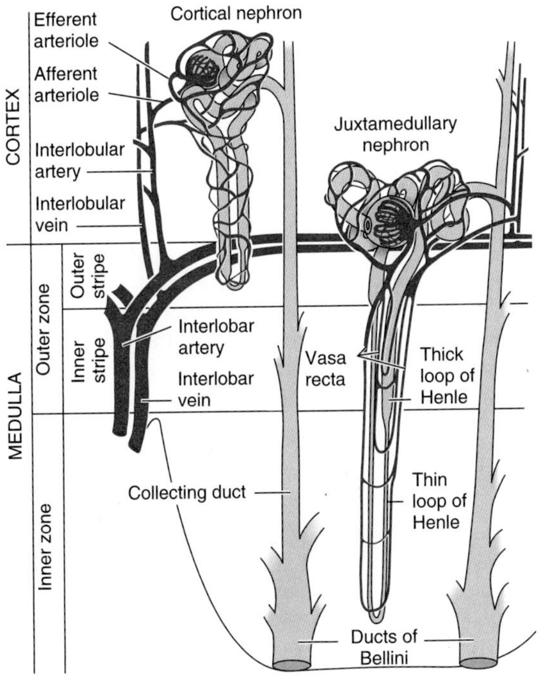

Renal Regulation of Blood Pressure

The kidney plays an important role in blood pressure regulation by virtue of its effect on Na^+ balance, a major determinant of blood pressure. First, the **macula densa** senses the Na^+ concentration in the

Figure 16–3. The vascular supply of the cortical and juxtamedullary nephrons. (Reproduced, with permission, from Pitts RF: *Physiology of the Kidney and Body Fluids,* 3rd ed. Year Book, 1963.)

Table 16–1. Characteristics of the different types of renal tubular acidosis.[1,2]

	Type 1 (Distal)	Type 2 (Proximal)	Type 4
Basic defect	Decreased distal acidification, eg, due to H^+-ATPase defect, reduced cortical Na^+ reabsorption, or increased membrane permeability.	Diminished proximal HCO_3^- reabsorption, eg, due to impaired Na^+-K^+ ATPase, Na^+-H^+ exchange, or carbonic anhydrase deficiency	Aldosterone deficiency or resistance
Urine pH during acidemia	> 5.3	Variable: > 5.3 if above reabsorptive threshold; < 5.3 if below	Usually < 5.3
Plasma [HCO_3^-], untreated	May be below 10 meq/L	Usually 14–20 meq/L	Usually above 15 meq/L
Fractional excretion of HCO_3^- at normal plasma [HCO_3^-]	< 3% in adults; may reach 5–10% in young children	> 15–20%	< 3%
Diagnosis	Response to $NaHCO_3$ or NH_4Cl	Response to $NaHCO_3$	Measure plasma aldosterone concentration
Plasma [K^+]	Usually reduced or normal; elevated with voltage defect	Normal or reduced	Elevated
Dose of HCO_3^- to normalize plasma [HCO_3^-], meq/kg per day	1–2 in adults; 4–14 in children	10–15	1–3; may require no alkali if hyperkalemia corrected
Nonelectrolyte complications	Nephrocalcinosis and renal stones	Rickets or osteomalacia	None

[1]Reproduced, with permission, from Rose BD: *Clinical Physiology of Acid-Base and Electrolyte Disorders*, 3rd ed. McGraw-Hill, 1989.
[2]What was once called type 3 RTA is actually a variant of type 1.

proximal tubular fluid (Figure 16–2). Likewise, an associated structure, the **juxtaglomerular apparatus,** assesses the perfusion pressure, an important indicator of intravascular volume status under normal circumstances. Through the action of these two sensors, either low Na^+ or low perfusion pressure acts as a stimulus to renin release. **Renin,** a protease made in the juxtaglomerular cells, cleaves angiotensinogen in the blood to generate **angiotensin I,** which is then cleaved to **angiotensin II** by **angiotensin-converting enzyme.** Angiotensin II raises blood pressure by triggering vasoconstriction directly and by stimulating aldosterone secretion, resulting in Na^+ and water retention by the collecting tubule. All of these effects raise proximal tubular Na^+ concentration and renal perfusion pressure and thus complete a homeostatic negative feedback loop that alleviates the initial stimulus for renin release.

Intravascular volume depletion also triggers vasopressin release. Receptors in the carotid body and elsewhere sense a fall in blood pressure and activate autonomic neural pathways, including fibers that go to the hypothalamus, where vasopressin release is controlled. Vasopressin is released and travels via the bloodstream throughout the body. At the collecting duct renal tubular apical plasma membrane, vasopressin facilitates vesicular fusion, thereby increasing the number of water channels. This results in reabsorption of free water. Further discussions of water balance and the role of vasopressin are presented in Chapter 19.

From rat studies, it appears that nephron number is programmed in utero. Some have speculated that low nephron number at birth (normal range: 0.3–1.4 million per kidney) predisposes an individual to development of essential hypertension in adulthood. Maternal malnutrition sufficiently severe to produce a small-for-gestational-age infant may also result in a nephron number at the lower end of the normal range, thus also predisposing to hypertension in adulthood.

Renal Regulation of Ca^{2+} Metabolism

The kidney plays a number of important roles in Ca^{2+} and phosphate homeostasis. First, the kidney is the site of 1α-hydroxylation or 24-hydroxylation of 25-hydroxycholecalciferol, the hepatic metabolite of vitamin D_3. This increases Ca^{2+} absorption from the gut. Second, the kidney is a site of action of **parathyroid hormone,** resulting in Ca^{2+} retention and phosphate wasting in the urine. Further discussion of the role of the kidney in Ca^{2+} and phosphate homeostasis is presented in Chapter 17.

Renal Regulation of Erythropoiesis

The kidney is the main site of production of the hormone **erythropoietin,** which stimulates bone marrow production and maturation of red blood cells. Thus, patients with end-stage renal disease typically display a profound anemia, with hematocrits in the range of 20–25%, and they improve in response to erythropoietin (epoetin alfa) administration.

Regulation of Renal Function

There are a variety of physical, hormonal, and neural mechanisms by which the functions of the kidney are controlled. Vasopressin, together with the physics of the countercurrent multiplier in the loop of Henle and the hypertonic medullary interstitium, make it possible to concentrate the urine under normal circumstances. This confers on the normal kidney the ability to maintain fluid homeostasis under widely diverse conditions (by generating either a concentrated or dilute urine, depending on whether the body needs to conserve or excrete salt and water).

Tubuloglomerular feedback refers to the ability of the kidney to regulate the glomerular filtration rate (GFR) in response to the solute concentration in the distal renal tubule. When an excessive concentration of Na^+ in the tubular fluid is sensed by the **macula densa,** afferent arteriolar vasoconstriction is triggered. This diminishes the GFR so that the renal tubule has a smaller solute load per unit time, allowing Na^+ to be more efficiently reclaimed from tubular fluid.

Another important challenge for the kidney is regulation of renal cortical versus medullary blood flow. Renal cortical blood flow needs to be sufficient to maintain a GFR high enough to clear renally excreted wastes efficiently without exceeding the capacity of the renal tubules for solute reabsorption. Likewise, medullary blood flow must be closely regulated. Excessive medullary blood flow can disrupt the osmolar gradient achieved by the countercurrent exchange mechanism. Insufficient medullary blood flow can result in anoxic injury to the renal tubule. From the perspective of individual nephrons, redistribution of blood flow from cortex to medulla involves preferentially supplying blood (and therefore oxygen) to those nephrons with long loops of Henle that dip down into the inner medulla.

Most medullary oxygen consumption goes to generate the ATP that fuels the array of active transporters involved in reabsorption of solute in the loop of Henle. Thus, when oxygen demand exceeds available supply, regulatory mechanisms tend to limit the workload of the ATP-consuming transporters. These regulatory mechanisms diminish the solute delivered to the loop of Henle, ie, by decreasing GFR (tubuloglomerular feedback). Renal blood flow is also preferentially shunted to medullary nephrons. In times of excessive oxygen demand, mediators are released which result in vasoconstriction of some vascular beds and vasodilation of others. This serves to both decrease GFR and, at the same time, redistribute blood flow from cortex to medulla. Table 16–2 lists some of these mediators and their proposed actions.

Adaptations of the kidney to injury can also be thought of as a form of regulation. Thus, loss of nephrons results in compensatory **glomerular hyperfiltration** (increased GFR per nephron) and renal hypertrophy. While hyperfiltration may be adaptive in the short term, allowing maintenance of the total renal GFR, it has been implicated as a common inciting event in further nephron destruction from a variety of causes. Once glomerular hyperfiltration occurs, an inexorable gradual progression to chronic renal failure is believed to begin.

There are other clinically important adaptations to injury. Poor renal perfusion from any cause results in responses that improve perfusion through afferent arteriolar vasodilation and efferent arteriolar vasoconstriction in response to hormonal and neural cues. These regulatory effects are reinforced by inputs sensing Na^+ balance. Alteration of Na^+ balance is another way to influence blood pressure and hence renal perfusion pressure.

Sympathetic innervation by the renal nerves influences renin release. Renal prostaglandins play an important role in vasodilation, especially in patients with chronically poor renal perfusion. Finally, the kidney is the source of various peptide hormones whose functions are poorly understood but which are likely to affect renal perfusion and GFR (eg, endothelins).

Table 16–2. Mechanisms regulating blood flow and tubular transport in the renal medulla.[1]

Medullary vasodilator
 Nitric oxide
 Prostaglandin E_2
 Adenosine
 Dopamine
 Urodilatin
Medullary vasoconstrictor
 Endothelin
 Angiotensin II
 Vasopressin
Inhibitor of transport in medullary thick limbs
 Prostaglandin E_2
 Adenosine
 Dopamine
 Platelet-activating factor
 Cytochrome P450-dependent arachidonate metabolites
Tubuloglomerular feedback

[1]Modified and reproduced, with permission, from Brezis M, Rosen S: Hypoxia of the renal medulla: Its implications for disease. N Engl J Med 1995;332:647.

3. What are the parts of the nephron, and what role do they play in renal function?
4. How is renal function regulated?
5. What are the nonexcretory functions of the kidney?
6. What are the relationships, if any, between each nonexcretory function named above and the kidney's role in fluid, electrolyte, and blood pressure regulation?

OVERVIEW OF RENAL DISEASE

ALTERATIONS OF KIDNEY STRUCTURE & FUNCTION IN DISEASE

Renal disease can be categorized either by the site of the lesion (eg, glomerulopathy versus tubulointerstitial disease) or by the nature of the factors that have led to kidney disease (eg, immunologic, metabolic, infiltrative, infectious, hemodynamic, or toxic).

Glomerular disease can be further categorized according to clinical presentation. Thus, some disorders present with profound proteinuria but no evidence of a cellular inflammatory reaction (nephrotic disorders), whereas others have variable degrees of proteinuria associated with red and white blood cells in the urine (nephritic disorders).

Nephrotic disorders typically show immune complex deposition at or under the epithelial cells, often with morphologic changes in the foot processes (Figure 16–4). This probably reflects damage to the selective nature of the glomerular filter, eg, by immune complex formation, or deposition of preformed complexes, in some cases with complement activation but without concomitant activation of a cellular immune response. While the lack of a cellular immune response may limit the damage done, it also slows the resolution of the disorder, with proteinuria taking months or years to resolve even when the underlying disease has been brought under control.

Nephritic disorders show immune complex deposits either in a subendothelial location or in the glomerular basement membrane or mesangium (Figure 16–4). The cellular immune system has ready access to all of these locations, and the resulting inflammatory reaction can be a two-edged sword. Thus, when the underlying process can be controlled, phagocytosis of the subendothelial deposits speeds recovery. On the other hand, an uncontrolled or prolonged inflammatory response can result in a greater degree of destruction of glomerular architecture, in part due to the local production and action of cytokines.

Certain regions of the kidney are particularly susceptible to certain kinds of injury: (1) The renal medulla is a low oxygen tension environment, which makes it more susceptible to ischemic injury. (2) The glomerulus is the initial filter of blood entering the kidney and thus is a prominent site of injury related to immune complex deposition and complement fixation. (3) Hemodynamic factors regulating blood flow have profound effects on the kidney both because the GFR, a primary determinant of renal function, depends on blood flow and because the kidney is susceptible to hypoxic injury.

One useful organizing scheme that combines a consideration of both the site and the cause of renal disease in approaching patients with new renal failure is to first categorize the cause of the patient's renal failure as prerenal, intrarenal, or postrenal and then to subdivide each of these categories according to specific causes and anatomic locations (Table 16–3).

Prerenal causes of renal failure are those resulting from inadequate blood flow to the kidney. These include intravascular volume depletion, structural lesions of the renal arteries, drug effects on renal blood flow, or hypotension from any cause that results in renal hypoperfusion.

Intrarenal causes are those disorders that result in damage to the nephron directly rather than indirectly as a secondary consequence of inadequate perfusion or obstruction. As mentioned earlier, intrarenal causes include specific disorders of the kidney as well as systemic diseases with prominent manifestations in the kidney. Some of these disorders are manifested as glomerular injury while others involve primarily the tubules. Within each category, disorders can be approached according to their specific cause or their phenotype and manifestations.

Postrenal causes are those related to urinary tract obstruction, either due to kidney stones, structural lesions (eg, tumors, prostatic hyperplasia, or strictures) or functional abnormalities (eg, spasm or drug effects).

MANIFESTATIONS OF ALTERED KIDNEY FUNCTION

The major manifestations of altered kidney function are the effects on excretion of urea and on maintenance of Na^+, K^+, water, and acid-base balance. Failure to excrete urea adequately, manifested as progressive elevation of BUN and serum creatinine, results in uremia (see Chronic Renal Failure, below). In the absence of adequate renal clearance mechanisms, ingestion of excess amounts of Na^+, K^+, water, or acids results in electrolyte, volume, and acid-base abnormalities that can be life-threatening. Furthermore, excess Na^+ ingestion in a patient with renal failure results in intravascular volume expan-

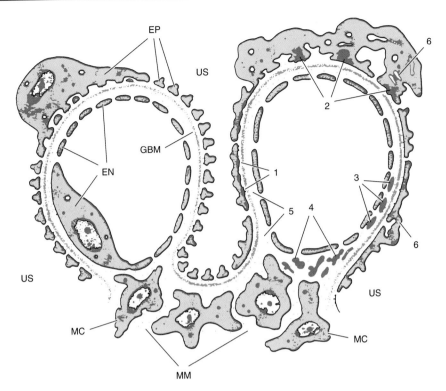

Figure 16–4. Anatomy of a normal glomerular capillary is shown on the left. Note the fenestrated endothelium (EN), glomerular basement membrane (GBM), and the epithelium with its foot processes (EP). The mesangium is composed of mesangial cells (MC) surrounded by extracellular matrix (MM) in direct contact with the endothelium. Ultrafiltration occurs across the glomerular wall and through channels in the mesangial matrix into the urinary space (US). Typical localization of immune deposits and other pathologic changes is depicted on the right. (1) Uniform subepithelial deposits as in membranous nephropathy. (2) Large, irregular subepithelial deposits or "humps" seen in acute postinfectious glomerulonephritis. (3) Subendothelial deposits as in diffuse proliferative lupus glomerulonephritis. (4) Mesangial deposits characteristic of IgA nephropathy. (5) Antibody binding to the glomerular basement membrane (as in Goodpasture's syndrome) does not produce visible deposits, but a smooth linear pattern is seen on immunofluorescence. (6) Effacement of the epithelial foot processes is common in all forms of glomerular injury with proteinuria. (Reproduced, with permission, from Luke RG et al: Nephrology and hypertension. In: *Medical Knowledge Self-Assessment Program IX.* American College of Physicians, 1992.)

sion, with complications of hypertension and congestive heart failure, while excess water ingestion results in peripheral edema.

7. What characteristics of various parts of the nephron make it particularly susceptible to certain types of injury?
8. What are the features that distinguish prerenal, intrarenal, and postrenal causes of renal failure?
9. What are the major categories of complications of inadequate renal function?

PATHOPHYSIOLOGY OF SELECTED RENAL DISEASES

ACUTE RENAL FAILURE

Clinical Presentation

Acute renal failure is a heterogeneous group of disorders that have in common the rapid deterioration of renal function, resulting in accumulation in the blood of nitrogenous wastes that would normally be excreted in the urine. The patient presents with a

Table 16-3. Major causes of kidney disease.[1]

Prerenal disease
  True volume depletion
    Gastrointestinal, renal, or sweat losses or bleeding
  Heart failure
  Hepatic cirrhosis (including the hepatorenal syndrome)
  Nephrotic syndrome (particularly after diuretic therapy for edema)
  Hypotension
  Nonsteroidal anti-inflammatory drugs
  Bilateral renal artery stenosis (particularly after therapy with an angiotensin-converting enzyme inhibitor)

Intrarenal disease
  Vascular disease
    Acute
      Vasculitis
      Malignant hypertension
      Scleroderma
      Thromboembolic disease
    Chronic
      Nephrosclerosis
  Glomerular disease
    Glomerulonephritis
    Nephrotic syndrome
  Tubular disease
    Acute
      Acute tubular necrosis
      Multiple myeloma
      Hypercalcemia
      Uric acid nephropathy
    Chronic
      Polycystic kidney disease
      Medullary sponge kidney
  Interstitial disease
    Acute
      Pyelonephritis
      Interstitial nephritis (usually drug-induced)
    Chronic
      Pyelonephritis (due primarily to vesicoureteral reflux)
      Analgesic abuse

Postrenal disease
  Obstructive uropathy
  Prostatic disease
  Malignancy
  Calculi
  Congenital abnormalities

[1] Reproduced, with permission, from Rose BD: Diagnostic approach to patient with renal disease. In: *Pathophysiology of Renal Disease,* 2nd ed. McGraw-Hill, 1987.

rapidly rising blood urea nitrogen and serum creatinine. Depending on the cause and on when the patient comes to medical attention, there may be other presenting features as well (Table 16-4). Thus, diminished urine volume (oliguria) is commonly but not always seen. Urine volume may be normal early, or indeed at any time in milder forms of acute renal injury. Patients presenting relatively late may display any of the clinical manifestations described below.

Etiology

The major causes of acute renal failure are presented in Table 16-5.

A. Prerenal Causes: Some patients who are dependent on prostaglandin-mediated vasodilation to maintain renal hypoperfusion can develop renal failure simply from ingestion of NSAIDs. Similarly, patients with renal hypoperfusion (eg, due to renal artery stenosis, congestive heart failure, or intrarenal small vessel disease) who are dependent on angiotensin II-mediated vasoconstriction of the efferent renal arteriole to maintain renal perfusion pressure may develop acute renal failure upon ingesting angiotensin-converting enzyme inhibitors.

B. Intrarenal Causes: The intrarenal causes can be further divided into specific **inflammatory diseases** such as vasculitis, glomerulonephritis, and drug-induced injury and **acute tubular necrosis** due to many causes (including ischemia, poisons, and hemolysis).

Notable among intrarenal causes are the toxic effects of aminoglycoside antibiotics and rhabdomyolysis, in which myoglobin, released into the bloodstream after crush injury to muscle, precipitates in the renal tubules. The former may be mitigated by close monitoring of renal function during antibiotic therapy, especially in elderly patients and those with some degree of underlying renal compromise. Rhabdomyolysis may be detected by obtaining a serum creatine kinase level in patients admitted to the hospital with trauma or altered mental status and may be mitigated by maintaining a vigorous alkaline diuresis to prevent myoglobin precipitation in the tubules.

C. Postrenal Causes: The postrenal causes are those that result in urinary tract obstruction, such as renal stones.

Sepsis is one of the most common causes of acute renal failure. As a complication of sepsis, acute renal failure involves a combination of prerenal and intrarenal factors. The prerenal factor is renal hypoperfusion as a consequence of the hypotensive, low systemic vascular resistance septic state. The intrarenal component may be a consequence of the cytokine dysregulation that characterizes the sepsis syndrome (Chapter 4), including elevated blood levels of tumor necrosis factor alpha, interleukin-1, and interleukin-6, which contribute to intrarenal inflammation, sclerosis, and obstruction. Patients with sepsis are often exposed also to nephrotoxic drugs such as aminoglycoside antibiotics.

Pathology & Pathogenesis

Regardless of their origin, all forms of acute renal failure, if untreated, result in acute tubular necrosis, with sloughing of cells that make up the renal tubule. Depending on the timing of intervention between onset of initial injury and eventual acute tubular necrosis, acute renal failure may be irreversible or reversible, with either prevention of—or recovery from—acute tubular necrosis.

The precise molecular mechanisms responsible for the development of acute tubular necrosis remain unknown. Theories favoring either a tubular or vascular basis have been proposed (Figure 16-5). According to the tubular theory, occlusion of the tubular lumen

Table 16–4. Initial clinical and laboratory data base for defining major syndromes in nephrology.[1]

Syndrome	Important Clues to Diagnosis	Common Findings Not of Diagnostic Value
Acute or rapidly progressive renal failure	Anuria Oliguria Documented recent decline in GFR	Hypertension Hematuria, proteinuria, pyuria, casts Edema
Acute nephritis	Hematuria, red cell casts Azotemia, oliguria Edema, hypertension	Proteinuria, pyuria Circulatory congestion
Chronic renal failure	Azotemia for > 3 months Prolonged symptoms or signs of uremia Symptoms or signs of renal osteodystrophy Kidneys reduced in size bilaterally Broad casts in urinary sediment	Hematuria, proteinuria, casts Oliguria, polyuria, nocturia Edema, hypertension Electrolyte disorders
Nephrotic syndrome	Proteinuria > 3.5 g/1.73 m^2 per 24 hours Hypoalbuminemia Hyperlipidemia Lipiduria	Casts Edema
Asymptomatic urinary abnormalities	Hematuria Proteinuria (below nephrotic range) Sterile pyuria, casts	
Urinary tract infection	Bacteriuria > 10^5 colonies/mL Other infectious agent documented in urine Pyuria, leukocyte casts Frequency, urgency Bladder tenderness, flank tenderness	Hematuria Mild azotemia Mild proteinuria Fever
Renal tubular defects	Electrolyte disorders Polyuria, nocturia Symptoms or signs of renal osteodystrophy Large kidneys Renal transport defects	Hematuria Mild azotemia Mild proteinuria Fever
Hypertension	Systolic/diastolic hypertension	Proteinuria Casts Azotemia
Nephrolithiasis	History of stone passage or removal Stone seen by x-ray Renal colic	Hematuria Pyuria Frequency, urgency
Urinary tract obstruction	Azotemia, oliguria, anuria Polyuria, nocturia, urinary retention Slowing of urinary stream Large prostate, large kidneys Flank tenderness, full bladder after voiding	Hematuria Pyuria Enuresis, dysuria

[1]Reproduced, with permission, from Coe FL, Brenner BM: Approach to the patient with diseases of the kidney and urinary tract. In: *Harrison's Principles of Internal Medicine,* 14th ed. Fauci AS et al (editors). McGraw-Hill, 1998.

with cellular debris forms a cast that increases intratubular pressure sufficiently to offset perfusion pressure and decrease or abolish net filtration pressure. Vascular theories propose that decreased renal perfusion pressure from the combination of afferent arteriolar vasoconstriction and efferent arteriolar vasodilation reduces glomerular perfusion pressure and therefore glomerular filtration. It may be that both mechanisms act to produce acute renal failure, varying in relative importance in different individuals depending on the cause and the time of presentation. Recent studies suggest that one consequence of hypoxia is disordered adhesion of renal tubular epithelial cells, resulting both in their exfoliation and subsequent adhesion to other cells of the tubule, thereby contributing to tubular obstruction (Figure 16–5). Renal damage, whether due to tubular occlusion or vascular hypoperfusion, is potentiated by the hypoxic state of the renal medulla, which increases the risk of ischemia (Table 16–6). Recent work has implicated cytokines and endogenous peptides such as endothelins and the regulation of their production as possible explanations for why, subjected to the same toxic insult, some patients develop acute renal

Table 16–5. Major causes of acute renal failure.[1]

Disorder	Examples
Hypovolemia	Volume loss via the skin, gastrointestinal tract, or kidney. Hemorrhage. Sequestration of extracellular fluid (burns, pancreatitis, peritonitis).
Cardiovascular failure	Impaired cardiac output (infarction, tamponade). Vascular pooling (anaphylaxis, sepsis, drugs).
Extrarenal obstruction	Urethral occlusion: Vesical, pelvic, prostatic, or retroperitoneal neoplasms. Surgical accident. Medication. Calculi. Pus, blood clots.
Intrarenal obstruction	Crystals (uric acid, oxalic acid, sulfonamides, methotrexate).
Bladder rupture	Trauma.
Vascular diseases	Vasculitis. Malignant hypertension. Thrombotic thrombocytopenia purpura. Scleroderma. Arterial or venous occlusion.
Glomerulonephritis	Immune complex disease. Anti-GBM disease.
Interstitial nephritis	Drugs. Hypercalcemia. Infections. Idiopathic.
Postischemic	All conditions listed above under hypovolemia and cardiovascular failure.
Pigment-induced	Hemolysis (transfusion reaction, malaria). Rhabdomyolysis (trauma, muscle disease, coma, heat stroke, severe exercise, potassium or phosphate depletion).
Poison-induced	Antibiotics. Contrast material. Anesthetic agents. Heavy metals. Organic solvents.
Pregnancy-related	Septic abortion. Uterine hemorrhage. Eclampsia.

[1]Reproduced, with permission, from Andersen RJ, Schrier RW: Acute renal failure. In: *Harrison's Principles of Internal Medicine*, 12th ed. Wilson JD et al (editors). McGraw-Hill, 1991.

failure whereas others do not and why some with acute renal failure recover whereas others do not. It appears that these products together with activation of complement and neutrophils increase vasoconstriction in the already ischemic renal medulla and in that way exacerbate the degree of hypoxic injury that occurs in acute renal failure.

Clinical Manifestations

The initial symptoms are typically fatigue and malaise—probably early consequences of loss of the ability to excrete water, salt, and wastes via the kidneys. Later, more profound symptoms and signs of loss of renal water and salt excretory capacity develop: dyspnea, orthopnea, rales, a prominent third heart sound (S_3), and peripheral edema. Altered mental status reflects the toxic effect of uremia on the brain, with elevated blood levels of nitrogenous wastes and fixed acids.

The clinical manifestations of acute renal failure depend not only on the cause but also on the stage in the natural history of the disease at which the patient comes to medical attention. Patients with renal hypoperfusion (prerenal causes of acute renal failure) first develop **prerenal azotemia** (elevated BUN without tubular necrosis), a direct physiologic consequence of a decreased GFR. With appropriate treatment, renal perfusion can typically be improved, prerenal azotemia can be readily reversed, and the development of acute tubular necrosis can be prevented. Without treatment, prerenal azotemia may progress to acute tubular necrosis. Recovery from acute tubular necrosis, if it occurs, will then follow a more protracted course, often requiring supportive dialysis before adequate renal function is regained.

A variety of clinical tests can help determine whether a patient with signs of acute renal failure is in the early phase of prerenal azotemia or has progressed to full-blown acute tubular necrosis. However, the overlap in clinical presentation along the continuum between prerenal azotemia and acute tubular necrosis is such that the results of any one of these tests must be interpreted in the context of other findings and the clinical history.

Perhaps the earliest manifestation of prerenal azotemia is an elevated ratio of BUN to serum creatinine. Normally 10–15:1, this ratio may rise to 20–30:1 in prerenal azotemia, with a normal or near-normal serum creatinine. If the patient proceeds to acute tubular necrosis, this ratio may return to normal but with a progressively elevated serum creatinine. Likewise, a fluctuating but not inexorably rising serum creatinine suggests prerenal azotemia.

Urinalysis may also be useful. There are no typical abnormal findings in simple prerenal azotemia, whereas granular casts, tubular epithelial cells, and epithelial cell casts are found in acute tubular necrosis. Casts are formed when debris in the renal tubules (protein, red cells, or epithelial cells) takes on the cylindric, smooth-bordered shape of the tubule. Likewise, since hypovolemia is a stimulus to vasopressin release (see Chapter 19), the urine is maximally concentrated (up to 1500 mosm/L) in prerenal azotemia. However, with progression to acute tubular necrosis, the ability to generate a concentrated urine is largely lost. Thus, a urine osmolality of less than 350 mosm/L is a typical finding in acute tubular necrosis.

Finally, the fractional excretion of Na^+

$$FE_{Na^+}[\%] = \frac{Urine_{Na^+}/Plasma_{Na^+}}{Urine_{Cr}/Plasma_{Cr}} \times 100$$

RENAL DISEASE / 393

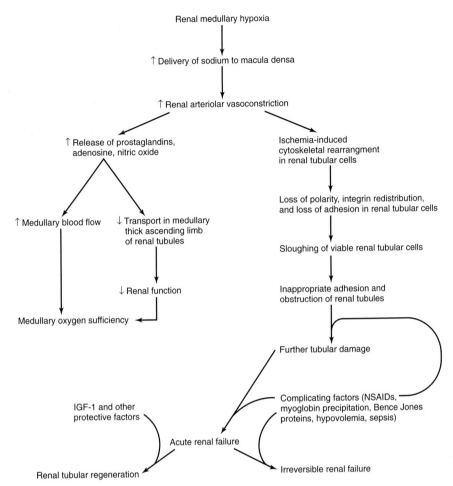

Figure 16–5. Pathophysiology of ischemia-induced acute renal failure. Mild or uncomplicated medullary hypoxia results in tubuloglomerular reflex adjustments that restore medullary oxygen sufficiency at the price of diminished renal function. However, in the event of extreme renal medullary hypoxia or when associated with complicating factors such as those indicated in the figure, full-blown acute renal failure develops. Whether acute renal failure is reversible or irreversible depends on a balance of reparative and complicating factors.

Table 16–6. Agents and events that ameliorate or exacerbate hypoxia in the renal medulla.[1]

Ameliorating effect
  Decreased tubular transport
  Decreased glomerular filtration rate
  Prostaglandin E_2
  Adenosine
  Bradykinin
  Nitric oxide
Exacerbating effect
  Polyene antibiotics (eg, amphotericin B)
  Renal hypertrophy
  Nonsteroidal anti-inflammatory drugs
  Angiotensin II
  Calcium
  Myoglobin
  Radiographic contrast agents

[1]Modified and reproduced, with permission, from Brezis M, Rosen S: Hypoxia of the renal medulla: Its implications for disease. N Engl J Med 1995;332:647.

Table 16–7. Causes of acute renal failure in which FE_{Na} may be below 1%.[1]

Prerenal disease
Acute tubular necrosis
  10% of nonoliguric cases
  Superimposed upon chronic prerenal state
    Hepatic cirrhosis
    Heart failure
    Severe burns
  Myoglobinuria or hemoglobinuria
  Radiocontrast media
  Sepsis
Acute glomerulonephritis or vasculitis
Acute obstructive uropathy
Acute interstitial nephritis

[1]Reproduced, with permission, from Rose BD: Acute renal failure—prerenal disease vs acute tubular necrosis. In: *Pathophysiology of Renal Disease,* 2nd ed. McGraw-Hill, 1987.

is an important indicator of whether a patient with acute renal failure has progressed from simple prerenal azotemia to frank acute tubular necrosis. In simple prerenal azotemia, over 99% of filtered Na$^+$ is reabsorbed. This value allows accurate identification of Na$^+$ retention states (such as prerenal azotemia) even when there is water retention due to vasopressin release. There are, however, some rare conditions in which the FE_{Na^+} is less than 1% in patients with acute tubular necrosis (Table 16–7).

10. What are the current theories for the development of acute tubular necrosis?
11. What clues are helpful in determining whether newly diagnosed renal failure is acute or chronic?
12. What is the natural history of acute renal failure?

CHRONIC RENAL FAILURE

Clinical Presentation

Patients with chronic renal failure and uremia show a constellation of symptoms, signs, and laboratory abnormalities in addition to those observed in acute renal failure. This reflects the long-standing and progressive nature of their renal impairment and its effects on many types of tissues (Table 16–8). Thus, osteodystrophy, neuropathy, bilateral small kidneys shown by abdominal x-ray or ultrasound, and anemia are typical initial findings that suggest a chronic course for a patient newly diagnosed with renal failure on the basis of elevated BUN and serum creatinine.

Etiology

The most common cause of chronic renal failure is diabetes mellitus (Chapter 18), followed closely by hypertension and glomerulonephritis (Table 16–9).

Table 16–8. Clinical abnormalities in uremia.[1,2]

Fluid and electrolyte	**Cardiovascular**
Volume expansion and contraction (I)	Arterial hypertension (I or P)
Hypernatremia and hyponatremia (I)	Congestive heart failure or pulmonary edema (I)
Hyperkalemia and hypokalemia (I)	Pericarditis (I)
Metabolic acidosis (I)	Cardiomyopathy (I or P)
Hypocalcemia (I)	Uremic lung (I)
Bone and mineral	Accelerated atherosclerosis (P or D)
Renal osteodystrophy (I or P)	Hypotension and arrhythmias (D)
Osteomalacia (D)	**Skin**
Metabolic	Skin pallor (I or P)
Carbohydrate intolerance (I)	Hyperpigmentation (I, P, or D)
Hypothermia (I)	Pruritus (P)
Hypertriglyceridemia (P)	Ecchymoses (I or P)
Protein-calorie malnutrition (I or P)	Uremic frost (I)
Impaired growth and development (P)	**Gastrointestinal**
Infertility and sexual dysfunction (P)	Anorexia (I)
Amenorrhea (P)	Nausea and vomiting (I)
Dialysis (amyloid, β_2-microglobulin) arthropathy (D)	Uremic fetor (I)
Neuromuscular	Gastroenteritis (I)
Fatigue (I)	Peptic ulcer (I or P)
Sleep disorders (P)	Gastrointestinal bleeding (I, P, or D)
Impaired mentation (I)	Hepatitis (D)
Lethargy (I)	Refractory ascites on hemodialysis (D)
Asterixis (I)	Peritonitis (D)
Muscular irritability (I)	**Hematologic**
Peripheral neuropathy (I or P)	Normocytic, normochromic anemia (P)
Restless legs syndrome (I or P)	Microcytic (aluminum-induced) anemia (D)
Paralysis (I or P)	Lymphocytopenia (P)
Myoclonus (I)	Bleeding diathesis (I or D)
Seizures (I or P)	Increased susceptibility to infection (I or P)
Coma (I)	Splenomegaly and hypersplenism (P)
Muscle cramps (D)	Leukopenia (D)
Dialysis disequilibrium syndrome (D)	Hypocomplementemia (D)
Dialysis dementia (D)	
Myopathy (P or D)	

[1]Virtually all the abnormalities contained in this table are completely reversed in time by successful renal transplantation. The response of these abnormalities to hemo- or peritoneal dialysis therapy is more variable. (I) denotes an abnormality that usually improves with an optimal program of dialysis and related therapy. (P) denotes an abnormality that tends to persist or even progress, despite an optimal program. (D) denotes an abnormality that develops only after initiation of dialysis therapy.
[2]Reproduced, with permission, from Lazarus JM, Brenner BM: Chronic renal failure. In: *Harrison's Principles of Internal Medicine,* 14th ed. Fauci AS et al (editors). McGraw-Hill, 1998.

Table 16–9. Primary diagnoses in patients with end-stage renal disease.[1,2]

Diabetic nephropathy	27.7%
Hypertension	24.5%
Glomerulonephritis	21.2%
Polycystic kidney disease	3.9%
Other, unknown	22.7%

[1]Number of new patients in 1985: 28,944.
[2]Source: Health Care Financing Administration, Bureau of Data Management and Strategy. Reproduced, with permission, from Brenner BM, Lazarus JM: Chronic renal failure. In: *Harrison's Principles of Internal Medicine,* 12th ed. Wilson JD et al (editors). McGraw-Hill, 1991.

Polycystic kidney disease, obstruction, and infection are among the less common causes of chronic renal failure.

Pathology & Pathogenesis

A. Development of Chronic Renal Failure: The pathogenesis of acute renal disease is very different from that of chronic renal disease. Whereas acute injury to the kidney results in death and sloughing of tubular epithelial cells, often followed by their regeneration with reestablishment of normal architecture, chronic injury results in irreversible loss of nephrons. As a result, a greater functional burden is borne by fewer nephrons, manifested as an increase in glomerular filtration pressure and hyperfiltration. For reasons not well understood, this compensatory hyperfiltration—which can be thought of as a form of "hypertension" at the level of the individual nephron—predisposes to fibrosis and scarring (**glomerular sclerosis**). As a result, the rate of nephron destruction and loss increases, thus speeding the progression to **uremia,** the complex of symptoms and signs that occurs when residual renal function is inadequate.

Owing to the tremendous functional reserve of the kidneys, up to 50% of nephrons can be lost without any short-term evidence of functional impairment. This is why individuals with two healthy kidneys are able to donate one for transplantation. When GFR is further reduced to the 30–50% range, leaving only about 20% of initial renal capacity, some degree of azotemia (elevation of blood levels of products normally excreted by the kidneys) is observed. Nevertheless, patients may be largely asymptomatic because a new steady state is achieved in which blood levels of these products are not high enough to cause overt toxicity. However, even at this apparently stable level of renal function, hyperfiltration-accelerated evolution to end-stage chronic renal failure is in progress. Furthermore, since patients with this level of GFR have little functional reserve, they can easily become uremic with any added stress (eg, infection, obstruction, dehydration, or nephrotoxic drugs) or with any catabolic state associated with increased turnover of nitrogen-containing products with reduction in GFR. Below approximately 20% of normal, renal excretory capacity is insufficient to prevent the development of frank uremia.

B. Pathogenesis of Uremia: The pathogenesis of chronic renal failure derives in part from a combination of the toxic effects of (1) retained products normally excreted by the kidneys (eg, nitrogen-containing products of protein metabolism); (2) normal products such as hormones now present in increased amounts; and (3) loss of normal products of the kidney (eg, loss of erythropoietin).

Excretory failure results also in fluid shifts, with increased intracellular Na^+ and water and decreased intracellular K^+. These alterations may contribute to subtle alterations in function of a host of enzymes, transport systems, etc.

Finally, uremia has a number of effects on metabolism that are currently not well understood, including (1) a decrease in basal body temperature (perhaps due to decreased Na^+-K^+ ATPase activity) and (2) diminished lipoprotein lipase activity with accelerated atherosclerosis.

Clinical Manifestations

A. Na^+ Balance and Volume Status: Patients with chronic renal failure typically have some degree of Na^+ and water excess, reflecting loss of the renal route of salt and water excretion. A moderate degree of Na^+ and water excess may occur without objective signs of extracellular fluid excess. However, continued excessive Na^+ ingestion will contribute to congestive heart failure, hypertension, ascites, and edema. On the other hand, excessive water ingestion contributes to hyponatremia, peripheral edema, and weight gain. A common recommendation for the patient with chronic renal failure is to avoid excess salt intake and to restrict fluid intake so that it equals urine output plus 500 mL (insensible losses). Further adjustments in volume status can be made either through the use of diuretics (in a patient who still makes urine) or at dialysis.

Because these patients also have impaired renal salt and water conservation mechanisms, they are more than normally sensitive to sudden extrarenal Na^+ and water losses (eg, vomiting, diarrhea, and increased sweating with fever). Under these circumstances, they will more easily develop ECF depletion, further deterioration of renal function (which may not be reversible), and even vascular collapse and shock. The symptoms and signs of dry oral and other mucous membranes, dizziness, syncope, tachycardia, and decreased jugular venous filling suggest progression of volume depletion.

B. K^+ Balance: Hyperkalemia is a serious problem in chronic renal failure for patients whose GFR has fallen below 5 mL/min. Above that GFR level, patients with chronic renal failure generally do not have difficulties in K^+ homeostasis because as GFR falls, aldosterone-mediated K$^+$ transport in the distal tubule increases in a compensatory fashion. However, this means that a patient whose GFR is between 50 mL/min and 5 mL/min is dependent on tubular transport to maintain K$^+$ balance. Treatment with K$^+$-sparing diuretics, angiotensin-converting enzyme inhibitors, or beta-blockers—drugs that may impair aldosterone-mediated K$^+$ transport—can therefore precipitate dangerous hyperkalemia in a patient with chronic renal failure.

Patients with diabetes mellitus (the leading cause of chronic renal failure) may have a syndrome of **hyporeninemic hypoaldosteronism.** This syndrome, also termed **type 4 renal tubular acidosis,** is a condition in which lack of renin production by the kidney diminishes the levels of angiotensin II and therefore impairs aldosterone secretion (Table 16–1). As a result, affected patients are unable to compensate for falling GFR by enhancing their aldosterone-mediated K$^+$ transport and therefore have relative difficulty handling K$^+$. This difficulty is usually manifested as extreme hyperkalemia even before GFR has fallen below 5 mL/min.

Finally, just as chronic renal failure patients are more susceptible to the effects of Na$^+$ or volume overload, so also are they at greater risk of hyperkalemia in the face of sudden loads of K$^+$ from either endogenous sources (eg, hemolysis, infection, trauma) or exogenous sources (eg, stored blood, K$^+$-rich foods, or K$^+$-containing medications).

C. Metabolic Acidosis: The diminished capacity to excrete acid and generate buffers in chronic renal failure results in metabolic acidosis. In most cases when the GFR is above 20 mL/min, only moderate acidosis develops before reestablishment of a new steady state of buffer production and consumption. The fall in blood pH in these individuals can usually be corrected with 20–30 mmol (2–3 g) of sodium bicarbonate by mouth daily. However, these patients are highly susceptible to acidosis in the event of a sudden acid load or the onset of disorders that increase the generated acid load.

D. Mineral and Bone: Several disorders of phosphate, Ca^{2+}, and bone metabolism are observed in chronic renal failure as a result of a complex series of events (Figure 16–6). The key factors in the pathogenesis of these disorders include (1) diminished absorption of Ca^{2+} from the gut, (2) overproduction of parathyroid hormone, (3) disordered vitamin D metabolism, and (4) chronic metabolic acidosis. All of these factors contribute to enhanced bone resorption. Hyperuricemia is also a common finding in chronic renal failure, though symptomatic gout is relatively rare. Hypophosphatemia and hypermagnesemia can occur through overuse of phosphate binders and magnesium-containing antacids, though hyperphos-

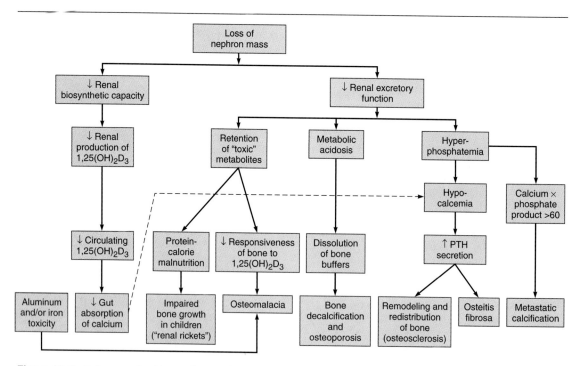

Figure 16–6. Pathogenesis of bone diseases in chronic renal failure. (Reproduced, with permission, from Brenner BM, Lazarus JM: Chronic renal failure. In: *Harrison's Principles of Internal Medicine,* 13th ed. Isselbacher KJ et al [editors]. McGraw-Hill, 1994.)

phatemia is more common. Hyperphosphatemia contributes to the development of hypocalcemia and thus serves as an additional trigger for secondary hyperparathyroidism, elevating blood PTH levels. The elevated blood PTH further depletes bone Ca^{2+} and contributes to osteomalacia and osteoporosis of chronic renal failure (see below).

E. Cardiovascular and Pulmonary Abnormalities: Congestive heart failure and pulmonary edema are most commonly due to volume and salt overload. However, a poorly understood syndrome involving increased permeability of the alveolar capillary membrane is also observed that can result in pulmonary edema even with normal or only slightly elevated pulmonary capillary wedge pressures.

Hypertension is a common finding in chronic renal failure, usually on the basis of fluid and Na^+ overload. However, hyperreninemia is also a recognized syndrome in which falling renal perfusion triggers the failing kidney to overproduce renin and thereby elevate systemic blood pressure.

Pericarditis resulting from irritation and inflammation of the pericardium by uremic toxins is a complication whose incidence in chronic renal failure is decreasing owing to the aggressive and early institution of renal dialysis.

Accelerated atherosclerosis is a complication seen in patients with chronic renal failure on long-term dialysis. It results in myocardial infarction, stroke, and peripheral vascular disease. Cardiovascular risk factors in these patients include hypertension, hyperlipidemia, glucose intolerance, chronic elevated cardiac output, and valvular and myocardial calcification as a consequence of elevated $Ca^{2+} \times$ phosphate product.

F. Hematologic Abnormalities: Patients with chronic renal failure have marked abnormalities in red blood cell count, white blood cell function, and clotting parameters. Normochromic, normocytic anemia, with symptoms of listlessness and easy fatigability and hematocrits typically in the range of 20–25%, is a consistent feature. The anemia is due chiefly to lack of production of erythropoietin and loss of its stimulatory effect on erythropoiesis. Thus, patients with chronic renal failure, regardless of dialysis status, show a dramatic improvement in hematocrit when treated with erythropoietin. Additional causes of anemia may include bone marrow suppressive effects of uremic poisons, bone marrow fibrosis due to elevated blood PTH, toxic effects of aluminum (from phosphate-binding antacids and dialysis solutions), and hemolysis and gastrointestinal blood loss related to dialysis (while the patient is anticoagulated with heparin).

Patients with chronic renal failure display abnormal hemostasis manifested as increased bruising, increased blood loss at surgery, and an increased incidence of spontaneous gastrointestinal and cerebrovascular hemorrhage (including both hemorrhagic strokes and subdural hematomas). Laboratory abnormalities include prolonged bleeding time, decreased platelet factor III, abnormal platelet aggregation and adhesiveness, and impaired prothrombin consumption—none of them reversible even in well-dialysed patients.

Uremia is associated with increased susceptibility to infections, believed to be due to leukocyte suppression by uremic toxins. The suppression seems to be greater for lymphoid cells than neutrophils and seems also to affect chemotaxis, the acute inflammatory response, and delayed hypersensitivity more than other leukocyte functions. Acidosis, hyperglycemia, malnutrition, and hyperosmolality also are believed to contribute to immunosuppression in chronic renal failure. The invasiveness of dialysis and the use of immunosuppressive drugs in renal transplant patients also contribute to an increased incidence of infections.

G. Neuromuscular Abnormalities: Central nervous system symptoms and signs may range from mild sleep disorders and impairment of mental concentration, loss of memory, errors in judgment, and neuromuscular irritability (manifested as hiccups, cramps, fasciculations, and twitching) to asterixis, myoclonus, stupor, seizures, and coma in end-stage uremia. Asterixis is manifested as involuntary flapping motions seen when the arms are extended and wrists held back to "stop traffic." It is due to altered nerve conduction in metabolic encephalopathy from a wide variety of causes including renal failure.

Peripheral neuropathy (sensory greater than motor, lower extremities greater than upper), typified by the "restless legs" syndrome (poorly localized sense of discomfort and involuntary movements of the lower extremities) is a common finding in chronic renal failure and an important indication for starting dialysis.

Patients receiving hemodialysis can develop aluminum toxicity, characterized by speech dyspraxia (inability to repeat words), myoclonus, dementia, and seizures. Likewise, aggressive acute dialysis can result in a disequilibrium syndrome characterized by nausea, vomiting, drowsiness, headache, and seizures in a patient with very high BUN levels. Presumably, this is an effect of rapid pH or osmolality change in extracellular fluid, resulting in cerebral edema.

H. Gastrointestinal Abnormalities: Up to 25% of patients with uremia have peptic ulcer disease, perhaps as a consequence of secondary hyperparathyroidism. A variety of other gastrointestinal abnormalities and syndromes are described as well, including uremic gastroenteritis, characterized by mucosal ulcerations with blood loss in the chronic renal failure patient, and a distinctive form of bad breath (uremic fetor) due to degradation of urea to ammonia by enzymes in the saliva.

Nonspecific gastrointestinal findings in uremic patients include anorexia, hiccups, nausea, vomiting, and diverticulosis. Although their precise pathogenesis is unclear, many of these findings improve with dialysis.

I. Endocrine and Metabolic Abnormalities: Women with uremia have low estrogen levels, which perhaps explains the high incidence of amenorrhea and the observation that they rarely are able to carry a pregnancy to term. Regular menses—but not a higher rate of successful pregnancies—typically return with frequent dialysis.

Similarly, low testosterone levels, impotence, oligospermia, and germinal cell dysplasia are common findings in men with chronic renal failure.

Finally, chronic renal failure eliminates the kidney as a site of insulin degradation, thereby increasing the half-life of insulin. This typically has a stabilizing effect on diabetic patients whose blood glucose was previously difficult to control.

J. Dermatologic Abnormalities: Skin changes arise from many of the effects of chronic renal failure already discussed. Patients with chronic renal failure may display pallor due to anemia, skin color changes due to accumulated pigmented metabolites or a gray discoloration due to transfusion-mediated hemochromatosis; ecchymoses and hematomas due to clotting abnormalities; and pruritus and excoriations due to Ca^{2+} deposits from secondary hyperparathyroidism. Finally, when urea concentrations are extremely high, evaporation of sweat leaves a residue of urea termed "uremic frost."

---

13. What is uremia?
14. What are the most prominent symptoms and signs of uremia?
15. What is the mechanism by which altered sodium, potassium, and volume status develop in chronic renal failure?
16. What are the most common causes of chronic renal failure?

GLOMERULONEPHRITIS & NEPHROTIC SYNDROME

Clinical Presentation

A number of disorders result in structural alterations of the glomerulus and present with some combination of the following findings: hematuria, proteinuria, reduced GFR, and hypertension. Some of these disorders are specific to the kidney, while others are systemic diseases in which the kidney is primarily or prominently involved.

Disorders resulting in glomerular disease, whether manifestations of systemic injury or otherwise, fall into five categories:

(1) **Acute glomerulonephritis,** in which there is an abrupt onset of hematuria and proteinuria with reduced GFR and renal salt and water retention, followed by full recovery of renal function. Patients with acute glomerulonephritis are a subset of those with an intrarenal cause of acute renal failure.

(2) **Rapidly progressive glomerulonephritis,** in which recovery from the acute disorder does not occur. Worsening renal function results in irreversible and complete renal failure over weeks to months. Early in the course of rapidly progressive glomerulonephritis, these patients can be categorized as having a form of acute renal failure. Later, with progression of their renal failure over time, they display all of the features described for chronic renal failure.

(3) **Chronic glomerulonephritis,** in which renal impairment following acute glomerulonephritis progresses slowly over a period of years but which eventually results in chronic renal failure.

(4) **Nephrotic syndrome,** manifested as marked proteinuria, particularly albuminuria (defined as 24-hour urine protein excretion > 3.5 g), hypoalbuminemia, edema, hyperlipidemia, and fat bodies in the urine. Nephrotic syndrome may be either isolated (eg, minimal change disease) or part of some other glomerular syndrome (eg, with hematuria and casts).

(5) **Asymptomatic urinary abnormalities,** including hematuria and proteinuria (usually in amounts below what is seen in nephrotic syndrome) but no functional abnormalities associated with reduced GFR, edema, or hypertension. Many patients with these findings will develop chronic renal failure slowly over decades.

Etiology

Acute glomerulonephritis occurs most typically in the setting of infectious diseases—classically pharyngeal or cutaneous infections with certain "nephritogenic" strains of group A beta-hemolytic streptococci but also other pathogens (Table 16–10).

Table 16–10. Causes of acute glomerulonephritis.[1,2]

Infectious diseases
  Poststreptococcal glomerulonephritis*
  Nonstreptococcal postinfectious glomerulonephritis
    Bacterial: infective endocarditis,* "shunt nephritis," sepsis,* pneumococcal pneumonia, typhoid fever, secondary syphilis, meningococcemia
    Viral: hepatitis B, infectious mononucleosis, mumps, measles, varicella, echovirus, coxsackievirus
    Parasitic: malaria, toxoplasmosis
Multisystem diseases: systemic lupus erythematosus,* vasculitis,* Henoch-Schönlein purpura,* Goodpasture's syndrome
Primary glomerular diseases: mesangiocapillary glomerulonephritis, Berger's disease (IgA nephropathy),* "pure" mesangial proliferative glomerulonephritis
Miscellaneous: Guillain-Barré syndrome, irradiation of Wilms' tumor, diphtheria-pertussis-tetanus vaccine, serum sickness

[1] Reproduced, with permission, from Glassock RJ, Brenner BM: The major glomerulopathies. In: *Harrison's Principles of Internal Medicine,* 12th ed. Wilson JD et al (editors). McGraw-Hill, 1991.
[2] Most common causes are marked with asterisks.

Rapidly progressive glomerulonephritis appears to be a heterogeneous group of disorders all of which display pathologic features common to various categories of necrotizing vasculitis (Table 16–11; and see below).

Chronic glomerulonephritis and nephrotic syndrome are also of unclear origin. For some reason, progressive renal deterioration in patients with chronic glomerulonephritis proceeds slowly but inexorably, resulting in chronic renal failure as many as 20 years after initial discovery of an abnormal urinary sediment.

Some cases of nephrotic syndrome are variants of acute glomerulonephritis, rapidly progressive glomerulonephritis, or chronic glomerulonephritis in which massive proteinuria is a presenting feature. Other cases of nephrotic syndrome fall into the category of **minimal change disease,** in which all of the pathologic consequences are due to proteinuria and progression to end-stage renal disease does not occur.

The most common cause of asymptomatic urinary abnormalities is **IgA nephropathy,** a poorly understood immune complex disease characterized by diffuse mesangial IgA deposition. Other causes are listed in Table 16–12.

Pathology & Pathogenesis

The different forms of glomerulonephritis and nephrotic syndrome probably represent differences in the nature, extent, and specific cause of immune-mediated renal damage. A number of cytokines—in particular transforming growth factor-1 (TGF-1) and platelet-derived growth factor (PDGF)—are synthesized by mesangial cells, inciting an inflammatory reaction in some forms of glomerular disease. Classic associations between the natural history and defining fluorescence and electron microscopic observations have been made (Figure 16–4; Table 16–13). However, because it is not known exactly how the various forms of immune-mediated renal damage occur, each category is described separately with its associated findings.

A. Acute Glomerulonephritis: Postinfectious acute glomerulonephritis is due to immune attack on the infecting organism in which there is cross-reactivity between an antigen of the infecting organism (eg, of group A beta-hemolytic streptococci) and a

Table 16–11. Causes of rapidly progressive glomerulonephritis.[1,2]

Infectious diseases
  Poststreptococcal glomerulonephritis*
  Infective endocarditis*
  Occult visceral sepsis
  Hepatitis B infection (with vasculitis or cryoimmunoglobulinemia)
  Human immunodeficiency virus infection (?)
Multisystem diseases
  Systemic lupus erythematosus*
  Henoch-Schönlein purpura*
  Systemic necrotizing vasculitis (including Wegener's granulomatosis)*
  Goodpasture's syndrome*
  Essential mixed (IgG/IgM) cryoimmunoglobulinemia
  Malignancy
  Relapsing polychondritis
  Rheumatoid arthritis (with vasculitis)
Drugs
  Penicillamine*
  Hydralazine
  Allopurinol (with vasculitis)
  Rifampin
Idiopathic or primary glomerular disease
  Idiopathic crescentic glomerulonephritis*
    Type I—with linear deposits of immunoglobulin (anti-GBM antibody-mediated)
    Type II—with granular deposits of immunoglobulin (immune complex-mediated)
    Type III—with few or no immune deposits of immunoglobulin ("pauci-immune")
    Anti-neutrophil cytoplasmic antibody-induced, ? "forme fruste" of vasculitis
  Superimposed on another primary glomerular disease
    Mesangiocapillary (membranoproliferative glomerulonephritis)* (especially type II)
    Membranous glomerulonephritis*
    Berger's disease (IgA nephropathy)*

[1]Reproduced, with permission, from Glassock RJ, Brenner BM: The major glomerulopathies. In: *Harrison's Principles of Internal Medicine,* 12th ed. Wilson JD et al (editors). McGraw-Hill, 1991.
[2]Most common causes are marked with asterisks.

Table 16–12. Glomerular causes of asymptomatic urinary abnormalities.[1,2]

Hematuria with or without proteinuria
  Primary glomerular diseases
    Berger's disease (IgA nephropathy)*
    Mesangiocapillary glomerulonephritis
    Other primary glomerular hematurias accompanied by "pure" mesangial proliferation, focal and segmental proliferative glomerulonephritis, or other lesions
    "Thin basement membrane" disease (?"forme fruste" of Alport's syndrome)
  Associated with multisystem or heredofamilial diseases
    Alport's syndrome and other "benign" familial hematurias
    Fabry's disease
    Sickle cell disease
  Associated with infections
    Resolving poststreptococcal glomerulonephritis*
    Other postinfectious glomerulonephritides*
Isolated nonnephrotic proteinuria
  Primary glomerular diseases
    "Orthostatic" proteinuria*
    Focal and segmental glomerulosclerosis*
    Membranous glomerulonephritis*
  Associated with multisystem or heredofamilial diseases
    Diabetes mellitus*
    Amyloidosis*
    Nail-patella syndrome

[1]Reproduced, with permission, from Glassock RJ, Brenner BM: The major glomerulopathies. In: *Harrison's Principles of Internal Medicine,* 12th ed. Wilson JD et al (editors). McGraw-Hill, 1991.
[2]Most common causes are marked with asterisks.

Table 16–13. Location of electron-dense deposits in glomerular disease.[1]

Subepithelial
  Amorphous (epimembranous) deposits
    Membranous nephropathy
    Systemic lupus erythematosus
  Humps
    Acute postinfectious glomerulonephritis, eg, poststreptococcal glomerulonephritis, bacterial endocarditis
Intramembranous
  Membranous nephropathy
  Membranoproliferative glomerulonephritis type II
Subendothelial
  Systemic lupus erythematosus
  Membranoproliferative glomerulonephritis type I
  Less commonly, bacterial endocarditis, IgA nephropathy, Henoch-Schönlein purpura, mixed cryoglobulinemia
Mesangial
  Focal glomerulonephritis
  IgA nephropathy
  Henoch-Schönlein purpura
  Systemic lupus erythematosus
  Mild or resolving acute postinfectious glomerulonephritis
Subepithelial and subendothelial
  Systemic lupus erythematosus
  Membranoproliferative glomerulonephritis, type III
  Postinfectious glomerulonephritis

[1]Reproduced, with permission, from Rose BD: Pathogenesis, clinical manifestations and diagnosis of glomerular disease. In: *Pathophysiology of Renal Disease.* McGraw-Hill, 1987.

host antigen. The result is deposition of immune complexes and complement (Figure 16–4; Table 16–14) in glomerular capillaries and the mesangium. Symptoms and signs typically occur 7–10 days after onset of the acute pharyngeal or cutaneous infection and resolve over weeks following treatment of the infection.

B. Rapidly Progressive Glomerulonephritis: Whereas the natural history of most cases of acute glomerulonephritis includes resolution of the underlying renal disease, some cases display—often abruptly—a form of renal disease that rapidly progresses to chronic renal failure over a period of weeks to months. It is unclear why this happens in some patients, but a distinctive pathologic feature in such cases is extracapillary cellular proliferation, which typically involves 70% of the glomeruli. Gaps and focal discontinuities in the glomerular basement membrane may also be observed. Immunofluorescence studies permit distribution into subgroups correlating with other features of the disease. Five to 20 percent of patients have linear anti-GBM antibody deposits in glomeruli and a tendency to hemoptysis reminiscent of Goodpasture's syndrome. Thirty to 40 percent have granular immunoglobulin deposits and an autoantibody pattern typical of Wegener's granulomatosis (antineutrophil cytoplasmic antibody). The latter patients are typically older, with more systemic constitutional symptoms.

C. Chronic Glomerulonephritis: Some patients with acute glomerulonephritis develop chronic renal failure slowly over a period of 5–20 years. Cellular proliferation, either in the mesangium or in the capillary, is a pathologic structural hallmark in some of these cases, while others are notable for obliteration of glomeruli (**sclerosing chronic glomerulonephritis,** which includes both focal and diffuse subsets), and yet others display irregular subepithelial proteinaceous deposits with uniform involvement of individual glomeruli (**membranous glomerulonephritis).**

D. Nephrotic Syndrome: In patients with nephrotic syndrome, the glomerulus may appear intact or only subtly altered, without a cellular infiltrate as a manifestation of inflammation. Immunofluorescence with antibodies to IgG often demonstrates deposition of antigen-antibody complexes in the glomerular basement membrane. In the subset of patients with minimal change disease, in which proteinuria is the sole urinary sediment abnormality and in which (often) no changes can be seen by light microscopy, electron microscopy reveals obliteration of epithelial foot processes (Table 16–15). In animal models, T cell-derived "permeability factors," as well as non-complement-fixing antibodies to glomerular epithelial cells, can mimic this process.

Clinical Manifestations

Damage to the glomerular capillary wall results in leakage of red blood cells and proteins, which are normally too large to cross the glomerular capillary, into the renal tubular lumen, giving rise to hematuria and proteinuria.

A fall in GFR results either because glomerular capillaries are infiltrated with inflammatory cells or because contractile cells (eg, mesangial cells) respond to vasoactive substances by restricting blood flow to many glomerular capillaries.

Edema and hypertension are a direct consequence

Table 16–14. Factors causing and mediators of glomerular injury.[1]

Factors affecting immune complex deposition
  Host immune response
  Rate of complex clearance
  In situ complex formation
  Antigenic or complex charge
  Renal hemodynamics
Mediators of glomerular damage
  Complement
  Neutrophils
  Macrophages
  Platelets
  Vasoactive amines
  Fibrin
  Lymphokines

[1]Modified and reproduced, with permission, from Rose BD: Pathogenesis, clinical manifestations and diagnosis of glomerular disease. In: *Pathophysiology of Renal Disease,* 2nd ed. McGraw-Hill, 1987.

Table 16–15. Clinical and histologic features of idiopathic nephrotic syndrome.[1]

Glomerular Disease	Distinguishing Clinical and Laboratory Findings	Characteristic Morphologic Features
Minimal change disease	Commonest cause in children (75%); steroid- or cyclophosphamide-sensitive (80% of cases); nonprogressive; normal renal function; scant hematuria.	**LM:** normal **IF:** negative to trace IgM **EM:** podocyte effacement; no immune deposits
Focal and segmental glomerulosclerosis	Early-onset hypertension; microscopic hematuria; progressive renal failure (75% of cases).	**LM:** early, segmental sclerosis in some glomeruli with tubular atrophy; late, sclerosis of most glomeruli **IF:** focal and segmental IgM, C3 **EM:** Foot process fusion, sclerosis, hyalin
Membranous nephropathy	Commonest cause in adults (40–50%); peak incidence fourth and sixth decades; male:female 2–3:1; microscopic hematuria (55%); early hypertension (30%); spontaneous remission (20%); progressive renal failure (30–40%).	**LM:** early, normal; late, GBM thickening **IF:** granular IgG and C3 **EM:** subepithelial deposits and GBM expansion
Membranoproliferative glomerulonephritis	Peak incidence second and third decades; mixed nephrotic-nephritic features; slowly progressive in most, rapid in some; hypocomplementemia.	**LM:** hypercellular glomeruli with duplicated GBM ("tramtracks") **IF:** type I, diffuse C3, variable IgG and IgM; type II, C3 capillary wall and mesangial nodules **EM:** type I, subendothelial immune deposits; type II, dense GBM

Key: LM = light microscopy; IF = immunofluorescence; EM = electron microscopy; GBM = glomerular basement membrane
[1]Reproduced, with permission, from Glassock RJ, Brenner BM: The major glomerulopathies. In: *Harrison's Principles of Internal Medicine,* 13th ed. Isselbacher KJ et al (editors). McGraw-Hill, 1994; and from Luke RG et al: Nephrology and hypertension: Clinical and histologic features of idiopathic nephrotic syndrome. In: *Medical Knowledge Self-Assessment Program IX.* American College of Physicians, 1992.

of fluid and salt overload secondary to the fall of GFR in the face of excess consumption of salt and water.

A transient fall in serum complement is observed as a result of immune complex and complement deposition in the glomerulus.

An elevation of titer of antibody to streptococcal antigens is observed in cases associated with group A beta-hemolytic streptococcal infections. Another characteristic of the clinical course in poststreptococcal acute glomerulonephritis is a lag between clinical signs of infection and the development of clinical signs of nephritis.

Patients with the nephrotic syndrome have profoundly decreased plasma oncotic pressures due to the loss of serum proteins in the urine. This results in intravascular volume depletion and activation of the renin-angiotensin-aldosterone system and the sympathetic nervous system. The secretion of vasopressin is also increased. Such patients also have altered renal responses to atrial natriuretic peptide. Nevertheless, they may develop signs of intravascular volume depletion, including syncope, shock, and acute renal failure.

Hyperlipidemia associated with nephrotic syndrome appears to be a result of decreased plasma oncotic pressure, which stimulates hepatic VLDL synthesis and secretion.

Loss of other plasma proteins besides albumin in nephrotic syndrome may present as any of the following: (1) A defect in bacterial opsonization and thus increased susceptibility to infections (eg, due to loss of IgG). (2) Hypercoagulability (eg, due to antithrombin III deficiency, reduced levels of protein C and protein S, hyperfibrinogenemia, and hyperlipidemia). (3) Vitamin D deficiency state and secondary hyperparathyroidism (eg, due to loss of vitamin D-binding proteins). (4) Altered thyroid function tests without any true thyroid abnormality (due to reduced levels of thyroxine-binding globulin).

17. What are the categories of glomerulonephritis and their common and distinctive features?
18. What are the pathophysiologic consequences of nephrotic syndrome?

RENAL STONES

Clinical Presentation

Patients with renal stones present with flank pain and hematuria with or without fever. Depending on the level of the stone and the patient's underlying anatomy (eg, if there is only a single functioning kid-

Table 16–16. Common mechanical causes of urinary tract obstruction.[1]

Ureter	Bladder outlet
Ureteropelvic junction narrowing or obstruction	Bladder neck obstruction
	Ureterocele
Ureterovesical junction narrowing or obstruction	Benign prostatic hypertrophy
	Cancer of prostate
Ureterocele	Cancer of bladder
Retrocaval ureter	Calculi
Calculi	Diabetic neuropathy
Inflammation	Spinal cord disease
Trauma	Carcinomas of cervix, colon
Sloughed papillae	Trauma
Tumor	**Urethra**
Blood clots	Posterior urethral valves
Uric acid crystals	Anterior urethral valves
Pregnant uterus	Stricture
Retroperitoneal fibrosis	Meatal stenosis
Aortic aneurysm	Phimosis
Uterine leiomyomas	Stricture
Carcinoma of uterus, prostate, bladder, colon, rectum	Tumor
	Calculi
	Trauma
Retroperitoneal lymphoma	
Accidental surgical ligation	

[1]Reproduced, with permission, from Seifter JL, Brenner BM: Urinary tract obstruction. In: *Harrison's Principles of Internal Medicine,* 14th ed. Fauci AS et al (editors). McGraw-Hill, 1998.

ney or significant preexisting renal disease), the presentation may be complicated by obstruction (Table 16–16) with decreased or absent urine production.

Etiology

While a variety of disorders may result in the development of renal stones (Table 16–17), at least 75% of renal stones contain calcium. Most cases of calcium stones are due to idiopathic hypercalciuria, with hyperuricosuria and hyperparathyroidism as other major causes. Uric acid stones are typically caused by hyperuricosuria, especially in patients with a history of gout or excessive purine intake (eg, a diet high in organ meat products). Defective amino acid transport, as occurs in cystinuria, can result in stone formation. Finally, struvite stones, made up of magnesium, ammonium, and phosphate salts, are a result of chronic or recurrent urinary tract infection by urease-producing organisms (typically *Proteus*).

Pathology & Pathogenesis

Renal stones result from alterations in the solubility of various substances in urine, such that there is nucleation and precipitation of salts. A number of factors can tip the balance in favor of stone formation.

Dehydration favors stone formation, and a high fluid intake to maintain a daily urine volume of 2 L or more appears to be protective. The precise mechanism of this protection is unknown. Hypotheses include dilution of unknown substances that predispose to stone formation and decreased transit time of Ca^{2+} through the nephron, minimizing the likelihood of precipitation.

A high-protein diet predisposes to stone formation in susceptible individuals. A dietary protein load causes transient metabolic acidosis and an increased GFR. While serum Ca^{2+} is not detectably elevated, there is probably a transient increase in calcium resorption from bone, an increase in glomerular calcium filtration, and inhibition of distal tubular calcium resorption. This effect appears to be greater in known stone-formers than in normal control subjects.

A high-Na^+ diet predisposes to Ca^{2+} excretion and calcium oxalate stone formation, whereas a low dietary Na^+ intake has the opposite effect. Furthermore, urinary Na^+ excretion increases the saturation of monosodium urate, which can act as a nidus for Ca^{2+} crystallization.

Despite the fact that most stones are calcium oxalate stones, oxalate concentration in the diet is generally too low to support a recommendation to avoid oxalate to prevent stone formation. Similarly, calcium restriction, formerly a major dietary recommendation to calcium stone formers, is beneficial only to the subset of patients whose hypercalciuria is diet-dependent. In others, decreased dietary calcium may actually increase oxalate absorption and predispose to stone formation.

An association between essential hypertension (Chapter 11), hypercalciuria, and renal stones has been noted for a number of years. However, the pathophysiologic basis for this association is unclear. One hypothesis is that a common genetic defect results in defective Ca^{2+} and Na^+ balance, initiating separate pathophysiologic processes resulting in renal stones or hypertension, or in some cases both.

A number of factors are protective against stone formation. In order of decreasing importance, fluids, citrate, magnesium, and dietary fiber appear to have a protective effect. Citrate may prevent stone formation by chelating calcium in solution and forming highly soluble complexes compared with calcium oxalate and calcium phosphate. While pharmacologic supplementation of the diet with potassium citrate has been shown to increase urinary citrate and pH and decrease the incidence of recurrent stone formation, the benefits of a naturally high-citrate diet have not been investigated. However, some studies suggest that vegetarians have a lower incidence of stone formation. Presumably, they avoid the stone-forming effect of high protein and Na^+ in the diet, combined with the protective effects of fiber and other factors.

Stone formation per se within the renal pelvis is painless until a fragment breaks off and travels down the ureter, precipitating ureteral colic. Hematuria and renal damage can occur in the absence of pain.

Clinical Manifestations

The pain associated with renal stones is due to distention of the ureter, renal pelvis, or renal capsule.

Table 16–17. Major causes of renal stones.[1]

Stone Type and Causes	All Stones (%)	Occurrence of Specific Causes[2]	M:F Ratio	Etiology	Diagnosis	Treatment[4]
Calcium stones	75–85%					
Idiopathic hypercalciuria		50–55%	2:1 to 3:1 2:1	Hereditary (?)	Normocalcemia, unexplained hypercalciuria[3]	Thiazide diuretic agents
Hyperuricosuria		20%	4:1	Diet	Urine uric acid > 750 mg/24 h (women), > 800 mg/24 h (men)	Allopurinol or diet
Primary hyperparathyroidism		5%	3:10	Neoplasia	Unexplained hypercalcemia	Surgery
Distal renal tubular acidosis		Rare	1:1	Hereditary	Hyperchloremic acidosis, minimum urine pH > 5.5	Alkali replacement
Intestinal hyperoxaluria		≈ 1–2%	1:1	Bowel surgery	Urine oxalate > 50 mg/24 h	Cholestyramine or oral calcium loading
Hereditary hyperoxaluria		Rare	1:1	Hereditary	Urine oxalate and glycolic or L-glyceric acid increased	Fluids and pyridoxine
Idiopathic stone disease		20%	2:1	Unknown	None of the above	Oral phosphate, fluids
Uric acid stones	5–8%					
Gout		≈ 50%	3:1 to 4:1	Hereditary	Clinical diagnosis	Alkali to raise urine pH
Idiopathic		≈ 50%	1:1	Hereditary (?)	Uric acid stones, no gout	Allopurinol if daily urine uric acid above 1000 mg
Dehydration		?	1:1	Intestinal, habit	History, intestinal fluid loss	Alkali, fluids, reversal of cause
Lesch-Nyhan syndrome		Rare	Men	Hereditary	Reduced hypoxanthine-guanine phosphoribosyl transferase level	Allopurinol
Malignant tumors		Rare	1:1	Neoplasia	Clinical diagnosis	Allopurinol
Cystine stones	1%	Rare	1:1	Hereditary	Stone type; elevated cystine excretion	Massive fluids, alkali, penicillamine if needed
Struvite stones	10–15%		2:10	Infection	Stone type	Antimicrobial agents and judicious surgery

[1] Reproduced, with permission, from Asplin, JR, Coe FL, Favus MJ: Nephrolithiasis. In: *Harrison's Principles of Internal Medicine*, 14th ed. Fauci AS et al (editors). McGraw-Hill, 1998.
[2] Values are percentages of patients within each category of stone who display each specific cause.
[3] Urine calcium above 300 mg/24 h (men), 250 mg/24 h (women), or 4 mg/kg/24 h (either sex). Hyperthyroidism, Cushing's syndrome, sarcoidosis, malignant tumors, immobilization, vitamin D intoxication, rapidly progressive bone disease, and Paget's disease all cause hypercalciuria and must be excluded in diagnosis of idiopathic hypercalciuria.
[4] Besides fluids and dietary protein restriction, which are a mainstay of therapy in most forms of stone disease.

The severity of pain is related to the degree of distention that occurs and thus is extremely severe in acute obstruction. Anuria and azotemia are suggestive of bilateral obstruction or unilateral obstruction of a single functioning kidney. The pain, hematuria, and even ureteral obstruction caused by a renal stone are typically self-limited. Passage of the stone usually requires only fluids, bed rest, and analgesia. The major complications are (1) hydronephrosis and permanent renal damage due to complete obstruction of a ureter, with resulting backup of urine and buildup of pressure; (2) infection or abscess formation behind a partially or completely obstructing stone, which can rapidly destroy the involved kidney; (3) renal damage subsequent to repeated kidney stones; and (4) hypertension due to increased renin production by the obstructed kidney.

---

19. How do patients with renal stones present?
20. Why do renal stones form?
21. What are the common categories of renal stones (by composition)?

REFERENCES

General
Andreoli SP: Renal manifestations of systemic diseases. Semin Nephrol 1998;18:270.
Brezis M, Rosen S: Hypoxia of the renal medulla: Its implications for disease. N Engl J Med 1995;332:647.
Brown WW, Wolfson M: Diet as culprit or therapy: Stone disease, chronic renal failure and nephrotic syndrome. Med Clin North Am 1993;77:783.
Hocher B et al: The paracrine endothelin system: Pathophysiology and implications in clinical medicine. Eur J Clin Chem Clin Biochem 1997;35:175.
Mackenzie HS, Brenner BM: Fewer nephrons at birth: A missing link in the etiology of essential hypertension? Am J Kidney Dis 1995;26:91.
Rose BD, Rennke HG: *Renal Pathophysiology—The Essentials.* Williams & Wilkins, 1994.
Rose BD: *Clinical Physiology of Acid-Base Disorders,* 4th ed. McGraw-Hill, 1994.
Waldo FB et al: Current concepts and controversies in IgA nephropathy. Pediatr Nephrol 1998;12:498.

Acute Renal Failure
Bennett WM: Drug nephrotoxicity: An overview. Ren Fail 1997;19:221.
Blantz RC: Pathophysiology of pre-renal azotemia [clinical conference]. Kidney Int 1998;53:512.
Morcos SK: Contrast media-induced nephrotoxicity—questions and answers. Br J Radiol 1998;71:357.
Thadhani R et al: Acute renal failure. N Engl J Med 1996;334:1448.
Zuk A et al: Polarity, integrin, and extracellular matrix dynamics in the postischemic rat kidney. Am J Physiol 1998;275(3 Part 1):C711.

Chronic Renal Failure
Abrass CK: Diabetic nephropathy: Mechanisms of mesangial matrix expansion. West J Med 1995;162:318.
Bankir L, Kriz W: Adaptation of the kidney to protein intake and to urine concentrating activity: Similar consequences in health and chronic renal failure. Kidney Int 1995;47:7.
Buckalew VM Jr: Pathophysiology of progressive renal failure. South Med J 1994;87:1028.
Eddy AA: Molecular insights into renal interstitial fibrosis [editorial]. J Am Soc Nephrol 1996;7:2495.
Fine RN: Pathophysiology of growth retardation in children with chronic renal failure. J Pediatr Endocrinol 1994;7:79.
Jehle PM et al: Renal osteodystrophy: New insights in pathophysiology and treatment modalities with special emphasis on the insulin-like growth factor system. Nephron 1998;79:249.
Preston RA, Epstein M: Renal parenchymal disease and hypertension. Semin Nephrol 1995;15:138.
Textor SC: Pathophysiology of renal failure in renovascular disease. Am J Kidney Dis 1994;24:642.

Glomerulonephritis and Nephrotic Syndrome
Eddy AA, Schnaper HW: The nephrotic syndrome: From the simple to the complex. Semin Nephrol 1998;18:304.
Hricik DE, Chung-Park M, Sedor JR: Glomerulonephritis. N Engl J Med 1998;339:888.

Renal Stones
Pak CY: Southwestern Internal Medicine Conference: Medical management of nephrolithiasis—a new, simplified approach for general practice. Am J Med Sci 1997;313:215.
Parivar F et al: The influence of diet on urinary stone disease. J Urol 1996;155:432.
Strazzullo P, Cappuccio FP: Hypertension and kidney stones: Hypotheses and implications. Semin Nephrol 1995;15:519.

Disorders of the Parathyroids & Calcium Metabolism

17

Dolores M. Shoback, MD, & Gordon J. Strewler, MD

This chapter presents a general overview of the key hormones involved in the regulation of calcium, phosphate, and bone mineral metabolism. These include **parathyroid hormone, vitamin D**—principally the 1,25-$(OH)_2$ vitamin D metabolite—and **calcitonin**. The cycle of bone remodeling is described as a basis for understanding normal mineral balance and the pathogenesis of mineral disorders and metabolic bone disease. The symptoms and signs caused by excess or deficiency of the calciotropic hormones are presented along with the natural histories of **primary hyperparathyroidism, familial (benign) hypocalciuric hypercalcemia, hypercalcemia of malignancy**, different forms of **hypoparathyroidism**, and **medullary carcinoma of the thyroid**. Two of the most commonly encountered causes of osteopenia—**osteoporosis** and **osteomalacia**—are reviewed along with current theories of their pathogenesis.

NORMAL REGULATION OF CALCIUM METABOLISM

PARATHYROID GLANDS

Anatomy

Normal parathyroid glands each weigh about 30–40 mg and are grayish tan to yellow gray in color. Each individual normally has four glands, so that the average total parathyroid tissue mass in the adult is about 120–160 mg.

The superior pair of parathyroid glands arises from the fourth branchial pouches. These glands are located near the point of intersection of the middle thyroid artery and the recurrent laryngeal nerve. The superior parathyroid glands may be attached to the thyroid capsule posteriorly or, rarely, embedded in the thyroid gland itself. Alternative locations include the tracheoesophageal groove and the retroesophageal space. The blood supply to the superior parathyroid glands is usually from the inferior thyroid artery or, in some cases, the superior thyroid artery.

The inferior parathyroid glands develop from the third branchial pouch, as does the thymus gland. These glands typically lie at or near the lower pole of the thyroid gland lateral to the trachea. The inferior glands receive their blood supply from the inferior thyroid arteries. The location of the inferior parathyroid glands is more variable. When there are ectopic glands, they are typically found in association with thymic remnants. A common site for ectopic glands is the anterior mediastinum. Less common ectopic locations are the carotid sheath, pericardium, and pharyngeal submucosa. About 10% of people have additional (supernumerary) parathyroid glands.

Histology

The parathyroid gland is composed of three different cell types: chief cells, clear cells, and oxyphil cells. Whether these cells serve specialized functions has not been established. **Chief cells** are thought to be responsible for the synthesis and secretion of **parathyroid hormone (PTH)**. Histologically, chief cells are small (4–8 μm in diameter), with central nuclei. In their active state, they have a prominent endoplasmic reticulum and dense Golgi regions where PTH is synthesized and packaged for secretion. **Clear cells** are probably chief cells with an increased glycogen content. **Oxyphil cells** appear in the parathyroid glands after puberty. They are larger than chief cells (6–10 μm), and their number increases with age. It is not clear whether these cells secrete PTH nor whether they are derived from chief cells.

The normal adult parathyroid gland contains fat. The relative contribution of fat to the glandular mass increases with age and may reach 60–70% of gland volume in the elderly. When the parathyroid gland undergoes hyperplasia or adenomatous changes, the component of the gland that is fat decreases dramatically.

Physiology

Approximately 99% of total body calcium is found in the skeleton and teeth, the remainder in the extracellular fluids. Calcium in these fluids exists in three forms—as ionized, protein-bound, and complexed calcium. Approximately 45–50% of total blood calcium is protein-bound, predominantly to albumin but also to globulins. A similar fraction is ionized. The remainder is complexed to organic ions such as citrate, phosphate, and bicarbonate. The ionized fraction of the serum calcium controls vital cellular functions such as muscle contraction, neuromuscular transmission, and blood clotting. The binding of calcium to albumin is pH-dependent, increasing with alkalosis and decreasing with acidosis. Thus, if the ionized calcium is low, acidosis tends to protect a subject from displaying the symptoms and signs of hypocalcemia. Conversely, alkalosis predisposes to symptomatic hypocalcemia.

Circulating levels of PTH can change within seconds after an alteration in serum calcium. PTH secretory rates are related to the serum ionized calcium by an inverse sigmoidal relationship (Figure 17–1). Low ionized calcium concentrations maximally stimulate secretion, while increases in calcium suppress the production and release of PTH. PTH secretion is exquisitely sensitive to very small changes in the calcium concentration, which have substantial effects on the rate of hormone synthesis and release.

A recently identified plasma membrane calcium receptor expressed by parathyroid cells detects changes in the extracellular calcium concentration. This receptor senses high calcium levels and couples to intracellular pathways that ultimately lead to inhibition of hormone secretion (Figure 17–2). In addition to the parathyroid gland, calcium receptors are expressed in the kidney, thyroid C cells, brain, and other tissues.

Chronic hypocalcemia is also a stimulus to the proliferation of parathyroid cells, which eventually results in glandular hyperplasia. The mechanism underlying this response to reduced calcium levels has not been clearly delineated.

PTH is produced in the parathyroid glands as a 115-amino-acid precursor molecule (preproPTH) that is successively cleaved within the cell to form the mature 84-amino-acid peptide PTH(1–84) (Figure 17–3). This form of the hormone is packaged into secretory granules and released into the circulation. PTH(1–84) is the biologically active form of PTH at target cells and has a very short half-life in vivo of approximately 10 minutes. PTH(1–84) is metabolized in the liver and other tissues to midregion and carboxyl terminal forms that are probably biologically inactive. These circulating fragments accumulate to very high levels in patients with renal failure, since the kidney is an important site for clearance of PTH from the body.

The assays most commonly used to assess PTH levels measure intact PTH(1–84). These are two-site immunoradiometric or immunochemiluminometric assays. They utilize antibodies directed against two

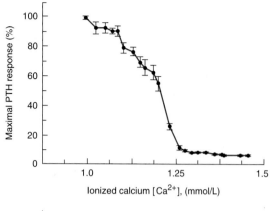

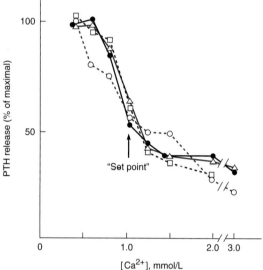

Figure 17–1. Inverse sigmoidal relationship between PTH release and the extracellular calcium concentration in human studies (upper panel) and in vitro in human parathyroid cells (bottom panel). Studies shown in the upper panel were performed by infusing calcium and the calcium chelator EDTA into normal subjects. Serum intact PTH was measured by a two-site immunoradiometric assay. In the lower panel, PTH was measured in the medium surrounding parathyroid cells in vitro by an assay for intact PTH. The midpoint between the maximal and minimal secretory rates is defined as the set-point for secretion. (Reproduced, with permission, from Brown E: Extracellular Ca^{2+} sensing, regulation of parathyroid cell function, and role of Ca^{2+} and other ions as extracellular [first] messengers. Physiol Rev 1991;71:371.)

different regions of the intact PTH(1–84) molecule (Figure 17–4). In the two-site assay, serum is incubated with the first antibody that is directed to the amino terminal portion of the molecule and which is also labeled. The second antibody, raised against the carboxyl terminal or the midregion of PTH (ie, PTH[39–84]) and conjugated to a bead, is added in a

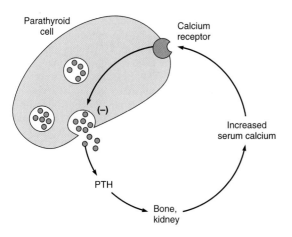

Figure 17–2. Sequence of events by which the calcium ion concentration is sensed by the parathyroid cell calcium receptor. Activation of this receptor is eventually linked through intracellular signal transduction pathways to the inhibition of PTH secretion. (Reproduced, with permission, from Taylor R: A new receptor for calcium ions. J NIH Res 1994:6:25.)

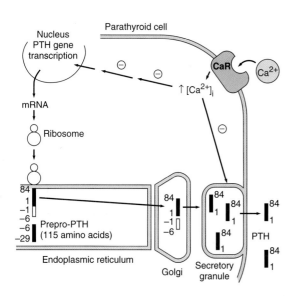

Figure 17–3. Biosynthetic events in the production of PTH within the parathyroid cell. PreproPTH gene is transcribed to its mRNA, which is translated on the ribosomes to preproPTH (amino acids –29 to +84). The presequence is removed within the endoplasmic reticulum, yielding proPTH (–6 to +84). An additional six-amino acid fragment is removed in the Golgi. Mature PTH(1–84) released from the Golgi is packaged in secretory granules and released into the circulation in the presence of hypocalcemia. The calcium receptor (CaR) is proposed to sense changes in extracellular calcium that affect both the release of PTH and the transcription of the preproPTH gene. (Modified and reproduced, with permission, from Habener JF et al: Biosynthesis of parathyroid hormone. Recent Prog Horm Res 1977;33:249.)

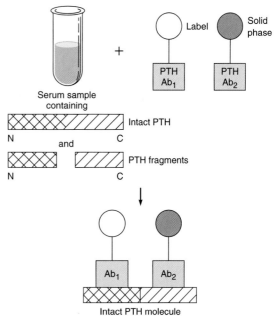

Figure 17–4. Schematic representation of the principle of the two-site assay for intact PTH. The label may be a luminescent probe or ^{125}I in the immunochemiluminometric or immunoradiometric assay, respectively. Two different region-specific antibodies are used (Ab_1 and Ab_2). Only the hormone species containing both immunodeterminants is counted in the assay.

second step. After the bead has been washed, the amount of bound label is determined by counting radioactivity or measuring luminescence. Only intact PTH(1–84) will be recognized by both antibodies, since it will be the only form of the peptide to have both immunodeterminants.

Some laboratories continue to perform the traditional midregion PTH assays, which typically detect those species of hormone containing amino acids 43–68 of the PTH molecule. These assays take advantage of the higher levels of the midregion fragments due to their longer half-life. The concentration of these fragments provides a reasonable—albeit indirect—assessment of glandular secretion in clinical situations where renal function and thus PTH clearance are normal. Reduced clearance of midregion PTH fragments occurs when the glomerular filtration rate (GFR) declines below about 40 mL/min. Thus, in renal insufficiency, measurements of PTH using midregion assays do not accurately reflect glandular secretion. For this reason, uremic secondary hyperparathyroidism is best monitored by use of the two-site assay for intact hormone, since PTH fragments, which accumulate when there is delayed renal clearance of PTH, do not cross-react in intact assays.

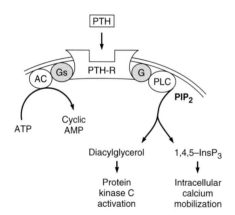

Figure 17–5. Signal transduction pathways activated by PTH binding to the PTH-1 receptor (PTH-R) in a target cell. PTH interacts with its receptor. This enhances GTP binding to the stimulatory G protein of adenylyl cyclase G_s, which activates the enzyme. cAMP (cyclic AMP) is formed. PTH also increases G protein-dependent activation of phospholipase C (PLC), which catalyzes the breakdown of the membrane phospholipid phosphatidylinositol 4,5-bisphosphate (PIP_2). This produces the second messengers inositol trisphosphate (1,4,5-$InsP_3$) and diacylglycerol. 1,4,5-$InsP_3$ mobilizes intracellular calcium, and diacylglycerol activates protein kinase C.

Mechanism of Parathyroid Hormone Action

Both PTH and parathyroid hormone-related peptide (PTHrP)—described below—bind to the PTH-1 receptor through residues in their amino terminals. This part of the molecule is also responsible for the activation of adenylyl cyclase and production of the second-messenger cAMP (Figure 17–5). PTH/PTHrP receptors also couple to the stimulation of phospholipase C activity, leading to the generation of inositol trisphosphate and diacylglycerol (Figure 17–5). Activation of this signal transduction pathway induces intracellular calcium mobilization and protein kinase C activation in PTH- and PTHrP-responsive cells. The exact pathways responsible for specific actions of PTH in its target cells continue to be a subject of intense investigation. The type 2 PTH receptor, which selectively binds PTH and not PTHrP, is expressed in nonclassic PTH target tissues (ie, brain, pancreas, testis, and placenta). This receptor is not thought to be involved in mineral balance, but its natural ligand and functions in vivo are unknown.

Effects of Parathyroid Hormone

The serum ionized calcium and phosphate concentrations reflect the net transfer of these ions from bone, gastrointestinal tract, and glomerular filtrate. PTH and 1,25-$(OH)_2D$ play key roles in the regulation of calcium and phosphate balance (Figure 17–6). When the serum calcium falls, PTH is rapidly released and acts quickly to promote calcium reabsorption in the distal tubule and the medullary thick ascending limb of Henle's loop. PTH also stimulates the release of calcium from a rapidly exchangeable pool of bone calcium. These actions serve to restore serum calcium levels to normal.

The renal action of PTH is rapid, occurring within minutes after an increase in the hormone. The overall effect of PTH on the kidney, however, depends on several factors. When hypocalcemia is present and PTH is elevated, urinary calcium excretion is low. This reflects the full expression of the primary renal effect of PTH to enhance renal calcium reabsorption. When PTH levels are high in primary hyperparathyroidism, hypercalcemia results from increased mobilization of calcium from bone and enhanced intestinal calcium absorption. These events increase the delivery of calcium to the glomerular filtrate. Because more calcium is filtered, more is excreted in the urine—despite the high PTH levels. If the filtered load of calcium is normal or low in a patient with primary hyperparathyroidism—because of a low dietary calcium intake or demineralized bone—urinary calcium excretion may be normal or even low. Thus, there may be considerable variability in calcium excretion among patients with hyperparathyroidism.

If kidney function is normal, chronic elevation in serum PTH increases renal 1,25-$(OH)_2D$ production. This steroid hormone stimulates both calcium and phosphate absorption across the small intestine (Figure 17–6). The effect requires at least 24 hours to develop fully and begin to restore normal calcium levels. Achievement of eucalcemia then leads to a downward readjustment in the PTH secretory rate. Any increase in 1,25-$(OH)_2D$ serves to inhibit further PTH synthesis.

The major effect of PTH on phosphate handling is to promote phosphate excretion by inhibition of sodium-dependent phosphate transport in the proximal and distal tubules. Serum phosphate levels are thought to affect PTH secretion rates directly. The mechanism is, however, unknown. Hypophosphatemia enhances the conversion of 25-(OH)D to 1,25-$(OH)_2D$ in the kidney, which through its intestinal and renal effects promotes phosphate retention. Hyperphosphatemia inhibits 1,25-$(OH)_2D$ production (see below), lowers serum calcium by complexing it, and thus indirectly stimulates PTH secretion.

PTH also increases urinary excretion of bicarbonate through its action on the proximal tubule. This can produce proximal renal tubular acidosis. These physiologic responses to PTH are the basis for the hypophosphatemia and hyperchloremic acidosis commonly observed in patients with hyperparathyroidism. Dehydration is also commonly seen in moderate to severe hypercalcemia of any origin. This is due to the effect of hypercalcemia on vasopressin action in the medullary thick ascending limb of the kidney. High calcium levels, presumably by interacting with

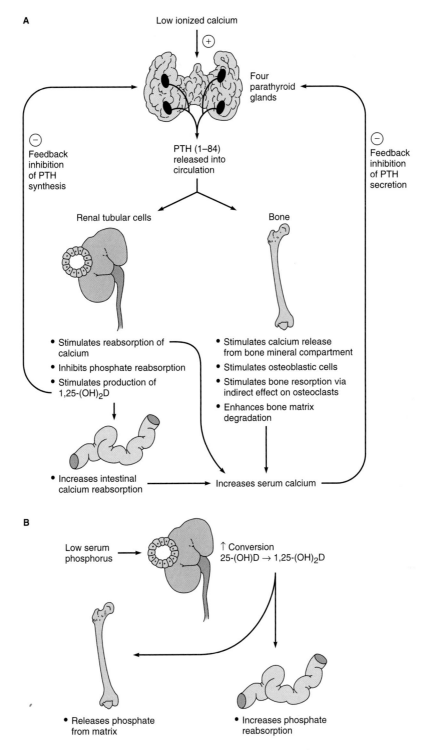

Figure 17–6. Main actions of PTH and 1,25-(OH)$_2$D in the maintenance of calcium and phosphate homeostasis. (Modified and reproduced, with permission, from Chandrasoma P, Taylor CE: *Concise Pathology,* 3rd ed. Appleton & Lange, 1998.)

the renal calcium receptor, blunt the ability of endogenous vasopressin to stimulate water reabsorption. Thus, hypercalcemia induces a form of vasopressin-resistant nephrogenic diabetes insipidus.

In conjunction with 1,25-$(OH)_2$D, PTH increases bone resorption to restore normocalcemia (see below). PTH acts on bone in two steps. The first is to mobilize calcium and phosphate rapidly from a compartment in direct contact with extracellular fluids. The second step of calcium mobilization results from bone matrix dissolution and alterations in the bone remodeling process. The initial skeletal response to PTH occurs within 2–3 hours. Later effects require several hours to develop. In its initial action on bone, PTH enhances osteoclastic activity and thus bone resorption. Subsequently, PTH stimulates bone formation, since the processes of resorption and formation are coupled. In primary and secondary hyperparathyroidism, when PTH production rates are excessive, net bone loss may occur over time—perhaps because even though the processes of formation and resorption are coupled, they may not occur with 100% efficiency.

PARATHYROID HORMONE-RELATED PEPTIDE (PTHrP)

Parathyroid hormone-related peptide (PTHrP) is a 141-amino-acid peptide which is homologous with PTH at its amino terminal (Figure 17–7) and is recognized by the type 1 PTH receptor. Consequently, PTHrP has effects on bone and kidney similar to those of PTH—it increases bone resorption, increases phosphate excretion, and decreases renal calcium excretion. PTHrP can be secreted by tumor cells and was originally identified as the cause of hypercalcemia of malignancy, a syndrome that can mimic primary hyperparathyroidism (see below).

Unlike PTH, which is exclusively the product of parathyroid cells, PTHrP is produced in many tissues and functions mainly as a tissue growth and differentiation factor at the local level and a regulator of smooth muscle tone. In the normal development of cartilage and bone, PTHrP stimulates the proliferation of chondrocytes and inhibits the mineralization of cartilage. Embryos without PTHrP are nonviable, with multiple abnormalities of bone and cartilage. PTHrP also appears to regulate the normal development of skin, hair follicles, teeth, and breasts. The list of normal functions of PTHrP is growing rapidly, and it is likely that ultimately it will be shown to regulate functions in many of the tissues in which it is expressed.

1. Describe the cellular composition of the parathyroid gland.
2. How do serum albumin concentration and blood pH influence the distribution of calcium into ionized and protein-bound fractions?
3. What is the advantage of two-site immunoassays for PTH?
4. What are the actions of PTH and 1,25-$(OH)_2$D on bone, kidney, and the gastrointestinal tract?
5. What is PTHrP? How is its action similar to and different from that of PTH?

BONE

Bone has two compartments. On the outside is **cortical** or **compact** bone, which makes up 80% of the skeletal mass. In this dense tissue, the resident

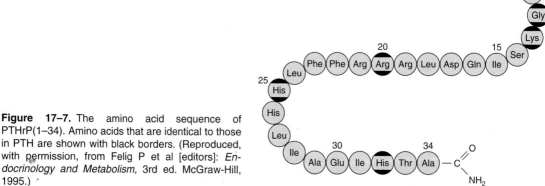

Figure 17–7. The amino acid sequence of PTHrP(1–34). Amino acids that are identical to those in PTH are shown with black borders. (Reproduced, with permission, from Felig P et al [editors]: *Endocrinology and Metabolism*, 3rd ed. McGraw-Hill, 1995.)

bone cells, called **osteocytes,** are deeply buried, communicating and receiving nutrients via a system of haversian canals. Osteocytes appear to function as mechanoreceptors, sensing strain on the bone and signaling for changes in bone remodeling. Because of the low ratio of surface to volume, cortical bone is remodeled only slowly.

Within the cortex lies the other compartment, **trabecular** or **cancellous** bone, which makes up 20% of skeletal mass. Trabecular bone consists of thin interconnected plates, the trabeculae, which are covered by bone cells. The spaces in this irregular honeycomb are filled with bone marrow—either red marrow, in which hematopoiesis is active, or white marrow, which is mainly fat. Because of its high surface-to-volume ratio and abundant cellular activity, trabecular bone is remodeled more rapidly than cortical bone. To understand the remodeling process, it is important to know something about bone cells.

The **osteoclast** is a multinucleated giant cell that is specialized for resorption of bone. Osteoclasts are terminally differentiated cells that arise continuously from hematopoietic precursors in the monocyte lineage and do not divide. The formation of osteoclasts requires hematopoietic growth factors such as macrophage colony-stimulating factor (M-CSF) and also requires a signal from marrow stromal cells. A cell surface molecule on marrow stromal cells named osteoclast differentiation factor (ODF; also known as receptor activator of NF-kappa B ligand, or RANKL, and as TNF-related activation-induced cytokine, or TRANCE) binds to a receptor (ODF receptor or RANK) on osteoclast precursors and transmits this signal. As they mature, osteoclast precursors acquire the capacity to produce osteoclast-specific enzymes and finally fuse to produce the mature multinucleated cell. The maturation process is accelerated by bone-resorbing hormones such as PTH and vitamin D.

To resorb bone, the motile osteoclast alights on a bone surface and seals off an area by forming an adhesive ring in which cellular integrins bind tightly to bone matrix proteins (Figure 17–8). Having isolated an area of bone surface, the osteoclast develops above the surface an elaborately invaginated plasma membrane structure called the **ruffled border.** The ruffled border is a distinctive organelle, but it acts essentially as a huge lysosome, which dissolves bone mineral by secreting acid onto the isolated bone surface, and simultaneously breaks down the bone matrix by secretion of collagenase and catheptic proteases. The resulting collagen peptides have pyridinoline cross-links that can be assayed in urine as a measure of bone resorption rates. Bone resorption can be controlled in two ways: by regulating the formation of osteoclasts to change their number and by regulating the activity of the mature osteoclast. The mature osteoclast has receptors for calcitonin but does not appear to have PTH or $1,25\text{-}(OH)_2D$ receptors.

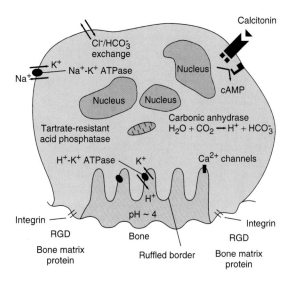

Figure 17–8. Schematic view of an active osteoclast. Calcitonin receptors, the ruffled border, and enzymes and channels involved in secretion of acid onto the bone surface are shown. Integrins are transmembrane-spanning receptors on osteoclasts which bind to determinants (RGD) in bone matrix proteins such as fibronectins. The integrins are responsible for the tight attachment of osteoclasts to the bone surface. (Reproduced, with permission, from Felig P et al [editors]: *Endocrinology and Metabolism,* 3rd ed. McGraw-Hill, 1995.)

The **osteoblast,** or bone-forming cell, arises from a mesenchymal precursor in the bone marrow stroma. When actively forming bone, the osteoblast is a tall, plump cell with an abundant Golgi apparatus. On active bone-forming surfaces, osteoblasts are found side by side, laying down bone matrix by secreting proteins and proteoglycans. The most important protein of bone matrix is type I collagen, which makes up 90% of bone matrix and is deposited in regular layers that serve as the main scaffold for deposition of minerals. There are many other constituents of bone matrix, including a protein called **osteocalcin** that is unique to bones and teeth and whose serum level is a clinical measure of the rate of bone formation.

Having laid down bone matrix, the osteoblast now mineralizes it, depositing hydroxyapatite crystals in an orderly array on the collagen layers to produce lamellar bone. The process of mineralization is poorly understood but requires an adequate supply of extracellular calcium and phosphate as well as the enzyme alkaline phosphatase, which is secreted in large amounts by active osteoblasts.

Bone remodeling occurs in an orderly cycle in which old bone is first resorbed and new bone then deposited. Cortical bone is remodeled from within by cutting cones (Figure 17–9), groups of osteoclasts

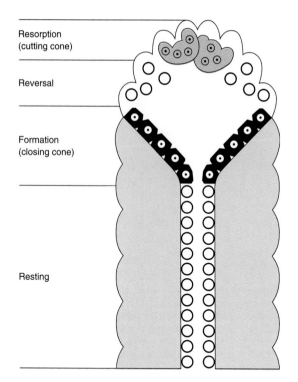

Figure 17–9. A cutting cone remodeling cortical bone. (Reproduced, with permission, from Felig P et al [editors]. *Endocrinology and Metabolism,* 3rd ed. McGraw-Hill, 1995.)

that the important signals are local, not systemic. Although they have not been identified with certainty, one very good candidate is osteoclast differentiation factor (ODF). ODF was described above as a cell surface molecule on stromal cells that sends a nurturing signal to osteoclast precursors; ODF also binds to receptors on mature osteoclasts and may mediate the coupling of bone formation and bone resorption. The process of bone remodeling does not absolutely require systemic hormones except to ensure an adequate supply of calcium and phosphate. For example, bone is quite normal in patients with hypoparathyroidism. However, systemic hormones use the bone pool as a source of minerals for regulation of extracellular calcium homeostasis. Osteoblasts have receptors for PTH and 1,25-$(OH)_2$ vitamin D but osteoclasts do not. Isolated osteoclasts do not respond to PTH or vitamin D except in the presence of osteoblasts. This coupling mechanism makes certain that when bone resorption is activated by PTH—eg, to provide calcium to correct hypocalcemia—bone formation will also increase, tending to replenish lost bone.

that cut tunnels through the compact bone. They are followed by trailing osteoblasts, lining the tunnels and laying down a cylinder of new bone on their walls, so that the tunnels are progressively narrowed until all that remains are the tiny haversian canals, by which the cells that are left behind as resident osteocytes are fed.

In trabecular bone, the remodeling process occurs on the surface (Figure 17–10). Osteoclasts first excavate a pit, and the pit is then filled in with new bone by osteoblasts. In a normal adult, this cycle takes 200 days. At each remodeling site, bone resorption and new bone formation are ordinarily well coupled, so that in a state of zero net bone balance, the amount of new bone formed is precisely equivalent to the amount of old bone resorbed. This state of perfection is only briefly attained, however. Until the age of 20–30, we are consolidating the gains in bone growth that were achieved during adolescence. After age 30, we begin to lose bone slowly.

How osteoclasts and osteoblasts communicate to achieve the coupling that assures perfect (or near-perfect) bone balance is not fully known. It appears

1. Osteoclast recruitment and activation

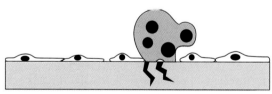

2. Resorption and osteoblast recruitment

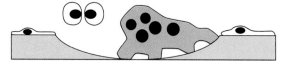

3. Osteoblastic bone formation

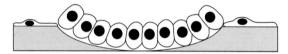

4. Completed remodeling cycle

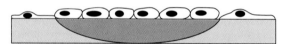

Figure 17–10. Sequential steps in remodeling of trabecular bone. (Reproduced, with permission, from Felig P et al [editors]: *Endocrinology and Metabolism,* 3rd ed. McGraw-Hill, 1995.)

6. Describe the two compartments of bone.
7. How is bone resorption by osteoclasts controlled?
8. What is the role of osteoblasts in bone formation?
9. How are the actions of osteoblasts and osteoclasts coupled?

VITAMIN D

Vitamin D is actually a hormone. With exposure to normal amounts of sunlight, we synthesize enough vitamin D in our skin to meet our needs. The only natural source of vitamin D in the diet is in the livers of meat-eating fish, who have simply stored vitamin D they ingested.

Physiology

Cholesterol in skin is metabolized to the vitamin D precursor 7-dehydrocholesterol, which is converted to vitamin D (cholecalciferol) by a nonenzymatic process when skin is subjected to tanning wavelengths of ultraviolet light (Figure 17–11). This step involves breakage of the B ring of cholesterol to produce a sterol; hormones with an intact cholesterol nucleus (eg, estrogen) are called steroids.

Although cutaneous synthesis of vitamin D is often adequate for our needs, persons in northern climates may be borderline deficient in vitamin D at the end of the winter months and the ill and infirm may not have adequate sunlight exposure. It is therefore recommended that the diet contain 400 IU of vitamin D per day (the RDA). In the United States, milk is supplemented with 400 IU of vitamin D per quart. Dietary supplements of vitamin D often consist of vitamin D_2 (ergocalciferol). Vitamin D_2 and vitamin D are metabolized identically and are equipotent.

Vitamin D formed in the skin is a lipophilic substance that is transported to the liver bound to a specific vitamin D-binding protein. In the liver, vitamin D is hydroxylated to produce 25-hydroxyvitamin D (25-[OH]D) (Figure 17–11). This process, like cutaneous synthesis of vitamin D, is not closely regulated. 25-(OH)D is still rather lipophilic, and it is transported by the serum binding protein to fat stores, where it is the principal storage form of vitamin D. Therefore, the clinical test for vitamin D deficiency is measurement of the serum level of 25-(OH)D.

The final metabolic processing step in the synthesis of the active hormone takes place in the kidney. But unlike previous steps, the conversion of 25-(OH)D to 1,25-$(OH)_2$D by the 25-(OH)D 1-hydroxylase in the renal cortex is tightly regulated. The synthesis of 1,25-$(OH)_2$D is increased by PTH, thus linking the formation of 1,25-$(OH)_2$D closely to PTH in the integrated control of calcium homeostasis. The

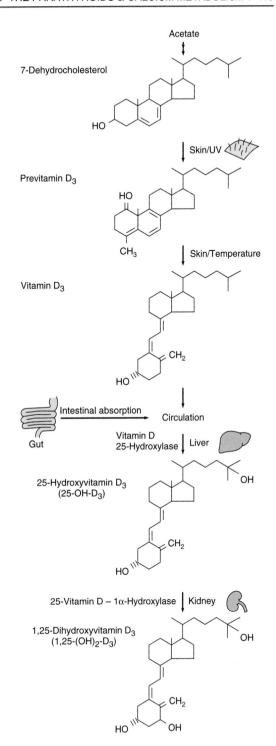

Figure 17–11. The formation and activation of vitamin D. (Reproduced, with permission, from Felig P et al [editors]: *Endocrinology and Metabolism,* 3rd ed. McGraw-Hill, 1995.)

production of 1,25-$(OH)_2$D is also stimulated by hypophosphatemia and probably by hypocalcemia. On the other hand, hypercalcemia, hyperphosphatemia, or an excess of 1,25-$(OH)_2$D will decrease the production of 1,25-$(OH)_2$D. The coordinated control by PTH, blood mineral levels, and the vitamin D supply is very efficient. Levels of 1,25-$(OH)_2$D vary little over an enormous range of vitamin D production rates but respond precisely to changes in the intake of calcium and phosphate within the normal range.

Vitamin D Action

The vitamin D receptor is a member of the steroid receptor superfamily of nuclear DNA-binding receptors. Upon ligand binding, the receptor attaches to enhancer sites in target genes and directly regulates their transcription. Thus, many of the effects of vitamin D involve new RNA and protein synthesis. Although many vitamin D metabolites are recognized by the receptor, 1,25-$(OH)_2$D has an affinity approximately 1000-fold greater than that of 25-(OH)D.

The primary target organs for 1,25-$(OH)_2$D are intestine and bone. The most essential action of 1,25-$(OH)_2$D is to stimulate the intestinal transport of calcium. Although some calcium can be absorbed passively over a paracellular route, most calcium absorbed at typical levels of dietary intake is actively transported through the microvilli of intestinal epithelial cells in a process that is induced by 1,25-$(OH)_2$D. 1,25-$(OH)_2$D also induces the active transport of phosphate, but passive absorption dominates this process and the net effect of 1,25-$(OH)_2$D is small.

In bone, 1,25-$(OH)_2$D activates osteoblast synthetic activities and is necessary for normal mineralization of osteoid. However, the defect in mineralization that occurs in vitamin D deficiency results mainly from decreased delivery of calcium and phosphate to sites of mineralization. 1,25-$(OH)_2$D also stimulates the osteoclast to resorb bone, releasing calcium to maintain extracellular calcium. This is an indirect effect of 1,25-$(OH)_2$D, probably involving stimulation of osteoblasts to release an osteoclast-activating substance.

Now consider a person who switches from a high normal to a low normal intake of calcium and phosphate—from 1200 mg to 300 mg per day of calcium (the equivalent of leaving three glasses of milk out of the diet). The net absorption of calcium falls sharply, causing a transient decrease in the serum calcium level. This activates a homeostatic response led by an increase in PTH. The increased PTH level stimulates the release of calcium from bone and the retention of calcium by the kidney. In addition, the increase in PTH, the fall in calcium, and the concomitant fall in the serum phosphate level (because of both decreased intake and PTH-induced phosphaturia) activate renal 1,25-$(OH)_2$D synthesis. 1,25-$(OH)_2$D increases the fraction of calcium that is absorbed, further increases calcium release from bone, and restores the serum calcium to normal.

---

10. How is vitamin D produced from cholesterol?
11. Where is vitamin D stored?
12. Where does the final step in activation of vitamin D take place, and how is it regulated?
13. What are the actions of vitamin D?

PARAFOLLICULAR CELLS (C Cells)

Anatomy & Histology

C cells of the thyroid gland secrete the peptide hormone calcitonin. They constitute 0.1% or less of thyroid cell mass and are distributed in the central parts of the lateral lobes of the thyroid, especially between the upper and middle third of the lobes. C cells are neuroendocrine cells and are derived from the ultimobranchial body. This structure fuses with the thyroid, and C cells are distributed throughout the gland.

C cells are small spindle-shaped or polygonal cells. They contain abundant granules, mitochondria, and Golgi. They may be present as single cells or arranged in nests, cords, and sheets within the thyroid parenchyma. They are often found within thyroid follicles, are larger than follicular cells, and stain positively for calcitonin.

Physiology

Calcitonin is a 32-amino-acid peptide hormone with a seven-membered amino terminal disulfide ring and carboxyl terminal prolineamide (Figure 17–12). Differential processing of the calcitonin gene can lead to the production of either calcitonin in C cells or calcitonin gene-related peptide in neurons. Although calcitonin gene-related peptide has cardiovascular and neurologic effects in pharmacologic doses, the function of the peptide in normal physiology is unknown. C cell tumors may release both peptides.

Hypercalcemia stimulates the release of calcitonin through the activation of calcium receptors, which appear to be highly homologous to parathyroid cell calcium receptors. Substantial changes in serum calcium are normally required to modulate the release of calcitonin. It is not known whether small physiologic changes in serum calcium can elicit significant changes in calcitonin levels. The gastrointestinal hormones cholecystokinin and gastrin are also secretagogues for calcitonin.

Calcitonin secretion in vivo is best assessed by measuring serum levels with a two-site radioimmunoassay. In some radioimmunoassays, basal calci-

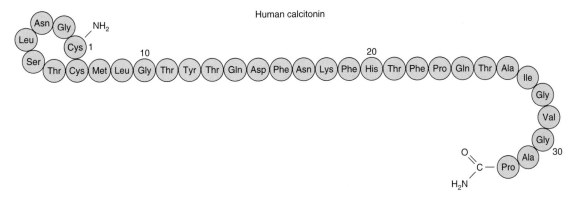

Figure 17–12. Amino acid sequence of human calcitonin, demonstrating its biochemical features, including an amino terminal disulfide bridge and carboxyl terminal prolineamide.

tonin levels are not detectable in normal people. Calcitonin typically rises to very high levels in patients with medullary carcinoma of the thyroid.

Actions of Calcitonin

Calcitonin interacts with receptors in kidney and bone. This interaction stimulates adenylyl cyclase activity and the generation of cAMP (as shown in Figure 17–5 for PTH). In the kidney, receptors for calcitonin are localized in the cortical ascending limb of Henle's loop, while in bone, calcitonin receptors are found on osteoclasts.

The main function of calcitonin is to lower serum calcium, and this hormone is rapidly released in response to hypercalcemia. Calcitonin inhibits osteoclastic bone resorption and rapidly blocks the release of calcium and phosphate from bone. The latter effect is apparent within minutes after the administration of calcitonin. This effect, along with the inhibition of resorption, ultimately leads to a fall in serum calcium and phosphate.

Calcitonin accomplishes its antiresorptive effect by acting directly on the osteoclast. Calcitonin blocks bone resorption induced by a variety of hormones, including PTH and vitamin D. The potency of calcitonin depends on the underlying rate of bone resorption. Calcitonin also has a modest effect on the kidney to produce mild phosphaturia. With prolonged administration of calcitonin, "escape" from its effects occurs.

The overall importance of calcitonin in the maintenance of calcium homeostasis is unclear. Serum calcium concentrations are normal in patients after thyroidectomy, which usually removes all functioning C cells.

---

14. What are the actions of calcitonin?
15. What is the effect of thyroidectomy on serum calcium?

PATHOPHYSIOLOGY OF SELECTED DISORDERS OF CALCIUM METABOLISM

PRIMARY & SECONDARY HYPERPARATHYROIDISM

Etiology

Primary hyperparathyroidism is due to excessive autonomous production and release of PTH by the parathyroid glands. The recognition of this disorder has increased substantially in the last 30 years as a result of the availability and routine performance of multichannel screening blood calcium analyses. The prevalence of hyperparathyroidism is approximately 1:1000 in the United States, and the incidence of the disease increases with age.

Primary hyperparathyroidism may be caused by any of the following: adenoma, carcinoma, or diffuse hyperplasia (Table 17–1). **Chief cell adenomas** are the most common cause, accounting for almost 85% of all cases. The vast majority of parathyroid adenomas occur sporadically and affect only a single gland.

Parathyroid hyperplasia classically refers to an enlargement or abnormality of all four glands. In atypical forms of hyperplasia, only one gland may be enlarged, but the other three glands typically show at least slight microscopic abnormalities such as increased cellularity and reduced fat content. The distinction between hyperplasia and multiple adenomas may be challenging to the pathologist, and all glands must be examined. The key characteristics for judging whether a gland is normal or not are its size, weight, and histologic features.

Parathyroid hyperplasia may be part of the autoso-

Table 17–1. Causes of primary hyperparathyroidism.

Solitary adenomas	80–85%
Hyperplasia	10%
Multiple adenomas	≈2%
Carcinoma	≈2–5%

mal dominant **multiple endocrine neoplasia (MEN)** syndromes (Table 17–2). In patients with MEN 1, there is high penetrance of hyperparathyroidism, affecting as many as 95% of patients. When their glands are examined microscopically, there are usually abnormalities in all four glands. Recurrent hyperparathyroidism, even after initially successful surgery, is common in these patients. Hyperparathyroidism also occurs in MEN 2a and MEN 2b, though at a much lower frequency in MEN 2a (about 20%) and rarely in MEN 2b. Familial hyperparathyroidism, without other features of MEN, characteristically involves all four glands. There is an increased risk of parathyroid cancer in these kindreds.

Parathyroid carcinoma is a rare malignancy, but the diagnosis should be considered in a patient with severe hypercalcemia and a palpable cervical mass. At surgery, cancers are firmer than adenomas and more likely to be attached to adjacent structures. It is sometimes difficult to distinguish parathyroid carcinomas from adenomas on histopathologic grounds. Vascular or capsular invasion by tumor cells is a good indicator of malignancy, but these features are not always present. In many cases, local recurrences or distant metastases to liver, lung, or bone are the clinical findings that support this diagnosis.

Secondary hyperparathyroidism implies diffuse glandular hyperplasia due to a defect outside the parathyroids. Secondary hyperparathyroidism in patients with normal kidney function may be observed in patients with severe calcium and vitamin D deficiency states (see below). In patients with chronic renal failure, there are many causative factors that contribute to the often dramatic enlargement of the parathyroid glands. These include decreased 1,25-$(OH)_2D$ production, reduced intestinal calcium absorption, skeletal resistance to PTH, and renal phosphate retention.

Pathogenesis

PTH secretion in primary hyperparathyroidism is excessive given the level of the serum calcium. At the cellular level, there is both increased cell mass and a secretory defect. The latter is characterized by reduced sensitivity of PTH secretion to suppression by the serum calcium concentration. This type of qualitative regulatory defect is more common than truly autonomous secretion. Thus, parathyroid glands from patients with primary hyperparathyroidism are typically enlarged and, in vitro, demonstrate a "shift to the right" in their calcium set-point for secretion (Figure 17–13). How these two potential defects interact in the pathogenesis of the disease remains to be fully elucidated.

Table 17–2. Clinical features of multiple endocrine neoplasia syndromes.

MEN 1
- Benign parathyroid tumors (very common)
- Pancreatic tumors (benign or malignant)
    - Gastrinoma
    - Insulinoma
    - Glucagonoma, VIPoma (both rare)
- Pituitary tumors
    - Growth hormone-secreting
    - Prolactin-secreting
    - ACTH-secreting
- Other tumors: lipomas, carcinoids, adrenal and thyroid adenomas

MEN 2a
- Medullary carcinoma of the thyroid
- Pheochromocytoma (benign or malignant)
- Hyperparathyroidism

MEN 2b
- Medullary carcinoma of the thyroid
- Pheochromocytoma
- Mucosal neuromas, ganglioneuromas
- Marfanoid habitus
- Hyperparathyroidism (very rare)

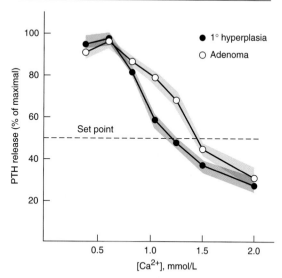

Figure 17–13. PTH secretion in vitro from human parathyroid cells from patients with parathyroid adenomas and hyperplasia. The set-point for secretion is the calcium concentration at which PTH release is suppressed by 50%. This is shifted to the right in the majority of parathyroid adenomas compared to normal tissues, in which the set-point is approximately 1.0 mmol/L ionized calcium. (Reproduced, with permission, from Brown EM et al: Dispersed cells prepared from human parathyroid glands: Distinct calcium sensitivity of adenomas vs primary hyperplasia. J Clin Endocrinol Metab 1978;46:267.)

The genetic defects responsible for primary hyperparathyroidism have received considerable attention. Genes that regulate the cell cycle are thought to be important in the pathogenesis of parathyroid tumors. The *PRAD1* gene (parathyroid rearrangement adenoma), whose product is a D1 cyclin, has been implicated in parathyroid tumor development. Cyclins are cell cycle regulatory proteins. The *PRAD1* gene is located on the long arm of chromosome 11, as is the gene encoding for PTH. Analysis of parathyroid tumor DNA suggests that a chromosome inversion event occurred which led to juxtaposition of the 5'-regulatory domain of the PTH gene upstream to the *PRAD1* gene (Figure 17–14). Because regulatory sequences in the PTH gene are responsible for its cell-specific transcription, this inversion could lead to abnormally regulated transcription of the *PRAD1* gene in a parathyroid cell-specific manner. Overproduction of the *PRAD1* gene product, a cyclin, would enhance the proliferative potential of the cell bearing this inversion. Increased proliferation could lead to a clonal outgrowth of the original cell with the inversion. Approximately 5% of sporadic parathyroid adenomas are thought to be related to overexpression of the *PRAD1* gene. *PRAD1* has also been implicated in the pathogenesis of B cell lymphomas, breast and lung cancers, and squamous cell cancers of the head and neck.

In 1988, linkage analysis of MEN 1 kindreds localized the responsible gene to chromosome 11q13. Further pedigree analysis led to a refinement of the responsible region on chromosome 11 and ultimately to an identification of the *MEN1* gene in 1997. The MEN 1 gene product, menin, is thought to be a tumor suppressor protein. In keeping with the "two-hit" hypothesis of oncogenesis, patients with MEN 1 inherit an abnormal or inactivated *MEN1* allele from one parent. This germline defect is present in all cells. During postnatal life, the other *MEN1* allele in a parathyroid cell (for example) undergoes spontaneous mutation or deletion. If this second mutation confers a growth advantage on the descendant cells, there is clonal outgrowth of cells bearing the second mutation, and eventually a tumor results. In approximately 25% of nonfamilial benign parathyroid adenomas, there is allelic loss of DNA from chromosome 11, where the *MEN1* gene is located.

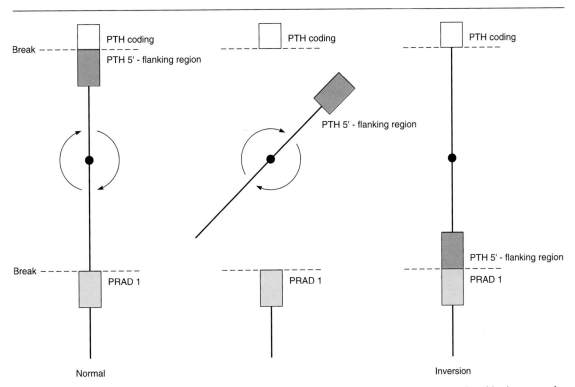

Figure 17–14. Proposed genetic rearrangement of chromosome 11 in a subset of sporadic parathyroid adenomas. An inversion of DNA sequence near the centromere of chromosome 11 places the 5'-regulatory region of the *PTH* gene (also on chromosome 11) adjacent to the *PRAD1* gene, whose product is involved in cell cycle control. This places the *PRAD1* gene under the control of *PTH* regulatory sequences, which would be predicted to be highly active in parathyroid cells. (Modified and reproduced, with permission, from Arnold A: Molecular genetics of parathyroid gland neoplasia. J Clin Endocrin Metabol 1993;77:1109.)

The MEN 1 gene product is the protein menin, which localizes to the nucleus. Little is known of the function of menin in normal physiology, and the mechanism by which it promotes tumor formation in the pituitary, pancreas, and parathyroid glands is unknown. Genetic testing to determine the presence of a mutation in the *MEN1* gene is not yet widely available. Mutations identified to date in families are scattered through the gene, which renders screening efforts more difficult.

The hyperparathyroidism in both MEN 2a and MEN 2b appears to be caused by mutations in the RET protein. RET clearly plays an important role in the pathogenesis of the other endocrine tumors in these syndromes as well as in familial medullary carcinoma of the thyroid (see below). How RET mutations alter parathyroid cell growth or PTH secretion has not been elucidated.

Clinical Manifestations

Hyperparathyroidism may present in a variety of ways. Patients with this disease may be truly asymptomatic, and their diagnosis is made by screening laboratory tests. Other patients may have skeletal complications or nephrolithiasis. Because calcium affects the functioning of nearly every organ system, the symptoms and signs of hypercalcemia are protean (Table 17–3). Depending on the nature of the complaints, the patient with primary hyperparathyroidism may be suspected of having a psychiatric disorder or even a malignancy.

Hyperparathyroidism is a chronic disorder in which long-standing PTH excess and hypercalcemia may produce increasing symptomatology, especially symptoms related to renal stones and worsening osteopenia. Recurrent stones containing calcium phosphate or calcium oxalate occur in 10–15% of patients with primary hyperparathyroidism. Nephrolithiasis may be complicated by urinary outflow tract obstruction, infection, and progressive renal insufficiency. Patients with significant PTH excess may experience increased bone turnover and progressive loss of bone mineral. This is reflected in subperiosteal resorption, osteoporosis (particularly of cortical bone), and even pathologic fractures.

A sizable proportion of patients with primary hyperparathyroidism, however, are asymptomatic. These patients may experience no clinical deterioration if their hyperparathyroidism is followed and not treated surgically. Because it is difficult to identify these patients with certainty when the diagnosis of hyperparathyroidism is made, regular follow-up is mandatory. A minority of asymptomatic patients experience skeletal or renal deterioration, which is an indication for surgery.

Radiologic features of primary hyperparathyroidism are caused by the chronic effects of excess PTH on bone and kidney. These include subperiosteal resorption (evident most strikingly in the clavicles and distal phalanges), generalized osteopenia, and the characteristic but now rare brown tumors. Uncommonly, osteosclerosis may result from excessive PTH action on bone. Abdominal films may show nephrocalcinosis or nephrolithiasis.

The complete differential diagnosis of hypercalcemia should be considered in all patients with this abnormality (Table 17–4). Primary hyperparathyroidism accounts for most cases of hypercalcemia in the outpatient setting. The diagnosis of primary hyperparathyroidism is confirmed by at least two simultaneous measurements of calcium and immunoreactive PTH, preferably by an assay for intact PTH. An elevated or inappropriately normal PTH in the setting of hypercalcemia is the key feature in making the diagnosis of primary hyperparathyroidism (Table 17–5).

Patients with secondary hyperparathyroidism may have normal or subnormal calcium levels (see below). If renal function is normal, serum phosphate is

Table 17–3. Symptoms and signs of primary hyperparathyroidism.

Systemic
  Weakness
  Easy fatigue
  Weight loss
  Anemia
  Anorexia
  Pruritus
  Ectopic calcifications
Neuropsychiatric
  Depression
  Poor concentration
  Memory deficits
  Peripheral sensory neuropathy
  Motor neuropathy
  Proximal and generalized muscle weakness
Ocular
  Band keratopathy
Cardiac
  Shortened Q–T interval
  Hypertension
Renal
  Stones
  Polyuria, polydipsia
  Metabolic acidosis
  Concentrating defects
  Nephrocalcinosis
Skeletal
  Osteopenia
  Pathological fractures
  Brown tumors of bone
  Bone pain
  Gout
  Pseudogout
  Chondrocalcinosis
  Osteitis fibrosa cystica
Gastrointestinal
  Peptic ulcer disease
  Pancreatitis
  Constipation
  Nausea
  Vomiting

Table 17-4. Differential diagnosis of hypercalcemia.

Primary hyperparathyroidism
   Adenoma
   Carcinoma
   Hyperplasia
Familial (benign) hypocalciuric hypercalcemia
Malignancy-associated hypercalcemia
   Solid tumors (majority with excess PTHrP production)
   Multiple myeloma
   Adult T cell leukemia and lymphoma
   Other lymphomas
Thyrotoxicosis
Drugs
   Thiazides
   Lithium
   Vitamin D or A intoxication
Granulomatous diseases
   Sarcoidosis
   Tuberculosis
   Histoplasmosis (and other fungal diseases)
Milk-alkali syndrome
Adrenal insufficiency

also often reduced. Although serum PTH is elevated, the demineralized state of the bone and the chronic vitamin D deficiency combine to produce a low filtered load of calcium. Hence, urinary calcium excretion is often quite low. The 25-(OH)D level will also be low or undetectable in vitamin D deficiency states due to a variety of causes.

FAMILIAL (BENIGN) HYPOCALCIURIC HYPERCALCEMIA

Etiology

In a substantial group of patients with asymptomatic hypercalcemia, the diagnosis of **familial (benign) hypocalciuric hypercalcemia** should be considered. Individuals with this condition typically have an elevated serum calcium and normal or even mildly elevated PTH levels. This disorder of calcium homeostasis is inherited in an autosomal dominant manner. In families with this form of benign hypercalcemia, there are rare occurrences of **neonatal severe primary hyperparathyroidism.**

It has been shown in the majority of kindreds studied that familial hypocalciuric hypercalcemia is due to a point mutation in the parathyroid calcium-sensing receptor gene. Those individuals with benign hypercalcemia typically have a single dose of a mutated calcium receptor gene. Infants with neonatal severe hyperparathyroidism, usually the result of consanguinity, have inherited two copies of mutant calcium receptor genes.

Pathogenesis

The calcium-sensing receptor, a member of the G protein-coupled receptor superfamily, is expressed in a variety of tissues, including the parathyroid gland and kidney. In the parathyroid, this molecule is thought to serve the function of detecting the ambient serum calcium concentration and then setting the rate of PTH secretion. In the kidney, the calcium receptor is thought to set the level of urinary calcium excretion, based on its perception of the serum calcium concentration.

In familial hypocalciuric hypercalcemia and neonatal hyperparathyroidism, the ability to detect serum calcium is faulty in both the kidney and parathyroid. Familial hypocalciuric hypercalcemia is due to a partial reduction, and neonatal hyperparathyroidism a marked reduction, in normal calcium receptor alleles. In the parathyroid, chief cells missense the serum calcium to be low, and PTH secretion occurs when it should be suppressed (Figure 17-2). This produces inappropriately normal or slightly high PTH levels. In the kidney, serum calcium concentrations are also detected (inappropriately) as low, and calcium is retained. This produces the hypocalciuria typical of this condition. Depending on the mutant gene dosage, the clinical symptoms tend to be mild in familial hypocalciuric hypercalcemia and severe in neonatal hyperparathyroidism.

Clinical Manifestations

Patients with familial hypocalciuric hypercalcemia typically have lifelong asymptomatic elevations in serum calcium. They do not, however, suffer the consequences of end-organ dysfunction that is character-

Table 17-5. Laboratory findings in hypercalcemia due to various causes.

	Serum Ca^{2+}	Serum PO_4^{3-}	Intact PTH	PTHrP	Urine Ca^{2+}
Primary hyperparathyroidism	↑	↓, N	↑	N, Und	N, ↑[1]
Malignancy-associated hypercalcemia	↑	↓, N	Und	↑[2]	↑
Familial (benign) hypocalciuric hypercalcemia	↑	N	N, ↑[3]	Und	↓

Key: N = normal; Und = undetectable
[1]Can also be low depending on the filtered load of calcium.
[2]In the 70–80% of patients with cancer and a humoral basis for hypercalcemia.
[3]Mild increases in PTH have been reported in some patients.

istic of hyperparathyroidism. These individuals are spared the nephrolithiasis, osteopenia, hypertension, and renal dysfunction that can occur with greater frequency in patients with primary hyperparathyroidism. Individuals with familial hypocalciuric hypercalcemia do not benefit from parathyroidectomy. Their hypercalcemia does not remit with surgery unless a total parathyroidectomy is performed. Surgery is not recommended, since the condition is benign.

In contrast, infants with neonatal hyperparathyroidism have marked hypercalcemia, dramatic elevations in serum PTH, bone demineralization at birth, hypotonia, and profound failure to thrive. These babies require immediate total parathyroidectomy in the newborn period for survival.

In the asymptomatic hypercalcemic patient, a careful family history should be obtained in an effort to document hypercalcemia or the occurrence of failed parathyroidectomies in other family members. Urinary calcium and creatinine excretion should be measured to rule out familial hypocalciuric hypercalcemia. In this condition, urinary calcium levels are typically low and almost always less than 100 mg/24 h (Table 17–5). The calcium:creatinine clearance ratio is usually below 0.01. Genetic testing is not yet widely available for this condition, since the point mutations responsible for it are dispersed over a large portion of the calcium receptor gene. This renders rapid screening difficult at present.

---

16. What is the most common cause of primary hyperparathyroidism?
17. What is the relationship of hyperparathyroidism to the multiple endocrine neoplasia (MEN) syndromes?
18. In what conditions does secondary hyperparathyroidism occur? By what symptoms and signs is it distinguished from primary hyperparathyroidism?
19. What are the common symptoms and signs of primary hyperparathyroidism?
20. How can primary hyperparathyroidism be distinguished from familial hypocalciuric hypercalcemia? What is the mechanism for this difference?

HYPERCALCEMIA OF MALIGNANCY

Etiology

Hypercalcemia occurs in approximately 10% of all malignancies. It is most commonly seen in solid tumors, particularly squamous cell carcinomas (lung, esophagus, etc), renal carcinoma, and breast carcinoma. Hypercalcemia occurs in over one-third of patients with multiple myeloma but is unusual in lymphomas and leukemias.

Pathogenesis

Solid tumors usually produce hypercalcemia by secreting PTHrP, whose properties have been described above. This is humoral hypercalcemia, which mimics primary hyperparathyroidism and results from a diffuse increase in bone resorption induced by high circulating levels of PTHrP and exacerbated by the effect of PTHrP to reduce renal excretion of calcium.

Multiple myeloma produces hypercalcemia by a different mechanism; myeloma cells induce local bone resorption or osteolysis in the bone marrow, probably by releasing cytokines with bone-resorbing activity, such as interleukin-1 and tumor necrosis factor. Rarely, lymphomas produce humoral hypercalcemia by secreting $1,25\text{-}(OH)_2D$.

Finally, even though many hypercalcemic patients have bone metastases, these may not contribute directly to the pathogenesis of hypercalcemia.

Clinical Manifestations

Unlike patients with primary hyperparathyroidism, who often are minimally symptomatic, patients with hypercalcemia of malignancy are typically very ill. Hypercalcemia typically occurs in advanced malignancy—the average survival of hypercalcemic patients is only 6 weeks—and the tumor is almost invariably obvious. In addition, hypercalcemia is often severe and symptomatic, with nausea, vomiting, dehydration, confusion, or coma. Biochemically, malignancy-associated hypercalcemia is characterized by a decreased serum phosphate and a suppressed level of intact PTH (Table 17–5). With most solid tumors, the serum level of PTHrP is increased. These findings, together with the differences in clinical presentation, usually make the differentiation of this syndrome from primary hyperparathyroidism relatively easy.

---

21. What tumors commonly result in hypercalcemia?
22. What are the mechanisms by which a tumor may cause hypercalcemia?
23. What are the clinical symptoms and signs of hypercalcemia of malignancy?

HYPOPARATHYROIDISM & PSEUDOHYPOPARATHYROIDISM

Etiology

The total serum calcium measured in the clinical setting includes the contribution from ionized, protein-bound, and complexed forms of calcium. It should be recognized, however, that symptoms of hypocalcemia occur only if the ionized fraction of calcium is reduced. Furthermore, only patients with low ionized calcium levels should be evaluated for the possibility of a hypocalcemic disorder.

A common cause of hypocalcemia in the clinical setting is hypoalbuminemia. A low serum albumin lowers only the protein-bound and not the ionized calcium. Thus, such patients need not be evaluated for mineral disorders. To determine whether a hypoalbuminemic patient has a low ionized calcium, this parameter can be measured directly. If this laboratory test is not readily available, a reasonable alternative is to correct the total serum calcium for the low serum albumin. This is done by adjusting the serum calcium upward by 0.8 mg/dL for each 1 g/dL reduction in serum albumin. This simple correction usually brings the adjusted serum calcium into the normal range.

The differential diagnosis of a low ionized calcium is lengthy (Table 17–6). Hypocalcemia can result from reduced PTH secretion due to **hypoparathyroidism** or hypomagnesemia. It can also be due to decreased end-organ responsiveness to PTH, despite adequate or even excessive levels of the hormone; this is termed **pseudohypoparathyroidism**.

Table 17–6. Differential diagnosis of hypocalcemia.

Failure to secrete PTH
Hypoparathyroidism (see Table 17–7)
Resistance to PTH action
Pseudohypoparathyroidism (types 1a, 1b, 2)
Sepsis-associated hypocalcemia
Failure to secrete PTH and resistance to PTH action
Chronic magnesium depletion due to—
Diarrhea, malabsorption
Alcoholism
Drugs: aminoglycoside antibiotics, loop diuretics, cisplatin, amphotericin B
Parenteral nutrition
Primary renal wasting
Failure to produce $1,25\text{-}(OH)_2D$
Vitamin D deficiency due to—
Nutritional causes
Liver disease
Cholestasis
Small intestinal disorders producing malabsorption
Renal failure
Vitamin D dependent rickets type 1: defective 1α-hydroxylase activity (very rare)
Tumor-induced osteomalacia
Resistance to $1,25\text{-}(OH)_2D$ action
Vitamin D-dependent rickets type 2: defect in vitamin D receptor (rare)
Acute challenges to the homeostatic mechanisms
Pancreatitis (formation of calcium salts in retroperitoneal fat)
Drug-induced (eg, EDTA, citrate, plicamycin, bisphosphonates, phosphate, foscarnet)
Liver transplantation (citrate is not metabolized, thereby forming calcium citrate complexes and lowering ionized calcium)
Rhabdomyolysis
Hungry bone syndrome (increased deposition into demineralized bone)
Osteoblastic metastases (eg, breast or prostate cancer)
Tumor lysis syndrome (acute phosphate load released from tumor cells due to cytolytic therapy)

Table 17–7. Causes of hypoparathyroidism.

Complication of thyroid or parathyroid surgery
Autoimmune
Post-^{131}I therapy for Graves' disease or thyroid cancer
Secondary to iron overload, Wilson's disease
DiGeorge syndrome: autosomal recessive disorder with congenital absence of parathyroid glands and thymic dysgenesis or agenesis
Hereditary forms of hypoparathyroidism: autosomal dominant or recessive and X-linked recessive
Activating mutations of the calcium receptor
Secondary to magnesium depletion
Tumor invasion (very rare)
Kearns-Sayre and Kenny syndromes
Hereditary nephrosis, nerve deafness, and hypoparathyroidism

All forms of hypoparathyroidism are uncommon (Table 17–7). Most cases are the result of inadvertent trauma to, removal of, or devascularization of the parathyroid glands during thyroid or parathyroid surgery. The incidence of postoperative hypoparathyroidism (range: 0.2–30%) depends on the extent of the antecedent surgery and the surgeon's skill in identifying normal parathyroid tissue and preserving its blood supply. Postoperative hypocalcemia may be transient or permanent. Some patients may also be left with diminished parathyroid reserve.

A variety of causes other than postsurgical complications may produce an absolute or relative state of PTH deficiency (Table 17–7). These include autoimmune glandular failure; magnesium depletion; autosomal dominant or recessive or X-linked hypoparathyroidism; hypoparathyroidism due to activating mutations of the calcium receptor; and hypoparathyroidism due to iron overload or Wilson's disease. Rarely, there is congenital absence of the parathyroid glands **(DiGeorge syndrome),** which presents in infancy or childhood accompanied by a defect in cell-mediated immunity.

Two syndromes of **autoimmune polyglandular failure** have been recognized. Patients with type 1 polyglandular failure commonly have mucocutaneous candidiasis, Addison's disease (adrenal insufficiency), and hypoparathyroidism. These disorders typically present by the teens or early twenties (Figure 17–15). Autoantibodies to adrenal and parathyroid tissue are seen in most of these patients. Eventually, other endocrine glands may become involved (eg, the gonads, thyroid, and pancreas). Type I polyglandular failure syndrome (autoimmune polyendocrinopathy candidiasis ectodermal dystrophy; APECED) is an autosomal recessive disorder and has recently been shown to be due to mutations in a gene termed the autoimmune regulator *(AIRE)*. This gene encodes a protein with biochemical features which suggest that it is a transcription factor. This is the first gene identified in which a mutation causes a systemic autoimmune disease.

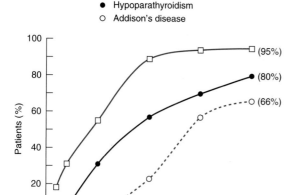

Figure 17–15. Cumulative incidence of three common manifestations of autoimmune polyglandular failure type 1 compared with age at onset in a cohort of 68 patients. The figures in parentheses reflect incidences at age 20. (Data plotted from Ahonen P et al: Clinical variation of autoimmune polyendocrinopathy-candidiasis-ectodermal dystrophy [APECED] in a series of 68 patients. N Engl J Med 1990;322:1829.)

Type 2 polyglandular failure syndrome (**Schmidt's syndrome**) is characterized by hypothyroidism and adrenal insufficiency and does not classically involve the parathyroid glands (see Chapter 21).

Pathogenesis

The pathogenesis of hypoparathyroidism in most cases is straightforward. The mineral disturbance occurs because the amount of PTH released is inadequate to maintain normal serum calcium concentrations, and hypocalcemia results. Hyperphosphatemia is also observed in these patients because the proximal tubular effect of PTH to promote phosphate excretion is lost. Since PTH is required to stimulate the renal production of 1,25-$(OH)_2$D, levels of 1,25-$(OH)_2$D are low in patients with hypoparathyroidism. Hyperphosphatemia further suppresses 1,25-$(OH)_2$D synthesis. Low 1,25-$(OH)_2$D levels lead to reduced intestinal calcium absorption. In the absence of adequate 1,25-$(OH)_2$D and PTH, the mobilization of calcium from bone is abnormal. Since less PTH is available to act in the distal nephron, urinary calcium excretion may be high, especially in view of the hypocalcemia. A combination of these mechanisms contributes to the mineral disturbances seen in hypoparathyroid patients.

Magnesium depletion is a common cause of hypocalcemia. The pathogenesis of hypocalcemia in this clinical setting relates to a functional and reversible state of hypoparathyroidism. There is also decreased renal and skeletal responsiveness to PTH. Magnesium depletion may occur from a variety of causes, including chronic alcoholism, diarrhea, and drugs such as loop diuretics, aminoglycoside antibiotics, amphotericin B, and cisplatin (Table 17–6). Magnesium is required to maintain normal PTH secretory responses. Once body magnesium stores are repleted, PTH levels rise appropriately in response to the hypocalcemia, and the mineral imbalance is corrected.

In **pseudohypoparathyroidism,** there are adequate levels of PTH in the circulation, but the ability of target tissues (kidney and bone) to respond to the hormone is subnormal. In type 1 pseudohypoparathyroidism, the ability of PTH to generate an increase in the second-messenger cAMP is reduced. In some patients, this is due to a deficiency in the cellular content of the alpha subunit of the stimulatory G protein ($G_{s-\alpha}$), which couples the PTH receptor to the adenylyl cyclase enzyme (type 1a). In other patients with pseudohypoparathyroidism, $G_{s-\alpha}$ protein levels are normal, and another as yet unidentified component in the PTH receptor-signal transduction complex is defective (type 1b). In patients with type 2 pseudohypoparathyroidism, urinary cAMP is normal but the phosphaturic response to infused PTH is reduced. The pathogenesis of this more rare form of PTH resistance remains obscure.

Patients with activating mutations of the calcium receptor present typically with autosomal dominant hypocalcemia and hypercalciuria. Both defects are due to overly sensitive calcium receptors, which turn off PTH secretion and renal calcium reabsorption at subnormal serum calcium levels. These individuals rarely experience symptoms of their often mild hypocalcemia, but if given vitamin D they are prone to development of marked hypercalciuria, nephrocalcinosis, and even renal failure.

Clinical Manifestations

The symptoms and signs of hypocalcemia are similar regardless of the underlying cause (Table 17–8). Patients may be asymptomatic or may have latent or overt tetany. **Tetany** is defined as spontaneous tonic muscular contractions. Painful carpal spasms and laryngeal stridor are striking manifestations of tetany. Latent tetany may be demonstrated by testing for Chvostek's and Trousseau's signs. **Chvostek's sign** is elicited by tapping on the facial nerve anterior to the ear. Twitching of the ipsilateral facial muscles indicates a positive test. A positive **Trousseau sign** is demonstrated by inflating the sphygmomanometer above the systolic blood pressure for 3 minutes. In hypocalcemic individuals, this causes painful carpal muscle contractions and spasms (Figure 17–16). If hypocalcemia is severe and unrecognized, airway compromise, generalized seizures, and even death may occur.

Table 17–8. Symptoms and signs of hypocalcemia.

Systemic	Confusion Weakness Mental retardation Behavioral changes
Neuromuscular	Paresthesias Psychosis Seizures Carpopedal spasms Chvostek's and Trousseau's signs Depression Muscle cramping Parkinsonism Irritability Basal-ganglia calcifications
Cardiac	Prolonged Q–T interval T wave changes Congestive heart failure
Ocular	Cataracts
Dental	Enamel hypoplasia of teeth Defective root formation Failure of adult teeth to erupt
Respiratory	Laryngospasm Bronchospasm Stridor

Chronic hypocalcemia can produce intracranial calcifications that have a predilection for the basal ganglia. These may be detectable by CT scanning or MRI or in some cases by plain skull radiographs. Chronic hypocalcemia may also enhance calcification of the lens and the formation of cataracts.

In addition to the symptoms and signs of hypocalcemia, patients with pseudohypoparathyroidism type 1a may have a constellation of features collectively known as **Albright's hereditary osteodystrophy.** These include short stature, obesity, mental retardation, brachycephaly, shortened fourth and fifth metacarpal and metatarsal bones, and subcutaneous ossifications. How these phenotypic features are related to the underlying molecular defect has not yet been explained.

In considering the differential diagnosis of hypocalcemia, one must be guided by the clinical setting. A positive family history is very important in supporting a diagnosis of pseudohypoparathyroidism, autoimmune polyglandular failure, or other hereditary forms of hypoparathyroidism. The patient with hypocalcemia, hyperphosphatemia, and a normal serum creatinine most likely has hypoparathyroidism. A history of neck surgery or radiation should be sought. Clearly, there may be a long latent period before symptomatic hypocalcemia presents, even in postsurgical hypoparathyroidism. The physical examination can be helpful if it is directed toward identifying signs of hypocalcemia, stigmas of Albright's hereditary osteodystrophy, or other features of autoimmune polyglandular failure (eg, vitiligo, mucocutaneous candidiasis). Patients with pseudohypoparathyroidism and Albright's hereditary osteodystrophy often have other endocrine abnormalities such as primary hypothyroidism or gonadal failure.

In the differential diagnosis of disorders that present with hypocalcemia, laboratory findings are extremely useful (Table 17–9). Serum phosphate is often (not invariably) elevated in hypoparathyroidism and pseudohypoparathyroidism. In magnesium depletion, serum phosphate is usually normal. In secondary hyperparathyroidism not due to renal failure, serum phosphate is typically low. Serum PTH levels are crucial in determining the cause of hypocalcemia. PTH is classically elevated in untreated pseudohypoparathyroidism but not in hypoparathyroidism or magnesium depletion. Intact PTH may be undetectable, low, or normal in patients with hypoparathyroidism depending on the parathyroid functional reserve. In patients with secondary hyperparathyroidism due to defects in the production or bioavailability of vitamin D, the clinical setting often suggests a problem with vitamin D (eg, regional enteritis, bowel resection, liver disease). The presence of a low 25-(OH)D level and an increased PTH confirms this diagnosis.

Measurement of serum magnesium is the first step in ruling out magnesium depletion as the cause of hypocalcemia and should be part of the initial evaluation. If urinary magnesium is inappropriately high relative to the serum magnesium, renal magnesium wasting is present. PTH levels in this setting are typically low or normal. Normal PTH levels, however, are inappropriate in the presence of hypocalcemia.

The diagnosis of pseudohypoparathyroidism can be confirmed by infusing synthetic human PTH(1–34) and measuring urinary cAMP and phosphate responses. This maneuver is designed to prove that there is end-organ resistance to PTH and to de-

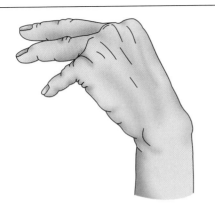

Figure 17–16. Position of fingers in carpal spasm due to hypocalcemic tetany. (Reproduced, with permission, from Ganong WF: *Review of Medical Physiology*, 19th ed. Appleton & Lange, 1999.)

Table 17-9. Laboratory findings in hypocalcemia.

	Serum Ca^{2+}	Serum PO$_4^{3-}$	Intact PTH	25-(OH)D$_3$	Urinary cAMP Response to PTH Infusion
Hypoparathyroidism	↓	↑, N	↓, N[1]	N	N
Pseudohypoparathyroidism	↓	↑, N	↑	N	↓
Magnesium depletion	↓	N	↓, N[1]	N	N
Secondary hyperparathyroidism[2]	↓	N, ↓	↑	↓	N

[1]May be normal, but inappropriate to level of serum calcium.
[2]Due to vitamin D deficiency, for example; urinary calcium excretion usually less than 50 mg/24 h.

termine whether the diagnosis is pseudohypoparathyroidism type 1 or type 2.

Hypoparathyroidism may vary in its severity and therefore in the need for therapy. In some patients with decreased parathyroid reserve, only situations of increased stress on the glands, such as pregnancy or lactation, induce hypocalcemia. In other patients, PTH deficiency is a chronic symptomatic disorder necessitating lifelong therapy with calcium supplements and vitamin D analogs. All patients so treated should have periodic monitoring of serum calcium, urinary calcium, and renal function. Patients with autoimmune hypoparathyroidism should also be examined regularly for the development of adrenal insufficiency, hypothyroidism, and diabetes mellitus as well as other complications of the type 1 polyglandular failure syndrome.

24. What are the causes of hypoparathyroidism?
25. What is the mechanism of pseudohypoparathyroidism?
26. What are the symptoms and signs of hypocalcemia?
27. How can laboratory studies be used to distinguish various causes of hypocalcemia?

MEDULLARY CARCINOMA OF THE THYROID

Etiology

Medullary carcinoma of the thyroid gland, a C cell neoplasm, accounts for only 5–10% of all thyroid malignancies. Approximately 80% are sporadic and 20% are familial, occurring in autosomal dominant MEN 2a and MEN 2b and in non-MEN syndromes. In sporadic cases, the tumor is usually unilateral. In hereditary forms, however, tumors are often bilateral and multifocal.

Pathogenesis

The growth pattern of medullary carcinoma is slow but progressive, and local invasion of adjacent structures is not uncommon. The tumor spreads hematogenously, with metastases typically to lymph nodes, bone, and lung. The clinical progression of this cancer is variable. While there may be early metastases to cervical and mediastinal lymph nodes in as many as 50–70% of patients, the tumor still usually behaves in an indolent fashion. In a minority of cases, a more aggressive pattern of tumor growth has been noted. Early detection in high-risk individuals, such as those with a family history of medullary carcinoma or MEN 2a or 2b, is crucial to prevent advanced disease and distant metastases. Overall survival is estimated to be 80% at 5 years and 60% at 10 years.

Patients with MEN 2 develop medullary carcinoma at frequencies approaching 100%. C cell hyperplasia typically precedes the development of cancer. In MEN 2a and 2b, the thyroid lesions are malignant. In contrast, pheochromocytomas associated with either MEN 2a or MEN 2b are infrequently malignant. Hyperparathyroidism in MEN 2a, which is uncommon, is usually due to diffuse hyperplasia and not to a malignancy. Chronic hypercalcitoninemia as a result of the tumor may also contribute to the pathogenesis of parathyroid hyperplasia. Parathyroid hyperplasia is rarely seen in patients with either MEN 2b or sporadic carcinoma. Germline mutations in the *RET* proto-oncogene on chromosome 10 are known to play a causal role in three forms of medullary carcinoma. These include cases of familial isolated medullary thyroid cancer, MEN 2a, and MEN 2b.

The RET protein is a membrane tyrosine kinase thought to be involved in the development of neural crest cells. A ligand for RET is glial cell-derived neurotrophic factor. Many of the mutations found in families with MEN 2a render the RET protein constitutively active, but how the pathways activated by RET eventually produce tumors in endocrine tissues is unknown.

Clinical Manifestations

Sporadic medullary carcinoma occurs with about equal frequency in males and females and is typically found in patients over 50 years of age. In MEN 2a or

2b, the tumor occurs at a much younger age, often in childhood. In fact, medullary carcinoma in a patient under age 40 should suggest that the patient may be an index case of familial medullary carcinoma or MEN 2a or 2b. Medullary carcinoma may present as a single nodule or as multiple thyroid nodules. Patients with sporadic medullary carcinoma often have palpable cervical lymphadenopathy.

Since C cells are neuroendocrine cells, these tumors have the capacity to release calcitonin and other hormones such as prostaglandins, serotonin, adrenocorticotropin, somatostatin, and calcitonin gene-related peptide. Serotonin, calcitonin, or the prostaglandins have been implicated in the pathogenesis of the secretory diarrhea observed in approximately 20–30% of patients with medullary carcinoma. If diarrhea is present, this usually indicates a large tumor burden or metastatic disease. Patients may also have flushing, which has been ascribed to the production by the tumor of substance P or calcitonin gene-related peptide, both of which are vasodilators.

In a patient suspected of having medullary carcinoma, a radionuclide thyroid scan may demonstrate one or more cold nodules. These nodules are solid by ultrasound. Fine-needle aspiration biopsy will show the characteristic C cell lesion with positive immunostaining for calcitonin. Surprisingly, the diagnosis of medullary carcinoma is not suspected preoperatively in most cases and is made instead by frozen section at the time of surgery. The tumor has the propensity to contain large calcifications, which can be seen on x-rays of the neck. Bone metastases may be lytic or sclerotic in their appearance, and pulmonary metastases may be surrounded by fibrotic reactions.

The most important laboratory test in determining the presence and extent of medullary carcinoma is the calcitonin level. Circulating calcitonin levels are typically elevated in most patients, and serum levels correlate with tumor burden. In C cell hyperplasia, basal calcitonin may or may not be elevated. These patients will usually, however, demonstrate abnormal provocative testing. Intravenous calcium gluconate (2 mg/kg of elemental calcium) is injected over 1 minute, followed by pentagastrin (0.5 μg/kg) over 5 seconds. Provocative testing is based on the ability of calcium and the synthetic gastrin analog pentagastrin to hyperstimulate calcitonin release in a patient with increased C cell mass, due either to hyperplasia or to carcinoma. A greater than twofold increase in serum calcitonin above the normal response is considered abnormal. It must be borne in mind that false-positive provocative testing for calcitonin can occur.

Serial calcitonin levels are a useful parameter for following therapeutic responses in patients with medullary carcinoma or for diagnosing a recurrence, along with clinical examination and imaging procedures. Calcitonin levels usually reflect the extent of disease. If the tumor becomes less differentiated, calcitonin levels may no longer reflect tumor burden. Another useful tumor marker for medullary carcinoma is carcinoembryonic antigen (CEA). This antigen is frequently elevated in patients with medullary carcinoma and is present at all stages of the disease. Rapid increases in CEA predict a worse clinical course.

Surgery is the mainstay of therapy for patients with medullary thyroid carcinoma. Total thyroidectomy is advocated because the tumors are often multicentric. Patients may also receive radioactive iodine ablation of any residual thyroid tissue, since any C cells remaining may undergo malignant degeneration. Patients should be monitored indefinitely for recurrences, because these tumors may be so indolent. All patients with medullary carcinoma of the thyroid, whether it is familial or sporadic, should be tested for *RET* oncogene mutations. This testing is now commercially available and has supplanted calcitonin provocative testing in patients from families with isolated medullary carcinoma or MEN 2a or 2b. Over 90% of patients with MEN 2 have been found to harbor *RET* mutations. Sporadic cases of medullary carcinoma of the thyroid should also be tested to detect the occurrence of a new mutation for which other family members can then be screened. Properly performed DNA testing is essentially unambiguous in predicting gene carrier status and can be used prospectively to recommend prophylactic thyroidectomy in young patients with MEN 2 prior to the development of C cell hyperplasia or frank carcinoma.

Patients with MEN 2a or 2b—even in the absence of symptoms—should undergo screening tests for the possibility of pheochromocytoma prior to thyroid surgery. These tests include the determination of urinary catecholamines and their metabolites and adrenal CT scanning. These tumors may be clinically silent at the time medullary carcinoma is diagnosed, and they should be removed before thyroidectomy.

---

28. How can you make the diagnosis of medullary carcinoma of the thyroid?
29. What is the treatment for medullary carcinoma?
30. Which patients are at higher risk for medullary carcinoma?

OSTEOPOROSIS

Etiology

Osteoporosis is defined as loss of bone mass. A slow loss of mineral from bone is a normal part of the aging process, commencing after age 30 (Figure 17–17). Thus, after age 30, the bone mass is determined by the level of peak bone mass that was attained and the subsequent rate of loss. Heredity

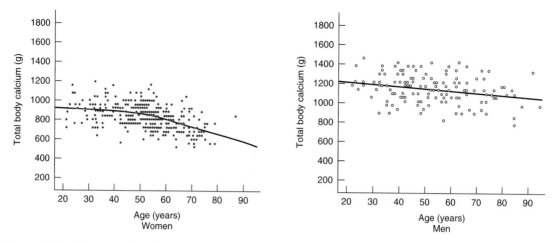

Figure 17–17. Total body calcium in women and men as a function of age. (Reproduced, with permission, from Aloia JF et al: A model for involutional bone loss. J Lab Clin Med 1985;106:630.)

is important in determining bone mass. It has long been recognized that blacks have greater peak bone mass than whites or Asians and are relatively protected from osteoporosis. It now appears that within a Caucasian population, more than half the variance in bone mass is genetically determined. However, a number of hormonal and environmental factors can reduce the genetically determined peak bone mass or hasten the loss of bone mineral and thus present important risk factors for osteoporosis (Table 17–10).

The most important etiologic factor in osteoporosis is sex steroid deficiency. The estrogen deficiency that occurs after menopause accelerates loss of bone; postmenopausal women consistently have lower bone mass than men and a higher incidence of osteoporotic fractures. With respect to bone, testosterone serves the same function in men as estrogen in women, and hypogonadal men also experience accelerated bone loss. Another important factor is the use of corticosteroids or endogenous cortisol excess in Cushing's syndrome. Glucocorticoid-induced osteoporosis is one of the most devastating complications of chronic therapy with these agents. Certain other medications—including thyroid hormone, anticonvulsants, and chronic heparin therapy—immobilization, alcohol abuse, and smoking, are also risk factors for osteoporosis. Diet is important as well. As discussed below, an adequate intake of calcium and vitamin D is necessary to build peak bone mass optimally and to minimize the rate of loss. Other dietary factors may also be important. Osteoporosis is most prevalent in Western societies, and it has been speculated that our high protein intake or related factors may predispose to osteoporosis, perhaps by enhancing urinary calcium losses.

Pathogenesis

Since bone remodeling involves the coupled resorption of bone by osteoclasts and the deposition of new bone by osteoblasts, bone loss could result from increased bone resorption, decreased bone formation, or a combination of the two. Postmenopausal osteoporosis is the consequence of accelerated bone re-

Table 17–10. Causes of osteoporosis.

Primary osteoporosis
  Aging (senile or involutional)
  Juvenile
  Idiopathic (young adults)
Connective tissue diseases
  Osteogenesis imperfecta
  Homocystinuria
  Ehlers-Danlos syndrome
  Marfan's syndrome
Drug-induced
  Corticosteroids
  Alcohol
  Thyroid hormone
  Chronic heparin
  Anticonvulsants
Hematologic
  Multiple myeloma
  Systemic mastocytosis
Immobilization
Endocrine
  Hypogonadism
  Hypercortisolism
  Hyperthyroidism
  Hyperparathyroidism
Gastrointestinal disorders
  Subtotal gastrectomy
  Malabsorption syndromes
  Obstructive jaundice
  Biliary cirrhosis

sorption. The urinary excretion of calcium and of bone collagen metabolites such as hydroxyproline and pyridinoline cross-links increases, the serum PTH level is somewhat suppressed, and if bone is biopsied resorption surfaces are found to be increased. The bone formation rate is also increased, with an increase in serum alkaline phosphatase and in the serum level of the bone matrix protein osteocalcin, both reflecting increased osteoblastic activity. This high-turnover state is the direct result of estrogen deficiency and can be reversed by estrogen replacement therapy.

The accelerated phase of estrogen-deficient bone loss begins immediately after menopause (natural or surgical). It is most evident in trabecular bone, the compartment which is remodeled most rapidly. As much as 5–20% of spinal trabecular bone mineral is lost yearly in postmenopausal women, and osteoporotic fractures in early postmenopausal women are often in the spine, a site of trabecular bone. After 5–15 years, the rate of bone loss slows, so that after age 65 the rates are similar in both sexes.

The cellular basis for the activation of bone resorption in estrogen- or androgen-deficient states is not fully understood. Osteoclasts have estrogen receptors and could respond directly to estrogen deficiency, but there is also evidence that osteoclast-stimulating cytokines such as interleukin-6 may be released from other bone cells in estrogen-deficient states.

The pathogenesis of age-related bone loss is less certain. It begins after age 30, is relatively slow, and occurs at a similar rate regardless of gender or race. It was once thought that elderly patients with osteoporosis ranged from low-turnover states, characterized by markedly decreased osteoblastic activity, to high-turnover states that resemble the accelerated phase of postmenopausal bone loss. It now appears that only a few such individuals are truly in a low-turnover state. For example, serum osteocalcin levels remain elevated throughout the latter decades of life, suggesting that osteoblast activity is not absolutely diminished. It is probable, however, that the balance of cellular activity is altered, with a reduced osteoblast response to continued bone resorption, so that resorption cavities are incompletely filled by new bone formation during the remodeling cycle.

One important factor in the pathogenesis of age-related bone loss (sometimes called senile osteoporosis) is a relative deficiency of dietary calcium and $1,25\text{-}(OH)_2D$. The capacity of the intestine to absorb calcium is diminished in the aged. Because renal losses of calcium are obligatory, a decreased efficiency of calcium absorption means that dietary calcium intake must be increased to prevent negative calcium balance. However, the typical woman has reduced—not increased—her dietary intake of calcium. It is estimated that about 1200 mg/d of elemental calcium is required to maintain calcium balance in people over age 65 (Table 17–11). American women in this age group ingest 500–600 mg of calcium daily; the calcium intakes in men are higher. In addition, some of the aged are deficient in vitamin D, further impairing their ability to absorb calcium. Particularly in northern climates, where sunlight exposure is reduced in the winter months, borderline low levels of 25-(OH)D and mild secondary hyperparathyroidism are evident by the end of winter.

Table 17–11. Calcium nutrition and osteoporosis.

Calcium requirements (to maintain balance)	
Children	800 mg daily
Adolescents	1200 mg daily
Adults	800 mg daily
Pregnant or lactating women	1200–1500 mg daily
Elderly (age > 60)	1200–1500 mg daily
Calcium intake (avg in women age > 65)	550 mg daily
Calcium sources:	
Dairy product-free diet	400 mg
Cow's milk (8 oz)	300 mg
Calcium carbonate (500 mg)	200 mg

The PTH level increases with age. This may be an example of secondary hyperparathyroidism that results from the following sequence of events: The well known decrease in the mass of functioning renal tissue with age could lead to decreased renal synthesis of $1,25\text{-}(OH)_2D$, which would directly release PTH secretion from its normal inhibition by $1,25\text{-}(OH)_2D$. The reduced $1,25\text{-}(OH)_2D$ level would also decrease calcium absorption, exacerbating an intrinsic inability of the aging intestine to absorb calcium normally. Secondary hyperparathyroidism would then result from the dual effects of $1,25\text{-}(OH)_2D$ deficiency on the parathyroid gland and the intestine. In addition, the responsiveness of the parathyroid gland to inhibition by calcium is reduced with aging. The hyperparathyroidism of aging may thus result from the combined effects of age on the kidney, the intestine, and the parathyroid gland itself.

One thing clear is that provision of a dietary supplement with adequate vitamin D will reduce the rate of age-related bone loss by at least 50%. This suggests that reduced calcium absorption and secondary hyperparathyroidism play significant roles in the pathogenesis of osteoporosis in the elderly. However, the loss of bone continues after calcium supplementation, albeit at a lower rate, and it is thus likely that intrinsic changes in bone remodeling—perhaps having to do with a reduced osteoblastic response to ongoing osteoclastic bone resorption—also contribute to senile osteoporosis.

In secondary osteoporosis associated with glucocorticoid administration or alcoholism, there is a marked reduction in bone formation rates and serum osteocalcin levels. It is likely that glucocorticoids produce a devastating osteoporotic syndrome because of the rapid loss of bone that results from frankly depressed bone formation in the face of normal or even increased bone resorption.

The form of secondary osteoporosis associated with immobilization is another example of a resorptive state with marked uncoupling of bone resorption and bone formation and is characterized by hypercalciuria and suppression of PTH. When individuals with a high preexisting state of bone remodeling are immobilized (eg, adolescents and patients with hyperthyroidism or Paget's disease), bone resorption may be accelerated enough to produce hypercalcemia.

Clinical Manifestations

Osteoporosis is asymptomatic until it produces fractures and deformity. Typical osteoporotic fractures occur in the spine, the hip, and the wrist (Colles' fracture). The vertebral bodies of the spine are predominantly trabecular bone, with a thin rim of cortex, and are thus prone to fracture relatively early in postmenopausal osteoporosis (Figure 17–18). The vertebral bodies may be crushed, resulting in loss of height, or may be wedged anteriorly, resulting in height loss and kyphosis. The dorsal kyphosis of elderly women ("dowager's hump") results from anterior wedging of multiple thoracic vertebrae. Spinal fractures may be acute and painful or may occur gradually and be manifested only as kyphosis or loss of height.

The worst complication of osteoporosis is hip fracture. Hip fractures typically occur in the elderly, with a sharply rising incidence in both sexes after age 80, because bone loss in the hip, with its large mass of cortical bone, is slower than in the spine. The personal and social costs of hip fracture are enormous. One-third of American women who survive past age 80 will suffer a hip fracture. The 6-month mortality rate is approximately 20%, much of it resulting from the complications of immobilizing frail persons in a hospital bed. The complications include pulmonary embolus and pneumonia. About half of elderly people with a hip fracture will never walk freely again. The long-term costs of chronic care for these persons are a major social concern.

The diagnosis of osteoporosis is sometimes made radiologically, but in general x-rays are a poor diagnostic tool. A chest x-ray will miss 30–50% of cases of spinal osteoporosis, and if overpenetrated may lead to the diagnosis of osteoporosis in someone with a normal bone mass. The best way to diagnose osteoporosis is with a quantitative measurement of bone density. The preferred method at present is dual-energy x-ray absorptiometry (DXA), which uses a measurement of fractional absorption of photons from an x-ray source to quantitate bone mineral content. The technique is precise, rapid, and relatively inexpensive. It delivers a considerably lower radiation dose than a chest x-ray.

In an osteoporotic person, there are three risk factors for fracture: bone density, bone quality, and falls. The ability of bone density measurements to predict the likelihood of fractures has only recently been clarified. For every standard deviation (SD) below the mean bone density for age, there is a twofold to threefold increase in the risk of fracture. Thus, the risk of fracture is increased fourfold in someone at the lower limit of normal bone density for age (2 SD below the mean). Because bone loss is systemic, measurements at a single site (eg, the spine) are nearly as good a predictor of fracture at other sites (eg, the hip) as measurements at the site itself. Thus, measurements of bone density offer prognostic information in an asymptomatic individual with osteoporosis. Of course, they also provide a means of assessing the efficacy of interventions.

Only a portion of the risk for fracture is captured by measurements of bone density because the mechanical strength of bone is also a function of bone quality—depending on the microarchitecture of a bone, its mechanical strength and its ability to withstand stress may be substantially different in two individuals with the same bone density. The assessment of bone quality is an active area of investigation.

Elderly persons with osteoporosis are unlikely to sustain a hip fracture unless they fall. Risk factors for falling include muscle weakness, impaired vision, impaired balance, sedative use, and environmental factors such as the necessity to climb stairs, negotiate loose carpeting, etc. Because we presently have a limited ability to intervene in osteoporosis with therapies that increase bone mass, strategies to prevent falls are an important part of the approach to the osteoporotic patient.

Most individuals at risk for osteoporosis benefit from calcium supplementation to a total intake of about 1200–1500 mg/d. This can be accomplished

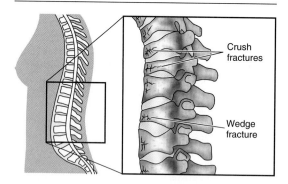

Figure 17–18. Types of vertebral osteoporotic fractures. (Reproduced, with permission, from Notelovitz M, Ware M: *Stand Tall: The Informed Women's Guide to Preventing Osteoporosis,* by Morris Notelovitz, MD, and Marsha Ware. Illustration © 1982 by Triad Publishing Company.)

with dairy products, the only rich dietary source of calcium, or with a calcium supplement such as calcium carbonate (Table 17–11). Vitamin D should be provided in approximately the multivitamin dose (400–800 IU). Calcium supplementation in younger individuals may increase peak bone mass and decrease premenopausal bone loss, but its optimal role in this age group has not been determined. Estrogen replacement is the recommended therapy for postmenopausal osteoporosis, though it requires concomitant use of progestins to prevent endometrial carcinoma and also increases the risk of breast cancer and venous thromboembolism. Other antiresorptive agents available for treatment of osteoporosis include alendronate, a bisphosphonate drug that directly inhibits osteoclastic bone resorption, and raloxifene, a selective estrogen response modifier that inhibits bone resorption as estrogen does, does not induce endometrial changes, and has estrogen antagonist actions in breast cells that may actually decrease the incidence of breast carcinoma.

Table 17–12. Causes of osteomalacia.

Vitamin D deficiency
  Nutritional (rare)
  Malabsorption
  Hereditary vitamin D-dependent rickets
    Type I (renal 1α-hydroxylase deficiency)
    Type II (absent or defective vitamin D receptor)
Phosphate deficiency
  Renal phosphate wasting
    X-linked hypophosphatemia
    Fanconi syndrome
    Renal tubular acidosis (type II)
    Oncogenic osteomalacia (acquired, associated with mesenchymal tumors)
  Phosphate-binding antacids
Deficient alkaline phosphatase: hereditary hypophosphatasia
Toxic
  Fluoride
  Aluminum (chronic renal failure)
  Etidronate disodium therapy
  Phosphate-binding antacids
Chronic renal failure

---

31. What is the relative importance of hereditary versus environmental or hormonal factors in contributing to osteoporosis?
32. What are the risk factors for osteoporosis?
33. What are the symptoms and signs of osteoporosis?
34. What are the risk factors for fracture in a patient with osteoporosis?
35. What treatments can prevent bone loss?

OSTEOMALACIA

Etiology

Osteomalacia is defined as a defect in the mineralization of bone. When it occurs in the young, it also affects the mineralization of cartilage in the growth plate, a disorder called **rickets**. Osteomalacia can result from a deficiency of vitamin D, a deficiency of phosphate, an inherited deficiency in alkaline phosphatase (hypophosphatasia), or from agents that have adverse effects on bone (Table 17–12). Surprisingly, dietary calcium deficiency rarely produces osteomalacia, though a few cases have been reported.

Dietary vitamin D deficiency is rare in the United States because of adequate sunlight exposure and dietary supplementation with vitamin D in milk and other products. When vitamin D deficiency is encountered, it is usually the result of malabsorption of this fat-soluble vitamin. Severe rickets also occurs as part of two heritable disorders of vitamin D action: renal 1α-hydroxylase deficiency, in which vitamin D is not converted to 1,25-(OH)$_2$D; and a vitamin D receptor defect.

Phosphate deficiency in osteomalacia is usually caused by heritable or acquired renal phosphate wasting. Osteomalacia has occasionally been seen in abusers of aluminum-containing antacids, which bind phosphate and prevent its absorption.

Pathogenesis

Vitamin D deficiency produces osteomalacia in stages. In the early stage, reduced calcium absorption produces secondary hyperparathyroidism, preventing hypocalcemia at the cost of increased renal phosphate excretion and hypophosphatemia. In later stages, hypocalcemia ensues and hypophosphatemia is progressive because of the combined effects of reduced absorption and the phosphaturic action of PTH. The poor delivery of minerals to bone (possibly coupled with the absence of direct effects of vitamin D on bone) impairs the mineralization of bone matrix, but osteoblasts actively form bone matrix. Thus, unmineralized matrix, or osteoid, accumulates at bone-forming surfaces.

Clinical Manifestations

Patients with vitamin D-deficient osteomalacia have bone pain, muscle weakness, and a waddling gait. Radiologically, they may have mild osteopenia, but the hallmark of the disorder is the pseudofracture—local bone resorption that has the appearance of a nondisplaced fracture, classically in the pubic rami, clavicles, or scapulas. In children with rickets, the leg bones are bowed (osteomalacia means "softening of bones"), the costochondral junctions are enlarged ("rachitic rosary"), and the growth plates are widened and irregular, reflecting the increase in unmineralized cartilage. Biochemically, the hallmarks of vitamin D-deficient osteomalacia are hypophosphatemia, hyperparathyroidism, variable hypocalcemia, and marked reductions in urinary calcium to less than 50 mg/d. The 25-(OH)D level is reduced, indicative of decreased body stores of vitamin D. In vitamin D deficiency and other forms of osteomalacia, the alkaline phosphatase level is increased.

Although the disorder can be suspected strongly on clinical grounds and the biochemical changes summarized above are confirmatory, a firm diagnosis of osteomalacia requires either the radiologic appearance of rickets or pseudofractures or else bone biopsy. If bone is biopsied for quantitative histomorphometry, thickened osteoid seams and a reduction in the mineralization rate are found. Treatment with vitamin D or aggressive phosphate replacement in patients with renal phosphate wasting will reverse osteomalacia or heal rickets.

36. What are the causes of osteomalacia?
37. What are the two stages in which vitamin D deficiency produces osteomalacia?
38. What are the symptoms and signs of osteomalacia?

REFERENCES

General Bone and Mineral Metabolism and Vitamin D

Bilezikian JP, Marcus R, Levine MA (editors): *The Parathyroids: Basic and Clinical Concepts.* Raven, 1994.

Bringhurst FR, Demay MB, Kronenberg HM: Hormones and disorders of mineral metabolism. In: *Williams Textbook of Endocrinology,* 9th ed. Wilson JD et al (editors). Saunders, 1998.

DeLuca HF, Zierold C: Mechanisms and functions of vitamin D. Nutr Rev 1998;56 (2 Part 2):S4.

Holick MF: Vitamin D and bone health. J Nutr 1996; 126:1159S.

Strewler GJ, Rosenblatt M: Mineral metabolism. In: *Endocrinology and Metabolism,* 3rd ed. Felig P, Baxter JD, Frohman L (editors). McGraw Hill, 1995.

Hyperparathyroidism

al Zahrani A, Levine MA: Primary hyperparathyroidism. Lancet 1997;349:1233.

Chanson P, Cadiot G, Murat A: Management of patients and subjects at risk for multiple endocrine neoplasia type 1: MEN 1. Horm Res 1997;47:211.

Hruska KA, Teitelbaum SL: Renal osteodystrophy. N Engl J Med 1995;333:166.

Marx S et al: Multiple endocrine neoplasia type 1: Clinical and genetic topics. Ann Intern Med 1998;129:484.

Potts JT Jr: Hyperparathyroidism and other hypercalcemic disorders. Adv Intern Med 1996;41:165.

Familial (Benign) Hypocalciuric Hypercalcemia & Neonatal Severe Primary Hyperparathyroidism

Brown EM: Mutations in the calcium-sensing receptor and their clinical implications. Horm Res 1997; 48:199.

Brown EM, Pollak M, Hebert SC: The extracellular calcium-sensing receptor: Its role in health and disease. Ann Rev Med 1998;49:15.

Pollak MR et al: Familial hypocalciuric hypercalcemia and neonatal severe hyperparathyroidism: Effects of mutant gene dosage on phenotype. J Clin Invest 1994;93:1108.

Hypercalcemia of Malignancy

Firkin F, Schneider H, Grill V: Parathyroid hormone-related protein in hypercalcemia associated with hematological malignancy. Leuk Lymph 1998;29:499.

Mundy GR, Guise TA: Hypercalcemia of malignancy. Am J Med 1997;103:134.

Philbrick WM et al: Defining the roles of parathyroid hormone-related protein in normal physiology. Physiol Rev 1996;76:127.

Rankin W, Grill V, Martin TJ: Parathyroid hormone-related protein and hypercalcemia. Cancer 1997;80(8 Suppl):1564.

Roodman GD: Mechanisms of bone lesions in multiple myeloma and lymphoma. Cancer 1997;80(8 Suppl): 1557.

Hypoparathyroidism and Hypocalcemia

Betterle C, Greggio NA, Volpato M: Autoimmune polyglandular syndrome type 1. J Clin Endocrinol Metabol 1998;83:1049.

Bjorses P et al: Gene defect behind APECED: A new clue to autoimmunity. Hum Molec Genet 1998;7:1547.

Li Y et al: Autoantibodies to the extracellular domain of the calcium sensing receptor in patients with acquired hypoparathyroidism. J Clin Invest 1996;97:899.

Mancilla EE, DeLuca F, Baron J: Activating mutations of the Ca^{2+}-sensing receptor. Molec Genet Metab 1998;64:198.

Mortensen L, Hyldstrup L, Charles P: Effect of vitamin D treatment in hypoparathyroid patients: A study on calcium, phosphate and magnesium homeostasis. Eur J Endocrinol 1997;136:52.

Reber PM, Heath H III: Hypocalcemic emergencies. Med Clin North Am 1995;79:93.

Rude RK: Hypocalcemia and hypoparathyroidism. Curr Ther Endocrinol Metab 1997;6:546.

Medullary Carcinoma of the Thyroid

Barbot N: Pentagastrin stimulation test and early diagnosis of medullary thyroid carcinoma using an immunoradiometric assay of calcitonin: Comparison with genetic screening in hereditary medullary thyroid carcinoma. J Clin Endocrinol Metab 1994; 78:114.

Berndt I et al: A new hot spot for mutations in the ret protooncogene causing familial medullary thyroid carcinoma and multiple endocrine neoplasia type 2A. J Clin Endocrinol Metab 1998;83:770.

Eng C: The RET proto-oncogene in multiple endocrine neoplasia type 2 and Hirschsprung's disease. N Engl J Med 1996;335:943.

Schuffenecker I et al: Risk and penetrance of primary hyperparathyroidism in multiple endocrine neoplasia type 2A families with mutations at codon 634 of the RET proto-oncogene. J Clin Endocrinol Metab 1998; 83:487.

Osteoporosis

Cummings SR et al: Risk factors for hip fracture in white women. Study of osteoporotic fractures research group. N Engl J Med 1995;332:767.

Dawson-Hughes B et al: Effect of calcium and vitamin D supplementation on bone density in men and women 65 years of age or older. N Engl J Med 1997; 337:670.

Eastell R: Treatment of postmenopausal osteoporosis. N Engl J Med 1998;338:736.

Meunier PJ (editor): *Osteoporosis: Diagnosis and Management.* Mosby, 1998.

Watts NB (editor): Osteoporosis. Endocrinol Metab Clin North Am 1998;27:255.

Osteomalacia

Bell NH, Key LL Jr: Acquired osteomalacia. Curr Ther Endocrinol Metab 1997;6:530.

Boutsen Y et al: Antacid-induced osteomalacia. Clin Rheumatol 1996;15:75.

Clark BL et al: Osteomalacia associated with adult Fanconi's syndrome: Clinical and diagnostic features. Clin Endocrinol 1995;43:479.

Nelson AE, Robinson BG, Mason RS: Oncogenic osteomalacia: Is there a new phosphate regulating hormone? Clin Endocrinol 1997;47:635.

Thomas MK et al: Hypovitaminosis D in medical inpatients. N Engl J Med 1998;338:777.

Schapira D et al: Tumor-induced osteomalacia. Semin Arthritis Rheum 1995;25:35.

18 Disorders of the Endocrine Pancreas

Kenneth R. Feingold, MD, & Janet L. Funk, MD

Insulin and **glucagon**, the two key hormones that orchestrate fuel storage and utilization, are produced by the islet cells in the pancreas. **Islet cells** are distributed in clusters throughout the exocrine pancreas. Taken all together, they comprise the endocrine pancreas. **Diabetes mellitus**, a heterogeneous disorder that affects 4% of the population and almost 20% of individuals between the ages of 65 and 74, is the most common disease associated with disordered secretion of hormones of the endocrine pancreas. Pancreatic tumors that secrete excessive amounts of specific islet cell hormones are far less common, but their clinical presentations underscore the important regulatory roles of each of the hormones secreted by the endocrine pancreas.

NORMAL STRUCTURE & FUNCTION OF THE PANCREATIC ISLETS

ANATOMY & HISTOLOGY

The endocrine pancreas is composed of nests of cells called the **islets of Langerhans** which are distributed throughout the exocrine pancreas. There are over 1 million islets in the human pancreas, many of which contain several hundred cells. The endocrine pancreas has great reserve capacity; over 70% of the B cells must be lost before dysfunction occurs. There are four cell types within the islets, each of which produces a different major secretory product (Table 18–1). The insulin-secreting **B cells** (β cells) are located in the central portion of the islets and are the predominant cell type (80% of cells) (Figure 18–1). The glucagon-secreting **A cells** (20% of the islet cells) are located mainly in the periphery. The **D cells**, which secrete somatostatin, are located between these two cell types and are few in number. The pancreatic polypeptide-secreting **F cells** are located mainly in the islets in the posterior lobe of the head of the pancreas, a region embryonically derived from the ventral rather than the dorsal bud and which therefore receives a different blood supply.

The islets are much more highly vascularized than the exocrine pancreatic tissues. Blood flow is thought to proceed from the center of the islet to the periphery, thereby allowing insulin produced by the central B cells to inhibit glucagon release by the peripheral A cells. Blood from the islets then drains into the hepatic portal vein. Thus, the islet cell secretory products pass directly into the liver, a major site of action of glucagon and insulin, before proceeding into the systemic circulation.

The islets are also abundantly innervated. Both parasympathetic and sympathetic axons enter the islets and either directly contact cells or terminate in the interstitial space between the cells. Neural regulation of islet cell hormone release, both directly through the sympathetic fibers and indirectly through stimulation of catecholamine release by the adrenal medulla, plays a key role in glucose homeostasis during stress.

Table 18–1. Cell types in pancreatic islets of Langerhans.[1]

Cell types	Secretory Products
A cell (α)	Glucagon
B cell (β)	Insulin, C peptide, proinsulin, amylin, γ-aminobutyric acid (GABA)
D cell (δ)	Somatostatin
F cell (PP cell)	Pancreatic polypeptide

[1]Modified and reproduced, with permission, from Greenspan FS, Baxter JD: *Basic & Clinical Endocrinology,* 4th ed. Appleton & Lange, 1994.

---

1. What percentage of islets must be lost before endocrine pancreatic dysfunction becomes manifest?
2. Describe the histologic and vascular organization of an islet of Langerhans.

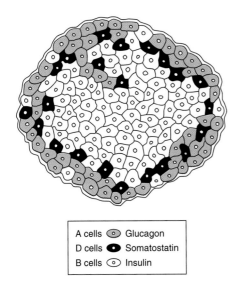

Figure 18–1. Schematic representation of a normal rat islet showing the topographical relationships of the major cell types. (Reproduced, with permission, from Orci L, Unger RH: Functional subdivision of islets of Langerhans and possible role of D cells. Lancet 1975;2:1243.)

PHYSIOLOGY

1. INSULIN

Synthesis & Metabolism

Insulin is a protein composed of two peptide chains (A and B chains) that are connected by two disulfide bonds (Figure 18–2). The precursor of insulin, **preproinsulin** (MW 11,500), is synthesized in the ribosomes and enters the endoplasmic reticulum of B cells, where it is promptly cleaved by microsomal enzymes to form proinsulin (MW 9000). **Proinsulin,** which consists of the A and B chains joined by a 31-amino-acid **C peptide,** is transported to the Golgi apparatus, where it is packaged into secretory vesicles. While in the secretory vesicle, proinsulin is cleaved at two sites to form insulin (51 amino acids; MW 5808) and the biologically inactive C peptide fragment (Figure 18–2). Secretion of insulin is therefore accompanied by an equimolar secretion of C peptide and also by small amounts of proinsulin that escape cleavage.

Human insulin differs by only one or three amino acids from pork and beef insulin, respectively. These preparations of the hormone were used to treat diabetes prior to the availability of recombinant human insulin. Insulin has a circulatory half-life of 3–5 minutes and is catabolized in both the liver and the kidney. The liver catabolizes approximately 50% of insulin on its first pass through the liver after it is secreted from the pancreas into the portal vein. In contrast, both C peptide and proinsulin are catabolized only by the kidney and therefore have half-lives three to four times longer than that of insulin itself.

Regulation of Secretion

Glucose is the primary physiologic stimulant of insulin release (Figure 18–3). Glucose enters B cells via a **glucose transporter (GLUT 2)** that has a low affinity for glucose, thereby allowing a graded response to glucose uptake. Once in the cell, it is thought that the metabolism of glucose—rather than glucose itself—stimulates insulin secretion. **Glucokinase,** an enzyme with low affinity for glucose whose activity is regulated by glucose, controls the first step in glucose metabolism—phosphorylation of glucose to form glucose 6-phosphate. It is thought that this enzyme may function as the **"glucose sensor"** in B cells. Metabolic coupling factors produced via glucose metabolism, such as ATP, then inhibit K^+ efflux from the B cell. This depolarizes the cell and allows Ca^{2+} to enter, which triggers exocytosis of insulin-containing granules.

Although glucose is the most potent stimulator of insulin release, other factors such as amino acids ingested with a meal or vagal stimulation can cause insulin release (Table 18–2). Glucose-induced insulin secretion can also be enhanced by several enteric hormones, such as glucagon-like peptide-1 (GLP-1[7–36]). Insulin secretion is inhibited by catecholamines and by somatostatin.

Mechanism of Action

Insulin exerts its effects by binding to **insulin receptors** present on the surfaces of target cells (Figure

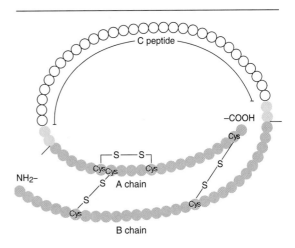

Figure 18–2. Amino acid sequence and covalent structure of human proinsulin. This structure is hydrolyted at the light-colored residues to form C peptide and insulin (dark-colored residues). (Modified from Kohler PO, Jordan RM [editors]: Clinical Endocrinology. Wiley, 1986.)

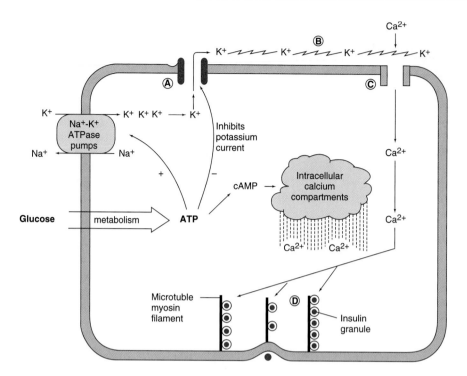

Figure 18–3. Schematic diagram of glucose-stimulated insulin release from B cell. Potassium (K+) efflux **(A)** polarizes the B cell membrane and prevents Ca^{2+} entry by closing a voltage-dependent Ca^{2+} channel **(B)**. When glucose is taken up by B cells, the metabolism of glucose is thought to inhibit K+ efflux, thus depolarizing the cell and allowing Ca^{2+} entry **(C)**. Ca^{2+} stimulates the secretion of insulin-containing vesicles **(D)**. (Reproduced, with permission, from Greenspan FS, Strewler GJ: *Basic and Clinical Endocrinology*, 5th ed. Appleton & Lange, 1997.)

Table 18–2. Regulation of islet cell hormone release.

	B Cell Insulin Release	D Cell Somatostatin Release	A Cell Glucagon Release
Nutrients			
Glucose	↑	↑	↓
Amino acids	↑	↑	↑
Fatty acids	—	—	↓
Ketones	—	—	↓
Hormones			
Enteric hormones	↑	↑	↑
Insulin	↓	↓?	↓
GABA	—	—	↓
Somatostatin	↓	—	↓
Glucagon	↑	↑	—
Cortisol	—	—	↑
Catecholamines	↓ (α-adrenergic)	—	↑ (β-adrenergic)
Neural			
Vagal	↑	—	↑
Beta-adrenergic	↑	—	↑
Alpha-adrenergic	↓	—	↓

Key: ↑ = increased; ↓ = decreased; — = no effect or no known effect.

18–4). Insulin receptors are present in liver, muscle, and fat—the classic insulin-sensitive tissues responsible for fuel homeostasis. In addition, insulin can mediate other effects in nonclassic target tissues, such as the ovary, via interaction with insulin receptors or by cross-reactivity with insulin-like growth factor-1 (IGF-1) receptors. Binding of insulin to its receptor causes activation of a tyrosine kinase region of the receptor and autophosphorylation of the receptor. The exact sequence of events following phosphorylation of the receptor is still being elucidated. However, binding of insulin to its receptor initiates a phosphorylation cascade within the cell—including phosphorylation of key cytosolic protein substrates (eg, insulin receptor substrate-1)—that ultimately mediate changes in the proteins responsible for the biologic effects of insulin (eg, translocation of GLUT 4 glucose transporter to the plasma membrane of muscle and fat).

Effects

Insulin plays a major role in fuel homeostasis (Table 18–3). Insulin mediates changes in fuel metabolism through its effects on three main tissues:

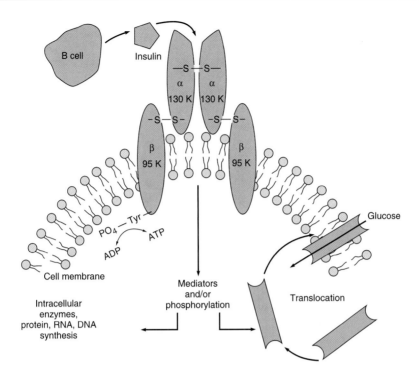

Figure 18–4. Model of insulin receptor. The insulin receptor is composed of two α and two β subunits linked by disulfide bonds. Binding of insulin to the extracellular α subunits activates a tyrosine kinase present in the cytoplasmic domain of the β subunit. The activated kinase autophosphorylates specific tyrosine residues in the β subunit. Kinase activation is a critical initial step in the poorly defined cascade of events that leads to the biologic effects of insulin, such as the translocation of glucose transporters to the cell surface. (Reproduced, with permission, from Rifkin H, Porte D Jr: In: *Ellenberg and Rifkin's Diabetes Mellitus: Theory and Practice,* 4th ed. Elsevier, 1990.)

liver, muscle, and fat. In these tissues, insulin promotes fuel storage (anabolism) and prevents the breakdown and release of fuel that has already been stored (catabolism). The total lack of insulin is incompatible with life, and the same is true of excess insulin.

In the liver, insulin promotes fuel storage by stimulation of glycogen synthesis and storage. Insulin inhibits hepatic glucose output by inhibiting gluconeogenesis (glucose synthesis) and glycogenolysis (glycogen breakdown). By also stimulating glycolysis (metabolism of glucose to pyruvate), insulin promotes the formation of precursors for fatty acid synthesis. Moreover, insulin stimulates lipogenesis, leading to the increased synthesis of very low density lipoproteins (VLDL), particles that deliver triglycerides to fat tissue for storage. Insulin also inhibits fatty acid oxidation and the production of ketone bodies (ketogenesis), an alternative fuel produced only in the liver that can be used by the brain when glucose is not available.

While hepatic uptake of glucose is not regulated by insulin, insulin does stimulate glucose uptake both in muscle and in fat by causing the rapid translocation of an insulin-sensitive glucose transporter (GLUT 4) to the surface of these cells. Uptake of glucose by muscle accounts for the vast majority (85%) of insulin-stimulated glucose disposal. In muscle, insulin promotes the storage of glucose by stimulating glycogen synthesis and inhibiting glycogen catabolism. Insulin also stimulates protein synthesis in muscle.

Insulin stimulates fat storage by stimulating lipoprotein lipase, the enzyme that hydrolyses the triglycerides carried in VLDL and other triglyceride-rich lipoproteins to fatty acids, which can then be taken up by fat cells. Increased glucose uptake caused by up-regulation of the GLUT 4 transporter also aids in fat storage since this increases the levels of α-glycerol phosphate, a substrate in the esterification of free fatty acids, which are then stored as triglycerides. In fat cells, insulin also inhibits lipolysis, preventing the release of fatty acids, a potential substrate for hepatic ketone body synthesis. Insulin exerts this effect by decreasing the activity of hormone-sensitive lipase, the enzyme that hydrolyzes stored triglycerides to releasable fatty acids. Together, these changes result in increased fat storage.

Table 18–3. Hormonal regulation of fuel homeostasis.

	Insulin	Somatostatin	Glucagon	Catecholamines	Cortisol	Growth Hormone
LIVER						
Fuel storage						
Glycogenesis	↑		↓			
Lipid synthesis	↑		↓			
Fuel breakdown						
Glycogenolysis	↓		↑	↑		↑
Gluconeogenesis	↓		↑	↑	↑	↑
Fatty acid oxidation or ketogenesis	↓		↑			
MUSCLE						
Fuel storage						
Glucose uptake or glycogenesis	↑			↓	↓	↓
Fuel breakdown						
Protein catabolism	↓				↑	
ADIPOSE TISSUE						
Fuel storage						
Lipoprotein lipolysis	↑					
Fatty acid esterification	↑					
Fuel breakdown						
Lipolysis of stored fat	↓			↑	↑	↑
PANCREAS						
Secretion of—						
Insulin (B cell)	↓	↓	↑	↓		
Glucagon (A cell)	↓	↓		↑	↑	↑
Somatostatin (D cell)	(↓ ?)	↓	↑			

Key: ↑ = increased, ↓ = decreased.

3. How does human insulin differ from pork and beef insulin?
4. What is the half-life of insulin? How is it catabolized? What percentage is extracted on first pass through the liver?
5. How do the half-lives of C peptide and proinsulin compare with that of insulin?
6. List the main substances that stimulate insulin secretion.
7. What characteristic of the B cell glucose transporter (GLUT 2) allows a graded response to glucose?
8. What is the probable "glucose sensor" in the B cell?
9. What are the major inhibitors of insulin secretion?
10. What are the current thoughts on the mechanisms of insulin action?
11. Which tissues are insulin-dependent for glucose uptake?
12. What are three ways in which insulin stimulates fat storage?

2. GLUCAGON

Synthesis & Metabolism

Glucagon, a 29-amino-acid peptide, is produced in the A cells of the pancreas by the proteolytic processing of preproglucagon, a larger precursor protein. In addition to the pancreas, preproglucagon, is also expressed in the intestine and brain. However, while glucagon is the major bioactive metabolite produced in the pancreatic A cell, the protein is differentially processed in the intestine such that glucagon-like peptide-1(7–36) (GLP-1[7–36]) and other peptides are produced in response to a meal (Figure 18–5). This tissue-specific processing results in two peptides that have opposing effects on carbohydrate metabolism; glucagon opposes the effects of insulin, while GLP-1(7–36) is a powerful stimulator of insulin synthesis and secretion. The physiologic roles of the other preproglucagon-derived peptides are not well understood.

The circulatory half-life of glucagon is 3–6 minutes. Like insulin, glucagon is metabolized in the liver and kidneys. However, the liver accounts for only 25% of glucagon clearance.

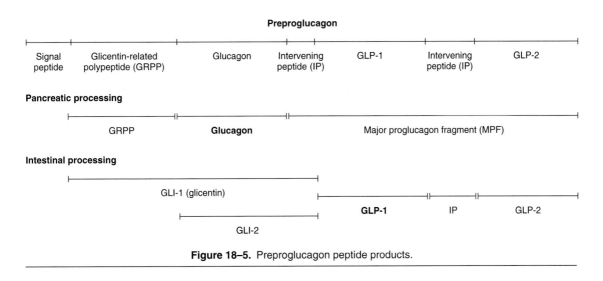

Figure 18–5. Preproglucagon peptide products.

Regulation of Secretion

In contrast to the stimulation of insulin secretion by glucose, glucagon secretion is inhibited by glucose (Table 18–2). It is not known whether glucose has a direct inhibitory effect on the A cell or whether its effect is mediated by the stimulation of insulin and somatostatin by B and D cells. Another B cell secretory product, **γ-aminobutyric acid (GABA)** is also thought to inhibit glucagon release. Like insulin, glucagon secretion is stimulated by amino acids, an important regulatory feature in the metabolism of protein meals. In contrast, fatty acids and ketones inhibit glucagon secretion. Counterregulatory hormones such as catecholamines (via a predominating beta-adrenergic effect) and cortisol stimulate glucagon release.

Mechanism of Action

The liver is the major target organ for glucagon action. Glucagon binds to a glucagon receptor present on the cell surface of hepatocytes. Binding of glucagon promotes interaction of the receptor with a stimulatory G protein, which in turn activates adenylyl cyclase. cAMP, generated by adenylyl cyclase, activates protein kinase A, which then phosphorylates enzymes responsible for the biologic activity of glucagon in the liver. There is also some evidence that the glucagon receptor may act via an adenylyl cyclase-independent mechanism by stimulation of phospholipase C.

Effects

Glucagon affects metabolism by its actions in the liver and elsewhere (Table 18–3). Glucagon is known as a **counterregulatory hormone**—one that counters the effects of insulin by acting in a catabolic fashion to maintain serum glucose levels. Glucagon maintains serum glucose levels by stimulating hepatic glucose output. This occurs by stimulating both the breakdown of hepatic glycogen stores (glycogenolysis) and hepatic glucose synthesis (gluconeogenesis). Glucagon also stimulates fatty acid oxidation and ketogenesis, thus providing an alternative fuel (ketone bodies) that can be used by the brain when glucose is not available. Lastly, glucagon stimulates hepatic uptake of amino acids which are then used to fuel gluconeogenesis.

3. SOMATOSTATIN

Synthesis, Metabolism, & Regulation of Secretion

Like preproglucagon, preprosomatostatin is synthesized in the pancreas, gastrointestinal tract, and brain, where it is differentially processed in a tissue-specific fashion to produce several biologically active peptides. Somatostatin-14 (SS-14), the first somatostatin to be isolated, is a 14-amino-acid peptide that was initially discovered in the hypothalamus as the factor responsible for the inhibition of growth hormone release. Only later was it appreciated that D cells of the pancreas also secrete SS-14. Somatostatin-28 (SS-28), an amino-terminally extended peptide that includes the 14-amino-acid sequence of SS-14, is also produced from preprosomatostatin and has a range of action comparable to that of SS-14 but a potency that is somewhat greater. The half-life of somatostatin (< 3 minutes) is shorter than that of insulin or glucagon. Octreotide, a synthetic eight-amino-acid analogue of somatostatin that is used clinically, is more potent than somatostatin and has a much longer half-life (hours).

The same secretagogues that stimulate insulin secretion also stimulate somatostatin (Table 18–2). These include glucose, amino acids, enteric hormones, and glucagon.

Mechanism of Action & Effects

Somatostatin exerts its effects via binding to a family of somatostatin receptors which are distributed in a tissue-specific fashion. Five members of this inhibitory G (G_i) protein-coupled receptor family have recently been cloned. In all of the tissues where somatostatin is produced, it acts primarily in an inhibitory fashion. In the endocrine pancreas, somatostatin is thought to act via paracrine effects on the other islet cells, inhibiting the release of insulin from B cells and glucagon from A cells (Table 18–3). In addition, somatostatin acts in an autocrine fashion to inhibit its own release from D cells. In the gastrointestinal tract, somatostatin retards the absorption of nutrients through multiple mechanisms, including the inhibition of gut motility, the inhibition of several enteric peptides, and the inhibition of pancreatic exocrine function. Consistent with the multiple inhibitory effects of this peptide, the synthetic somatostatin analog octreotide has multiple clinical uses, including inhibition of hormone production by pituitary adenomas, inhibition of certain types of chronic diarrhea, inhibition of tumor growth, and inhibition of bleeding from esophageal varices.

4. PANCREATIC POLYPEPTIDE

Little is known about the biosynthesis and physiologic function of **pancreatic peptide (PP).** This 36-amino-acid peptide is produced by the F cells in the islets of the posterior lobe of the head of the pancreas. PP is released in response to a mixed meal, an effect that appears to be mediated by protein and vagal stimulation. PP is a member of the polypeptide family that includes neuropeptide Y (NPY), a peptide produced in sympathetic neurons and in the brain, where it stimulates appetite.

---

13. What are some important stimulators and inhibitors of glucagon secretion?
14. What is the major target organ for glucagon? What are the mechanisms of glucagon action?
15. What metabolic pathways are sensitive to glucagon, and how are they affected?
16. What hormone antagonizes glucagon's effect on metabolic pathways?
17. Where else in the body besides the islets of Langerhans is glucagon made?
18. What is the role of somatostatin in the islets of Langerhans?

---

5. HORMONAL CONTROL OF CARBOHYDRATE METABOLISM

Carbohydrate metabolism is controlled by the relative amounts of insulin and glucagon that are produced by the endocrine pancreas (Table 18–3; Figure 18–6). When plasma glucose levels are high, plasma glucagon levels are suppressed and the actions of insulin predominate. Fuel storage is promoted by insulin stimulation of glycogen storage in the liver; glucose uptake, glycogen synthesis, and protein synthesis by muscle; and fat storage by adipose tissue. Insulin inhibits the mobilization of substrates from peripheral tissues and opposes any effects of glucagon on the stimulation of hepatic glucose output.

In contrast, when glucose levels are low, plasma insulin levels are suppressed and the effects of glucagon predominate in the liver (ie, increased hepatic glucose output and ketone body formation). In the absence of insulin, muscle glucose uptake is markedly decreased; muscle protein is catabolized; and fat is mobilized from adipose tissue. Therefore, with insulinopenia, glucose loads cannot be cleared, and substrates for hepatic gluconeogenesis (amino acids, glycerol) and ketogenesis (fatty acids)—processes that are stimulated by glucagon—are increased.

Fasting State

After an overnight fast, blood glucose is maintained by the liver, which produces glucose at the same rate at which it is utilized by resting tissues

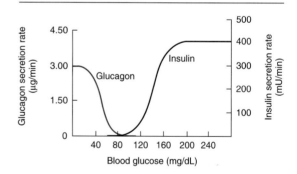

Figure 18–6. Mean rates of insulin and glucagon delivery from an artificial pancreas at various blood glucose levels. The device was programmed to establish and maintain normal blood glucose in insulin-requiring diabetic humans, and the values for hormone output approximate the output of the normal human pancreas. The shape of the insulin curve also resembles the insulin response of incubated B cells to graded concentrations of glucose. (Reproduced, with permission, from Mariles EB et al: Normalization of glycemia in diabetics during meals with insulin and glucagon delivery by the artificial pancreas. Diabetes 1977;26:663.)

Table 18–4. Insulin: glucagon (I:G) molar ratios in blood in various conditions.[1]

Condition	Hepatic Glucose Storage (S) or Production (P)[2]	I:G
Glucose availability		
Large carbohydrate meal	++++ (S)	70
IV glucose	++ (S)	25
Small meal	+ (S)	7
Glucose need		
Overnight fast	+ (P)	2.3
Low-carbohydrate diet	++ (P)	1.8
Starvation	++++ (P)	0.4

[1]Courtesy of RH Unger. Reproduced, with permission, from Ganong WF: *Review of Medical Physiology,* 19th ed. Appleton & Lange, 1999.
[2]+ to ++++ indicate relative magnitude.

(Table 18–4). Glucose uptake and utilization occur predominantly in tissues that do not require insulin for glucose uptake, such as the brain. Hepatic glucose output is stimulated by glucagon and is primarily due to glycogenolysis. The low levels of insulin that are present (basal secretion of 0.25–1.0 unit/h) allow the release of fatty acids from fat to provide fuel for muscles (fatty acid oxidation) and substrate for hepatic ketogenesis. However, these levels of insulin are sufficient to prevent excessive lipolysis, ketogenesis, and gluconeogenesis, thus preventing hyperglycemia and ketoacidosis.

With prolonged fasting (> 24–60 hours), liver glycogen stores are depleted. Glucagon levels rise slightly, and insulin levels decline further. Gluconeogenesis becomes the predominant source of hepatic glucose production, utilizing substrates such as amino acids that are mobilized from the periphery at a greater rate. With starvation, a switch occurs from gluconeogenesis to the production of ketones, an alternative fuel source for the brain. In this manner, survival is prolonged as muscle protein is conserved in favor of increased mobilization of fatty acids from adipose tissue, a process made possible by increased insulinopenia. The liver then converts fatty acids to ketone bodies, a process that is stimulated by glucagon.

Fed State

With ingestion of a carbohydrate load, insulin secretion is stimulated and glucagon is suppressed (Table 18–4). Hepatic glucose production and ketogenesis are suppressed by the high ratio of insulin to glucagon. Insulin stimulates hepatic glycogen storage. Insulin-mediated glucose uptake, which occurs primarily in muscle, is also stimulated, as is muscle glycogen synthesis. Fat storage occurs in adipose tissue.

With ingestion of a protein meal, both insulin and glucagon are stimulated. In this way, insulin stimulates amino acid uptake and protein formation by muscle. However, stimulation of hepatic glucose output by glucagon counterbalances the tendency of insulin to cause hypoglycemia.

Conditions of Stress

During severe stress, when fuel delivery to the brain is in jeopardy, **counterregulatory hormones**—in addition to glucagon—act synergistically. They maintain blood glucose levels by maximizing hepatic output of glucose and peripheral mobilization of substrates and by minimizing fuel storage (Table 18–3). **Glucagon** and **epinephrine** act within minutes to elevate blood glucose, while the counterregulatory effects of **cortisol** and **growth hormone** are not seen for several hours. Epinephrine, cortisol, and growth hormone all stimulate glucagon release while epinephrine inhibits insulin, thus maximally increasing the glucagon:insulin ratio. In addition, these three hormones act directly on the liver to increase hepatic glucose production and peripherally to stimulate lipolysis and inhibit insulin-sensitive glucose uptake. During severe stress, hyperglycemia may actually result from the combined effects of counterregulatory hormones.

Similar but less marked effects occur in response to exercise when glucagon, catecholamines, and to a lesser extent cortisol help supply exercising muscle with glucose and fatty acids by increasing hepatic glucose output and lipolysis of fat stores, effects that are made possible by a lowering of insulin levels. Low insulin levels also allow muscles to utilize glycogen stores for energy.

---

19. In insulinopenic states, why are substrates for hepatic gluconeogenesis and ketogenesis increased?
20. What is the effect of a protein meal on insulin versus glucagon secretion?
21. What is the difference in time course of action of the various counterregulatory hormones?

PATHOPHYSIOLOGY OF SELECTED ENDOCRINE PANCREATIC DISORDERS

DIABETES MELLITUS

Clinical Presentation

Diabetes mellitus is a heterogeneous disorder defined by the presence of **hyperglycemia.** Diagnostic criteria for diabetes include (1) a fasting plasma glucose ≥ 126 mg/dL; (2) symptoms of diabetes plus a random plasma glucose ≥ 200 mg/dL; or (3) a plasma glucose level ≥ 200 mg/dL after an oral dose of 75 g of glucose (oral glucose tolerance test).

Hyperglycemia in all cases is due to a functional deficiency of insulin action. Deficient insulin action can be due to a decrease in insulin secretion by the B cells of the pancreas, a decreased response to insulin by target tissues **(insulin resistance),** or an increase in the counterregulatory hormones that oppose the effects of insulin. The relative contributions of each of these three factors not only form the basis of classification of this disorder into subtypes but also help to explain the characteristic clinical presentations of each subtype (Table 18–5).

Over 90% of cases of diabetes are regarded as primary processes for which individuals have a genetic predisposition and are classified as either **type 1 or type 2** (Tables 18–5 and 18–6). Type 1 diabetes mellitus is less common than type 2, accounting for fewer than 10% of cases of primary diabetes. Type 1 diabetes, which is characterized by B cell destruction with severe insulin deficiency, is caused by autoimmune destruction of pancreatic B cells. In a minority of patients, the cause of type 1 diabetes is unknown. The disease commonly affects individuals under age 30 (juvenile-onset diabetes), with peak incidence occurring at puberty. Although autoimmune destruction of the B cells does not occur acutely, clinical symptoms do. Patients present after only days or weeks of polyuria, polydipsia, and weight loss with markedly elevated serum glucose concentrations. **Ketone bodies** are also increased because of the marked lack of insulin, resulting in severe, life-threatening acidosis **(diabetic ketoacidosis).** Patients with type 1 diabetes require treatment with insulin.

Type 2 diabetes differs from type 1 in several distinct ways (Table 18–6): It is ten times more common, has a stronger genetic component (Table 18–7), occurs most commonly in adults, increases in prevalence with age (eg, 20% prevalence over the age of 65), occurs more commonly in Native Americans,

Table 18–5. Etiologic classification of diabetes mellitus.[1]

I. Type 1 diabetes[2] (B cell destruction, usually leading to absolute insulin deficiency)
   A. Immune-mediated
   B. Idiopathic
II. Type 2 diabetes[2] (may range from predominantly insulin resistance with relative insulin deficiency to a predominantly secretory defect with insulin resistance)
III. Other specific types
   A. Genetic defects of B cell function
      1. Chromosome 12, HNF-1α (MODY 3)
      2. Chromosome 7, glucokinase (MODY 2)
      3. Chromosome 20, HNF-4α (MODY 1)
      4. Mitochondrial DNA
      5. Others
   B. Genetic defects in insulin action
      1. Type A insulin resistance
      2. Leprechaunism
      3. Rabson-Mendenhall syndrome
      4. Lipoatrophic diabetes
      5. Others
   C. Diseases of the exocrine pancreas
      1. Pancreatitis
      2. Trauma, pancreatectomy
      3. Neoplasia
      4. Cystic fibrosis
      5. Hemochromatosis
      6. Fibrocalculous pancreatopathy
      7. Others
   D. Endocrinopathies
      1. Acromegaly
      2. Cushing's syndrome
      3. Glucagonoma
      4. Pheochromocytoma
      5. Hyperthyroidism
      6. Somatostatinoma
      7. Aldosteronoma
      8. Others
	E. Drug- or chemical-induced
	      1. Vacor
	      2. Pentamidine
	      3. Nicotinic acid
	      4. Glucocorticoids
	      5. Thyroid hormone
	      6. Diazoxide
	      7. β-Adrenergic agonists
	      8. Thiazides
	      9. Phenytoin
	     10. α-Interferon
	     11. Others
	F. Infections
	      1. Congenital rubella
	      2. Cytomegalovirus
	      3. Others
	G. Uncommon forms of immune-mediated diabetes
	      1. "Stiff-man" syndrome
	      2. Anti-insulin receptor antibodies
	      3. Others
	H. Other genetic syndromes sometimes associated with diabetes
	      1. Down's syndrome
	      2. Klinefelter's syndrome
	      3. Turner's syndrome
	      4. Wolfram's syndrome
	      5. Friedreich's ataxia
	      6. Huntington's chorea
	      7. Laurence-Moon-Biedl syndrome
	      8. Myotonic dystrophy
	      9. Porphyria
	     10. Prader-Willi syndrome
	     11. Others
	IV. Gestational diabetes mellitus (GDM)

[1]Modified and reproduced, with permission, from Expert Committee on the Diagnosis and Classification of Diabetes Mellitus: Report of the Expert Committee on the Diagnosis and Classification of Diabetes Mellitus. Diabetes Care 1998;21(1 Suppl):7.
[2]Patients with any form of diabetes may require insulin treatment at some stage of the disease. Such use of insulin does not, of itself, classify the patient.

Table 18-6. Some features distinguishing type 1 from type 2 diabetes mellitus.[1]

	Type 1	Type 2
Synonym	IDDM	NIDDM
Age at onset	Usually < 30	Usually > 40
Ketosis	Common	Rare
Body weight	Nonobese	Obese (80%)
Prevalence	0.2–0.3%	5%

Genetics
  HLA association
  Monozygotic twin studies
	
	Yes
	30–50% concordance rate
		
		No
		35–80% concordance rate

Circulating islet cell antibodies	Yes	No
Associated with other autoimmune phenomena	Occasionally	No
Treatment with insulin	Always necessary	Usually not necessary
Complications	Frequent	Frequent
Insulin secretion	Severe deficiency	Variable: moderate deficiency to hyperinsulinemia
Insulin resistance	Occasional—with poor control or excessive insulin antibodies	Usual—due to receptor and postreceptor defects

[1]Modified, with permission, from Wyngaarden JB, Smith LH Jr, Bennett JC (editors): *Cecil Textbook of Medicine*, 19th ed. Saunders, 1992.

Mexican-Americans, and African-Americans (particularly in women), and is associated with increased resistance to the effects of insulin at its sites of action as well as a decrease in insulin secretion by the pancreas. It is often (80% of cases) associated with obesity, an additional factor that increases insulin resistance. **Insulin resistance** is the hallmark of this disorder. Because these patients often have varying amounts of residual insulin secretion that prevent severe hyperglycemia or ketosis, they often are asymptomatic and are diagnosed long after the actual onset of disease by the discovery of an elevated fasting glucose on routine screening tests. Population screening surveys show that a remarkable 50% of cases of type 2 diabetes in the United States are undiagnosed. Once they are identified, these individuals can usually be managed with diet alone or with diet and medications that enhance endogenous insulin secretion (eg, sulfonylureas or benzoic acid derivatives), decrease insulin resistance in hepatic (eg, biguanides) or peripheral (eg, thiazolidinediones) tissues, or interfere with intestinal absorption of carbohydrates (eg, intestinal α-glycosidase inhibitors). These patients therefore do not require insulin treatment for survival. However, some patients with type 2 diabetes are treated with insulin to achieve optimal glucose control.

Other causes of diabetes, accounting for less than 5% of cases, include processes that inhibit insulin secretion by destroying the pancreas (eg, pancreatitis), specific inhibition of insulin secretion (eg, drug-induced diabetes), or increases in counterregulatory hormones (eg, Cushing's syndrome) (Table 18–5: III). Clinical presentations in these cases depend on the exact nature of the process and are not discussed here.

Gestational diabetes mellitus occurs in 4% of pregnant women (Table 18–5: IV); may recur with subsequent pregnancies; and tends to resolve at parturition. It is associated with a markedly increased risk—up to 50% in obese women—for the subsequent development of diabetes (predominantly type 2 diabetes). Because of its adverse effects on fetal outcome, gestational diabetes should be diagnosed or ruled out by routine screening with an oral glucose load at 24 weeks of gestation, particularly in high-risk populations (obese, over 25 years of age, family history of diabetes, or member of an ethnic group with a high prevalence of diabetes). Gestational diabetes usually occurs in the second half of gestation, precipitated by the increasing levels of hormones such as chorionic somatomammotropin, progesterone, cortisol, and prolactin that have counterregulatory anti-insulin effects.

Etiology

A. Type 1 Diabetes: Type 1 diabetes is caused by selective T lymphocyte-mediated autoimmune destruction of the B cells of the pancreatic islets. Macrophages are thought to be among the first inflammatory cells present in the islets. Later, the islets are infiltrated with activated, cytokine-secreting mononuclear cells. CD8 suppressor T lymphocytes comprise the majority of these cells and are thought to be the primary cell responsible for B cell destruc-

Table 18-7. Incidence of diabetes mellitus in the United States.

	Type 1	Type 2
In population	0.2–0.3%	5%
If proband with the disease is:		
Sibling	6%	38%[1]
Monozygotic twin	23–53%	34–72%
Parent	2–6%	33%[1]
Mother	2–3%	. . .
Father	5–6%	. . .

[1]Incidence of diabetes mellitus *or* abnormal glucose tolerance test.

tion. CD4 helper T lymphocytes and B lymphocytes are also present in the islets. Autoimmune destruction of the B cell, a process that is thought to be mediated by cytokines, occurs gradually over several years until sufficient B cell mass is lost to cause symptoms of insulin deficiency. At the time of diagnosis, ongoing inflammation is present in some islets, while other islets are atrophic and consist only of glucagon-secreting A cells and somatostatin-secreting D cells.

Genetic susceptibility appears to play a somewhat more important role in the development of type 2 than type 1 diabetes, as evidenced by a comparison of the concordance rates in monozygotic twins. The risk for development of type 1 diabetes is also clearly increased in first-degree relatives of individuals with type 1 diabetes (Table 18–7). Genetic susceptibility has been linked to the genes of the major histocompatibility complex (MHC) that encode class II human leukocyte antigens (HLA), molecules that are expressed on the surface of specific antigen-presenting cells such as macrophages. Class II molecules form a complex with processed foreign antigens or autoantigens which then activates CD4 T lymphocytes via interaction with the T cell receptor (Figure 18–7). Alleles at the class II HLA gene locus (known as the D locus) conferring risk for the development of diabetes vary with racial group and can be associated with amino acid substitutions in the antigen-binding domain of the encoded class II molecules. Identification of HLA haplotypes remains a research tool at this time.

Although B cell destruction is thought to be a cell-mediated and not a humoral process, **autoantibodies** are associated with the development of type 1 diabetes and have been used in research studies to predict disease onset. It is hypothesized that these antibodies serve as markers of immune destruction of the islets and may be directed against the B cell antigen that initiates the immune response. **Islet cell antibodies (ICA)** are measured by exposing serum to sections of pancreas, an assay that is commercially available but difficult to standardize. They are present in more than 50% of individuals at the time of diagnosis and are predictive of disease onset in both first-degree relatives and in the general population. Antibodies against insulin **(insulin autoantibody [IAA])** are also present in 50% of newly diagnosed individuals. The combination of islet cell antibodies and insulin autoantibody is highly predictive for the development of type 1 diabetes (70% of first-degree relatives positive for both antibodies develop disease within 5 years). In addition to insulin, a number of other islet cell antigens have been identified. In particular, **glutamic acid decarboxylase (GAD),** an enzyme that converts glutamate to GABA, has attracted attention because GAD antibodies are present early and are more highly predictive of disease than are islet cell antibodies or insulin autoantibodies.

The low concordance rate for type 1 diabetes in twin studies suggests that environmental factors may also play a role in the development of type 1 diabetes. Evidence suggests that viral infections may precipitate disease, particularly in genetically susceptible individuals. It is hypothesized that an immune response to foreign antigens may incite B cell destruction if these foreign antigens have some homology with islet cell antigens **(molecular mimicry).** For example, one identified islet cell antigen (GAD) shares homology with a coxsackievirus protein and another with bovine serum albumin, a protein present in cow's milk, whose consumption in early childhood may be associated with an increased incidence of type 1 diabetes.

In the development of diabetes, the appearance of islet cell antibodies is followed by progressive impairment of insulin release in response to glucose (Figure 18–8). These two criteria have been used with great success to identify first-degree relatives at risk for the development of diabetes with the ultimate goal of intervening to prevent the development of diabetes. However, since only 10% of individuals newly diagnosed with type 1 diabetes have a family history of diabetes, such screening methods will not identify the vast majority of individuals developing diabetes. Given the low incidence of type 1 diabetes in the population, current screening methods do not

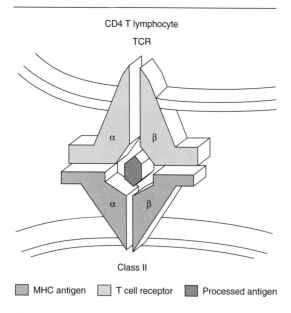

Figure 18–7. Presentation of processed antigen by HLA class II molecule to the T cell receptor. (Reproduced, with permission, from Muir A, Schatz DA, Maclaren NK: The pathogenesis, prediction, and prevention of insulin-dependent diabetes mellitus. Endocrinol Metab Clin North Am 1992;21:199.)

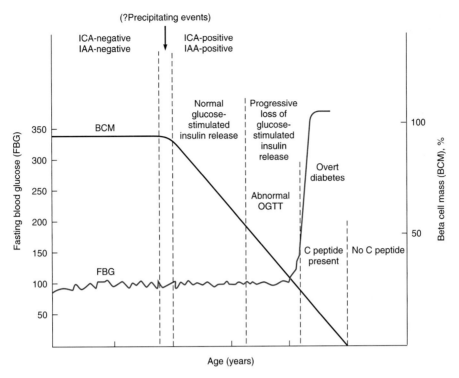

Figure 18–8. Stages in development of type 1 diabetes. (BCM, basal cell mass; FBG, fasting blood glucose; ICA, islet cell antibodies; IAA, insulin autoantibodies; OGTT, oral glucose tolerance test.) (Reproduced, with permission, from Wilson JD, Foster DW [editors]: *Williams Textbook of Endocrinology,* 8th ed. Saunders, 1992.)

have sufficient sensitivity to identify most individuals at risk in the general population.

B. Type 2 Diabetes: Although type 2 diabetes is ten times more prevalent than type 1 diabetes and has a much stronger genetic predisposition, the specific molecular defect or defects causing type 2 diabetes remain largely unknown, due in part to the heterogeneous nature of the disorder as well as to its probable polygenic origin. While type 1 diabetes is caused by insulin deficiency, both defective insulin secretion and insulin resistance are present in type 2 diabetes and are required in the majority of cases for the disease to be clinically manifest. Individuals with type 2 diabetes secrete a decreased amount of insulin in response to glucose and have a characteristic decrease in the early release of insulin (first-phase insulin release). In addition, type 2 diabetics are resistant to the effects of insulin.

It is not known with certainty whether abnormal islet cell insulin release or insulin resistance is the primary lesion in type 2 diabetes. Several decades prior to the onset of clinical diabetes, both insulin resistance and high insulin levels are present. This has led researchers to hypothesize that **insulin resistance** could be the primary lesion, resulting in a compensatory increase in insulin secretion that ultimately cannot be maintained by the pancreas. When the pancreas becomes "exhausted" and cannot keep up with insulin demands, clinical diabetes results. Others have proposed that **hyperinsulinemia,** a primary B cell defect, could initiate the disease process. Elevated insulin levels down-regulate the number of insulin receptors, leading to insulin resistance and to the eventual common pathway of B cell exhaustion. In this scenario, hyperinsulinemia is thought to be the expression of a "thrifty genotype" that offers a selective advantage to populations with inconstant food supplies but which leads to obesity and resultant increased insulin resistance in settings of abundant food. Others have proposed that **impaired early secretion of insulin** by islet cells in response to glucose (first-phase insulin release) may be the primary defect, resulting in hyperglycemia. Hyperglycemia and compensatory hyperinsulinemia could then contribute to the development of insulin resistance.

Candidate genes whose defective gene product could explain resistance to insulin action would include insulin itself, the insulin receptor, or other gene products responsible for the postreceptor effects of insulin. Reports of insulin resistance due to defects in insulin, such as mutations causing lack of processing of proinsulin to insulin, are rare. Proinsulin levels are elevated in many individuals with type 2 diabetes; the significance of this finding is unknown. Specific syndromes of severe insulin resistance that are caused either by **insulin receptor defects** (type A insulin resistance; Table 18–5: III.B.1) or by autoantibodies to the insulin receptor (type B syndrome) have been identified. These are distinct from type 2 diabetes. To date, however, there is no compelling evidence that defects in the insulin receptor are the primary lesion causing insulin resistance in type 2 diabetes. Therefore, insulin resistance is commonly thought to be due to a postreceptor defect. The defect could be in signaling intermediates distal to the insulin receptor kinases or the ultimate gene products regulated by insulin, such as glucose transporters or enzymes. For example, the gene for **GLUT 4**, the insulin-sensitive glucose transporter present in muscle and fat, has been studied as a possible candidate gene. Similarly, since muscle, the tissue responsible for the bulk of postprandial glucose disposal, appears to exhibit insulin resistance early in the prediabetic state owing to a defect in glycogen synthesis, the genes for enzymes responsible for glycogen synthesis—eg, **glycogen synthetase** or the phosphatases that activate this enzyme—have been studied as possible candidate genes.

Gene products capable of altering B cell insulin secretion are also being evaluated. For example, a defect in the gene encoding glucokinase has been identified in a subset of type 2 diabetics (**maturity-onset diabetes of the young [MODY 2; Table 18–5: III.A.2]**). **Glucokinase,** the enzyme catalyzing the first step in glucose metabolism in the B cell, is thought to be the B cell glucose sensor. Individuals with MODY have mild diabetes consistent with type 2 disease but are much younger than the average adult type 2 patient and inherit the disease in an autosomal dominant pattern. However, alterations in glucokinase do not appear to play a role in most cases of type 2 diabetes. Another candidate gene product that may alter B cell function is the newly identified **islet amyloid polypeptide (IAPP; amylin),** which is cosecreted with insulin. Its physiologic role is not yet well understood, but amyloid deposits composed of IAPP occur in the islets of individuals with type 2 diabetes. Because examination of specific candidate genes for genetic mutations has yet to identify any major causes of type 2 diabetes, genetic mapping studies are now also under way in specific pedigrees or populations (eg, Pima Indians) to attempt to identify the chromosomal location of the genetic defects underlying type 2 diabetes.

The majority of type 2 diabetics are obese. Obesity, particularly central abdominal obesity, is associated with increased insulin resistance. Obese nondiabetics have increased insulin levels and downregulation of insulin receptors. Obese type 2 diabetics often have elevated insulin levels relative to nonobese controls. However, for a given level of glucose, insulin levels in obese type 2 diabetics are lower than those seen in obese controls. This suggests that type 2 diabetics have a relative insulin deficiency and cannot compensate for the increased insulin resistance caused by obesity. Obesity, therefore, plays a role in the development of type 2 diabetes. The importance of obesity in type 2 diabetes is underscored by the fact that weight loss in obese type 2 diabetics can ameliorate or even prevent the disorder.

---

22. What are the key characteristics of type 1 and type 2 diabetes mellitus?
23. What is the role of heredity versus the environment in each of the two major types of diabetes mellitus?
24. What are two possible mechanisms of insulin resistance in type 2 diabetes mellitus?
25. What is the role of obesity in type 2 diabetes mellitus?

Pathology & Pathogenesis

No matter what the origin, all types of diabetes result from a relative deficiency of insulin action. In addition, in both type 1 and type 2 diabetes, glucagon levels appear to be inappropriately high. This high **glucagon:insulin ratio** creates a state similar to that seen in fasting and results in a "super-fasting" milieu that is inappropriate for maintenance of normal fuel homeostasis (Table 18–3).

The resulting metabolic derangements depend on the degree of loss of insulin action. Adipose tissue is most sensitive to insulin action. Therefore, low insulin activity is capable of suppressing lipolysis and enhancing fat storage. Higher levels of insulin are required to oppose glucagon effects on the liver and block hepatic glucose output. In normal individuals, basal levels of insulin activity are capable of mediating these responses. However, the ability of muscle and other insulin-sensitive tissues to respond to a glucose load with insulin-mediated glucose uptake requires the stimulated secretion of insulin from the pancreas.

Mild deficiencies in insulin action are therefore manifested first by an inability of insulin-sensitive tissues to clear glucose loads. Clinically, this results in **postprandial hyperglycemia.** Such individuals, most commonly type 2 diabetics with residual insulin secretion but increased insulin resistance, will have abnormal oral glucose tolerance tests. However, fasting glucose levels remain normal since sufficient insulin action is present to counterbalance the glucagon-mediated hepatic glucose output that maintains them. When a further loss of insulin action occurs, glucagon's effects on the liver are not sufficiently counterbalanced. Individuals therefore have both postprandial and **fasting hyperglycemia.**

While type 2 diabetics usually have some degree

of residual endogenous insulin action, type 1 diabetics have none. Therefore, untreated or inadequately treated type 1 diabetics manifest the most severe signs of insulin deficiency. In addition to fasting and postprandial hyperglycemia, they also develop **ketosis** since a marked lack of insulin allows maximal lipolysis of fat stores to supply substrates for unopposed glucagon stimulation of ketogenesis in the liver.

Fatty acids liberated from increased lipolysis, in addition to being metabolized by the liver into ketone bodies, can also be reesterified and packaged into VLDL. Furthermore, insulin deficiency causes a decrease in lipoprotein lipase, the enzyme responsible for hydrolysis of VLDL triglycerides in preparation for fatty acid storage in adipose tissue, thereby slowing VLDL clearance. Therefore, both type 1 and type 2 diabetics can have elevations in VLDL levels due both to an increase in VLDL production and a decrease in VLDL clearance.

Since insulin stimulates amino acid uptake and protein synthesis in muscle, the decrease in insulin action in diabetes results in decreased muscle protein synthesis. Marked insulinopenia, such as occurs in type 1 diabetics, can cause negative nitrogen balance and marked protein wasting. Amino acids not taken up by muscle are instead diverted to the liver where they are used to fuel gluconeogenesis.

In type 1 or type 2 diabetics, the superimposition of stress-induced counterregulatory hormones on what is already an insulinopenic state exacerbates the metabolic manifestations of deficient insulin action. The stress of infection, for example, can therefore induce diabetic ketoacidosis in both type 1 and some type 2 diabetics.

In addition to the metabolic derangements discussed above, diabetes causes other chronic complications that are responsible for the high morbidity and mortality rates associated with this disease. Diabetic complications are largely the result of vascular disease affecting both the microvasculature (retinopathy, nephropathy, and some types of neuropathy) and the macrovasculature (coronary artery disease, peripheral vascular disease).

Clinical Manifestations

A. Acute Complications:

1. Hyperglycemia—When elevated glucose levels exceed the renal threshold for reabsorption of glucose, **glucosuria** results. This causes an osmotic diuresis manifested clinically by **polyuria**, including **nocturia**. Dehydration results, stimulating thirst that results in **polydipsia**. A significant loss of calories can result from glucosuria, since urinary glucose losses can exceed 75 g/d (75 g × 4 kcal/g = 300 kcal/d). **Polyphagia** results because of decreased activity of the satiety center in the hypothalamus. The three "polys" of diabetes—polyuria, polydipsia, and polyphagia—are common presenting symptoms in both type 1 and symptomatic type 2 patients. Weight loss can also occur due both to dehydration and loss of calories in the urine. Severe weight loss is most apt to occur in patients with severe insulinopenia (type 1 diabetes) and is due both to caloric loss and to muscle wasting. Increased protein catabolism also contributes to the growth failure seen in children with type 1 diabetes.

Elevated glucose levels raise plasma osmolality:

$$\text{Osmolality (mosm/L)} = 2[Na^+(meq/L) + K^+(meq/L)] + \frac{\text{Glucose (mg/dL)}}{18} + \frac{\text{BUN (mg/dL)}}{2.8}$$

Changes in the water content of the lens of the eye in response to changes in osmolality can cause blurred vision.

In women, glucosuria can lead to an increased incidence of candidal vulvovaginitis. In some cases, this may be their only presenting symptom. In uncircumcised men, candidal balanitis (a similar infection of the glans penis) can occur.

2. Diabetic ketoacidosis—A profound loss of insulin activity leads not only to increased serum glucose levels due to increased hepatic glucose output and decreased glucose uptake by insulin-sensitive tissues but also to ketogenesis. In the absence of insulin, lipolysis is stimulated, providing fatty acids that are preferentially converted to ketone bodies in the liver by unopposed glucagon action. Typically, profound hyperglycemia and ketosis (diabetic ketoacidosis) occurs in type 1 diabetes, individuals who lack endogenous insulin. However, diabetic ketoacidosis can also occur in type 2 diabetes—particularly during infections, severe trauma, or other causes of stress that increase levels of counterregulatory hormones, thus producing a state of profound inhibition of insulin action.

Severe hyperglycemia with glucose levels reaching an average of 500 mg/dL can occur if compensation for the osmotic diuresis associated with hyperglycemia fails. Initially, when elevated glucose levels cause an increase in osmolality, a shift of water from the intracellular to the extracellular space and increased water intake stimulated by thirst help to maintain intravascular volume. If polyuria continues and these compensatory mechanisms cannot keep pace with fluid losses—particularly decreased intake due to the nausea and increased losses due to the vomiting that accompany ketoacidosis—the depletion of intravascular volume leads to decreased renal blood flow. The kidney's ability to excrete glucose is therefore reduced. Hypovolemia also stimulates counterregulatory hormones. Therefore, glucose levels rise acutely owing to increased glucose production stimulated by these hormones and decreased clearance by the kidney—an important source of glucose clearance in the absence of insulin-mediated glucose uptake.

In diabetic ketoacidosis, coma occurs in a minority of patients (10%). Hyperosmolality (not acidosis) is the cause of coma. Profound cellular dehydration occurs in response to the marked increase in plasma osmolality. A severe loss of intracellular fluid in the brain leads to coma. Coma occurs when the effective plasma osmolality reaches 340 mosm/L (normal: 280–295 mosm/L). Since urea is freely diffusible across cell membranes, BUN is not used to calculate the effective plasma osmolality:

Effective osmolality = $2[Na^+(meq/L) + K^+(meq/L)]$
$$+ \frac{\text{Glucose (mg/dL)}}{18}$$

The increase in **ketogenesis** caused by a severe lack of insulin action results in increased serum levels of ketones and ketonuria. Insulinopenia is also thought to decrease the ability of tissues to utilize ketones, thus contributing to the maintenance of ketosis. **Acetoacetate** and **β-hydroxybutyrate**, the chief ketone bodies produced by the liver, are strong organic acids and therefore cause metabolic acidosis, decreasing blood pH and serum bicarbonate (Figure 18–9). Respiration is stimulated, which partially compensates for the metabolic acidosis by reducing PCO_2. When the pH is lower than 7.20, characteristic deep, rapid respirations occur (**Kussmaul breathing**). Although acetone is a minor product of ketogenesis (Figure 18–9), its fruity odor can be detected on the breath during diabetic ketoacidosis.

Na^+ is lost in addition to water during the osmotic diuresis accompanying diabetic ketoacidosis. Therefore, total body Na^+ is depleted. Serum levels of Na^+ are usually low owing to the osmotic activity of the elevated glucose, which draws water into the extracellular space and in that way decreases the Na^+ concentration (Na^+ falls approximately 1.6 mmol/L for every 100 mg/dL increase in glucose).

Total body stores of K^+ are also depleted by diuresis and vomiting. However, acidosis, insulinopenia, and elevated glucose levels cause a shift of K^+ out of cells, thus maintaining normal or even elevated serum K^+ levels until acidosis and hyperglycemia are corrected. With administration of insulin and correction of acidosis, serum K^+ falls as K^+ moves back into cells. Without treatment, K^+ can fall to dangerously low levels, leading to potentially lethal cardiac arrhythmias. Therefore, K^+ supplementation is routinely given in the treatment of diabetic ketoacidosis. Similarly, phosphate depletion accompanies diabetic ketoacidosis, though acidosis and insulinopenia can cause serum phosphorus levels to be normal prior to treatment. Phosphate replacement is only provided in cases of extreme depletion given the risks of phosphate administration. (Intravenous phosphate may complex with Ca^{2+}, resulting in hypocalcemia and Ca^{2+} phosphate deposition in soft tissues.)

Marked **hypertriglyceridemia** frequently accompanies diabetic ketoacidosis because of the increased production and decreased clearance of VLDL that accompany insulin-deficient states. Increased production is due to the increased hepatic flux of fatty acids, which, in addition to fueling ketogenesis, can be repackaged and secreted as VLDL; decreased clearance is due to decreased lipoprotein lipase activity. Although serum Na^+ levels can be decreased owing to the osmotic effects of glucose, hypertriglyceridemia can interfere with some of the older procedures used to measure serum Na^+. This causes pseudohyponatremia, ie, falsely low Na^+ values.

Nausea and vomiting often accompany diabetic ketoacidosis, contributing to further dehydration. Abdominal pain, present in 30% of patients, may be due to gastric stasis and distention. Amylase is frequently elevated (90% of cases), in part due to elevations of salivary amylase, but it is usually not associated with other symptoms of pancreatitis. Leukocytosis is frequently present and does not necessarily indicate the presence of infection. However, since infections can precipitate diabetic ketoacidosis in type 1 and type 2 diabetes, other manifestations of infection should be sought—such as fever, a finding that cannot be attributed to diabetic ketoacidosis.

Diabetic ketoacidosis is treated by replacement of water and electrolytes (Na^+ and K^+) and administration of insulin. With fluid and electrolyte replacement, renal perfusion is increased, restoring renal clearance of elevated blood glucose; and counterregulatory hormone production is decreased, thus decreasing hepatic glucose production. Insulin administration also corrects hyperglycemia by restoring insulin-sensitive glucose uptake and inhibiting hepatic glucose output. Rehydration is a critical component of the treatment of hyperosmolality. If insulin is administered in the absence of fluid and electrolyte

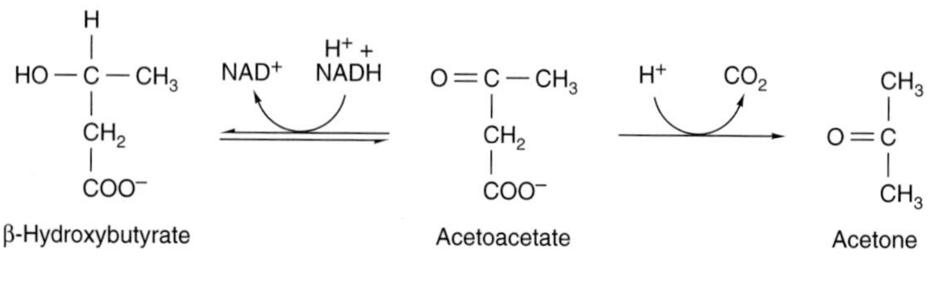

Figure 18–9. Interconversion of ketone bodies. (Reproduced, with permission, from Stryer L: *Biochemistry*, 3rd ed. Freeman, 1988.)

replacement, water will move from the extracellular space back into the cells with correction of hyperglycemia, leading to vascular collapse. Insulin administration is also required to inhibit further lipolysis, thus eliminating substrates for ketogenesis, and to inhibit hepatic ketogenesis, thereby correcting ketoacidosis.

During treatment of diabetic ketoacidosis, measured serum ketones may transiently rise instead of showing a steady decrease. This is an artifact due to the limitations of the nitroprusside test that is usually used to measure ketones in both serum and urine. Nitroprusside only detects acetoacetate and not β-hydroxybutyrate. During untreated diabetic ketoacidosis, accelerated fatty acid oxidation generates large quantities of NADH in the liver, which favors the formation of β-hydroxybutyrate over acetoacetate (Figure 18–9). With insulin treatment, fatty acid oxidation decreases and the redox potential of the liver shifts back in favor of acetoacetate formation. Therefore, while the absolute amount of hepatic ketone body production is decreasing with treatment of diabetic ketoacidosis, the relative amount of acetoacetate production is increasing, leading to a transient increase in measured serum ketones by the nitroprusside test.

3. Hyperosmolar coma–Severe hyperosmolar states in the absence of ketosis can occur in type 2 diabetes. These episodes are frequently precipitated by decreased fluid intake such as can occur during an intercurrent illness or in older debilitated patients who lack sufficient access to water and have abnormal renal function hindering the clearance of excessive glucose loads. The mechanisms underlying the development of hyperosmolality and **hyperosmolar coma** are the same as in diabetic ketoacidosis. However, since only minimal levels of insulin activity are required to suppress lipolysis, these individuals have sufficient insulin to prevent the ketogenesis that results from increased fatty acid flux. Because of the absence of ketoacidosis and its symptoms, patients often present later and therefore have more profound hyperglycemia and dehydration, with glucose levels ranging as high as 800–2400 mg/dL. Therefore, the effective osmolality exceeds 340 mosm/L more frequently in these patients than in those presenting with diabetic ketoacidosis, resulting in a higher incidence of coma.

Although ketosis is absent, mild ketonuria can be present if the patient has not been eating. K^+ losses are less severe than in diabetic ketoacidosis. Treatment is similar to that of diabetic ketoacidosis. Mortality is ten times higher than in diabetic ketoacidosis, because the type 2 diabetics who develop hyperosmolar nonketotic states are older and often have other serious precipitating or complicating illnesses. For example, myocardial infarction can precipitate hyperosmolar states, or it can result from the alterations in vascular blood flow and other stressors that accompany severe dehydration.

4. Hypoglycemia–Hypoglycemia is a complication of insulin treatment in both type 1 and type 2 diabetes, but it can also occur with oral hypoglycemic drugs that stimulate endogenous insulin secretion (eg, sulfonylureas or benzoic acid derivatives). Hypoglycemia often occurs during exercise or with fasting, states that normally are characterized by slight elevations in counterregulatory hormones and depressed insulin levels. Low insulin levels in these conditions are permissive for the counterregulatory hormone-mediated mobilization of fuel substrates, increased hepatic glucose output, and inhibition of glucose disposal in insulin-sensitive tissues. These responses normally would increase blood glucose. However, hypoglycemia is precipitated in diabetic patients in these circumstances by inappropriate dosing with exogenous insulin or by induction of endogenous insulin.

The acute response to hypoglycemia is mediated by the counterregulatory effects of glucagon and catecholamines (Table 18–8). Initial symptoms of hypoglycemia occur secondary to **catecholamine release** (shaking, sweating, palpitations). As glucose drops further, **neuroglycopenic symptoms** also occur from the direct effects of hypoglycemia on central nervous system function (confusion, coma). A characteristic set of symptoms (night sweats, nightmares, morning headaches) also accompanies hypoglycemic episodes that occur during sleep (**nocturnal hypoglycemia**).

Type 1 diabetics are especially prone to hypoglycemia. After several years of diabetes, the glucagon response to hypoglycemia can become inadequate though the catecholamine response is still effective. If in later years the catecholamine response

Table 18–8. Symptoms and signs of hypoglycemia.[1]

Secondary to catecholamine release (adrenergic)	
Sweating	Tremor
Shakiness	Hunger
Anxiety	Faintness
Palpitations	Tachycardia
Weakness	

Secondary to central nervous system dysfunction (neuroglycopenic)	
Confusion	Diplopia
Irritability	Inappropriate affect
Headaches	Motor incoordination
Abnormal behavior	Convulsion
Weakness	Coma

Nocturnal hypoglycemia (usually due to excessive insulin therapy; symptoms do not usually awaken the patient)	
Morning headaches	Difficulty in awakening
Lassitude	Psychologic changes
Night sweats	Restlessness during sleep
Nightmares	Loud respirations

[1]Reproduced, with permission, from Andreoli TE et al (editors): *Cecil Essentials of Medicine,* 3rd ed. Saunders, 1993.

is lost as a consequence of autonomic neuropathy—a chronic complication of diabetes—these individuals will have no acute defense against hypoglycemia. In addition, even a single episode of hypoglycemia can cause a transient decrease in the catecholamine response to hypoglycemia, thus increasing the risk of recurrent hypoglycemia (Chapter 12).

Type 1 or type 2 patients with autonomic neuropathy who have a deficient catecholamine response to hypoglycemia and patients who are being treated with beta-adrenergic blockade for other conditions will not experience the catecholamine-mediated warning signs that precede neuroglycopenic symptoms (with the exception of sweating, which is preserved). Therefore, they are especially at risk for serious hypoglycemia.

Acute treatment of hypoglycemia in diabetic individuals consists of rapid oral or intravenous administration of glucose at the onset of warning symptoms, or the administration of glucagon intramuscularly. Rebound hyperglycemia can occur following hypoglycemia due to the actions of counterregulatory hormones (**Somogyi phenomenon**), an effect that can be aggravated by excessive glucose administration.

B. Chronic Complications: Over time, diabetes results in damage and dysfunction in multiple organ systems (Table 18–9). Vascular disease is a major cause of many of the sequelae of this disease. Both **microvascular disease** (retinopathy, nephropathy) and **macrovascular disease** (coronary artery disease, peripheral vascular disease) contribute to the high morbidity and mortality rates associated with diabetes. **Neuropathy** also causes increased morbidity, particularly by virtue of its role in the pathogenesis of foot ulcers.

Although type 1 and type 2 diabetics both suffer from the complete spectrum of diabetic complications, the incidence varies with each type. Macrovascular disease is the major cause of death in type 2 diabetes, while renal failure secondary to **nephropathy** is the most common cause in type 1. Although blindness occurs in both types, proliferative changes in retinal vessels (**proliferative retinopathy**) are a major cause of blindness in type 1 while macular edema is the most important cause in type 2 diabetes. **Autonomic neuropathy,** one of the manifestations of diabetic neuropathy, is more common in type 1 diabetics.

1. Role of glycemic control in preventing complications–There has been controversy for many years about whether the chronic complications of diabetes could be directly attributed to the effects of elevated glucose or to other genetic factors. This question has important implications for the treatment of diabetes, since a causative role for elevated glucose would suggest that normalization of glucose should be the goal of treatment (**tight or intensive diabetic control**). In 1993, publication of the results of the Diabetes Control and Complications Trial (DCCT) provided the first compelling evidence that intensive treatment (versus conventional treatment) could reduce both the development and the progression of retinopathy (by 50–80%); could reduce the occurrence of nephropathy, as measured by effects on proteinuria (by 40–50%); and could reduce the occurrence of neuropathy (by 60%) in type 1 diabetes. Recent studies have also shown that improved glycemic control prevents microvascular complications in type 2 diabetics. In contrast, the role of glycemic control in preventing macrovascular disease is less clear, perhaps because atherosclerosis is a multifactorial disease that is also strongly influenced by other risk factors such as hypercholesterolemia, hypertension, and tobacco use.

Three other interesting findings emerged from the DCCT: (1) Despite best therapeutic efforts, complete normalization of blood glucose did not occur; (2) intensive treatment carried a threefold increased risk of hypoglycemia requiring assistance or resulting in seizures or coma; and (3) intensively treated patients experienced weight gain, a finding which underscores the anabolic effect of insulin. In type 2 diabetes, hypoglycemia can also occur with aggressive treatment, but this occurs much less commonly than in type 1 diabetes. Weight gain occurs frequently in type 2 diabetics who are treated with insulin or drugs that induce endogenous insulin, a troublesome side effect in patients who are already obese.

While glycemic control clearly influences the occurrence of microvascular complications, genetic factors may also play a role. For example, evidence from a variety of studies suggests that approximately 20–40% of type 1 diabetics may be particularly susceptible to the development of severe microvascular complications. The reason for this increase is not known.

2. Microvascular complications–Although microvascular complications are thought to be related to raised glucose levels, the pathogenesis of diabetic microvascular disease is not completely understood. Basement membranes in small vessels are

Table 18–9. Chronic complications of diabetes mellitus.[1]

Microvascular disease
    Retinopathy
    Nephropathy
Macrovascular disease
    Coronary artery disease
    Cerebrovascular disease
    Peripheral vascular disease
Neuropathic disease
    Peripheral symmetric polyneuropathy
    Autonomic neuropathies
    Mononeuropathies
Foot ulcers
Infections

[1]Reproduced, with permission, from Andreoli TE et al (editors): *Cecil Essentials of Medicine,* 3rd ed. Saunders, 1993.

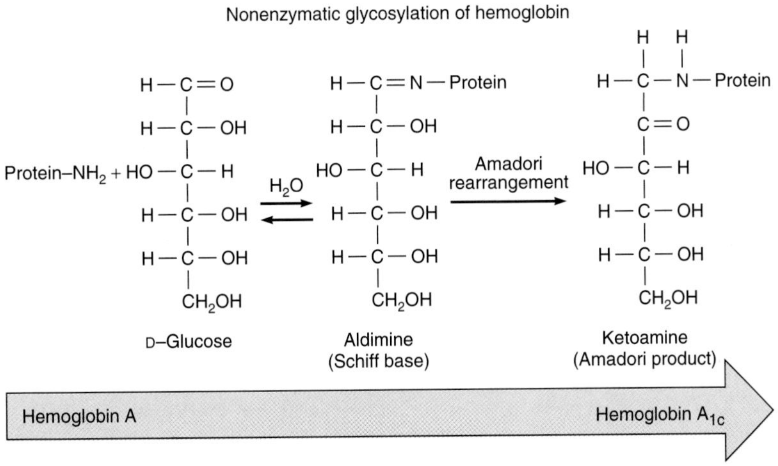

Figure 18–10. Amadori product. (Reproduced, with permission, from Wyngaarden JB, Smith LH Jr, Bennett JC [editors]: *Cecil Textbook of Medicine,* 19th ed. Saunders, 1992.)

thickened in diabetes and contain increased amounts of collagen and decreased amounts of proteoglycan, of which heparan sulfate is the major component.

One biochemical mechanism that has been proposed to account for the pathogenesis of microvascular lesions in diabetes is the formation of irreversibly glycated proteins called **advanced glycosylation end products (AGE).** When present in high concentrations, glucose can react nonenzymatically with amino groups in proteins to form an unstable intermediate, a Schiff base, that then undergoes an internal rearrangement to form a stable glycated protein, also known as an early glycosylation product (**Amadori product**) (Figure 18–10). Such a reaction accounts for the formation of **glycated HbA,** also known as HbA_{1c}. In diabetics, elevated glucose leads to increased glycation of HbA within red blood cells. Since red blood cells circulate for 120 days, measurement of HbA_{1c} in diabetic patients serves as an index of glycemic control over the preceding 2–3 months. Early glycosylation products can undergo a further series of chemical reactions and rearrangements, leading to the formation of AGE, which are covalently and irreversibly linked by glucose-derived imidazole- and pyrrole-based cross-links (Figure 18–11). AGE can bind to the matrix components of the basement membrane. Both small and large vessels in diabetics show a continuous accumulation of plasma proteins. It is hypothesized that this may be due to the accumulation of AGE or to the capture by accumulated AGE of other normal plasma proteins, such as LDL. In addition, binding of AGE to specific receptors on macrophages causes the release of cytokines that can in turn affect the proliferation and function of vascular cells. AGE receptors are also present on endothelial cells.

Another biochemical pathway that has been extensively studied in diabetic nerve cells but which is also present in endothelial cells is the **polyol pathway** (Figure 18–12). Many cells contain aldose reductase, an enzyme that converts aldohexoses, such as glucose, to their respective alcohols (polyol pathway). Hyperglycemia provides increased substrate for this enzyme. The excess **sorbitol** produced from this reaction cannot exit the cell but instead is converted to fructose, a step that is rate-limiting. Therefore, sorbitol tends to accumulate in the cells in the presence of hyperglycemia. Sorbitol accumulation has been demonstrated in nerve and endothelial cells and in the lens of the eye, where it is associated with cataract formation. Sorbitol, perhaps through an increase in cell osmolality, is thought to decrease cellular myoinositol content. Hyperglycemia may also directly contribute to intracellular myoinositol depletion by inhibiting its uptake. Decreased myoinositol in turn alters inositol phosphate metabolism, ultimately leading to a protein kinase C-mediated decrease in cellular Na^+-K^+ ATPase activity. In nerve cells, these sorbitol-mediated effects are thought to be responsible for decreased nerve conduction. The effect of this pathway on vascular biology is not known.

a. Retinopathy–(Figure 18–13.) Diabetes is the leading cause of new blindness among United States adults. Diabetic retinopathy occurs in two distinct stages: nonproliferative and proliferative.

Nonproliferative retinopathy occurs frequently in both type 1 and type 2 diabetics. **Microaneurysms** of the retinal capillaries, appearing as tiny red dots, are the earliest clinically detectable sign of diabetic retinopathy (**background retinopathy**). These outpouchings in the capillary wall are thought to be re-

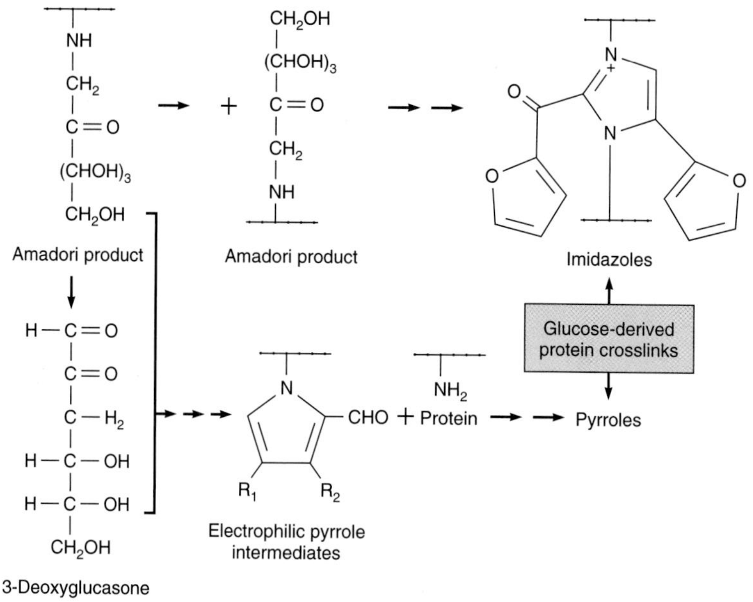

Figure 18–11. Formation of irreversible advanced glycosylation end products (AGE) from Amadori products. Through a complex series of chemical reactions, Amadori products can form families of imidazole-based and pyrrole-based glucose-derived cross-links. (Reproduced, with permission, from Kohler PO, Jordan RM [editors]: *Clinical Endocrinology.* Wiley, 1986.)

lated to loss of the pericytes that surround and support the capillary walls. Vascular permeability is increased. Fat that has leaked from excessively permeable capillary walls appears as shiny yellow spots with distinct borders **(hard exudates)** forming a ring around the area of leakage. The appearance of hard exudates in the area of the macula is often associated with macular edema, the most common cause of visual impairment in type 2 diabetes. As retinopathy progresses, signs of ischemia appearing as background retinopathy worsen **(preproliferative stage).** Occlusion of capillaries and terminal arterioles causes areas of retinal ischemia that appear as hazy yellow areas with indistinct borders **(cotton wool spots** or **soft exudates)** due to the accumulation of axonoplasmic debris at areas of infarction. Retinal hemorrhages can also occur, and retinal veins develop segmental dilation.

Retinopathy can progress to a second, more severe stage characterized by the proliferation of new vessels **(proliferative retinopathy).** Neovascularization is more prevalent in type 1 than in type 2 diabetes (60% versus 10% after 20 years) and is a major cause of blindness. It is hypothesized that retinal ischemia stimulates the release of growth-promoting factors, resulting in new vessel formation. However, these capillaries are abnormal, and traction between new fibrovascular networks and the vitreous can lead to **vitreous hemorrhage** or **retinal detachment,** two potential causes of blindness.

b. Nephropathy–In the United States, diabetes is the leading cause of end-stage renal disease requiring kidney dialysis or transplantation. Although end-stage renal disease occurs more frequently in type 1 than in type 2 diabetes (20–30% versus < 5%), type 2 accounts for half of the diabetic population with end-stage renal disease because of its greater prevalence.

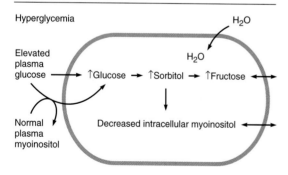

Figure 18–12. The sorbitol pathway. Hyperglycemia increases intracellular sorbitol, which in turn is associated with depletion of intracellular myoinositol levels. Hyperglycemia may also decrease myoinositol directly by inhibiting its uptake. (Modified and reproduced, with permission, from Wyngaarden JB, Smith LH Jr, Bennett JC (editors): *Cecil Textbook of Medicine,* 19th ed. Saunders, 1992.)

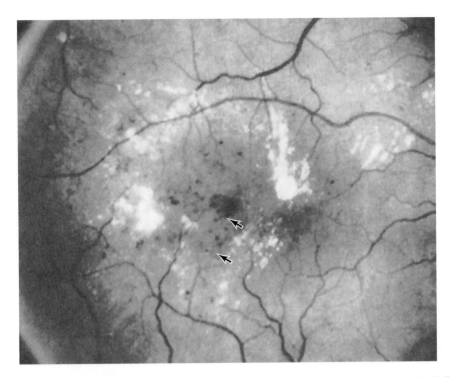

Figure 18–13. Diabetic retinopathy. A hard caudate ring 1.5 disk diameters in diameter is centered 1.0 disk diameter superotemporal to the center of the macula in this right eye. Part of the ring is a plaque of hard exudate just above the center of the macula. Within the ring, many large microaneurysms can be seen, some with visible walls (arrows). They are slightly out of focus because the retina here is thickened (edematous) and the camera is focused on the surrounding retina. With stereoscopic viewing, retinal thickening was obvious and could be seen to extend into the center of the macula. (Courtesy of the ETDRS Research Group. Reproduced, with permission, from Davis MD: Diabetic retinopathy: A clinical overview. Diabetes Care 1992;15:1844.)

End-stage renal disease also occurs more frequently in Native Americans, African-Americans, and Hispanic-Americans than in non-Hispanic whites with type 2 diabetes.

Diabetic nephropathy results primarily from disordered glomerular function (Figure 18–14). Histologic changes in glomeruli are indistinguishable in type 1 and type 2 diabetes and occur to some degree in the majority of individuals. Basement membranes of the glomerular capillaries are thickened and can obliterate the vessels; the mesangium surrounding the glomerular vessels is increased owing to the deposition of basement membrane-like material and can encroach on the glomerular vessels; and the afferent and efferent glomerular arteries are also sclerosed. **Glomerulosclerosis** is usually diffuse, but in 50% of cases it is associated with nodular sclerosis. This nodular component, called **Kimmelstiel-Wilson nodules** after the investigators who first described the pathologic changes in diabetic kidneys, is pathognomonic for diabetes.

In type 1 diabetics, glomerular changes are pre-

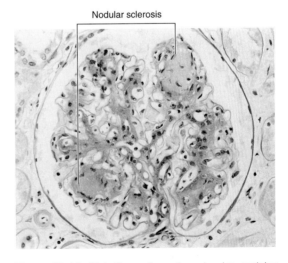

Figure 18–14. Diabetic nephropathy, showing nodular glomerulosclerosis (Kimmelstiel-Wilson disease). (Reproduced, with permission, from Chandrasoma P, Taylor CR: *Concise Pathology,* 3rd ed. Appleton & Lange, 1998.)

ceded by a phase of **hyperfiltration** due to vasodilation of both the afferent and efferent glomerular arterioles, an effect perhaps mediated by two of the counterregulatory hormones, glucagon and growth hormone, or by hyperglycemia. It is unclear whether this early hyperfiltration phase occurs in type 2 diabetes. It has been proposed that the presence of atherosclerotic lesions in older type 2 diabetics may prevent hyperfiltration and thus account for the lower incidence of overt clinical nephropathy in these individuals.

Early in the course of the disease, the histologic changes in renal glomeruli are accompanied by **microalbuminuria,** a urinary loss of albumin that cannot be detected by routine urinalysis dipstick methods (Figure 18–15). Albuminuria is thought to be due to a decrease in the heparan sulfate content of the thickened glomerular capillary basement membrane. Heparan sulfate, a negatively charged proteoglycan, can inhibit the filtration of other negatively charged proteins, such as albumin, through the basement membrane; its loss therefore allows for increased albumin filtration.

If glomerular lesions worsen, **proteinuria** increases and overt nephropathy develops (Figure 18–15). Diabetic nephropathy is defined clinically by the presence of over 300–500 mg of urinary protein per day, an amount that can be detected by routine urinalysis. In diabetic nephropathy (unlike other renal diseases), proteinuria continues to increase as renal function decreases. Therefore, end-stage renal disease is preceded by massive, nephrotic-range proteinuria (> 4 g/d). The presence of hypertension speeds this process. While type 2 diabetics often already have hypertension at the time of diagnosis, type 1 patients usually do not develop hypertension until after the onset of nephropathy. In both cases, hypertension worsens as renal function deteriorates. Therefore, control of hypertension is critical in preventing the progression of diabetic nephropathy.

Retinopathy, a process that is also worsened by the presence of hypertension, usually precedes the development of nephropathy. Therefore, other causes of proteinuria should be considered in diabetic individuals who present with proteinuria in the absence of retinopathy.

3. **Macrovascular complications**—Atherosclerotic macrovascular disease occurs with increased frequency in diabetes, resulting in an increased incidence of myocardial infarction, stroke, and claudication and gangrene of the lower extremities. Although macrovascular disease accounts for significant morbidity and mortality in both types of diabetes, the effects of large vessel disease are particularly devastating in type 2 diabetes and are responsible for approximately 60% of deaths. The protective effect of gender is lost in women with diabetes; their risk of atherosclerosis is equal to that of men.

Reasons for the increased risk of **atherosclerosis** in diabetes are threefold: (1) The incidence of other known risk factors, such as hypertension and hyperlipidemia, is increased; (2) diabetes itself is an independent risk factor for atherosclerosis; and (3) diabetes appears to act synergistically with other known

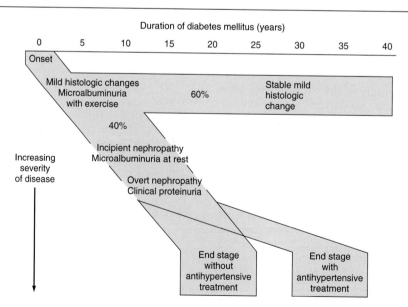

Figure 18–15. Development of renal failure in type 1 diabetes. (Reproduced, with permission, from Omachi R: The pathogenesis and prevention of diabetic nephropathy. West J Med 1986;145:222.)

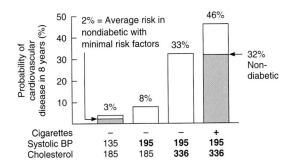

Figure 18–16. Relative importance of risk factors for coronary artery disease in a 40-year-old diabetic man. (Reproduced, with permission, from Siperstein MD: Diabetic microangiopathy, genetics, environment, and treatment. Am J Med 1988;85[Suppl 5A]:119.)

risk factors to markedly increase the risk of atherosclerosis. The elimination of other risk factors therefore can greatly reduce the risk of atherosclerosis in diabetes (Figure 18–16).

Hypertension occurs with increased frequency in type 1 and type 2 diabetes and is associated with an increase in total body extracellular Na^+ content, causing volume expansion and suppression of renin. Despite these similar findings, the epidemiology of hypertension in the two subtypes suggests that different pathophysiologic mechanisms may be operative. In type 1 diabetes, hypertension usually occurs after the onset of nephropathy, when renal insufficiency impairs the ability to excrete water and solutes. In type 2 diabetes, hypertension is often present at the time of diagnosis in these older, obese, insulin-resistant individuals. It has been proposed that insulin resistance and hyperinsulinemia may play a central role both in diabetes and in hypertension. Insulin resistance and hyperinsulinemia have been reported in nondiabetics with essential hypertension. A cluster of metabolic abnormalities associated with an increased risk of cardiovascular disease in nondiabetic individuals—insulin resistance, hyperinsulinemia, glucose intolerance, hypertension, hypertriglyceridemia, and low levels of high-density lipoprotein (HDL)—has been called **syndrome X,** or insulin resistance syndrome. It is hypothesized that the metabolic abnormalities in syndrome X are caused by insulin resistance (see Chapter 11). Type 2 diabetes—with its overt hyperglycemia occurring in the setting of these same metabolic abnormalities—may lie at the extreme end of a continuum of metabolic derangements described by these signs.

The principal lipid abnormality in poorly controlled type 1 and type 2 diabetes is **hypertriglyceridemia,** which is due to increased VLDL. Hypertriglyceridemia, particularly in type 2 diabetes, can also be associated with decreased HDL cholesterol.

LDL cholesterol may also be elevated both because of increased production (VLDL is catabolized to LDL) and decreased clearance (insulin deficiency may reduce LDL receptor activity). VLDL levels are increased because of insufficient insulin action in adipose tissue. This results in decreased VLDL clearance due to decreased lipoprotein lipase activity and in increased VLDL production due to increased fatty acid flux from adipose tissue to the liver (ie, increased lipolysis). Hypertriglyceridemia, low HDL cholesterol, and high LDL cholesterol are all risk factors for atherosclerosis. Insulin treatment usually corrects lipoprotein abnormalities in type 1 diabetes. In contrast, treatment of hyperglycemia often does not normalize lipid profiles in obese, insulin-resistant individuals with type 2 diabetes unless accompanied by weight reduction (ie, by a concomitant reduction in insulin resistance).

Possible reasons that diabetes may be an independent risk factor for atherosclerosis and may also act synergistically with other risk factors include the following: (1) alterations in lipoprotein composition in diabetes that make the particles more atherogenic (ie, increased small dense LDL, increased levels of Lp[a], enhanced oxidation and glycation of lipoproteins); (2) the occurrence of a relative procoagulant state in diabetes, including an increase in certain clotting factors and increased platelet aggregation; (3) proatherogenic alterations in the vessel walls caused either by the direct effects of hyperinsulinemia in type 2 diabetes or by boluses of exogenously administered insulin (versus hepatic first-pass clearance of endogenously secreted insulin) in type 1 diabetics. These include promotion of smooth muscle proliferation, alteration of vasomotor tone, and enhancement of foam cell formation (cholesterol-laden cells that characterize atherogenic lesions); and (4) proatherogenic alterations in the vessel walls caused by the direct effects of hyperglycemia, including deposition of glycated proteins, just as occurs in the microvasculature.

4. Neuropathy—(Table 18–10.) Neuropathy occurs commonly in both type 1 and type 2 diabetes and is a major cause of morbidity. Diabetic neuropathy can be divided into three major types: (1) a distal, primarily sensory, symmetric polyneuropathy that is by far the most common; (2) autonomic neuropathy, occurring frequently in individuals with distal polyneuropathy; and (3) the less common transient, asymmetric neuropathies involving specific nerves, nerve roots, or plexuses.

a. Symmetric distal polyneuropathy—Demyelination of peripheral nerves, which is a hallmark of diabetic polyneuropathy, affects distal nerves preferentially and is usually manifested clinically by a symmetric sensory loss in the distal lower extremities **(stocking distribution)** that is preceded by numbness, tingling, and paresthesias. These symptoms, which begin distally and move proximally, can also

Table 18–10. Classification of diabetic neuropathy.

Symmetric distal polyneuropathy (sensory >> motor)
Autonomic neuropathy
Asymmetric mononeuropathy or mononeuropathy multiplex
  (motor >> sensory)
    Cranial nerves
      Ocular (III >> VI > IV)
      Bell's palsy (VII)
    Peripheral nerves
      Femoral
      Obturator
      Sciatic
      Median
      Ulnar

---

occur in the hands **(glove distribution)**. Pathologic features of affected peripheral somatic nerves include demyelination and loss of nerve fibers with reduced axonal regeneration accompanied by microvascular lesions, including thickening of basement membranes. Activation of the polyol pathway in nerve cells is thought to play a major role in inducing symmetric distal polyneuropathy in diabetes. In addition, evidence suggests that the microvascular disease which accompanies these neural lesions may also contribute to nerve damage.

b. Autonomic neuropathy–Autonomic neuropathy often accompanies symmetric peripheral neuropathy, occurs more frequently in type 1 diabetes, and can affect all aspects of autonomic functioning, most notably those involving the cardiovascular, genitourinary, and gastrointestinal systems. Less information is available regarding the morphologic changes occurring in affected autonomic nerves, but similarities to somatic nerve alterations suggest a common pathogenesis.

Fixed, resting **tachycardia** and **orthostatic hypotension** are signs of cardiovascular involvement that can be easily ascertained on physical examination. Orthostatic hypotension can be quite severe. **Impotence** occurs in over 50% of diabetic men and is due both to neurogenic (parasympathetic control of penile vasodilation) and vascular factors. Sexual dysfunction in diabetic women has not been well studied. Loss of bladder sensation and difficulty in emptying the bladder (neurogenic bladder) lead to overflow **incontinence** and an increased risk of urinary tract infections due to residual urine. Motor disturbances can occur throughout the gastrointestinal tract, resulting in delayed gastric emptying (gastroparesis), constipation, or diarrhea. Anhidrosis in the lower extremities can lead to excessive sweating in the upper body as a means of dissipating heat, including increased sweating in response to eating **(gustatory sweating)**. Autonomic neuropathy can also result in decreased glucagon and epinephrine responses to hypoglycemia.

c. Mononeuropathy and mononeuropathy multiplex–The abrupt, usually painful onset of motor loss in isolated cranial or peripheral nerves **(mononeuropathy)** or in multiple isolated nerves **(mononeuropathy multiplex)** occurs less frequently than does symmetric polyneuropathy or autonomic neuropathy. Vascular occlusion and ischemia is thought to play a central role in the pathogenesis of these asymmetric focal neuropathies, which are usually of limited duration and occur more frequently in type 2 diabetics.

The third nerve is the most frequent cranial nerve involved, causing ipsilateral headache followed by ptosis and ophthalmoplegia with sparing of the pupil. Peripheral nerves are usually involved at sites of possible compression (eg. ulnar nerve at elbow; median nerve at the wrist).

5. Diabetic foot ulcers–Symmetric polyneuropathy, manifested on clinical examination by decreased vibratory and cutaneous pressure sensation and absence of ankle reflexes, is the leading cause of diabetic foot ulcers and is present in 75–90% of diabetics with foot ulcers. Diabetic foot ulcers often lead to **amputations** because of ischemia due to macrovascular disease (present in 30–40% of diabetics with foot ulcers) and to microvascular disease, infections due to alterations in neutrophil function and vascular insufficiency, and faulty wound healing due to unknown factors. The 3-year mortality rate for diabetics who have undergone amputations is 50%.

6. Infection–Neutrophil chemotaxis and phagocytosis are defective in poorly controlled diabetes. Cell-mediated immunity may also be abnormal. In addition, vascular lesions can hinder blood flow, preventing inflammatory cells from reaching wounds (eg, foot ulcers) or other possible sites of infection. Therefore, individuals with diabetes are more prone to develop infections and may have more severe infections. As a result, certain common infections (eg, **candidal infections, periodontal disease**) occur more frequently in diabetics. A number of unusual infections also are seen in diabetics, ie, **necrotizing papillitis; mucormycosis** of the nasal sinuses, invading the orbit and cranium; and **malignant otitis externa** caused by *Pseudomonas aeruginosa*.

---

26. How does type 1 diabetes mellitus result in negative nitrogen balance and protein wasting?
27. What are some acute clinical manifestations of diabetes mellitus?
28. Describe the pathophysiologic mechanisms at work in diabetic ketoacidosis.
29. Explain why ketones may appear to be increasing with appropriate treatment of ketoacidosis.
30. Explain why hyperosmolar coma without ketosis is a more common presentation than ketoacidosis in type 2 diabetes mellitus.

31. What chronic complication of diabetes mellitus can exacerbate iatrogenic hypoglycemia?
32. What are the most common microvascular and macrovascular complications of long-standing diabetes mellitus, and what are their pathophysiologic mechanisms?
33. What were the major conclusions from the DCCT?
34. What are the proposed roles of nonenzymatic glycosylation and the polyol pathway in the development of complications of diabetes mellitus?
35. What are the characteristics of nonproliferative and proliferative retinopathy in diabetes mellitus?
36. What are the anatomic and physiologic changes observed during the progression of diabetic nephropathy?
37. Does nephropathy usually precede retinopathy in patients with diabetes mellitus?
38. Suggest three reasons for increased risk of atherosclerosis in diabetes mellitus.
39. What are the probable differences in the pathophysiology of hypertension in type 1 versus type 2 diabetes mellitus?
40. What three major types of neuropathy are observed in long-standing diabetes mellitus? What are the common symptoms and signs of each?
41. Which types of infections occur with increased frequency in patients with diabetes mellitus, and why?

INSULINOMA

Clinical Presentation

The occurrence of fasting hypoglycemia in an otherwise healthy individual is usually due to an insulin-secreting tumor of the B cells of the islets of Langerhans (**insulinoma**; Table 18-11). Although insulinoma is the most common islet cell tumor, it is still a rare disorder. Insulinomas occur most frequently in the fourth to seventh decades, though they can occur earlier, particularly when associated with multiple endocrine neoplasia type 1 (MEN 1), a neoplastic syndrome characterized by tumors of the parathyroids, pituitary, and endocrine pancreas (see Chapter 17). The diagnosis of hypoglycemia is based on Whipple's triad: (1) symptoms and signs of hypoglycemia, (2) an associated low plasma glucose level, and (3) reversibility of symptoms upon administration of glucose.

Etiology

In the great majority of cases, insulinomas are benign solitary lesions composed of whorls of insulin-secreting B cells. Multiple tumors, though infrequent (< 10%), are seen most often in patients with MEN 1. Fewer than 10% of the tumors are malignant, as determined by the presence of metastases.

Pathology & Pathogenesis

Inappropriately high levels of insulin in situations normally characterized by a lowering of insulin secretion (eg, fasting and exercise) result in hypoglycemia. Normally, in the postabsorptive and fasting state, insulin levels decline, leading to an increase in glucagon-stimulated hepatic glucose output and a decrease in insulin-mediated glucose disposal in the periphery which maintain normal serum glucose levels. With exercise, low insulin allows muscles to utilize glycogen; glucagon and other counterregulatory hormones to increase hepatic glucose output; and counterregulatory hormones to mobilize fatty acids for ketogenesis and fatty acid oxidation by muscle. With an insulinoma, insulin levels remain high during fasting or exercise. In this circumstance, glucagon-mediated hepatic glucose output is suppressed while insulin-mediated peripheral glucose uptake continues, and insulin stimulates hepatic fatty acid synthesis and peripheral fatty acid storage while suppressing fatty acid mobilization and hepatic ketogenesis. The result is fasting or exercise-induced hypoglycemia in the absence of ketosis.

Clinical Manifestations

Individuals with insulinomas often are symptomatic for years prior to diagnosis and are self-treated with frequent food intake. Not all patients experience fasting hypoglycemia in the morning (only 30% of insulinoma patients develop hypoglycemia after a diagnostic 12-hour fast). Often they experience late afternoon hypoglycemia, particularly when precipitated by exercise. Since alcohol, like insulin, inhibits gluconeogenesis, alcohol ingestion can also precipitate symptoms. A high percentage of individuals with insulinoma experience neuroglycopenic as well as autonomic symptoms (Table 18-8). Confusion (80%), loss of consciousness (50%), and seizures (10%) often lead to misdiagnoses of psychiatric or neurologic disorders.

Fasting hypoglycemia can be due either to elevated insulin, as occurs in insulinoma, or to non-insulin-mediated effects such as loss of counterregulatory hormones (eg, loss of cortisol in Addison's disease), severe hepatic damage that prevents hepatic glucose production, loss of peripheral stores of substrates for hepatic glucose production (eg, cachexia), or some states of markedly increased glucose utilization (eg, sepsis, cancer). To distinguish **insulin-mediated** from **non-insulin-mediated fasting hypoglycemia,** patients suspected of having insulinoma are subjected to a diagnostic fast during which glucose, insulin, and C peptide levels are measured. Elevated insulin levels in the setting of hypoglycemia is

Table 18–11. Syndromes associated with islet cell tumors.[1]

Tumor	Major Findings	Minor Findings	Other Hormones in Tumor or Plasma	Percent Malignancy	Hyperplasia	MEN Syndrome
Insulinoma	Adrenergic: palpitations, tremor, hunger, sweating Neuroglycopenic: confusion, seizures, transient focal deficit, coma	Ischemic cardiovascular disease, permanent neurologic deficits	Gastrin, glucagon, PP, somatostatin, GRH	10%	Occasional	10%
Gastrinoma	Peptic ulcers, enhanced acid secretion	Diarrhea, malabsorption, weight loss, dumping	ACTH, insulin, glucagon, VIP, 5-HIAA, MSH, somatostatin, calcitonin, PP	40–60%	10%	25%
VIPoma	Watery diarrhea, hypokalemia, hypochlorhydria	Hypercalcemia, hyperglycemia, weakness, hypomagnesemia	PHM, PP, prostaglandins(?), GRH, gastrin	40%	20%	Rare
Glucagonoma	Rash, diabetes, weight loss, anemia	Diarrhea, abdominal pain, thromboembolic disease	PP, VIP, 5-HIAA, gastrin, insulin	60%	Occasional	Occasional
Somatostatinoma	Diabetes, cholelithiasis, steatorrhea, malabsorption, weight loss	Indigestion, abdominal pain, anemia, diarrhea, ductal obstruction, hypoglycemia	ACTH, gastrin, calcitonin, PGE_2, glucagon, GRH, PP, VIP, 5-HIAA, substance P	66%	None reported	One case (MEN 3)
PPoma	None	Watery diarrhea, hypocalcemia, achlorhydria, abdominal pain, weight loss	Glucagon, insulin, somatostatin, VIP	40%	Occasional	25%

[1]Reproduced, with permission, from Wyngaarden JB, Smith LH Jr, Bennett JC (editors): *Cecil Textbook of Medicine,* 19th ed. Saunders, 1992.

Key: ACTH = adrenocorticotropic hormone
GRH = growth hormone-releasing hormone
5-HIAA = 5-hydroxyindoleacetic acid
MEN = multiple endocrine neoplasia
MSH = melanocyte-stimulating hormone
PGE_2 = prostaglandin E_2
PHM = peptide histidine methionine
PP = pancreatic polypeptide
VIP = vasoactive intestinal polypeptide

diagnostic of an insulin-mediated cause of hypoglycemia.

Causes of insulin-mediated hypoglycemia other than insulinoma include **surreptitious injection of insulin** or ingestion of oral hypoglycemic medications that stimulate endogenous insulin (**sulfonylureas**) or the presence of **insulin antibodies.** Binding of insulin to the antibodies prevents insulin action but still allows detection of insulin by most assays; release of insulin at an inappropriate time results in hypoglycemia. Surreptitious insulin administration can be ruled out by C peptide measurements. Since insulin and C peptide are cosecreted, insulinomas will cause elevations in both, while elevated levels of exogenous insulin will not be matched by elevations of C peptide in surreptitious injections of insulin. Similarly, insulin antibodies do not result in elevated C peptide levels. Since sulfonylurea drugs stimulate endogenous insulin (and therefore C peptide) secretion, insulinoma and inappropriate ingestion of these agents can only be differentiated by measuring drug levels.

42. What are the common clinical manifestations of insulinoma?
43. How can surreptitious insulin injection be ruled out?

OTHER HORMONE-SECRETING PANCREATIC TUMORS

1. GLUCAGONOMA

Glucagonomas are usually diagnosed by the appearance of a characteristic rash in middle-aged individuals with mild diabetes mellitus (Table 18–11). Glucagon levels are usually increased tenfold relative to normal values but can even be increased 100-fold.

Necrolytic migratory erythema begins as an erythematous rash on the face, abdomen, perineum, or lower extremities. Following the development of induration with central blistering, the lesions crust over and then resolve, leaving an area of hyperpigmentation. These lesions may be the result of nutritional deficiency, such as the hypoaminoacidemia that occurs due to excessive glucagon stimulation of hepatic amino acid uptake and utilization as fuel for gluconeogenesis, rather than the direct effect of glucagon on the skin. Appearance of the rash is a late manifestation of the disease.

Diabetes mellitus or glucose intolerance is present in the vast majority of patients due to increased stimulation of hepatic glucose output by the inappropriately high glucagon levels. Insulin levels are secondarily increased. Diabetes is therefore mild and is not accompanied by glucagon-stimulated ketosis, since sufficient insulin is present to suppress lipolysis, thus limiting potential substrates for ketogenesis.

Anemia and a variety of nonspecific gastrointestinal symptoms related to decreased intestinal motility also can accompany glucagonomas.

While these tumors are solitary and their growth is slow, they are usually large and have often metastasized by the time of diagnosis, making surgical resection difficult. Octreotide, the synthetic somatostatin analogue, can be used to ameliorate symptoms via its suppression of glucagon secretion.

2. SOMATOSTATINOMA

Somatostatinomas present with a variety of gastrointestinal symptoms in individuals with mild diabetes. However, these extremely rare tumors are almost uniformly found incidentally during operations for cholelithiasis or other abdominal complaints since the presenting symptoms are both nonspecific and commonplace in an adult population. Documentation of elevated somatostatin levels confirms the diagnosis.

A **classic triad** of symptoms frequently occurs with excessive somatostatin secretion: **diabetes mellitus,** due to its inhibition of insulin and glucagon secretion; **cholelithiasis,** due to its inhibition of gallbladder motility; and **steatorrhea,** due to its inhibition of pancreatic exocrine function. Hypochlorhydria, diarrhea, and anemia can also occur.

In type 1 and type 2 diabetes, the effects of insulin insufficiency are aggravated by the occurrence of elevated glucagon levels. In contrast, with somatostatinomas, both insulin and glucagon are suppressed. Therefore, the hyperglycemia resulting from insulinopenia is tempered by the absence of glucagon stimulation of hepatic glucose output. Although low insulin levels are permissive for lipolysis, glucagon deficiency prevents hepatic ketogenesis. The diabetes associated with somatostatinomas is therefore mild and not ketosis-prone.

While the majority of somatostatinomas occur in the pancreas, a significant number are found in the duodenum or jejunum. Like glucagonomas, somatostatinomas are often solitary and large and have frequently metastasized by the time of diagnosis.

---

44. What are the characteristic findings in a patient with glucagonoma?
45. What is the classic triad of findings in a patient with somatostatinoma?

REFERENCES

General
Cryer PE: Hierarchy of physiological responses to hypoglycemia. Horm Metab Res 1997;29:92.

Diabetes Mellitus
The Diabetes Control and Complications Trial Research Group: The effect of intensive treatment of diabetes on the development and progression of long-term complications in insulin-dependent diabetes mellitus. N Engl J Med 1993;329:973.

Aiello LP et al: Diabetic retinopathy. Diabetes Care 1998;21:143.

Caputo GM et al: Assessment and management of foot disease in patients with diabetes. N Engl J Med 1994;331:854.

DeFronzo RA: Diabetic nephropathy: Etiologic and therapeutic considerations. Diabetes Rev 1995;3:510.

Expert Committee on the Diagnosis and Classification of Diabetes Mellitus: Report of the Expert Committee on the Diagnosis and Classification of Diabetes Mellitus. Diabetes Care 1998;21:S5.

Goldberg RB: Prevention of type 2 diabetes. Med Clin North Am 1998;82:805.

Haffner SM: The insulin resistance syndrome revisited. Diabetes Care 1996;19:275.

Haffner, SM: Management of dyslipidemia in adults with diabetes. Diabetes Care 1998;21:160.

Harris MI et al: Prevalence of diabetes, impaired fasting glucose, and impaired glucose tolerance in U.S. adults: The Third National Health and Nutrition Examination Survey, 1988–1994. Diabetes Care 1998; 21:518.

Howard BV et al: Adverse effects of diabetes on multiple cardiovascular disease risk factors in women: The Strong Heart Study. Diabetes Care 1998;21:1258.

Kuhl C: Etiology and pathogenesis of gestational diabetes. Diabetes Care 1998;21(Suppl 2):B19.

Lebovitz HE: Diabetic ketoacidosis. Lancet 1995;345: 767.

Moller DE, Bjorbaek C, Vidal-Puig A: Candidate genes for insulin resistance. Diabetes Care 1996;19:396.

Porte D, Sherwin RS (editors): *Ellenberg and Rifkin's Diabetes Mellitus: Theory and Practice,* 5th ed. Elsevier, 1997.

Rabinovitch A, Skyler JA: Prevention of type 1 diabetes. Med Clin North Am 1998;82:739.

UK Prospective Diabetes Study (UKPDS) Group: Intensive blood glucose control with sulphonylureas or insulin compared with conventional treatment and risk of complications in patients with type 2 diabetes (UKPDS 33). Lancet 1998;352:837.

Insulinoma, Glucagonoma, and Somatostatinoma

Drucker DJ: Glucagon-like peptides. Diabetes 1998;47: 159.

Lamberts SW et al: Octreotide. N Engl J Med 1996;334: 246.

Lefèbvre PJ: Glucagon and its family revisited. Diabetes Care 1995;18:715.

Perry RR, Vinik AI: Clinical review 72: Diagnosis and management of functioning islet cell tumors. J Clin Endocrinol Metab 1995;80:2273.

Reisine T, Bell GI: Molecular properties of somatostatin receptors. Neuroscience 1995;67:777.

Service FJ: Insulinoma and other islet-cell tumors. Cancer Treat Res 1997;89:335.

Disorders of the Hypothalamus & Pituitary Gland

19

Vishwanath R. Lingappa, MD, PhD

The hypothalamus is the part of the brain where activity of the autonomic nervous system and endocrine glands, which directly control various organ systems of the body, is integrated with input from higher centers that give rise to emotions and behavior. The hypothalamus thus serves to ensure (1) that the organism responds appropriately to deviations from various internal set points (including set points for temperature, volume, osmolality, satiety, and body fat content); (2) that the responses to such deviations from a set point include coordinated activity of the nervous and endocrine systems; and (3) that the emotions and behavior being manifested are appropriate for reflex responses being triggered to correct the deviations from internal set points. For example, in response to intravascular volume loss due to any cause, autonomic neural responses retain fluid and electrolytes, maintain blood pressure through vascular smooth muscle contraction, and maintain cardiac output by increasing heart rate. The effect of these immediate neural responses is reinforced by the action of hormones (vasopressin and aldosterone in retaining fluid and electrolytes and catecholamines in maintaining blood pressure and cardiac output). In this instance, a fully appropriate response depends on whether the intravascular volume loss was due to dehydration from fluid deprivation or from bleeding after an attack by a predator. Both would be associated with feelings of thirst, but in the latter instance the desire to search for something to drink would probably be suppressed either by fear and the desire to escape or by anger and the desire to fight.

The pituitary gland is the partner to the hypothalamus on the body side of the mind-body interface. Once viewed as the "master gland" in regulation of neuroendocrine systems, the pituitary is now known to be a "middle manager" responding to input from both the brain (via the hypothalamus) and the body (via the various peripheral endocrine glands).

The basic framework for hypothalamic-pituitary function is the **neuroendocrine axis,** a cascade of interacting products from regions of the central nervous system to the hypothalamus, the anterior pituitary gland, endocrine end organs, and peripheral target tissues, in that order. Some neuroendocrine axes involve hormones released by the hypothalamus that stimulate cells in the anterior pituitary to secrete other hormones into the systemic circulation. Each of these anterior pituitary hormones travels to a distant endocrine gland to stimulate secretion of yet other hormones that affect various target tissues. Thus, disorders of the hypothalamus and pituitary have important consequences for the pathophysiologic mechanisms of a wide range of disorders involving many different tissues and organs.

This chapter focuses on five clinical entities. The first, obesity, is one in which the hypothalamus plays a crucial role and which has enormous implications for diseases involving many other organ systems. The remaining four problems reflect the diversity of pituitary disease: pituitary adenomas, panhypopituitarism, vasopressin excess, and vasopressin deficiency.

NORMAL STRUCTURE & FUNCTION OF THE HYPOTHALAMUS & PITUITARY GLAND

Anatomy, Histology, & Cell Biology

The hypothalamus is a poorly demarcated region located in the floor and lateral walls of the third ventricle and comprising about 1% of the mass of the brain (Figure 19–1). Hypothalamic nuclei are clusters of neurons whose cell bodies lie in discrete regions (Figure 19–2). From these nuclei, hypothalamic neurons send projections to other parts of the central and peripheral nervous systems and secrete hormones that make possible the hierarchical control of various physiologic processes (see Table 19–1).

The hypothalamus is connected to the pituitary

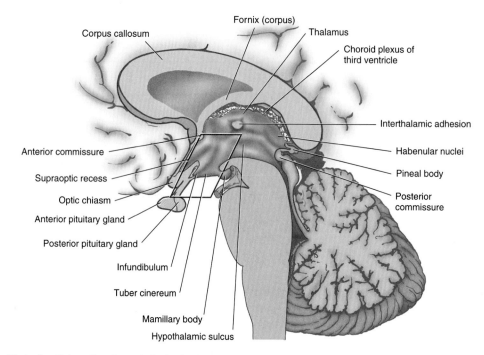

Figure 19–1. Sagittal section through the brain showing the diencephalon. (Reproduced, with permission, from Chusid JG: *Correlative Neuroanatomy and Functional Neurology,* 19th ed. Lange, 1985.)

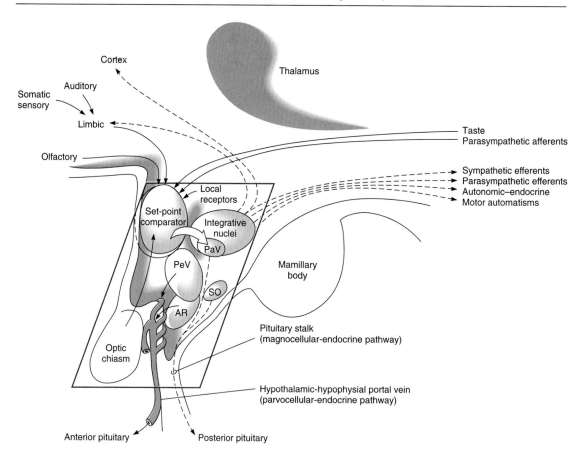

Figure 19–2. Functional organization of the hypothalamus. AR, arcuate nucleus; PaV, paraventricular nucleus; PeV, periventricular nucleus; SO, supraoptic nucleus. (Reproduced, with permission, from Saper CB: Hypothalamus. In: *Neurobiology of Disease.* Pearlman AL, Collins RC [editors]. Oxford Univ Press, 1990.)

Table 19–1. Functions of hypothalamic nuclei.[1]

Hypothalamic Region	Location and Description	Function
Periventricular zone	Most medial part of the hypothalamus; adjacent to third ventricle	Production of releasing factors for anterior pituitary hormones
Paraventricular and supraoptic nuclei	Medial zone (just lateral to periventricular zone)	Production of oxytocin and vasopressin stored in posterior pituitary
Medial preoptic nucleus, dorsomedial, ventromedial, premamillary, anterior and posterior hypothalamic nuclei	Medial zone	Controlling behavior for homeostasis
Medial forebrain bundle	Lateral zone tracts	Connect cells of the hypothalamic nuclei to both the brain stem and the forebrain
Anterior hypothalamic and preoptic areas	Anterior third of the hypothalamus	Integration of fluid and electrolyte, thermoregulatory, and nonendocrine reproductive functions
Tuberal region	Middle third of hypothalamus just posterior to the anterior area; gives rise to the pituitary stalk	Contain nuclei responsible for the endocrine and autonomic regulatory mechanisms and integration of energy, metabolic, and reproductive responses
Posterior, lateral, and premamillary nuclei	Posterior third of the hypothalamus	Involved in thermoregulatory and emergency response integration

[1]Reproduced, with permission, from Saper CB: Hypothalamus. In: *Neurobiology of Disease.* Pearlman AL, Collins RC (editors). Oxford Univ Press, 1990.

gland by a stalk at the base of the brain. Axons of some hypothalamic neurons travel down the pituitary stalk, and their endings comprise the posterior pituitary gland. Embryologically distinct from the anterior lobe (Figures 19–3 and 19–4), the posterior pituitary neurons secrete the peptide hormones, oxytocin and vasopressin, directly into the systemic circulation. The distinct anterior and posterior lobes of the pituitary gland are encased in a tough fibrous capsule, the sella turcica. The pituitary gland is bounded above by the optic chiasm and laterally by the cavernous sinus and the structures that traverse it (internal carotid artery, cranial nerves III, IV, first and second divisions of V, and VI).

In parts of the hypothalamus, the capillaries are fenestrated. As a result, the blood-brain barrier is not intact at all locations, and the brain has unimpeded access to blood. Some hypothalamic neurons are involved in sensing various specific chemical stimuli in the bloodstream. These sensory neurons transmit the information regarding changes in stimuli (eg, change in temperature, osmolality, volume) to other hypothalamic neurons involved in a variety of specific types of secretory activities.

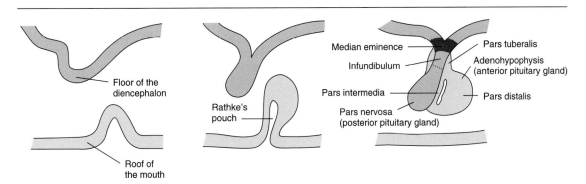

Figure 19–3. Diagram of the development of the adenohypophysis and neurohypophysis. The ectoderm of the roof of the mouth and its derivatives is shown in light color (lower portion). The upper portion (dark color) shows the neural ectoderm from the floor of the diencephalon. (Reproduced, with permission, from Junqueira LC, Carneiro J, Kelley RO: *Basic Histology,* 9th ed. Appleton & Lange, 1998.)

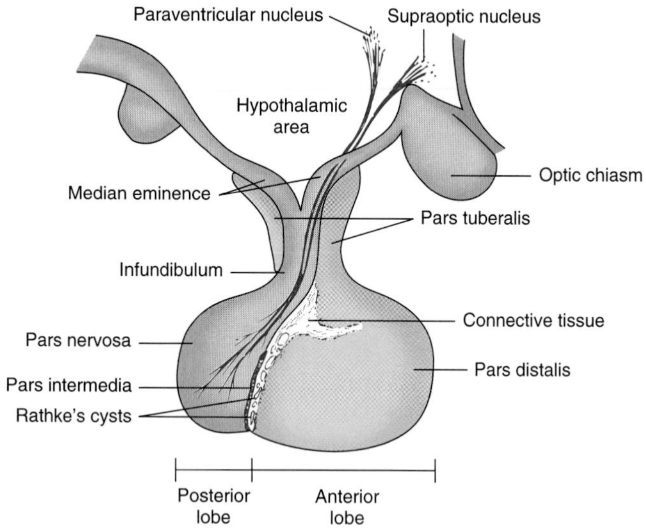

Figure 19–4. The component parts of the pituitary and their relationship to the hypothalamus. The pars tuberalis, pars distalis, and pars intermedia, which is rudimentary in humans, form the adenohypophysis. The infundibulum and pars nervosa form the neurohypophysis. (Modified, redrawn, and reproduced, with permission, from the *Ciba Collection of Medical Illustrations,* by Frank H. Netter, MD.)

Other hypothalamic neurons secrete peptide hormones into a specialized capillary bed termed the **pituitary portal system** (Figure 19–5). Blood in this capillary system flows directly from the median eminence to the anterior pituitary gland, where specific cells that display receptors for the various hypothalamic hormones are found. Thus, the secretion of specific anterior pituitary hormones is stimulated. The cells of the anterior pituitary are thus bathed in blood rich in the hypothalamic hormones, without the dilution that would occur in the systemic circulation. This intimate connection between hypothalamus and pituitary has important pathophysiologic consequences (see below).

Once secreted, the anterior pituitary hormones travel via the bloodstream throughout the body and trigger the release of yet other hormones from particular endocrine glands. These hormones in turn have effects on target tissues that influence growth, reproduction, metabolism, and response to stress. In addition to their effects on target tissues, hormones secreted in response to stimulation by pituitary hormones also feed back and inhibit secretion of the corresponding pituitary and hypothalamic hormones.

The posterior pituitary hormones are involved in a very different type of neuroendocrine axis, one that bypasses the pituitary and the peripheral endocrine glands and affects peripheral target tissues directly.

While most peptide factors secreted by the hypothalamus cause release of a pituitary hormone, some are inhibitory factors that block or diminish secretion of particular hormones. The anterior pituitary consists of cells each of which produces and secretes one of five families of hormones: pro-opiomelanocortin and adrenocorticotropic hormone (ACTH), thyrotropin (TSH), growth hormone (GH), prolactin (PRL), and the gonadotropins (LH and FSH).

In addition to their roles in regulation of neuroendocrine axes, some hypothalamic and pituitary hormones are important—but poorly understood—regulators of immune functions and the inflammatory response. Furthermore, secretion of hypothalamic and pituitary hormones can be significantly influenced by cytokines that regulate the immune response.

1. What is the role of the hypothalamus?
2. What are the neuroendocrine axes, and how do they work?
3. What structures surround the pituitary?
4. Where do the neurons whose axons comprise the posterior pituitary originate?

PHYSIOLOGY OF THE HYPOTHALAMUS & PITUITARY GLAND

1. ANTERIOR PITUITARY HORMONES

Pro-opiomelanocortin & ACTH

In response to a variety of indicators of stress, the hypothalamus releases corticotropin-releasing hormone (CRH) into the pituitary portal system. CRH triggers synthesis and intracellular transport of a large protein termed pro-opiomelanocortin (POMC). During intracellular transport, POMC is processed by proteases to release smaller peptides, including a 39-amino-acid residue peptide, adrenocorticotropin hormone (ACTH) (Figure 19–6). ACTH triggers synthesis and secretion of the corticosteroids from the adrenal cortex: glucocorticoids, androgens, and, to some extent, mineralocorticoids (see Chapter 21).

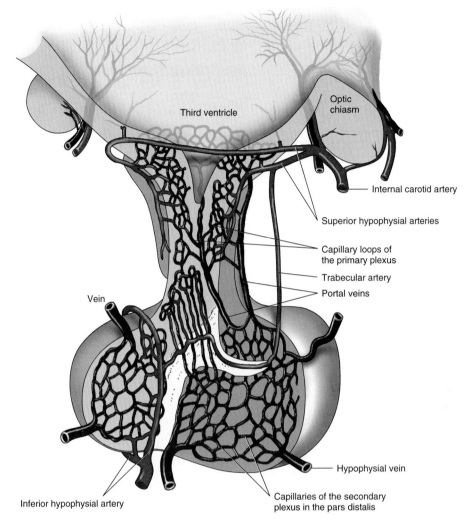

Figure 19–5. Diagram of the blood circulation in the pituitary, including the portal system. (Redrawn and reproduced, with permission, from the *Ciba Collection of Medical Illustrations,* by Frank H. Netter, MD.)

These steroid hormones in turn have complex effects on many tissues to protect the animal from stress— they raise blood pressure and blood glucose, alter responsiveness of the immune system, etc. Glucocorticoids also feed back to the hypothalamus, where they inhibit CRH secretion, and to the pituitary, where they further inhibit ACTH secretion. In the absence of unusual stress, there is a daily diurnal rhythm of CRH, ACTH, and adrenal steroid release.

In addition to stimulating synthesis and secretion of corticosteroids, ACTH stimulates growth of the glucocorticoid and androgen-secreting layers of the adrenal cortex. Thus, conditions in which there are large amounts of circulating CRH or ACTH produce hypertrophy of the target organ (adrenal cortex). Conversely, conditions that down-regulate the axis (eg, oral glucocorticoids) result in atrophy of the adrenal cortex because they reduce ACTH secretion to less than its normal diurnal levels (Chapter 21). On the other hand, ACTH has little or no effect on the growth of mineralocorticoid-secreting tissues of the adrenal cortex, despite the fact that it does trigger acute release of mineralocorticoids.

Thyrotropin (TSH)

Thyrotropin is released from specific cells in the pituitary upon stimulation by thyrotropin-releasing hormone (TRH) from the hypothalamus. TSH in turn travels via the systemic bloodstream to the thyroid gland, where it stimulates synthesis and secretion of the thyroid hormones thyroxine and triiodothyronine. Thyroid hormone has effects on nearly every tissue in the body but especially the cardiovascular, respiratory, skeletal, and central nervous systems. Thyroid

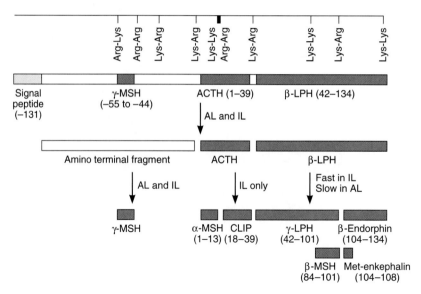

Figure 19–6. Schematic representation of the prepro-opiomelanocortin molecule formed in pituitary cells, neurons, and other tissues. The numbers in parentheses identify the amino acid sequences in each of the polypeptide fragments. For convenience, the amino acid sequences are numbered from the amino terminal of ACTH and read toward the carboxyl terminal portion of the parent molecule, whereas the amino acid sequences in the other portion of the molecule read to the left to –131, the amino terminal of the parent molecule. The locations of Lys-Arg and other pairs of basic amino acids residues are also indicated; these are the sites of proteolytic cleavage in the formation of the smaller fragments of the parent molecule. AL, anterior lobe; IL, intermediate lobe. (Reproduced, with permission, from Ganong WF: *Review of Medical Physiology,* 19th ed. Appleton & Lange, 1999.)

hormones are critical at key points in development, and their deficiency during development has effects—such as severe mental retardation and short stature—that are not reversible by subsequent thyroid hormone administration (Chapter 20).

Thyroxine undergoes an important metabolic modification in peripheral tissues, ie, removal of one of the four covalently attached iodine molecules. Depending on which iodine is removed, thyroid hormone activity is increased tenfold (removal of an iodine in the 5' position of thyroxine to form triiodothyronine [T_3]) or abolished (removal of an iodine in the 5 position to form the biologically inactive reverse T_3). In severe illness, patients can have depressed T_4 and T_3 levels, with increased conversion to other thyroid hormone metabolites. This appears to be a physiologic response and does not require thyroid hormone replacement therapy. Besides its target tissue effects, thyroid hormone feeds back onto the pituitary and hypothalamus to inhibit secretion of TSH and TRH. TSH also triggers growth of thyroid tissue, resulting in goiter under conditions of chronic TSH stimulation (see Chapter 20).

Gonadotropins

LH and FSH are glycoprotein hormones each containing two subunits that are released by specific cells of the anterior pituitary termed gonadotrophs. The alpha subunits of LH and FSH (and TSH) and the placental hormone hCG are identical, while the beta subunits differ from each other and are responsible for the biologic differences between these hormones.

The role of the gonadotropins is to regulate the reproductive system's neuroendocrine axis. Thus, a releasing factor from the hypothalamus termed gonadotropin-releasing hormone (GnRH) stimulates LH and FSH secretion, which stimulates steroidogenesis within the ovaries and testes. The steroids produced by the ovaries (estrogens) and by the testes (testosterone) inhibit GnRH, LH, and FSH production and have target tissue effects on developing follicles within the ovary itself, on the uterus (controlling the menstrual cycle), on breast development, on spermatogenesis, and on many other tissues and physiologic processes (see Chapters 22 and 23).

As is the case with all neuroendocrine axes, the simple feedback loop is complicated by other inputs (eg, from the central nervous system) that modify responsiveness (Chapter 7). A notable feature for many hypothalamic releasing factors—but particularly GnRH—is that secretion occurs in pulsatile fashion and that changes in the rate and amplitude of secretion result in altered pituitary responsiveness due to down- or up-regulation of the receptors for the hypothalamic releasing factors found on the surface of the pituitary cells.

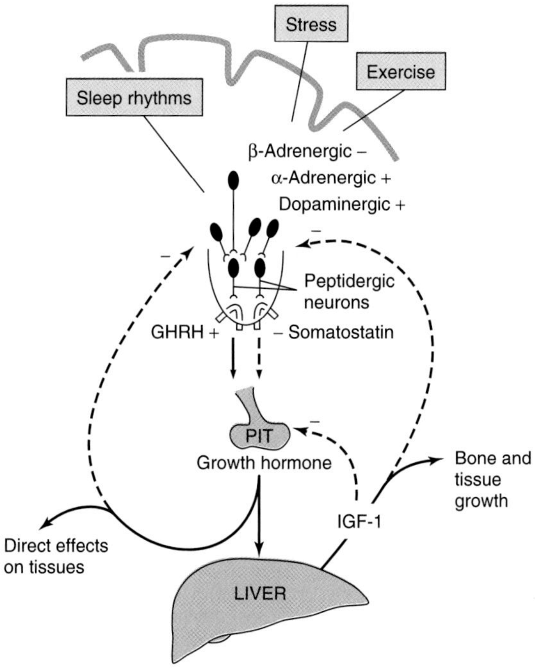

Growth Hormone & Prolactin

Growth hormone and prolactin are structurally related single-chain polypeptides with different spectrums of action.

A. Growth Hormone: Growth hormone (GH), regulated by hypothalamic growth hormone-releasing hormone (GHRH) and somatostatin, triggers growth-promoting effects in a wide range of tissues (Figure 19–7). GH has direct actions (eg, stimulating the growth of cartilage) as well as indirect ones (eg, via insulin-like growth factor-1 [IGF-1], a polypeptide secreted by the liver and other tissues (Figures 19–8 and 19–9). IGF-1 has insulin-like effects of promoting fuel storage in various tissues. IGF-1 in turn inhibits GHRH and GH secretion. As in the other neuroendocrine feedback axes, the central nervous system and other factors can significantly influence the simple regulatory axis (Figure 19–7; Table 19–2).

Many of the direct actions of GH appear to have a "counterregulatory" character in that they raise blood glucose levels and antagonize the action of insulin. In contrast, the indirect actions of GH via IGF-1 are insulin-like. This apparent contradiction makes sense when you consider that promoting growth requires first raising blood levels of substrates and then using them for synthesis and growth (Figure 19–9). To do the latter without the former would simply make the individual hypoglycemic without promoting long-term growth.

Figure 19–7. Schematic diagram of the hypothalamic control of growth hormone secretion. Inhibitory arrows are dashed; stimulating ones are solid. (Modified from Reichlin S: Neuroendocrinology. In: *Williams Textbook of Endocrinology,* 9th ed. Wilson JD et al [editors]. Saunders, 1998.)

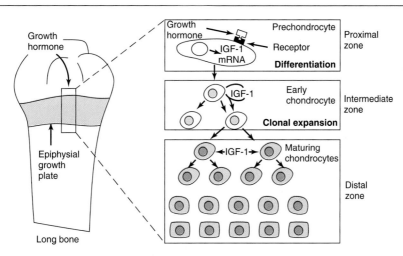

Figure 19–8. Growth hormone acts directly at the epiphysial plate to stimulate linear growth. Growth hormone stimulates differentiation of prechondrocytes into early chondrocytes, which then secrete IGF-1. In turn, IGF-1 stimulates clonal expansion and maturation of chondrocytes. (Modified by Thorner MO et al: The anterior pituitary. In: *Williams Textbook of Endocrinology,* 9th ed. Wilson JD et al [editors]. Saunders, 1998; and from Isakson OPG et al: Direct action of growth hormone. In: *Basic and Clinical Aspects of Growth Hormone.* Plenum, 1988.)

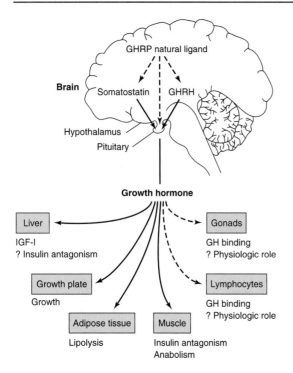

Figure 19–9. Schematic representation of multiple sites of GH action. (Reproduced, with permission, from Thorner MO et al: The anterior pituitary. In: *Williams Textbook of Endocrinology,* 9th ed. Wilson JD et al [editors]. Saunders, 1998.)

B. Prolactin: The primary role of prolactin in humans is to stimulate breast development and milk synthesis. It is discussed in greater detail in Chapter 22. Prolactin secretion is regulated by the neurotransmitter dopamine from the hypothalamus rather than by a peptide. Furthermore, dopamine acts to inhibit rather than to stimulate prolactin secretion. Pathologic processes that result in separation of the pituitary gland from the hypothalamus cause loss of all pituitary hormones except prolactin (**panhypopituitarism** from lack of the hypothalamic releasing hormones). Loss of dopamine results instead in an increase in prolactin secretion from specific anterior pituitary cells now freed of inhibition by dopamine.

Prolactin may also play a role as a regulator of immune functions.

2. POSTERIOR PITUITARY HORMONES

Vasopressin & Oxytocin

The peptide hormones vasopressin and oxytocin are synthesized in the supraoptic and paraventricular nuclei of the hypothalamus. The axons of the neurons in these nuclei form the posterior pituitary, where these peptide hormones are stored. Thus there is no need for a separate set of hypothalamic releasing factors to trigger vasopressin or oxytocin release.

A. Vasopressin: In response to physiologic stimuli (eg, a small increase in blood osmolality), the hypothalamic "osmostats" responds by triggering the

Table 19–2. Factors influencing normal growth hormone secretion.[1]

Factor	Augmented Secretion	Inhibited Secretion
Neurogenic	Stage III and stage IV sleep Stress (traumatic, surgical, inflammatory, psychic) Alpha-adrenergic agonists Beta-adrenergic antagonists Dopamine agonists Acetylcholine agonists	REM sleep Alpha-adrenergic antagonists Beta-adrenergic agonists Acetylcholine antagonists
Metabolic	Hypoglycemia Fasting Falling fatty acid level Amino acids Uncontrolled diabetes mellitus Uremia Hepatic cirrhosis	Hyperglycemia Rising fatty acid level Obesity
Hormonal	GHRH Low insulin-like growth factor Estrogens Glucagon Arginine vasopressin	Somatostatin High insulin-like growth factor Hypothyroidism High glucocorticoid levels

[1]Reproduced, with permission, from Thorner MO et al: The anterior pituitary. In: *Williams Textbook of Endocrinology,* 9th ed. Wilson JD et al (editors). Saunders, 1998.

subjective sense of thirst and at the same time the release of vasopressin. Vasopressin increases the number of active water channels in the renal collecting tubules, allowing conservation of free water that would otherwise be lost in the urine, thus increasing the concentration of the urine. Conservation of free water and stimulation of thirst have the net effect of correcting the small change in blood osmolality. While the minute-to-minute function of vasopressin is to maintain blood osmolality, its secretion is also increased by large decreases in intravascular volume.

Vasopressin binds to at least three classes of receptors. One of these classes of vasopressin receptors (V_{1A}) is found on smooth muscle. Its major effect is to trigger vasoconstriction. V_{1B} receptors are found on corticotrophs, and they mediate increased ACTH secretion. The other class of receptors (V_2) is found in the distal nephrons in the kidneys; its major action is to mediate vasopressin's effects on osmolality. Because of its V_2-mediated actions, vasopressin is also known as **antidiuretic hormone (ADH).** The combination of peripheral vasoconstriction and water retention can be understood as a way of ensuring that perfusion of critical organs is maintained in the face of major intravascular volume deficits—even if the volume and osmolar composition of the perfusing blood is not ideal. The relationship between osmotic forces, volume, and vasopressin secretion is illustrated in Figure 19–10).

Another possible effect of vasopressin is alteration of immune functions.

B. Oxytocin: Like vasopressin, this peptide is stored in nerve terminals of hypothalamic neurons in the posterior pituitary. It plays an important role in smooth muscle contraction both on a minute-to-minute basis during breast feeding and in contraction of the uterus during parturition.

---

5. How do neuroendocrine feedback loops of the anterior and posterior pituitary differ?
6. How can two polypeptide hormones whose mature forms have no sequence in common be derived from the same precursor?
7. Describe the distinguishing features of each pituitary neurendocrine feedback axis.
8. What is the significance of receptor down-regulation for hypothalamic control of pituitary function?

PHYSIOLOGY OF THE NEUROENDOCRINE AXIS

A number of features of neuroendocrine axis physiology have important implications for the pathophysiology of disease.

First, the hypothalamic hormones that traverse the pituitary portal system are short-lived. They also have relatively low affinities for their receptors. These properties are generally more characteristic of neurotransmitters in the nervous system than of hormones in the bloodstream. Some of these hormones—and the receptor systems with which they interact—have evolved in ways that take advantage of the unique features of a neuroendocrine axis. For example, in the case of GnRH, secretion is markedly pulsatile in character, with a particular rate and amplitude of hypothalamic hormone secretion being crucial for a proper response by the receptor-bearing gonadotrophs. If the pulse rate or amplitude is too high, the receptors are down-regulated.

Second, for some of the neuroendocrine axes, measurement of a random blood level of the end-organ hormone is not generally clinically useful. A more reliable approach to assessment of neuroendocrine axis function is often to assess the secretory response to a provocative stimulus, or **challenge test.** Thus, an adequate increase in blood cortisol 1 hour after an intravenous injection of ACTH provides far more compelling evidence for an intact adrenal gland than does a randomly drawn, unprovoked normal blood level of cortisol. Measurement of growth hormone is similarly best done after a provocative stimulus.

Finally, besides stimulating end-organ hormone secretion, most of the pituitary hormones exert trophic

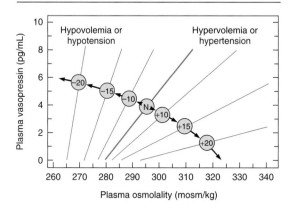

Figure 19–10. The influence of hemodynamic status on the osmoregulation of vasopressin in otherwise healthy humans. The numbers in the center circles refer to the percentage change in volume or pressure: N refers to the normovolemic normotensive subject. Note that the hemodynamic status affects both the slope of the relationship between the plasma vasopressin and osmolality and the osmotic threshold for vasopressin release. (Adapted from Robertson GL, Shelton RL, Athar S: The osmoregulation of vasopressin. Kidney Int 1976;10:25. Adapted by Rose BD in: *Clinical Physiology of Acid-Base and Electrolyte Disorders*, 3rd ed. McGraw-Hill, 1989. Reprinted with permission from Kidney International.)

effects on the hormone-secreting cells of the end organ. Thus, excess of pituitary hormone results in end-organ hypertrophy and lack of the pituitary hormone results in end-organ atrophy.

4. PHYSIOLOGY OF BODY WEIGHT CONTROL

Various physiologic control mechanisms integrated by the hypothalamus work to maintain body weight over the short and long term (Figure 19–11).

The key parameters of short-term regulation of body weight are (1) the amount and composition of food; (2) nutrient absorption and assimilation; and (3) satiety, the sense of having eaten enough food. Satiety is a complex response to food intake that has mechanical, neural, and hormonal components. Thus, we feel a sense of fullness in response to mechanical distention of the stomach, which triggers afferent neural pathways to the hypothalamus. In addition, hormones such as cholecystokinin are secreted in response to food ingestion and absorption and have direct effects on the hypothalamus to induce satiety.

In contrast to short-term control of body weight, long-term regulation is largely influenced by the degree of obesity. Fat cells secrete a protein hormone called leptin in proportion to the amount of triglyceride they have stored. Thus, over the long term, excess ingestion of calories resulting in increased fat deposition triggers an increase in leptin secretion.

Leptin impinges on its receptors in the hypothalamus to alter the set point at which satiety is reached, so that the individual eats less and therefore assimilates fewer calories. Another response to leptin is to increase sympathetic nervous system activity so that more calories are burned. There may also be effects of leptin outside of the brain that reinforce the central effects and thereby contribute to the body's corrective response to weight gain.

Conversely, when caloric intake is insufficient to maintain body weight, fat is mobilized, leptin secretion goes down, and set points in the hypothalamus are changed in ways that promote food-seeking behavior, diminish sympathetic neural activity, and generally conserve calories to offset the tendency toward weight loss. As a result of this feedback loop, further decrease in body weight is resisted. It is likely that this system evolved primarily as a defense against starvation, but it also serves to defend against obesity.

How these signals are normally integrated in the hypothalamus to achieve satiety in the short term and maintain normal body weight in the long term is an area of ongoing investigation. It appears that two regions of the hypothalamus are involved: Lesions in the ventromedial region result in obesity, and lesions in the lateral hypothalamus result in weight loss. One hypothesis attempting to integrate current information on the regulation of fuel homeostasis proposes different responses by the body to falling versus rising leptin concentrations—as would be seen in

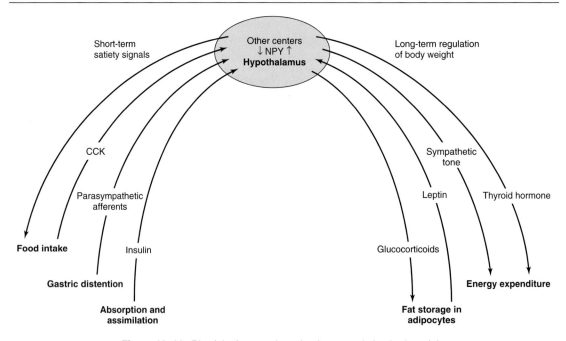

Figure 19–11. Physiologic control mechanisms regulating body weight.

weight loss versus weight gain, respectively. Thus, in response to falling leptin levels, neuropeptide Y is secreted from leptin receptor-bearing cells of the arcuate nucleus in the ventromedial hypothalamus. Neuropeptide Y is believed to mediate hypothalamic responses to starvation (see below).

A different set of neuropeptides is released in response to rising leptin concentrations, as would normally occur in response to weight gain. It appears that a subtype of melanocortin (MC) receptors (MC-4) responds to elevated leptin either by increased agonist peptides such as melanocyte-stimulating hormone or by decreased antagonist peptides. Increased signaling through the MC-4 receptor then mediates hypothalamic responses such as decreased food intake, increased sympathetic nervous system activity, and increased energy expenditure through pathways that affect glucocorticoids and thyroid hormone.

Exactly how these two feedback loops—one responding to rising leptin concentrations and the other to falling leptin concentrations—are normally integrated remains to be determined. Furthermore, it is believed that many other neuropeptides, including bombesin, insulin, and a group of peptides termed orexins, have complex effects on the hypothalamus that affect feeding, satiety, energy balance, and other parameters relevant for weight control. The orexins appear to be ligands for previously "orphan" G protein-coupled receptors in the brain. How the effects of these peptides are integrated with those of leptin and neuropeptide Y is currently unknown.

---

9. What are the short- and long-term factors involved in normal control of body weight?
10. What is the significance of the short half-life, low affinity, and restricted circulation of most hypothalamic hormones?
11. Why are challenge tests particularly important in assessing function of a neuroendocrine axis?
12. What happens to an end organ in the absence of the pituitary hormone that normally triggers its secretion?

PATHOPHYSIOLOGY OF SELECTED HYPOTHALAMIC & PITUITARY DISEASES

New studies have implicated the hypothalamus or pituitary gland in the pathophysiology of a variety of complex diseases with major behavioral components. These include anxiety disorders, where abnormalities of the hypothalamic-pituitary-growth hormone axis appear to be a specific pathologic marker; alcoholism, where neuropeptide Y has been implicated in mouse models of this condition; and obesity, where a host of hypothalamic neuropeptides are affected and in turn affect parameters of fuel homeostasis. We will focus our discussion on obesity, the disorder about which our understanding is most advanced.

OBESITY

Changes in body weight can occur through alteration of several variables, including (1) the amount and type of food ingested, (2) the central control of satiety, (3) hormonal control of assimilation or storage, and (4) physical activity or metabolic rate.

Clinical Presentation & Etiology

Obesity can be defined as excess body weight sufficient to increase overall morbidity and mortality. While extreme obesity is associated with dramatically increased mortality, the risks of mild to moderate obesity are less clear. When individuals are assessed with respect to height and weight in a way that some believe measures "fatness"—body mass index (BMI) = weight (in kilograms) divided by height (in meters squared), with normal being $18.5–25$ kg/m^2—and clinically significant obesity being a BMI > 30 kg/m^2, it is observed that over 20% of the United States population is obese. Individuals with a BMI 150% of normal have an overall twofold risk of premature death, while those that are 200% of normal BMI have a tenfold risk. Table 19–3 lists some important causes of morbidity and mortality associated with obesity, and Figure 19–12 shows possible pathophysiologic mechanisms involved in their production.

Pathophysiology

Recognition that obesity plays a role in the pathophysiology of disease comes from epidemiologic studies identifying obesity as a risk factor without providing insight into the mechanism of the risk.

Table 19–3. Some disorders associated with obesity.

Hypertension
Diabetes mellitus
Coronary artery disease
Gallstones
Sudden death
Cardiomyopathy
Sleep apnea
Hirsutism
Osteoarthritis
Gout
Stroke
Cancer (breast, endometrial, ovarian, cervical, gallbladder in women; prostatic, colorectal in men)

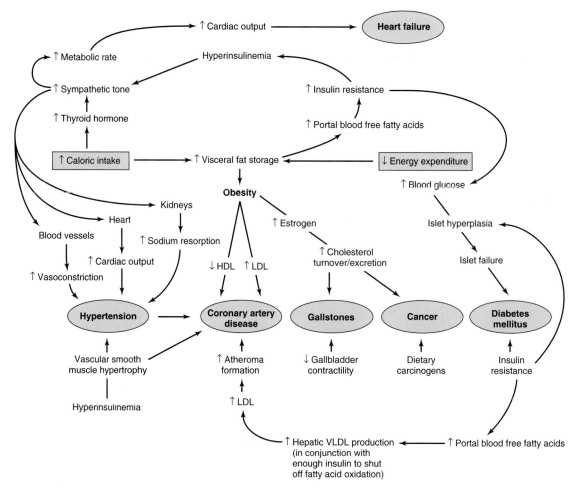

Figure 19–12. Role of obesity in the pathophysiology of disease. Some ways by which obesity contributes to disease. Short arrows refer to a change in the indicated parameter, and long arrows indicate a consequence of that change. In some cases, evidence is epidemiologic; in others, it is experimental. (Modified and reproduced, with permission, from Bray GA: Pathophysiology of obesity. Am J Clin Nutr 1992;55:488S.)

There appear to be multiple mechanisms by which obesity can develop. Thus, obesity may be either a cause or a consequence of disease, depending on the disorder. For example, non-insulin-dependent diabetes mellitus is sometimes first manifested clinically by sudden weight gain, and this disorder can be difficult to control without weight loss—reflecting the insulin-resistant character of the obese state. Moreover, if the weight can be lost, the diabetes may once again become latent, controlled by diet and exercise alone. In such cases, obesity seems clearly to be an etiologic factor in the development of diabetes mellitus. Yet insulin injections, which may be necessary to control the symptoms of diabetes in such a patient, further exacerbates the weight gain that precipitated the disorder in the first place. Such "chicken-or-egg" relationships make the pathophysiology of obesity particularly difficult to dissect. Nevertheless, important progress has been made in recent years toward developing a coherent framework in which to view obesity as both cause and consequence of disease. Some of these observations are noted below.

First, the number of fat cells in the body is probably established during infancy. One hypothesis is that obesity appearing during adulthood results from enlargement of individual fat cells (hypertrophy) rather than an increased number of fat cells (hyperplasia). Obesity due to fat cell hypertrophy appears to be much more easily controlled than obesity due to fat cell hyperplasia. Perhaps feedback signals in response to the degree of fat cell hypertrophy are important to the hypothalamic "lipostat."

Second, it is now recognized that *where* fat is deposited is more important than *how much* is deposited. Thus, so-called visceral or central obesity (omental fat in the distribution of blood flow draining into the portal vein) seems far more important as a risk factor for obesity-related morbidity and mortality than so-called subcutaneous (gynecoid, lower body) or peripheral fat. It appears that visceral fat is more sensitive to catecholamines and less sensitive to insulin, making it a marker of insulin resistance. Consistent with these findings is the observation that obese individuals who engage in vigorous physical activity and whose obesity is largely due to high caloric intake (eg, sumo wrestlers) have subcutaneous rather than visceral fat and do not demonstrate substantial increased insulin resistance. In contrast, the obesity associated with a sedentary lifestyle is believed to be largely visceral obesity—it carries a much higher risk and is associated with a greater degree of insulin resistance in patients both with and without a diagnosis of diabetes mellitus.

Third, the cell bodies of neuropeptide Y-secreting neurons lie in the arcuate nucleus of the hypothalamus, near where at least some GnRH-secreting neurons that control the reproductive neuroendocrine axis are located in humans. Falling leptin concentrations during prolonged starvation result in increased neuropeptide Y secretion. This triggers a starvation response, including increased appetite, decreased sympathetic nervous system activity and energy expenditure, decreased GnRH secretion, and diminished reproductive function, and increases in both parasympathetic tone and CRH secretion (stress response).

Fourth, it has been demonstrated that the genetically obese mice of the *ob/ob* strain have a defective leptin gene. The resulting loss of a normal hormonal cue to long-term satiety seems to be a critical feature of this particular model of excessive weight gain. When these animals are treated with leptin, they lose weight—and gain fertility.

Mutated leptin genes are also associated with obesity in some humans. However, in the vast majority of obese humans, excessive rather than deficient leptin levels are observed. Thus, it appears that the most common form of human obesity involves leptin resistance in the face of high endogenous leptin levels rather than defective leptin secretion as observed in *ob/ob* mice. An animal model for this condition is the obese *db/db* mouse, in which there is a defective leptin receptor. A variety of mechanisms, including diminished signaling through the leptin receptor and diminished transport across the blood-brain barrier, could account for leptin resistance in different individuals. There is great interest in the development of drugs that alter these pathways (eg, neuropeptide Y antagonists) in ways that would promote weight loss as a treatment for obesity.

Psychologic factors also make an important contribution to the development of obesity. For example, obese individuals appear to regulate their desire for food by greater reliance on external cues (eg, time of day, appeal of the food) rather than internal signals (eg, feeling hungry).

13. Define obesity.
14. What diseases are associated with obesity?
15. Outline several pathophysiologic mechanisms by which obesity contributes to disease.

PITUITARY ADENOMA

An adenoma is a benign tumor of epithelial cell origin. Pituitary adenomas are of particular significance (1) because the pituitary is in an enclosed space with very limited capacity to accommodate an expanding mass; and (2) because they may arise from cells that secrete hormones, giving rise to hormone overproduction syndromes.

Clinical Presentation

Patients with adenomas or other tumors of the pituitary come to medical attention either with symptoms and signs related to an expanding intracranial mass (headaches, vision changes, diabetes insipidus, cranial nerve impingement) or with manifestations of excess or deficiency of one or more pituitary hormones. Hormone deficiency results from destruction of the normal pituitary by the expanding adenoma. Hormone excess occurs when the adenoma secretes a particular hormone. **Microadenomas** (< 10 mm) are more likely to present with complaints related to hormone excess than to local mass effects, since they are small. Conversely, whether or not they secrete hormones, **macroadenomas** (> 10 mm) can impinge on the optic chiasm above the sella turcica or the cavernous sinuses laterally.

Etiology

Any cell type in the pituitary gland can undergo hyperplasia or give rise to a tumor. Whether the patient with a pituitary tumor presents with a mass effect or symptoms referable to pituitary hormones depends on the size, growth rate, and secretory characteristics of the tumor. Which (if any) hormones the tumor secretes is generally a reflection of the cell type from which the tumor originated. **Gigantism** and **acromegaly** are due to oversecretion of growth hormone. **Cushing's disease** is a syndrome of glucocorticoid excess due to oversecretion of ACTH. TSH-, LH-, and FSH-secreting tumors are rare. **Galactorrhea** occurs in prolactin-secreting tumors.

Pathophysiology

Most pituitary adenomas are clonal in origin: A single cell with altered growth control and feedback regulation gives rise to the adenoma. In a number of cases of pituitary adenomas, a point mutation has occurred in the alpha subunit of a cytosolic GTP-binding protein (G_s) that normally regulates growth-stimulatory signal transduction. As a result of this mutation, the G protein is "on" much longer. This is functionally analogous to the G protein activation that causes cholera. In the case of cholera, the G protein controls fluid secretion into the gut lumen, and G protein activation is due to a cholera toxin-mediated posttranslational modification of genetically normal G proteins. Thus, the disease is cured when the cholera bacterium is eliminated and the individual modified G protein polypeptides are degraded and replaced by newly synthesized G protein molecules. In the case of pituitary adenomas, the alteration is at the genetic level, and all cells of that clone thus need to be destroyed to eradicate the aberrant G protein.

Clinical Manifestations

Clinical manifestations related to mass effects are summarized in Figure 19–13. Bitemporal hemianopia is the classic visual field defect in a patient with an expanding pituitary mass (see Figure 19–13, panel C). It occurs because the crossing fibers of the optic tract, which lie directly above the pituitary gland and innervate the part of the retina responsible for temporal vision, are compressed by the tumor. However, in practice, a wide variety of visual field defects are seen, reflecting the unpredictable nature of the direction and extent of tumor growth as well as anatomic variability. The clinical manifestations of hormone excess are discussed under specific syndromes below.

Regardless of whether a pituitary tumor is producing hormones or not, infarction of or hemorrhage into the expanding mass can destroy the normal pituitary gland. This leaves the patient without one or more of the pituitary hormones. The resulting clinical manifestations are considered below in the discussion of panhypopituitarism.

A. Prolactinoma: Hyperprolactinemia is the most common anterior pituitary disorder and has many causes (Table 19–4). Pathologic hyperprolactinemia, including that due to prolactin-secreting adenomas (prolactinomas), excess dopamine-receptor blocking drugs, and primary hypothyroidism, must all be distinguished from the physiologic hyperprolactinemia of pregnancy and lactation. Prolactinomas are found in approximately one-fourth of all patients who come to autopsy, and they account for 60% of all primary pituitary tumors. Most of the patients had no symptoms from microadenomas and died of unrelated causes.

Patients with macroadenomas generally present with mass effect symptoms while those with microadenomas may develop symptoms related to hormonal effects, either due to the direct actions of prolactin (galactorrhea in 30–80% of women and up to one-third of men) or to prolactin's indirect effect of suppressing gonadal function (by decreasing GnRH secretion and perhaps by blocking gonadotropin actions at the ovary and testis). The resulting reproduc-

Headaches

A. Stretching of dura by tumor

B. Hydrocephalus (rare)

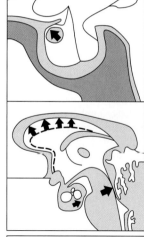

Visual field defects

C. Nasal retinal fibers compressed by tumor

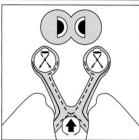

Cranial nerve palsies and temporal lobe epilepsy

D. Lateral extension of tumor

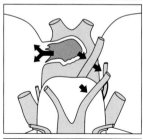

Cerebrospinal fluid rhinorrhea

E. Downward extension of tumor

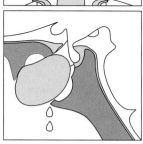

Figure 19–13. Various symptoms of pituitary tumor. Headaches are rarely caused by hydrocephalus. Visual field defects caused by extension of the tumor are plotted with the Goldmann perimeter. (From Wass JAH: Hypopituitarism. In: *Clinical Endocrinology: An Illustrated Text.* Besser GM et al [editors]. Gower, 1987.)

Table 19–4. Causes of hyperprolactinemia.[1]

Physiologic causes
  Pregnancy
  Lactation
Hypothalamic disease
  Tumor, eg, metastases, craniopharyngioma, germinoma, cyst, glioma, hamartoma
  Infiltrative disease, eg, sarcoidosis, tuberculosis, histiocytosis X, granuloma
  Pseudotumor cerebri
  Cranial radiation
Pituitary disease
  Prolactinoma
  Acromegaly
  Cushing's disease
  Pituitary stalk section
  Empty sella syndrome
  Other tumors, eg, metastases, nonfunctioning adenoma, gonadotroph adenoma, meningioma
  Intrasellar germinoma
  Infiltrative disease, eg, sarcoidosis, giant cell granuloma, tuberculosis
Drugs
  Dopamine receptor antagonists, eg, chlorpromazine, fluphenazine, haloperidol, perphenazine, promazine, domperidone, metoclopramide, sulpiride
  Other drugs
    Antihypertensives, eg, methyldopa, reserpine, verapamil
    Estrogens
    Opioids
    Cimetidine
Primary hypothyroidism
Chronic renal failure
Cirrhosis
Neurogenic, eg, breast manipulation, chest wall lesions, spinal cord lesions
Stress, eg, physical, psychologic
Idiopathic

[1]Modified and reproduced, with permission, from Thorner MO et al: The anterior pituitary. In: *Williams Textbook of Endocrinology,* 9th ed. Wilson JD et al (editors). Saunders, 1998.

tive dysfunction presents variably: amenorrhea, irregular menses, or menses with infertility in women and decreased libido and partial or complete impotence or infertility in men.

Decreased bone density is another common consequence of hyperprolactinemia—due both to hypogonadism and perhaps also to poorly understood direct effects of prolactin on bone.

B. Growth Hormone-Secreting Adenoma: GH-secreting tumors give rise to the syndromes of **gigantism** or **acromegaly** depending on whether they develop before or after closure of the epiphyses. Clinical findings in gigantism and acromegaly are summarized in Tables 19–5 and 19–6 and reflect a combination of the insulin-like effects of the hormone, promoting visceromegaly, and the counterregulatory effects, promoting glucose intolerance.

C. ACTH-Secreting Pituitary Adenoma (Cushing's Disease): Secretion of excess cortisol due to overproduction of ACTH by a pituitary adenoma is the most common cause of spontaneous Cushing's syndrome (Chapter 21). ACTH-secreting pituitary adenomas are eight times more common in women than in men and must be distinguished from the effects caused by CRH or ACTH arising from outside the hypothalamus and pituitary gland, respectively, and from adrenal adenomas and carcinomas. As with the other types of pituitary adenomas, those secreting ACTH can be divided into micro- and macroadenomas. For microadenomas, transsphenoidal microsurgery is generally quite successful. For macroadenomas, which have a far poorer prognosis, radiation and medical therapy are often employed to inhibit adrenal cortisol production or ACTH secretion.

The symptoms and signs of ACTH-secreting pituitary adenomas are a consequence of both local mass effects, similar to those discussed above for other types of pituitary tumors, and effects from overproduction of cortisol by the adrenal gland, as discussed in Chapter 21. **Nelson's syndrome** is the rapid progression of an ACTH-secreting pituitary adenoma which is often observed after bilateral adrenalectomy to control the symptoms of cortisol excess. With the advent of transsphenoidal hypophysectomy and radiation therapy, the incidence of this complication has greatly diminished.

---

16. What is a pituitary adenoma?
17. What brings patients with pituitary adenomas to medical attention?
18. What are the most common forms of pituitary adenoma?
19. How does a pituitary adenoma develop?

HYPOPITUITARISM

Panhypopituitarism is the syndrome resulting from complete loss of all of the hormones secreted by the pituitary gland. Hypopituitarism refers to the loss of one or more pituitary hormones.

Clinical Presentation

The complex of symptoms in hypopituitarism varies depending on the extent and duration of disease. In some cases panhypopituitarism is of sudden onset (eg, due to pituitary infarction or trauma). These patients may rapidly develop two potentially life-threatening situations as a consequence of loss of ACTH and vasopressin. First, since the patient is unable to mount a stress response due to lack of ACTH-stimulated glucocorticoid secretion, even relatively mild stress may be lethal. Second, a patient unable to maintain water intake will be unable to compensate for the massive diuresis associated with vasopressin deficiency (**diabetes insipidus**). Thus, the patient will quickly become comatose as a result of profound water loss and the complications of dehydration and hypernatremia.

Table 19–5. Effects of growth hormone excess.[1]

Location	Symptoms	Signs
General	Fatigue Increased sweating Heat intolerance Weight gain Possible increased malignancy risk	Glucose intolerance Hypertriglyceridemia
Skin and subcutaneous tissue	Enlarging hands, feet Coarsening facial features Oily skin Hypertrichosis	Moist, warm, fleshy, doughy handshake Skin tags Acanthosis nigricans Increased heel pad
Head	Headaches	Parotid enlargement Frontal bossing
Eyes	Decreased vision	Visual field defects
Ears		Otoscope speculum cannot be inserted
Nose, throat, paranasal sinuses	Sinus congestion Increased tongue size Malocclusion Voice change	Enlarged furrowed tongue Tooth marks on tongue Widely spaced teeth Prognathism
Neck		Goiter Obstructive sleep apnea due to visceromegaly
Cardiorespiratory system	Congestive heart failure	Hypertension Cardiomegaly, cardiomyopathy Left ventricular hypertrophy
Genitourinary system	Decreased libido Impotence Oligomenorrhea Infertility Renal colic	Urolithiasis
Neurologic system	Paresthesias Hypersomnolence	Carpal tunnel syndrome Nerve root compression due to bone and cartilage growth
Muscles	Weakness	Proximal myopathy
Skeletal system	Joint pains (shoulders, back, knees)	Osteoarthritis Increased 1,25-$(OH)_2D_3$ due to increased 1α-hydroxylase, resulting in increased Ca^{2+} absorption from gut and excretion in urine, increased bone density and turnover

[1]Modified and reproduced, with permission, from Daniels GH, Martin JB: Neuroendocrine regulation and diseases of the anterior pituitary and hypothalamus. In: *Harrison's Principles of Internal Medicine,* 13th ed. Isselbacher KM et al (editors) McGraw-Hill, 1994.

In other cases, pituitary insufficiency develops more insidiously (eg, due to progressive destruction of the pituitary gland by a nonsecreting tumor or subsequent to pituitary radiation therapy). In many of these slowly developing cases of panhypopituitarism, the patient comes to medical attention with complaints related to reproductive functions (amenorrhea in women or infertility or impotence in men) due to LH and FSH deficiency. Other patients have nonspecific complaints (eg, lethargy or altered bowel habits), perhaps related to the gradual development of hypothyroidism (due to TSH deficiency). Panhypopituitarism may be unmasked only when the patient does poorly during some other unrelated medical emergency because of inability to mount a protective stress response due to an ACTH and consequent glucocorticoid deficiency.

Etiology

Panhypopituitarism of sudden onset is usually due to traumatic disruption of the pituitary stalk, infarction and hemorrhage into a pituitary tumor, or ischemic destruction of the pituitary following systemic hypotension (eg, **Sheehan's syndrome** or postpartum hypopituitarism following massive blood loss in childbirth). A number of rare genetic causes have also been reported (Table 19–7). Gradually acquired hypopituitarism is most often due to extension

Table 19–6. Clinical and laboratory findings in 57 patients with acromegaly.[1]

Finding	%
Recent acral growth	100
Arthralgias	72
Excessive sweating	91
Weakness	88
Malocclusion	68
New skin tags	58
Hypertension (> 150/90)	37
Carpal tunnel syndrome	44
Fasting blood glucose > 6 mmol/L	30
Abnormal glucose tolerance test (blood glucose > 6.1 mmol/L [>110 mg/dL])	68
Heel pad thickness > 22 mm	91
Serum prolactin > 25 μg/L	16
Serum phosphorus > 1.5 mmol/L (> 4.5 mg/dL)	48
Sella volume > 1300 mm^3	96
Serum T$_4$ < 53 nmol/L (< 3 ng/mL)	0[2]
Serum testosterone (men) < 10 nmol/L (< 3 ng/mL)	23
8:00 AM serum cortisol < 200 nmol/L (< 8 μg/dL)	4

[1]Modified and reproduced, with permission, from Clemmons DR et al: Evaluation of acromegaly by radioimmunoassay of somatomedin-C. N Engl J Med 1979;301:1138.
[2]Eleven patients were receiving T$_4$ replacement at the time of the study.

of pituitary tumors or occurs as a complication of radiation therapy for brain tumors.

Pathophysiology

The biochemical hallmark of hypopituitarism is low levels of pituitary hormones in the face of low end-organ products of one or more components of the neuroendocrine axes involving the pituitary. By contrast, primary end-organ failure results in high levels of the relevant pituitary hormones.

Table 19–7. Causes of hypopituitarism.[1]

Ischemic necrosis of the pituitary
  Postpartum necrosis (Sheehan's syndrome)
  Head injury
  Vascular disease, commonly associated with diabetes mellitus
Neoplasms involving the sella turcica
  Nonfunctioning adenoma
  Craniopharyngioma
  Suprasellar chordoma
  Histiocytosis X (eosinophilic granuloma; Hand-Schüller-Christian disease)
Intrasellar cysts
Chronic inflammatory lesions
  Tuberculosis, syphilis, sarcoidosis
Infiltrative diseases
  Amyloidosis
  Hemochromatosis
  Mucopolysaccharidoses

[1]Modified and reproduced, with permission, from Chandrasoma P, Taylor CR: *Concise Pathology*, 3rd ed. Appleton & Lange, 1998.

Another biochemical difference between primary end-organ failure and end-organ failure secondary to hypopituitarism is that not all end-organ functions are equally controlled by the pituitary. In the case of the adrenal cortex, for example, mineralocorticoid secretion is only partly under the control of ACTH.

Both of the biochemical distinctions between primary end-organ failure and pituitary failure have important clinical implications. For example, hyperpigmentation occurs in primary adrenal insufficiency because melanocyte-stimulating hormone (MSH) is, like ACTH, a by-product of pro-opiomelanocortin precursor processing; its overproduction does not occur in adrenal insufficiency secondary to pituitary or hypothalamic disease. Similarly, the symptoms of adrenal insufficiency secondary to pituitary disease may be more subtle than in the case of primary adrenal failure, since a significant fraction of mineralocorticoid production is preserved even in the absence of ACTH (Chapter 21).

In the case of trauma and pituitary stalk transection, it is notable that hypopituitarism in general and vasopressin deficiency in particular may improve over time as local edema diminishes and some degree of integrity of the pituitary stalk with its connection to the hypothalamus is reestablished. Sometimes, however, these symptoms and signs may worsen over time as the few residual intact cells or connections are lost.

Clinical Manifestations

The symptoms and signs of hypopituitarism depend on the extent and duration of specific pituitary hormone deficiencies and the patient's overall clinical status. Thus, a relative deficiency of vasopressin can be compensated for by increasing water intake; adrenal insufficiency may not be manifest until the patient needs to mount a stress response. Hypothyroidism may become manifest gradually over months because of the relatively long half-life and large reservoir of thyroid hormone normally available in the gland.

The clinical manifestations of hypopituitarism are those of the end-organ deficiency syndromes. Most important are adrenal insufficiency, hypothyroidism, and diabetes insipidus. Less crucial but often the most sensitive clue to the presence of pituitary disease are amenorrhea in women and infertility or impotence in men.

---

20. What are the most common causes of panhypopituitarism?
21. How do patients with panhypopituitarism come to medical attention?
22. How would you determine what replacement therapy is required for a patient with panhypopituitarism?

DIABETES INSIPIDUS

Diabetes insipidus is a syndrome of polyuria resulting from the inability to concentrate urine and therefore to conserve water as a result of lack of vasopressin action.

Clinical Presentation

The initial clinical presentation of diabetes insipidus is polyuria that persists in the face of circumstances which would normally lead to diminished urine output (eg, dehydration), accompanied by thirst. Adults may complain of frequent urination at night (nocturia), and children may present with bed-wetting (enuresis). No further symptoms develop if the patient is able to maintain a water intake commensurate with water loss. The volume of urine produced in the total absence of vasopressin may reach 10–20 L/d. Thus, should the patient's ability to maintain this degree of fluid intake be compromised (eg, by whatever accident or process led to the development of diabetes insipidus in the first place), dehydration can develop and may rapidly progress to coma.

Etiology

Diabetes insipidus can be due to (1) diseases of the central nervous system (**central diabetes insipidus**), affecting the synthesis or secretion of vasopressin; (2) diseases of the kidney (**nephrogenic diabetes insipidus**), with loss of the kidney's ability to respond to circulating vasopressin by retaining water (Table 19–8); or (3) in pregnancy, probable increased metabolic clearance of vasopressin. In both central and nephrogenic diabetes insipidus, urine is hypotonic. The most common central causes are accidental head trauma, intracranial tumor, and the post-intracranial surgery state. Less common causes are listed in Table 19–8. Nephrogenic diabetes insipidus may be familial or due to renal damage from a variety of drugs (Table 19–8). Diabetes insipidus-like syndromes may result from mineralocorticoid excess, pregnancy, and other causes. True nephrogenic diabetes insipidus must be distinguished from an osmotic (and hence vasopressin-resistant) diuresis. Likewise, washout of the medullary interstitial osmotic gradient (which is necessary for the concentration of urine) may occur with prolonged diuresis due to any cause and may be confused with true diabetes insipidus. In both cases (osmotic diuresis and medullary washout), the urine is hypertonic or isotonic rather than hypotonic. Finally, extreme primary polydipsia (drinking excessive amounts of water, often due to a psychiatric disorder) results in an appropriately large volume of dilute urine and a low plasma vasopressin level, thus mimicking true diabetes insipidus.

Pathophysiology

A. Central Diabetes Insipidus: Central diabetes insipidus can be either permanent or transient, reflecting the natural history of the underlying disorder (Table 19–8). Only about 15% of the vasopressin-secreting cells of the hypothalamus need to be intact to maintain fluid balance under normal conditions. Simple destruction of the posterior pituitary does not cause sufficient neuronal loss to result in permanent diabetes insipidus. Rather, destruction of the hypothalamus or at least some of the supraoptic-hypophysial tract must also occur.

A more common finding is transient disease resulting from acute injury with neuronal shock and edema (eg, postinfarction or posttrauma), leading to cessation of vasopressin secretion with subsequent resumption of sufficient vasopressin secretion to resolve symptoms, either due to neuronal recovery or resolution of edema with reestablishment of hypothalamic-pituitary neurovascular integrity.

B. Nephrogenic Diabetes Insipidus: Familial nephrogenic diabetes insipidus appears to be the result of a generalized defect in either the V_2 class of vasopressin receptors or the aquaporin-2 water channel of the renal collecting tubules.

Drug-induced nephrogenic diabetes insipidus appears to result from sensitivity of the vasopressin receptor to lithium, fluoride, and other salts. This occurs in about 12–30% of patients treated with these drugs. It is generally reversible upon termination of exposure to the offending drug (Table 19–8).

C. Mineralocorticoid Excess: In the case of mild hypernatremia associated with mineralocorticoid excess, it appears that chronic hypervolemia due

Table 19–8. Causes of central and nephrogenic diabetes insipidus.[1]

Central diabetes insipidus
Hereditary, familial (autosomal dominant)
Acquired
Idiopathic
Traumatic or postsurgical
Neoplastic disease: craniopharyngioma, lymphoma, meningioma, metastatic carcinoma
Ischemic or hypoxic disorder: Sheehan's syndrome, aneurysms, cardiopulmonary arrest, aortocoronary bypass, shock, brain death
Granulomatous disease: sarcoidosis, histiocytosis X
Infections: viral encephalitis, bacterial meningitis
Autoimmune disorder
Nephrogenic diabetes insipidus
Hereditary, familial (two types)
Acquired
Hypokalemia
Hypercalcemia
Postrenal obstruction
Drugs: lithium, demeclocycline, methoxyflurane
Sickle cell trait or disease
Amyloidosis
Pregnancy

[1]Modified and reproduced, with permission, from Reeves BW, Bichet DG, Andreoli TE: The posterior pituitary and water metabolism. In: *Williams Textbook of Endocrinology,* 9th ed. Wilson JD et al (editors). Saunders, 1998.

to mineralocorticoid-induced sodium retention results in resetting of the osmotic threshold for vasopressin release. Correction of the volume overload with diuretics is sufficient to reset the osmostat and correct the hypernatremia.

D. Pregnancy: Diabetes insipidus is a rare complication of pregnancy. Occurring in this setting, it can have features of both central and nephrogenic diabetes insipidus. It appears to be due to excessive vasopressinase in plasma. This enzyme, which selectively degrades vasopressin, is presumably released from the placenta. Normally, its level falls after delivery. The pathophysiology of excessive vasopressinase release is unclear. A hallmark of this entity is that it is reversed by administration of the vasopressin analog desmopressin acetate, which is resistant to degradation by the enzyme.

Clinical Manifestations

Diabetes insipidus must be distinguished from other causes of polyuria and hypernatremia (Table 19–9). The hallmark of diabetes insipidus is dilute urine, even in the face of hypernatremia. Dipstick testing of the urine for glucose distinguishes diabetes mellitus. Conditions in which **osmotic diuresis** is responsible for polyuria can be distinguished from diabetes insipidus by their normal or elevated urine osmolality. Primary polydipsia is distinguished by the presence of hyponatremia, whereas in diabetes insipidus the serum sodium should be normal or elevated. In primary polydipsia, uncontrolled excess water ingestion drives the polyuria, whereas in diabetes insipidus, hypertonicity stimulates thirst.

Distinguishing central from nephrogenic diabetes insipidus depends ultimately on a determination of responsiveness to injected vasopressin, with a dramatic decrease in urine volume and increase in urine osmolality in the former and little or no change in the latter. In central diabetes insipidus, circulating vasopressin levels are low for a given plasma osmolality while in nephrogenic diabetes insipidus they are high.

Polyuria in nephrogenic diabetes insipidus results from an inability to conserve water in the distal nephron due to lack of vasopressin-dependent water channels. These channels, which reside within vesicles just under the renal tubular cell surface, are normally inserted into the apical plasma membrane in response to vasopressin stimulation and allow conservation of water. Up to 13% of the volume of the glomerular filtrate can be reclaimed in this manner.

In diabetes insipidus of either central or nephrogenic origin, if the patient is unable to maintain sufficient water intake to offset polyuria, dehydration with consequent hypernatremia develops. Hypernatremia leads to a number of neurologic manifestations, including progressive obtundation (decreased responsiveness to verbal and physical stimuli), myoclonus, seizures, focal deficits, and coma. These neurologic manifestations result from cell shrinkage and volume loss due to osmotic forces, sometimes complicated by intracranial hemorrhage due to stretching and rupture of small blood vessels. Barring structural changes such as those leading to hemorrhage, the neurologic consequences of hypernatremia are reversible upon resolution of the underlying metabolic disorder.

The time course of hypernatremia is an important variable in the development of neurologic symptoms in that over time, neurons generate "idiogenic osmoles," ie, amino acids and other metabolites that serve to raise intracellular osmolality to the level in the blood and thereby minimize fluid shifts out of the cells of the brain. Thus, the more slowly hypernatremia develops, the less the likelihood of neurologic complications due to fluid shifts in the brain or of a vascular catastrophe.

Table 19–9. Major causes of hypernatremia.[1]

Impaired thirst
  Coma
  Essential hypernatremia
Excessive water losses
  Renal
    Central diabetes insipidus
    Nephrogenic diabetes insipidus
    Impaired medullary hypertonicity
  Extrarenal
    Sweating
    Osmotic diarrhea
    Burns
Solute diuresis
  Glucose
    Diabetic ketoacidosis
    Nonketotic hyperosmolar coma
  Other
    Mannitol administration
    Glycerol administration
Sodium excess
  Administration of hypertonic NaCl
  Administration of hypertonic $NaHCO_3$

23. What clues would suggest diabetes insipidus in a new patient?
24. How would you make a definitive diagnosis of diabetes insipidus?
25. What are the pathophysiologic differences between central and nephrogenic diabetes insipidus?

[1]Modified and reproduced, with permission, from Reeves BW, Bichet DG, Andreoli TE: The posterior pituitary and water metabolism. In: *Williams Textbook of Endocrinology*, 9th ed. Wilson JD et al (editors). Saunders, 1998.

Table 19–10. The hypotonic syndromes.[1]

Excessive water ingestion
Decreased water excretion
  Decreased solute delivery to diluting segments
    Starvation
    Beer potomania
  Vasopressin excess
    Syndrome of inappropriate antidiuretic hormone
    Drug-induced vasopressin secretion
  Vasopressin excess with decreased distal solute delivery
    Congestive heart failure
    Cirrhosis of the liver
    Nephrotic syndrome
    Cortisol deficiency
    Hypothyroidism
    Diuretic use
    Renal failure

[1]Modified and reproduced, with permission, from Reeves BW, Bichet DG, Andreoli TE: The posterior pituitary and water metabolism. In: *Williams Textbook of Endocrinology*, 9th ed. Wilson JD et al (editors). Saunders, 1998.

Table 19–11. Causes of SIADH.[1]

Tumors
  Bronchial carcinoma (particularly small-cell type)
  Other carcinomas: duodenum, pancreas, bladder, ureter, prostate
  Leukemia, lymphoma
  Thymoma, sarcoma
Central nervous system disorders
  Mass lesions: tumors, abscess, hematoma
  Infections: encephalitis, meningitis
  Cerebrovascular accident
  Senile cerebral atrophy
  Hydrocephalus
  Trauma
  Delirium tremens
  Acute psychosis
  Demyelinating and degenerative disease
  Inflammatory disease
Pulmonary disorders
  Infections: tuberculosis, pneumonia, abscess
  Acute respiratory failure
  Positive pressure ventilation
Drugs
  Vasopressin, desmopressin acetate
  Chlorpropamide
  Clofibrate
  Carbamazepine
  Others: vincristine, vinblastine, tricyclic antidepressants, phenothiazines
Idiopathic
  Diagnosis of exclusion

[1]Reproduced, with permission, from Chauvreau ME: Pathology of posterior pituitary. In: *Pathophysiologic Foundations of Critical Care*. Pinsky MR, Dhainaut JA (editors). Williams & Wilkins, 1993.

SYNDROME OF INAPPROPRIATE VASOPRESSIN SECRETION (SIADH)

The syndrome of inappropriate ADH (vasopressin) secretion (SIADH) is one of several causes of a hypotonic state (Table 19–10). SIADH is due to the secretion of vasopressin in excess of what is appropriate for hyperosmolality or intravascular volume depletion.

Clinical Presentation

The cardinal clinical presentation of SIADH is hyponatremia without edema. Depending on the rapidity of onset and the severity, the neurologic consequences of hyponatremia include confusion, lethargy and weakness, myoclonus, asterixis, generalized seizures, and coma.

Etiology

A variety of vasopressin-secreting tumors, central nervous system disorders, pulmonary disorders, and drugs have been associated with SIADH (Table 19–11). Several metabolic disorders can produce hyponatremia and must be investigated and ruled out before the diagnosis of true SIADH is made. In particular, adrenal insufficiency and hypothyroidism are often associated with hyponatremia. In these conditions, sodium deficiency and subsequent volume depletion trigger vasopressin secretion.

Pathophysiology

The serum sodium level is normally determined by the balance of water intake, renal solute delivery (a necessary step in water excretion), and vasopressin-mediated distal renal tubular water retention. Disorders in any one of these features of normal sodium balance—or factors controlling them—can result in hyponatremia. Hyponatremia occurs when the magnitude of the disorder exceeds the capacity of homeostatic mechanisms to compensate for dysfunction. Thus, simple excess water ingestion is generally compensated for by renal water diuresis. The exceptions are (1) when water ingestion is extreme (greater than the approximately 18 L daily that can be excreted via the kidney) or (2) when renal solute delivery is limited (eg, in salt depletion), thereby limiting the ability of the kidney to excrete free water.

In hypoadrenal states, renal sodium loss due to lack of aldosterone has two consequences. First, diminished renal solute delivery impairs the ability of the kidney to excrete a water load—in the case where ingestion of water exceeds nonrenal water loss. Second, volume depletion as a consequence of renal sodium loss results in an appropriate stimulus for vasopressin secretion.

In hypothyroidism, both renal solute delivery and function of the osmostat to which vasopressin secretion is coupled appear to be impaired, resulting in hyponatremia.

True causes of hyponatremia, including SIADH, must also be distinguished from so-called pseudohyponatremia. **Pseudohyponatremia** occurs in two groups of conditions (Table 19–12). First, there are

Table 19–12. Causes of pseudohyponatremia.[1]

Elevated plasma osmolality
  Hyperglycemia
  Mannitol administration
  Glycerol administration

Normal plasma osmolality
  Hyperproteinemia (eg, multiple myeloma)
  Hyperlipidemia
  Prostate surgery, with use of irrigant fluid containing glycine or sorbitol

[1]Modified and reproduced, with permission, from Reeves BW, Bichet DG, Andreoli TE: The posterior pituitary and water metabolism. In: *Williams Textbook of Endocrinology,* 9th ed. Wilson JD et al (editors). Saunders, 1998.

those in which infusion of hyperosmolar solutions (eg, glucose) pulls water out of cells, thereby diluting the sodium. The key feature of these conditions is hyponatremia without hypo-osmolality. Secondly, pseudohyponatremia occurs when the nonaqueous fraction of plasma is larger than normal. Sodium only equilibrates with—and is regulated in—the aqueous fraction of plasma, and calculations of serum sodium concentration typically correct for total plasma volume since the nonaqueous fraction of plasma volume is normally negligible. In those relatively rare conditions where the nonaqueous fraction is significant (eg, severe hyperlipidemic states, multiple myeloma, and other conditions with higher than normal serum lipid or protein concentrations), the calculated sodium concentration will therefore be misleadingly low.

The pathophysiologic mechanisms behind most cases of SIADH are not well understood. It has been proposed that baroreceptor input from the lung is impaired in those pulmonary disorders that result in SIADH. Central nervous system lesions causing SIADH are presumed to interrupt the vasopressin-inhibiting neural pathways. Regardless of the mechanism, in most cases the hyponatremia of SIADH is partially limited by secretion of atrial natriuretic peptide. Thus, severe hyponatremia develops only when water intake is relatively increased, and edema formation is rare. The simplest therapy is restriction of free water intake and, in the case of central nervous system or pulmonary lesions, treatment of the underlying disease.

Clinical Manifestations

The clinical manifestations of SIADH are in part determined by the nature and course of any underlying disorder (eg, central nervous system or pulmonary disease), by the severity of hyponatremia, and by the rapidity with which hyponatremia develops. Regardless of its cause, SIADH can have neurologic manifestations, including confusion, asterixis, myoclonus, generalized seizures, and coma. These occur as a result of osmotic fluid shifts and resulting brain edema and elevated intracranial pressures, with brain swelling limited by the size of the skull. Physiologic mechanisms to counter this swelling include depletion of intracellular osmoles—especially potassium ions. The more rapid the progression of hyponatremia, the more likely it is that brain edema and increased intracranial pressure will develop and that the neurologic complications and herniation will lead to permanent damage. However, even when hyponatremia develops slowly, it can in extreme cases (eg, serum sodium < 110 meq/L) result in seizures and altered mental status. **Central pontine myelinolysis** can develop and cause permanent neurologic damage in patients whose hyponatremia is corrected too rapidly.

26. What conditions are associated with SIADH?
27. How would you distinguish SIADH from other causes of hyponatremia?
28. What are the neurologic consequences of SIADH, and how may they be prevented?

REFERENCES

General

Chickens IC, Groomsman AS: Hypothalamic-pituitary mediated immunomodulation: Arginine vasopressin is a neuroendocrine immune mediator. Br J Rheum 1998;37:131.

Greenspan FS, Strewler GJ: *Basic and Clinical Endocrinology,* 5th ed. Appleton & Lange, 1997.

Sullivan GM, Coplan JD, Gorman JM: Psychoneuroendocrinology of anxiety disorders. Psychiatr Clin North Am 1998;21:397.

Veldhuis JD et al: Estrogen and testosterone, but not a nonaromatizable androgen, direct network integration of the hypothalamo-somatotrope (growth hormone)-insulin-like growth factor I axis in the human: Evidence from pubertal pathophysiology and sex-steroid hormone replacement. J Clin Endocrinol Metab 1997;82:3414.

Wong M et al: Interleukin (IL) 1beta, IL-1 receptor antagonist, IL-10, and IL-13 gene expression in the central nervous system and anterior pituitary during systemic inflammation: Pathophysiological implications. Proc Natl Acad Sci U S A 1997;94:227.

Obesity

Bray GA, York DA: The MONA LISA hypothesis in the time of leptin. Recent Prog Horm Res 1998;53:95.

Friedman JM, Halaas JL: Leptin and the regulation of body weight in mammals. Nature 1998;395:763.

Matsuzawa Y: Pathophysiology and molecular mechanisms of visceral fat syndrome: The Japanese experience. Diabetes Metab Rev 1997;13:3.

Pi-Sunyer FX: Medical hazards of obesity. Ann Intern Med 1993;119:665.

Speroff L et al: Obesity. In: *Clinical Gynecologic Endocrinology and Infertility,* 6th ed. Williams & Wilkins, 1999.

Pituitary Adenoma

Aron DC et al: Pituitary tumors: Current concepts in diagnosis and management. West J Med 1995;162:340.

Hypopituitarism

Donovan LE, Corenblum B: The natural history of the pituitary incidentaloma. Arch Intern Med 1995;155:181.

Diabetes Insipidus

Robertson GL: Diabetes insipidus. Endocrinol Metab Clin North Am 1995;24:549.

Syndrome of Inappropriate ADH Secretion

Sorensen JB et al: Syndrome of inappropriate secretion of antidiuretic hormone (SIADH) in malignant disease. J Intern Med 1995;238:97.

Spigset O, Hedenmalm K: Hyponatremia and the syndrome of inappropriate antidiuretic hormone secretion (SIADH) induced by psychotropic drugs. Drug Saf 1995;12:209.

Thyroid Disease 20

Stephen J. McPhee, MD, & Douglas C. Bauer, MD

The thyroid gland synthesizes the hormones **thyroxine (T_4)** and **triiodothyronine (T_3),** iodine-containing amino acids that regulate the body's metabolic rate. Adequate levels of thyroid hormone are necessary in infants for normal development of the central nervous system; in children for normal skeletal growth and maturation; and in adults for normal function of multiple organ systems. Thyroid dysfunction is one of the most common endocrine disorders encountered in clinical practice. While abnormally high or low levels of thyroid hormones may be tolerated for long periods of time, usually there are symptoms and signs of thyroid dysfunction.

NORMAL STRUCTURE & FUNCTION

ANATOMY

The normal thyroid gland is a firm, reddish brown, smooth gland consisting of two lateral lobes and a connecting central isthmus (Figure 20–1). A pyramidal lobe of variable size may extend upward from the isthmus. The normal weight of the thyroid ranges from 30 g to 40 g. It is surrounded by an adherent fibrous capsule from which multiple fibrous projections extend deeply into its structure, dividing it into many small lobules. The thyroid is highly vascular and has one of the highest rates of blood flow per gram of tissue of any organ.

HISTOLOGY

Histologically, the thyroid gland consists of many closely packed acini, called **follicles,** each surrounded by capillaries and stroma. Each follicle is roughly spherical, lined by a single layer of cuboidal epithelial cells and filled with **colloid,** a proteinaceous material composed mainly of **thyroglobulin** and stored thyroid hormones. When the gland is inactive, the follicles are large, the lining cells are flat, and the colloid is abundant. When the gland is active, the follicles are small, the lining cells are cuboidal or columnar, the colloid is scanty, and its edges are scalloped, forming **"reabsorption lacunae"** (Figure 20–2). Scattered between follicles are the **parafollicular cells (C cells),** which secrete **calcitonin,** a hormone that inhibits bone resorption and lowers the plasma calcium level (see Chapter 17).

The ultrastructure of a follicular epithelial cell is

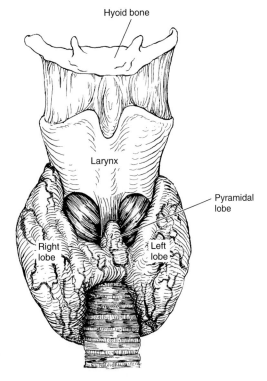

Figure 20–1. The human thyroid. (Reproduced, with permission from Ganong WF: *Review of Medical Physiology,* 19th ed. Appleton & Lange, 1999.)

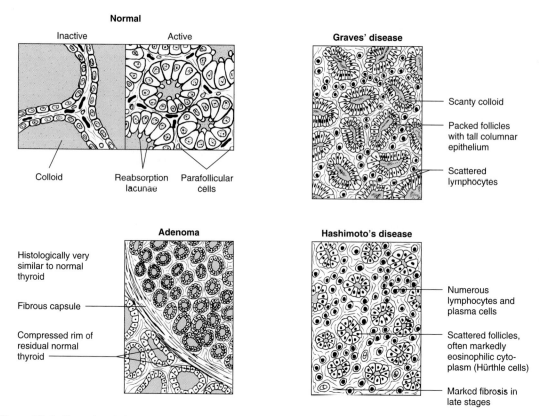

Figure 20–2. Normal and abnormal thyroid histology. (Reproduced, with permission, from Ganong WF: *Review of Medical Physiology,* 19th ed. Appleton & Lange, 1999; from Chandrasoma P, Taylor CE: *Concise Pathology,* 3rd ed. Appleton & Lange, 1997; and from Greenspan FS, Baxter JD (editors): *Basic and Clinical Endocrinology,* 5th ed. Appleton & Lange, 1997.)

diagrammed in Figure 20–3. The cells vary in appearance with the degree of gland activity. The follicular cell rests on a basal lamina. The nucleus is round and centrally located. The cytoplasm contains mitochondria, rough endoplasmic reticulum, and ribosomes. The apex has a discrete Golgi apparatus, small secretory granules containing thyroglobulin, and abundant lysosomes and phagosomes. At the apex, the cell membrane is folded into microvilli.

PHYSIOLOGY

Formation & Secretion of Thyroid Hormones

A. T_4, T_3, and Thyroglobulin: Thyroid follicular cells have three functions: (1) to collect and transport iodine to the colloid; (2) to synthesize **thyroglobulin,** a glycoprotein (MW 660,000) made up of two subunits and containing many tyrosine residues, and secrete it into the colloid; and (3) to release thyroid hormones from thyroglobulin and secrete them into the circulation. The structures of the two thyroid hormones, T_3 and T_4, are shown in Figure 20–4. T_3 and T_4 are synthesized in the colloid by iodination and condensation of tyrosine molecules bound together in thyroglobulin.

B. Iodine Metabolism and Trapping: For normal thyroid hormone synthesis, an adult requires a minimum daily intake of 150 μg of iodine. In the USA, the average intake is about 500 μg/d. Iodine ingested in food is first converted to **iodide,** which is absorbed and taken up by the thyroid. The follicular cells transport iodide from the circulation to the colloid ("iodide trapping," or "iodide pump"). The transporter is a 65-kDa cell membrane protein. This iodide transport is an example of secondary active transport dependent on Na^+-K^+ ATPase for energy; it is stimulated by thyroid-stimulating hormone (TSH). At the normal rate of thyroid hormone synthesis, about 120 μg/d of iodide enters the thyroid. About 80 μg/d is secreted in T_3 and T_4 and the rest diffuses into the extracellular fluid and is excreted in the urine.

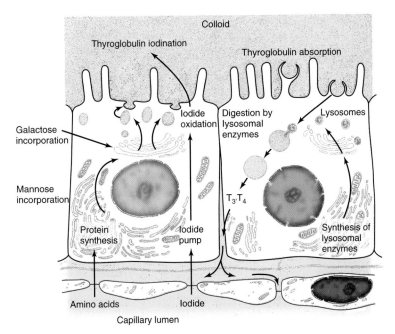

Figure 20–3. Thyroid cell ultrastructure (schematic). The processes of synthesis and iodination of thyroglobulin are shown on the left and its reabsorption and digestion on the right. (Reproduced, with permission, from Junqueira LC, Carneiro J, Kelley R: *Basic Histology,* 9th ed. Appleton & Lange, 1998.)

C. Thyroid Hormone Synthesis and Secretion: Thyroid hormones are synthesized in the colloid, near the apical cell membrane of the follicular cells. Catalyzed by the enzyme thyroidal peroxidase, iodide in the thyroid cell is oxidized to iodine. The iodine enters the colloid and is rapidly bound at the 3 position (Figure 20–4) to tyrosine molecules attached to thyroglobulin, forming **monoiodotyrosine (MIT).** MIT is next iodinated at the 5 position, forming **diiodotyrosine (DIT).** Two DIT molecules then condense in an oxidative process ("coupling reaction") to form one **thyroxine (T_4)** molecule. Some T_3 is probably formed within the thyroid gland by condensation of MIT with DIT. A small amount of reverse T_3 is also formed. Figure 20–4 shows the structures of MIT, DIT, T_4, T_3, and reverse T_3. In the normal thyroid, the average distribution of iodinated compounds is 23% MIT, 33% DIT, 35% T_4, 7% T_3, and 2% reverse T_3 (rT_3).

The thyroid secretes about 80 μg (103 nmol) of T_4 and 4 μg (7 nmol) of T_3 per day. The folds of the apical cell membrane (lamellipodia) encircle a bit of colloid and bring it into the cytoplasm by endocytosis, forming **endosomes.** This process is accelerated by TSH. The endosomes fuse with lysosomes containing proteases that break peptide bonds between the iodi-

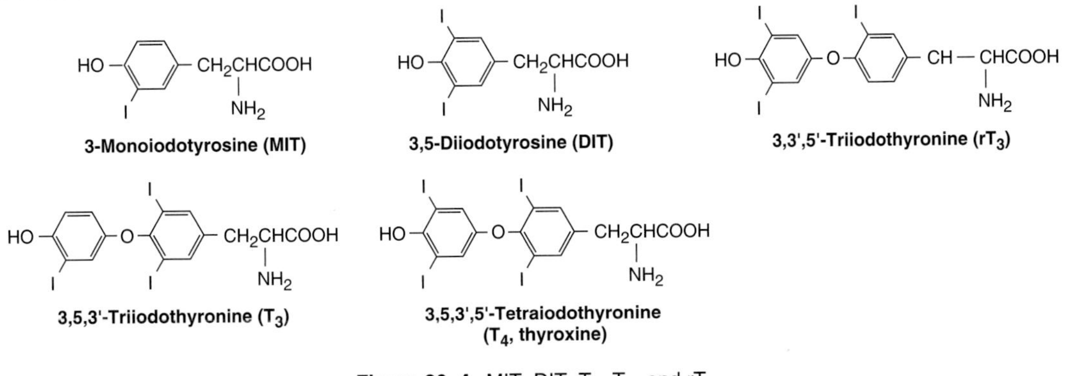

3-Monoiodotyrosine (MIT)

3,5-Diiodotyrosine (DIT)

3,3',5'-Triiodothyronine (rT_3)

3,5,3'-Triiodothyronine (T_3)

3,5,3',5'-Tetraiodothyronine (T_4, thyroxine)

Figure 20–4. MIT, DIT, T_3, T_4, and rT_3.

nated residues and thyroglobulin, releasing T_4, T_3, DIT, and MIT into the cytoplasm. The free T_4 and T_3 then cross the cell membrane and enter adjacent capillaries. The MIT and DIT are enzymatically degraded in the cell by thyroid deiodinase (iodotyrosine dehalogenase) to iodine and tyrosine, which are reused in colloid synthesis.

D. Thyroid Hormone Transport and Metabolism: The normal plasma level of T_4 is approximately 8 μg/dL (103 nmol/L) (range: 5–12 μg/dL or 65–156 nmol/L), and the normal plasma level of T_3 is approximately 0.15 μg/dL (2.3 nmol/L) (range: 0.08–0.22 μg/dL, or 1.2–3.3 nmol/L). Both hormones are bound to plasma proteins, including albumin, **transthyretin** (formerly called thyroxine-binding prealbumin [TBPA]), and **thyroxine-binding globulin (TBG)**. The thyroid hormone-binding proteins serve mainly to transport T_4 and T_3 in the serum and to facilitate uniform distribution of hormones within tissues.

Physiologically, it is the free (unbound) T_4 and T_3 in plasma that are active and inhibit pituitary secretion of TSH. The free T_4 and T_3 are in equilibrium with the protein-bound hormones in plasma and tissue and circulate in much lower concentrations. Tissue uptake of the free hormones is proportionate to their plasma concentrations.

Almost all (99.98%) of the circulating T_4 is bound to TBG (thyroxine-binding globulin) and other plasma proteins, so that the free T_4 level is approximately 2 ng/dL and the biologic half-life of T_4 is long (about 6–7 days). Somewhat less T_3 (99.8%) is protein-bound. Therefore, compared with T_4, T_3 acts more rapidly and has a shorter half life (about 30 hours). It is also three to five times more potent on a molar basis.

T_4 and T_3 are metabolized in the liver, the kidneys, and many other tissues by deiodination and by conjugation to **glucuronides**. Normally, one-third of circulating T_4 is converted to T_3 by 5′-deiodination, and 45% is converted to the metabolically inert **reverse triiodothyronine (rT$_3$)** by 5-deiodination. About 87% of circulating T_3 derives from peripheral conversion of T_4 to T_3 and only 13% from thyroid secretion. Both T_4 and T_3 are conjugated to glucuronides in the liver and excreted into the bile. Upon passage into the intestine, the conjugates are hydrolyzed, and a small amount of T_4 and T_3 are reabsorbed (enterohepatic circulation). The rest is excreted in the stool.

Regulation of Thyroid Secretion

Thyroid hormone secretion is stimulated by pituitary **thyroid-stimulating hormone (TSH, thyrotropin)**. Pituitary TSH secretion is in turn stimulated by **thyrotropin-releasing hormone (TRH)**, a tripeptide secreted by the hypothalamus that also increases the biologic activity of TSH, by altering its glycosylation.

TSH is a two-subunit glycoprotein containing 211 amino acids. The alpha subunit is identical to that of pituitary follicle-stimulating hormone (FSH) and luteinizing hormone (LH) and placental human chorionic gonadotropin (hCG). The beta subunit confers the specific binding properties and biologic activity of TSH. The gene encoding the alpha subunit is located on chromosome 6, and the gene for the beta subunit is on chromosome 1.

TSH has a biologic half-life of about 60 minutes. The average plasma level of TSH is 2 mU/L (normal range: 0.4–4.8 mU/L). Although the phenomenon is not clinically important, normal TSH secretion exhibits a circadian pattern, rising in the afternoon and evening, peaking after midnight, and declining during the day.

Circulating free T_4 and T_3 inhibit TSH secretion by the pituitary both directly and indirectly, by regulating biosynthesis of TRH in the hypothalamus. TSH secretion is inhibited by stress, perhaps via glucocorticoid inhibition of TRH secretion. In infants—but not in adults—TSH secretion is increased by cold and inhibited by warmth. Dopamine and somatostatin also inhibit pituitary secretion of TSH. In animals, there is a pituitary-specific form of the thyroid hormone receptor that may be selectively regulated by thyroid hormone. Figure 20–5 illustrates the hypothalamic pituitary-thyroid axis and various stimulatory and inhibitory factors.

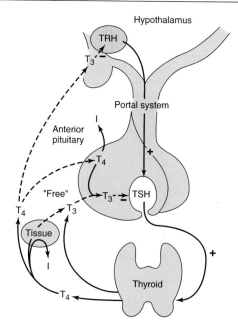

Figure 20–5. Hypothalamic-pituitary-thyroid axis. (Modified and reproduced, with permission, from Greenspan FS, Strewler GJ [editors]: *Basic and Clinical Endocrinology*, 5th ed. Appleton & Lange, 1997.)

When TSH is secreted or administered, it binds to a specific **TSH receptor (TSH-R)** in the thyroid cell membrane, activating the GTP-binding (G_s) protein-adenylyl cyclase-cAMP cascade. The increase in intracellular cAMP mediates immediate increases in uptake and transport of iodide, iodination of thyroglobulin, and synthesis of iodotyrosines, T_3, and T_4. Within a few hours, there is an increase in mRNA for thyroglobulin and thyroidal peroxidase, enhanced lysosomal activity, increased secretion of thyroglobulin into colloid, more endocytosis of colloid, and increased secretion of T_4 and T_3 from the gland.

TSH binding to TSH-R also stimulates membrane phospholipase C, which leads to thyroid cell hypertrophy. With chronic TSH stimulation, the entire gland hypertrophies, increases in vascularity and becomes a **goiter**.

The TSH receptor (TSH-R) has been cloned. It is a single-chain glycoprotein composed of 744 amino acids. Two specific amino acid sequences are thought to represent different binding sites for TSH and for the **TSH receptor-stimulating antibody (TSH-R [stim] Ab)** found in Graves' disease (see below).

The amount of thyroid hormone needed to maintain normal organ system function in thyroidectomized individuals is defined as the amount necessary to maintain the plasma TSH within the normal range (0.5–5.0 mU/L). About 80% of orally administered levothyroxine is absorbed from the gastrointestinal tract, and 100–125 μg/d usually maintains a normal plasma TSH in individuals of average size.

Mechanism of Action of Thyroid Hormones

Thyroid hormones enter cells either by passive diffusion or specific transport through the cell membrane and cytoplasm. Within the cell cytoplasm, most of the T_4 is converted to T_3. The nuclear receptor for T_3 has been cloned and found to be similar to the nuclear receptors for glucocorticoids, mineralocorticoids, estrogens, progestins, vitamin D_3, and retinoic acid. For reasons that are presently unclear, at least two different T_3 receptors, coded by different genes, exist in human tissues. The two biologically active human thyroid hormone receptors (hTR) are labeled hTR-α1 and hTR-β1. The gene for the alpha form is on chromosome 17 and that for the beta form is on chromosome 3. The two different receptor forms may help to explain both the normal variation in thyroid hormone responsiveness of various organs and the selective tissue abnormalities found in various thyroid resistance syndromes. For example, the brain contains mostly alpha receptors, the liver contains mostly beta receptors, and the heart contains both. Point mutations in the *hTR-β1* gene result in abnormal T_3 receptors and the syndrome of **generalized resistance to thyroid hormone (Refetoff's syndrome)**.

When the T_3-receptor complex binds to DNA, it increases expression of specific genes, with the induction of messenger RNAs. A wide variety of enzymes must be produced to account for the many effects of thyroid hormones on cell function.

Effects of Thyroid Hormones

The effects of thyroid hormones in various organs are summarized in Table 20–1. Thyroid hormones increase the activity of membrane-bound Na^+-K^+ ATPase, increase heat production, and stimulate oxygen consumption ("calorigenesis"). Thyroid hormones also affect tissue growth and maturation, help regulate lipid metabolism, increase cardiac contractility by stimulating the expression of myosin protein, and increase intestinal absorption of carbohydrates.

The effects of T_4 and T_3 and of the catecholamines epinephrine and norepinephrine are closely interrelated. Both increase the metabolic rate and stimulate the nervous system and heart. In humans, the transcriptional effects of T_3 include production of increased β-adrenergic receptors; in animals, incubation of thyroid cells in a medium containing TSH increases the number of $α_1$-adrenergic receptors, presumably by inducing their biosynthesis.

Table 20–1. Physiologic effects of thyroid hormones.

Target Tissue	Effect	Mechanism
Heart	Chronotropic	Increase number and affinity of beta-adrenergic receptors.
	Inotropic	Enhance responses to circulating catecholamines. Increase proportion of alpha myosin heavy chain (with higher ATPase activity).
Adipose tissue	Catabolic	Stimulate lipolysis.
Muscle	Catabolic	Increase protein breakdown.
Bone	Developmental and metabolic	Promote normal growth and skeletal development; accelerate bone turnover.
Nervous system	Developmental	Promote normal brain development.
Gut	Metabolic	Increase rate of carbohydrate absorption.
Lipoprotein	Metabolic	Stimulate formation of LDL receptors.
Other	Calorigenic	Stimulate oxygen consumption by metabolically active tissues (exceptions: adult brain, testes, uterus, lymph nodes, spleen, anterior pituitary). Increase metabolic rate.

1. Describe a thyroid follicle and its change with activity versus inactivity of the gland.
2. What forms of thyroid hormone does the thyroid gland secrete? What are the normal proportions of the different forms? What are the relative potencies of each hormone?
3. To what is thyroid hormone bound during its transport in plasma?
4. How are thyroid hormone levels regulated?
5. What is the mechanism of action of thyroid hormone?
6. What are the most prominent organ system-specific effects of thyroid hormone?

OVERVIEW OF THYROID DISEASE

The symptoms and signs of thyroid disease in humans are predictable consequences of the physiologic effects of thyroid hormones discussed above. The clinician commonly encounters patients with one of five types of thyroid dysfunction: (1) **hyperthyroidism** (thyrotoxicosis), caused by an excess of thyroid hormone; (2) **hypothyroidism** (myxedema), caused by a deficiency of thyroid hormone; (3) **goiter**, a diffuse enlargement of the thyroid gland, caused by prolonged elevation of TSH; (4) **thyroid nodule**, a focal enlargement of a portion of the gland, caused by a benign or malignant neoplasm; and (5) **abnormal thyroid function tests in a clinically euthyroid patient.**

Several laboratory tests are useful in the initial evaluation of patients suspected of having thyroid dysfunction. The first is plasma TSH measured by a sensitive assay (usually defined by a lower detection limit of 0.1 mU/L or less). TSH is below normal in hyperthyroidism and above normal in hypothyroidism (except in the rare instances of pituitary or hypothalamic disease). The second useful laboratory test is measurement of non-protein-bound thyroxine. Most clinical laboratories are now able to accurately measure free thyroxine (FT_4) directly. Alternatively, an estimate of non-protein-bound thyroxine is provided by the free thyroxine index (FT_4I), the product of the total plasma thyroxine (TT_4) and the T_4 resin uptake (RT_4U) (ie, $FT_4I = TT_4 \times RT_4U$). The TT_4 by itself often reflects the functional state of the thyroid hormone-binding proteins. The RT_4U is an indicator of thyroid-binding globulin and serves to correct for alterations in the concentration of binding protein. Some laboratories instead measure T_3 resin uptake (RT_3U).

Although total and free T_3 levels can be measured, they have a short half life and are technically difficult assays. Therefore, under most circumstances, circulating levels of T_3 correlate less well with clinical hyper- or hypothyroidism.

A variety of thyroid autoantibodies are detectable in patients with thyroid dysfunction, including (1) **thyroidal peroxidase antibody (TPO Ab)**, formerly termed antimicrosomal antibody; (2) **thyroglobulin antibody (Tg Ab)**; and (3) **TSH receptor antibody**, either **stimulating (TSH-R [stim] Ab)** or **blocking (TSH-R [block] Ab)**. Thyroglobulin and thyroidal peroxidase antibodies are commonly found in hypothyroidism due to Hashimoto's thyroiditis and occasionally in hyperthyroidism due to Graves' disease (see below). TSH-R [stim] Ab is present in most individuals with hyperthyroidism due to Graves' disease. Detection of TSH-R [block] Ab in maternal serum is predictive of congenital hypothyroidism in newborns of mothers with autoimmune thyroid disease.

Other procedures such as thyroid scans and the thyrotropin-releasing hormone (TRH) test are discussed below.

PATHOPHYSIOLOGY OF SELECTED THYROID DISEASES

The pathogenesis of the most common thyroid diseases probably involves an autoimmune process with sensitization of the host's own lymphocytes to various thyroidal antigens. Three major thyroidal antigens have been documented: thyroglobulin (Tg), thyroidal peroxidase (TPO), and the TSH receptor (TSH-R). Both environmental factors (eg, viral or bacterial infection or high iodine intake) and genetic factors (eg, defect in suppressor T lymphocytes) may be responsible for initiating autoimmune thyroid disease.

HYPERTHYROIDISM

Etiology

The causes of hyperthyroidism are listed in Table 20–2. Most commonly, thyroid hormone overproduction is due to Graves' disease. In Graves' disease, the TSH receptor autoantibody TSH-R [stim] Ab stimulates the thyroid follicular cells to produce excessive amounts of T_4 and T_3. Less commonly, patients with multinodular goiter may become thyrotoxic without circulating antibodies if given inorganic iodine (eg, potassium iodide) or organic iodine compounds (eg, the antiarrhythmic drug amiodarone, which contains 37% iodine by weight). Multinodular goiters may also develop one or more nodules that become au-

Table 20–2. Hyperthyroidism: Causes and pathogenetic mechanisms.

Etiologic Classification	Pathogenetic Mechanism
Thyroid hormone overproduction	
Graves' disease	Thyroid-stimulating hormone receptor-stimulating antibody (TSH-R [stim] Ab)
Toxic multinodular goiter	Autonomous hyperfunction
Follicular adenoma	Autonomous hyperfunction
Pituitary adenoma	TSH hypersecretion (rare)
Pituitary insensitivity	Resistance to thyroid hormone (rare)
Hypothalamic disease	Excess TRH production
Germ cell tumors: choriocarcinoma, hydatidiform mole	hCG stimulation
Struma ovarii (ovarian teratoma)	Functioning thyroid elements
Metastatic follicular thyroid carcinoma	Functioning metastases
Thyroid gland destruction	
Lymphocytic thyroiditis	Release of stored hormone
Granulomatous (subacute) thyroiditis	Release of stored hormone
Hashimoto's thyroiditis	Transient release of stored hormone
Other	
Thyrotoxicosis medicamentosa, thyrotoxicosis factitia	Ingestion of excessive exogenous thyroid hormone

tonomous from TSH regulation and secrete excessive quantities of T_4 or T_3. Patients from regions where goiter is endemic may develop thyrotoxicosis when given iodine supplementation (jodbasedow phenomenon). Large follicular adenomas (> 3 cm in diameter) may produce excessive thyroid hormone.

Occasionally, TSH overproduction (eg, from a pituitary adenoma) or hypothalamic disease may cause excessive thyroid hormone production. The diagnosis is suggested by clinically evident hyperthyroidism with elevated serum T_4 and T_3 and *elevated* serum TSH levels. Neuroradiologic procedures such as CT scans or MRI of the sella turcica confirm the presence of a pituitary tumor. Even more rarely, hyperthyroidism results from TSH overproduction due to pituitary (but not peripheral tissue) resistance to the suppressive effects of T_4 and T_3. The diagnosis is suggested by finding elevated serum T_4 and T_3 levels with an inappropriately normal serum TSH level.

Hyperthyroidism may be precipitated by germ cell tumors (choriocarcinoma and hydatidiform mole), which secrete large quantities of human chorionic gonadotropin (hCG). The large quantities of hCG secreted by these tumors bind to the follicular cell TSH receptor and stimulate overproduction of thyroid hormone. Rarely, hyperthyroidism can be produced by ovarian teratomas containing thyroid elements (struma ovarii). Patients with large metastases from follicular thyroid carcinomas may produce excess thyroid hormone, particularly following iodide administration.

Transient hyperthyroidism is occasionally observed in patients with lymphocytic or granulomatous (subacute) thyroiditis (Hashimoto's thyroiditis). In such cases, the hyperthyroidism is due to destruction of the thyroid with release of stored hormone.

Finally, patients who consume excessive amounts of exogenous thyroid hormone (accidentally or deliberately) may present with symptoms, signs, and laboratory findings of hyperthyroidism.

Pathogenesis

Whatever the cause of hyperthyroidism, serum thyroid hormones are elevated. Both the free thyroxine (FT_4) and the free thyroxine index (FT_4I) are elevated. In about 5–10% of patients, T_4 secretion is normal while T_3 levels are high (so-called **T_3 toxicosis**). Total serum T_4 and T_3 levels are not always definitive because of variations in concentrations of thyroid-hormone binding proteins.

Hyperthyroidism due to Graves' disease is characterized by a suppressed serum TSH level as determined by sensitive immunoenzymometric or immunoradiometric assays. However, TSH levels may also be suppressed in some acute psychiatric and other nonthyroidal illnesses. In the rare TSH-secreting pituitary adenomas (so-called **secondary hyperthyroidism**) and in hypothalamic disease with excessive TRH production (so-called **tertiary hyperthyroidism**), hyperthyroidism is accompanied by elevated plasma TSH.

The radioactive iodine (RAI) uptake of the thyroid gland at 4, 6, or 24 hours is increased when the gland produces an excess of hormone (eg, Graves' disease); it is decreased when the gland is leaking stored hormone (eg, thyroiditis), when hormone is produced elsewhere (eg, struma ovarii), or when excessive exogenous thyroid hormone is being ingested (eg, factitious hyperthyroidism). Technetium Tc 99m scanning can provide information similar to that obtained with RAI and is quicker and entails less radiation exposure.

The TRH test is sometimes helpful in diagnosis when patients have confusing results of thyroid function tests. In normal individuals, administration of TRH (500 μg intravenously) produces an increase in serum TSH of at least 6 mU/L within 15–30 minutes. In primary hyperthyroidism, TSH levels are low and TRH administration induces little or no rise in the TSH level.

Graves' Disease

A. Pathology: Graves' disease is the most common cause of hyperthyroidism. In this condition, the thyroid gland is symmetrically enlarged and its vascularity markedly increased. The gland may double or triple in weight. Microscopically, the follicular epithelial cells are columnar in appearance and increased in number and size (Figure 20–2). The follicles are small and closely packed together. The colloid is scanty, with the edges scalloped in appearance secondary to the rapid proteolysis of thyroglobulin. The gland's interstitium is diffusely infiltrated with lymphocytes and may contain lymphoid follicles with germinal centers.

B. Pathogenesis: The serum of more than 90% of patients with Graves' disease contains TSH-R [stim] Ab, an antibody directed against the TSH receptor site in the thyroid follicular epithelial membrane. This antibody was formerly called long-acting thyroid stimulator (LATS) or thyroid-stimulating immunoglobulin (TSI). When it binds to the cell membrane TSH receptors, TSH-R [stim] Ab stimulates hormone synthesis and secretion in somewhat the same way as TSH. While serum levels of TSH-R [stim] Ab correlate poorly with disease severity, its presence can be helpful diagnostically, and although controversial, its disappearance may be helpful in deciding when antithyroid drug therapy can be withdrawn without precipitating a relapse.

The genesis of TSH-R [stim] Ab in patients with Graves' disease is uncertain. However, Graves' disease is familial. In Caucasians, it is associated with the HLA-B8 and HLA-DR3 histocompatibility antigens; in Asians, with HLA-Bw46 and HLA-B5; and in blacks, with HLA-B17. Furthermore, patients with Graves' disease frequently suffer from other autoimmune disorders (Table 20–3). The precipitating cause of this antibody production is unknown, but an immune response against a viral antigen that shares homology with TSH-R may be responsible. Another theory of the pathogenesis of Graves' disease is a defect of suppressor T lymphocytes, which allows helper T lymphocytes to stimulate B lymphocytes to secrete antibodies directed against follicular cell membrane antigens, including the TSH receptor (Figure 20–6).

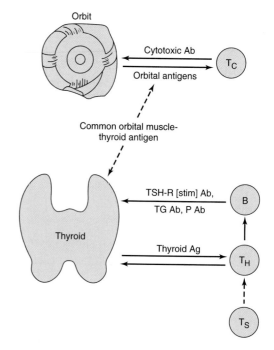

Figure 20–6. Proposed pathogenesis of Graves' disease. A defect in suppressor T lymphocytes (T_s) allows helper T lymphocytes (T_H) to stimulate B lymphocytes (B) to synthesize thyroid autoantibodies. The thyroid receptor-stimulating antibody (TSH-R [stim] Ab) is the driving force for thyrotoxicosis. Inflammation of the orbital muscles may be due to sensitization of cytotoxic T lymphocytes (T_c), or killer cells, to orbital antigens linked to an antigen in the thyroid. What triggers this immunologic cascade is not known. (Tg Ab, thyroglobulin antibody; P Ab, peroxidase or microsomal antibody; Ag, antigen.) (Reproduced, with permission, from Greenspan FS, Strewler GJ: *Basic and Clinical Endocrinology,* 5th ed. Appleton & Lange, 1997.)

Moderate titers of other autoantibodies (thyroidal peroxidase antibody and TSH-R [block] Ab) can be found in patients with Graves' disease. Their significance is uncertain. In some cases, TSH-R [block] Ab) appears following ^{131}I radioiodine therapy of Graves' disease.

Patients with hyperthyroidism from Graves' disease may later develop hypothyroidism by one of several mechanisms: (1) thyroid ablation by surgery or ^{131}I radiation treatment; (2) autoimmune thyroiditis, leading to thyroid destruction; and (3) development of antibodies that block TSH stimulation (TSH-R [block] Ab).

Table 20–3. Autoimmune disorders associated with Graves' disease and Hashimoto's thyroiditis.

Endocrine disorders
  Diabetes mellitus
  Hypoadrenalism, autoimmune (Addison's disease)
  Orchitis or oophoritis, autoimmune
  Hypoparathyroidism, idiopathic
Nonendocrine disorders
  Pernicious anemia
  Vitiligo
  Systemic lupus erythematosus
  Rheumatoid arthritis
  Immune thrombocytopenic purpura
  Myasthenia gravis
  Sjögren's syndrome
  Primary biliary cirrhosis
  Chronic active hepatitis

7. What are the five categories of thyroid dysfunction most commonly observed in patients?
8. What are seven different pathophysiologic mechanisms by which a patient might develop hyperthyroidism?
9. What are the most useful initial tests of thyroid function in hyperthyroidism? What results would you expect compared to normal?
10. How can thyroid scanning help confirm the suspected cause of hyperthyroidism?
11. Describe the mechanism of hyperthyroidism in Graves' disease.

Clinical Manifestations

The clinical consequences of thyroid hormone excess (Table 20–4) are exaggerated expressions of the physiologic activity of T_3 and T_4.

An excess of thyroid hormone causes enough extra heat production to result in a slight rise in body temperature and to activate heat-dissipating mechanisms, including cutaneous vasodilation and a decrease in peripheral vascular resistance and increased sweating. The increased basal metabolic rate leads to weight loss, especially in older patients with poor appetite. In younger patients, food intake typically increases, and some patients have seemingly insatiable appetites.

The apparent increased catecholamine effect of hyperthyroidism is probably multifactorial in origin. Thyroid hormones increase beta-adrenergic receptors in many tissues, including heart muscle, skeletal muscle, adipose tissue, and lymphocytes. They also decrease alpha-adrenergic receptors in heart muscle and may amplify catecholamine action at a postreceptor site. Thus, thyrotoxicosis is characterized by an increased metabolic and hemodynamic sensitivity of the tissues to catecholamines. However, circulating catecholamine levels are normal. Drugs that block beta-adrenergic receptors (eg, propranolol) reduce or eliminate the tachycardia, arrhythmias, sweating, and tremor of hyperthyroidism.

Thyroid hormone excess causes rapid mentation, nervousness, irritability, emotional lability, restlessness, and even mania and psychosis. Patients complain of poor concentration and reduced performance at work or in school. Tremor is common and deep tendon reflexes are brisk, with a rapid relaxation phase. Muscle weakness and atrophy (**thyrotoxic myopathy**) commonly develops in hyperthyroidism, particularly if severe and prolonged. Proximal muscle weakness may interfere with walking, climbing, rising from a deep knee bend, or weight lifting. Such muscle weakness may be due to increased protein catabolism and muscle wasting, to decreased muscle efficiency, or to changes in myosin. Despite an increased number of beta-adrenergic receptors in muscle, the increased proteolysis is apparently not mediated by beta receptors, and muscle weakness and wasting are not affected by beta-adrenergic blockers. Myasthenia gravis or periodic paralysis may accompany hyperthyroidism.

Vital capacity and respiratory muscle strength are reduced. Extreme muscle weakness may cause respiratory failure.

In hyperthyroidism, cardiac output is increased as a result of increased heart rate and contractility and reduced peripheral vascular resistance. Pulse pressure is increased, and circulation time is shortened in the hyperthyroid state. Tachycardia, usually supraventricular, is frequent and thought to be related to the direct effects of thyroid hormone on the cardiac conducting system. Atrial fibrillation may occur, particularly in elderly patients. Continuous 24-hour electrocardiographic monitoring of thyrotoxic patients shows persistent tachycardia but preservation of the normal circadian rhythm of the heart rate, suggesting that normal adrenergic responsiveness persists. Myocardial calcium uptake is increased in thyrotoxic rats; in humans, calcium channel-blocking agents (eg, diltiazem) can decrease the heart rate, the number of premature ventricular beats, and the number of bouts of supraventricular tachycardia, paroxysmal atrial fibrillation, and ventricular tachycardia. Long-standing hyperthyroidism may lead to cardiomegaly and a "high-output" congestive heart failure. Flow murmurs are common and extracardiac sounds occur, generated by the hyperdynamic heart.

Hyperthyroidism leads to increased hepatic gluconeogenesis, enhanced carbohydrate absorption, and increased insulin degradation. In nondiabetic pa-

Table 20–4. Clinical findings in hyperthyroidism (thyrotoxicosis).

Symptoms
Alertness, emotional lability, nervousness, irritability
Poor concentration
Muscular weakness, fatigability
Palpitations
Voracious appetite, weight loss
Hyperdefecation (increased frequency of bowel movements)
Heat intolerance

Signs
Hyperkinesia, rapid speech
Proximal muscle (quadriceps) weakness, fine tremor
Fine, moist skin; fine, abundant hair; onycholysis
Lid lag, stare, chemosis, periorbital edema, proptosis
Accentuated first heart sound, tachycardia, atrial fibrillation (resistant to digitalis), widened pulse pressure, dyspnea

Laboratory findings
Suppressed serum TSH level
Elevated serum free thyroxine, elevated serum total T_4, elevated resin T_3 or T_4 uptake, elevated free thyroxine index
Increased radioiodine uptake by thyroid gland (some causes)
Increased basal metabolic rate (BMR)
Decreased serum cholesterol level

tients, after ingestion of carbohydrate, the blood glucose rises rapidly, sometimes causing glycosuria, then falls rapidly. There may be an adaptive increase in insulin secretion, perhaps explaining the normal glycemic, glycogenolytic, glycolytic, and ketogenic sensitivity to epinephrine. Diabetic patients have an increased insulin requirement in the hyperthyroid state.

Metabolically, the total plasma cholesterol is usually low, related to an increase in the number of hepatic LDL receptors. Lipolysis is increased, and adipocytes show an increase in beta-adrenergic receptor density and increased responsiveness to catecholamines. With the rise in metabolic rate, there is also an increased need for vitamins; if dietary sources are inadequate, vitamin deficiency syndromes may occur. Bone resorption exceeds bone formation in hyperthyroidism, leading to hypercalciuria and sometimes hypercalcemia. Long-standing hyperthyroidism may lead to osteopenia.

There is an increase in frequency of bowel movements (hyperdefecation) due to increased gastrointestinal motility. Accelerated small bowel transit may be caused by increased frequency of bowel contractions and of giant migrating contractions. In severe thyrotoxicosis, abnormal liver function tests may be observed, reflecting malnutrition.

In women, hyperthyroidism may lead to oligomenorrhea and decreased fertility. In the follicular phase of the menstrual cycle, there is an increased basal plasma LH and an increased LH and FSH response to GnRH (Chapter 22). There is an increase in sex hormone-binding globulin, leading to increased levels of total estradiol. In men, hyperthyroidism may cause decreased fertility and impotence from altered steroid hormone metabolism. Serum levels of total testosterone, total estradiol, sex hormone-binding globulin, LH, and FSH and gonadotropin response to GnRH are significantly greater than normal. However, the ratio of free testosterone to free estradiol is lower than normal. Mean sperm counts are normal, but the percentage of forward progressive sperm motility is lower than normal (Chapter 23). These hormone and semen abnormalities are reversible with successful treatment of the hyperthyroidism. Gynecomastia may occur despite high normal serum testosterone levels secondary to increased peripheral conversion of androgens to estrogens (Chapter 23).

There is an increased plasma concentration of atrial natriuretic peptide (ANP) and its precursors. The plasma ANP concentration correlates with the serum thyroxine level and heart rate and decreases to normal with successful antithyroid therapy.

The wide-eyed stare of hyperthyroid patients may be due to increased sympathetic tone. In addition, proptosis develops in 25–50% of patients with Graves' disease due to infiltration of orbital soft tissues and extraocular muscles with lymphocytes, mucopolysaccharides, and edema fluid (Figure 20–7). This may lead to fibrosis of the extraocular muscles,

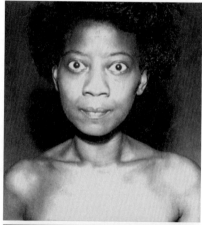
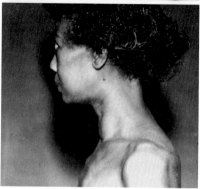

Figure 20–7. Graves' disease. (Courtesy of PH Forsham.)

restricted ocular motility, and diplopia. In severe Graves' ophthalmopathy, pressure on the optic nerve or keratitis due to corneal exposure may lead to blindness. The pathogenesis of Graves' ophthalmopathy may involve cytotoxic lymphocytes (killer cells) and cytotoxic antibodies to an antigen common to orbital fibroblasts, orbital muscle, and thyroid tissue (Figure 20–6). It is postulated that cytokines released from these sensitized lymphocytes cause inflammation of orbital tissues, resulting in the proptosis, diplopia, and edema. For unknown reasons, Graves' ophthalmopathy is worse in smokers and may be exacerbated by radioiodine therapy.

The skin is warm, sweaty, and velvety in texture. There may be onycholysis (ie, retraction of the nail from the nail plate). In Graves' disease, the pretibial skin may become thickened, resembling an orange peel (**pretibial myxedema** or **thyrotoxic dermopathy**). The dermopathy is usually a late manifestation of Graves' disease, and affected patients invariably have ophthalmopathy. The most common form of the dermopathy is nonpitting edema, but nodular, plaque-like, and even polypoid forms also occur. The pathogenesis of thyroid dermopathy may also involve lymphocyte cytokine stimulation of fibroblasts. Thyroid dermopathy is associated with a very high serum titer of TSH-R [stim] Ab.

Untreated hyperthyroidism may decompensate into a state called **thyroid storm.** Patients so affected have tachycardia, fever, agitation, nausea, vomiting, diarrhea, and restlessness or psychosis. The condition is usually precipitated by an intercurrent illness or by a surgical emergency.

---

12. Describe the physiologic consequences of hyperthyroidism and identify their mechanism (as is best known) on the following systems:
    Heart
    Liver
    Lungs
    GI tract
    Kidney
    Eyes
    Skin
    Brain
    Bone
    Reproductive system

HYPOTHYROIDISM

Etiology

The causes of hypothyroidism are listed in Table 20–5. The most common cause is Hashimoto's thyroiditis, which probably results from an autoimmune destruction of the thyroid, though the precipitating cause and exact mechanism of the autoimmunity and subsequent destruction are unknown. Hypothyroidism may also be caused by lymphocytic thyroiditis following a transient period of hyperthyroidism. Thyroid ablation, whether by surgical resection or by therapeutic radiation, commonly results in hypothyroidism.

Diseases of the pituitary or hypothalamus may cause diminished TSH secretion, producing hypothyroidism as a secondary or tertiary result. In some cases of hypothyroidism caused by hypothalamic disease, the TSH secreted by the pituitary lacks biologic activity and exhibits impaired binding to its receptor. This defect can be reversed by administration of TRH. Thus, TRH may regulate not only the secretion of TSH but also the specific molecular and conformational features that enable it to act at its receptor.

Finally, a host of drugs, including the thioamide antithyroid medications propylthiouracil and methimazole, may produce hypothyroidism. The thioamides inhibit thyroid peroxidase and block the synthesis of thyroid hormone. In addition, propylthiouracil (but not methimazole) blocks the peripheral conversion of T_4 to T_3. Deiodination of iodine-containing compounds such as amiodarone, releasing large amounts of iodide, may also cause hypothyroidism by blocking iodide organification, an effect known as the Wolff-Chaikoff block. Lithium is concentrated by the thyroid and inhibits the release of hormone from the gland. Most patients treated with lithium compensate by increasing TSH secretion, but some become hypothyroid.

Table 20–5. Hypothyroidism: Causes and pathogenetic mechanisms.

Etiologic Classification	Pathogenetic Mechanism
Congenital	Aplasia or hypoplasia of thyroid gland
	Defects in hormone biosynthesis or action
Acquired	
Hashimoto's thyroiditis	Autoimmune destruction
Severe iodine deficiency	Diminished hormone synthesis, release
Lymphocytic thyroiditis	Diminished hormone synthesis, release
Thyroid ablation	Diminished hormone synthesis, release
Thyroid surgery	
^{131}I radiation treatment of hyperthyroidism	
External beam radiation therapy of head and neck cancer	
Drugs	Diminished hormone synthesis, release
Iodine, inorganic	
Iodine, organic (amiodarone)	
Thioamides (propylthiouracil,[1] methimazole)	
Potassium perchlorate	
Thiocyanate	
Lithium	
Hypopituitarism	Deficient TSH secretion
Hypothalamic disease	Deficient TRH secretion

[1] Also blocks peripheral conversion of T_4 to T_3.

Pathogenesis

Hypothyroidism is characterized by abnormally low serum T_4 and T_3 levels. Free thyroxine levels are always depressed. The serum TSH level is elevated in hypothyroidism (except in cases of pituitary or hypothalamic disease). TSH is the most sensitive test for early hypothyroidism, and marked elevations of serum TSH (> 20 mU/L) are found in frank hypothyroidism. Modest TSH elevations (5–20 mU/L) may be found in euthyroid individuals with normal serum T_4 and T_3 levels and indicate impaired thyroid reserve and incipient hypothyroidism. In patients with primary hypothyroidism (end organ failure), the nocturnal TSH surge is intact. In patients with central (pituitary or hypothalamic) hypothyroidism, the serum TSH level is low and the normal nocturnal TSH surge is absent.

In hypothyroidism due to end-organ failure, administration of TRH produces a prompt rise in the TSH level, the magnitude of which is proportionate to the baseline serum TSH level. The hypernormal response is caused by absence of feedback inhibition by T_4 and T_3. However, the TRH test is not usually performed in patients with primary hypothyroidism, since the elevated basal serum TSH level suffices to make the diagnosis. The test is useful in the clinically hypothyroid patient with an unexpectedly low serum TSH level in establishing a central (pituitary or hypothalamic) origin. Pituitary disease is suggested by the failure of TSH to rise following TRH administration; hypothalamic disease is suggested by a delayed TSH response (at 60–120 minutes rather than 15–30 minutes) with a normal increment.

Hashimoto's Thyroiditis

A. Pathology: In the early stages of Hashimoto's thyroiditis, the gland is diffusely enlarged, firm, rubbery, and nodular. As the disease progresses, the gland becomes smaller. In the late stages, the gland is atrophic and fibrotic, weighing as little as 10–20 g. Microscopically, there is destruction of thyroid follicles and lymphocytic infiltration with lymphoid follicles. The surviving thyroid follicular epithelial cells are large, with abundant pink cytoplasm (Hürthle cells). As the disease progresses, there is an increasing amount of fibrosis.

B. Pathogenesis: The pathogenesis of Hashimoto's thyroiditis is unclear. Again, it is possible that a defect in suppressor T lymphocytes allows helper T lymphocytes to interact with specific antigens on the thyroid follicular cell membrane. Once these lymphocytes become sensitized to thyroidal antigens, autoantibodies are formed that react with these antigens. Cytokine release and inflammation then cause glandular destruction. The most important thyroid autoantibodies in Hashimoto's thyroiditis are thyroglobulin antibody (Tg Ab), thyroidal peroxidase antibody (TPO Ab) (formerly termed antimicrosomal antibody), and the TSH receptor blocking antibody (TSH-R [block] Ab). During the early phases, Tg Ab is markedly elevated and TPO Ab only slightly elevated. Later, Tg Ab may disappear, but TPO Ab persists for many years. TSH-R [block] Ab is found in patients with atrophic thyroiditis and myxedema and in mothers who give birth to infants with no detectable thyroid tissue (**athyreotic cretins**). Serum levels of these antibodies do not correlate with the severity of the hypothyroidism, but their presence is helpful in diagnosis. In general, high antibody titers are diagnostic of Hashimoto's thyroiditis; moderate titers are seen in Graves' disease, multinodular goiter, and thyroid neoplasm; and low titers are found in the elderly.

Patients with Hashimoto's thyroiditis have an increased frequency of the HLA-DR5 histocompatibility antigen, and the disease is associated with a host of other autoimmune diseases (Table 20–3). A **polyglandular failure syndrome** has been defined in which two or more endocrine disorders mediated by autoimmune mechanisms occur (Chapter 17). Affected patients frequently have circulating organ- and cell-specific autoantibodies that lead to organ hypofunction.

---

13. What are some drugs that cause hypothyroidism?
14. What are the most useful initial tests of thyroid function in hypothyroidism? What results would you expect compared to normal?
15. What are the key pathophysiologic findings in Hashimoto's thyroiditis?

Clinical Manifestations

The clinical consequences of thyroid hormone deficiency are summarized in Table 20–6.

Hypothermia is common, and the patient may complain of cold intolerance. The decreased basal metabolic rate leads to weight gain despite reduced food intake.

Thyroid hormones are required for normal development of the nervous system. In hypothyroid infants, synapses develop abnormally, myelination is defective, and mental retardation occurs. Hypothyroid adults have slowed mentation, forgetfulness, decreased hearing, and ataxia. Some patients have severe mental symptoms, including reversible dementia or overt psychosis ("myxedema madness"). The cerebrospinal fluid protein level is abnormally high. However, total cerebral blood flow and oxygen consumption are normal. Deep tendon reflexes are sluggish, with a slowed ("hung-up") relaxation phase. Paresthesias are common, often caused by compression neuropathies due to accumulation of myxedema (carpal tunnel syndrome and tarsal tunnel syndrome).

Hypothyroidism is associated with muscle weakness, cramps, and stiffness. The serum creatine kinase (CK) level may be elevated. The pathophysiol-

Table 20–6. Clinical findings in adult hypothyroidism (myxedema).

Symptoms
  Slow thinking
  Lethargy, decreased vigor
  Dry skin; thickened hair; hair loss; broken nails
  Diminished food intake; weight gain
  Constipation
  Menorrhagia; diminished libido
  Cold intolerance

Signs
  Round puffy face; slow speech; hoarseness
  Hypokinesia; generalized muscle weakness; delayed relaxation of deep tendon reflexes
  Cold, dry, thick, scaling skin; dry, coarse, brittle hair; dry, longitudinally ridged nails
  Periorbital edema
  Normal or faint cardiac impulse; indistinct heart sounds; cardiac enlargement; bradycardia
  Ascites; pericardial effusion; ankle edema
  Mental clouding, depression

Laboratory findings
  Increased serum TSH level
  Decreased serum free thyroxine, decreased serum total T_4 and T_3; decreased resin T_3 or T_4 uptake; decreased free thyroxine index
  Decreased radioiodine uptake by thyroid gland
  Diminished basal metabolic rate (BMR)
  Macrocytic anemia
  Elevated serum cholesterol level
  Elevated serum CK level
  Decreased circulation time; low voltage of QRS complex on ECG

ogy of the muscle disease in hypothyroidism is poorly understood. Study of the bioenergetic abnormalities in hypothyroid muscle suggests a hormone-dependent, reversible mitochondrial impairment. Changes in energy metabolism are not found in hyperthyroid muscle.

Patients rendered acutely hypothyroid by total thyroidectomy exhibit a decreased cardiac output, decreased stroke volume, decreased diastolic volume at rest, and an increased peripheral resistance. However, the pulmonary capillary wedge pressure, right atrial pressure, heart rate, left ventricular ejection fraction, and left ventricular systolic pressure-volume relation (a measure of contractility) are not significantly different from the euthyroid state. Thus, in early hypothyroidism, alterations in cardiac performance are probably primarily related to changes in loading conditions and exercise-related heart rate rather than to changes in myocardial contractility.

In chronic hypothyroidism, echocardiography shows bradycardia and features that suggest cardiomyopathy, including increased thickening of the intraventricular septum and ventricular wall, decreased regional wall motion, and decreased global left ventricular function. These changes may be due to deposition of excessive mucopolysaccharides in the interstitium between myocardial fibers, leading to fiber degeneration, decreased contractility, low cardiac output, cardiac enlargement, and congestive heart failure. Pericardial effusion (with high protein content) may lead to findings of decreased electrocardiographic voltage and flattened T waves, but cardiac tamponade is rare.

Hypothyroid patients exhibit decreased ventilatory responses to hypercapnia and hypoxia. There is a high incidence of sleep apnea in untreated hypothyroidism; such patients sometimes demonstrate myopathy of upper airway muscles. Weakness of the diaphragm also occurs frequently and, when severe, can cause chronic alveolar hypoventilation (CO_2 retention). Pleural effusions (with high protein content) may occur.

In hypothyroidism, the plasma cholesterol and triglyceride levels increase, related to decreased lipoprotein lipase activity and decreased formation of hepatic LDL receptors. In hypothyroid children, bone growth is slowed and skeletal maturation (closure of epiphyses) is delayed. Pituitary secretion of growth hormone may also be depressed, because thyroid hormone is needed for its synthesis. Hypothyroid animals demonstrate decreased width of epiphysial growth plate and articular cartilage and decreased volume of epiphysial and metaphysial trabecular bone. These changes are not solely due to lack of pituitary growth hormone, since administering exogenous growth hormone does not restore normal cartilage morphology or bone remodeling, whereas administering T_4 does. If unrecognized, prolonged juvenile hypothyroidism results in a permanent height deficit.

A normochromic, normocytic anemia may occur as a result of decreased erythropoiesis. Alternatively, a moderate macrocytic anemia can occur as a result of decreased absorption of cyanocobalamin (vitamin B_{12}) from the intestine and diminished bone marrow metabolism. Frank megaloblastic anemia suggests coexistent pernicious anemia.

Constipation is common and reflects decreased gastrointestinal motility. Achlorhydria occurs when hypothyroidism is associated with pernicious anemia. Ascitic fluid with high protein content may accumulate.

The skin in hypothyroidism is dry and cool. Normally, the skin contains a variety of proteins complexed with polysaccharides, chondroitin sulfuric acid, and hyaluronic acid. In hypothyroidism, these complexes accumulate, promoting sodium and water retention and producing a characteristic diffuse, nonpitting puffiness of the skin (myxedema). The patient's face appears puffy, with coarse features (Figure 20–8). Similar accumulation of mucopolysaccharides in the larynx may lead to hoarseness. The hair is brittle and lacking in luster, and there is frequently loss of body hair, particularly over the scalp and lateral eyebrows. If thyroid hormone is administered, the protein complexes are mobilized, a diuresis ensues, and myxedema resolves.

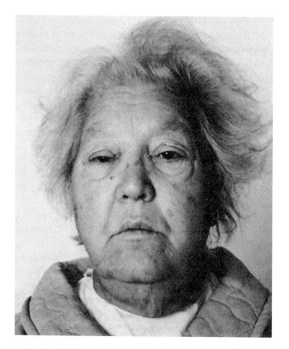

Figure 20–8. Myxedema. (Reproduced, with permission, from Greenspan FS, Strewler GJ [editors]: *Basic and Clinical Endocrinology,* 5th ed. Appleton & Lange, 1997.)

usually precipitated by an intercurrent illness such as an infection or stroke or by a medication such as a sedative-hypnotic. The mortality rate approaches 100% unless myxedema coma is recognized and treated promptly.

16. Describe and explain the physiologic consequence of hypothyroidism (as is best known) on the following:
    Nervous system
    Muscle
    Cardiovascular system
    Lungs
    Liver
    Blood
    GI tract
    Skin
    Reproductive system
    Kidney

Carotenemia (manifested as yellow-orange discoloration of the skin) may occur in hypothyroidism because thyroid hormones are needed for hepatic conversion of carotene to vitamin A. In the absence of sufficient hormone, carotene accumulates in the bloodstream and skin.

In women, hypothyroidism may lead to menorrhagia from anovulatory cycles. Alternatively, menses may become scanty or disappear secondary to diminished secretion of gonadotropins. Since thyroid hormone normally has an inhibitory effect on prolactin secretion, hypothyroid patients may exhibit hyperprolactinemia, with galactorrhea and amenorrhea. In men, hypothyroidism can cause infertility and gynecomastia from enhanced release of prolactin. Hyperprolactinemia occurs because TRH stimulates prolactin release.

There is reduced renal blood flow and a decreased glomerular filtration rate. The vasoconstriction may be due to decreased concentrations of plasma ANP. The consequent reduced ability to excrete a water load may cause hyponatremia. However, the serum creatinine level is usually normal.

Long-standing severe untreated hypothyroidism may lead to a state called **myxedema coma.** Affected patients have typical myxedematous facies and skin, bradycardia, hypothermia, alveolar hypoventilation, and severe obtundation or coma. This condition is

GOITER

Etiology

Diffuse thyroid enlargement most commonly results from prolonged stimulation by TSH (or a TSH-like agent). Such stimulation may be the result of one of the causes of hypothyroidism (eg, TSH in Hashimoto's thyroiditis) or of hyperthyroidism (eg, TSH-R [stim] Ab in Graves' disease, hCG in germ cell tumors, or TSH in pituitary adenoma). Alternatively, goiter may occur in a clinically euthyroid patient. Table 20–7 lists the causes and pathogenetic mechanisms.

Iodine deficiency is the most common cause of goiter in developing nations. A diet that contains less than 10 µg/d of iodine hinders the synthesis of thyroid hormone, resulting in an elevated TSH level and thyroid hypertrophy. Iodination of salt has eliminated this problem in much of the developed world.

A goiter may also develop from ingestion of **goitrogens** (factors that block thyroid hormone synthesis) either in food or in medication. Dietary goitrogens are found in vegetables of the Brassicaceae family (rutabagas, cabbage, turnips, cassava, etc). A goitrogenic hydrocarbon has been found in the water supply in some locations. Medications that act as goitrogens include thioamides and thiocyanates (propylthiouracil, methimazole, nitroprusside, etc), sulfonylureas, and lithium. Lithium inhibits thyroid hormone release and perhaps also iodide organification. Most patients remain clinically euthyroid because TSH production increases.

A congenital goiter associated with hypothyroidism (**sporadic cretinism**) may occur as a result of a defect in any of the steps of thyroid hormone synthesis (Table 20–5). All of these defects are rare.

Table 20–7. Goiter: Causes and pathogenetic mechanisms.

Causes	Pathogenetic Mechanism
I. Goiter associated with hypothyroidism or euthyroidism	
Iodine deficiency	Interferes with hormone biosynthesis
Iodine excess	Blocks secretion of hormone
Goitrogen in diet or drinking water	Interferes with hormone biosynthesis
Goitrogenic medication Thioamides: propylthiouracil, methimazole, carbimazole Thiocyanates: nitroprusside Aniline derivatives: sulfonylureas, sulfonamides, aminosalicylic acid, phenylbutazone, aminoglutethimide	Interferes with hormone biosynthesis
Lithium	Blocks secretion of hormone
Congenital disorders Defective transport of iodide Defective organification of iodide due to absence or reduction of peroxidase or production of an abnormal peroxidase Synthesis of an abnormal thyroglobulin Abnormal interrelationships of iodotyrosine Impaired proteolysis of thyroglobulin Defective deiodination of iodotyrosine	Various defects in hormone biosynthesis
Pituitary and peripheral resistance to thyroid hormone	? Receptor defects
II. Goiter associated with hyperthyroidism	
Graves' disease	TSH-R [stim] Ab stimulation of gland
Toxic multinodular goiter	Autonomous hyperfunction
Germ cell tumor	hCG stimulation of gland
Pituitary adenoma	TSH overproduction
Thyroiditis	Enlargement due to "injury," infiltration, and edema

Goiter with hyperthyroidism is usually due to Graves' disease. In Graves' disease, the gland is enlarged because of stimulation by TSH-R [stim] Ab and other antibodies rather than by TSH.

Pathogenesis & Pathology

In goiter due to impaired thyroid hormone synthesis, there is a progressive fall in serum T_4 and a progressive rise in serum TSH. As the TSH increases, iodine turnover by the gland is accelerated and the ratio of T_3 secretion relative to T_4 secretion is increased. Consequently, the serum T_3 may be normal or increased, and the patient may remain clinically euthyroid. If there is more marked impairment of hormone synthesis, goiter formation is associated with a low T_4, low T_3, and elevated TSH, and the patient becomes clinically hypothyroid.

In the early stages of goiter, there is diffuse enlargement of the gland, with cellular hyperplasia caused by the TSH stimulation. Later, there are enlarged follicles with flattened follicular epithelial cells and accumulation of thyroglobulin. This accumulation occurs particularly in iodine deficiency goiter, perhaps because poorly iodinated thyroglobulin is less easily digested by proteases. As TSH stimulation continues, multiple nodules may develop in some areas and atrophy and fibrosis in others, producing a multinodular goiter (Figure 20–9).

In patients with severe iodine deficiency or inherited metabolic defects, a nontoxic goiter develops because impaired hormone secretion leads to an in-

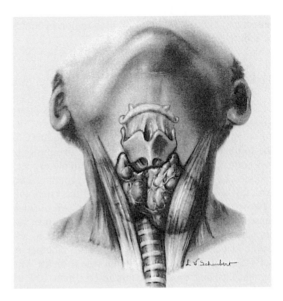

Figure 20–9. Multinodular goiter. (Reproduced, with permission, from Greenspan FS, Strewler GJ [editors]: *Basic and Clinical Endocrinology,* 5th ed. Appleton & Lange, 1997.)

crease in TSH secretion. The elevation in serum TSH level results in diffuse thyroid hyperplasia. If TSH stimulation is prolonged, the diffuse hyperplasia is followed by focal hyperplasia with necrosis, hemorrhage, and formation of nodules. These nodules often vary from "hot" nodules that can trap iodine and synthesize thyroglobulin to "cold" ones that cannot. In early goiters, the hyperplasia is TSH-dependent, but in later stages the nodules become TSH-independent **autonomous nodules.** Thus, over a period of time there may be a transition from a nontoxic, TSH-dependent, diffuse hyperplasia to a toxic or nontoxic, TSH-independent, multinodular goiter.

The exact mechanism underlying this transition to autonomous growth and function is unknown. However, mutations of the *gsp* oncogene have been found in nodules from many patients with multinodular goiter. Such mutations presumably occur during TSH-induced cell division. The *gsp* oncogene is responsible for activation of regulatory GTP-binding (G_s) protein in the follicular cell membrane. Chronic activation of this protein and its effector, adenylyl cyclase, is postulated to result in thyroid cell proliferation, hyperfunction, and independence from TSH.

Clinical Manifestations

With decades of TSH stimulation, enormous hypertrophy and enlargement of the gland can occur. The enlarged gland may weigh 1–5 kg and may produce respiratory difficulties secondary to obstruction of the trachea or dysphagia secondary to obstruction of the esophagus. More modest enlargements pose cosmetic problems.

Some patients with multinodular goiter also develop hyperthyroidism late in life **(Plummer's disease),** particularly following administration of iodide or iodine-containing drugs.

THYROID NODULES & NEOPLASMS

Tumors of the thyroid usually present as a solitary mass in the neck. The commonest neoplasm, accounting for 30% of all solitary thyroid nodules, is the **follicular adenoma.** It is a solitary, firm, gray or red nodule, up to 5 cm in diameter, completely surrounded by a fibrous capsule. The surrounding normal thyroid tissue is compressed by the adenoma. Microscopically, the adenoma consists of normal-appearing follicles of varying size, sometimes associated with hemorrhage, fibrosis, calcification, and cystic degeneration. Occasionally, only ribbons of follicular cells are present, without true follicles. Malignant change probably occurs in less than 10% of follicular adenomas.

Thyroid cancers are infrequent. Most are derived from the follicular epithelium and, depending on their microscopic appearance, are classified as **papillary** or **follicular carcinoma.** The major risk factor predisposing to epithelial thyroid carcinoma is exposure to radiation, but genetic factors have also been recognized recently. Most papillary and follicular cancers pursue a prolonged clinical course (15–20 years). Papillary carcinoma typically metastasizes to regional lymph nodes in the neck, while follicular cancer tends to spread via the bloodstream to distant sites such as bone or lung. **Medullary carcinoma** is an uncommon neoplasm of the C cells (parafollicular cells) of the thyroid that produce calcitonin (see Chapter 17). Approximately 25–35% of all medullary thyroid carcinomas are a manifestation of multiple endocrine neoplasia type 2 (MEN 2), inherited in an autosomal dominant fashion.

ABNORMAL THYROID FUNCTION TESTS IN CLINICALLY EUTHYROID INDIVIDUALS

Increases & Decreases in Hormone-Binding Proteins

Sustained increases or decreases in the concentration of TBG and other thyroid-binding proteins in the plasma are produced by several normal and disordered physiologic states and by medications. These are summarized in Table 20–8. For example, TBG levels are elevated during pregnancy and by estrogen and oral contraceptive therapy. TBG levels are depressed in the nephrotic syndrome and by glucocorticoid or androgen therapy.

When a sustained increase in the concentration of TBG and other binding proteins occurs, the concentration of free thyroid hormones falls temporarily. This fall stimulates TSH secretion, which then results in an increase in the production of free hormone. Eventually, a new equilibrium is reached in which the levels of total plasma T_4 and T_3 are elevated, but the concentrations of free hormones, the rate of hormone degradation, and the rate of TSH secretion are normal. Therefore, individuals manifesting sustained increases in TBG and other binding proteins remain euthyroid. When a sustained decrease in the concentration of TBG and other binding proteins occurs, equivalent changes occur in the opposite direction, and again the individuals remain euthyroid.

Abnormal Hormone-Binding Proteins

Changes in serum concentrations of the hormone-binding proteins transthyretin or albumin alone usually do not cause significant changes in thyroid hormone levels. However, several unusual syndromes of **familial euthyroid hyperthyroxinemia** have been described. In the first, a familial syndrome called **euthyroid dysalbuminemic hyperthyroxinemia,** there is abnormal binding of T_4 (but not T_3) to albumin. In the second, there is an increased serum level of

Table 20–8. Effects of normal and disordered physiologic states and medications on plasma thyroid-binding proteins and thyroid hormone levels.[1]

Condition	Concentrations of Binding Proteins	Total Plasma T_4, T_3, RT_3	Free Plasma T_4, T_3, RT_3	Plasma TSH	Clinical State
Primary hyperthyroidism	Normal	High	High	Low	Hyperthyroid
Primary hypothyroidism	Normal	Low	Low	High	Hypothyroid
Drugs (estrogens, methadone, heroin, perphenazine, clofibrate), pregnancy, acute and chronic hepatitis, acute intermittent porphyria, estrogen-producing tumors, idiopathic, hereditary	High	High	Normal	Normal	Euthyroid
Drugs (glucocorticoids, androgens, danazol, asparaginase), acromegaly, nephrotic syndrome, hypoproteinemia, chronic liver disease (cirrhosis), testosterone-producing tumors, hereditary	Low	Low	Normal	Normal	Euthyroid

[1]Modified and reproduced, with permission, from Ganong WF: *Review of Medical Physiology,* 19th ed. Appleton & Lange, 1999.

transthyretin. In the third, there are alterations in transthyretin, a tetrameric protein that transports 15–20% of circulating T_4. The alterations in transthyretin structure produced by different point mutations can markedly increase its affinity for T_4. In some families, these mutations in transthyretin are transmitted by autosomal dominant inheritance. In all three of these syndromes, total T_4 is elevated, but free T_4 is normal and the patients are euthyroid. A fourth syndrome has also been described in which there is both pituitary and peripheral resistance to thyroid hormone. As noted above, this condition may be due to point mutations in the human thyroid receptor *(hTR-β1)* gene, resulting in abnormal nuclear T_3 receptors.

Effects of Nonthyroidal Illness & Drugs

Several nonthyroidal illnesses and various drugs inhibit the 5'-deiodinase that converts T_4 to T_3, resulting in a fall in plasma T_3. Illnesses that depress 5'-deiodinase include severe burns or trauma, surgery, advanced cancer, cirrhosis, renal failure, myocardial infarction, prolonged fever, and caloric deprivation (fasting, anorexia nervosa, malnutrition). The decreased serum T_3 in nonthyroidal illnesses is thought to be an adaptive physiologic change, enabling the sick patient to conserve energy and protein. Drugs which depress 5'-deiodinase include glucocorticoids, propranolol, amiodarone, propylthiouracil, and cholecystography dyes (eg, ipodate, iopanoic acid).

Since T_3 is the major active thyroid hormone at the tissue level, it is surprising that patients with mild to moderate nonthyroidal illness exhibit normal TSH levels despite low T_3 levels and do not appear hypothyroid. However, such patients retain the ability to respond to a further reduction (or to an increase) in serum T_3 by increasing (or decreasing) pituitary TSH secretion. Patients with severe illnesses (eg, patients undergoing bone marrow transplantation for leukemia) may manifest impaired TSH secretion.

Most patients with nonthyroidal illnesses have low serum T_3 levels related to the decreased peripheral conversion of T_4 to T_3. However, in some patients, the primary cause of the low serum T_3 is reduced secretion of T_4 by the gland. In others, the binding of T_4 and T_3 by serum thyroid-binding proteins is impaired because of the decreased concentrations of thyroid-binding proteins (Table 20–8) and the presence of circulating inhibitors of binding.

The low T_3 state generally disappears with recovery from the illness or cessation of the drug. Because low T_3 levels are difficult to interpret during acute illness, the diagnostic approach should be based primarily on serum TSH levels.

Subclinical Thyroid Disease

With the development of more sensitive tests of thyroid function, it is increasingly recognized that some clinically euthyroid individuals have subclinical thyroid disease, defined as low or high TSH levels but normal circulating T_4 and T_3 levels. Many individuals with subclinical thyroid disease have abnormal TRH stimulation tests, but the clinical significance of these biochemical abnormalities is not known.

Subclinical hypothyroidism is defined as an elevated TSH (> 5 mU/L) but normal circulating thyroid hormone levels. In the presence of circulating thyroid autoantibodies, approximately 5% of individuals with subclinical hypothyroidism will progress to overt hypothyroidism each year. Subclinical hypothyroidism may be associated with subtle neuropsychiatric abnormalities, and some individuals report an improved sense of well-being when given sufficient thyroxine to normalize serum TSH.

Subclinical hyperthyroidism is defined as a low TSH (< 0.1 mU/L) but normal circulating thyroid hormone levels. Although the natural history of subclinical hyperthyroidism is not well understood, autonomous thyroid nodules are believed to account for many cases. Several studies have demonstrated subtle abnormalities of cardiac contractility in individuals with subclinical hyperthyroidism, and one prospective study found that individuals over age 65 with TSH < 0.1 mU/L had a threefold greater risk of developing atrial fibrillation than those with normal TSH levels. Subclinical hyperthyroidism may also be associated with bone loss and fractures in postmenopausal women, but this has not been well studied. The natural history of subclinical hyperthyroidism is not well known, but in one study of postmenopausal women with endogenous subclinical hyperthyroidism over 50% had normal TSH levels after 1 year of follow-up.

17. What is a goiter?
18. What are the causes and mechanisms of goiter formation?
19. What is the basis for transition from nontoxic, TSH-dependent diffuse hyperplasia to a toxic or nontoxic TSH-independent multinodular goiter?
20. How large can the thyroid gland become with decades of stimulation?
21. What are the different types of thyroid cancer and their characteristics?
22. What are some physiologic and pathophysiologic conditions in which thyroid metabolism is altered? How and with what effects?
23. What is the overall thyroid status of a patient with a sustained decrease in thyroid-binding globulin?
24. What are some of the factors which depress 5'-deiodinase activity?
25. How does nonthyroidal illness typically affect thyroid hormone levels?

REFERENCES

General

Braverman LE, Utiger RD (editors): *Werner and Ingbar's The Thyroid: A Fundamental and Clinical Text,* 7th ed. Lippincott-Raven, 1996.

Brent GA: The molecular basis of thyroid hormone action. N Engl J Med 1994;331:847.

Davies TF: T-cell receptor gene expression in autoimmune thyroid disease: Some observations and possible mechanisms. Ann N Y Acad Sci 1995;756:331.

Greenspan FS: The thyroid gland. In: *Basic and Clinical Endocrinology,* 5th ed. Greenspan FS, Strewler GJ (editors). Appleton & Lange, 1997.

Grossman M, Weintraub BD, Szkudlinski MW: Novel insights into the molecular mechanisms of human thyrotropin action: Structural, physiological and therapeutic implications for the glycoprotein hormone family. Endocr Rev 1997;18:476.

Larsen PT, Davies TF, Hay ID: The thyroid gland. In: *Williams Textbook of Endocrinology,* 9th ed. Wilson JD et al (editors). Saunders, 1998.

Mariotti S et al: The aging thyroid. Endocr Rev 1995; 16:686.

Hyperthyroidism

Bertelsen JB, Hegedus L: Cigarette smoking and the thyroid. Thyroid 1994;4:327.

Burch HB, Wartofsky L: Life-threatening thyrotoxicosis: Thyroid storm. Endocrinol Metab Clin North Am 1993;22:263.

Davies TF et al: Thyroid controversy: Stimulating antibodies. J Clin Endocrinol Metab 1998;83:3777.

Dremier S et al: Thyroid autonomy: Mechanism and clinical effects. J Clin Endocrinol Metab 1996;81:4187.

Fatourechi V, Pajouhi M, Fransway AF: Dermopathy of Graves' disease (pretibial myxedema): Review of 150 cases. Medicine 1994;73:1.

Gomberg-Maitland M, Frishman WH: Thyroid hormone and cardiovascular disease. Am Heart J 1998;135:187.

Heufelder AE: Involvement of the orbital fibroblast and TSH receptor in the pathogenesis of Graves' ophthalmopathy. Thyroid 1995;5:331.

McIver B et al: Lack of effect of thyroxine in patients with Graves' hyperthyroidism who are treated with an antithyroid drug. N Engl J Med 1996;334:220.

Wall J: Extrathyroidal manifestations of Graves' disease. J Clin Endocrinol Metab 1995;80:3427.

Hypothyroidism

Bayan CM, Daniels GH: Chronic autoimmune thyroiditis. N Engl J Med 1996;335:99.

Comtois R, Faucher L, Lafleche L: Outcome of hypothyroidism caused by Hashimoto's thyroiditis. Arch Intern Med 1995;155:1404.

Heufelder AE: Involvement of the orbital fibroblast and TSH receptor in the pathogenesis of Graves' ophthalmopathy. Thyroid 1995;5:331.

LiVolsi VA: The pathology of autoimmune thyroid disease: A review. Thyroid 1994;4:333.

Wall J: Extrathyroidal manifestations of Graves' disease. J Clin Endocrinol Metab 1995;80:3427.

Goiter

Gharib H: Diffuse nontoxic and multinodular goiter. Curr Ther Endocrinol Metab 1994;5:99.

Studer H, Derwahl M: Mechanisms of nonneoplastic endocrine hyperplasia—a changing concept: A review focused on the thyroid gland. Endocr Rev 1995;16:411.

Trimarchi F, Benvenga S, Vermiglio F: Endemic goiter. Curr Ther Endocrinol Metab 1994;5:89.

Weetman AP: Is endemic goiter an autoimmune disease? (Editorial.) J Clin Endocrinol Metab 1994;5:89.

Thyroid Nodules & Neoplasms

Boyd CM, Baker JR Jr: The immunology of thyroid cancer. Endocrinol Metab Clin North Am 1996;25:159.

Gagel RF, Goepfert H, Callender DL: Changing concepts in the pathogenesis and management of thyroid carcinoma. CA Cancer J Clin 1996;46:261.

Gharib H, Mazzaferri EL: Thyroxine suppressive therapy in patients with nodular thyroid disease. Ann Intern Med 1998;128:386.

Houlston RS, Stratton MR: Genetics of non-medullary thyroid cancer. Q J Med 1995;88:685.

Santoro M et al: Molecular defects in thyroid carcinomas: Role of the *RET* oncogene in thyroid neoplastic transformation. Eur J Endocrinol 1995;133:513.

Singer PA et al: Treatment guidelines for patients with thyroid nodules and well-differentiated thyroid cancer. American Thyroid Association. Arch Intern Med 1996;156:2165.

Abnormal Thyroid Function Tests in Clinically Euthyroid Individuals

Bodenner DL, Lash RW: Thyroid disease mediated by molecular defects in cell surface and nuclear receptors. Am J Med 1998;105:524.

Brucker-Davis F et al: Genetic and clinical features of 42 kindreds with resistance to thyroid hormone. The National Institutes of Health Prospective Study. Ann Intern Med 1995;123:572.

Chopra IJ: Simultaneous measurement of free thyroxine and free 3,5,3'-triiodothyronine in undiluted serum by direct equilibrium dialysis/radioimmunoassay: Evidence that free triiodothyronine and free thyroxine are normal in many patients with the low triiodothyronine syndrome. Thyroid 1998;8:249.

Howland RH: Thyroid dysfunction in refractory depression: Implications for pathophysiology and treatment. J Clin Psychiatry 1993;54:47.

Kopp P, Kitajima K, Jameson JL: Syndrome of resistance to thyroid hormone: Insights into thyroid hormone action. Proc Soc Exper Biol Med 1996;211:49.

Sawin CT et al: Low serum thyrotropin concentrations as a risk factor for atrial fibrillation in older persons. N Engl J Med 1994;331:1249.

Surks M, Ocampo E: Subclinical thyroid disease. Am J Med 1996;100:217.

Yeo PB, Loh KC: Subclinical thyrotoxicosis. Adv Intern Med 1998;43:501.

21

Disorders of the Adrenal Cortex

Stephen J. McPhee, MD

The adrenal gland is actually two endocrine organs, one wrapped around the other. The outer **adrenal cortex** secretes many different steroid hormones, including glucocorticoids such as cortisol, mineralocorticoids such as aldosterone, and sex hormones, chiefly androgens. The glucocorticoids help to regulate carbohydrate, protein, and fat metabolism. The mineralocorticoids help to regulate Na^+ and K^+ balance and extracellular fluid volume. The glucocorticoids and mineralocorticoids are essential for survival, but the adrenal androgens have only a minor role in reproductive function. The inner **adrenal medulla,** discussed in Chapter 12, secretes catecholamines (epinephrine, norepinephrine, and dopamine). The catecholamines help prepare the individual to deal with emergency situations.

The major disorders of the adrenal cortex (Table 21–1) are characterized by excessive or deficient secretion of each type of adrenocortical hormone: **hypercortisolism (Cushing's syndrome), adrenal insufficiency (Addison's disease), hyperaldosteronism (Conn's syndrome), hypoaldosteronism,** and **androgen excess (adrenogenital syndrome).**

NORMAL STRUCTURE & FUNCTION OF THE ADRENAL CORTEX

ANATOMY

The adrenal glands are paired organs located in the retroperitoneal area near the superior poles of the kidneys (Figure 21–1). They are flattened, crescent-shaped structures which together normally weigh about 8–10 g. They are covered by tight fibrous capsules and surrounded by fat. The blood flow to the adrenals is copious.

Grossly, each gland consists of two concentric layers: the yellow peripheral layer is the **adrenal cortex,** and the reddish brown central layer is the **adrenal medulla.** Adrenal cortical tissue is sometimes found at other sites, usually near the kidney or along the path taken by the gonads during their embryonic descent (Figure 21–1).

HISTOLOGY

The adrenal cortex can be subdivided into three concentric layers: the zona glomerulosa, the zona fasciculata, and the zona reticularis (Figure 21–2). The **zona glomerulosa** is the outermost layer, situated immediately beneath the capsule. Zona glomerulosa cells are columnar or pyramidal in appearance and are arranged in closely packed, rounded or arched clusters surrounded by capillaries. They secrete **mineralocorticoids,** primarily **aldosterone.** The **zona fasciculata** is the middle layer of cortex. Zona fasciculata cells are polyhedral in shape and arranged in straight cords or columns, one or two cells thick, running at right angles to the capsule with capillaries between them. The **zona reticularis,** the innermost layer of the cortex, lies between the zona fasciculata and the adrenal medulla; it accounts for 7% of the mass of the adrenal gland. Zona reticularis cells are smaller than the other two types and are arranged in irregular cords or interlaced in a network. Zona fasciculata and zona reticularis cells secrete both **glucocorticoids,** primarily **cortisol** and **corticosterone,** and **sex hormones,** primarily **androgens** such as **dehydroepiandrosterone.** The ultrastructure of all three types of adrenocortical cells is similar to that of other steroid-synthesizing cells in the body. The steroid hormones produced are low-molecular-weight lipid-soluble molecules able to diffuse freely across cell membranes.

Table 21–1. Principal diseases of the adrenal glands.

Hyperfunction of cortex
  Bilateral hyperplasia
    ACTH excess (affects mainly zona fasciculata and reticularis)
    Enzyme deficiencies
  Adenoma
    Primary hyperaldosteronism (Conn's syndrome) (zona glomerulosa)
    Hypercortisolism (Cushing's syndrome) (zona fasciculata)
    Virilization (zona reticularis)
  Carcinoma
    Cushing's syndrome
    Virilization
    Feminization (rare)
Hypofunction of cortex
  Bilateral adrenal gland destruction (Addison's disease)
    Autoimmune
    Infection
      Tuberculosis
      Histoplasmosis
      AIDS-related (CMV, disseminated *Mycobacterium avium* complex)
    Ischemia, shock
      Bacteremia (meningococcus, pseudomonas)
    Hemorrhage, anticoagulation
    Metastatic tumor (lung carcinoma, other carcinomas, Kaposi's sarcoma)
Hyperfunction of medulla
  Pheochromocytoma
  Hyperplasia (rare)
  Other: ganglioneuroma, neuroblastoma
Hypofunction of medulla

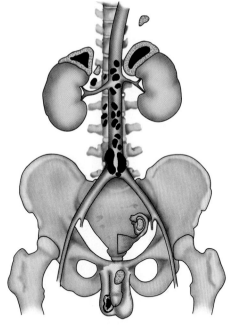

Figure 21–1. Human adrenal glands. Adrenocortical tissue is stippled; adrenal medullary tissue is black. Note location of adrenal at superior pole of each kidney. Also shown are extra-adrenal sites at which cortical and medullary tissue is sometimes found. (Reproduced, with permission, from Forsham PH: The adrenal cortex. In: *Textbook of Endocrinology,* 4th ed. Williams RH [editor]. Saunders, 1968.)

PHYSIOLOGY OF NORMAL ADRENAL CORTEX

1. GLUCOCORTICOIDS

Glucocorticoid Synthesis, Protein Binding, & Metabolism

Cortisol and corticosterone are referred to as glucocorticoids because they increase hepatic glucose output by stimulating the catabolism of peripheral fat and protein to provide substrate for hepatic gluconeogenesis. The glucocorticoids help regulate the metabolism of carbohydrates, proteins, and fat. They act on virtually all cells of the body.

A. Synthesis and Binding to Plasma Proteins: The major glucocorticoids secreted by the adrenal cortex are cortisol and corticosterone. Biosynthetic pathways for these hormones are illustrated in Figure 21–3.

Both cortisol and corticosterone are secreted in an unbound state but circulate bound to plasma proteins. They bind mainly to **corticosteroid-binding globulin (CBG)** (or **transcortin**) and to a lesser extent to albumin. Protein binding serves mainly to distribute and deliver the hormones to target tissues, but it may also delay their metabolic clearance and prevent marked fluctuations of glucocorticoid levels during episodic secretion by the gland.

B. Corticosteroid-Binding Globulin (CBG): CBG (MW about 50,000) is an α-globulin synthesized in the liver. Its production is increased by pregnancy, estrogen or oral contraceptive therapy, hyperthyroidism, diabetes, certain hematologic disorders, and familial CBG excess. When the CBG level rises, more cortisol is bound, and the free cortisol level falls temporarily. This fall stimulates pituitary ACTH secretion and more adrenal cortisol production. Eventually, the free cortisol level and the ACTH secretion return to normal, but with an elevated level of protein-bound cortisol. CBG production is decreased in cirrhosis, nephrotic syndrome, hypothyroidism, multiple myeloma, and familial CBG deficiency. When the CBG level falls, changes in the opposite direction occur.

C. Free and Bound Glucocorticoid: Normally, about 90% of the circulating cortisol is bound to CBG and 10% is free (unbound). The bound hormone is inactive. The free hormone is physiologically active. The normal AM total plasma cortisol is

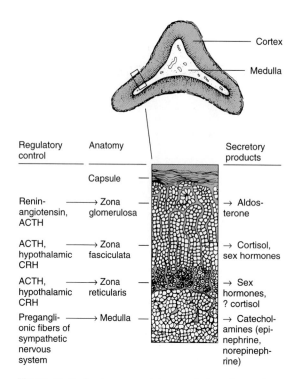

Figure 21–2. Anatomy, regulatory control, and secretory products of the adrenal gland. (Modified and reproduced, with permission, from Chandrasoma P, Taylor CE: *Concise Pathology,* 2nd ed. Appleton & Lange, 1994.)

5–20 µg/dL (140–550 nmol/L). Because cortisol is protein-bound to a greater degree than corticosterone, its half-life in the circulation is longer (about 60–90 minutes) than that of corticosterone (about 50 minutes).

D. Metabolism: The glucocorticoids are metabolized in the liver and conjugated to glucuronide or sulfate groups. The inactive conjugated metabolites are excreted in the urine and stool. The metabolism of cortisol is decreased in infancy, old age, pregnancy, chronic liver disease, hypothyroidism, anorexia nervosa, surgery, starvation, and other major physiologic stress. Catabolism of cortisol is increased in thyrotoxicosis. Because of its avid protein binding and extensive metabolism before excretion, less than 1% of secreted cortisol appears in the urine as free cortisol.

Regulation of Secretion

A. Adrenocorticotropic Hormone (ACTH) and Corticotropin-Releasing Hormone (CRH): Glucocorticoid secretion is regulated primarily by ACTH, a 39-amino-acid polypeptide secreted by the anterior pituitary. Its half-life in the circulation is very short (about 10 minutes). The site of its catabolism is unknown. ACTH regulates both basal secretion of glucocorticoids and increased secretion provoked by stress.

ACTH, in turn, is regulated by the central nervous system and hypothalamus by CRH, a 41-amino-acid polypeptide secreted in the median eminence of the hypothalamus. CRH secretion by the hypothalamus is regulated by a variety of neurotransmitters (Figure 21–4). The hypothalamus is subject to regulatory influences from other parts of the brain, particularly the limbic system. CRH is transported in the portal-hypophysial vessels to the anterior pituitary. There, CRH causes a prompt increase in ACTH secretion. This in turn leads to a transient increase in cortisol secretion by the adrenal.

The control of ACTH and CRH secretion involves three components: episodic secretion and diurnal rhythm of ACTH, stress responses of the hypothalamic-pituitary-adrenal axis, and negative feedback inhibition of ACTH secretion by cortisol.

B. Episodic and Diurnal Rhythm of ACTH Secretion: ACTH is secreted in episodic bursts throughout the day, following a diurnal (circadian) rhythm, with bursts most frequent in the early morning and least frequent in the evening (Figure 21–5). The peak level of cortisol in the plasma normally occurs between 6:00 and 8:00 AM (during sleep, just before awakening) and the nadir at around 12:00 MN. The diurnal rhythm of ACTH secretion persists in patients with adrenal insufficiency who are receiving maintenance doses of glucocorticoids but is lost in Cushing's syndrome. The diurnal rhythm is altered also by changes in patterns of sleep, light-dark exposure, or food intake; physical stress such as major illness, surgery, trauma, or starvation; psychologic stress, including severe anxiety, depression, and mania; central nervous system and pituitary disorders; liver disease and other conditions that affect cortisol metabolism; chronic renal failure; alcoholism; and antiserotonergic drugs such as cyproheptadine.

Normally, the morning plasma ACTH concentration is about 25 pg/mL (5.5 pmol/L). Plasma ACTH and cortisol values in various normal and abnormal states are shown in Figure 21–6.

C. Stress Response: Plasma ACTH and cortisol secretion are also triggered by various forms of stress. Emotional stress (such as fear and anxiety) and bodily injury (such as surgery or hypoglycemia) release CRH from the hypothalamus and thus ACTH from the pituitary. This in turn results in a transient increase in cortisol secretion (Figure 21–7). If the stress is prolonged, it may abolish the normal diurnal rhythm of ACTH and cortisol secretion.

The stress response of plasma ACTH and cortisol is abolished in Cushing's syndrome but is exaggerated following adrenalectomy. The circulating catecholamines, epinephrine and norepinephrine, do not increase ACTH secretion.

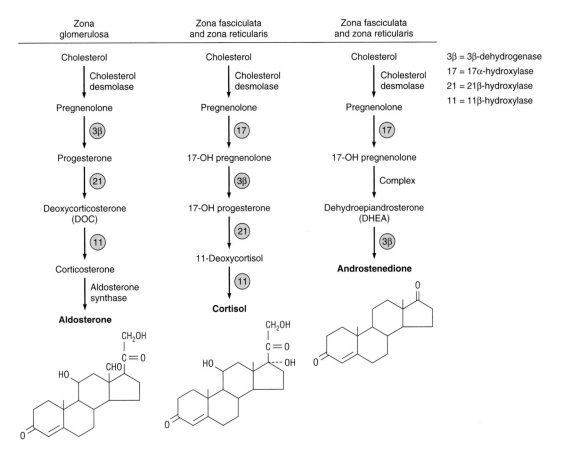

Figure 21–3. Simplified pathways of steroid synthesis in the different zones of the adrenal cortex. Note the differences in the types of enzyme necessary and the different order of enzymatic reactions in the different zones.

D. Negative Feedback: ACTH secretion is inhibited in a negative feedback fashion by high circulating levels of free cortisol. This feedback inhibition occurs at both the pituitary and the hypothalamus (Figure 21–4).

A rising level of plasma cortisol inhibits release of ACTH from the pituitary, both by inhibiting CRH release from the hypothalamus and by interfering with the stimulatory action of CRH on the pituitary. The fall in plasma ACTH leads to a decline in adrenal secretion of cortisol. Conversely, a drop in plasma cortisol level stimulates ACTH secretion. In chronic adrenal insufficiency, there is a marked increase in the rate of ACTH synthesis and secretion.

ACTH secretion is also inhibited by chronic treatment with exogenous corticosteroids in proportion to their glucocorticoid potency. When prolonged corticosteroid treatment is stopped, the adrenal is atrophic and unresponsive and the patient is at risk for acute adrenal insufficiency. The pituitary may not be able to secrete normal amounts of ACTH for as long as a month, presumably due to diminished ACTH synthesis. Thereafter, there is a slow rise in ACTH to higher than normal levels (Figure 21–8). The higher than normal level of ACTH in turn stimulates adrenal glucocorticoid output, and feedback inhibition gradually reduces the ACTH level to normal. The risk of acute adrenal insufficiency following sudden cessation of corticosteroid therapy can be avoided by slowly tapering the corticosteroid dosage over a long period of time (or by switching to alternate-day steroid regimens before tapering).

E. Effects of ACTH on the Adrenal: Circulating ACTH binds to high-affinity receptors on adrenocortical cell membranes, activating adenylyl cyclase, increasing intracellular cAMP, and promoting synthesis of the enzyme that converts cholesterol to steroid hormone precursors. Increased glucocorticoid synthesis and secretion result within minutes.

Prolonged hypersecretion or administration of ACTH causes adrenocortical hyperplasia and hypertrophy. Conversely, prolonged ACTH deficiency results in adrenocortical atrophy.

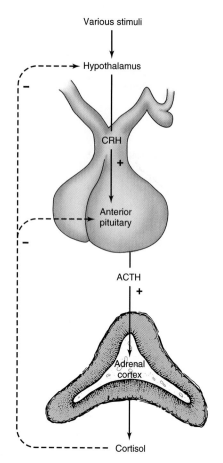

Figure 21–4. Feedback mechanism of ACTH-glucocorticoid secretion. Solid arrows indicate stimulation; dashed arrows, inhibition. (Reproduced, with permission, from Junqueira LC, Carneiro J, Kelley RO: *Basic Histology*, 9th ed. Appleton & Lange, 1998.)

Mechanism of Action

The physiologic effects of glucocorticoids in various tissues are the result of their binding to cytosolic glucocorticoid receptors. The hormone-receptor complexes then enter the nucleus, bind to nuclear DNA, and promote the transcription of DNA, the production of mRNAs, and the synthesis of proteins. The enzymes and other proteins thus produced mediate the glucocorticoid response, which may be inhibitory or stimulatory depending on the tissue involved. The cytosolic glucocorticoid receptors present in virtually all tissues are quite similar. However, the proteins produced vary widely as a result of the expression of different genes in specific target tissue cells. The regulation of this expression is not well understood.

Effects

The physiologic effects of glucocorticoids on target tissues are summarized in Table 21–2. In most tissues, glucocorticoids have a catabolic effect, promoting degradation of protein and fat to provide substrate for intermediary metabolism. In the liver, however, glucocorticoids have a synthetic effect, promoting the uptake and use of carbohydrates (in synthesis of glucose and glycogen), amino acids (in synthesis of RNA and protein enzymes), and fatty acids (as an energy source).

During fasting, glucocorticoids help to maintain plasma glucose levels by several mechanisms (Table 21–2). In peripheral tissues, glucocorticoids antagonize the effects of insulin. Glucocorticoids inhibit glucose uptake in muscle and adipose tissue. The brain and heart are spared this antagonism, and the extra supply of glucose helps these vital organs to cope with stress. In diabetics, the insulin antagonism may worsen control of blood sugar, raise plasma lipid levels, and increase the formation of ketone bodies. However, in nondiabetics, the rise in blood glucose stimulates a compensatory increase in insulin secretion that prevents these sequelae.

Small amounts of glucocorticoids must be present for other metabolic processes to occur (**permissive action**). For example, glucocorticoids must be present for catecholamines to produce their calorigenic, lipolytic, pressor, and bronchodilator effects and for glucagon to increase hepatic gluconeogenesis.

Glucocorticoids are also required to resist various stresses. Indeed, the increased secretion of pituitary ACTH and consequent increase in circulating glucocorticoids following injury are essential to survival. Hypophysectomized or adrenalectomized individuals treated with only maintenance doses of glucocorticoids may die when exposed to such stress. The reasons for this are unclear but may be related to interactions between glucocorticoids and catecholamines in maintaining vascular reactivity and in mobilizing free fatty acids as an emergency energy supply.

2. MINERALOCORTICOIDS

Synthesis, Protein Binding, & Metabolism

The primary function of the mineralocorticoids is to regulate Na^+ excretion and maintain a normal intravascular volume. However, other factors affect Na^+ excretion besides the mineralocorticoids, such as the glomerular filtration rate, atrial natriuretic peptide, the presence of an osmotic diuretic, and changes in tubular reabsorption of Na^+ that are not regulated by mineralocorticoid.

A. Synthesis: Aldosterone is the principal mineralocorticoid secreted by the adrenal. Deoxycorticosterone also has minor mineralocorticoid activity, and so does corticosterone. (See Figure 21–3.)

B. Protein Binding: Aldosterone is bound to plasma proteins (albumin and corticosteroid-binding globulin) to only a slight extent. The amount of al-

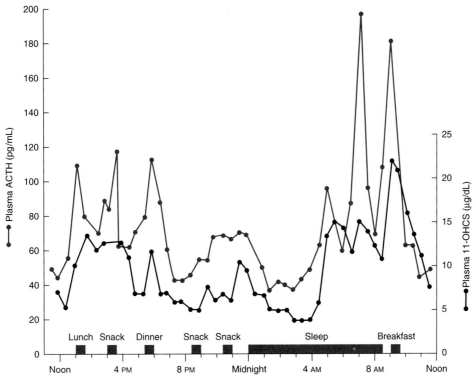

Figure 21–5. Fluctuations in plasma ACTH and glucocorticoids (11-OHCS) throughout the day. Note the greater ACTH and glucocorticoid rises in the morning before awakening. (Reproduced, with permission, from Krieger DT et al: Characterization of the normal temporal pattern of plasma corticosteroid levels. J Clin Endocrinol Metab 1971;32:266.)

dosterone secreted under normal circumstances is small (about 0.15 mg/24 h). The normal average plasma concentration of (free and bound) aldosterone is 0.006 μg/dL (0.17 nmol/L). Free (unbound) aldosterone comprises 30–40% of the total.

C. Metabolism: The half-life of aldosterone is short (about 20–30 minutes). Aldosterone is catabolized principally in the liver, and its metabolites are excreted in the urine. Less than 1% of secreted aldosterone is excreted in urine in the free form.

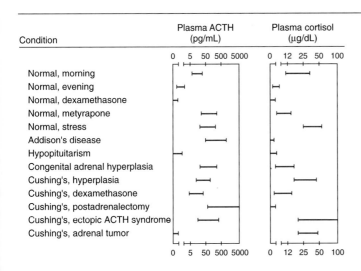

Figure 21–6. Plasma concentrations of ACTH and cortisol in various clinical states. (Reproduced, with permission, from Liddle G: The adrenal cortex. In: *Textbook of Endocrinology*, 5th ed. Williams RH [editor]. Saunders, 1974.)

1. What are the histologic layers of the adrenal cortex, and what steroids does each secrete?
2. What three roles are proposed for steroid-binding proteins?
3. In what conditions is corticosteroid-binding globulin increased? Decreased?
4. In what conditions is cortisol metabolism increased? Decreased?
5. Describe the diurnal rhythm of ACTH secretion, and name the conditions in which it is altered.
6. What stress responses trigger ACTH secretion?
7. Describe the negative feedback control of the hypothalamic-pituitary-adrenal axis.
8. Describe the major physiologic effects of glucocorticoids.

Regulation

Aldosterone secretion is regulated primarily by the renin-angiotensin system but also by pituitary ACTH and by the plasma electrolytes, Na^+ and K^+.

A. Regulation by Renin-Angiotensin System: The **renin-angiotensin system** regulates aldosterone secretion in a feedback fashion (Figure 21–9). **Renin** is a proteolytic enzyme produced from a larger protein, **prorenin.** In humans, prorenin contains 406 amino acid residues, whereas renin has 292 amino acid residues and a molecular weight of 37,325. Renin is excreted by the juxtaglomerular cells of the kidney in response to changes in renal perfusion pressure and reflex increases in renal nerve discharge. Once in the circulation, renin acts on **an-**

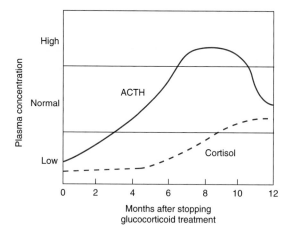

Figure 21–8. Pattern of plasma ACTH and cortisol values in patients recovering from prior long-term daily treatment with large doses of glucocorticoids. (Courtesy of R Ney. Reproduced, with permission, from Ganong WF: *Review of Medical Physiology,* 19th ed. Appleton & Lange, 1999.)

giotensinogen, an α_2-globulin produced in the liver, to form **angiotensin I,** a decapeptide. In the lung and elsewhere, angiotensin I is converted by **angiotensin-converting enzyme (ACE)** to **angiotensin II,** an octapeptide. Angiotensin II binds to zona glomerulosa cell membrane receptors and stimulates synthesis and secretion of aldosterone. The aldosterone promotes Na^+ and water retention, causing plasma volume expansion, which then shuts off renin secretion. In the supine state, there is a diurnal rhythm of aldosterone and renin secretion, with the highest values in the early morning before awakening.

The physiologic stimuli for the renin-angiotensin system to increase aldosterone secretion are factors which reduce renal perfusion and include extracellular fluid volume depletion, dietary Na^+ restriction, and decreases in intra-arterial vascular pressure (eg, due to hemorrhage or upright posture). Disease states that less commonly cause reduced renal perfusion include renal artery stenosis, salt-losing disorders, congestive heart failure, and hypoproteinemic states (cirrhosis of the liver, or nephrotic syndrome). These disorders increase renin secretion, producing **secondary hyperaldosteronism.**

B. Regulation by ACTH: ACTH also stimulates mineralocorticoid output. More ACTH is needed to stimulate mineralocorticoid than glucocorticoid secretion, but the amount required is still within the range of normal ACTH secretion. The effect of ACTH on aldosterone secretion is transient, however. Even if ACTH secretion remains elevated, aldosterone production declines to normal within 48

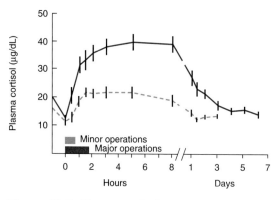

Figure 21–7. Plasma cortisol responses to major surgery (continuous line) and minor surgery (broken line) in normal subjects. Mean values and standard errors for 20 patients are shown in each case. (Reproduced, with permission, from Plumpton FS, Besser GM, Cole P: Anesthesia 1969;24:3.)

Table 21–2. Effects of glucocorticoids.

Target Tissue	Effect	Mechanism
Muscle	Catabolic	Inhibit glucose uptake and metabolism Decrease protein synthesis Increase release of amino acids, lactate
Fat	Lipolytic	Stimulate lipolysis Increase release of FFAs and glycerol
Liver	Synthetic	Increase gluconeogenesis Increase glycogen synthesis, storage Increase glucose-6-phosphatase activity Increase blood glucose
Immune system	Suppression	Reduce number of circulating lymphocytes, monocytes, eosinophils, basophils Inhibit T lymphocyte production of interleukin-2 Interfere with antigen processing, antibody production and clearance
	Anti-inflammatory	Decrease migration of neutrophils, monocytes, lymphocytes to sites of injury
	Other	Stimulate release of neutrophils from marrow Interfere with neutrophil migration out of vascular compartment
Cardiovascular	Increase cardiac output Increase peripheral vascular tone	
Renal	Increase glomerular filtration rate Aid in regulating water, electrolyte balance	
Other	Permissive action Resistance to stress Insulin antagonism	Increase blood glucose

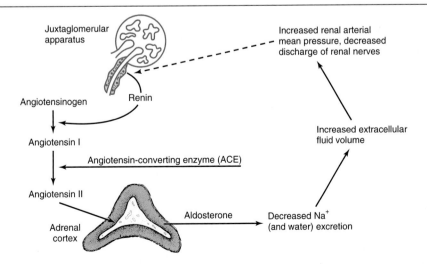

Figure 21–9. Feedback mechanism regulating aldosterone secretion. The dashed arrow indicates inhibition. (Redrawn and reproduced, with permission, from Ganong WF: *Review of Medical Physiology,* 19th ed. Appleton & Lange, 1999.)

hours, perhaps because renin secretion decreases in response to hypervolemia.

C. Regulation by Plasma Electrolytes: An increase in plasma K^+ concentration—or a fall in plasma Na^+—stimulates aldosterone release. Conversely, a fall in plasma K^+ level—or a rise in plasma Na^+—inhibits its release. While minor changes of plasma K^+ (1 meq/L or less) have an effect, major changes in plasma Na^+ (drops of about 20 meq/L) are needed to stimulate aldosterone secretion. Na^+ depletion increases the affinity and number of angiotensin II receptors on adrenocortical cells.

Mechanism of Action

The mechanism of action of aldosterone is complex and incompletely understood.

Aldosterone, like other steroid hormones, acts by binding to a mineralocorticoid receptor in the cytosol. The steroid-receptor complex then moves into the nucleus of the target cell and increases transcription of DNA, induction of mRNA, and stimulation of protein synthesis by ribosomes. The proteins that are formed act to increase active transport of Na^+ via the Na^+ pump (Figure 21–10).

In addition, functional studies have been conducted on extrarenal, nonepithelial cells such as smooth muscle cells and circulating mononuclear leukocytes. High-affinity binding sites for aldosterone have been found in mononuclear leukocytes. In these cells, aldosterone produces effects in vitro on intracellular Na^+, K^+, and Ca^{2+} concentrations and cell volume. These effects on transmembrane electrolyte movements are quite rapid, with onset within 1–2 minutes. They have been shown to involve activation of the cell membrane Na^+-proton exchanger at very low physiologic concentrations of aldosterone. The inositol 1,4,5-trisphosphate-calcium messenger cascade, which responds over the same rapid time course, may also be involved. The rapid response of the Na^+-proton exchanger of the cell membrane cannot be explained by a mechanism of action involving the interaction of a steroid receptor complex with nuclear DNA, since it is too fast. Instead, the rapid direct membrane effects of aldosterone might indicate distinct membrane receptors with a high affinity for aldosterone. Genomic mechanisms are presumably responsible for later effects of aldosterone.

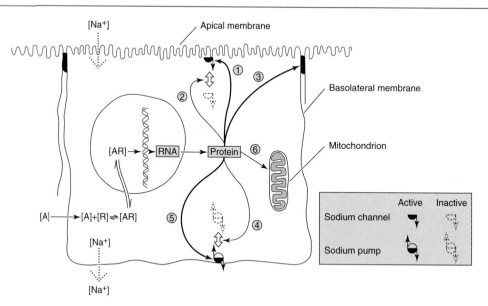

Figure 21–10. Model of the mechanisms of action of aldosterone in an epithelial cell. Aldosterone (A) crosses the plasma membrane and links to its cytosolic receptor (R). The complex (AR) is activated, enters the nucleus, and links to nuclear chromatin sites. Following this interaction, RNA transcription is induced or repressed. Induced or repressed proteins mediate an increased transepithelial ion transport at different sites. Sites 1, 3, and 5 are a constitutive pathway for Na^+ transport, and sites 2, 4, and 6 are a regulatory pathway for Na^+ transport across the apical membrane (locus of the amiloride-sensitive Na^+ channel), the basolateral membrane (locus of the ouabain-sensitive Na^+ pump), and the tight junction apparatus. (Reproduced, with permission, from Truscello A, Gaggler HP, Rossier BC: Thyroid hormone antagonizes an aldosterone-induced protein: A candidate mediator for the late mineralocorticoid response. J Membr Biol 1986;89:173.)

Effects

The target cells for the mineralocorticoids are the kidney, colon, duodenum, salivary glands, and sweat glands. In the distal renal tubules and collecting ducts, aldosterone acts to promote the exchange of Na^+ for K^+ and H^+, causing Na^+ retention, K^+ diuresis, and increased urine acidity (Figure 21–10). Elsewhere, it acts to increase the reabsorption of Na^+ from the colonic fluid, saliva, and sweat. The mineralocorticoids may also increase K^+ and decrease Na^+ concentrations in muscle and brain cells.

> 9. How is aldosterone secretion regulated?
> 10. How does the effect of ACTH on aldosterone secretion differ from the effect on glucocorticoid secretion?
> 11. What are the overall effects of aldosterone?

PATHOPHYSIOLOGY OF SELECTED ADRENOCORTICAL DISORDERS

Characteristic syndromes are produced by excessive or deficient secretion of each type of adrenal hormone. Excessive glucocorticoid secretion (**Cushing's syndrome**) results in a moon-faced, plethoric appearance, with truncal obesity, purple abdominal striae, hypertension, osteoporosis, mental aberrations, protein depletion, and glucose intolerance or frank diabetes mellitus.

Excessive mineralocorticoid secretion (**Conn's syndrome**) leads to Na^+ retention, usually without edema, and K^+ depletion, resulting in hypertension, muscle weakness, polyuria, hypokalemia, metabolic alkalosis, and sometimes hypocalcemia and tetany.

Excessive androgen secretion causes masculinization (**adrenogenital syndrome**) and precocious pseudopuberty or female pseudohermaphroditism.

Deficient glucocorticoid secretion due to autoimmune or other destruction of the adrenal glands (**Addison's disease**) causes symptoms of weakness, fatigue, malaise, anorexia, nausea and vomiting, weight loss, hypotension, hypoglycemia, and marked intolerance of physiologic stress (eg, infection). Elevation of plasma ACTH may produce hyperpigmentation.

Associated mineralocorticoid deficiency leads to renal Na^+ wasting and K^+ retention and can produce manifestations of severe dehydration, hypotension, decreased cardiac size, hyponatremia, hyperkalemia, and metabolic acidosis. Deficient mineralocorticoid secretion also occurs in patients with renal disease and low circulating renin levels (**hyporeninemic hypoaldosteronism**).

CUSHING'S SYNDROME

Cushing's syndrome is the clinical condition resulting from chronic exposure to excessive circulating levels of glucocorticoids (Figure 21–11). It is also called **hyperadrenocorticalism, hyperadrenal corticalism**, and **hypercortisolism**. The most common cause of the syndrome is excess secretion of ACTH from the anterior pituitary gland (**Cushing's disease**). This condition was originally described by Harvey Cushing. Other conditions causing the syndrome are described below.

Etiology

Cushing's syndrome may occur either spontaneously or as the result of chronic corticosteroid administration (iatrogenic Cushing's syndrome). The overall incidence of spontaneous Cushing's syndrome is approximately two to four cases per million population. It is nine times more common in women than in men. The major causes of Cushing's syndrome are summarized in Table 21–3. Unusual causes are discussed below.

A. Cushing's Disease: Cushing's disease is the most common cause of noniatrogenic hypercortisolism. It is four to six times more prevalent in women than in men. Over 90% of patients with Cushing's disease have a pituitary adenoma causing excessive secretion of ACTH (Figure 21–12). Such adenomas are located in the anterior pituitary, are usually less than 10 mm in diameter (**microadenomas**), and are composed of basophilic corticotroph cells containing ACTH in secretory granules. **Macroadenomas** are less common and carcinomas extremely rare. Use of molecular biology techniques to determine the clonal origin of corticotroph tumors has shown that ACTH-secreting pituitary adenomas are monoclonal, arising from a single progenitor cell. Presumably, somatic mutation is required for tumorigenesis.

Much less commonly, patients with Cushing's disease have **diffuse hyperplasia of pituitary corticotroph cells** responsible for ACTH hypersecretion. The hyperplasia is probably due to hypersecretion of CRH by the hypothalamus or CRH-secreting tumors. Chronic CRH hypersecretion does not cause pituitary adenomas.

In Cushing's disease, the chronic ACTH hypersecretion causes bilateral hyperplasia of the adrenal cortex. Combined adrenal weights (normal: 8–10 g) range from 12 g to 24 g. The adrenal hyperplasia is most typically micronodular, but in some patients, particularly those with long-standing Cushing's disease, macronodular hyperplasia develops.

B. Ectopic ACTH Syndrome: In the **ectopic ACTH syndrome**, a nonpituitary tumor synthesizes and hypersecretes biologically active ACTH or an ACTH-like peptide (Figure 21–12). The neoplasms most frequently responsible are small cell carcinoma

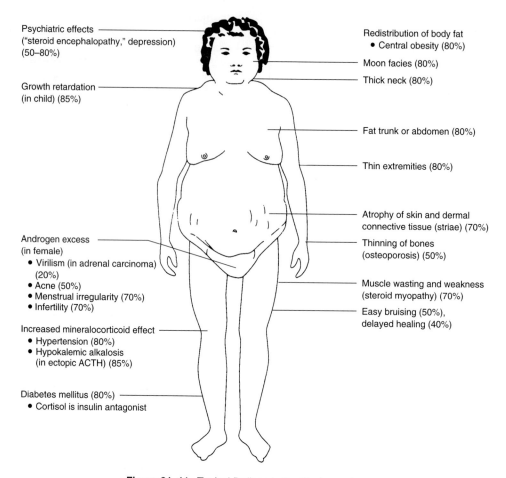

Figure 21–11. Typical findings in Cushing's syndrome.

of the lung and bronchial carcinoid tumors. Ectopic ACTH hypersecretion is more common in men, largely owing to the more frequent occurrence of these lung tumors in men. Other associated tumors are listed in Table 21–3. CRH-secreting tumors have also been described (see below).

Chronic ACTH hypersecretion causes marked bilateral adrenocortical hyperplasia, with combined adrenal weights ranging from 24 g to 50 g or more. The ACTH secreted by the nonpituitary tumor causes adrenal hyperfunction, and the high circulating cortisol levels suppress hypothalamic secretion of CRH and the pituitary secretion of ACTH. Pituitary corticotroph cells have a decreased ACTH content.

C. Ectopic CRH Syndrome: The ectopic CRH syndrome is a very rare cause of Cushing's syndrome (see Figure 21–12). Most cases have been associated with bronchial carcinoid tumors.

D. Functioning Adrenocortical Tumors: Both **adrenocortical adenomas** and **carcinomas** may cause Cushing's syndrome by elaborating cortisol autonomously (Figure 21–12). Adenomas are usually 1–6 cm in diameter, weigh 10–70 g, are encapsulated, and consist predominantly of zona fasciculata cells. Because they are relatively inefficient in cortisol synthesis, adrenal carcinomas are usually quite large, weighing 100 g to several kilograms, and are often palpable as an abdominal mass by the time Cushing's syndrome becomes clinically manifest. Grossly, they are highly vascular, with areas of necrosis, hemorrhage, cystic degeneration, and calcification. They are highly malignant lesions, tending to invade adrenal capsule and blood vessels and to metastasize to the kidney, retroperitoneum, liver, and lung.

E. Adrenal Micronodular Hyperplasia: Adrenal micronodular hyperplasia is a rare cause of Cushing's syndrome. Pathologically, it is characterized by multiple small, pigmented, usually bilateral cortisol-secreting adenomas. About half of cases occur sporadically in children and young adults. The remainder occur as an autosomal dominant disorder in association with blue nevi; pigmented lentigines (freckles) of the skin and mucosal surfaces of the

Table 21–3. Major causes of Cushing's syndrome.

NONIATROGENIC

ACTH-Dependent
1. **Cushing's disease (ACTH-secreting pituitary adenoma):**
   - *Epidemiology:* 68% of cases of noniatrogenic Cushing's syndrome. More common in women (F:M ratio of approximately 8:1). Age at diagnosis usually 20–40 years.
   - *Clinical features:* Hyperpigmentation and hypokalemic alkalosis are rare; androgenic manifestations limited to acne and hirsutism. Secretion of cortisol and adrenal androgens is only moderately increased.
   - *Course:* Slow progression over several years.
2. **Ectopic ACTH syndrome:**
   - *Epidemiology:* 15% of cases of spontaneous Cushing's syndrome. More common in men (M:F ratio of approximately 3:1). Age at diagnosis usually 40–60 years. Occurs most commonly in patients with small cell carcinoma of lung and bronchial carcinoid tumors. Rarely, other tumors secrete ACTH; these include carcinoid tumors of the thymus, gut, pancreas, or ovary; pancreatic islet cell tumors; ovarian cancer; medullary thyroid carcinoma; pheochromocytoma; small cell carcinoma of vagina or uterine cervix.
   - *Clinical features:* Frequently limited to weakness, hypertension, and glucose intolerance, due to the rapid onset of hypercortisolism. Weight loss and anemia are common effects of malignancy. Primary tumor usually apparent. Hyperpigmentation, hypokalemia, and alkalosis may occur from the mineralocorticoid effects of cortisol and other steroids secreted.
   - *Course:* With underlying carcinoma, hypercortisolism is of rapid onset, steroid hypersecretion is frequently severe, with equally elevated levels of glucocorticoids, androgens, and deoxycorticosterone (DOC). With underlying benign tumor, more slowly progressive course.

ACTH-Independent
3. **Functioning adrenocortical tumor:**
   - *Epidemiology:* 17% of cases of Cushing's syndrome. Adrenal ademoma in 9%, adrenal carcinoma in 8%. More common in women. Adrenal carcinoma occurs in about 2 per million population per year. Age at diagnosis usually 35–40 years.
   - *Clinical features and course:* Adenoma: Onset is gradual. Usually secretes only cortisol. Hypercortisolism is mild to moderate. Androgenic effects absent. Carcinoma: Rapid onset, rapidly progressive. Marked elevations of glucocorticoids, androgens, and mineralocorticoids. Hypokalemia, abdominal pain, abdominal masses, hepatic and pulmonary metastases.

IATROGENIC
4. **Exogenous glucocorticoid administration:** Glucocorticoid administered in high doses in the treatment of nonendocrine disorders.

---

head and face; cutaneous, mammary, and atrial myxomas; pituitary somatotroph adenomas; and tumors of peripheral nerves, testes, and other endocrine glands (Carney complex).

F. Adrenal Macronodular Hyperplasia: Another rare cause of Cushing's syndrome is bilateral adrenal macronodular hyperplasia. In this condition, both glands are markedly enlarged, with bulging nodules found at cut section. Microscopically, the nodules reveal a variegated histologic pattern characterized by trabecular, adenoid, and zona glomerulosa-like structures. Occasionally, the hyperplasia may be unilateral. Some patients with macronodular hyperplasia do not show typical cushingoid features. In these cases, the macronodular hyperplasia is most often discovered incidentally on ultrasound or CT examination of the abdomen.

Pathophysiology

The various causes of Cushing's syndrome can be divided into two categories: ACTH-dependent and ACTH-independent. The causes of ACTH-dependent Cushing's syndrome include Cushing's disease (80% of ACTH-dependent cases), ectopic ACTH hypersecretion (20%), and ectopic CRH secretion (rare), all of which are characterized by chronic ACTH hypersecretion and increased secretion of cortisol. Causes of ACTH-independent Cushing's syndrome include glucocorticoid-secreting adrenocortical adenomas and carcinomas and adrenal micronodular and macronodular hyperplasia, all of which are characterized by autonomous secretion of cortisol and suppression of pituitary ACTH (Figures 21–12 and 21–13).

A. Cushing's Disease: In Cushing's disease, there is a persistent overproduction of ACTH by the pituitary adenoma. The ACTH hypersecretion is disorderly, episodic, and random; the normal diurnal rhythm of ACTH and cortisol secretion is usually absent. Plasma levels of ACTH and cortisol vary and may at times be within the normal range (Figure 21–13). However, a **24-hour urine free cortisol** measurement confirms hypercortisolism. The excessive cortisol does not suppress ACTH secretion by the pituitary adenoma.

Patients with Cushing's disease typically have exaggerated plasma ACTH and cortisol responses to CRH stimulation and incompletely suppressed secretion of ACTH and cortisol by exogenous glucocorticoids (eg, dexamethasone). While these findings suggest that the pituitary adenoma cells are unusually sensitive to CRH and relatively resistant to glucocorticoids, the findings may simply be due to the increased number of ACTH-secreting cells. About 10%

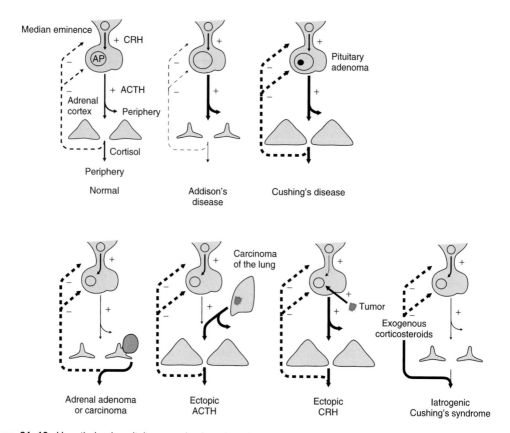

Figure 21–12. Hypothalamic, pituitary, and adrenal cortical relationships. Solid arrows indicate stimulation; dashed arrows, inhibition. **Normal:** Corticotropin-releasing hormone (CRH) elaborated by the median eminence of the hypothalamus stimulates secretion of adrenocorticotropic hormone (ACTH) by the anterior pituitary (AP). ACTH triggers the synthesis and release of cortisol, the principal glucocorticoid of the adrenal cortex (AC). A rising level of cortisol inhibits the stimulatory action of CRH on ACTH release (or cortisol may inhibit CRH release), completing a negative feedback loop. **Addison's disease:** In primary destructive disease of the adrenal cortex, the level of plasma cortisol is very low, and the effect of CRH on the anterior pituitary proceeds without inhibition, causing a marked increase in the secretion of ACTH. High levels of ACTH produce characteristic skin pigmentary changes. **Cushing's disease:** The primary lesion may be at the level of the pituitary or hypothalamus. In either case, production of ACTH and cortisol is excessive. The former causes bilateral adrenal hyperplasia and the latter causes clinical manifestations of hypercortisolism. Cells of the anterior pituitary are relatively resistant to the high levels of circulating cortisol. **Adrenal adenoma or carcinoma:** An adenoma or carcinoma of the adrenal cortex may produce cortisol autonomously. When the rate of production exceeds physiologic quantities, Cushing's syndrome results; the effect of CRH on the anterior pituitary is inhibited by the high levels of circulating cortisol, with resultant diminished ACTH secretion and atrophy of normal adrenal tissue. **Ectopic ACTH:** In this syndrome, ACTH or an ACTH-like peptide is elaborated by a tumor such as carcinoma of the lung. The adrenals are stimulated; circulating cortisol is increased; and pituitary ACTH secretion is inhibited. **Ectopic CRH:** In this rare syndrome, CRH is elaborated by a tumor such as a bronchial carcinoid. The pituitary is stimulated, and there is elaboration of excess ACTH. The adrenals are stimulated, and circulating cortisol is increased. The hypercortisolism causes diminished hypothalamic CRH production; however, the negative feedback on the pituitary production of ACTH is overcome by the ectopic CRH. **Iatrogenic Cushing's syndrome:** Exogenous corticosteroid administration in excess of physiologic quantities of cortisol leads directly to peripheral manifestations of hypercortisolism and inhibits the effect of CRH on the anterior pituitary, with resultant diminished ACTH secretion, diminished cortisol production, and atrophy of normal adrenal tissue. (Modified and reproduced, with permission, from Burns TW, Carlson HE: Endocrinology. In: *Pathologic Physiology: Mechanisms of Disease.* Sodeman WA, Sodeman TM [editors]. Saunders, 1985.)

of patients with pituitary microadenomas do not exhibit major increases in plasma ACTH in response to CRH. Presumably, the clonal cells of such patients have a receptor or postreceptor defect.

Despite ACTH hypersecretion, the pituitary and adrenals fail to respond normally to stress. Stimuli such as hypoglycemia or surgery fail to increase ACTH and cortisol secretion, probably because chronic hypercortisolism has suppressed CRH secretion by the hypothalamus. Hypercortisolism also in-

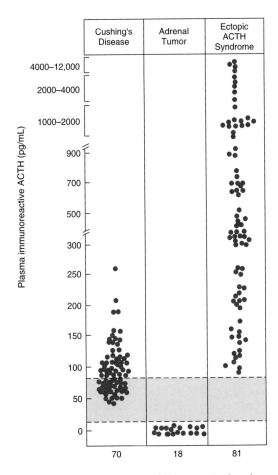

Figure 21–13. Basal plasma ACTH concentrations in patients with various types of noniatrogenic Cushing's syndrome. The colored zone represents the normal range. (Reproduced, with permission, from Scott AP et al: Pituitary adrenocorticotropin and the melanocyte stimulating hormones. In: *Peptide Hormones.* Parsons JA [editor]. University Park Press, 1979.)

hibits other normal pituitary and hypothalamic functions, affecting thyrotropin, growth hormone, and gonadotropin release.

Surgical removal of the ACTH-producing pituitary adenoma reverses these abnormalities.

B. Ectopic ACTH Syndrome: In the ectopic ACTH syndrome, hypersecretion of ACTH and cortisol is random and episodic and quantitatively greater than in patients with Cushing's disease (Figure 21–13). Indeed, plasma levels and urinary excretion of cortisol, adrenal androgens, and other steroids are often markedly elevated. Ectopic ACTH secretion by tumors is usually not suppressible by exogenous glucocorticoids such as dexamethasone (Figure 21–14).

C. Ectopic CRH Syndrome: Clinically, the ectopic CRH syndrome is indistinguishable from the ectopic ACTH syndrome. Biochemically, however, plasma CRH concentrations are elevated (not suppressed), and CRH-stimulated secretion of ACTH is suppressible with high doses of dexamethasone (not so in the ectopic ACTH syndrome). Sometimes, nonpituitary tumors produce both CRH and ACTH ectopically.

D. Adrenal Tumors: Primary adrenal adenomas and carcinomas are not under hypothalamic-pituitary control and thus autonomously hypersecrete cortisol. The hypercortisolism suppresses pituitary ACTH production, resulting in atrophy of the uninvolved adrenal cortex (Figure 21–12). Steroid secretion is random and episodic and not usually suppressible by dexamethasone. With adrenal carcinomas, overproduction of androgenic precursors is common, resulting in hirsutism or virilization of adult women or children of either sex. On the other hand, with adrenal adenomas, production of androgenic precursors is relatively limited. Thus, their clinical manifestations are chiefly those of cortisol excess.

It is not known why adrenal adenomas develop, but activating mutations of receptors for corticotropic factors have been found. Although structural mutations of the ACTH-receptor gene have not been detected, some tumors have recently been found to have aberrant expression of receptors for a variety of hormones (eg, gastrointestinal inhibitory peptide and somatostatin receptors), neuropeptides (vasopressin and β-adrenergic receptors), and even cytokines (interleukin-1 receptors). For example, patients with food-induced ACTH-independent Cushing's syndrome have been identified. In these patients, cortisol secretion by a unilateral adrenal adenoma is stimulated by the gut hormone gastrointestinal inhibitory peptide (GIP). Abnormal expression of GIP receptors on the adrenal tumor cells allows them to respond to food intake with an increase in cAMP and subsequent cortisol production.

E. Bilateral Micronodular Hyperplasia: ACTH levels are low, and cortisol is not suppressed by high doses of dexamethasone.

F. Bilateral Macronodular Hyperplasia: Again, hypercortisolism, low plasma ACTH, loss of diurnal rhythm of ACTH, and lack of suppression with high doses of dexamethasone are found.

Clinical Manifestations

The clinical manifestations of Cushing's syndrome (Figure 21–11) are predictable consequences of the physiologic effects of cortisol discussed above and in Table 21–2.

Glucocorticoid excess leads to glucose intolerance in several ways. First, cortisol excess promotes synthesis of glucose in the liver from amino acids liberated by protein catabolism. The increased hepatic gluconeogenesis occurs via stimulation of the enzymes glucose-6-phosphatase and phosphoenolpyruvate carboxykinase. Second, there is an increase in hepatic synthesis of glycogen and ketone bodies.

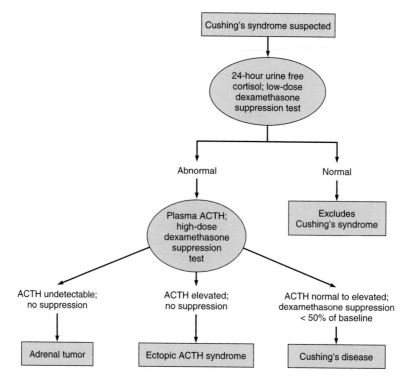

Figure 21–14. Diagnostic evaluation of Cushing's syndrome and procedures for determining the cause. Boxes enclose clinical decisions, and ovals enclose diagnostic tests. (Redrawn and reproduced, with permission, from Baxter JD, Tyrrell JB: The adrenal cortex. In: *Endocrinology and Metabolism,* 2nd ed. Felig P, Baxter JD [editors]. McGraw-Hill, 1987.)

Third, cortisol antagonizes the action of insulin in peripheral glucose utilization, perhaps by inhibiting glucose phosphorylation. The glucose intolerance and hyperglycemia are signaled by thirst and polyuria. Overt diabetes mellitus occurs in about 10–15% of patients with Cushing's syndrome. The diabetes is characterized by insulin resistance, ketosis, and hyperlipidemia, but acidosis and microvascular complications are rare.

With chronic cortisol excess, muscle wasting occurs as a result of excess protein catabolism, decreased muscle protein synthesis, and induction of insulin resistance in muscle via a post-insulin receptor defect. Proximal muscle weakness occurs in about 60% of cases. It is usually manifested by difficulty in climbing stairs or rising from a chair or bed without use of the arms or fatigue when combing or drying the hair.

Obesity and redistribution of body fat are probably the most recognizable features of Cushing's syndrome. Weight gain is often the initial symptom. The obesity is centralized, with relative sparing of the extremities. The redistribution of adipose tissue affects mainly the face, neck, trunk, and abdomen, producing the characteristic "moon" facies, "buffalo hump," supraclavicular fat pads, truncal obesity, and abdominal striae. Thickening of facial fat rounds the facial contour, producing the "moon facies." An enlarged dorsocervical fat pad ("buffalo hump") can occur with weight gain due to any cause; increased fat pads that fill and bulge above the supraclavicular fossae are more specific for Cushing's syndrome. Abdominal fat deposition results in centripetal obesity, with an elevated waist-to-hip circumference ratio (> 1.0 in men and > 0.8 in women), in 50% of patients with Cushing's syndrome. This fat deposition occurs both subcutaneously and intra-abdominally, most prominently around the viscera, perhaps because intra-abdominal fat appears to have a higher density of glucocorticoid receptors than other fat tissue.

The reason for the abnormal fat distribution is unknown. However, plasma leptin levels are significantly elevated in patients with Cushing's syndrome compared with both nonobese healthy individuals and obese individuals with a similar percentage body fat but no endocrine or metabolic disorder. Leptin, the obese *(ob)* gene product, is an adipocyte-derived satiety factor that helps to regulate appetite and body weight. The elevated leptin in patients with Cushing's syndrome is probably a result of the visceral obesity. Glucocorticoids may act—at least in part—directly on adipose tissue to increase leptin synthesis and secretion. Chronic hypercortisolism may also have an indirect effect via the associated hyperinsulinemia or insulin resistance.

Given the known lipolytic effects of glucocorticoids, the increased fat deposition caused by glucocorticoid excess seems paradoxical. It may be explained by the increase in appetite or by the lipogenic effects of the hyperinsulinemia the cortisol excess causes.

Glucocorticoid excess inhibits fibroblasts, leading to loss of collagen and connective tissue. Thinning of the skin, abdominal striae, easy bruisability, poor wound healing, and frequent skin infections are the result. Atrophy leads to a translucent appearance of the skin. Cutaneous atrophy is best appreciated as a fine "cigarette paper" wrinkling or tenting of the skin over the dorsum of the hand or over the elbow.

On the face, corticosteroid excess causes perioral dermatitis, characterized by small follicular papules on an erythematous base around the mouth, and a rosacea-like eruption, characterized by central facial erythema. Facial telangiectases and plethora over the cheeks may result from loss of subcutaneous tissue with hypercortisolism. Steroid acne, characterized by numerous pustular lesions reflecting androgenic effects or papular lesions reflecting glucocorticoid effects, sometimes occurs on the face, chest, or back. **Acanthosis nigricans,** a dark, soft, velvety skin with fine folds and papillae, may occur in intertriginous areas, such as under the breasts and in the groin, or at sites of friction, such as the neck or belt line. Acanthosis nigricans is thought to result from two changes in the skin's extracellular matrix: decreased viscosity caused by altered glycosaminoglycan formation and abnormal deposition of the extracellular matrix in papillae that protrude from the dermis.

Prominent reddish purple **striae** occur in 50–70% of patients, most commonly over the abdominal wall, breasts, hips, buttocks, thighs, and axillae. The striae result from increased subcutaneous fat deposition, which stretches the thin skin and ruptures the subdermal tissues. These striae are depressed below the skin surface because of loss of underlying connective tissue and are wider (not infrequently 0.5–2 cm) than the pinkish-white striae of pregnancy or rapid weight gain. Easy bruisability occurs in about 40% of cases. Ecchymoses occur following minimal trauma, resulting in purpura. Wound healing is delayed, and surgical incisions sometimes undergo dehiscence. Fungal infections of the skin and mucous membranes are frequent, including tinea versicolor, seborrheic dermatitis, onychomycosis, and oral candidiasis.

In the ectopic ACTH syndrome, hyperpigmentation of the skin occurs owing to the markedly elevated level of circulating ACTH, which has some melanocyte-stimulating hormone (MSH)-like activity. However, hyperpigmentation is rare in Cushing's disease or adrenal tumors except after total adrenalectomy (Nelson's syndrome).

In about 80% of female patients, hirsutism from increased secretion of adrenal androgens occurs over the face, abdomen, breasts, chest, and upper thighs. Acne often accompanies the hirsutism.

While the physiologic role of glucocorticoids in bone and Ca^{2+} metabolism is not well understood, excessive glucocorticoid production inhibits bone formation and accelerates bone resorption (see Chapter 17). Glucocorticoids directly inhibit bone formation by decreasing cell proliferation and synthesis of RNA, protein, collagen, and hyaluronic acid. Glucocorticoids decrease the rate of production of osteoclasts from progenitor cells in bone. They directly stimulate osteoclasts, leading to osteolysis and increased urinary hydroxyproline excretion. They potentiate the actions of PTH and $1,25\text{-}(OH)_2$ vitamin D on bone.

Furthermore, glucocorticoid excess decreases intestinal Ca^{2+} absorption and increases urinary Ca^{2+} excretion (hypercalciuria), resulting in a negative Ca^{2+} balance. Glucocorticoids impair intestinal absorption and renal tubular reabsorption of Ca^{2+} both by inhibiting the effects of vitamin D on the intestine and renal tubules and by inhibiting hydroxylation of vitamin D in the liver. There is a secondary increase in PTH secretion, accelerating bone resorption.

As a result of the hypercalciuria, kidney stones occur in about 15% of patients. Such patients may present with renal colic. Glucocorticoids also reduce the renal tubular reabsorption of phosphate, leading to phosphaturia and reduced serum phosphorus concentrations.

The combination of decreased bone formation and increased bone resorption ultimately leads to a generalized loss in bone mass (**osteoporosis**) and an increased risk of bony fracture. Osteoporosis is present in most patients; back pain is an initial complaint in 58% of cases. X-rays frequently reveal vertebral compression fractures (16–22% of cases), rib fractures, and sometimes multiple stress fractures. For unknown reasons, avascular (aseptic) necrosis of bone (usually of the femur or humerus) occurs sometimes with exogenous (iatrogenic) corticosteroids but is rare with endogenous hypercortisolemia.

Glucocorticoid excess alters the normal inflammatory response to infection or injury by several mechanisms. Glucocorticoids inhibit the action of phospholipase A_2 in releasing arachidonic acid from tissue phospholipids, thereby reducing formation of leukotrienes, which are powerful mediators of inflammation; they also decrease formation of thromboxanes, prostaglandins, and prostacyclin. They stabilize lysosomal membranes, inhibiting the release of interleukin-1 (endogenous pyrogen) from granulocytes. They suppress antibody formation and inhibit the accumulation and migration of polymorphonuclear neutrophils to sites of inflammation. They inhibit fibroblastic activity, preventing the walling off of bacterial and other infections. And they decrease local swelling and block the systemic effects of bacterial toxins. Cell-mediated immunity may also be adversely affected by the immune dysregulation in Cushing's syndrome. Patients with hypercortisolemia have a decrease in CD4 T lymphocytes, an increase in CD8 T lymphocytes, and diminished NK cell activity.

Glucocorticoid excess also suppresses manifestations of allergic disorders that are due to the release of histamine from tissues.

Hypertension occurs in about 75–85% of patients with spontaneous Cushing's syndrome. The exact pathogenesis of the hypertension is unclear. It may be related to salt and water retention from the mineralocorticoid effects of the excess glucocorticoid. Alternatively, it may be due to increased secretion of angiotensinogen. While plasma renin activity and concentrations are generally normal or suppressed in Cushing's syndrome, angiotensinogen levels are elevated to approximately twice normal because of a direct effect of glucocorticoids on its hepatic synthesis, and angiotensin II levels are increased by about 40%. Administration of the angiotensin II antagonist saralasin to patients with Cushing's syndrome causes a prompt 8- to 10-mm Hg drop in systolic and diastolic blood pressure. Studies in experimental animals have demonstrated that glucocorticoids exert permissive effects on vascular tone by a variety of mechanisms. Some involve vascular smooth muscle cells, including an increased secretion of the vasoconstrictor endothelin, an increase in Ca^{2+} uptake and Ca^{2+} channel antagonist binding, and an increase of α_{1B}-adrenergic receptors. In addition, glucocorticoids cause a decrease in atrial natriuretic peptide (ANP)-mediated cGMP formation, leading to decreased vasodilation by ANF. Glucocorticoids inhibit nitric oxide synthase in vascular endothelial cells, predisposing to vasoconstriction. Glucocorticoids also sensitize arterioles to the pressor effects of catecholamines.

Gonadal dysfunction occurs commonly in Cushing's syndrome and is the result of increased secretion of adrenal androgens (in females) and cortisol (in males and females). In premenopausal women, the androgens may cause hirsutism, acne, amenorrhea, and infertility. Hypercortisolism appears to affect the hypothalamic GnRH pulse generator to inhibit normal LH and FSH pulsatility and pituitary responsiveness to GnRH. The high levels of cortisol can thus suppress pituitary LH secretion. In women, this results in menstrual irregularities, including amenorrhea, oligomenorrhea, or polymenorrhea. In men, this results in decreased testosterone secretion by the testis, for which the increased adrenal secretion of weak androgens does not compensate. Decreased libido, loss of body hair, small and soft testes, and impotence ensue.

Excess glucocorticoids frequently produce mental symptoms, including euphoria, increased appetite, irritability, emotional lability, and decreased libido. Many patients experience impaired cognitive function, with poor concentration and poor memory, and disordered sleep, with decreased REM sleep and early morning awakening. Glucocorticoid excess also accelerates the basic electroencephalographic rhythm. Significant psychiatric illness—mainly depression but also anxiety, psychosis with delusions or hallucinations, paranoia, or hyperkinetic (even manic) behavior—occurs in 51–81% of patients with Cushing's syndrome. The pathogenesis of these central nervous system effects is not well understood.

Glucocorticoid excess inhibits growth in children, in part by directly inhibiting bone cells and in part by decreasing growth hormone and TSH secretion and somatomedin generation. Glucocorticoids suppress growth also by exerting direct effects on the growth plate, including inhibition of mucopolysaccharide production, resulting in reduced cartilaginous bone matrix and epiphysial proliferation.

With long-standing hypercortisolism, there may be mild to moderate elevations of intraocular pressure and glaucoma, perhaps related to swelling of collagen strands in the trabecular meshwork, which interferes with aqueous humor drainage. Posterior subcapsular cataracts may develop. About half of patients will develop exophthalmos, which is often asymptomatic. Visual field defects occur in 40% of patients with pituitary macroadenomas related to pressure on the optic chiasm; field defects do not occur with microadenomas.

Routine laboratory tests in Cushing's syndrome usually demonstrate a high normal hemoglobin, hematocrit, and red cell number. Polycythemia occurs rarely, secondary to androgen excess. The total white blood cell count is usually normal; however, the percentages of lymphocytes and eosinophils and the total lymphocyte and eosinophil counts are frequently subnormal.

Serum electrolytes are usually normal. Hypokalemic metabolic alkalosis sometimes occurs as a result of mineralocorticoid hypersecretion in patients with ectopic ACTH syndrome or adrenocortical carcinoma. Fasting hyperglycemia occurs in about 10–15% of patients; postprandial hyperglycemia and glucosuria are more common. Most patients with Cushing's syndrome have secondary hyperinsulinemia and abnormal glucose tolerance tests. The serum Ca^{2+} is generally normal; the serum phosphorus is low normal or slightly low. Hypercalciuria can be demonstrated in 40% of cases.

Routine x-rays may reveal cardiomegaly due to hypertensive or atherosclerotic heart disease, vertebral compression fractures, rib fractures, and renal calculi.

The ECG may show left ventricular hypertrophy (LVH) from hypertension, ischemia, or ST–T wave changes from electrolyte disturbances (eg, flattening of T waves from hypokalemia).

Diagnosis

Suspected hypercortisolism can be investigated by several approaches (Figure 21–14).

Measurement of free cortisol in a 24-hour urine specimen collected on an outpatient basis demonstrates excessive excretion of cortisol (24-hour urinary free cortisol levels > 150 μg/24 h). Urinary free cortisol values are rarely normal in Cushing's syndrome. Urinary free cortisol measurement is the most sensitive and specific test to screen for and to confirm the presence of Cushing's syndrome.

Performance of an overnight 1 mg dexamethasone suppression test will demonstrate lack of the normal suppression of adrenal cortisol production by exogenous corticosteroid (dexamethasone). The overnight dexamethasone suppression test is accomplished by prescribing 1 mg of dexamethasone at 11:00 PM, and then obtaining a plasma cortisol level the following morning at 8:00 AM. In normal individuals, the dexamethasone suppresses the early morning surge in cortisol, resulting in plasma cortisol levels of < 5 μg/dL (0.14 μmol/L); in Cushing's syndrome, cortisol secretion is not suppressed to as great a degree, and values are > 10 μg/dL (0.28 μmol/L).

If the overnight dexamethasone suppression test is normal, the diagnosis is very unlikely; if the urine free cortisol is also normal, Cushing's syndrome is excluded. If both tests are abnormal, hypercortisolism is present and the diagnosis of Cushing's syndrome can be considered established if conditions causing false positives (pseudo-Cushing's syndrome) are excluded (acute or chronic illness, obesity, high-estrogen states, drugs, alcoholism, and depression). The CRH test is a useful adjunct in patients with borderline elevated urinary cortisol levels due to probable pseudo-Cushing's state.

In patients with equivocal or borderline results, a 2-day low-dose dexamethasone suppression test is often performed (0.5 mg every 6 hours for eight doses). Normal responses to this test exclude the diagnosis of Cushing's syndrome. Normal responses are an 8:00 AM plasma cortisol less than 5 μg/dL (138 nmol/L); a 24-hour urinary free cortisol less than 10 μg/24 h (< 28 μmol/24 h); and a 24-hour urinary 17-hydroxycorticosteroid level less than 2.5 mg/24 h (6.9 μmol/24 h) or 1 mg/g creatinine (0.3 mmol/mol creatinine).

Confirmation of the diagnosis of Cushing's syndrome entails measurement of plasma ACTH level and a high-dose dexamethasone suppression test (Figure 21–14). Assay of the plasma ACTH level helps to differentiate ACTH-dependent from ACTH-independent causes of Cushing's syndrome. The high-dose dexamethasone suppression test is useful for differentiating pituitary from ectopic ACTH secretion. These tests are then followed by imaging procedures (eg, thin section CT scan or MRI) to determine the location of a suspected pituitary, adrenal, lung, or other tumor.

---

12. What are the symptoms and signs of excess of each class of adrenal steroids?
13. What are the major causes of Cushing's syndrome?
14. How is the regulation of glucocorticoid secretion altered in patients with Cushing's disease? With ectopic ACTH secretion? With autonomous adrenal tumors?
15. What are the symptoms and signs of glucocorticoid excess?
16. Name some different ways to make the diagnosis of Cushing's disease in a patient with suggestive symptoms and signs.

ADRENOCORTICAL INSUFFICIENCY

Adrenocortical insufficiency generally occurs either because of destruction or dysfunction of the adrenal cortex (**primary adrenocortical insufficiency**) or because of deficient pituitary ACTH secretion (**secondary adrenocortical insufficiency**). However, congenital defects in any one of several enzymes occurring as "inborn errors of metabolism" can lead to deficient cortisol secretion. Enzyme deficiencies can also result from treatment with various drugs, such as metyrapone, amphenone, and mitotane.

The causes of adrenocortical insufficiency are shown in Table 21–4. No matter what the origin, the clinical manifestations of adrenocortical insufficiency are a consequence of deficiencies of cortisol, aldosterone, and (in women) androgenic steroids.

Etiology

A. Primary Adrenocortical Insufficiency: Primary adrenocortical insufficiency (Addison's disease) is most often due to autoimmune destruction of the adrenal cortex (about 80% of cases). In the past, tuberculosis involving the adrenals was the most common cause, but it now accounts for about 20% of cases. Less common causes include other granulomatous diseases such as histoplasmosis, adrenal hemorrhage or infarction, metastatic carcinoma, and AIDS-related (cytomegalovirus) adrenalitis.

Primary adrenal insufficiency is rare, with reported prevalence rates of 39–60 cases per million population. However, as the number of patients with AIDS increases and as patients with malignancies live longer, more cases of adrenocortical insufficiency may be encountered. Addison's disease is somewhat more common in women, with a female:male ratio of 1.25:1. It usually occurs in the third to fifth decades.

Table 21–4. Causes of adrenocortical insufficiency.[1]

Primary adrenocortical insufficiency (Addison's disease)
   Major causes
      Autoimmune (about 80%)
      Tuberculosis (about 20%)
   Uncommon causes
      Adrenal hemorrhage and infarction
      Histoplasmosis and other granulomatous infections
      Metastatic carcinoma and lymphoma (non-Hodgkin's)
      HIV, AIDS-related opportunistic infection
      Amyloidosis
      Sarcoidosis
      Hemochromatosis
      Radiation therapy
      Antiphospholipid syndrome
      Surgical adrenalectomy
      Enzyme inhibitors (metyrapone, aminoglutethimide, trilostane, ketoconazole)
      Cytotoxic and chemotherapeutic agents (mitotane, megestrol)
      Congenital defects (X-linked adrenoleukodystrophy, enzyme defects, adrenal hypoplasia, familial glucocorticoid deficiency)

Secondary adrenocortical insufficiency
   Major cause
      Chronic exogenous glucocorticoid therapy
   Uncommon causes
      Pituitary tumor
      Hypothalamic tumor
      Acquired hypothalamic isolated CRH deficiency

[1]Modified and reproduced, with permission, from Greenspan FS, Strewler GJ (editors): *Basic and Clinical Endocrinology*, 5th ed. Appleton & Lange, 1997.

1. Autoimmune adrenocortical insufficiency–Autoimmune destruction of the adrenal glands is thought to be related to generation of **antiadrenal antibodies.** Circulating adrenal autoantibodies can be detected in over 80% of patients with autoimmune adrenal insufficiency, either isolated or associated with autoimmune polyglandular syndrome type 1 or type 2 (see below). These antibodies are of two types: adrenal cortex antibodies (ACA) and antibodies to the steroid 21-hydroxylase enzyme (cytochrome P450c21). The latter antibodies inhibit the ability of 21-hydroxylase to convert progesterone to deoxycorticosterone (see Figure 21–3), potentially contributing to the onset of adrenocortical failure. 21-Hydroxylase antibodies are highly specific for Addison's disease. In asymptomatic patients, these antibodies may also be important predictors for the subsequent development of adrenal insufficiency. In adults with other organ-specific autoimmune disorders (eg, premature ovarian failure), researchers have found that detection of adrenal cortex or 21-hydroxylase antibodies was associated with progression to overt Addison's disease in 21% and to subclinical hypoadrenalism in 29%. In children, the risk was even higher—in children with other organ-specific autoimmune diseases (eg, hypoparathyroidism), detection of adrenal autoantibodies was associated with a 90% risk of development of overt Addison's disease and a 10% risk of subclinical hypoadrenalism.

Autoantibodies to other tissue antigens are frequently found in patients with autoimmune adrenocortical insufficiency as well. Thyroid antibodies have been found in 45%, gastric parietal cell antibodies in 30%, intrinsic factor antibodies in 9%, parathyroid antibodies in 26%, gonadal antibodies in 17%, and islet cell antibodies in 8%.

It is not surprising, therefore, that autoimmune adrenal insufficiency is frequently associated with other autoimmune endocrine disorders. Two distinct polyglandular syndromes involving the adrenal glands have been described. **Autoimmune polyendocrine syndrome type 1 (APS-1)** is a rare autosomal recessive, non-HLA-associated disorder with onset in childhood. The diagnosis requires at least two of the following: adrenal insufficiency, hypoparathyroidism, and mucocutaneous candidiasis. Other endocrine disorders are sometimes associated, including gonadal failure and type 1 diabetes mellitus. There is also an increased incidence of other nonendocrine immunologic disorders, including alopecia, vitiligo, pernicious anemia, chronic hepatitis, and gastrointestinal malabsorption. The autoimmune pathogenesis of this condition involves antibody formation against cytochrome P450 cholesterol-side chain cleavage enzyme (P450-ssc). This enzyme converts cholesterol to pregnenolone, an initial step in cortisol synthesis (see Figure 21–3). P450-ssc is found in both the adrenal glands and gonads but not in other tissues involved in APS-1.

Autoimmune polyendocrine syndrome type 2 (APS-2) consists of adrenal insufficiency, Hashimoto's thyroiditis, and type 1 diabetes mellitus. It is associated with HLA-B8 (DW3) and HLA-DR3. Its pathogenesis involves antibody formation against the 21-OH enzyme mentioned above. The autoantibody against 21-hydroxylase does not explain the autoantibodies to other tissues.

Pathologically, the adrenal glands are small and atrophic, and the capsule is thickened. There is an intense lymphocytic infiltration of the adrenal cortex. Cortical cells are absent or degenerating, surrounded by fibrous stroma and lymphocytes. The adrenal medulla is preserved.

2. Adrenal tuberculosis–Tuberculosis causes adrenal failure by total or near-total destruction of both glands. Such destruction usually occurs gradually and produces a picture of chronic adrenal insufficiency. Adrenal tuberculosis usually results from hematogenous spread of systemic tuberculous infection (lung, gastrointestinal tract, or kidney) to the adrenal cortex. Pathologically, the adrenal is replaced with caseous necrosis; both cortical and medullary tissue are destroyed. Calcification of the adrenals can be detected radiographically in about 50% of cases.

3. Bilateral adrenal hemorrhage–Bilateral adrenal hemorrhage leads to rapid destruction of the adrenals and precipitates acute adrenal insufficiency. In children, hemorrhage is usually related to fulminant meningococcal septicemia **(Waterhouse-Friderichsen syndrome)** or pseudomonas septicemia. In adults, hemorrhage is related to anticoagulant therapy of other disorders in one-third of cases. Other causes in adults include sepsis, coagulation disorders, adrenal vein thrombosis, adrenal metastases, traumatic shock, severe burns, abdominal surgery, and obstetric complications.

Pathologically, the adrenal glands are often massively enlarged. The inner cortex and medulla are almost entirely replaced by hematomas. There is ischemic necrosis of the outer cortex, and only a thin rim of subcapsular cortical cells survives. There is often thrombosis of the adrenal veins. In surviving patients, the hematomas may later calcify.

The pathogenesis of adrenal insufficiency is thought to be related to a stress-induced increase in ACTH levels, which markedly increases adrenal blood flow to such a degree that it exceeds the capacity for adrenal venous drainage. Thrombosis may then lead to hemorrhage.

4. Adrenal metastases–Metastases to the adrenals occur frequently from lung, breast, and stomach carcinomas, melanoma, lymphoma, and many other malignancies. However, metastatic disease seldom produces adrenal insufficiency because over 90% of the adrenal must be destroyed before overt adrenal insufficiency develops. On pathologic examination, the adrenal glands are often massively enlarged.

5. AIDS-related adrenal insufficiency–Adrenal insufficiency in AIDS usually occurs in the later stages of HIV infection. The adrenal gland is commonly affected by opportunistic infection (especially cytomegalovirus, disseminated *Mycobacterium avium-intracellulare*, *M tuberculosis*, *Cryptococcus neoformans*, *Pneumocystis carinii*, and *Toxoplasma gondii*) or by Kaposi's sarcoma. Although pathologic involvement of the adrenal glands is frequent, clinical adrenal insufficiency is uncommon. More than half of AIDS patients have necrotizing adrenalitis (most commonly due to CMV infection), but it is usually limited in extent to less than 50–70% of the gland. Because adrenal insufficiency does not occur until over 90% of the gland is destroyed, clinical adrenal insufficiency occurs in less than 5% of patients with AIDS.

In addition, medications used by AIDS patients can alter steroid secretion and metabolism. Ketoconazole interferes with steroid synthesis by the adrenals and gonads. Rifampin, phenytoin, and opioids increase steroid metabolism.

Finally, various cytokines (including TNF-α and interferon) released by macrophages in AIDS may inhibit the hypothalamic-pituitary-adrenal axis.

In AIDS-related adrenal insufficiency, researchers have demonstrated a shift from mineralocorticoid and androgen production to glucocorticoid production, perhaps in response to the stress of severe illness. However, the hyponatremia frequently found in AIDS patients is most often due to the syndrome of inappropriate ADH (vasopressin) secretion rather than to adrenal insufficiency.

6. Antiphospholipid syndrome–Primary adrenal insufficiency is sometimes caused by the antiphospholipid syndrome (recurrent spontaneous abortion, cerebrovascular occlusion, multiple arterial and venous thromboses, and thrombocytopenia, accompanied and perhaps caused by circulating antiphospholipid antibody). In this syndrome, the antiphospholipid antibody (also known as the lupus anticoagulant) and thrombocytopenia are causes of adrenal thrombosis or adrenal hemorrhage.

7. Familial glucocorticoid deficiency–Familial glucocorticoid deficiency is a rare autosomal recessive disorder of hereditary adrenocortical unresponsiveness to ACTH. This unresponsiveness causes both decreased adrenal secretion of glucocorticoids and androgens and increased pituitary secretion of ACTH. Responsiveness to angiotensin II is normal. Affected infants and young children come to medical attention because of symptoms of cortisol deficiency, especially cutaneous hyperpigmentation, growth retardation, hypoglycemia, and recurrent infections. Older children may later manifest tall stature related to advanced bone age. The diagnosis is suggested when cortisol secretion does not respond to either endogenous or exogenous ACTH stimulation. On histologic examination, there is preservation of the zona glomerulosa but degeneration of the zona fasciculata and zona reticularis. In some patients, the resistance to ACTH is caused by a mutation in the ACTH receptor.

8. X-linked adrenoleukodystrophy–Adrenoleukodystrophy is an X-linked disorder characterized by adrenal insufficiency and progressive demyelination of the nervous system. Two different patterns have been described—cerebral adrenoleukodystrophy and adrenomyeloneuropathy. In cerebral adrenoleukodystrophy, adrenal insufficiency and neurologic symptoms occur in boys (onset by age 5–15 years). The neurologic symptoms are due to central nervous system demyelination: seizures, cortical blindness, dementia, coma, and death, often before puberty. Adrenomyeloneuropathy occurs in young men (onset by age 15–30 years). Adrenal insufficiency is often accompanied by hypogonadism. The neurologic involvement includes demyelination of the spinal cord and peripheral nervous system (sensory and motor peripheral neuropathy, bladder dysfunction) and sometimes of the central nervous system (color blindness, spastic paralysis).

The pathogenesis of both types of adrenoleukodystrophy involves deficiency of a peroxisomal enzyme, very long chain fatty acid acyl-CoA. This enzyme normally catalyzes very long chain fatty acids to ketones; in its absence, these very long chain fatty acids accumulate in circulating cholesterol esters. Accumulation of very long chain fatty acids and esterified cholesterol in the adrenal is thought to be responsible for adrenal cell death and adrenal insufficiency.

B. Secondary Adrenocortical Insufficiency: Secondary adrenocortical insufficiency most commonly results from ACTH deficiency due to chronic exogenous glucocorticoid therapy. Rarely, ACTH deficiency results from pituitary or hypothalamic tumors or from isolated CRH deficiency.

Pathophysiology

A. Primary Adrenocortical Insufficiency: Gradual adrenocortical destruction, such as occurs in the autoimmune, tuberculous, and other invasive forms, results initially in a decreased adrenal glucocorticoid reserve. Basal glucocorticoid secretion is normal but does not increase in response to stress and surgery; trauma or infection can precipitate acute adrenal crisis. With further loss of cortical tissue, even basal secretion of glucocorticoids and mineralocorticoids becomes deficient, leading to the clinical manifestations of chronic adrenal insufficiency. The fall in plasma cortisol reduces the feedback inhibition of pituitary ACTH secretion (Figure 21–12), and the plasma level of ACTH rises (Figure 21–15).

Rapid adrenocortical destruction such as occurs in septicemia or adrenal hemorrhage results in sudden loss of both glucocorticoid and mineralocorticoid secretion, leading to acute adrenal crisis.

B. Secondary Adrenocortical Insufficiency: Secondary adrenocortical insufficiency occurs when large doses of glucocorticoids are given for their anti-inflammatory and immunosuppressive effects in treatment of asthma, rheumatoid arthritis, ulcerative colitis, and other diseases. If such treatment is extended beyond 4–5 weeks, it produces prolonged suppression of CRH, ACTH, and endogenous cortisol secretion (Figure 21–12). Should the exogenous steroid treatment be abruptly discontinued, the hypothalamus and pituitary are unable to respond normally to the reduction in level of circulating glucocorticoid. The patient may develop symptoms and signs of chronic adrenocortical insufficiency or, if subjected to stress, acute adrenal crisis. Prolonged suppression of the hypothalamic-pituitary-adrenal axis can be avoided by using alternate-day steroid regimens whenever possible.

ACTH deficiency is the primary problem in secondary adrenocortical insufficiency. The ACTH deficiency leads to diminished cortisol and adrenal androgen secretion, but aldosterone secretion generally remains normal. In the early stages, there is a decreased pituitary ACTH reserve. Basal ACTH and cortisol secretion may be normal but do not increase in response to stress. With progression, there is further loss of ACTH secretion, atrophy of the adrenal cortex, and decreased basal cortisol secretion. At this stage, there is decreased responsiveness not only of pituitary ACTH to stress but also of adrenal cortisol to stimulation with exogenous ACTH.

Clinical Manifestations

The clinical manifestations of glucocorticoid deficiency are nonspecific symptoms: weakness, lethargy, easy fatigability, anorexia, nausea, and occasionally vomiting. Hypoglycemia occurs occasionally. In primary adrenal insufficiency, hyperpigmentation of skin and mucous membranes also occurs. In secondary adrenal insufficiency, hyperpigmentation does not occur, but arthralgias and myalgias may occur.

Other clinical features of adrenocortical insufficiency are listed in Table 21–5 and detailed below.

Impaired gluconeogenesis predisposes to hypoglycemia. Severe hypoglycemia may occur spontaneously in children. In adults, the blood glucose level is normal provided there is adequate intake of calories, but fasting causes severe (and potentially fatal) hypoglycemia. In acute adrenal crisis, hypoglycemia may also be provoked by fever, infection, or nausea and vomiting.

In primary adrenal insufficiency, the persistently low or absent plasma cortisol level results in marked hypersecretion of ACTH by the pituitary. Because ACTH has intrinsic MSH activity, a variety of pig-

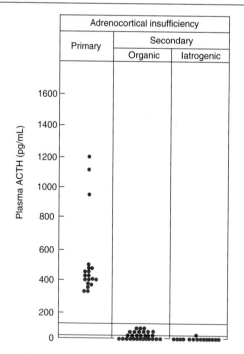

Figure 21–15. Basal plasma ACTH levels in primary and secondary adrenocortical insufficiency. (Reproduced, with permission, from Irvine WJ, Toft AD, Feek CM: Addison's disease. In: *The Adrenal Gland.* James VHT [editor]. Raven Press, 1979.)

Table 21-5. Clinical features of adrenocortical insufficiency.[1]

Primary and secondary adrenal insufficiency
   Tiredness, weakness, mental depression
   Anorexia, weight loss
   Dizziness, orthostatic hypotension
   Nausea, vomiting, abdominal cramps, diarrhea
   Hyponatremia
   Hypoglycemia
   Normocytic anemia, lymphocytosis, eosinophilia
Primary adrenal insufficiency
   Hyperpigmentation of skin, mucosa
   Salt craving
   Hyperkalemia
Secondary adrenal insufficiency
   Pallor
   Amenorrhea, decreased libido, impotence
   Scanty axillary and pubic hair
   Small testes
   Prepubertal growth deficit, delayed puberty
   Headache, visual symptoms

[1]Modified and reproduced, with permission, from Oelkers W: Current Concepts: adrenal insufficiency. N Engl J Med 1996; 335:1206.

mentary changes can occur. These include generalized hyperpigmentation (diffuse darkening of the skin); increased pigmentation of skin creases, nail beds, nipples, areolae, pressure points (such as the knuckles, toes, elbows, and knees), and scars formed after the onset of ACTH excess; increased tanning and freckling of sun-exposed areas; and hyperpigmentation of the buccal mucosa, gums, and perivaginal and perianal areas.

Vitiligo occurs in 4–17% of patients with the autoimmune form of adrenal insufficiency but is rare in insufficiency due to other causes.

In primary adrenal insufficiency, aldosterone deficiency results in renal loss of Na$^+$ and retention of K$^+$, causing hypovolemia and hyperkalemia. The hypovolemia in turn leads to prerenal azotemia and hypotension. Salt craving has been documented in about 20% of patients with adrenal insufficiency.

Patients may also be unable to excrete a water load. Hyponatremia may develop, reflecting retention of water in excess of Na$^+$. The defective water excretion is probably related to increases in posterior pituitary vasopressin secretion; these can be reduced by glucocorticoid administration. In addition, the glomerular filtration rate (GFR) is low. Treatment with mineralocorticoids raises the GFR by restoring plasma volume, and treatment with glucocorticoids improves the GFR even further.

The inability to excrete a water load may predispose to water intoxication. A dramatic example of this sometimes occurs when untreated patients with adrenal insufficiency are given a glucose infusion and subsequently develop high fever (**"glucose fever"**), collapse, and death. The pathogenesis of this condition is related to metabolism of the glucose and release of free water to dilute plasma. This dilution results in an osmotic gradient between plasma and cells of the hypothalamic thermoregulatory center which causes cells to swell and malfunction.

In secondary adrenal insufficiency, aldosterone secretion by the zona glomerulosa is usually preserved. Thus, clinical manifestations of mineralocorticoid deficiency, such as volume depletion, dehydration, hypotension, and electrolyte abnormalities, generally do not occur. Hyponatremia may occur as a result of inability to excrete a water load but is not accompanied by hyperkalemia.

Hypotension occurs in about 90% of patients. It frequently causes orthostatic symptoms and occasionally syncope or recumbent hypotension. Hyperkalemia may cause cardiac arrhythmias, which are sometimes lethal. Refractory shock may occur in glucocorticoid-deficient individuals who are subjected to stress. Vascular smooth muscle becomes less responsive to circulating epinephrine and norepinephrine, and capillaries dilate and become permeable. These effects impair vascular compensation for hypovolemia and promote vascular collapse.

Cortisol deficiency commonly results in loss of appetite, weight loss, and gastrointestinal disturbances. Weight loss is common and, in chronic cases, may be profound (15 kg or more). Nausea and vomiting occur in most patients; diarrhea is less frequent. Such gastrointestinal symptoms often intensify during acute adrenal crisis.

In women with adrenal insufficiency, loss of pubic and axillary hair may occur as a result of decreased secretion of adrenal androgens. Amenorrhea occurs commonly—in most cases related to weight loss and chronic illness but sometimes due to ovarian failure or hyperprolactinemia.

Central nervous system consequences of adrenal insufficiency include personality changes (irritability, apprehension, inability to concentrate, and emotional lability), increased sensitivity to olfactory and gustatory stimuli, and the appearance of electroencephalographic waves slower than the normal alpha rhythm.

Patients with **acute adrenal crisis** have symptoms of high fever, weakness, apathy, and confusion. Anorexia, nausea, and vomiting may lead to volume depletion and dehydration. Abdominal pain may mimic that of an acute abdominal process. Recent evidence suggests that the symptoms of acute glucocorticoid deficiency are mediated by significantly elevated plasma levels of cytokines, particularly IL-6 and, to a lesser extent, IL-1 and TNF-α. Hyponatremia, hyperkalemia, lymphocytosis, eosinophilia, and hypoglycemia occur frequently. Acute adrenal crisis can occur in patients with undiagnosed ACTH deficiency or in patients receiving corticosteroids who are not given increased steroid dosage during periods of stress. Precipitants include infection, trauma, surgery, and dehydration. If unrecognized and untreated, coma, severe hypotension, or shock unresponsive to vasopressors may rapidly lead to death.

Table 21–6. Typical plasma electrolyte levels in normal humans and in patients with adrenocortical diseases.[1]

	Na+ (meq/L)	K+ (meq/L)	Cl− (meq/L)	HCO_3^- (meq/L)
Normal	142	4.5	105	25
Adrenal insufficiency	120	6.7	85	45
Primary hyperaldosteronism	145	2.4	96	41
Hypoaldosteronism	145	6.7	105	25

[1]Modified and reproduced, with permission, from Ganong WF: *Review of Medical Physiology,* 19th ed. Appleton & Lange, 1999.

Laboratory findings in primary adrenocortical insufficiency include hyponatremia, hyperkalemia, hypoglycemia, and mild azotemia (Table 21–6). The hyponatremia and hyperkalemia are manifestations of mineralocorticoid deficiency. The azotemia, with elevations of blood urea nitrogen (BUN) and serum creatinine, is due to volume depletion and dehydration. Mild acidosis is frequently present. Hypercalcemia of mild to moderate degree occurs infrequently.

In secondary adrenocortical insufficiency, mineralocorticoid secretion is usually normal. Thus, serum Na+, K+, creatinine, bicarbonate, and BUN are usually normal. Plasma glucose may be low, though severe hypoglycemia is unusual.

Hematologic manifestations of adrenal insufficiency include normocytic, normochromic anemia, neutropenia, lymphocytosis, monocytosis, and eosinophilia. Hyperprolactinemia occurs when serum cortisol levels are low. Abdominal x-rays demonstrate adrenal calcification in about 50% of patients with Addison's disease due to adrenal tuberculosis and in a smaller percentage of patients with bilateral adrenal hemorrhage. CT scans detect adrenal calcification even more frequently in such cases and may also reveal bilateral adrenal enlargement in cases of adrenal hemorrhage; tuberculous, fungal, or cytomegalovirus infection; metastases; and other infiltrative diseases. Electrocardiographic findings include low voltage, a vertical QRS axis, and nonspecific ST–T wave changes related to electrolyte abnormalities (eg, peak T waves from hyperkalemia).

Diagnosis

A. Primary Adrenal Insufficiency: To establish the diagnosis of primary adrenal insufficiency, the physician must demonstrate a low level of plasma cortisol (< 3 μg/dL; 84 nmol/L) and an inability of the adrenal glands to respond normally to ACTH stimulation. This is usually done by performing an ACTH stimulation test (Figure 21–16). To do so, the physician obtains an 8:00 AM plasma cortisol, then administers 250 μg of synthetic ACTH (cosyntropin) intravenously or intramuscularly. Repeat plasma cortisol levels are obtained 60 and 120 minutes later. Normal subjects have a normal 8:00 AM plasma cortisol and usually a twofold or greater increase in plasma cortisol following cosyntropin. In Addison's disease, there is a low 8:00 AM plasma cortisol and virtually no increase in plasma cortisol following cosyntropin.

B. Secondary Adrenocortical Insufficiency: The diagnosis of ACTH deficiency due to exogenous glucocorticoids is suggested by obtaining a history of chronic glucocorticoid therapy or by finding cushingoid features on physical examination. Hypothalamic or pituitary tumors leading to ACTH deficiency usually produce symptoms and signs of other endocrinopathies. Deficient secretion of other pituitary hormones such as LH and FSH or TSH may produce hypogonadism or hypothyroidism. Excessive secretion of growth hormone or prolactin from a pituitary adenoma may produce acromegaly or amenorrhea and galactorrhea. Unfortunately, the conventional ACTH stimulation test uses a dose (250 μg ACTH) that is supraphysiologic and capable of transiently stimulating the adrenal cortex in some patients with secondary (pituitary or hypothalamic) adrenal insufficiency. Therefore, in evaluating patients with suspected central causes, experts now recommend using a much lower dose (1 μg) of ACTH in the ACTH stimulation test.

17. What are the major causes of glucocorticoid deficiency?
18. With what other autoimmune disorders is autoimmune adrenal failure associated?
19. What are the major causes of adrenal hemorrhage?
20. What are the clinical symptoms and signs of adrenal failure?
21. Name some different ways to make the diagnosis of adrenal insufficiency in a patient with suggestive symptoms and signs.

HYPERALDOSTERONISM (EXCESSIVE PRODUCTION OF MINERALOCORTICOIDS)

Primary hyperaldosteronism occurs because of excessive unregulated secretion of aldosterone by the adrenal cortex. **Secondary hyperaldosteronism** occurs because aldosterone secretion is stimulated by excessive secretion of renin by the juxtaglomerular apparatus of the kidney.

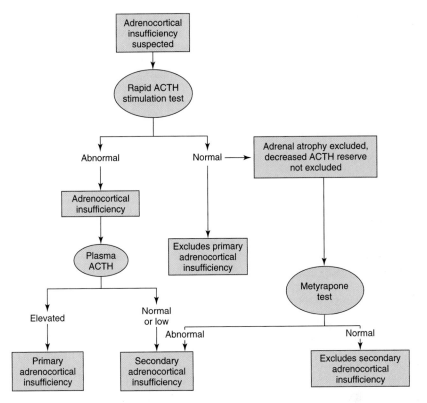

Figure 21–16. Diagnostic evaluation of suspected primary or secondary adrenocortical insufficiency. Boxes enclose clinical decisions, and ovals enclose diagnostic tests. (Redrawn and reproduced, with permission, from Miller WL, Tyrrell JB: The adrenal cortex. In: *Endocrinology and Metabolism,* 3rd ed. Felig P, Baxter JD, Frohman LA [editors]. McGraw-Hill, 1995.)

Etiology

The causes of hyperaldosteronism are listed in Table 21–7.

A. Primary Hyperaldosteronism: Primary hyperaldosteronism (Conn's syndrome) is rare and usually results from an aldosterone-secreting tumor of the adrenal cortex, most often a solitary **adenoma** (Figure 21–17). Bilateral tumors are unusual. Small satellite adenomas are sometimes found. Adenomas are readily identified by their characteristic golden yellow color. The adjacent adrenal cortex may be compressed. Adenomas producing excessive aldosterone are indistinguishable from those producing excessive cortisol except that they tend to be smaller (usually < 2 cm in diameter).

Bilateral adrenal hyperplasia accounts for most of the remaining cases of primary hyperaldosteronism (idiopathic hyperaldosteronism). Affected patients have bilateral nonadenomatous hyperplasia of the zona glomerulosa.

Table 21–7. Causes of hyperaldosteronism.

Primary hyperaldosteronism (Conn's syndrome)
   Aldosterone-secreting adrenocortical adenoma
   Bilateral hyperplasia of zona glomerulosa
   Glucocorticoid-remediable hyperaldosteronism
   Aldosterone-secreting adrenocortical carcinoma (rare)
   Idiopathic
Secondary hyperaldosteronism
   Renal ischemia
      Renal artery stenosis
      Malignant hypertension
   Decreased intravascular volume
      Congestive heart failure
      Chronic diuretic or laxative use
      Hypoproteinemic states (cirrhosis, nephrotic syndrome)
   Sodium-wasting disorders
      Chronic renal failure
      Renal tubular acidosis
   Juxtaglomerular cell hyperplasia (Bartter's syndrome)
   Surreptitious vomiting or diuretic ingestion (pseudo-Bartter's syndrome)
   Oral contraceptives
   Renin-secreting tumors (rare)

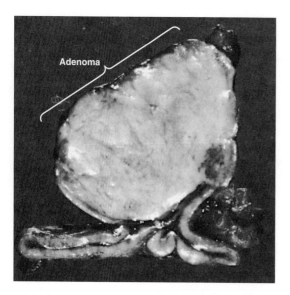

Figure 21–17. Cross section of adrenal, showing an adrenocortical adenoma in a patient with primary hyperaldosteronism. The gross and microscopic features do not permit differentiation of aldosterone- and cortisol-secreting adenomas in most cases. (Reproduced, with permission, from Chandrasoma P, Taylor CE: *Concise Pathology,* 3rd ed. Appleton & Lange, 1997.)

Adrenocortical carcinomas producing only aldosterone are extremely rare. Such tumors are generally large, and there is no diurnal rhythm in aldosterone production.

A dominantly inherited form of hyperaldosteronism—**glucocorticoid-remediable aldosteronism (GRA)**, or **familial hyperaldosteronism type I (FH-I)**—has recently been identified. As noted in Chapter 11, affected patients have a "hybrid" 11β-hydroxylase-aldosterone synthase gene in which the 11β-hydroxylase gene's regulatory elements are fused to the coding region of the aldosterone synthase gene. Therefore, ACTH stimulates aldosterone synthase activity. The hybrid *CYP11B1/CYP11B2* gene is thought to arise from an unequal crossing over between the two *CYP11B* genes during meiosis. The hybrid gene can be detected in peripheral blood leukocyte DNA by Southern blot or polymerase chain reaction methods. The clinical phenotype varies from severe early-onset hypertension to much milder blood pressure elevation; hypokalemia is usually mild. Affected individuals apparently have an increased risk of premature stroke. Because expression of the hybrid gene is stimulated by ACTH, leading to increased production of aldosterone and other steroids, the hyperaldosteronism is glucocorticoid-suppressible. Treatment with low doses of dexamethasone inhibits ACTH secretion and reverses the biochemical and clinical features of the disorder.

Familial hyperaldosteronism type II (FH-II) is clinically and genetically distinct from FH-I. It is characterized by autosomal dominant inheritance and hypersecretion of aldosterone due to adrenocortical hyperplasia or an aldosterone-producing adenoma. Unlike FH-I, the hyperaldosteronism in FH-II is not suppressible by dexamethasone therapy. Although its genetic basis has yet to be determined, studies have shown that the *CYP11B1/CYP11B2* hybrid gene is not responsible for FH-II.

In some cases, no definite abnormality is detected in the gland despite evident hyperaldosteronism.

B. Secondary Hyperaldosteronism: Secondary hyperaldosteronism is common. It results from excessive renin production by the juxtaglomerular apparatus of the kidney. The high renin output occurs in response to (1) renal ischemia (eg, renal artery stenosis or malignant hypertension); (2) decreased intravascular volume (eg, congestive heart failure, cirrhosis, nephrotic syndrome, or laxative or diuretic abuse); (3) Na^+-wasting disorders (eg, chronic renal failure or renal tubular acidosis); (4) hyperplasia of the juxtaglomerular apparatus (Bartter's syndrome); or (5) renin-secreting tumors. In these states, stimulation of the zona glomerulosa by the renin-angiotensin system leads to increased aldosterone production.

Pathologically, in secondary hyperaldosteronism, the adrenals may appear grossly normal; but microscopically there may be hyperplasia of the zona glomerulosa.

Pathophysiology

In primary hyperaldosteronism, there is a primary (autonomous) increase in aldosterone production by the abnormal zona glomerulosa tissue (adenoma or hyperplasia). However, circulating levels of aldosterone are still modulated to some extent by variations in ACTH secretion. The chronic aldosterone excess results in expansion of the extracellular fluid volume and plasma volume. In turn, this expansion is registered by stretch receptors of the juxtaglomerular apparatus and Na^+ flux at the macula densa, leading to suppression of renin production and low circulating plasma renin activity.

Patients with secondary hyperaldosteronism also produce excessively large amounts of aldosterone but—in contrast to patients with primary hyperaldosteronism—have elevated plasma renin activity.

Clinical Consequences of Mineralocorticoid Excess

The major consequences of chronic aldosterone excess are Na^+ retention and K^+ and H^+ wasting by the kidney.

The excess aldosterone initially stimulates Na^+ reabsorption by the renal collecting and distal tubules, causing the extracellular fluid volume to expand and the blood pressure to rise. When the extracellular fluid expansion reaches a certain point, however, Na^+ excretion resumes despite the continued action of aldosterone on the renal tubule. This **"escape" phenomenon** is probably due to increased secretion of **atrial natriuretic peptide.** Because the escape phenomenon causes the excretion of excess salt, affected patients are not edematous. Such escape from the action of aldosterone does not occur in the distal tubules. There, the elevated aldosterone levels promote continued exchange of Na^+ for K^+ and H^+, causing K^+ depletion and alkalosis. Affected patients are not markedly hypernatremic because water is retained along with the Na^+.

The chronic aldosterone excess also produces a prolonged K^+ diuresis. Total body K^+ stores are depleted, and hypokalemia develops. Patients may complain of tiredness, loss of stamina, weakness, nocturia, and lassitude—all symptoms of K^+ depletion. Prolonged K^+ depletion damages the kidney **(hypokalemic nephropathy),** causing resistance to antidiuretic hormone (vasopressin). The resultant loss of concentrating ability causes thirst and polyuria (especially nocturnal).

When the K^+ loss is marked, intracellular K^+ is replaced by Na^+ and H^+. The intracellular movement of H^+, along with increased renal secretion of H^+, causes metabolic alkalosis to develop.

Hypertension—related to Na^+ retention and expansion of plasma volume—is a characteristic finding. Hypertension can range from borderline to severe, but it is usually mild or moderate. Accelerated (malignant) hypertension is extremely rare. Because the hypertension is sustained, however, it may produce retinopathy, renal damage, or left ventricular hypertrophy. For example, patients with primary hyperaldosteronism due to aldosterone-producing adenomas have increased wall thickness and mass and decreased early diastolic filling of the left ventricle compared with patients who have essential hypertension. Thus, the chance of curing hypertension with resection of an adrenal adenoma is less predictable than the likelihood of correcting the related biochemical abnormalities. Only 50% of patients with adenomas are normotensive 5 years after adrenalectomy; older patients in particular are more likely to require postoperative antihypertensive medications.

The heart may be mildly enlarged as a result of plasma volume expansion and left ventricular hypertrophy. Severely K^+-depleted patients may develop blunting of baroreceptor function, manifested by postural falls in blood pressure without reflex tachycardia, or even malignant arrhythmias and sudden cardiac death.

The K^+ depletion causes a minor but detectable degree of carbohydrate intolerance (demonstrated by an abnormal glucose tolerance test). The decrease in glucose tolerance is corrected following K^+ repletion.

In addition, the alkalosis accompanying severe K^+ depletion may lower the plasma ionized Ca^{2+} to the point where latent or frank tetany occurs (see Chapter 17). The hypokalemia may cause severe muscle weakness, muscle cramps, and intestinal atony. Paresthesias may develop as a result of the hypokalemia and alkalosis. A positive Trousseau or Chvostek sign is suggestive of alkalosis and hypocalcemia (see Chapter 17).

Laboratory findings in hyperaldosteronism include hypokalemia and alkalosis (Table 21–6). Typically, the serum K^+ is below 3.6 meq/L (3.6 mmol/L), serum Na^+ is normal or slightly elevated, serum HCO_3^- is increased, and serum Cl^- is decreased (hypokalemic, hypochloremic metabolic alkalosis). There is an inappropriately large amount of K^+ in the urine.

The hematocrit may be reduced because of hemodilution by the expanded plasma volume. Affected patients may fail to concentrate urine and may have abnormal glucose tolerance tests.

The plasma renin level is suppressed in primary hyperaldosteronism and elevated in secondary hyperaldosteronism. Adrenal cortisol production is normal or low.

The ECG may show changes of modest left ventricular hypertrophy and K^+ depletion (flattening of T waves and appearance of U waves).

Diagnosis of Hyperaldosteronism

A. Primary Hyperaldosteronism: The diagnosis of primary hyperaldosteronism is usually suggested by finding hypokalemia in an untreated patient with hypertension (ie, one not taking diuretics). Thus, screening such patients for hyperaldosteronism is most easily accomplished by determining the serum K^+ level (Table 21–6). However, a low-Na^+ intake, by diminishing renal K^+ loss, may mask total body K^+ depletion. In patients with normal renal function, dietary salt loading will unmask hypokalemia as a manifestation of total body K^+ depletion. Thus, finding a low serum K^+ in a hypertensive patient on a high-salt intake and not receiving diuretics warrants further evaluation for hyperaldosteronism.

If hypokalemia is documented, the next step should be to assess the renin-angiotensin system by determining the random **plasma renin activity.** If the random plasma renin activity level is low, primary hyperaldosteronism is likely. However, if plasma renin activity is normal or high, it is very unlikely. If the renin activity is high, secondary hyperaldosteronism must be considered.

Subsequent workup entails measuring the 24-hour urinary aldosterone excretion and the plasma aldosterone level with the patient on a diet containing more than 120 meq of Na^+ per day. The urinary aldosterone excretion exceeds 14 μg/d, and the plasma aldosterone is usually greater than 90 pg/mL in primary hyperaldosteronism.

Measurement of the plasma aldosterone level can also help to differentiate between **adrenal adenoma** and **adrenal hyperplasia.** This distinction is important because surgery is indicated for treatment of adenoma but not hyperplasia. It is made by examining both the degree of plasma aldosterone elevation and its response to assumption of the upright posture. First, the 8:00 AM plasma aldosterone level is measured after the patient has been given at least 4 days of high Na$^+$ intake (exceeding 120 meq daily) and has been supine overnight (at least 6 hours). A plasma aldosterone level of greater than 20 ng/dL (554 pmol/L) indicates adrenal adenoma, and less than 20 ng/dL usually indicates hyperplasia. Then, after the patient has been erect for 2–4 hours, the plasma aldosterone level is again measured. Normally, the upright posture stimulates the renin-angiotensin system, causing a rise in plasma aldosterone. In most patients with adrenal hyperplasia, the erect plasma aldosterone level rises, owing to an enhanced sensitivity of the hyperplastic gland to the increased renin and angiotensin. In contrast, in most patients with adrenal adenoma, the erect plasma aldosterone level shows either no change or a decrease, due to profound suppression of renin by the high circulating aldosterone level and to a decreased number and affinity of angiotensin II receptors in the adenoma tissue.

B. Secondary Hyperaldosteronism: Patients with secondary hyperaldosteronism due to malignant hypertension, renal artery stenosis, or chronic renal disease also excrete large amounts of aldosterone but—in contrast to primary hyperaldosteronism—have elevated plasma renin activity.

---

22. What are the causes of hyperaldosteronism?
23. What are the presenting symptoms and signs of hyperaldosteronism?
24. How is the diagnosis of hyperaldosteronism made?

HYPOALDOSTERONISM (DEFICIENT PRODUCTION OF MINERALOCORTICOIDS)

Primary mineralocorticoid deficiency (hypoaldosteronism) may result either from destruction of adrenocortical tissue or from defective mineralocorticoid synthesis. Hypoaldosteronism is characterized by Na$^+$ loss, with hyponatremia, hypovolemia, and hypotension, and impaired secretion of both K$^+$ and H$^+$ in the renal tubules, resulting in hyperkalemia and metabolic acidosis. Renin activity is typically increased.

A **secondary deficiency** of endogenous mineralocorticoids may occur when renin production is suppressed or deficient. Renin production may be suppressed by the Na$^+$ retention and volume expansion resulting from exogenous mineralocorticoids (fludrocortisone acetate) or mineralocorticoid-like substances (licorice). When this happens, hypertension, hypokalemia, and metabolic alkalosis result. When renin production is deficient and unable to stimulate mineralocorticoid production, Na$^+$ loss, hyperkalemia, and metabolic acidosis occur.

Etiology

Acute and chronic adrenocortical insufficiency are discussed above. In long-standing **hypopituitarism,** atrophy of the zona glomerulosa occurs, and the increase in aldosterone secretion normally produced by surgery or other stress is absent. **Hyporeninemic hypoaldosteronism (type IV renal tubular acidosis)** is a disorder characterized by hyperkalemia and acidosis in association with (usually mild) chronic renal insufficiency. Typically, affected individuals are men in the fifth to seventh decades of life who have underlying pyelonephritis, diabetes mellitus, or gout. The chronic renal insufficiency is usually not severe enough to account for the hyperkalemia. Plasma and urinary aldosterone levels and plasma renin activity are consistently low and unresponsive to stimulation by ACTH administration, upright posture, dietary Na$^+$ restriction, or furosemide administration. The syndrome is thought to be due to impairment of the juxtaglomerular apparatus associated with the underlying renal disease. Finally, two genetic disorders may produce the symptoms and signs of hypoaldosteronism. In **congenital adrenal hypoplasia,** there are enzymatic abnormalities in mineralocorticoid biosynthesis. Aldosterone levels are low. In **pseudohypoaldosteronism,** there is renal tubular resistance to mineralocorticoid hormones, presumably due to a deficiency of mineralocorticoid hormone receptors. Affected patients manifest symptoms and signs of hypoaldosteronism, but aldosterone levels are high.

Clinical Consequences of Mineralocorticoid Deficiency

Patients undergoing bilateral adrenalectomy, if not given mineralocorticoid replacement therapy, will develop profound urinary Na$^+$ losses resulting in hypovolemia, hypotension, and, eventually, shock and death. In adrenal insufficiency, these changes can be delayed by increasing the dietary salt intake. However, the amount of dietary salt needed to prevent them entirely is so large that collapse and death are inevitable unless mineralocorticoid treatment is also initiated. Secretion of both K$^+$ and H$^+$ are impaired in the renal tubule, resulting in hyperkalemia and metabolic acidosis (Table 21–6).

DISORDERS OF ADRENAL ANDROGEN PRODUCTION

The adrenal cortex also secretes androgens, principally **androstenedione, dehydroepiandrostenedione (DHEA),** and **dehydroepiandrostenedione** sulfate (**DHEAS**). In general, the secretion of adrenal androgens parallels that of cortisol. ACTH is the major factor regulating androgen production by the adrenal cortex. The adrenal androgens are secreted in an unbound state but circulate weakly bound to plasma proteins, chiefly albumin. They are metabolized either by degradation and inactivation or by peripheral conversion to the more potent androgens testosterone and dihydrotestosterone. The androgen metabolites are conjugated either as glucuronides or sulfates and excreted in the urine.

Dehydroepiandrosterone has both masculinizing and anabolic effects. However, it is less than one-fifth as potent as the androgens produced by the testis. Consequently, it has very little physiologic effect under normal conditions. In women, the androgenic steroids (adrenal and ovarian) are thought to be required for the maintenance of libido and the capacity to achieve orgasm, perhaps through a trophic action on the clitoris.

Excessive secretion of adrenal androgens may occur as an associated phenomenon with Cushing's syndrome, particularly that due to adrenocortical neoplasms (particularly carcinomas). Excessive production of adrenal androgens has little effect in mature males but may cause hirsutism in mature females. It may result in precocious pseudopuberty in prepubertal boys and in masculinization in prepubertal girls.

Excessive secretion of adrenal androgens may also be congenital, resulting from one of several enzymatic defects in steroid metabolism (such as **congenital adrenal hyperplasia** caused by 21-hydroxylase or 11-hydroxylase deficiency [Figure 21–3]). With these inborn errors of steroidogenesis, there is insufficient cortisol production by the adrenal cortex. All of these enzyme defects are autosomal recessive traits.

Congenital adrenal hyperplasia is a relatively common disease, occurring in 1:15,000–1:5000 births. Most cases are due to deficiency of the enzyme steroid 21-hydroxylase. The 21-hydroxylase enzyme (cytochrome P450c21) is encoded by the gene *CYP21*. The active *CYP21* gene is on the short arm of chromosome 6; there is a neighboring pseudogene (an inactive gene that is transcribed but not translated). Most *CYP21* mutations are caused by conversion of a portion of the active *CYP21* gene sequence into a pseudogene sequence, resulting in a less active or inactive gene (gene conversion).

Impaired *CYP21* activity causes deficient production of both cortisol and aldosterone. The low serum cortisol stimulates ACTH production; adrenal hyperplasia occurs; and precursor steroids—in particular 17-hydroxyprogesterone—accumulate. The accumulated precursors cannot enter the cortisol synthesis pathway and for that reason spill over into the androgen synthesis pathway, forming androstenedione and testosterone. Prenatal exposure to excessive androgens results in masculinization of the female fetus, leading to ambiguous genitalia at birth. Newborn males have normal genitalia.

During the newborn period, there are two classic presentations of congenital adrenal hyperplasia due to classic 21-hydroxylase deficiency: salt-wasting and non-salt-wasting (also called "simple virilizing"). Neonates with the salt-wasting form have severe cortisol and aldosterone deficiencies and, if undiagnosed and untreated, will develop potentially lethal adrenal crisis and salt wasting at 2–3 weeks of age. Those with the simple virilizing form have sufficient cortisol and aldosterone production to avoid both adrenal crisis and salt wasting and are usually diagnosed because of virilization between birth and 5 years of age. Postnatally, both sexes present with virilization, reflecting the continuing androgen excess. The excess androgens during childhood can produce pseudo-precocious puberty, premature growth acceleration, early epiphysial fusion, and adult short stature. Variability in the phenotype occurs, depending on the severity of the 21-hydroxylase deficiency.

Analysis of DNA obtained by chorionic villus sampling in early pregnancy permits prenatal diagnosis. Administration of dexamethasone to the mother of an affected female fetus can prevent genital ambiguity. Postnatally, lifelong hormonal replacement with hydrocortisone (a glucocorticoid) and fludrocortisone (a mineralocorticoid) can ensure normal puberty and fertility. Antiandrogen therapy (with flutamide) plus inhibition of androgen-to-estrogen conversion (with testolactone) permits reduction in the dose of hydrocortisone sometimes required to suppress androgen levels.

Deficiency of adrenal sex hormones usually has little effect in the presence of normal testes or ovaries. In mature women, minor menstrual abnormalities may occur.

---

25. What are the causes of hypoaldosteronism?
26. What are the clinical manifestations of hypoaldosteronism?
27. What is the effect of excess or deficiency of adrenal androgens on otherwise normal adult men and women (ie, individuals with normal gonads)?

REFERENCES

General

Besser GM, Rees LH: The pituitary-adrenocortical axis. Clin Endocrinol Metab 1985;14:765.

Buckingham JC, Smith T, Loxley HD: Control of adrenocortical hormone secretion. In: *The Adrenal Gland,* 2nd ed. James VHT (editor). Raven Press, 1992.

Chrousos GP: Regulation and dysregulation of the hypothalamic-pituitary-adrenal axis: The corticotropin-releasing hormone perspective. Endocrinol Metab Clin North Am 1992;21:833.

Findling JW, Aron DC, Tyrrell JB: Glucocorticoids and adrenal androgens. In: *Basic and Clinical Endocrinology,* 5th ed. Greenspan FS, Strewler GJ (editors). Appleton & Lange, 1997.

Fraser R: Biosynthesis of adrenocortical steroids. In: *The Adrenal Gland,* 2nd ed. James VHT (editor). Raven Press, 1992.

Fuller PJ: Aldosterone and its mechanism of action: More questions than answers. Aust N Z J Med 1995;25:800.

Imura H: Adrenocorticotropic hormone. In: *Endocrinology,* 3rd ed. DeGroot LJ et al (editors). Saunders, 1995.

Miller WL, Tyrell JB: The adrenal cortex. In: *Endocrinology and Metabolism,* 3rd ed. Felig P, Baxter JD, Frohman LA (editors). McGraw-Hill, 1995.

Wilkinson CW, Peskind ER, Raskind MA: Decreased hypothalamic-pituitary-adrenal axis sensitivity to cortisol feedback inhibition in human aging. Neuroendocrinology 1997;65:79.

Cushing's Syndrome

Becker M, Aron DC: Ectopic ACTH syndrome and CRH-mediated Cushing's syndrome. Endocrinol Metab Clin North Am 1994;23:585.

N'Diaye N et al: Hormone receptor abnormalities in adrenal Cushing's syndrome. Horm Metab Res 1998;30(6–7):440.

Nieman LK: Cushing's syndrome. Curr Ther Endocrinol Metab 1997;6:161.

Orth DN: Cushing's syndrome. N Engl J Med 1995;332:791.

Tsigos C, Papanicolaou DA, Chrousos GP: Advances in the diagnosis and treatment of Cushing's syndrome. Bailliere's Clin Endocrinol Metab 1995;9:315.

Willenberg HS et al: Aberrant interleukin-1 receptors in a cortisol-secreting adrenal adenoma causing Cushing's syndrome. N Engl J Med 1998;339:27.

Yanovski JA, Cutler GB Jr: Glucocorticoid action and the clinical features of Cushing's syndrome. Endocrinol Metab Clin North Am 1994;23:487.

Adrenocortical Insufficiency

Carey RM: The changing clinical spectrum of adrenal insufficiency. Ann Intern Med 1997;127:1103.

Furmaniak J et al: Autoimmune Addison's disease–evidence for a role of steroid 21-hydroxylase autoantibodies in adrenal insufficiency. J Clin Endocrinol Metab 1994;79:1517.

Oelkers W: Adrenal insufficiency. N Engl J Med 1996;335:1206.

Orth DN: Adrenal insufficiency. Cur Ther Endocrinol Metab 1994,5:124.

Werbel SS, Ober KP: Acute adrenal insufficiency. Endocrinol Metab Clin North Am 1993;22:303.

Hyperaldosteronism

Blumenfeld JD et al: Diagnosis and treatment of hyperaldosteronism. Ann Intern Med 1994;121:877.

Connell JM et al: Dexamethasone-suppressible hyperaldosteronism: clinical, biochemical and genetic relations. J Hum Hypertens 1995;9:505.

Litchfield WR, Dluhy RG: Primary aldosteronism. Endocrinol Metab Clin North Am 1995;24:593.

Torpy DJ et al: Familial hyperaldosteronism type II: Description of a large kindred and exclusion of the aldosterone synthase *(CYP11B2)* gene. J Clin Endocrinol Metab 1998;83:3214.

Vallotton MB: Primary aldosteronism. Part I. Diagnosis of primary hyperaldosteronism. Clin Endocrinol 1996;45:47.

Vallotton MB: Primary aldosteronism. Part II. Differential diagnosis of primary hyperaldosteronism and pseudoaldosteronism. Clin Endocrinol 1996;45:53.

Weinberger MH: Mineralocorticoids and blood pressure. Curr Opin Nephrol Hypertens 1994;3:550.

Hypoaldosteronism

Holland OB: Hypoaldosteronism: Disease or normal response? (Editorial.) N Engl J Med 1991;324:488.

Horton R, Nadler J: Hypoaldosteronism. Curr Ther Endocrinol Metab 1997;6:164.

Polsky FI, Roque D, Hill PE: Hyporeninemic hypoaldosteronism complicating primary autonomic insufficiency. West J Med 1993;159:185.

Williams GH: Hyporeninemic hypoaldosteronism. (Editorial.) N Engl J Med 1986;314:1041.

Disorders of Adrenal Androgen Production (Congenital Adrenal Hyperplasia)

Hughes IA: Congenital adrenal hyperplasia: A continuum of disorders. Lancet 1998;352:752.

Merke DP, Cutler GB: New approaches to the treatment of congenital adrenal hyperplasia. JAMA 1997; 277:1073.

New MI: Diagnosis and management of congenital adrenal hyperplasia. Annu Rev Med 1998; 49:311.

Sciarra F, Tosti-Croce C, Toscano V: Androgen-secreting adrenal tumors. Minerva Endocrinol 1995;20:63.

Disorders of the Female Reproductive Tract

22

Vishwanath R. Lingappa, MD, PhD

Disorders of the female reproductive system typically occur either as a result of disease involving one of the reproductive organs (ovaries, uterus, uterine [fallopian] tubes, vagina, breast) or involving organs whose functions affect reproductive organs (eg, brain, hypothalamus, pituitary, thyroid, adrenals, kidney, liver). Many reproductive system disorders present during the reproductive years as **altered menstruation** or as **infertility**.

Disorders of reproductive function that are a consequence of disease in other systems (eg, hypothyroidism) are typically painless. Intrinsic disease of the reproductive organs can present either with or without pain. Pain may not occur until disease is far-advanced depending upon the location and anatomic features of reproductive organs. Some of these organs are deep and relatively inaccessible (eg, the ovaries) while others contain large amounts of adipose tissue (eg, the breast) or have a relative paucity of sensory nerve endings (eg, the ovaries, the uterine tubes). These features contribute significantly, for example, to the high mortality rates and the high incidence of widespread metastases associated with certain female reproductive system cancers. The widespread availability of the Papanicolaou smear as an early diagnostic test dramatically reduced the mortality rate of cervical cancer. However, the mortality rate from ovarian cancer has remained high.

The reproductive system and its hormones are involved in other functions besides reproduction, including maintenance and health of various tissues. Thus, besides menstrual disorders and infertility, the consequences of disorders of reproductive function can include **osteoporosis** (loss of bone mass), atrophy and inflammation of estrogen-deprived tissues (eg, atrophic vaginitis), an increased risk of some forms of cancer (eg, endometrial and breast cancer as a consequence of estrogen excess), and unique variants of systemic disorders. The latter include gestational diabetes and the hypertensive syndrome of **preeclampsia-eclampsia**.

1. How do female reproductive system disorders present during the reproductive years?
2. To what might you ascribe the *lack* of reduction in mortality rate from ovarian cancer in contrast to cervical cancer?
3. What are some consequences of reproductive system dysfunction?

NORMAL STRUCTURE & FUNCTION OF THE FEMALE REPRODUCTIVE TRACT

ANATOMY

The two **ovaries** house **oocytes** and produce estrogen and progesterone when appropriately stimulated. The ovaries contain thousands of **follicles**—oocytes with surrounding **granulosa cells,** which are steroid-producing cells that nourish and maintain the developing oocyte—embedded in a steroid-producing matrix of thecal cells. The ovary produces a wide range of endocrine and paracrine products besides steroids, which are likely to be important in follicular maturation and coordination of events in reproduction. However, currently the paracrine actions remain poorly understood (Table 22–1).

The **uterus** is a muscular pelvic organ with a hormone-responsive endometrial lining into which implantation of a fertilized egg occurs (Figure 22–1). Menstrual bleeding is the culmination of monthly cycles of endometrial growth, development, and sloughing in response to changes in blood levels of estrogen and progesterone (Figure 22–2). Besides proliferation and maturation, the role of the endometrium includes production of a wide variety of

Table 22–1. Endocrine and paracrine products of the ovary in addition to steroids.[1]

Products	Compartment	Regulatory Factors
Inhibin	Granulosa, theca, corpus luteum	FSH, EGF, IGF-1, GnRH, VIP, TGF
Activin	Granulosa	FSH
Müllerian-inhibiting substance	Granulosa, cumulus oophorus	LH, FSH
Follistatin	Follicles	LH, FSH
Relaxin	Corpus luteum, theca	n.d.
	Placenta, uterus	?PRL, LH, oxytocin, PGs
Oocyte meiosis inhibitor	Follicular fluid	n.d.
Follicle regulatory protein	Follicular fluid, granulosa, luteal	FSH, GnRH
Plasminogen activator	Granulosa	n.d.
Extracellular membrane proteins	Granulosa, follicular fluid	FSH, GnRH
Insulin-like growth factor-1	Granulosa	LH, FSH, GH, EGF, TGF, PDGF, estrogen
Epidermal growth factor-like	Granulosa, theca	Gonadotropins
Transforming growth factor-α	Theca, interstitial	FSH
Basic fibroblast growth factor	Corpus luteum	n.d.
Transforming growth factor-β	Theca, interstitial, granulosa	Fibronectin, FSH, TGF-β
Platelet-derived growth factor	Granulosa	n.d.
Nerve growth factor	Ovary	n.d.
Pro-opiomelanocortin	Corpus luteum, interstitial, luteal, granulosa	n.d.
Enkephalin	Ovary	n.d.
Dynorphin	Ovary	n.d.
Gonadotropin-releasing hormone	Ovary, follicular fluid, ?granulosa	n.d.
Oxytocin	Corpus luteum, granulosa	LH, FSH, $PGF_{2\alpha}$
Vasopressin	Ovary, follicular fluid	n.d.
Renin	Follicular fluid, theca, luteal	LH, FSH
Angiotensin II	Follicular fluid	n.d.
Atrial natriuretic factor	Corpus luteum, ovary, follicular fluid	n.d.
Luteinization inhibitor and luteinization stimulator	Follicular fluid	n.d.
Gonadotropin surge-inhibiting factor	Granulosa	n.d.
Luteinizing hormone receptor-binding inhibitor	Corpus luteum	n.d.
Neuropeptide Y, calcitonin gene-related peptide, substance P, peptide histidine methionine, somatostatin	Nerve fibers	n.d.
Vasoactive intestinal peptide	Nerve fibers	n.d.
c-mos	Oocytes	Developmental

Key: EGF = epidermal growth factor; FSH = follicle-stimulating hormone; GH = growth hormone; GnRH = gonadotropin-releasing hormone; IGF = insulin-like growth factor; LH = luteinizing hormone; n.d. = not determined; PDGF = platelet-derived growth factor; PG = prostaglandin; PGF = prostaglandin F; PRL = prolactin; TGF = transforming growth factor; VIP = vasoactive intestinal peptide.
[1]Modified and reproduced, with permission, from Ackland JF et al: Nonsteroidal signals originating in the gonads. Physiol Rev 1992;72:731.

DISORDERS OF THE FEMALE REPRODUCTIVE TRACT / 531

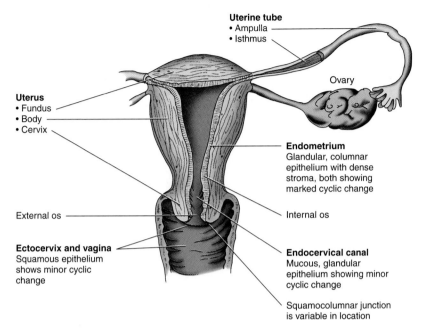

Figure 22–1. Anatomic landmarks of the uterus and adjacent organs. (Reproduced, with permission, from Chandrasoma P, Taylor CE: *Concise Pathology,* 3rd ed. Appleton & Lange, 1998.)

endocrine and paracrine products (Table 22–2). Beneath the endometrium is a muscle layer termed the myometrium whose contraction is necessary to expel the fetus at parturition.

The **uterine tubes** connect the uterine lining, peritoneal space, and ovaries. The **vagina** is the muscular tube connecting the vulva with the uterine cervix (Figure 22–1).

The **breasts** produce, store, and eject milk upon appropriate hormonal and physical stimulation (Figure 22–3).

SEXUAL DIFFERENTIATION & MATURATION OF ESTROGEN-DEPENDENT TISSUES

Embryonic Sexual Differentiation

Normal human somatic cells have 46 chromosomes, including two sex chromosomes. In the case of females, both sex chromosomes are X chromosomes; males have one X and one Y chromosome. This distribution determines the **chromosomal sex** of an individual.

A gene on the Y chromosome determines whether the individual will develop male gonads (testes). In the absence of the influence of this Y chromosome gene, the individual will develop female gonads (ovaries). The presence of testes versus ovaries, normally a consequence of chromosomal sex, determines the **gonadal sex** of the individual.

In the weeks of embryonic development that follow germ cell migration, secretions of the male gonads (müllerian inhibitory substance, testosterone, and dihydrotestosterone) determine development of male internal and external genitalia. In the absence of these secretions, female internal and external genitalia develop. Thus, the male represents the induced phenotype. No ovarian secretions are necessary for expression of the female phenotype. This development constitutes the **phenotypic sex** of the individual. The development of phenotypic sex involves events during embryogenesis as well as events during puberty.

Before the eighth week of gestation, the sex of the embryo cannot be recognized. Appropriately, this period is termed the **indifferent phase** of sexual development. The embryo acquires a dual genital duct system within the primitive kidney. The first to form is the wolffian duct. Subsequently, the müllerian duct forms, dependent on prior wolffian duct development. These two duct systems have different embryologic derivations. After 8 weeks of gestation, the müllerian ducts regress in the male as a result of the production of **müllerian inhibitory substance** by Sertoli cells of the fetal testes, and the wolffian duct gives rise to the prostate, epididymis, and seminal vesicles. In the female, the internal reproductive organs are formed from the müllerian ducts, while the wolffian structures degenerate. External genitalia of both males and females develop from common em-

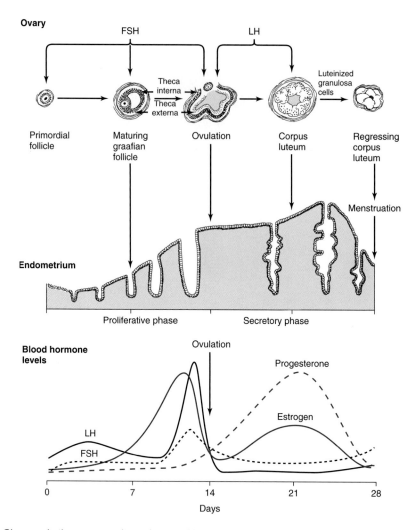

Figure 22–2. Changes in the ovary, endometrium, and blood hormone levels during the menstrual cycle. (Reproduced, with permission, from Chandrasoma P, Taylor CR: *Concise Pathology,* 3rd ed. Appleton & Lange, 1998.)

Table 22–2. Endocrine and paracrine products of the endometrium.[1]

Lipids	Cytokines	Peptides
Prostaglandins Thromboxanes Leukotrienes	Interleukin-1α Interleukin-1β Interleukin-6 Interferon-γ Colony-stimulating factor-1	Prolactin Relaxin Renin Endorphin Epidermal growth factor Insulin-like growth factors (IGFs) Fibroblast growth factor Platelet-derived growth factor Transforming growth factor IGF binding proteins Corticotropin-releasing hormone Fibronectin Tumor necrosis factor Parathyroid hormone-like peptide

[1] Reproduced, with permission, from Speroff L, Glass RH, Kase NG: *Clinical Gynecologic Endocrinology and Infertility,* 6th ed. Williams & Wilkins, 1999.

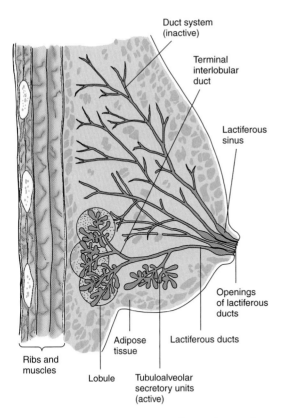

Figure 22–3. Schematic drawing of female breast showing the mammary glands with ducts that open in the nipple. The outlines of the lobules do not exist in vivo but are shown for instructional purposes. The stippling indicates the loose intralobular connective tissue. (Reproduced, with permission, from Junqueira LC, Carneiro J, Kelley RO: *Basic Histology,* 9th ed. Appleton & Lange, 1998.)

bryologic structures under different hormonal influences. Thus, exposure to androgens results in virilization of the external genitalia of female embryos, whereas androgen deficiency results in defective male development (Figure 22–4).

The embryonic germ cells originate in the endoderm of the yolk sac, allantois, and hindgut of the embryo. By week 5–6 of gestation, they migrate to the genital ridge and multiply. By 24 weeks of gestation, there are about 7 million oogonia in the primitive ovaries. They continue to multiply, but most die around this time, so that only about 1 million primary oocytes are left at birth. This decreases to about 400,000 by puberty. The surviving oogonia are arrested at the prophase of meiosis. Completion of the first division of meiosis does not occur until the time of ovulation. Only about 400 of these oocytes actually mature and are released by ovulation in a woman's lifetime; the others die at various stages of development.

Puberty

The secondary sexual characteristics develop at puberty (when maturation of the capacity for adult reproductive function occurs). Poorly understood changes occur in the brain and hypothalamus with the onset of puberty, resulting in the establishment first of sleep-dependent and later of truly pulsatile release of gonadotropin-releasing hormone from the hypothalamus. Prior to about age 10 in girls, gonadotropin secretion is at low levels and does not display a pulsatile character. At this age, pulsatile release of GnRH is set in motion and initiates the cyclic maturation and atresia of cohorts of follicles and the corresponding cyclic changes in estrogen and progesterone levels. The cyclic changes in estrogen and progesterone levels allow estrogen-dependent tissues to complete their maturation and manifest cyclic changes corresponding to the systemic hormonal environment. The appearance of the first menstrual period is termed the **menarche.**

Estrogen-Dependent Tissues

The major estrogen-dependent tissues include the brain, hypothalamus, pituitary, ovary, breasts, vagina, and the epithelium in the uterus and uterine tubes. The vagina is lined with a squamous epithelium. Under the influence of estrogen, the vaginal epithelium accumulates glycogen, which is deposited in the vaginal lumen as epithelial cells **desquamate** (slough). Fermentation of this glycogen to lactate by normal vaginal bacteria maintains a low pH barrier to pathogenic microorganisms. Although the vagina lacks glands, fluid can extravasate through the epithelium upon appropriate stimulation.

---

4. What is the difference between the chromosomal, gonadal, and phenotypic sex of an individual?
5. Approximately what percentage of the total number of oocytes present in the ovaries of a female at birth complete their maturation and are released upon ovulation over the course of her reproductive life?
6. Describe some changes that occur in the female with onset of puberty.

THE MENSTRUAL CYCLE

Normal female reproductive function involves a coordinated interaction of the hypothalamus, pituitary, ovary, and uterus under the influence of other organs such as the liver (which makes steroid-binding globulin), adrenals, and thyroid gland. The functional anatomy of the female reproductive system is best approached as a neuroendocrine feedback axis (Figure 22–5). The most striking feature of the fe-

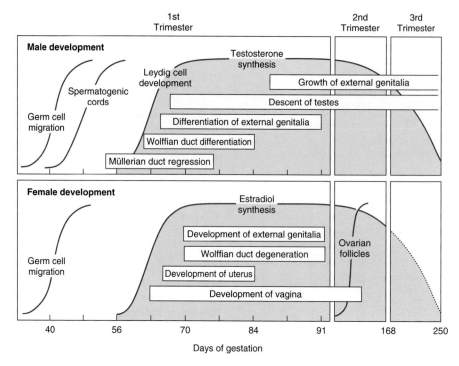

Figure 22–4. Timing of male and female human sexual differentiation. (Reproduced, with permission, from Griffin JE, Ojeda SR: *Textbook of Endocrine Physiology,* 2nd ed. Oxford Univ Press, 1992.)

male reproductive neuroendocrine axis is that its functions fluctuate approximately monthly with the **menstrual cycle.**

The peptide **gonadotropin-releasing hormone (GnRH)** is secreted in a pulsatile manner from the hypothalamus into the pituitary portal circulation. Upon reaching the anterior pituitary, GnRH stimulates certain cells termed **gonadotrophs.** Gonadotrophs respond to GnRH by secreting two polypeptide hormones (gonadotropins) termed **luteinizing hormone (LH)** and **follicle-stimulating hormone (FSH).** The target tissues for LH and FSH are the ovaries, which respond in two general ways.

One ovarian response to gonadotropins—in particular to FSH—is maturation of oocytes (Figure 22–6). Under the influence of FSH, a cohort of follicles starts to mature. Normally, only one follicle in this cohort survives to complete the process, culminating in release of a fertilizable egg (**ovulation**). The other activated follicles succumb during the course of maturation to a process of degeneration and death termed **atresia.**

A second ovarian response to both LH and FSH is synthesis, modification, and secretion of steroid hormones (Figure 22–2). Steroid hormone production by the ovary occurs in two phases. Early in each ovarian cycle, the major steroids secreted are androgens and estrogens. Androgens are made in the thecal cells and diffuse into the follicles, where they are converted (by an enzymatic reaction termed aromatization) into estrogens in the granulosa cells. Over the first half of the cycle, termed the **follicular phase,** the level of estrogens rises. LH stimulates androgen production in thecal cells, while FSH stimulates aromatase activity in granulosa cells. Estrogen and FSH trigger the

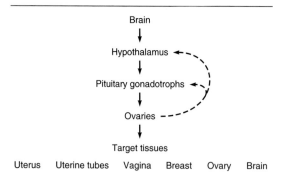

Figure 22–5. Female reproductive neuroendocrine feedback axis. Solid arrows indicate stimulation; dashed arrows indicate inhibition.

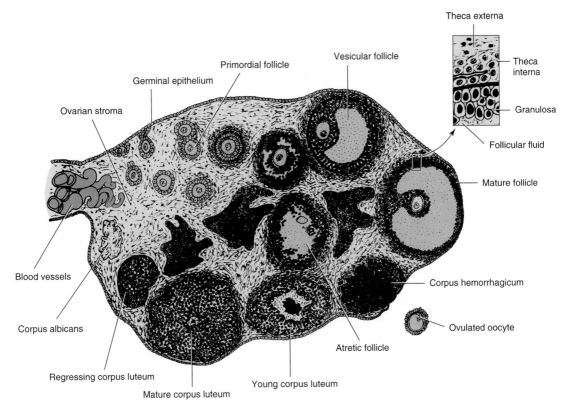

Figure 22-6. Diagram of mammalian ovary, showing the sequential development of a follicle and the formation of the corpus luteum. An atretic follicle is shown in the center, and the structure of the wall of the mature follicle is detailed at the upper right. (Reproduced, with permission, from Gorbman A, Bern H: *Textbook of Comparative Endocrinology*. Wiley, 1962.)

eventual appearance of LH receptors on the surface of granulosa cells. Stimulation of these receptors by LH activates production of progesterone by the end of the follicular phase, which lasts for 12–18 days. A midcycle surge of LH and FSH secretion, induced by the high levels of estrogen followed by ovulation, marks the end of the follicular phase. At ovulation, the mature follicle ruptures through the wall of the ovary, releasing the egg, which enters one of the uterine tubes and travels toward the endometrium. Fertilization, if it occurs, takes place along this path.

After release of the egg, what is left of the follicle develops into a structure termed the **corpus luteum** that synthesizes and releases large amounts of both estrogen and progesterone. During the second half of the cycle, termed the **luteal phase,** plasma estrogens and progesterone rise dramatically. The high levels of estrogen and progesterone promote maturation of the endometrium, which had proliferated in the follicular phase with straight glands and thin secretions. Under the influence of progesterone, the endometrium develops tortuous glands engorged with thick secretions (Figure 22–2). By itself, the corpus luteum is able to sustain progesterone production for only a limited period of time. This is because the high levels of estrogen, perhaps potentiated by progesterone, rapidly inhibit LH secretion, on which the survival of the corpus luteum depends. Thus, the luteal phase lasts 14 days.

In the absence of fertilization and implantation, the corpus luteum degenerates, and the levels of estrogen and progesterone decrease dramatically. The end of the menstrual cycle is marked by sloughing of the endometrium, which can no longer be maintained in the absence of estrogen (Figure 22–2). The onset of menstruation marks the nadir of estrogen and progesterone levels, ending the preceding cycle and initiating maturation of a cohort of new follicles for the next cycle.

If fertilization and implantation do occur, the developing placenta produces an LH-like hormone termed **human chorionic gonadotropin (hCG).** Unlike LH secretion by the gonadotrophs of the anterior pituitary, placental secretion of hCG is not inhibited

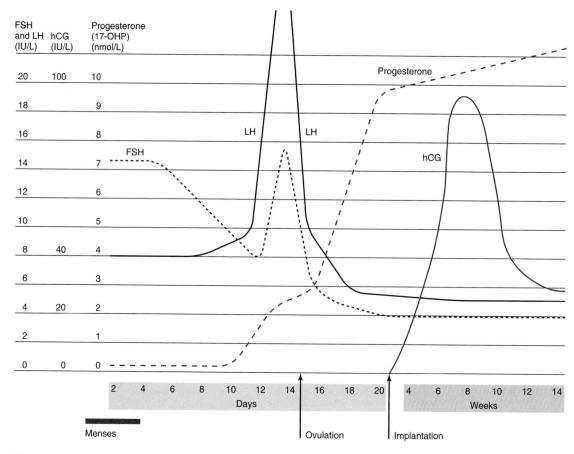

Figure 22–7. Steroid production during pregnancy. (Reproduced, with permission, from Speroff L, Glass RH, Kase NG: *Clinical Gynecologic Endocrinology and Infertility,* 6th ed. Williams & Wilkins, 1999.)

even by the high levels of estrogen and progesterone. hCG maintains the corpus luteum for a period of 8–10 weeks until the full progesterone-producing capacity of the placenta has developed. At that point, hCG levels fall and the placenta becomes the major producer of progesterone, working in concert with both mother and fetus to maintain the pregnancy (Figure 22–7).

The ovarian steroid hormones have a wide range of effects on their target tissues, including (1) paracrine effects in the ovary itself; (2) feedback (inhibitory) effects on the brain, hypothalamus, and pituitary; and (3) feed-forward (stimulatory) effects on the end-organ target tissues of the axis: uterus, breast, vagina, and uterine tubes.

The developing dominant follicle secretes many other products besides steroids, and many of these products act in a paracrine manner (Table 22–1).

Ovarian products drive not only the cyclic changes that occur in the ovary but also the cyclic changes in the end-organ target tissues. The transition from follicular to luteal phases of the cycle corresponds to the optimum environment in the uterus and uterine tubes for sperm and egg transport. Subsequently, the endometrial changes of the luteal phase are optimal for implantation and render the endometrium inhospitable for sperm transport to the uterine tube.

When perfectly coordinated with each other, the cyclic changes in structure during the course of the menstrual cycle allow the reproductive organs to perform different functions at different points in the cycle to optimize the chances for successful reproduction. When these mechanisms malfunction, the result may be infertility, altered menstrual bleeding, amenorrhea, or even cancer.

PHYSIOLOGY OF OVARIAN STEROIDS & CONTRACEPTION

Like the adrenal gland, the ovary is a steroid factory. The ovary secretes three types of steroids: **progesterone,** containing 21 carbons; **androgens,** containing 19 carbons; and **estrogens,** containing 18 carbons. Outside of the ovary it is possible to convert the 19-carbon androgens to 18-carbon estrogens, but the reverse is not the case. Steroid synthesis occurs by conversion from cholesterol in a series of biochemical reactions catalyzed by enzymes in the mitochondria and in the endoplasmic reticulum (see Chapter 21). Generally, the rate-limiting step in steroid production is side chain cleavage of cholesterol within the mitochondrion to generate the basic steroid nucleus that is further modified in the endoplasmic reticulum to generate the various steroids. Because steroids are synthesized by a cascade of enzyme reactions in various pathways, a block in one step (eg, due to a congenital enzyme defect or inhibition by certain drugs) can result in lack of synthesis of one steroid and "spillover" of precursors into another. Conversely, induction of new enzyme activities can convert progestins to androgens or androgens to estrogens.

The major mechanism of steroid hormone action involves diffusion across the plasma membrane, binding of the steroid to receptor proteins in the cytoplasm or nucleus, and activation of transcription of certain genes by binding of the steroid-receptor complex to specific regions of DNA. In this way the pattern of gene expression is changed in complex ways in the various steroid-responsive tissues (ie, those that contain steroid receptors).

While steroids are physiologic modulators of tissue phenotype through gene expression, modern medicine often uses them as pharmacologic agents. When used in this manner, certain steroid-mediated effects are viewed as desirable while others are considered undesirable "side effects." One of the common desirable pharmacologic uses of the ovarian steroids is contraception. Undesirable side effects of large doses include immediate consequences such as nausea and an increased risk of thrombosis and long-term consequences such as an increased risk of certain cancers.

Birth control pills are a pharmacologic means of inducing infertility by disrupting the precise timing of hormone-directed events necessary for reproduction. Formulations include estrogens alone, progestins alone, and combinations of estrogens and progestins. Most preparations of estrogen and progesterone block the LH/FSH surge at midcycle, thereby preventing ovulation. However, their contraceptive actions also include effects on other estrogen- and progesterone-sensitive tissues, such as inducing changes in cervical mucus and the endometrial lining that are unfavorable to sperm transport and implantation. Over the years, the amount of estrogen contained in birth control pills has been decreased and progestins have been added, with considerable mitigation of unpleasant and dangerous side effects.

7. What are the target tissues for GnRH? For gonadotropins? For ovarian steroids?
8. Why is pulsatile secretion of GnRH important?
9. What are some specialized features of GnRH action?
10. What are the specific effects of gonadotropins on the ovary?
11. How does the structure of the uterus differ in the midfollicular versus the late luteal stages, and for what reproduction-related events is each stage optimized?
12. What products are made by a granulosa cell in the dominant follicle over the course of its lifetime?

PREGNANCY

Prerequisites for a Successful Pregnancy

A number of changes must occur in reproductive and other organs for establishment and successful completion of a pregnancy. Fertilization requires not only successful ovulation but also effective transport of viable sperm into the uterine tube. This in turn is dependent on characteristics of the surface of the endometrium described above (Figure 22–2).

The uterine tubes allow the mature egg released upon ovulation to be captured and transported into the uterus, during which time fertilization may occur. If properly implanted in the wall of the uterus, the embryo will develop a placenta to support fetal growth and development. If fertilization or proper implantation does not occur, the endometrium is sloughed, only to regrow in response to the estrogen produced by the ovary during the next menstrual cycle (Figure 22–2).

The placenta is composed of three layers: the cytotrophoblast, the syncytiotrophoblast, and the decidual layer (Figure 22–8). The first two are derived from the embryo, the third from the maternal endometrium. The placenta allows close apposition of maternal and fetal circulations for exchange of nutrients, oxygen, and other substances. Moreover, the placenta develops the capacity to secrete a variety of important products, including human chorionic gonadotropin (hCG), progesterone, and a growth hormone-like protein termed **human chorionic somatomammotropin (hCS),** also known as **placental lactogen (hPL)** (Table 22–3).

Placental hCG serves to maintain stimulation to the corpus luteum for progesterone secretion and thus to maintain the high levels of progesterone necessary for successful pregnancy. hCG production continues until the placenta has fully developed, a period of approximately 8–10 weeks, after which the corpus luteum at-

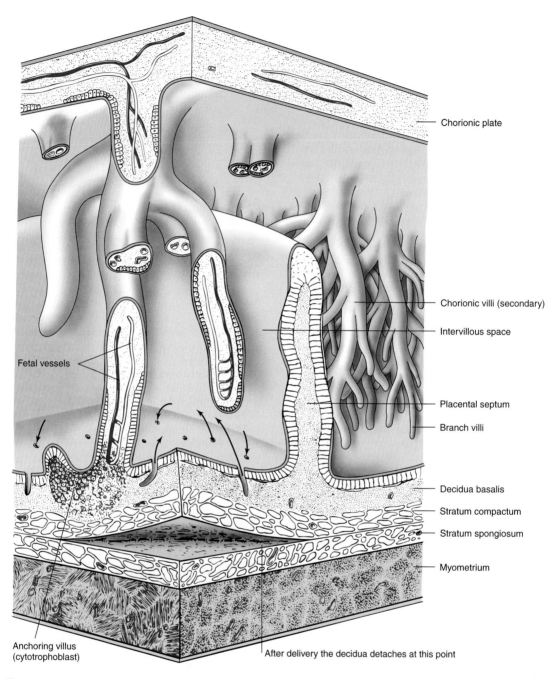

Figure 22–8. Placental anatomy. (Reproduced, with permission, from Copenhaver WM, Kelly DE, Wood RL: *Bailey's Textbook of Histology,* 17th ed. Williams & Wilkins, 1978.)

rophies, perhaps due to down-regulation of receptors by the high levels of hCG. By then, the mature placenta, working in concert with both the mother (who supplies the cholesterol) and the developing fetus, has developed the capacity to produce progesterone directly. During most of pregnancy, the fetus provides the placenta with androgens, which are used to make estrogens by the maternal compartment (Figure 22–9). This reflects the action of a special zone in the fetal adrenal cortex engaged in androgen production. Toward the end of pregnancy, the onset of ACTH secretion by the fetal pituitary triggers the fetal adrenal to produce cortisol rather than androgen. This switch may play a role in triggering onset of labor.

Table 22–3. Endocrine and paracrine products in pregnancy other than steroids.[1]

Fetal Compartment	Placental Compartment	Maternal Compartment

Alpha-fetoprotein	Hypothalamic-like hormones
	  GnRH
	  CRH
	  TRH
	  Somatostatin
	Pituitary-like hormones
	  hCG
	  hCS
	  hGH
	  hCT
	  ACTH
	Growth factors
	  IGF-1
	  Epidermal growth factor
	  Platelet-derived growth factor
	  Fibroblast growth factor
	  Transforming growth factor-β
	  Inhibin
	  Activin
	Cytokines
	  Interleukin-1
	  Interleukin-6
	  Colony-stimulating factor
	Other
	  Opioids
	  Prorenin
	  Pregnancy-specific β-glycoprotein
	  Pregnancy-associated plasma protein A
		Decidual proteins
		  Prolactin
		  Relaxin
		  IGFBP-1
		  Interleukin-1
		  Colony-stimulating factor-1
		  Progesterone-associated endometrial protein
		Corpus luteum proteins
		  Relaxin
		  Prorenin

[1]Reproduced, with permission, from Speroff L, Glass RH, Kase NG: *Clinical Gynecologic Endocrinology and Infertility*, 6th ed. Williams & Wilkins, 1999.

In addition to the changes in organs with pregnancy-specific functions, a number of physiologic changes occur in other maternal organ systems. These include increased blood volume (increased by more than 40% by the middle of the third trimester), increased total body water (increased by 6–8 L), and increased cardiac output due both to increased stroke volume (increased by 30%) and heart rate (increased by 15%). A striking increase in minute ventilation (increased by 50% over nonpregnant) without any change in respiratory rate is observed as a result of increased tidal volume (Chapter 9). Dramatic increases in renal blood flow and glomerular filtration rate (increased by 40%) are also seen. Most of these effects are related in complex ways to the effects of steroids in pregnancy.

Role of Steroids in Pregnancy

The precise role of various steroids in pregnancy is incompletely understood. The demonstrated and proposed roles of progesterone in pregnancy include (1) promotion of implantation; (2) suppression of the maternal immune response to fetal antigens, thus preventing rejection of the fetus; (3) provision of substrate for manufacture by the fetal adrenal of glucocorticoids and mineralocorticoids; (4) maintenance of uterine quiescence through gestation; and (5) a role in parturition.

Human Chorionic Somatomammotropin & Fuel Homeostasis in Pregnancy

Another example of fetal-placental-maternal interactions is seen in the actions of hCS (Figure 22–10). This "counterregulatory" hormone—ie, a hormone whose actions oppose those of insulin—appears to serve as a defense against fetal hypoglycemia. From a metabolic standpoint, pregnancy is a form of "accelerated starvation" characterized by fasting hypoglycemia, as fuel substrates produced by the mother are used by the growing fetus. hCS produced by the placenta in response to hypoglycemia serves to increase lipolysis, thereby raising maternal free fatty acid levels and ultimately blood glucose and ketone levels. This "diabetogenic" role of hCS is a major additional burden on the maternal compartment and contributes to the tendency for diabetes mellitus to emerge in susceptible individuals during pregnancy. Normally, glucose is the major fuel source for the fetus. However, in the event of glucose deprivation, ketones provide a ready emergency fuel supply (as they do in starvation) for both the mother and—via the placenta—for the fetus.

---

13. How is the corpus luteum maintained until the placenta has developed adequately?
14. What are some possible roles of steroids during pregnancy?
15. Why is new-onset diabetes mellitus a common complication of pregnancy?

LACTATION

Breast Structure & Development

The mature adult female breast consists of a cluster of 15–25 lactiferous ducts, each emerging independently at the nipple (Figure 22–3). The rudiments for breast development are established during embryonic development. During puberty, rising estrogen levels stimulate breast growth as one of a number of female secondary sexual characteristics. Finally, during pregnancy, the hormones progesterone, prolactin, and chorionic somatomammotropin play a dominant

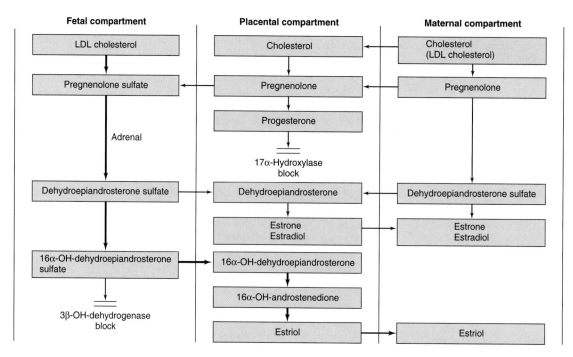

Figure 22–9. Fetal-placental-maternal cooperation in steroidogenesis. (Reproduced, with permission, from Speroff L et al: Regulation of the menstrual cycle. In: *Clinical Gynecologic Endocrinology and Infertility*, 6th ed. Williams & Wilkins, 1999.)

role in stimulating breast growth and the capacity for milk synthesis. However, the presence of high levels of estrogen and progesterone during pregnancy block actual milk synthesis. Subsequent to delivery, with the fall in estrogen and progesterone levels, this block is removed. Both the pubertal and pregnant phases of breast growth require the permissive influence of glucocorticoids, thyroxine, and insulin for full development, and their actions are potentiated by estrogen and progesterone.

Breast growth involves both proliferation and branching of lactiferous ducts as well as accumulation of adipose and connective tissue. In the mature breast, each terminal lactiferous duct drains clusters of tubulo-alveolar secretory units lined by milk-secreting epithelial cells and is suspended in connective and adipose tissue well populated with lymphocytes.

Initiation & Maintenance of Milk Synthesis & Secretion

Although prolactin stimulates breast growth and milk synthesis, actual lactation, ie, milk release, is inhibited by the high levels of estrogen and progesterone prior to birth. After delivery of the placenta, estrogen and progesterone levels fall dramatically, removing this block. Maintenance of milk secretion requires the joint action of both anterior and posterior pituitary factors as well as of infant and mother (Figure 22–11).

Suckling stimulates afferent neural pathways that suppress dopamine levels in the hypothalamus, thereby maintaining high levels of prolactin necessary for milk synthesis. At the same time, suckling (as well as other stimuli such as the baby's cry, etc) triggers afferent sensory nerve fibers that stimulate synthesis, transport, and secretion of oxytocin from the posterior pituitary. Oxytocin stimulates contraction of mammary myoepithelial cells, thereby triggering ejection of milk from the mammary epithelial alveoli and out the nipple.

Toward the end of pregnancy, there is an increase in the IgA-secreting lymphocyte population in the vasculature and connective tissue of the breast. These lymphocytes secrete IgA into the local bloodstream, from which it is taken up by the mammary epithelial cells. By the process of transcytosis, IgA crosses the mammary epithelial cells to be deposited into the luminal secretion (milk). This mechanism is responsible for conferring passive immunity on the newborn. Indeed, the earliest mammary gland secretion after birth, termed colostrum, has a particularly high immunoglobulin content.

The high level of prolactin maintained during lactation also has a contraceptive effect, primarily by inhibition of pulsatile secretion of GnRH. The precise mechanism is not known but may involve a short feedback loop by which prolactin stimulates dopamine release, which in turn elevates endogenous opi-

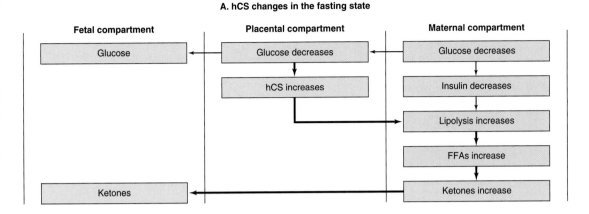
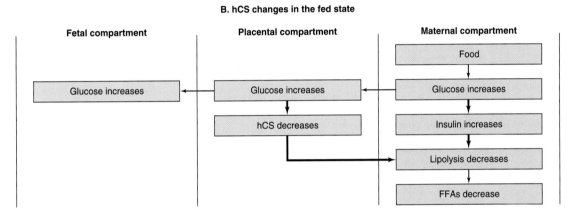

Figure 22–10. Fetal-placental-maternal cooperation in fuel homeostasis. (Reproduced, with permission, from Speroff L, Glass RH, Kase NG: *Clinical Gynecologic Endocrinology and Infertility*, 6th ed. Williams & Wilkins, 1999.)

oid release, which inhibits GnRH secretion. There may also be effects of prolactin directly on the ovary that contribute to lactational amenorrhea and anovulation. However, it should be noted that the contraceptive effect of prolactin is only moderate and therefore of low reliability.

---

16. Which hormones are involved in breast development?
17. Why is milk rarely secreted prior to parturition?
18. What is the probable mechanism of lactational amenorrhea?

MENOPAUSE

Menopause is the point in a woman's life when, as a result of exhaustion of the supply of functioning follicles within the ovary, menstrual cycles cease. After approximately age 40, even before menopause actually occurs, reproductive function starts to diminish. This is manifested as a decreased frequency of ovulation and atrophy of the reproductive organs. During this time, culminating in menopause, GnRH-stimulated LH and FSH secretion does not result in as much estrogen secretion as in earlier reproductive years because of the relative paucity of follicles. Hence the cyclic changes in estrogen-dependent tissues diminish and estrogen-dependent tissues atrophy as a consequence of estrogen deficiency. This period of diminished reproductive function approaching menopause is termed the **climacteric.**

During the climacteric transition from a cyclic high-estrogen state to the low-estrogen postmenopausal state, **vasomotor symptoms** such as hot flushes, sweating, and chills as well as psychologic symptoms such as irritability, tension, anxiety, and depression may be observed. Later, after the menopause, other more gradual changes can occur. In addition to atrophy of estrogen-dependent tissues

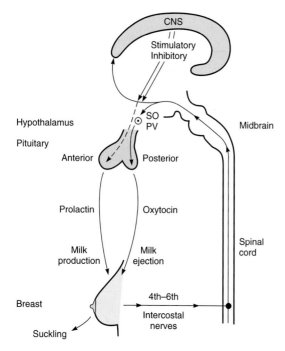

Figure 22–11. The role of anterior and posterior pituitary factors in milk synthesis and secretion. (SO, supraoptic nucleus; PV, paraventricular nucleus.) (Reproduced, with permission, from Rebar RW: The breast and physiology of lactation. In: *Maternal-Fetal Medicine: Principles and Practice.* Creasy RK, Resnick R [editors]. Saunders, 1984.)

such as the vaginal epithelium, these include a gradual loss in bone density termed **osteoporosis**. Since lack of estrogen also results in an inability to inhibit gonadotropin secretion in a negative-feedback fashion, LH and FSH levels are typically very high in the postmenopausal woman.

A significant degree of androgen production from thecal cells of the residual ovarian stroma continues even in the absence of follicles. Even in postmenopausal women, ovarian and adrenal androgens can be aromatized into estrogens by adipose tissue and hair follicles. The significance of peripheral aromatization in relation to severity of symptoms of menopause may vary in different individuals.

---

19. What are the symptoms of menopause?
20. What is the source of the estrogen found in the bloodstream of postmenopausal women not on estrogen replacement therapy?
21. Compare LH and FSH levels before puberty, during the reproductive years, and after the menopause.

OVERVIEW OF FEMALE REPRODUCTIVE TRACT DISORDERS

Many female reproductive disorders can be traced back to a particular level of the neuroendocrine feedback axis and thus can be categorized as resulting from central (pituitary, hypothalamus, or higher brain centers with influence over the hypothalamus), or end organ (ovarian or target tissue, eg, uterine) dysfunction.

DISORDERS OF CENTRAL-HYPOTHALAMIC-PITUITARY FUNCTION

Any change in the precise rate and amplitude of GnRH secretion by the hypothalamus can result in altered pituitary responsiveness (eg, down-regulation of GnRH receptors or altered gonadotropin secretion). The alteration in pituitary function in turn results in altered ovarian function (eg, inadequate steroidogenesis with or without anovulation) and altered target tissue response (eg, menstrual abnormalities). Many central (eg, psychic stress) and peripheral (eg, body fat content) inputs affecting pulsatile GnRH release are integrated in the hypothalamus. Thus, altered GnRH release from the hypothalamus is an extremely common cause of amenorrhea (eg, in athletic young women).

DISORDERS OF THE OVARY

Proper ovarian function involves responsiveness to gonadotropins, intrinsic viability of follicles, and a host of paracrine interactions within and between individual follicles. The polycystic ovary syndrome is an example of ovarian dysfunction due to a self-perpetuating cycle of altered feedback relationships and altered ovarian structure (see below). Polycystic ovary syndrome is manifested by anovulation, hirsutism, infertility, and either abnormal uterine bleeding or amenorrhea.

DISORDERS OF THE UTERUS & UTERINE TUBES & VAGINA

Since normal menstrual bleeding is most directly a function of the growth state of the uterine endometrium, disorders of the uterus, including myomas (fibroids), benign tumors of the underlying myometrium, and cancer of the endometrium itself, often present with abnormal vaginal bleeding.

Pelvic infections can produce adhesions and scarring of the uterus or uterine tubes that result in chronic pain and infertility.

Estrogen deficiency in postmenopausal women may present as dryness, irritation, and inflammation of estrogen-dependent tissues, including the vagina, with increased susceptibility to infection.

DISORDERS OF PREGNANCY

The normal events of pregnancy set the stage for a wide array of localized and systemic disorders. Abnormalities in the process of implantation, for example, appear to set in motion events leading to preeclampsia-eclampsia (see below). Inadequacy of the normal events of pregnancy (eg, insufficient steroidogenesis by the placenta) is also believed to contribute to spontaneous abortions or premature labor. In addition, genetic predispositions to disease that might otherwise remain latent for decades may be manifested first—often transiently—during pregnancy.

A good example of the latter is the genetic predisposition to development of diabetes mellitus. As discussed above, pregnancy is a counterregulatory state, with elevation of multiple blood glucose-elevating hormones, especially hCS. Because of these counterregulatory features of pregnancy, blood glucose control in pregnant diabetics (pregestational diabetes mellitus) is more difficult. Many patients without known diabetes mellitus first develop the disease during pregnancy (gestational diabetes mellitus). Gestational diabetes mellitus is six to ten times more common than pregestational diabetes mellitus and involves 2–5% of all pregnancies in the United States. Many individuals who go on to manifest type 2 diabetes mellitus later in life first manifest the disease during pregnancy.

Poor control of blood glucose during pregnancy has prominent effects on the mother, on the course of the pregnancy, and on the fetus. Retinopathy and nephropathy may first appear in the mother with known diabetes during pregnancy, though the long-term severity of the mother's disease is probably not altered by pregnancy. There is a higher incidence of acute complications of diabetes, including ketoacidosis, hypoglycemia, and infections during pregnancy. Patients with gestational and pregestational diabetes mellitus are at greater risk for preeclampsia-eclampsia. Since a long-term consequence of diabetes mellitus is small blood vessel damage, it has been proposed that preeclampsia-eclampsia results from endothelial cell injury as a consequence of ischemia. Poor glucose control also increases the rate and risk of cesarean section with associated anesthetic and surgical morbidity.

The effects of poor glucose control on the fetus are even more profound. **Congenital anomalies** and **macrosomia** (large body size) are increased, as are unexplained fetal deaths and spontaneous abortions. Just how gestational diabetes increases the risk of congenital anomalies is not well understood. Some studies have implicated altered myoinositol and prostaglandin metabolism. Other studies have demonstrated embryopathic effects of oxygen free radicals generated at elevated levels in diabetic pregnancies.

Macrosomia increases the risk of complications of birth trauma and of cesarean section. High maternal blood glucose triggers increased fetal insulin secretion and therefore results in a larger fetus. As the fetus becomes larger, the risk of fetopelvic disproportion increases. Fetopelvic disproportion contributes to inability to deliver vaginally, therefore requiring cesarean section. Neonatal hypoglycemia, hypocalcemia, polycythemia, and hyperbilirubinemia also occur.

The high levels of steroids and other products in the pregnant state can lead to a range of other serious medical complications. Thus, pregnancy is paradoxically associated with both hemorrhage and thrombosis. Both are related to the special functions of the placenta and its adaptations in the course of mammalian evolution.

Separation of the placenta from the wall of the uterus at birth poses a threat of massive, life-threatening hemorrhage given the intimate apposition of the placenta and the maternal blood supply. Perhaps as an adaptation to reduce this risk, pregnancy is also a hypercoagulable state. Physiologically, this increased tendency to coagulation and decreased activity of the fibrinolytic system may serve to control postpartum hemorrhage. Pathologically, these same factors pose a risk of inappropriate thrombosis and disseminated intravascular coagulation. It has been calculated that the risk of thrombophlebitis is increased nearly 50 times in the first month postpartum compared with before pregnancy. The risk of thromboembolism in pregnancy increases with age and with the presence of hypertension. Table 22–4 indicates some of the diverse ways in which pregnancy

Table 22–4. Factors predisposing to thrombosis in pregnancy.

Factor	Mechanism
Estrogen effects	Alterations in blood flow resulting in increased stasis
	Increased blood viscosity due to impaired erythrocyte deformability
	Activation of coagulation due to elevated factors I (fibrinogen), VII, VIII, IX, X, and XII and decreased antithrombin III
Nonestrogen effect	Depressed fibrinolytic activity

may predispose to inappropriate coagulation. When thrombosis does occur, therapy is complicated by the fact that the standard treatment with warfarin is contraindicated owing to the risks of teratogenicity in early pregnancy and of fetal hemorrhage in the third trimester. Thus, pregnant patients with thrombosis are given subcutaneous heparin injection therapy.

One—but not the only—facet of the increased risk for thrombosis associated with pregnancy is the high-estrogen state. Thus, an increased risk of thrombosis is also seen in pharmacologic estrogen use, as in oral contraceptives. The observation of enhanced cardiovascular mortality with birth control pills is probably due to these thrombogenic effects. The use of low-dose estrogen combination pills reduces but may not eliminate this risk. Progestins have also been implicated.

Threatened Abortion & Placental Disorders

At least 15% of all pregnancies terminate spontaneously as a result of genetic or environmental factors prior to the period when extrauterine life is possible (about 20 weeks of gestation and 500 g of body weight). Abortion is threatened when painless uterine bleeding occurs with a closed, uneffaced cervix. Heavy bleeding, pain, and dilation of the internal os are signs of inevitable abortion. In patients presenting with these symptoms, abortion must be distinguished from ectopic pregnancy, which typically is associated with more severe abdominal pain, and from hydatidiform mole. The differential diagnosis relies on the rate of rise of serum β-hCG on serial determinations and on the findings on ultrasound.

Third-trimester bleeding is typically associated with **placenta previa** (implantation of trophoblastic tissue on the lower uterine segment obstructing all or part of the internal cervical os) or **placental abruption** (premature separation of a normally implanted placenta after more than 20 weeks of gestation).

Women who have had multiple prior pregnancies are at increased risk of placenta previa, which is believed to be due to scar tissue formation from previous implantations. Placental abruption is due to hemorrhage into the decidual plate secondary to vascular rupture and is associated with hypertension, smoking, and multiple pregnancies, all of which would be expected to affect the condition of the placental vasculature. Hemorrhage can be massive and life-threatening.

Trophoblastic Malignancies

Molar pregnancies are abnormal growths due to trophoblastic proliferation (**hydatidiform mole**). Rarely, they are coexistent with a fetus (**partial mole**). The incidence in the USA is approximately 1:1500 pregnancies, but in certain areas of Asia it is as high as 1:125 pregnancies. The tissue in complete moles has higher malignant potential and is purely of paternal origin, while that of partial moles is usually benign and may simply contain an excess of paternal chromosomes. Most moles present with vaginal bleeding and are diagnosed during evaluation of threatened abortion by (1) the lack of a fetus and (2) the presence of trophoblastic tissue by ultrasound. Particularly severe nausea of pregnancy, a uterus larger than expected for gestational age, and an extremely elevated hCG level are suggestive but not diagnostic of molar pregnancy.

The complications of hydatidiform mole include high risks of (1) **choriocarcinoma**, a highly malignant, trophoblastic neoplasm with high potential for metastasis, especially to lung and brain; (2) hyperthyroidism with added risk of thyroid storm during induction of anesthesia; and (3) severe hemorrhage or trophoblastic tissue pulmonary embolism during suction curettage procedure to remove the molar products. Approximately 5% of women with hydatidiform mole subsequently develop choriocarcinoma. The serum β-hCG can be used as a sensitive test to detect the continued presence of malignant tissue. The exquisite sensitivity of choriocarcinoma to chemotherapy has made it a readily curable malignancy if detected early. The extremely high levels of β-hCG that occur with molar pregnancy and choriocarcinoma can result in cross-activation of the TSH receptor and trigger hyperthyroidism in some patients.

DISORDERS OF THE BREAST

Intrinsic disorders of the breast are either malignant (breast cancer) or benign (eg, fibrocystic disease). Breast disease can also occur as a result of the effects of other disorders or drug therapy, as in galactorrhea in women or gynecomastia in men. In females, the breast, like the uterus and other estrogen- and progesterone-responsive tissues, displays cyclic changes in concert with alterations in the level of ovarian steroids through the menstrual cycle. Subtle imbalances in the relative levels of estrogen and progesterone have been considered a possible basis for endometrial dysfunction (infertility due to inadequate luteal phase progesterone support of the secretory endometrium). Such hormonal imbalances may be the cause of so-called **benign breast disease** as well. This term refers to abnormalities ranging from normal premenstrual breast tenderness relieved with menstruation at one extreme to so-called fibrocystic disease at the other. In fibrocystic disease, there are both fibrosis and cysts in association with mammary epithelial hyperplasia. Normal breast tissue may have either fibrosis or cysts but not epithelial cell hyperplasia. True fibrocystic disease with epithelial cell hyperplasia is a risk factor for breast cancer in much the same way that endometrial hyperplasia due to unopposed estrogen action is a risk factor for endometrial cancer.

> 22. What are some central causes of menstrual disorders?
> 23. Why might you suspect some patients with choriocarcinoma to develop hyperthyroidism?
> 24. Are fibrocystic changes a risk factor for breast cancer?

DISORDERS OF SEXUAL DIFFERENTIATION

Under certain circumstances, aberrations can occur during embryogenesis that alter the normal course of events in chromosomal, gonadal, or phenotypic sexual development. An example of an aberration in chromosomal sex is **Turner's syndrome** (45,X). Individuals with Turner's syndrome are phenotypic females with primary amenorrhea, absent secondary sexual characteristics, short stature, multiple congenital anomalies, and bilateral streak gonads.

An example of altered gonadal sex is the syndrome of pure **gonadal dysgenesis.** Affected individuals have bilateral streak gonads and an immature female phenotype, but unlike those with Turner's syndrome they are of normal height, have no associated somatic defects, and have a normal male or female karyotype.

Disorders of phenotypic sex include female and male **pseudohermaphroditism.** These syndromes result from exposure of female embryos to excessive androgens during sexual differentiation or from defects in androgen synthesis or tissue sensitivity in male embryos.

PATHOPHYSIOLOGY OF SELECTED FEMALE REPRODUCTIVE TRACT DISORDERS

MENSTRUAL DISORDERS

Disorders of the menstrual cycle involve either (1) **amenorrhea** (lack of menstrual bleeding), which may be primary amenorrhea, ie, the failure of onset of menstrual periods by age 16; or secondary amenorrhea, ie, the lack of menstrual periods for 6 months in a previously menstruating woman; (2) **dysmenorrhea** (pain) and other symptoms accompanying menstruation; or (3) **menorrhagia** or **metrorrhagia**, excessive or irregular vaginal bleeding.

Etiology

A. Amenorrhea: The cause of amenorrhea can be traced to one of four broad categories of conditions (Table 22–5):

1. Normal physiologic processes such as pregnancy and menopause.

2. Disorders of the uterus or the pathway of menstrual flow such as destruction of the endometrium following excessive postpartum curettage, which can cause scarring and adhesion formation (**Asherman's syndrome**).

3. Disorders of the ovary such as gonadal failure due to a range of chromosomal, developmental, and structural abnormalities, autoimmune disorders, premature loss of follicles, and poorly understood syndromes in which ovaries with follicles are resistant to gonadotropin stimulation.

4. Disorders of the hypothalamus or pituitary resulting in either lack of or disordered GnRH secretion and, as a consequence, insufficient gonadotropin secretion to maintain ovarian steroid production. The causes of hypothalamic and pituitary dysfunction include prolactin-secreting tumors of the pituitary gland, hypothyroidism, excessive stress and exercise, and weight loss.

Within these categories, amenorrhea can have very diverse specific causes.

B. Dysmenorrhea: Dysmenorrhea is pain, typically cramping in character and lower abdominal in location, occurring in the days just before and during menstrual flow. Dysmenorrhea can occur as a primary disorder in the absence of identifiable pelvic disease or may be secondary to underlying pelvic disease, or as part of the premenstrual syndrome (Table 22–6).

C. Abnormal Vaginal Bleeding: Vaginal bleeding is abnormal if it occurs in childhood; if it occurs at the time of usual menses but is of longer than usual duration (metrorraghia); if it occurs at the time of usual menses but is heavier than usual (menorraghia); if it occurs between menstrual periods (dysfunctional uterine bleeding); or if it occurs after menopause in the absence of pharmacologic treatment with estrogen and progesterone (postmenopausal bleeding). The categories of abnormal vaginal bleeding and some specific causes are set forth in Table 22–7.

Pathology & Pathogenesis

A. Amenorrhea: The pathogenesis of amenorrhea depends on the level of the neuroendocrine reproductive axis from which the disorder stems and, at each level of the axis, whether it is due to a structural problem at that level or to a functional problem of hormonal control (Table 22–5). In a previously menstruating patient presenting with amenorrhea, it is important first to rule out pregnancy and then to assess thyroid function (serum TSH level) and pituitary function (serum prolactin level) before approaching

Table 22–5. Causes of amenorrhea.

Category	Common Causes	Pathophysiologic Mechanisms	How to Make a Diagnosis	Intervention
Normal physiologic processes	Pregnancy	Sustained high estrogen and progesterone	Serum β-hCG, history	Prenatal care
	Menopause	Lack of estrogen	Clinical diagnosis	Recommendations for osteoporosis prevention
Disorders of the uterus and outflow tract	Disorders of sexual development	Excessive androgen exposure	Physical examination	Surgical treatment
	Congenital anomalies (eg, imperforate hymen)		Physical examination	Surgical treatment
	Asherman's syndrome	Endometrial destruction, eg, by vigorous curettage	Lack of response to estrogen-progestin trial; direct visualization of endometrium	
Disorders of the ovary	Gonadal dysgenesis	Deletion of genetic material from the X chromosome	Karyotype	Remove streak gonads if Y chromosome is present in view of high risk of germ cell cancer
	Premature ovarian failure	Lack of viable follicles	Check gonadotropins	
	Polycystic ovary disease	Altered intraovarian hormone relationships	Clinical diagnosis in patients with chronic anovulation and androgen excess	Decrease ovarian androgen secretion (wedge resection, oral contraceptives); increase FSH secretion
Disorders of the hypothalamus or pituitary	Stress, athletic endeavor, underweight	Altered GnRH pulses	Check serum TSH, PRL, gonadotropins	Replacement if deficient; search for tumor if excessive

Table 22–6. Categories of dysmenorrhea.

Categories	Etiology	Distinguishing Features
Primary dysmenorrhea	Prostaglandins	Lack of organic pelvic disease
Secondary dysmenorrhea		
Endometriosis	Ectopic endometrium, including intramyometrial endometrial tissue	Finding of endometrial tissue on laparoscopy
Pelvic inflammatory disease	Infection	Positive culture
Anatomic lesions (imperforate hymen, intrauterine adhesions, leiomyomas, polyps)	Congenital, inflammatory, or neoplastic	Findings on physical examination, ultrasound
Premenstrual syndrome (PMS)	Unknown	Association with emotional, behavioral, and other symptoms

the workup of amenorrhea compartment by compartment.

1. Uterine disorders—Menstruation results from cyclic changes in the estrogen- and progesterone-sensitive endometrium. Thus, lack of an endometrium, or lack of cyclic estrogen-progesterone stimulation of the endometrium, results in amenorrhea. This is most commonly an iatrogenic problem occurring after overly vigorous **curettage** (scraping of the endometrium) either for severe postpartum bleeding or for dysfunctional uterine bleeding. Amenorrhea in such cases is due to scarring and destruction of the underlying stem cells from which the endometrium proliferates.

Renewed vaginal bleeding in an amenorrheic patient after a challenge with either progesterone alone or the sequential combination of estrogen and progesterone, followed by cessation of hormone therapy, suggests that the endometrium is intact. This response also indicates that the cause of amenorrhea lies elsewhere (ie, is due to something causing lack or insufficiency of endogenous cyclic estrogen and progesterone stimulation).

2. Ovarian failure—Amenorrhea due to ovarian failure can be either primary or secondary to dysfunction higher in the female neuroendocrine repro-

Table 22–7. Causes of abnormal vaginal bleeding.[1]

Childhood
  Genital lesions
    Vaginitis
    Foreign body
    Trauma
    Tumors
  Endocrine changes
    Estrogen ingestion
    Precocious puberty
    Ovarian tumors

Adolescents and adults
  Dysfunctional uterine bleeding
    Estrogen breakthrough
    Estrogen withdrawal
  Diseases of the genital tract
    Benign conditions
      Uterine leiomyoma
      Cervical polyp
      Endometrial polyp
      Genital laceration
      Endometrial hyperplasia
    Malignant diseases
      Endometrial cancer
      Cervical cancer
      Vaginal cancer
  Pregnancy
    Ectopic pregnancy
    Threatened abortion
    Death of embryo
  Other causes
    Thyroid disease
    von Willebrand's disease
    Thrombocytopenia

[1]Reproduced, with permission, from Cowan BD, Morrison JC: Management of abnormal genital bleeding in girls and women. (Current Concepts.) N Engl J Med 1991;324:1710.

ductive axis. Primary ovarian failure may occur as a result of genetic disorders (chromosomal aberrations) or premature loss of all follicles. The latter, excessive atresia, is due to structural abnormalities, which impede the normal paracrine interactions within the ovary (eg, thickening of the basement membrane between thecal and granulosa cells). Secondary ovarian failure results from lack of gonadotropin stimulation of otherwise normal ovaries, resulting in failure to produce the estrogen and progesterone needed for menstrual cycles.

a. Genetic causes–Genetic causes of ovarian failure include Turner's syndrome (abnormality in or absence of an X chromosome) and mosaicism (multiple cell lines of varying sex chromosome composition). Approximately 40% of patients who appear to have Turner's syndrome (short stature, webbed neck, shield chest, and hypergonadotropic hypoestrogenic amenorrhea) prove to be mosaics. The presence of any Y chromosome in the karyotype of these individuals carries a high risk of development of germ cell tumors and is an indication for surgery. Thus, a karyotype should be performed on any amenorrheic individual under the age of 30 with high FSH and LH levels.

b. Premature ovarian failure–Premature ovarian failure occurs when atresia of follicles is accelerated in an ovary of a woman of reproductive age. It presents with symptoms and signs of menopause due to estrogen deficiency at an inappropriately young age. LH and FSH levels are elevated. There is a lack of estrogen production and an absence of viable follicles. In some instances, premature ovarian failure is just one manifestation of an autoimmune polyglandular failure syndrome in which autoantibodies destroy a number of different tissues, including the ovary. These patients may also have associated hypothyroidism, adrenal insufficiency, or pernicious anemia (Chapters 17 and 21).

c. Chronic anovulation–Other patients are found to have adequate numbers of follicles that fail to mature and ovulate. This condition is known as **chronic anovulation** and is manifested as amenorrhea with intermittent bleeding between the expected time of menstrual periods (due to overgrowth of the endometrium in response to stimulation by estrogen alone). Left untreated, the high estrogen level places these women at increased risk for the development of endometrial and breast carcinomas. Among the causes of chronic anovulation is thyroid dysfunction (Table 22–8). Both hyperthyroidism and hypothyroidism can alter ovarian function and the metabolism of androgens and estrogens, resulting in a variety of menstrual disorders. Another cause of chronic anovulation is hyperprolactinemia. It has been proposed that progressively more severe hyperprolactinemia presents first as an inadequate luteal phase with recurrent abortion, then as anovulation with intermittent bleeding, and finally as amenorrhea.

d. Hormonal feedback disorders–Given the importance of hormone feedback in the menstrual cycle, it is not surprising that a prominent syndrome of menstrual dysfunction is one in which key features of feedback are disordered. This condition, termed **polycystic ovary syndrome**, presents as hirsutism and infertility (Table 22–9). It affects 2–5% of women of reproductive age. Patients are often obese, and workup reveals elevated LH with exaggerated pulses, depressed FSH with few and small pulses, elevated plasma androgens, elevated plasma estrogens (estrone derived from peripheral aromatization of adrenal androgens but not estradiol generated by granulosa cell aromatase activity), anovulation (with associated amenorrhea, and estrogen-induced endometrial hyperplasia with breakthrough bleeding), and hyperinsulinemia with insulin resistance (Table 22–10).

The hyperinsulinemia is believed to be a key factor in development of the other abnormalities. Any cause of insulin resistance, including obesity and insulin receptor defects, results in hyperinsulinemia. This is because insulin resistance means that a higher blood insulin level is necessary to maintain (or, in a patient with overt diabetes mellitus, at least try to

Table 22–8. Causes and mechanisms of chronic anovulation.[1]

Causes	Mechanisms

Thyroid disease
  Hyperthyroidism
  Hypothyroidism
	Increased estrogen clearance
	Decreased androgen clearance with resulting increased peripheral aromatization to estrogen

Hyperprolactinemia	Altered GnRH pulses
Obesity	Increased peripheral aromatization of androgens to estrogens Decreased steroid hormone-binding globulin, resulting in increased free estrogen and testosterone Increased insulin resistance, resulting in increased secretion of insulin which increases ovarian stromal production of androgens
Primary ovarian failure	Genetic disorders (eg, Turner's syndrome)
Secondary ovarian failure	Cytotoxic drugs Irradiation Autoimmune disorders

[1]Modified and reproduced, with permission, from Speroff L, Glass RH, Kase NG: *Clinical Gynecologic Endocrinology and Infertility,* 6th ed. Williams & Wilkins, 1999.

maintain) a normal blood glucose. But as the blood insulin level rises, it has other actions besides its effects on fuel metabolism. For one, insulin results in a decreased hepatic synthesis of steroid hormone-binding globulin (SHBG) and insulin-like growth factor-1 (IGF-1) (Figure 22–12). A decrease in levels of binding protein results in an increase in free androgens, estrogens, and IGF-1.

Androgens worsen insulin resistance through effects on both the liver and the periphery and are a substrate for peripheral aromatization to further increase blood estrogens. Elevated estrogen levels at the wrong time in the menstrual cycle can inhibit the rise in FSH just before menses that is believed to be crucial to activating development of a new cohort of ovarian follicles. Elevated estrogen levels are also implicated in development of endometrial cancer and possibly breast cancer.

IGF-1 increases thecal androgen production in response to LH, contributing to the hyperandrogenemic state. At high enough levels, insulin also stimulates the IGF-1 receptor, further increasing thecal androgen production. The high androgens favor atresia of developing follicles and disruption of the feedback relationships that would normally result in selection of a dominant follicle for ovulation (Figure 22–12).

Events occurring in the brain, the ovary, and the bloodstream of these patients work together to constitute a vicious circle that maintains the aberrant feedback relationships.

In the brain (hypothalamus), GnRH pulses appear abnormal, perhaps as a result of chronic deprivation of progesterone due to persistent anovulation. FSH levels are diminished to the point that they are no longer sufficient to support the aromatase activity needed to complete follicular development. LH levels are high but lack the characteristic midcycle surge. As a result of excessive overall LH stimulation, there is thecal hypertrophy and androgen oversecretion by the ovary. Together these effects result in lack of ovarian follicular development, accelerated follicular atresia, and increased inhibin secretion.

The ovary develops a thickened fibrous capsule that itself may somehow contribute to maintenance

Table 22–9. Manifestations of polycystic ovary syndrome.[1,2]

Hirsutism	95%
Large ovaries	95%
Infertility	75%
Amenorrhea	55%
Obesity	40%
Dysmenorrhea	28%
Persistent anovulation	20%

[1]Reproduced, with permission, from Beaulieu EE, Kelly PA (editors): *Hormones: From Molecules to Disease,* Chapman & Hall, 1990.
[2]Figures are percentage of patients with syndrome manifesting each symptom or sign.

Table 22–10. Clinical consequences of chronic anovulation.[1]

Infertility
Menstrual dysfunction (either amenorrhea or dysfunctional uterine bleeding)
Hirsutism and acne (androgen excess state)
Increased risk of endometrial cancer
Possible increased risk of breast cancer
Increased risk of cardiovascular disease
Increased risk of diabetes mellitus (hyperinsulinemia)

[1]Assembled from materials in Speroff L, Glass RH, Kase NG: *Clinical Gynecologic Endocrinology and Infertility,* 6th ed. Williams & Wilkins, 1999.

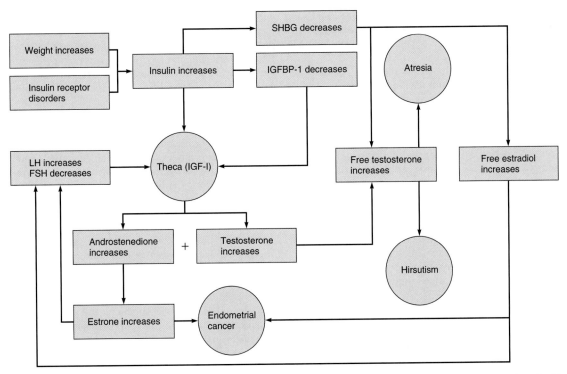

Figure 22–12. Pathogenesis of the various clinical manifestations of the polycystic ovary syndrome. (Reproduced, with permission, from Halki IT: *Menopause and Climacteric in Clinical Medicine: Selected Problems With Pathophysiologic Correlations.* Year Book, 1988.)

of the abnormal feedback relationships. The high levels of androgens in the bloodstream are responsible for hirsutism. Furthermore, as a result of conversion of these androgens to estrogens by peripheral aromatase activity (eg, in fat and hair follicles, both of which are increased in these patients), a variety of hormonal abnormalities may occur. These include exaggerated pituitary LH secretion but without a midcycle peak. Patients with elevated androgens from totally different causes (eg, Cushing's disease and congenital adrenal hyperplasia) also display amenorrhea associated with polycystic ovaries, suggesting that the structural changes in the ovaries are secondary to the disordered feedback.

e. Pituitary and hypothalamic disorders– Trauma resulting in stalk transection with loss of hypothalamic-pituitary communication should be considered in patients with new-onset infertility with amenorrhea. The same is true of vascular accidents such as **Sheehan's syndrome,** in which postpartum hemorrhage causes hypotension and consequent ischemic necrosis of the pituitary. Enlargement of the anterior pituitary during pregnancy may predispose to ischemia under conditions of hypotension. The pituitary approximately doubles in size, largely due to hypertrophy and hyperplasia of prolactin-secreting lactotrophs.

f. Stress–Inputs from many different central pathways impinge on the mediobasal portion of the hypothalamus (including the arcuate nucleus) from which GnRH pulses originate. Thus, any of a wide range of factors that alter this pulsatile release of GnRH can influence female reproductive physiology. Some of the most prominent pathogenic factors include a variety of forms of stress, including psychic stress, weight loss (decreased body fat), and vigorous exercise. Lack of menstrual periods due to a change in one of these factors is termed **hypothalamic amenorrhea.** It is a common cause of infertility and can be treated with pulsatile GnRH therapy, thereby reestablishing normal patterns of stimulation, receptor-mediated responsiveness, and feedback. Many different neurotransmitters affect GnRH secretion (opioids, dopaminergics, and norepinephrine), and for that reason a wide range of drugs that affect release or action of these neurotransmitters also have effects on GnRH secretion. This underscores the importance of a careful history in the workup of this common condition.

g. Indirect influences–In addition to factors that work directly on the GnRH-secreting neurons, indirect influences must be considered as well. Thus, primary hypothyroidism and primary or secondary hyperprolactinemia can result in altered GnRH pulse frequency and amplitude and therefore diminished gonadotropin secretion and secondary ovarian failure and amenorrhea.

Examples of conditions that result in secondary hyperprolactinemia include lactation, treatment with drugs that have dopamine-blocking effects (eg, antipsychotic agents), and stalk transection that results in loss of endogenous dopamine.

h. Amenorrhea associated with other functional or organic disorders—Finally, a number of complex syndromes are observed in which amenorrhea occurs in association with other findings. In patients with **anorexia nervosa,** distorted eating habits are associated with psychologic dysfunction, a distorted body image, weight loss, and a variety of medical problems including amenorrhea. Amenorrhea in these patients can occur even before onset of weight loss, implicating the psychiatric disorder rather than the stress of starvation as the initiating event.

---

25. Name four kinds of stress that can cause hypothalamic amenorrhea.
26. What are the consequences of untreated amenorrhea?

B. Dysmenorrhea: Primary dysmenorrhea is due to disordered or excessive prostaglandin production by the secretory endometrium of the uterus in the absence of a structural lesion. Prostaglandin $F_{2\alpha}$ ($PGF_{2\alpha}$) stimulates myometrial contractions of the nonpregnant uterus, while prostaglandins of the E series inhibit its contraction. It appears that patients with severe dysmenorrhea generally have excessive production of $PGF_{2\alpha}$ rather than increased sensitivity to this prostaglandin as a cause of excessive myometrial contraction. Excessive contractions of the myometrium result in ischemia of uterine muscle, which stimulates uterine pain fibers of the autonomic nervous system. Anxiety, fear, and stress may lower the pain threshold and thereby exaggerate the prominence of these symptoms from one patient to another and over time in a given patient.

Among the secondary causes of dysmenorrhea is **endometriosis,** a disorder in which ectopic endometrial tissue responds cyclically to estrogen and progesterone (Table 22–6). This is a common disorder affecting 10–25% of women of reproductive age. The presenting symptoms of patients with endometriosis can range from pain and cramping during menstruation to adhesions with frank bowel obstruction in severe cases. Typical locations for ectopic endometrial tissue include the pelvic portion of the peritoneal space and ovaries. Establishment of endometrial tissue in these locations is believed to occur by either or both of two mechanisms: (1) by transport of sloughed endometrial tissue by retrograde menstruation through the uterine tubes; or (2) by metaplasia of undifferentiated celomic epithelial mesenchyme in the peritoneum, perhaps under the influence of growth factors present in retrograde menstrual efflux. Recent work supports the hypothesis of a vicious circle involving peritoneal inflammation with elevated cytokines in peritoneal fluid and secretion of angiogenic factors that maintain ectopic endometrial tissue. A characteristic feature of endometriosis is amelioration after a pregnancy and after menopause. This observation provides a therapeutic rationale for the most common modes of medical therapy, which include birth control pills; synthetic androgens (danazol), which block the midcycle LH surge; and long-acting GnRH analogs that down-regulate the reproductive neuroendocrine axis. Some of these drugs may also work by down-regulation of cytokine production. It is unclear whether endometriosis causes infertility directly or simply as a consequence of resultant adhesions and scarring.

Other prominent causes of secondary dysmenorrhea are chronic pelvic infection or the adhesions resulting from prior pelvic infections and ectopic pregnancies. Infections of the pelvis typically present with abdominal and pelvic (cervical and adnexal) pain and with either fever, an elevated white blood cell count, or a positive endocervical culture. Common infectious agents include gonorrhea, anaerobic bacteria, and chlamydia. Multiple organisms are usually involved. Aggressive antibiotic therapy is important in treating these infections in order to limit the damage to sensitive reproductive structures. Pelvic infections can develop into tubo-ovarian abscesses requiring surgical drainage.

Especially if untreated or inadequately treated, pelvic infections can result in scarring of the epithelial lining of the uterus or uterine tubes. Subsequently, these changes can impede transit of either the mature ovulated egg—or of sperm—through the uterine tube. If fertilization occurs with impeded transport of the fertilized egg out of the uterine tube, implantation into the lining of the tube can occur, resulting in an ectopic pregnancy. In this location, the embryo is not viable. Moreover, growth of the embryo results in rupture and potentially life-threatening hemorrhage unless it is surgically removed. Diagnosis is made by a failure of β-hCG to rise appropriately in the first several weeks of pregnancy and by ultrasonographic localization of the ectopic conceptus.

The symptoms of **premenstrual syndrome** (see below), with which dysmenorrhea is often associated, have been hypothesized to be due to escape of prostaglandins and their metabolites into the systemic circulation.

C. Abnormal Vaginal Bleeding: The pathogenesis of abnormal vaginal bleeding depends on the cause, as summarized and described in the following paragraphs.

1. Functional disorders—In these cases, depending on individual variables, the disorder results in altered amounts and timing of menstrual flow rather than a complete cessation of menses.

2. **Structural lesions**—Examples would be a benign or malignant tumor of the endometrium or myometrium, a foreign body, or a superimposed process (eg, pelvic infection). The most common cancers of the female genital tract involve the uterus. Two forms of uterine cancer are most prominent: endometrial and cervical. Cancer of the endometrium is generally believed to be a consequence of excessive or unopposed estrogen stimulation of this tissue, which normally proliferates in response to the cyclic presence of estrogen levels. Unopposed estrogen stimulation can occur because of an ovarian disorder (eg, chronic anovulation); enhanced peripheral aromatization of adrenal androgens; or estrogen therapy (eg, postmenopausal replacement for prevention of osteoporosis) without a progestin. Endometrial cancer is largely a peri- and postmenopausal disease, with only 5% of cases occurring during the reproductive years. Endometrial cancer spreads by direct involvement of lymphatics with distant metastases to the lung, brain, skeleton, and abdominal organs. Patients with endometrial cancer typically present with abnormal vaginal bleeding. As with ovarian cancer, ascites, bowel obstruction, and associated pleural effusions occur in widespread disease.

In cancer of the uterine cervix, the pathophysiologic process is quite different. The major epidemiologic risk factors appear to be multiple sexual partners and onset of intercourse before age 20. Infection with human papillomavirus (HPV), herpesvirus type 2, and other sexually transmitted pathogens predisposes to development of cervical cancer. HPV infection is found in approximately 25% of cases of severe cervical dysplasia (carcinoma in situ). Condylomas (viral warts), which are caused by HPV, are often seen adjacent to areas of severe dysplasia on pathology specimens. Likewise, carcinogens in tobacco and mutagens in sperm have been suspected of contributing to cervical dysplasia.

Unlike other female reproductive organ cancers, cervical cancer can be readily detected by the Papanicolaou smear performed during a simple pelvic examination. As a result, there has been a dramatic decrease in the mortality rate associated with cervical cancer over the last 4 decades. A Papanicolaou smear allows detection of both preneoplastic changes and cancer itself prior to metastasis, at which point it can be cured. If untreated, cervical cancer spreads directly into the pelvis, with death often occurring through hemorrhage, infection, or renal failure secondary to ureteral obstruction.

3. **Systemic conditions with altered coagulation**—Normal blood clotting involves both coagulation factors and platelets. Thus, disorders affecting the production, quality, and survival of either clotting factors or platelets can cause abnormal vaginal bleeding (Table 22–11).

Table 22–11. Disorders of coagulation.[1]

Disorders resulting in thrombocytopenia
Suppressed platelet production
Splenic sequestration
Accelerated platelet destruction
Nonimmunologic (eg, prosthetic valves)
Immunologic
Viral and bacterial infections
Drugs
Autoimmune mechanisms (eg, idiopathic thrombocytopenic purpura)
Disorders resulting in clotting factor deficiency
Congenital disorders of coagulation
Acquired disorders of coagulation
Vitamin K deficiency
Liver disease
Disseminated intravascular coagulation

[1]Assembled from materials in Handin RI: Disorders of the platelet and vessel wall. In: *Harrison's Principles of Internal Medicine,* 14th ed. Faucci A et al (editors). McGraw-Hill, 1998.

27. What are effective medical therapies for endometriosis, and how do they work?
28. What factors predispose to cervical cancer?

Clinical Manifestations

A. Amenorrhea: The clinical symptoms and signs that accompany amenorrhea depend on its category (Table 22–5). In genetic disorders—particularly in disorders of sexual development—various degrees of delayed puberty, such as lack of breast development and absence of pubic hair, may accompany amenorrhea. In outflow tract disorders (eg, imperforate hymen), pain from occult menstruation occurs on a cyclic basis. Generally, disorders of the uterus and of the hypothalamic-pituitary axis that result in amenorrhea are painless. Ovarian failure resulting in amenorrhea is often preceded by symptoms referable to altered estrogen and progesterone production. These include hot flushes and other vasomotor symptoms and emotional lability and irritability.

The most common complication in the nonpregnant patient with amenorrhea is infertility. Additional complications depend on the specific cause of lack of menstruation. Osteoporosis is a major potential long-term complication of inadequate estrogen stimulation. Inadequate estrogen can also be associated with thinning of estrogen-dependent epithelia, such as that of the vagina, resulting in atrophic vaginitis. The vaginitis usually responds to topical estrogen creams. In the case of inadequate progesterone production—typically associated with irregular vaginal bleeding but seen also in some cases of amenorrhea—the risk of endometrial cancer is greatly increased. Endometrial cancer is the most common cancer of the female genital tract, with 34,000 new cases annually in the United States. Risk factors for endometrial cancer include late menopause, nulliparity, obesity, hypertension, and diabetes mellitus.

B. Dysmenorrhea: Dysmenorrhea may be accompanied by a variable constellation of symptoms including sweating, weakness and fatigue, insomnia, nausea, vomiting, diarrhea, back pain, headache (including both migraine and tension headaches; see Chapter 7), dizziness, and even syncope.

In the **premenstrual syndrome,** dysmenorrhea is accompanied by additional symptoms including a sensation of bloating, weight gain, edema of the hands and feet, breast tenderness, acne, anxiety, aggression, mood swings, irritability, food cravings, and change in libido. An initial approach should be to encourage changes in lifestyle if indicated by the history (eg, more sleep, exercise, improved diet, less tobacco, alcohol, and caffeine). Approximately half of patients with premenstrual syndrome are not responsive to such measures and may benefit from monthly pharmacotherapy with prostaglandin synthesis inhibitors (non-steroidal anti-inflammatory agents).

C. Abnormal Vaginal Bleeding: The symptoms and signs that accompany abnormal vaginal bleeding vary with the cause. In children, vulvovaginitis is the most frequent disorder, accompanied by a mucopurulent discharge that may become bloody with mucosal erosion. Other prominent causes, including foreign objects and tumors, can be assessed by physical examination. In adolescents and adults, dysfunctional uterine bleeding is most common, but other causes must be considered, including pregnancy (assessed by serial serum β-hCG determinations and ultrasound examination), trauma (by history and physical examination), cancer (by hysteroscopy), and systemic disorders such as a hemorrhagic diathesis (by platelet, prothrombin, and partial thromboplastin time determinations) and thyroid disease (by serum TSH, total and free T_4 determinations). In postmenopausal women, one-fifth of cases of vaginal bleeding prove to be endometrial cancer.

INFERTILITY

The infertile patient presents with a history of at least 1 year of unprotected regular sexual intercourse without conception. Inability to become pregnant must be distinguished from inability to carry the pregnancy to term.

Etiology

In approximately 30% of cases, the cause of infertility is due to factors involving the male (eg, inadequate sperm count) (see Chapter 23). When the defects are in the female, about 40% are due to ovulatory failure, about 40% are due to endometrial or tubal disease, about 10% are due to rarer causes

Table 22–12. Causes of female infertility.[1,2]

Cause	Incidence in Patients With Infertility
Ovulatory failure	40%
Tubal or pelvic pathology	40%
Thick mucus	
Scarring and adhesions (from pelvic inflammatory disease, chronic infection, tubal surgery, ectopic pregnancy, or ruptured appendix)	
Miscellaneous	10%
Thyroid disease	
Pituitary disease (hyperprolactinemia)	
Unexplained	10%

[1]Modified and reproduced, with permission, from Speroff L, Glass RH, Kase NG: *Clinical Gynecologic Endocrinology and Infertility,* 6th ed. Williams & Wilkins, 1999.
[2]In infertile couples, problems in the male account for 30% of the total.

(eg, thyroid disease or hyperprolactinemia), and about 10% remain undefined after full workup (Table 22–12).

Pathology & Pathogenesis

A. Ovulatory Causes: Infertility referable to ovarian dysfunction can result from disorders of the hypothalamus or pituitary, resulting in inadequate gonadotropic stimulation of the ovary; or from ovarian disorders, resulting either in inadequate secretory products or failure to ovulate; or from both types of disorders occurring at the same time. The most common ovarian disorders are age-related and can involve both the oocytes themselves and the secretory products of the ovary.

There is accelerated loss of follicles with the approach of menopause. Loss of all follicles from the ovaries (ie, ovarian failure) results in permanent anovulation and menopause. With the approach of ovarian failure, FSH levels tend to rise, reflecting inadequate production of inhibin. In principle, this could result either from an inadequate number of follicles, diminished competence of the remaining follicles, diminished steroidogenesis by the aging ovary, or some combination of these factors. Regardless of the specific reason, the net effect is a shortened follicular phase and is associated with increased rates of infertility. Treatment with clomiphene citrate, a weak estrogen antagonist, is a means of diminishing negative feedback and in that way further increasing gonadotropin stimulation of the ovary. In some cases this appears to result in ovulation, perhaps due to prolongation of the follicular phase.

In some cases, infertility is due to a shortened or inadequate luteal phase manifested as an inadequate quantity or duration of progesterone production. One possible mechanism is excess estrogen in the follicular phase. Estrogen elevates $PGF_{2\alpha}$, which antagonizes the effect of LH, thereby decreasing progesterone production by the corpus luteum and shortening the luteal phase. This mechanism has a clinical correlation in the efficacy of postcoital high-dose estrogen as a contraceptive. The technique is effective only in the week subsequent to coitus, because hCG production upon implantation overcomes the antagonism of LH action caused by the elevated $PGF_{2\alpha}$.

Treatment with progesterone, either directly or indirectly by clomiphene or gonadotropin stimulation, can correct infertility due to a shortened luteal phase.

B. Tubal and Pelvic Causes: Given normal follicles and reproductive neuroendocrine axis function, the major cause of infertility is abnormality of the endometrium and uterine tubes. Prior or ongoing pelvic infections, with scarring and adhesions or inflammation, can result in failure of sperm or egg transport, failure of implantation, or implantation in an inappropriate location (ectopic pregnancy). Since sperm are viable for only about 24 hours after insemination and a freshly released mature egg is only viable for about 12 hours, any impediment to transport of either sperm or egg or of implantation of a fertilized egg can greatly diminish the likelihood of pregnancy.

Endometriosis, with cyclic proliferation and sloughing of ectopic endometrial tissue, resulting in inflammation, scarring, and adhesions, should be suspected when infertility is associated with dysmenorrhea.

C. Other Causes of Female Infertility: Most of the less common causes of infertility can be grouped into (1) those that affect the production of GnRH by the hypothalamus or the hormone's effect on the pituitary (eg, thyroid disease and hyperprolactinemia) and (2) those that affect ovarian feedback (eg, hyperandrogenism and the polycystic ovary syndrome).

> 29. What are the most common causes of infertility in couples?
> 30. How do postcoital high-dose estrogens work as a contraceptive?
> 31. What feature of the history suggests a tubal or uterine cause of infertility?

PREECLAMPSIA-ECLAMPSIA

Pregnancy is associated with a host of medical complications whose principles of clinical management are grounded in the underlying physiology of pregnancy and the pathophysiology of the particular disorder. The syndrome of preeclampsia-eclampsia, characterized by hypertension, proteinuria, and edema, is chosen for focus for several reasons: First, because preeclampsia-eclampsia is the most important cause of maternal death in the USA and much of Western Europe; second, because it illustrates how pathophysiologic mechanisms in pregnancy may be far more complex—and the clinical consequences far more serious—than would have been expected from a simple consideration of each of the presenting symptoms in isolation; and third, because recent advances have significantly altered current thinking about the pathogenesis of this disorder.

Clinical Presentation

Hypertension is the most common medical complication of pregnancy and can be of two general forms. First, patients who either have or do not have a history of elevated blood pressure may develop asymptomatic essential hypertension (see Chapter 11), typically early in pregnancy. A distinguishing feature of essential hypertension of pregnancy is that even slight overtreatment, which would be inconsequential in the nonpregnant state, may result in **placental insufficiency** (due to underperfusion), and fetal distress. The major complication of untreated essential hypertension in pregnancy, which typically appears before the 20th week of gestation, is the risk of placental damage and insufficiency and an increased risk of fetal distress later in gestation. Placental insufficiency in untreated essential hypertension results from loss of placental capacity due to small vessel infarction and hemorrhage.

A second, far more ominous syndrome of hypertension known as preeclampsia-eclampsia occurs in approximately 5% of pregnancies in the United States. Preeclampsia-eclampsia is associated with proteinuria (> 3 g/24 h) and edema and results in a cascade of changes that in its most dramatic form leads to hemorrhage, seizures, renal failure, disseminated intravascular coagulation (DIC), and death. Table 22–13 summarizes the symptoms and signs of preeclampsia-eclampsia.

Etiology

The underlying causes of both essential hypertension and preeclampsia-eclampsia remain largely unknown. However, important progress has been made in understanding the cause of preeclampsia-eclampsia. It now appears that preeclampsia-eclampsia is a disorder of endothelial cell function caused by faulty implantation (see below). As such, it is likely to be fundamentally different from essential hypertension. Strongly suggestive of this etiologic distinction is the occurrence of a variant of preeclampsia-eclampsia, known as the HELLP syndrome (hemolysis, elevated liver enzymes, low platelets), in which hypertension is not even present.

Pathology & Pathogenesis

The placenta in both essential hypertension of pregnancy and preeclampsia shows signs of prema-

Table 22–13. Symptoms and signs of preeclampsia-eclampsia.[1]

Maternal syndrome
  Pregnancy-induced hypertension
  Excessive weight gain (>1 kg/wk)
  Generalized edema
  Ascites
  Hyperuricemia
  Proteinuria
  Hypocalciuria
  Increased plasma von Willebrand factor concentration
  Increased plasma cellular fibronectin
  Reduced plasma antithrombin III concentration
  Thrombocytopenia
  Increased packed cell volume
  Increased serum liver enzyme levels

Fetal syndrome
  Intrauterine growth retardation
  Intrauterine hypoxemia

[1]Reproduced, with permission, from Roberts JM, Redman CWG: Preeclampsia: More than pregnancy-induced hypertension. Lancet 1993;341:1447.

ture aging, including degeneration, hyaline deposition, calcification, and congestion. In preeclampsia, the maternal half of the placenta also shows hemorrhage and necrosis with thrombosis of spiral arteries and infarcts.

Predisposing factors for the development of preeclampsia include first pregnancy, multiple pregnancy, excess amniotic fluid, preexisting diabetes or hypertension, hydatidiform mole, malnutrition, and a family history of preeclampsia.

Normally, the blood vessels of the uterine wall at the site of implantation undergo striking morphologic changes such as increase in diameter of the spiral arteries and loss of their muscular and elastic components. These changes facilitate placental perfusion. This is believed to be related to an increase in production of the strong vasodilator prostacyclin and a concomitant decrease in the vasoconstrictor thromboxanes. For unknown (perhaps immune-mediated) reasons, these early changes of implantation do not occur—or at least not fully—in patients who develop preeclampsia-eclampsia. As a result, a condition of relative placental ischemia is established, with release of as yet unknown factors that damage vascular endothelium at first locally, within the placenta, and later throughout the body. Oxidative injury, analogous to that which triggers atherosclerosis, is believed to work together with maternal factors (eg, obesity, diabetes, diet, genes) to cause endothelial cell damage.

Endothelial damage has two important pathophysiologic consequences. First, the balance between vasodilation and vasoconstriction is altered, specifically by diminished production of vasodilatory products such as prostacyclin, increased production of vasoconstrictive thromboxane, and production of new vasoconstrictive products such as platelet-derived growth factor. As a result there is increased vasoconstriction of small blood vessels, with hypoperfusion and ischemia of downstream tissues and systemic hypertension. Second, the endothelial cell barrier between platelets and the collagen of basement membranes is breached.

As a result of these changes, additional events are set in motion including increased platelet aggregation, activation of the clotting cascade, and production of vasoactive substances causing capillary leak. This results in further tissue hypoperfusion, edema formation, and proteinuria, the hallmarks of preeclampsia-eclampsia. Because these processes result in further vascular endothelial damage, a vicious circle is established. Delivery of the fetus terminates the sequence of pathologic events by removing the ischemic placenta, the presumed source of the unknown products causing systemic endothelial damage.

Without treatment, preeclampsia can proceed to eclampsia, a condition characterized by maternal seizures due to cerebral ischemia and petechial hemorrhage; hepatic periportal necrosis, congestion, and hemorrhage; and renal changes, including glomerular endothelial cell swelling, mesangial proliferation, and marked narrowing of glomerular capillary lumens. The renal cortex displays significant cortical ischemia that may progress to frank necrosis. Endothelial thickening, hemorrhage, and edema may occur in other tissues along with DIC (Table 22–14).

Clinical Manifestations

The clinical manifestations of preeclampsia-eclampsia fall on a continuum in which hypertension is the earliest manifestation, typically after the 20th week of gestation, followed by edema, proteinuria, muscle twitching, generalized tonic muscle contraction, seizures, and DIC (Table 22–13). Early delivery of the fetus appears to be a definitive cure for this syndrome, which otherwise carries a high mortality rate.

Table 22–14. Complications of preeclampsia-eclampsia.[1]

Cerebral hemorrhage
Cortical blindness
Retinal detachment
HELLP syndrome (hemolysis, elevated liver enzymes, low platelets)
Hepatic rupture
Disseminated intravascular coagulation (DIC)
Pulmonary edema
Laryngeal edema
Acute renal cortical necrosis
Acute renal tubular necrosis
Abruptio placentae
Intrauterine fetal asphyxia and death

[1]Reproduced, with permission, from Roberts JM, Redman CWG: Pre-eclampsia: More than pregnancy-induced hypertension. Lancet 1993;341:1447.

Unless prevented by early delivery, the risks of preeclampsia-eclampsia to the fetus are a consequence of placental deterioration and insufficiency, resulting in intrauterine growth retardation and hypoxia. The risks to the mother include development of malignant hypertension, placental abruption with serious hemorrhage, cerebrovascular accidents, renal failure, seizures, and death (Table 22–14).

The pathophysiology of preeclampsia appears to be quite similar to that of thrombotic thrombocytopenic purpura and the hemolytic uremic syndrome. In those conditions, similar morphologic and biochemical changes consistent with endothelial cell dysfunction are observed, including diminished prostacyclin activity and increased thromboxane synthesis.

---

32. What are the hallmarks of preeclampsia-eclampsia?
33. What are the risks to the fetus of untreated maternal hypertension?
34. What other disorders in nonpregnant individuals have features in common with preeclampsia-eclampsia?

REFERENCES

General
Speroff, L, Glass RH, Kase NG: *Clinical Gynecologic Endocrinology and Infertility,* 6th ed. Williams & Wilkins, 1999.

Disorders of Pregnancy: Gestational Diabetes Mellitus, Hypertension, and Preeclampsia-Eclampsia
Bernheim J: Hypertension in pregnancy [clinical conference]. Nephron 1997;6:254.

Bick RL: Disseminated intravascular coagulation: Objective laboratory diagnostic criteria and guidelines for management. Clin Lab Med 1994;14:729.

Boden G: Fuel metabolism in pregnancy and in gestational diabetes mellitus. Obstet Gynecol Clin North Am 1996;23:1.

Lesser KB, Carpenter MW: Metabolic changes associated with normal pregnancy and pregnancy complicated by diabetes mellitus. Semin Perinatol 1994;18:399.

Reece EA, Eriksson UJ: The pathogenesis of diabetes-associated congenital malformations. Obstet Gynecol Clin North Am 1996;23:29.

Roberts JM: Endothelial dysfunction in preeclampsia. Semin Reprod Endocrinol 1998;16:5.

Suevo DM: The infant of the diabetic mother. Neonatal Network 1997;16:25.

Zamorski MA; Green LA: Preeclampsia and hypertensive disorders of pregnancy. Am Fam Phys 1996;53:1595.

Menstrual Disorders
Guzick D: Polycystic ovary syndrome: Symptomatology, pathophysiology, and epidemiology. Am J Obstet Gynecol 1998;179(6 Part 2):S89.

Marshall LA: Clinical evaluation of amenorrhea in active and athletic women. Clin Sports Med 1994;13:371.

Taylor AE: Understanding the underlying metabolic abnormalities of polycystic ovary syndrome and their implications. Am J Obstet Gynecol 1998;179 (6 Part 2): S94.

Infertility
Ryan IP, Taylor RN: Endometriosis and infertility: New concepts. Obstet Gynecol Surv 1997;52:365.

Zreik TG, Olive DL: Pathophysiology of endometriosis. Obstet Gynecol Clin North Am 1997;24:259.

23 Disorders of the Male Reproductive Tract

Stephen J. McPhee, MD

The male reproductive tract has two major functions: (1) the production of androgenic hormones needed for embryonic differentiation of male external and internal genitalia, development of male secondary sexual characteristics at puberty, and maintenance of libido and potency during adult life; and (2) the production of approximately 30 million spermatozoa per day during male reproductive life (from puberty to death). These functions are interrelated, and both require an intact hypothalamic-pituitary-testicular axis. Thus, disorders of the hypothalamus, pituitary, testes, or accessory glands may result in abnormalities of androgen production (producing hypogonadism) or sperm production (producing infertility). In addition, testicular androgens play an important role in the development of prostatic hyperplasia in older men. This chapter considers two common disorders of the male reproductive tract: male infertility and benign prostatic hyperplasia.

NORMAL STRUCTURE & FUNCTION OF THE MALE REPRODUCTIVE TRACT

ANATOMY & HISTOLOGY

The male reproductive tract is composed of the testes, genital ducts, accessory glands, and penis (Figure 23–1).

The **testes** are the two primary sex glands of the male. They are normally ovoid in shape, measuring about $4.5 \times 3 \times 2.5$ cm in size. The testes have two functions: (1) to manufacture the male reproductive cells, the **spermatozoa;** and (2) to produce the androgenic hormones, **testosterone** and **dihydrotestosterone.** Anatomically, the testes are composed of loops of convoluted tubules, called **seminiferous tubules** (Figure 23–2). The spermatozoa are produced from primitive germ cells along the seminiferous tubule walls, deep in folds of cytoplasm of the **Sertoli cells,** in a process known as **spermatogenesis.** Between the tubules are the nests of **interstitial (Leydig) cells,** which manufacture testosterone and dihydrotestosterone and secrete them into the bloodstream.

The testes are normally found in the scrotum, which serves both to envelop and protect the testes and to maintain the testicular temperature at approximately 1.5–2 °C below abdominal temperature. Testicular spermatogenesis is sensitive to body temperature, occurring optimally at the lower temperature and being diminished or abolished at higher temperatures.

The genital ducts include the **epididymis** and **vas deferens.** Both ends of each seminiferous tubule loop drain into the head of the epididymis. The spermatozoa move from the seminiferous tubule to the epididymis, then into the vas deferens. During ejaculation, the sperm enter the urethra through the ejaculatory ducts located in the body of the prostate.

The accessory glands include the **seminal vesicles, Cowper's bulbourethral glands, urethral glands,** and **prostate** (Figure 23–3). These glands produce secretions that help to nourish and transport the spermatozoa to the outside.

The **prostate** is a muscular gland, roughly triangular in shape, situated in the pelvis at the posterior and inferior surface of the bladder, close to the rectum. It surrounds the upper (prostatic) urethra (Figure 23–3). The prostate has an anterior, middle, posterior and two lateral lobes. A shallow median posterior groove, readily palpated on digital rectal examination, separates the lateral lobes. Histologically, the prostate is a compound tubuloalveolar gland with a stroma composed of smooth muscle. The function of the prostate gland is to secrete **prostatic fluid,** a cloudy, alkaline fluid that is a major component of **semen,** the fluid that is ejaculated at orgasm.

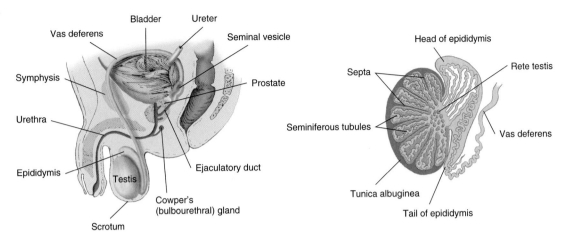

Figure 23–1. Anatomy of male reproductive system (left) and duct system of testis (right). (Reproduced, with permission, from Ganong WF: *Review of Medical Physiology,* 19th ed. Appleton & Lange, 1999.)

PHYSIOLOGY

Androgen Synthesis, Protein Binding & Metabolism

The testes secrete two steroid hormones that are essential to male reproductive function: testosterone and dihydrotestosterone. The pathways for testicular androgen biosynthesis are illustrated in Figure 23–4.

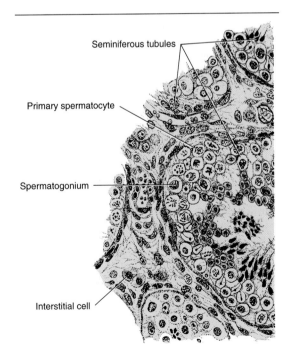

Figure 23–2. Schematic section of testis. (Reproduced, with permission, from Ganong WF: *Review of Medical Physiology,* 19th ed. Appleton & Lange, 1999.)

Testosterone, a C_{19} steroid, is synthesized from cholesterol by the interstitial (Leydig) cells of the testes and from androstenedione secreted by the adrenal cortex. In normal adult males, the testosterone secretion rate is 4–9 mg/d (13.9–31.2 nmol/d). In the blood, testosterone exists in both protein-bound and free (unbound) states. Ninety-eight percent of the testosterone in plasma is protein-bound: About 60% is bound to a beta-globulin called **sex-hormone binding globulin (SHBG)** (or gonadal steroid-binding globulin), and about 38% is bound to albumin. SHBG is similar in structure to, but not identical to, the androgen-binding protein secreted by the Sertoli cells (see below). SHBG is synthesized in the liver, and its gene is located on chromosome 17. Serum concentrations of SHBG are increased by hyperthyroidism, cirrhosis, and administration of various drugs, including estrogens, tamoxifen, phenytoin, and thyroid hormone, and decreased by hypothyroidism, obesity, acromegaly, and administration of exogenous androgens, glucocorticoids, or growth hormone. About 2% of the circulating testosterone is unbound and can enter cells to exert its metabolic action. In addition, some protein-bound testosterone can dissociate from its binding protein to enter the cells of target tissues. The normal plasma testosterone level for the adult male (including both free and bound testosterone) is 300–1100 ng/dL (10.4–38.2 nmol/L) (Table 23–1). The plasma testosterone level declines somewhat with age, as illustrated in Figure 23–5. The normal plasma free testosterone is 50–210 ng/dL (1.7–7.28 nmol/L).

Dihydrotestosterone (DHT) is derived both from direct secretion by the testes (about 20%) and from conversion in peripheral tissues of testosterone and other androgen (and estrogen) precursors secreted by the testes and adrenals (about 80%). DHT circulates in the bloodstream. The normal plasma DHT level

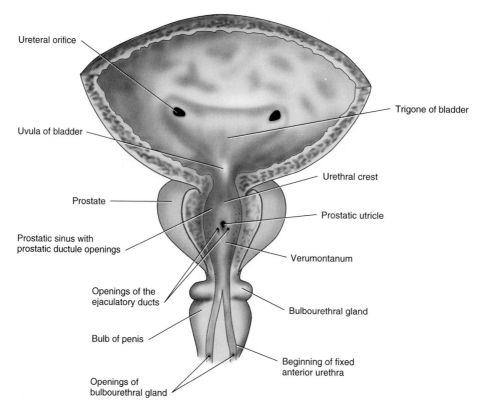

Figure 23–3. Anatomic relationships of the prostate. (Reproduced, with permission, from Lindner HH: *Clinical Anatomy.* Appleton & Lange, 1989.)

for the adult male is 27–75 ng/dL (0.9–2.6 nmol/L) (Table 23–1).

Regulation of Androgen Secretion & Control of Testicular Function

The endocrine mechanisms controlling male reproduction are diagrammed in Figure 23–6. The pituitary controls both testosterone production and spermatogenesis through the production of two gonadotropic hormones, **luteinizing hormone (LH)** and **follicle-stimulating hormone (FSH)**. LH stimulates the testicular interstitial (Leydig) cells to produce testosterone. FSH acts on the testicular Sertoli cells to facilitate spermatogenesis. The normal ranges for plasma LH and FSH levels are given in Table 23–1.

A. Hypothalamic-Pituitary-Testicular (Leydig Cell) Axis: The hypothalamus controls the pituitary production of gonadotropins through secretion of a decapeptide, **gonadotropin-releasing hormone (GnRH)**. The hypothalamus releases GnRH in a pulsatile fashion every 90–120 minutes into the portal circulation connecting the hypothalamus and anterior pituitary. When GnRH binds to the gonadotrophs in the anterior pituitary, it stimulates release of LH and, to a lesser extent, FSH into the general circulation. In the testes, LH binds to specific membrane receptors on the Leydig cells. This binding causes activation of adenylyl cyclase and generation of cAMP, which in turn results in secretion of androgens.

As depicted in Figure 23–6, hormones secreted by the testes exert a negative feedback influence on the hypothalamus and pituitary. Both the hypothalamus and the pituitary have androgen and estrogen receptors. Experimentally, administration of androgens such as DHT reduces LH pulse frequency, and administration of estrogens such as estradiol reduces LH pulse amplitude. In vivo, testosterone inhibits LH secretion directly by acting on the anterior pituitary and indirectly by inhibiting the secretion of GnRH from the hypothalamus. Estradiol, derived from the aromatization of testosterone (Figure 23–4), also exerts a major inhibitory effect on the hypothalamus.

B. Hypothalamic-Pituitary-Testicular (Seminiferous Tubule) Axis: Stimulation of the pituitary gonadotrophs by GnRH also causes them to secrete FSH into the systemic circulation. In the testes, FSH acts on the Sertoli cells to produce **testicular fluid,** which helps to transport spermatozoa to the epididymis, and to promote synthesis and secretion of

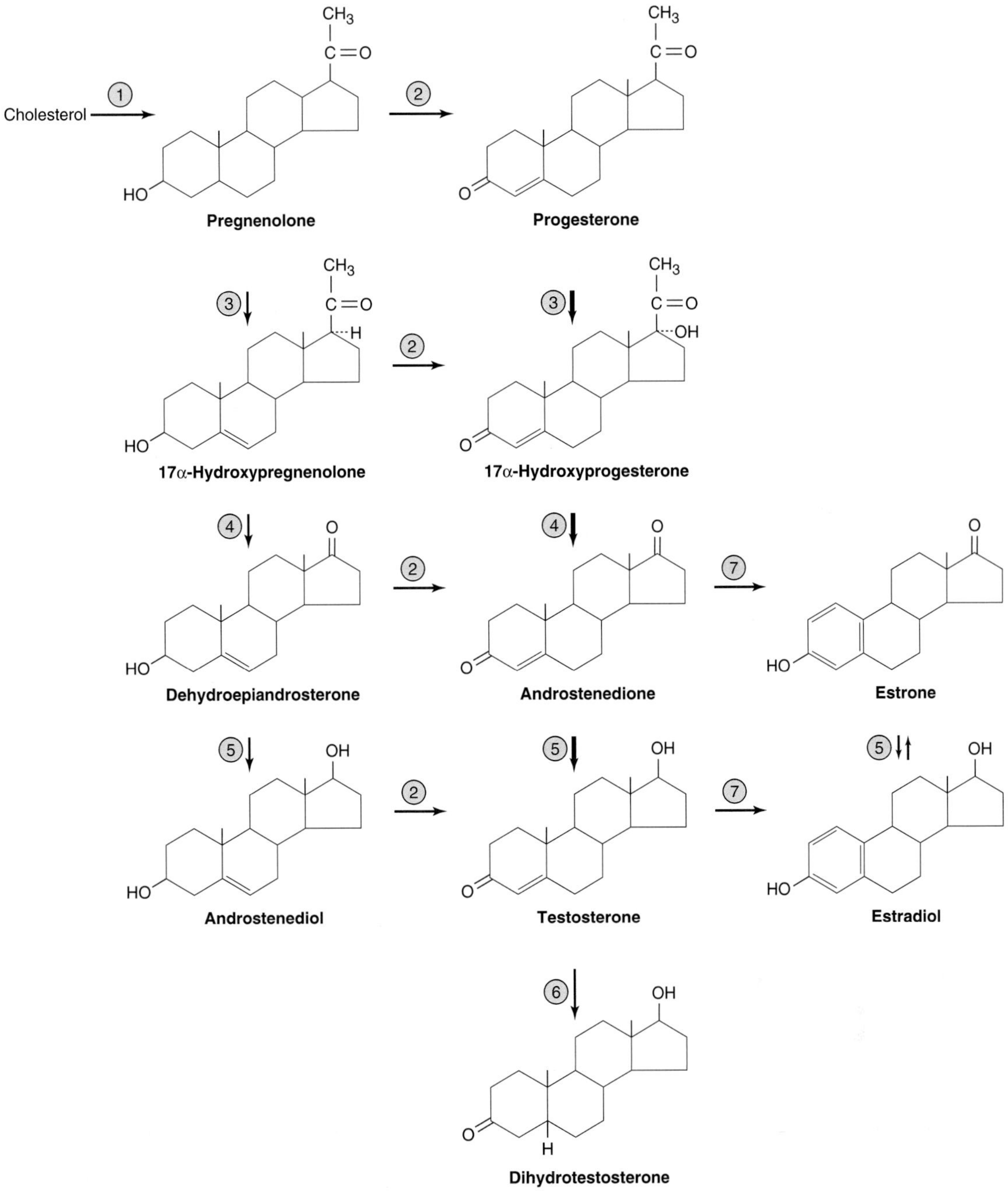

Figure 23–4. Biosynthesis and metabolism of testosterone. Heavy arrows indicate major pathways. (Circled numbers represent enzymes as follows: ①, 20,22-desmolase (P450scc); ②, 3β-hydroxysteroid dehydrogenase and Δ^{4,5}-isomerase; ③, 17-hydroxylase (P450c17); ④, 17,20-desmolase (P450c17); ⑤, 17-ketoreductase; ⑥, 5α-reductase; ⑦, aromatase.) (Reproduced, with permission, from Greenspan FS, Strewler GJ [editors]: *Basic and Clinical Endocrinology*, 5th ed. Appleton & Lange, 1997.)

Table 23–1. Normal plasma levels for pituitary and gonadal hormones in men.[1]

Hormone	Conventional Units	SI Units
Testosterone, total	300–1100 ng/dL	10.4–38.2 nmol/L
Testosterone, free	50–210 pg/mL	173–729 pmol/L
Dihydrotestosterone	27–75 ng/dL	0.9–2.6 nmol/L
Androstenedione	50–200 ng/dL	1.7–6.9 nmol/L
Estradiol	15–40 pg/mL	55–150 pmol/L
Estrone	15–65 pg/mL	55.5–240 pmol/L
FSH	2–15 mIU/mL	2–15 IU/L
LH	2–15 mIU/mL	2–15 IU/L
Prolactin	4–18 ng/mL	4–18 µg/L

[1]Modified and reproduced, with permission, from Greenspan FS, Strewler GJ [editors]: *Basic and Clinical Endocrinology,* 5th ed. Appleton & Lange, 1997.

two proteins, androgen-binding protein and inhibin. **Androgen-binding protein** binds to testosterone and transports it into the lumen of the seminiferous tubules. In so doing, it guarantees a high local concentration of testosterone in the tubular fluid, which is necessary for normal spermatogenesis by the Sertoli cells. **Inhibin** acts directly on the anterior pituitary to inhibit FSH secretion without affecting LH release. Two forms of inhibin have been identified, and three genes have been found to direct its synthesis. Inhibin is probably the major physiologic regulator of pituitary FSH secretion along with the gonadal steroids testosterone, DHT, and estradiol.

Mechanism of Androgen Action

Testosterone acts much like other steroid hormones. When it leaves the circulation, it rapidly

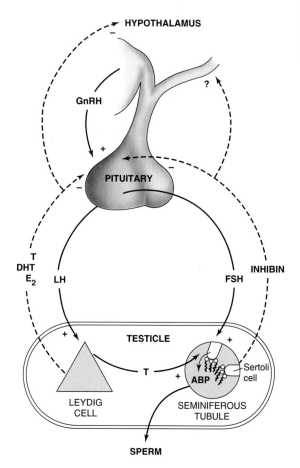

Figure 23–6. Endocrine control of male reproductive system. (APB, androgen-binding protein; GnRH, gonadotropin-releasing hormone; T, testosterone; E_2, estradiol; DHT, dihydrotestosterone.) (Modified and reproduced, with permission, from Greenspan FS, Strewler GJ [editors]: *Basic and Clinical Endocrinology,* 5th ed. Appleton & Lange, 1997.)

crosses the cell membrane (Figure 23–7). In the cytoplasm of most androgen target cells, testosterone is then converted to the more potent DHT by 5α-reductase. Both testosterone and DHT bind to an intracytoplasmic receptor protein (labeled R_c in Figure 23–7) that is distinct from both androgen-binding protein and SHBG. The gene encoding this protein is located on the X chromosome. Although DHT binds to the same intracellular receptor as testosterone, the DHT-receptor complexes are more stable than the testosterone-receptor complexes. Thus, DHT formation serves to amplify the action of testosterone in target tissues.

The testosterone- or DHT-receptor protein complex then traverses the nuclear membrane, where it undergoes transformation (to $T\text{-}R_n$ or $DHT\text{-}R_n$ in

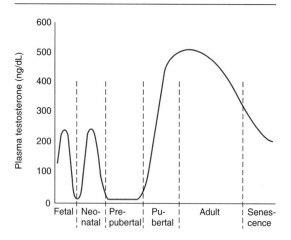

Figure 23–5. Plasma testosterone levels at various ages in males. (Reproduced, with permission, from Ganong WF: *Review of Medical Physiology,* 19th ed. Appleton & Lange, 1999.)

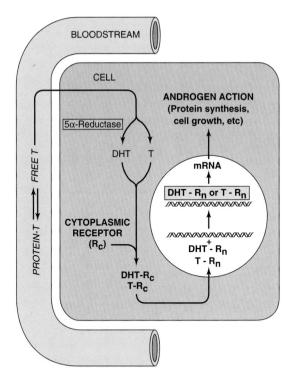

Figure 23–7. Mechanism of androgen action. (DHT, dihydrotestosterone; T, testosterone; R_c, cytoplasmic receptor, which becomes the nuclear receptor, R_n, in the nucleus.) (Reproduced, with permission, from Greenspan FS, Strewler GJ [editors]: *Basic and Clinical Endocrinology*, 5th ed. Appleton & Lange, 1997.)

deferens, seminal vesicles, prostate, and penis. During adolescence, androgens cause rapid growth of skeletal muscle and bone. Androgenic stimulation of the epiphysial cartilaginous plates initially causes rapid growth of the skeleton but eventually causes the epiphyses to fuse to the long bones, ultimately stopping further growth. Androgens are also responsible for development of the secondary sex characteristics summarized in Table 23–2. During adult life, androgens are necessary for normal male reproductive function. Androgens also stimulate erythropoiesis.

1. What is the difference between the temperature in the scrotum and core body temperature?
2. In what conditions does the serum concentration of steroid hormone-binding globulin (SHBG) increase?
3. In what conditions does it decrease?
4. What are the two testicular androgenic steroids, and what is their source?
5. How much of blood dihydrotestosterone is derived from peripheral conversion of testosterone?
6. How is testosterone secretion regulated?
7. Since there is only a single androgen receptor, how do you account for the differences in the effects of testosterone and dihydrotestosterone?
8. What are the effects of androgens?

Figure 23–7), enabling it to bind to DNA in the nuclear chromatin. The binding of the hormone-receptor complex to the nuclear chromatin results in synthesis of messenger RNA (mRNA). The mRNA is then transported to the cytoplasm, where it facilitates transcription of various genes, permitting synthesis of new proteins responsible for androgenic effects.

Effects of Androgens

In general, androgens act to promote growth and development, to promote spermatogenesis (see above), to develop and maintain the male secondary sex characteristics, and to inhibit pituitary secretion of LH. Their **anabolic effects** are mediated by an increase in the rate of synthesis and a decrease in the rate of breakdown of proteins.

In the fetus, androgens are necessary for normal differentiation and development of the internal and external male genitalia. During puberty, the androgens are needed for normal growth of the male genital structures, including the scrotum, epididymis, vas

Table 23–2. Pubertal development of male secondary sex characteristics.[1]

External genitalia	Penis increases in length and width; scrotum becomes pigmented and rugose
Internal genitalia	Seminal vesicles enlarge and secrete
Larynx	Larynx enlarges, vocal cords increase in length and thickness, voice deepens
Hair	Beard appears; scalp hairline recedes anterolaterally; pubic hair appears with male pattern (triangle with apex up); axillary, chest, and perianal hair appears
Musculoskeletal	Shoulders broaden; skeletal muscles enlarge
Skin	Sebaceous gland secretions increase and thicken
Mental	More aggressive, active attitude appears; libido develops

[1]Modified from from Ganong WF: *Review of Medical Physiology*, 19th ed. Appleton & Lange, 1999.

PATHOPHYSIOLOGY OF SELECTED MALE REPRODUCTIVE TRACT DISORDERS

MALE INFERTILITY

Infertility—defined as the failure to conceive after 6–12 months of regular sexual intercourse without contraception—affects about 15–20% of married couples. About one-third of cases are due to male, one-third to female, and one-third to combined male-female reproductive tract disorders. Thus, up to 10% of otherwise healthy men are infertile.

Male infertility is due to a heterogeneous group of disorders. Recognizable causes account for only 30–50% of cases. The remainder are idiopathic.

Etiology

Table 23–3 lists the most common causes of male infertility. They can be classified into one of three etiologic categories:

A. Pretesticular Causes: These include endocrine disorders such as hypothalamic or, more commonly, pituitary disorders—in which failure of gonadotropic hormone secretion leads to testicular failure. Other causes include androgen insensitivity states, thyroid disorders, and adrenal disorders. In addition, some medications (eg, phenytoin) may lower FSH levels.

B. Testicular Causes: Varicocele, trauma, infection, drugs and toxins (including medications, ingestants, and environmental exposures), chromosomal abnormalities such as the 47,XXY karyotype (Klinefelter's syndrome), and developmental abnormalities such as cryptorchism may be responsible for male factor infertility (Table 23–3). Chromosomal abnormalities account for approximately 2% of all cases of male infertility and approximately 15% of cases of azoospermia. **Testicular atrophy** can result in end-organ failure and infertility. Conditions associated with testicular atrophy are listed in Table 23–4.

C. Posttesticular Causes: The most common posttesticular problem is bilateral obstruction to the outflow of spermatozoa, resulting in absence of sperm in semen (**azoospermia**). Obstruction is responsible for up to 50% of cases of male infertility and may be surgically correctable. The diagnosis is established by vasography, in which radiographic dye is used to visualize the vas deferens and to localize the obstruction, and by testicular biopsy, which demonstrates normal spermatogenesis. Other conditions producing posttesticular causes of infertility in-

Table 23–3. Etiology of male infertility.

Pretesticular	Testicular	Posttesticular

Hypothalamic-pituitary disorders
  Panhypopituitarism
  Gonadotropin deficiency
    Isolated LH deficiency (fertile eunuch)
    Biologically inactive LH
    Combined LH and FSH deficiency
      (eg, Kallmann's syndrome)
  Prader-Willi syndrome
  Laurence-Moon-Biedl syndrome
  Cerebellar ataxia
  Pituitary tumors (eg, prolactinoma)
  Systemic illness (eg, cirrhosis, uremia)
Thyroid disorders (eg, hyperthyroidism, hypothyroidism)
Adrenal disorders (eg, adrenal insufficiency, congenital adrenal hyperplasia)
Drugs (eg, phenytoin, androgens)
	Varicocele
	Trauma
	  Testicular torsion
	  Orchiopexy
	Infection
	  Mumps orchitis
	Drugs and toxins
	  Medications (eg, sulfasalazine, cimetidine, nitrofurantoin, cyclophosphamide, chlorambucil, vincristine, methotrexate, procarbazine)
	  Ingestants (eg, alcohol, marijuana)
	  Environmental exposures (eg, pesticides, radiation, thermal exposure)
	Chromosomal abnormalities (eg, Klinefelter's syndrome [XXY seminiferous tubule dysgenesis], Y chromosome deletions)
	Developmental abnormalities
	  Cryptorchidism
	  Congenital absence of vas deferens, seminal vesicles
	  Immotile cilia syndrome
	  Bilateral anorchia (vanishing testes syndrome)
	  Leydig cell aplasia
	  Noonan's syndrome (male Turner's syndrome)
	  Myotonic dystrophy
	  Defective androgen biosynthesis (eg, 5α-reductase deficiency)
		Ductular obstruction, scarring
		  Pelvic, retroperitoneal, inguinal, or scrotal surgery (eg, retroperitoneal lymphadenectomy, hemiorrhaphy, Y-V plasty, transurethral resection of prostate, vasectomy)
		  Genital tract infections (eg, venereal disease, prostatitis, tuberculosis)
		  Cystic fibrosis
		Retrograde ejaculation (eg, diabetic autonomic neuropathy, postsurgical, medications)
		Antibodies to sperm or seminal plasma
		Developmental abnormalities
		  Penile anatomic defects (eg, hypospadias, epispadias, chordee)
		  Congenital absence or obstruction of vas deferens
		Androgen insensitivity (eg, androgen receptor deficiency, testicular feminization syndrome)
		Poor coital technique
		Sexual dysfunction, impotence
		Idiopathic

Table 23–4. Causes of testicular atrophy.[1]

Trauma
Testicular torsion
Hypopituitarism
Cryptorchidism
Klinefelter's syndrome (47,XXY)
Alcoholism and cirrhosis
Infection, eg, mumps orchitis, gonococcal epididymitis
Malnutrition and cachexia
Radiation
Obstruction to ouflow of semen
Aging
Drugs, eg, estrogen therapy for prostatic cancer

[1]Modified, with permission, from Chandrasoma P, Taylor CR: *Concise Pathology,* 3rd ed. Appleton & Lange, 1998.

clude retrograde ejaculation (often resulting from diabetic neuropathy), absence of seminal emission (often from radical pelvic or retroperitoneal surgery, producing damage to sympathetic nerves), antibodies to sperm or seminal plasma, developmental anomalies, sexual dysfunction, and poor coital technique (failure to deposit semen in the vagina during sexual intercourse).

D. Idiopathic: In many men there may be a genetic basis for male infertility currently classified as idiopathic. Among the approximately 10% of 46,XY men who have severe oligospermia or azoospermia in the absence of ductal obstruction, researchers have shown that between 8% and 15% carry one or another microdeletion in the long arm of the Y chromosome. The microdeletion, by loss of specific DNA segments, leads to loss of vital genes for sperm production. First discovered by cytogenetic screening, these deletions have more recently been detected by DNA analysis of the Y chromosome using sequence-tagged site-polymerase chain reaction assays. For example, microdeletions in a family of genes mapping to Yq11.23 (also called the Yq6 deletion interval) are thought to be important in causing azoospermia. Two genes in particular have been implicated: *DAZ* (deleted in azoospermia) and *RBM* (RNA-binding motif; previously known as *YRRM,* Y chromosome RNA recognition motif). These genes seem to encode for RNA binding proteins, but their function in spermatogenesis is unknown. These microdeletions appear to arise de novo in the infertile patient. Further investigation is needed to understand the distribution and activity of the Y-linked genes that control spermatogenesis.

Pathology

Percutaneous or open testicular biopsy specimens may show any of several lesions involving the entire testes or only portions. The most common lesion is **"maturation arrest,"** defined as failure to complete spermatogenesis beyond a particular stage. There can be early or late arrest patterns, with cessation of development at either the primary spermatocyte or the spermatogonial stage of the spermatogenic cycle. The second most common and least severe lesion is **"hypospermatogenesis,"** in which all stages of spermatogenesis are present but there is a reduction in the number of germinal epithelial cells per seminiferous tubule. Peritubular fibrosis may be present. **"Germ cell aplasia"** is a more severe lesion characterized by complete absence of germ cells, with only Sertoli cells lining the seminiferous tubules (**"Sertoli-cell-only"** syndrome). The most severe lesion (eg, in Klinefelter's syndrome) is hyalinization, fibrosis, and sclerosis of the tubules. These findings usually indicate irreversible damage. The testicular biopsy appearance varies in patients with Yq6 microdeletions and includes findings of germ cell arrest, severe hypospermatogenesis, and Sertoli cell-only syndrome.

Recent studies have found an increased frequency of apoptotic bodies (markers of programmed cell death) in testes with maturation arrest and hypospermatogenesis compared with those of men with obstructive azoospermia. This finding suggests that altered regulation of programmed cell death may be a mediator of abnormal spermatogenesis. Specific gene mediators of apoptosis *(Bax, Bcl, CREM)* have been identified in animal models.

Pathogenesis

For conception to occur, the following conditions must be met: (1) The testes must have normal spermatogenesis; (2) the spermatozoa must complete their maturation; (3) the ducts for sperm transport must be patent; (4) the prostate and seminal vesicles must supply adequate amounts of seminal fluid; (5) the coital technique must enable the male partner to deposit his semen near the female's cervix; (6) the spermatozoa must be able to penetrate the cervical mucus and reach the uterine tubes; and (7) the spermatozoa must undergo capacitation and the acrosome reaction, fuse with the oolemma, and be incorporated into the ooplasm. Any defect in this pathway can result in infertility.

Failure of gonadotropic hormone secretion (**hypogonadotropic hypogonadism**) produces defective spermatogenesis. Men with isolated gonadotropin-releasing hormone (GnRH) deficiency typically fail to develop normally during puberty. However, an adult-onset form of idiopathic hypogonadotropic hypogonadism causes infertility that develops after puberty. Hypogonadotropic hypogonadism can be overcome by chorionic gonadotropin, combined chorionic gonadotropin and FSH, or intermittent GnRH pulsatile therapy. **Hypergonadotropic hypogonadism** refers to primary gonadal (end-organ) failure and is indicated by elevated serum FSH and LH levels due to the absence of negative feedback effects of testosterone and DHT on the pituitary and hypothalamus. Unfortunately, parenteral testosterone therapy does not usually result in adequate intratesticular testosterone levels to maintain spermatogenesis. Future approaches may involve direct intratesticular injection of testosterone-laden microspheres; in experimental animals, such an approach has been found to restore testosterone concentrations and subsequent sperm production and fertility.

An elevated serum prolactin (PRL) level can inhibit the normal release of pituitary gonadotropins, probably through an effect on the hypothalamus (eg, patients with elevated prolactin levels have been found to have a reduced LH pulse frequency). Thus, a serum PRL measurement should be obtained in any patient with hypogonadotropic hypogonadism. If an elevated PRL level is found, the patient should be evaluated by radiographic imaging of the sella turcica to exclude a prolactinoma or other pituitary tumor. Other causes of hyperprolactinemia are discussed in Chapter 19.

Other **endocrine disorders** such as hyperthyroidism, hypothyroidism, adrenal insufficiency, and congenital adrenal hyperplasia are found in about 4% of men evaluated for infertility. Both hyperthyroidism and hypothyroidism can alter spermatogenesis. Hyperthyroidism affects both pituitary and testicular function by altering steroid hormone metabolism. In hyperthyroidism, there is increased conversion of androgens to estrogens which in turn leads to inappropriate feedback and consequent alterations in secretion of LH and FSH. In hypothyroidism, infertility results from enhanced release of prolactin (TRH simulates prolactin release). Similarly, primary adrenal insufficiency causes a reversible elevation of the serum prolactin level.

Testicular disorders, including cryptorchism (undescended testes), adult seminiferous tubule failure, and sex chromosome abnormalities, are found in about 15% of infertile men.

Varicoceles are varicose enlargement of the veins of the spermatic cord. They are very common, being found in 8–20% of men in the general population and in 25–40% of patients with otherwise unexplained infertility. They are often (50–70%) bilateral. Among men in infertility clinics, varicoceles affect 11% of men with normal semen analyses but 25% of men with abnormal semen analyses. It is hypothesized that varicoceles may lead to oligospermia by increasing testicular temperature (see below). The incidence of varicoceles is much lower in men who have never fathered a child (primary male factor infertility) than in currently infertile men who were able to father a child in the past (secondary male factor infertility) (35% versus 81%). This finding suggests that varicoceles may cause a progressive decline in fertility and that prior fertility in men with varicoceles does not confer resistance to the varicocele-induced impairment of spermatogenesis. Prophylactic surgery remains controversial, but studies of the efficacy of varicocelectomy have demonstrated significant increases in sperm count, motility, and sometimes morphology and a marked improvement in pregnancy rates over nonoperated individuals. Of men so treated, about 50–75% show improvement in semen quality, and 30–40% initiate a pregnancy. Men with larger varicoceles appear to have greater postoperative improvement than those with small or subclinical varicoceles.

Chemotherapy or radiation therapy for malignancies may also impair spermatogenesis by their direct cytotoxic effects on the germ cells. For example, more than 80% of men who are cured of testicular cancer are infertile. The infertility is usually multifactorial, secondary to the chemotherapeutic agents, retroperitoneal lymph node dissection, and radiation therapy these patients receive.

A variety of **drugs and environmental toxins** may interfere with spermatogenesis, either directly or indirectly through alterations in the endocrine system. Recreational drugs (marijuana, alcohol), toxins (lead and arsenic), and medications (sulfasalazine, cimetidine, antimetabolites, phenytoin, monoamine oxidase inhibitors, and nitrofurantoin) have all been reported to interfere with spermatogenesis. Exogenous androgens and anabolic steroids can depress gonadotropin secretion. Discontinuation of these agents may restore sperm concentrations in semen to normal.

Men who are born with undescended testes (**cryptorchism**) have poorer semen quality than normal men regardless of the timing of corrective orchiopexy (fixation of the testes in the scrotum by sutures). Approximately 30% of men with unilateral cryptorchism and 50% with bilateral cryptorchism will have low sperm counts. Experimental studies in animals have shown that there is a temperature differential between the abdomen and the scrotum of 1.5–2 °C (2.7–3.6 °F) and that the increase in testicular temperature in cryptorchism can result in depression of spermatogenesis.

Other defects in spermatogenesis—eg, those produced by **chromosomal abnormalities** or associated with the **immotile cilia syndrome**—are not correctable.

Genital tract infections can impair fertility. Mumps orchitis can cause testicular atrophy, presumably as a consequence of inflammation, swelling, and pressure necrosis. Among men who develop mumps after onset of puberty, approximately 13% develop unilateral orchitis and 65% bilateral orchitis. Acute gonococcal epididymitis, chronic epididymo-orchitis, tuberculosis, or bacterial prostatitis can produce scarring and obstruction of the epididymis, vas deferens, or ejaculatory ducts and thus impair fertility. Prior venereal disease may also be associated with urethral strictures. Epididymovasostomy to relieve epididymal obstruction, vasovasotomy to correct localized obstruction of the vas deferens, and transurethral resection of the ejaculatory ducts or urethral stricture have all been associated with increases in ejaculate volume, sperm density and motility, and pregnancy rates. In addition, in cases of irreparable vasal obstruction and nonobstructive azoospermia due to anejaculation, microepididymal sperm retrieval by aspiration for in vitro fertilization (IVF) by intracytoplasmic sperm injection (ICSI) is possible. ICSI has the potential to overcome many of the causes of male infertility. However, ICSI may transmit to the male offspring chromosomal or gene defects (such as Y chromosome microdeletions or *CFTR* gene mutations) that might otherwise be lost or eliminated by natural means. Therefore, genetic counseling is recommended for couples contemplating ICSI.

Retrograde ejaculation of semen into the urinary bladder may occur with autonomic neuropathy (eg, from diabetes mellitus), with disruption of the internal bladder sphincter (eg, from corrective Y-V plasty of the bladder neck during childhood or from transurethral resection of the prostate), with disruption or dysfunction of sympathetic nerves (eg, following radical pelvic or retroperitoneal surgery), or with certain medications.

About 3% of infertile couples are suspected of having immunologic infertility, with more than 10% of mobile spermatozoa coated with antibody. The role and mechanism of **antibodies to sperm** (or to seminal plasma) in producing infertility remains controversial. The antibodies may be associated with premature onset of capacitation and the acrosome reaction. A variety of autoimmune disorders can result in production of antisperm antibodies by the female partner. Such antibodies in the female genital tract can lead to agglutination or immobilization of sperm and can be responsible for failure of sperm to penetrate the ovum. However, this mechanism probably rarely causes infertility. Factors that cause antisperm antibody production by the male partner include vasectomy, ejaculatory duct obstruction, infection, varicocele, cryptorchism, and testicular trauma, torsion, or cancer. Antisperm antibodies can be measured in serum or semen by a variety of techniques. The sperm mucus-penetration test is most useful for assessing the significance of positive sperm antibody tests. Spermatozoa must be unable to penetrate cervical mucus before the amount of sperm antibodies is considered clinically significant. Immunosuppressive doses of systemic corticosteroids can significantly improve fertility. Alternatively, corticosteroids can be used to reduce antibody titers before IVF.

About 1–2% of infertile men have congenital bilateral absence of the vas deferens. This defect also occurs in 95% of men with cystic fibrosis. Yet while 50–70% of men with congenital absence of the vas have mutations in the transmembrane conductance regulator gene *CFTR* responsible for cystic fibrosis, most infertile men found to have congenital bilateral absence of the vas deferens have no respiratory symptoms. The most common cause of congenital absence of the vas appears to be a mutation in *CFTR* combined with a variant in a noncoding region of *CFTR* (the 5T allele) which causes reduced levels of the normal CFTR protein.

Infertility can also occur in patients with anatomic defects of the penis, such as **hypospadias** (urethral opening on the penile under surface), **epispadias** (urethral opening on the penile dorsal surface), and **chordee** (painful erection with penile curvature due to nondistensibility of one corpus cavernosum). These abnormalities may lead to an improper placement of the ejaculate in the vagina.

Poor coital technique and **improper timing of intercourse** can interfere with fertility. Too frequent masturbation in the periovulatory period can deplete the sperm reserve, particularly in an oligospermic male. Several commonly used lubricants (eg, K-Y Jelly, Surgilube, Keri Lotion, and even saliva) can be spermatotoxic, causing a deterioration in sperm motility.

Finally, sexual dysfunction can be responsible for male factor infertility. Male sexual dysfunction can be categorized into several problem areas. **Impotence** is defined as the consistent inability to maintain an erect penis with sufficient rigidity to allow sexual intercourse **(loss of erections).** Such erectile dysfunction may be the result of arterial, venous, neurogenic, or psychogenic causes. Impotence should be clearly distinguished from problems with libido, ejaculation, and orgasm. A **loss of libido** (sexual desire) may be the direct consequence of androgen deficiency, whether on the basis of hypothalamic, pituitary, or testicular disease. **Loss of emission** (lack of seminal fluid during ejaculation) may result from retrograde ejaculation (as noted above) or from androgen deficiency (which decreases prostatic and seminal vesicle secretions). **Premature ejaculation** is usually an anxiety-related disorder. **Loss of orgasm** is usually of psychologic origin.

---

9. What are the categories of male infertility? Name several specific causes for each category.
10. From the perspective of the male reproductive system, what are the steps that must occur for conception?
11. What drugs commonly interfere with spermatogenesis?
12. What are the causes of impotence?

Clinical Manifestations

A. Symptoms and Signs: Infertility is often the only complaint. However, depending on the cause of the infertility, there may be other symptoms and signs. For example, with hypogonadotropic hypogonadism, there may be decreased libido and potency, emotional instability, fatigue, decreased mental concentration, and vasomotor instability (palpitations, hot flushes, diaphoresis). If hypogonadism occurs before onset of puberty, there may be other signs of androgen deficiency, such as decreased body hair, gynecomastia, and eunuchoid proportions (narrow shoulders, little muscle development). Galactorrhea in a male strongly suggests an anterior pituitary prolactinoma. Neurologic or ophthalmologic abnormalities suggest suprasellar extension of a pituitary tumor, and profuse polyuria consistent with diabetes insipidus suggests destruction of the posterior pituitary. Anosmia and a history of delayed sexual maturation are key features of **Kallmann's syndrome,** with associated hypogonadotropic hypogonadism. In Kallmann's syndrome, isolated gonadotropin deficiency is associated with abnormalities of the olfactory cortex. During embryonic life, GnRH-producing neurons fail to migrate from the olfactory area to the medial basal hypothalamus. Affected patients may have undescended testes, gynecomastia, and obesity in addition to delays in reaching adult height and in sexual maturation during puberty. Recently, a deletion of a single gene, *Kalig-2,* has been found in the X-linked form of the disease. On the other hand, a history of precocious puberty suggests congenital adrenal hyperplasia.

Patients with the immotile cilia (Kartagener's) syndrome have severe asthenospermia (poor sperm motility) due to missing dynein arms, in association with mucociliary transport defects in the lower airways that result in chronic obstructive pulmonary disease. The occurrence of chronic respiratory disease, particularly bronchiectasis and chronic sinusitis, also suggests infertility due to congenital absence of the vas deferens (cystic fibrosis) or epididymal obstructions (Young syndrome).

Physical examination of the male genitalia is very important in diagnosis of infertility. Measurement of testicular size (**orchidometry**) may be helpful since spermatogenic disorders are often associated with abnormally small testes. Testicular atrophy is diagnosed when the physical examination finds the testes to be smaller than the normal $4.5 \times 3 \times 2.5$ cm. Careful palpation of the spermatic cord may reveal a varicocele, palpable as a boggy intrascrotal mass. Elicited increase in intra-abdominal pressure (eg, by Valsalva's maneuver: forced expiratory effort against a closed airway) will sometimes produce a palpable impulse in the mass. Varicoceles are more easily detected if the patient is examined in the standing position. They are more common on the left side. Infections of the epididymis may be associated with epididymal induration, irregularity, and cystic changes. There may be absence of the vas deferens or nodularity along its course suggestive of obstruction. An enlarged, boggy, or tender prostate suggests prostatitis. Finally, the penis must be carefully inspected for abnormal position of the urethral opening or abnormal penile angulation or curvature. The penile shaft should be palpated for fibrosis suggestive of Peyronie's disease, a disorder in which deposition of fibrous tissue around the corpus cavernosum of the penis causes deformity and painful erections.

B. Laboratory Tests and Evaluation: Figure 23–8 outlines an approach to the diagnosis of male infertility. Determination of serum levels of testosterone, FSH, and LH and performance of semen analysis allow the clinician to classify patients as having either primary or secondary gonadal failure. Patients with primary gonadal failure have an abnormal semen analysis, low or low normal testosterone levels, and elevated FSH or LH levels. Those with secondary gonadal failure have an abnormal semen analysis, low serum testosterone level, and low or inappopriately normal FSH or LH levels.

Semen analysis involves examination of semen collected by masturbation (using a special plastic condom) after 72 hours of sexual abstinence. The analysis entails determination of the volume, sperm count, sperm motility, and sperm morphology. The reference standards for semen analysis are presented in Table 23–5. The average volume of ejaculate is 2.5–5 mL after 72 hours without intercourse. Volumes less than 1.5 mL may result in inadequate buffering of vaginal acidity to enable sperm survival and are usually caused by either retrograde ejaculation or androgen deficiency. There are normally about 100 million sperm per milliliter of semen. Both **azoospermia** (absence of sperm) and **oligospermia** (usually defined as < 20 million sperm per milliliter of semen) result in infertility. Men with poor sperm production frequently have poorly functioning sperm as well. Normal sperm motility and morphology are defined as at least 60% motile sperm and more than 60% with normal morphology. Abnormal motility may result from infection or antisperm antibodies. Abnormal morphology may be the result of varicocele, infection, or exposure to a toxin. Semen analysis is sometimes limited in its usefulness. A significant proportion of men with "normal" semen analyses will be infertile because of defects in sperm function, and a significant number of men with "abnormal" semen quality will nonetheless have normal sperm function.

Fructose is produced in the seminal vesicles, and its absence in the semen implies obstruction of the ejaculatory ducts. **Leukospermia** (excessive numbers of leukocytes in the semen) may adversely affect sperm movement and fertilization ability, due perhaps to excessive generation of reactive oxygen species by the leukocytes. The finding of leukospermia should prompt further investigations to exclude a subclinical genital tract infection.

Several functional assays of spermatozoa are now available to assess the ability of the sperm to reach and penetrate the ova. The **postcoital test** assesses sperm interaction with cervical mucus. It is performed by examining the cervical mucus for the

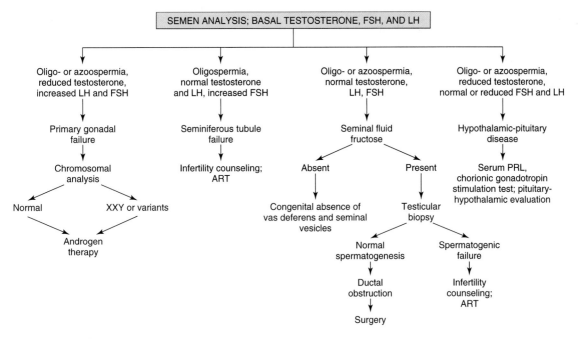

Figure 23–8. Approach to diagnosis of male infertility. (ART, assisted reproduction technologies.) (Reproduced, with permission, from Greenspan FS, Strewler GJ [editors]: *Basic and Clinical Endocrinology,* 5th ed. Appleton & Lange, 1997.)

presence of viable sperm within a few hours after intercourse. The test is best conducted during the preovulatory phase of the menstrual cycle when cervical mucus is least viscous. The test is considered normal if there are at least 10–20 sperm per high power field and most of them demonstrate forward motility. Causes of an abnormal test include the presence of antibodies to sperm or seminal plasma in the cervical mucus or semen, anatomic abnormalities, poor coital technique, abnormal semen (demonstrable on semen analysis), and improper timing of the test. The test is simple and inexpensive yet provides a measure of sperm function. Failure of spermatozoa to penetrate the mucus predicts poor fertilization rates at in vitro fertilization.

A variety of in vitro tests have been developed to assess sperm function in an attempt to explain previously hidden male factors in couples with unexplained infertility. These couples have significantly lower in vitro fertilization rates when compared with those in whom simple uterine tubal problems can be identified. These tests are designed to uncover defects in sperm capacitation and motion, in binding to the zona pellucida, in acrosome reaction, and in ability to penetrate the oocyte. The **sperm mucus-penetration test** assesses the capacity of spermatozoa to move through a column of midcycle cervical mucus and aids in detection of impaired motility caused by antibodies.

In the **sperm penetration assay,** the infertile man's sperm are processed, allowed to capacitate, and then incubated with hamster oocytes that have had the zona pellucida removed enzymatically to allow penetration. Results are reported as either the percentage of ova that have been penetrated (normal is 10–30%) or as the number of sperm penetrations per ovum (normal is more than five).

The **hemizona assay** assesses the fertilizing capability of sperm using the zona pellucida from a nonfertilizable, nonliving human oocyte. The zona is divided in half. One half is incubated with the infertile man's sperm, while the other half is incubated with

Table 23–5. Normal values for semen analysis.[1]

Characteristic	Reference Standard
Ejaculate volume	1.5–5.0 mL
Sperm count	>20 million/mL
Sperm motility	>60%
Sperm morphology	>60% normal
Sperm forward progression	>2 (scale 0–4)
Sperm agglutination	Absent
Leukospermia	Absent
Hyperviscosity	Absent

[1]Reproduced, with permission, from Fisch H, Lipshultz LI: Diagnosing male factors of infertility. Arch Pathol Lab Med 1992;116:398.

sperm from a known fertile donor. The number of sperm penetrations is compared and expressed as a ratio. However, a major problem with this assay is the limited availability of human ova. Recent identification of zona pellucida glycoprotein 3 (ZP3) as the primary determinant of sperm-zona binding has led to exploring use of recombinant human ZP3 rather than the zona itself for testing sperm-zona interactions.

High-resolution **transrectal ultrasonography** can be used to evaluate the seminal vesicles for dysplasia or obstruction; the ejaculatory ducts for scarring, cysts, or calcifications; and the prostate for calcifications. **Venography** is occasionally useful to demonstrate testicular venous reflux in a man with a suspected varicocele when the physical examination is difficult or in a man with a suspected recurrence following surgical repair. Finally, **testicular biopsy** is useful in azoospermic (and sometimes oligospermic) men to distinguish intrinsic testicular abnormalities from ductal obstruction. Testicular biopsy can recover some spermatozoa for ICSI in over 90% of azoospermic men. However, to do so may require more than one testicular biopsy in men with germ cell aplasia and maturation arrest. In men with lesser degrees of defective sperm production (eg, Sertoli cell-only syndrome), biopsy often demonstrates foci of spermatogenesis.

BENIGN PROSTATIC HYPERPLASIA

Benign prostatic hyperplasia (BPH) is a nonmalignant neoplasm of the prostate stroma and epithelial glands that causes enlargement of the prostate gland. Growing slowly over decades, the gland can eventually reach up to ten times the normal adult prostate size in severe cases. Benign prostatic hyperplasia is a common age-related disorder. Most men are asymptomatic, but clinical symptoms and signs occur in up to one-third of men over age 65, and each year more than 400,000 men in the United States undergo transurethral resection of the prostate.

Etiology

The cause of benign prostatic hyperplasia is unknown. However, aging and hormonal factors are both clearly important. Age-related increases in prostate size are evident at autopsy, and the development of symptoms is age-related. Data from autopsy studies show pathologic evidence of benign prostatic hyperplasia in less than 10% of men in their thirties, in 40% of men in their fifties, more than 70% of men in their sixties, and almost 90% of men in their eighties. Clinical symptoms of bladder outlet obstruction are seldom found in men younger than 40 years but are found in about one-third of men over age 65 and in up to three-fourths of men at age 80. Prostatic androgen levels, particularly dihydrotestosterone (DHT) levels, play an important role in development of the disorder. These factors are discussed below.

Pathology

The normal prostate is composed of both stromal (smooth muscle) and epithelial (glandular) elements. Each of these elements—alone or in combination—can give rise to hyperplastic nodules and ultimately the symptoms of benign prostatic hyperplasia. Pathologically, the hyperplastic gland is enlarged, with a firm, rubbery consistency. While small nodules are often present throughout the gland, benign prostatic hyperplasia arises most commonly in the periurethral and transition zones of the gland (Figure 23–9). With advancing age, there is an increase in the overall size

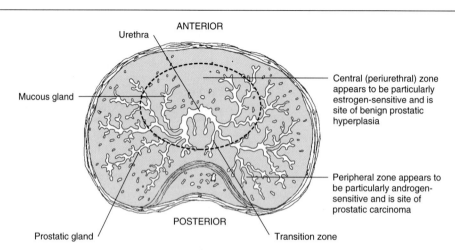

Figure 23–9. Structure of the prostate. (Reproduced, with permission, from Chandrasoma P, Taylor CE: *Concise Pathology,* 3rd ed. Appleton & Lange, 1998.)

of the transition zone as well as an increase in the number—and later the size—of nodules. The urethra is compressed and has a slit-like appearance.

Histologically, benign prostatic hyperplasia is a true hyperplastic process since studies document an increase in prostatic cell number. The prostatic nodules are composed of both hyperplastic glands and hyperplastic stromal muscle. Most periurethral nodules are stromal in character, but transition zone nodules are most often glandular tissue. The glands become larger than normal, with stromal muscle between the proliferative glands. Perhaps as much as 40% of the hyperplastic prostate is smooth muscle. The cellular proliferation leads to a tight packing of glands within a given area. There is an increase in the height of the lining epithelium, and the epithelium often shows papillary projections (Figure 23–10). There is also some hypertrophy of individual epithelial cells.

In men with benign prostatic hyperplasia, the bladder shows both detrusor smooth muscle hypertrophy and trabeculation associated with an increase in collagen deposition.

Pathogenesis

While the actual cause of benign prostatic hyperplasia is undefined, several factors are known to be involved in the pathogenesis. These include age-related prostatic growth, prostatic capsule, androgenic hormones and their receptors, prostatic smooth muscle and adrenergic receptors, stromal-epithelial interactions and growth factors, and detrusor responses.

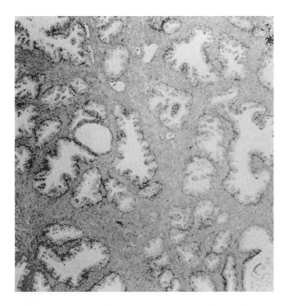

Figure 23–10. Benign prostatic hyperplasia. (Reproduced, with permission, from Chandrasoma P, Taylor CE: *Concise Pathology,* 3rd ed. Appleton & Lange, 1998.)

A. Age-Related Prostatic Growth: The size of the prostate does not always correlate with the degree of obstruction. The amount of periurethral and transition zone tissue may relate more to the degree of obstruction than the overall prostate size. However, the idea that the clinical symptoms of benign prostatic hyperplasia are due simply to a mass-related increase in urethral resistance is probably too simplistic. Instead, some of its symptoms may be due to obstruction-induced detrusor dysfunction and neural alterations in the bladder and prostate.

B. Prostatic Capsule: The presence of a capsule around the prostate is thought to play a role in development of obstructive symptoms. Besides man, the dog is the only animal known to develop benign prostatic hyperplasia. However, the canine prostate lacks a capsule, and dogs do not develop obstructive symptoms. In men, the capsule presumably causes the "pressure" created by the expanded periurethral-transition zone tissue to be transmitted to the urethra, leading to an increase in urethral resistance. Surgical incision of the prostatic capsule or removal of the obstructing portion of the prostate—whether by transurethral resection or by open prostatectomy—is effective in relieving symptoms.

C. Hormonal Regulation of Prostatic Growth: Development of benign prostatic hyperplasia requires testicular androgens as well as aging. There are several lines of evidence for this relationship. First, men who are castrated before puberty or who have disorders of impaired androgen production or action do not develop benign prostatic hyperplasia. Second, the prostate—unlike other androgen-dependent organs—maintains its ability to respond to androgens throughout life. Androgens are required for normal cell proliferation and differentiation in the prostate. They may also actively inhibit cell turnover and death. Finally, androgen deprivation at various levels of the hypothalamic-pituitary-testicular axis can reduce prostate size and improve obstructive symptoms (Table 23–6).

While androgenic hormones are clearly required for the development of benign prostatic hyperplasia, testosterone is not the major androgen in the prostate. Instead, 80–90% of prostatic testosterone is converted to the more active metabolite dihydrotestosterone (DHT) by the enzyme 5α-reductase. Recently, two subtypes of 5α-reductase (type 1 and type 2) have been described. Both type 1 and type 2 isoenzymes are found in skin and liver, but only the type 2 isoenzyme is found in the fetal and adult urogenital tract, including both basal epithelial cells and stromal cells in the prostate, and only the type 2 isoenzyme is inhibited by the drug finasteride (see below). In the prostate, it appears that DHT synthesis largely depends on the type 2 enzyme and that once it is synthesized, the DHT acts in a paracrine fashion on androgen-dependent epithelial cells. The nuclei of these cells contain large numbers of androgen receptors

Table 23–6. Mechanisms and side effects of antiandrogenic treatment for benign prostatic hyperplasia.[1]

Agent	Mechanism	Side Effects[2]
Androgen ablation GnRH agonists (eg, nafarelin, leuprolide, buserelin, goserelin)	Inhibits pituitary LH secretion, decreases T and DHT. Reduces prostate volume by ≈35%.	Hot flushes, loss of libido, impotence, gynecomastia.
True antiandrogens (eg, flutamide, bicalutamide, Zanoterone)	Androgen receptor inhibition.	Gynecomastia or nipple tenderness, no significant incidence of impotence.
5α-Reductase inhibitors (eg, finasteride, episteride)	Decreases DHT, no alteration in T or LH. Reduces prostate volume by ≈20%.	Three to 4% incidence of impotence and decreased libido.
Mixed mechanism of action Progestins (eg, megestrol acetate, hydroxyprogesterone caproate, medrogestone)	Inhibits pituitary LH secretion, decreases T and DHT, androgen receptor inhibition.	Loss of libido, impotence, heat intolerance.
Cyproterone acetate	Androgen receptor inhibition, inhibits pituitary LH secretion, variable decreases in T and DHT.	Loss of libido, impotence (variable).

[1]Modified and reproduced, with permission, from McConnell JD: Benign prostatic hyperplasia: Hormonal treatment. Urol Clin North Am 1995;22:387.
[2]Other than gastrointestinal, hematologic, and central nervous system reactions.

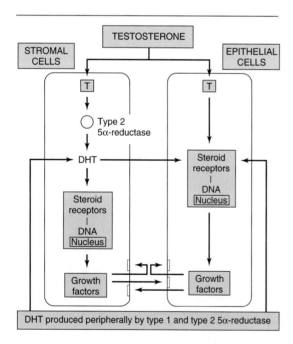

Figure 23–11. Mechanism of androgen action on prostatic stromal and epithelial cells. After testosterone (T) diffuses into the cell, it can interact directly with the androgen (steroid) receptors bound to the promoter region of androgen-related genes. In the stromal cell, a majority of T is converted into dihydrotestosterone (DHT), which acts in an autocrine fashion in the stromal cell and in a paracrine fashion after diffusing into nearby epithelial cells. DHT produced peripherally in skin and liver can also diffuse into the prostate and act in an endocrine fashion.

(Figure 23–11). DHT levels are the same in hyperplastic and normal glands. However, prostatic levels of DHT remain high with aging despite the fact that peripheral levels of testosterone decrease. These decreases in plasma androgen levels are further amplified by an age-related increase in the plasma sex-hormone binding globulin (SHBG) level, resulting in relatively greater decreases in free testosterone than in total testosterone levels.

Suppression of androgens leads to reduction in prostate size and relief of symptoms of bladder outlet obstruction. True antiandrogens, which block the action of testosterone and DHT in the prostate, should be distinguished from agents that impair androgen production (Table 23–6). Gonadotropin-releasing hormone (GnRH) agonists work by down-regulating GnRH receptors in the pituitary, producing a transient increase and subsequent long-term reduction in concentrations of LH. A variety of antiandrogen treatment approaches have been used successfully, including GnRH agonists (nafarelin, leuprolide, buserelin), androgen receptor inhibitors (cyproterone acetate, flutamide), progestogens, and 5α-reductase inhibitors (finasteride, episteride) (Figure 23–12). Most of these agents are associated with intolerable adverse effects, such as impotence, flushing, and loss of libido. However, the 5α-reductase inhibitor finasteride suppresses plasma DHT levels by 65% and prostatic DHT levels by approximately 80–90%. Treatment with this agent has been shown to induce significant decreases in the size of the prostate as a whole and in the size of the periurethral zone. Finasteride has fewer adverse side effects than other antiandrogen medications, but it must be given for at

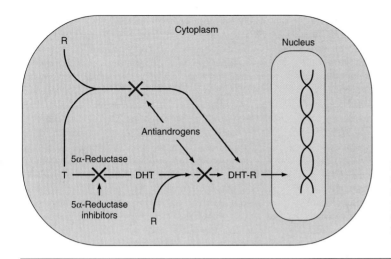

Figure 23–12. Site of action of antiandrogens and 5α-reductase inhibitors. (X, site of blockade.) (Adapted, with permission, from Oesterling JE: Endocrine therapies for symptomatic benign prostatic hyperplasia. Urology 1994;3[2 Suppl]:7.)

least 6–12 months to have a beneficial effect and must be continued indefinitely thereafter. Both GnRH agonists and finasteride have been shown to be effective in improving symptoms and urinary flow rates in patients with benign prostatic hyperplasia, particularly in men with larger (> 40 g) prostates. Finasteride is less effective than GnRH agonists in reducing the size of the prostate, but it causes fewer side effects.

Androgen receptor levels remain high with aging, thus maintaining the mechanism for androgen-dependent cell growth. Nuclear androgen receptor levels have been found to be higher in prostatic tissue from men with benign prostatic hyperplasia than in that from normal controls. The regulation of androgen receptor expression in benign prostatic hyperplasia is now being studied at the transcriptional level.

Finally, androgens are not the only important hormones contributing to the development of benign prostatic hyperplasia. Estrogens appear to be involved in induction of the androgen receptor. Serum estrogen levels increase in men with age—absolutely or relative to testosterone level. Age-related increases in estrogens may thus increase androgen receptor expression in the prostate, leading to increases in cell growth (or decreases in cell death). Intraprostatic levels of estrogen are increased in men with benign prostatic hyperplasia. Patients with benign prostatic hyperplasia who have larger prostatic volumes tend to have higher plasma levels of estradiol. Studies of prostatic specimen tissue have documented an accumulation of DHT, estradiol, and estrone that correlates with patient age. The results show a dramatic increase of the estrogen:androgen ratio with increasing age, particularly in the stroma of prostatic tissue.

Recent investigations suggest a role for estradiol in particular, demonstrating powerful cell-specific, nontranscriptional effects of estradiol on the human prostate. Estradiol, acting in concert with SHBG, has been found to produce an eightfold increase in intracellular cAMP in hyperplastic prostatic tissue. This increase in cAMP does not occur with estrogens such as diethylstilbestrol, which do not bind to SHBG, and is not blocked by antiestrogen such as tamoxifen. Both of these findings suggest that the classic estrogen receptor is not involved. On the other hand, DHT, which blocks the binding of estradiol to SHBG, completely negates the effect of estradiol on cAMP. Finally, the SHBG-estradiol-responsive second-messenger system has been primarily localized to the prostatic stromal cells and not to the epithelial cells.

Thus, estrogens may be causally linked to the onset of benign prostatic hyperplasia and may have an important supportive role in its maintenance. Aromatase inhibitors such as atamestane can result in marked reductions in both serum levels and intraprostatic concentrations of estrogens, including estradiol and estrone. However, to date, clinical trials with aromatase inhibitors for benign prostatic hyperplasia have been disappointing.

D. Growth Factors: Recent evidence suggests that prostatic growth is under the direct control of specific growth factors and only indirectly modulated by androgens. According to this evidence, growth factors from both the fibroblast growth factor (FGF) family and the TGF (transforming growth factor) "superfamily" act together to regulate growth. These growth factors are polypeptides that modulate cell proliferation. The FGF family stimulates cell division and growth: Basic fibroblast growth factor (bFGF) stimulates both growth of stroma and blood vessels (angiogenesis), and fibroblast growth factor 7 (FGF7, also known as keratinocyte growth factor [KGF]) stimulates growth of epithelial cells. On the other hand, members of the transforming growth factor-beta (TGF-β) family inhibit cell division. TGF-$β_1$

primarily inhibits growth of stroma and TGF-β_2 growth of epithelial cells. In the normal prostate, the rate of cell death is equaled by the rate of cell production. It is hypothesized that a balance exists in the stroma between the stimulatory effects of bFGF and the inhibitory effects of TGF-β_1 and in the epithelial glands between FGF7 stimulation and TGF-β_2 inhibition. In benign prostatic hyperplasia, when excess growth of stroma predominates, bFGF is overproduced relative to its regulator TGF-β_1; when excess growth of epithelial glands occurs, FGF7 is overproduced relative to TGF-β_2.

Other growth factors, including epidermal growth factor and insulin-like growth factors (IGF-I and IGF-II) are also known to stimulate prostatic tissue growth. Growth factors undoubtedly also play a role in the development of bladder hypertrophy in response to outflow obstruction (see below). TGF-β is known to stimulate collagen synthesis and deposition in the bladder.

Targeting peptide growth factors offers a potential means of regulating prostatic enlargement and relieving symptoms associated with benign prostatic hyperplasia. Preliminary clinical trials of growth factor antagonists have led to significant improvements in urinary symptoms, maximal flow rates, and residual volumes.

E. Prostatic Smooth Muscle and Adrenergic Receptors: Prostatic smooth muscle represents a significant proportion of the gland. Undoubtedly, both resting and dynamic prostatic smooth muscle tone play a major role in the pathophysiology of benign prostatic hyperplasia. Smooth muscle cells in the prostate—at the bladder neck and in the prostatic capsule—are richly populated with alpha-adrenergic receptors. Contraction of the prostate and bladder neck are mediated by α_1-adrenergic receptors. Stimulation of these receptors results in a dynamic increase in prostatic urethral resistance. Alpha$_1$-adrenergic receptor blockade clearly diminishes this response and has been found to improve symptoms, urinary flow rates, and residual urine volumes in patients with benign prostatic hyperplasia within 2–4 weeks after start of therapy. The selective α_1-blockers prazosin, terazosin, doxazosin, and alfuzosin have been extensively studied and found to be effective (Table 23–7). Because the bladder's smooth muscle cells do not contain a significant number of α_1 receptors, alpha-blocker therapy can selectively diminish urethral resistance without affecting detrusor smooth muscle contractility.

Recent studies have suggested that the α_1 receptors involved in the contraction of prostate smooth muscle appear to be α_{1a} receptors (previously called α_{1c} receptors). Clinical studies involving subtype-selective α_{1a} antagonists such as tamsulosin are under way.

Alpha-blockers may also work by changing the balance between prostate cell growth and death. Some investigators hypothesize that benign prostatic hyperplasia occurs as a result of a decrease in apoptosis (programmed cell death), allowing more cells to accumulate in the prostate, hence causing its enlargement. One alpha-blocker, doxazosin, has been shown to induce apoptosis in the stroma of the prostate.

F. Possible Mechanisms of Bladder Outlet Obstruction: There are several ways in which benign prostatic hyperplasia might cause obstruction of the bladder neck. The prominent median lobe may simply act as a ball valve, restriction may occur from the nondistensible capsule, static obstruction may result from the enlarged prostate surrounding the prostatic urethra, and dynamic obstruction may occur related to contraction of prostatic smooth muscle. In fact, there are clinical data supporting a role for each of these proposed factors. For example, transurethral resection of the prostate (TURP) frequently relieves obstructive symptoms, as does simple surgical incision of the prostatic capsule. Medications that shrink the prostate or relax smooth muscle also relieve bladder outlet obstruction and increase urinary flow rates.

Recently, various thermal therapies have been investigated as less invasive surgical procedures than TURP for benign prostatic hyperplasia—including transurethral microwave, high-intensity focused ultrasound, laser-delivered interstitial thermal therapies, and transurethral needle ablation of the prostate (TUNA). These procedures use different forms of energy such as microwave, ultrasound, laser, and radiofrequency to produce the thermal injury. It is unclear if these procedures work by anatomic shrinkage or debulking of the obstructing enlarged prostate or by physiologic alteration of voiding function. In pathologic studies of TUNA, for example, coagulative necrosis gradually changes to retractile fibrous scar. This could cause decrease in the volume of the treated area even without significant decrease in prostatic volume. Alternatively, severe thermal damage to intraprostatic nerve fibers may reduce the dynamic component of the bladder outlet obstruction by denervation of alpha receptors or sensory nerves.

Table 23–7. Alpha receptor blockade for benign prostatic hyperplasia.

Agent	Site and Mechanism of Action	Side Effects
Phenoxybenzamine	Pre- and postsynaptic α_1, α_2 blockade	Hypotension
Prazosin Terazosin Doxazosin Alfuzosin	Postsynaptic α_1 blockade	Hypotension (especially postural hypotension leading to syncope)
Tamsulosin	Postsynaptic α_{1a} blockade	

G. Bladder Response to Obstruction: Many of the clinical symptoms of benign prostatic hyperplasia are related to obstruction-induced changes in bladder function rather than to outflow obstruction per se. Thus, one-third of men continue to have significant voiding problems even after surgical relief of obstruction. Obstruction-induced changes in bladder function are of two basic types. First, there are changes that lead to **detrusor overactivity (instability).** These are clinically manifested by frequency and urgency. Second, there are changes that lead to **decreased detrusor contractility.** These are clinically manifested by symptoms of decreased force of the urinary stream, hesitancy, intermittency, increased residual urine, and, in a minority of cases, **detrusor failure.**

The bladder's response to obstruction is largely an adaptive one (Figure 23–13). The initial response is the development of detrusor smooth muscle hypertrophy. It is hypothesized that this increase in muscle mass, although an adaptive response to increased intravesical pressure and one that maintains urinary outflow, is associated with significant intra- and extracellular changes in smooth muscle cells that predispose to detrusor instability. In experimental animal models, unrelieved obstruction results in significant increases in detrusor extracellular matrix (collagen).

In addition to obstruction-induced changes in the smooth muscle cells and extracellular matrix of the bladder, there is increasing evidence that chronic obstruction in patients with untreated benign prostatic hyperplasia may alter neural responses as well, occasionally predisposing to detrusor failure.

Traditional therapies for symptoms associated with bladder obstruction have been directed toward relief of bladder outflow resistance. New treatments of obstructive detrusor instability have been suggested using drugs that are autonomically active (such as α_1 antagonists) and drugs that stabilize muscle cell membranes (such as anticholinergic agents).

The effects of chronic obstruction on the bladder are still not well understood. Future studies must examine the importance of changes in receptor density, affinity and distribution, and agonist release and degradation that occur during chronic obstruction and the ultrastructural and physiologic changes that occur with relief of obstruction.

Clinical Manifestations

A. Symptoms and Signs: Obstruction to urinary outflow and bladder dysfunction are responsible for the major symptoms and signs of benign prostatic hyperplasia. Prostatic enlargement may cause either acute or chronic urinary retention. With **acute urinary retention,** there is painful dilation of the bladder, with inability to void. Acute urinary retention is often precipitated by swelling of the prostate caused by infarction of a nodule or by certain medications. With **chronic urinary retention,** there are both obstructive and irritative voiding symptoms.

There are two types of symptoms. The irritative ones are related to bladder filling and the obstructive ones to bladder emptying. **Irritative symptoms** occur as a consequence of bladder hypertrophy and dysfunction and include urinary frequency, nocturia, and urgency. The patient commonly complains of difficulty initiating urination and decreased flow, causing decreased caliber and force of the urinary stream. **Obstructive symptoms** result from distortion and narrowing of the bladder neck and prostatic urethra, leading to incomplete emptying of the bladder. Obstructive symptoms include difficulty in initiating urination, decreased force and caliber of the urinary stream, intermittency of the urinary stream, urinary hesitancy, and dribbling.

To evaluate objectively the severity and complexity of symptoms in benign prostatic hyperplasia, a symptom index has been developed by the American Urologic Association. The self-administered questionnaire evaluates patient symptoms, such as bladder emptying, frequency, intermittency, urgency, and nocturia, and quality of life. The symptom index has been validated and found to have good test-retest reliability and to discriminate well between affected patients and controls. In clinical trials, there have been good correlations between urinary symptoms and the total score, and the instrument has proved useful to describe changes in symptoms over time and following treatment.

Complications of the chronic bladder dilation include hypertrophy of the bladder wall musculature and development of diverticula; urinary tract infec-

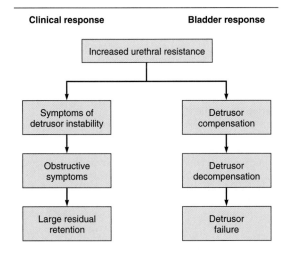

Figure 23–13. Schematic of natural history of benign prostatic hyperplasia. (Adapted, with permission, from McConnell JD: The pathophysiology of benign prostatic hyperplasia. J Androl 1991;11:356.)

tion of the stagnant bladder urine; hematuria, particularly with infarction of a prostatic nodule; and chronic renal failure and azotemia from bilateral hydroureter and hydronephrosis.

Digital rectal examination may reveal either focal or diffuse enlargement of the prostate. However, the size of the prostate as estimated by digital rectal examination does not correlate well with either the symptoms or signs of benign prostatic hyperplasia or the need for treatment. Examination of the lower abdomen may reveal a distended bladder, consistent with urinary retention, which may occur silently in the absence of severe symptoms.

B. Laboratory Tests and Evaluation: Laboratory tests performed to evaluate patients with benign prostatic hyperplasia include BUN and serum creatinine to exclude renal failure and urinalysis and urine culture to exclude urinary tract infection. **Intravenous pyelography (IVP)** or **ultrasonography (US)** is usually not performed in patients with normal findings on these simple laboratory tests. Instead, it is generally reserved for patients with hematuria or suspected hydronephrosis. When an IVP or US is done in men with benign prostatic hyperplasia, it typically shows elevation of the bladder base by the enlarged prostate; trabeculation, thickening, and diverticula of the bladder wall; elevation of the ureters; and poor emptying of the bladder. Uncommonly, the IVP or US shows hydronephrosis. The most useful technique for assessing the significance of benign prostatic hyperplasia is **urodynamic evaluation** with **uroflowmetry** and **cystometry**. In these tests, the patient voids and various measurements are made. In uroflowmetry, the maximal urinary flow rate is recorded. If the peak flow rate is less than 10 mL/s, the patient is considered to have significant bladder outlet obstruction. However, the patient must void at least 150 mL for the measurement to be considered reliable. **Pressure-flow studies** are simultaneous recordings of urinary bladder pressure and urinary flow rates, which provide information about urethral resistance. **Cystourethroscopy** is usually reserved for patients who have hematuria that remains unexplained despite an IVP or US, or preoperatively for patients who require transurethral resection of the prostate.

---

13. Which is the major androgen controlling prostate size?
14. What are some of the different ways in which androgens can be suppressed in order to decrease prostate size and obtain at least temporary relief of obstructive symptoms?
15. What are the effects of antiestrogen treatment on males with benign prostatic hyperplasia?
16. What is the role of (α_1-adrenergic receptors in benign prostatic hyperplasia?
17. What are some bladder changes that occur in patients with benign prostatic hyperplasia?
18. What are some symptoms and signs of benign prostatic hyperplasia?
19. How is the diagnosis of benign prostatic hyperplasia made?

REFERENCES

General
Chandrasoma P, Taylor CE: *Concise Pathology,* 3rd ed. Appleton & Lange, 1998.
Ganong WF: *Review of Medical Physiology,* 19th ed. Appleton & Lange, 1999.
Greenspan FS, Strewler GJ: *Basic and Clinical Endocrinology,* 5th ed. Appleton & Lange, 1997.
McClure RD: Male infertility. In: *Smith's General Urology,* 14th ed. Tanagho EA, McAninch JW (editors). Appleton & Lange, 1995.

Male Infertility
Barratt CL, St John JC: Diagnostic tools in male infertility. Hum Reprod 1998;13(Suppl 1):51.
Bhasin S, de Kretser DM, Baker HW: Pathophysiology and natural history of male infertility. J Clin Endocrinol Metab 1994;79:1525.
Chandley AC: Chromosome anomalies and Y chromosome microdeletions as causal factors in male infertility. Hum Reprod 1998;13(Suppl 1):45.
de Kretser DM: Male infertility. Lancet 1997;349:787.
Irvine DS: Epidemiology and aetiology of male infertility. Hum Reprod 1998;13(Suppl 1):33.
Nachtigall LB et al: Adult-onset idiopathic hypogonadotropic hypogonadism: A treatable form of male infertility. N Engl J Med 1997;336:410.

Benign Prostatic Hyperplasia
Agency for Health Care Policy and Research: Benign prostatic hyperplasia: Diagnosis and treatment. J Am Geriatr Soc 1998;46:1163.
Algaba F: Pathophysiology of benign prostatic hyperplasia. Eur Urol 1994;25(Suppl 1):3.
Beduschi MC, Beduschi R, Oesterling JE: Alpha-blockade therapy for benign prostatic hyperplasia: From a nonselective to a more selective alpha$_{1A}$-adrenergic antagonist. Urology 1998;51:861.
Desgrandchamps F: Clinical relevance of growth factor antagonists in the treatment of benign prostatic hyperplasia. Eur Urol 1997;32(Suppl 1):28.
Elbadawi A: Voiding dysfunction in benign prostatic hyperplasia: Trends, controversies and recent revela-

tions. I. Symptoms and urodynamics. Urology 1998;51(5A Suppl):62.

Elbadawi A: Voiding dysfunction in benign prostatic hyperplasia: Trends, controversies and recent revelations. II. Pathology and pathophysiology. Urology 1998;51(5A Suppl):73.

Kuritzky L: Benign prostatic hyperplasia. Compr Ther 1998;24:130.

Lawson RK: Role of growth factors in benign prostatic hyperplasia. Eur Urol 1997;32(Suppl 1):22.

Lepor H: The pathophysiology of lower urinary tract symptoms in the ageing male population. Br J Urol 1998;81(Suppl 1):29.

Mauroy B: Bladder consequences of prostatic obstruction. Eur Urol 1997;32(Suppl 1):3.

24 Inflammatory Rheumatic Diseases

Eric L. Greidinger, MD, & Antony Rosen, MD

Although the rheumatic diseases are highly variable in their expression, many of them have in common the presence of inflammation and consequent damage to connective tissues. The specific clinical and pathologic features of each entity in this category reflect the stimuli that initiate and propagate the inflammatory response, the particular tissues targeted, and the inflammatory effector mechanisms that predominate. Although the spectrum of inflammatory rheumatic diseases is broad, some general principles provide a framework within which to discuss the pathophysiology of all.

OVERVIEW OF INFLAMMATORY RHEUMATIC DISEASES

Diseases have discrete kinetics: initiation, propagation, and flares.

1. ACUTE DISEASES

The initiating force of acute diseases (eg, gout, immune complex vasculitis) is often exogenous and clearly recognizable (eg, crystal deposition or streptococcal skin infection). The disease is self-limited owing to the success of the inflammatory response in removing the initiating stimulus (eg, crystals in gout; decreasing the load of external antigen; see Figure 24–1). Flares occur upon reexposure to the initiating stimulus.

2. CHRONIC DISEASES

The initiating force in chronic diseases (eg, systemic lupus erythematosus) is often remote and no longer recognizable once the unique disease phenotype becomes fully established and the diagnosis clear. Propagation of the disease typically occurs as a result of an autoimmune response, inducing a self-amplifying cycle of damage. While initiation is rare, flares are frequent, probably reflecting the vast capacity of the immune system to "remember" previously encountered antigens and to respond to them with greater vigor and at lower concentrations when it encounters them again (Figure 24–1).

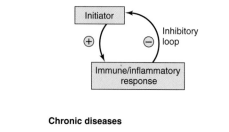
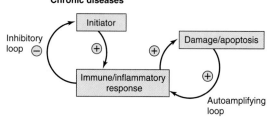

Figure 24–1. Kinetics of acute and chronic inflammatory rheumatic diseases.

Different tissues are affected in various diseases (eg, specific synovial joints in gout; skin, joints, kidney, nervous system, blood elements in SLE).

Recruitment and activation of specific subsets of inflammatory and immune cells is an essential determinant of the pathologic features. In this regard, the role of activation of regional blood vessel endothelium by proinflammatory cytokines (eg, TNF-α, IL-1) must be emphasized. Several cytokines induce the expression on endothelial cells of ligands for the adhesion-promoting receptors of inflammatory cells (integrins and selectins) and allow neutrophils and monocytes to adhere to the vessel wall in the inflamed area and migrate into the underlying tissues.

The pathologic features of the chronic inflammatory disorders reflect the combination of inflammatory damage and the consequences of healing.

Immune complex formation and deposition is an important pathophysiologic mechanism in autoimmune rheumatic diseases. Any antigen that elicits a humoral immune response may give rise to circulating immune complexes if the antigen remains present in significant quantities once antibody is generated. Immune complexes are efficiently cleared by the reticuloendothelial system and are rarely pathogenic. Pathogenicity is a function of the relative amounts of antigen and antibody and of the intrinsic features of the complex that determine overall composition, size, and solubility. Of particular significance in terms of pathogenicity are immune complexes formed at slight antigen excess that are soluble, are not effectively cleared by the reticuloendothelial system, and are of a size which allows them to gain access to and be deposited at subendothelial and extravascular sites (Figure 24–2). Thus, if foreign antigens (eg, drugs or infectious organisms) induce an antibody response and significant numbers of immune complexes of the appropriate size are formed, these complexes may be deposited (in skin, joints, kidney, blood vessel walls) where they activate several effector pathways (eg, FcR receptor, classic complement cascade) and where they may lead to skin rashes, arthritis, small vessel vasculitis, and glomerulonephritis. Clinical conditions in which this situation might arise include drug reactions, serum sickness, and infections (including infective endocarditis, streptococcal skin and pharyngeal infections, and others). Autoimmune diseases are characteristically antigen-driven, but in this case the humoral response is directed against self antigens (eg, nucleosomes in SLE). Under conditions leading to the liberation of significant amounts of self antigen from host tissue (cell damage or death), immune complex formation, Fc receptor binding, and complement activation may result. The consequences of immune complex formation and deposition are the same whether caused by foreign or self antigens.

Recent studies have emphasized the role of immunoglobulin Fc receptors in the activation of myelomonocytic cell effector function that results in tissue damage. Indeed, these receptors play a critical role in generating the pathologic picture characteristic of immune complex-mediated diseases (see below). For example, the immune complex-mediated renal disease and vasculitis that occur in several murine models of SLE are completely absent in the FcγR knockout mouse.

PATHOGENESIS OF INFLAMMATION

The nature of tissue damage and joint injury is determined in part by the inflammatory and immune effector functions that predominate.

1. CYTOKINES

Distinct classes of immune effector function are activated depending upon the pattern of cytokines that predominate during initiation of the inflammatory response. For example, some cytokines (eg, IL-12) produced by infected monocyte-macrophages skew the lymphocyte response toward TH1 cells (which generate the TH1 cytokines IL-2, interferon-γ, TNF-α) that are associated with activation of macrophage killing functions. In contrast, the presence of IL-4 during the initial response induces the differentiation of TH2 lymphocytes, which generate TH2 cytokines (eg, IL-4, IL-5, IL-6, and IL-10).

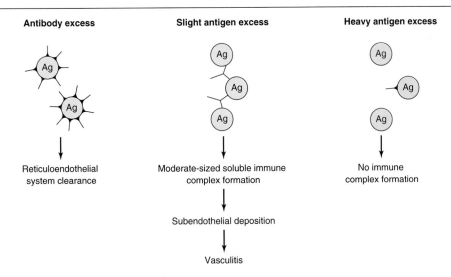

Figure 24–2. Immune complex formation. Impact of concentrations of antigens and antibodies.

These cytokines have their predominant function in the activation of B cells and antibody generation. Although significant overlap exists, specific pathologic features tend to accompany the different cytokine patterns (eg, granulomas for TH1 versus immune complex disease for TH2).

2. COMPLEMENT PATHWAY

The classic complement pathway is activated when antibody binds to its specific antigen. Activation of the complement cascade induces inflammatory cell recruitment and activation (with all the consequences mentioned above) as well as other features of the acute inflammatory response (eg, increased capillary permeability).

3. MYELOMONOCYTIC CELLS (MACROPHAGES & NEUTROPHILS)

While macrophages and neutrophils have numerous effector pathways that function to rid the host of foreign invaders, some of the products that normally serve this purpose can damage healthy tissue if released in large amounts. These include free radical species generated during the respiratory burst as well as a variety of secretory products contained in the granules of these inflammatory cells. Important granule contents include a variety of proteases such as cathepsins, elastase, and collagenase. These products are liberated into the extracellular medium in the inflammatory locus, where they accumulate and may have damaging effects on normal connective tissue. In addition, numerous proinflammatory mediators released in this environment (including TNF-α, IL-1, IL-6, prostaglandins, and leukotrienes) attract further inflammatory cells to the area.

4. CELLULAR CYTOTOXICITY

Lymphocyte-Mediated Cytotoxicity

Some T lymphocytes are capable of killing target cells. When target cell destruction exceeds the capacity for renewal, tissue hypofunction can result. As with other lymphocyte function, this effector function is activated only upon ligation of the T cell receptor by a specific peptide (bound within the cleft of an MHC molecule). Upon recognition of antigen on the surface of a target cell, cytotoxic T lymphocytes induce the death of those cells, using several distinct mechanisms. One prominent mechanism involves the Fas-Fas-ligand pathway, where FasL present on activated lymphocytes binds to the Fas receptor on target cells and activates target cell apoptosis. The second prominent mechanism involves the release of cytotoxic T lymphocyte secretory granules. These granules contain at least two distinct classes of proteins. One, called **perforin,** polymerizes to generate transmembrane pores in cell membranes. These pores allow water, salt, and proteins (including the second class of granule protein, the granzymes) to enter the target cell. The **granzymes,** a family comprising several proteases, target a number of critical cellular substrates and appear to activate the process of apoptosis (programmed cell death) within the target cell.

Antibody-Dependent Cellular Cytotoxicity

The destruction of antibody-coated target cells by natural killer cells is called antibody-dependent cellular cytotoxicity (ADCC) and occurs when the Fc receptor of an NK cell binds to the Fc portion of the surface-bound antibody. The cytotoxic mechanism involves the release of cytoplasmic granules containing perforin and granzymes into the cytoplasm of the antibody-coated cell (similar to cytotoxic T lymphocyte-mediated killing, described above). This mechanism has been implicated in many autoantibody-mediated syndromes, where the autoantigen is either at the cell surface or appears there following some insult. An example of this would be the photosensitive skin disease that occurs in patients with SLE who have the Ro autoantibody.

---

1. What is the hallmark of rheumatic diseases?
2. What three features account for the specific clinical and pathologic characteristics of different rheumatic diseases?
3. What are the six general principles of the pathogenesis of rheumatic diseases? Give an example of a disease that illustrates each.

PATHOPHYSIOLOGY OF SELECTED RHEUMATIC DISEASES

GOUT

Clinical Presentation

Gout is the classic example of crystal-induced inflammation of synovial joints. Deposition of crystals of monosodium urate causes episodes of intense acute pain and swelling (particularly in the great toe, foot, and ankle) which tend to resolve completely and spontaneously within a week even without treatment. If not properly treated, this completely resolving form of the disease can give way over many years to a chronic, destructive pattern resulting in significant joint deformity. Accumulations of uric acid crystals elsewhere in the body can lead to subcutaneous deposits known as tophi.

Etiology

The critical initiating factor in gout is the formation and deposition of monosodium urate crystals in the synovia of joints. This occurs when body fluids become supersaturated with uric acid (generally at serum levels > 7 mg/dL). Indeed, the level of serum hyperuricemia correlates well with the development of gout, with annual incidence rates of about 5% for serum uric acid levels of > 9 mg/dL. Increased levels of serum uric acid result from either underexcretion (90% of patients) or overproduction (10%) of uric acid. Decreased glomerular filtration rate is the most frequent cause of decreased excretion of uric acid and may be due to numerous causes (see Chapter 16). Diuretic usage is also a frequent cause of decreased excretion of uric acid. Overproduction defects can result from primary defects in the purine salvage pathway (eg, HPRT deficiency), leading to an increase in de novo purine synthesis, and high flux through the purine breakdown pathway. Diseases causing increased cell turnover (eg, myeloproliferative disorders) and DNA degradation are secondary causes of hyperuricemia.

Pathophysiology

Although the concentration of monosodium urate in joint fluid slowly equilibrates with that in the serum, formation of crystals is markedly influenced by physical factors such as temperature and blood flow. The propensity for gout to involve distal joints (eg, great toes and ankles), which are cooler than other body parts, probably reflects the presence of local physical conditions at these sites that favor crystal formation.

Monosodium urate crystals are not biologically inert, and their highly negatively charged surfaces function as efficient initiators of the acute inflammatory response. The crystals are potent activators of the classic complement pathway, generating complement cleavage products (eg, C3a, C5a) that are strong chemoattractants for neutrophil influx (Figure 24–3). The crystals also activate the kinin system and in that way induce local vasodilation, pain, and swelling. Phagocytosis of crystals by synovial macrophages stimulates the release of proinflammatory products (eg, TNF-α, IL-1, IL-8, PGE_2). These products increase adhesion molecule expression on local vessel endothelium to facilitate neutrophil adhesion and migration and are also potent chemoattractants for neutrophils. Neutrophils also amplify their own recruitment by releasing leukotriene B4 upon phagocytosis of urate crystals (Figure 24–3).

The intense inflammatory response of gout typically resolves spontaneously and completely over the course of several days even without therapy. This down-modulation of the inflammatory response is a typical fea-

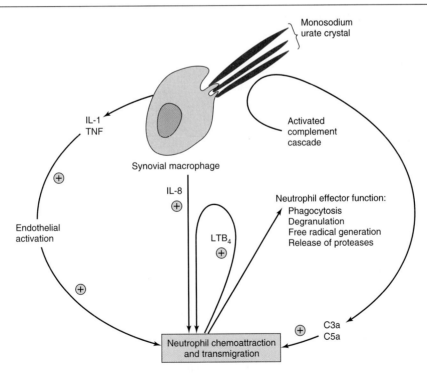

Figure 24–3. Mechanisms in initiation and amplification of the acute inflammatory response in gout involve both cytokines and humoral mediators.

Table 24–1. Mechanisms causing down-modulation of the inflammatory response in gout.

Efficient phagocytosis of crystals
Increased heat and fluid influx, favoring solubilization
Coating of crystals with serum proteins, shielding their pro-inflammatory surfaces
Secretion of anti-inflammatory cytokines (eg, TGF-β) by activated joint macrophages
Phagocytosis of apoptotic neutrophils, enhancing anti-inflammatory effects

---

ture of acute inflammation, where the inflammatory response itself successfully removes the proinflammatory stimulus (Table 24–1). Numerous mechanisms appear to be responsible: (1) efficient phagocytosis of crystals, preventing them from activating newly recruited inflammatory cells; (2) increased heat and fluid influx, altering local physicochemical conditions to favor crystal solubilization; (3) coating of crystals with serum proteins that leak into the joint during inflammation, rendering the surface of the crystals less inflammatory; (4) secretion of a variety of anti-inflammatory cytokines (eg, TGF-β) by activated joint macrophages; and (5) phagocytosis of previously activated apoptotic neutrophils by macrophages in the joint, altering the balance of cytokines secreted by these macrophages in such a way that secretion of proinflammatory cytokines is inhibited while anti-inflammatory cytokine secretion is enhanced.

Thus, gout represents a good example of an acute inflammatory response initiated by a proinflammatory initiating force. The response is acute, highly focused, self-limited rather than self-sustaining, and associated with little tissue destruction in the acute phase. Flares of disease represent recurrence of crystals in a proinflammatory form in the joints. Myelomonocytic cells and humoral factors (eg, cytokines and the complement and kinin cascades) are critical mediators of the acute syndrome.

Clinical Manifestations

A. Podagra and Episodic Oligoarticular Arthritis: Podagra, severe inflammatory arthritis at the first metatarsophalangeal joint, is the most frequent manifestation of gout. Patients typically describe waking in the middle of the night with dramatic pain, redness, swelling, and warmth at the area. Flares of gout typically produce one of the most intense forms of inflammatory arthritis. The toes—and, to a lesser extent, the ankles and knees—are the most common sites for gout flares. Gout flares frequently occur in circumstances that increase serum uric acid levels, such as metabolic stressors leading to increased DNA or ATP turnover (eg, sepsis or surgery) or dehydration. Agents that reduce prostaglandin synthesis (eg, nonsteroidal anti-inflammatory drugs), that reduce neutrophil immigration to the joints (eg, colchicine), or that decrease the activation of myelomonocytic cells (eg, corticosteroids) reduce the duration of a gouty flare.

Gouty arthritis can be diagnosed by examination of synovial fluid from an actively affected joint under a polarizing microscope. Monosodium urate crystals can be seen as negatively birefringent needle-like structures engulfed by myelomonocytic cells.

B. Formation of Tophi: Firm, irregular subcutaneous deposits of monosodium urate crystals occur in patients with chronic gout. Tophi most often form along tendinous tissues on the extensor surfaces of joints as well as on the outer helix of the ear.

C. Chronic Erosive Polyarthritis: In some patients, the total body burden of uric acid increases greatly over years, with deposits of monosodium urate crystals developing in multiple joints and resulting in a persistent but more indolent inflammatory arthritis. Joint deformities due to bone and cartilage erosions can develop. Renal tubular injury and nephrolithiasis can also develop under these conditions. Chronic drug therapy to decrease uric acid production (eg, xanthine oxidase inhibitors) or increase uric acid excretion (eg, uricosuric agents) can be used to avoid the chronic sequelae of gout.

---

4. What physical factors other than uric acid concentration influence crystal formation in gout?
5. What are some proinflammatory products released by synovial macrophages upon phagocytosis of urate crystals?
6. Suggest five reasons why the intense acute inflammatory response in gout typically resolves spontaneously over the course of several days even in the absence of therapy.
7. What are three metabolic conditions that can precipitate a gout flare?
8. Name three chronic sequelae of recurrent gout flares.

IMMUNE COMPLEX VASCULITIS

Clinical Presentation

Immune complex vasculitis is an acute inflammatory disease of small blood vessels that occurs in the setting of ongoing antigen load and an established humoral immune response. Tissues affected include skin, joints, and kidney, which demonstrate leukocytoclastic vasculitic rash, inflammatory arthritis of small and medium-sized synovial joints, and immune complex glomerulonephritis, respectively.

Etiology

Antigens are frequently derived from exogenous sources, including infections (eg, streptococcal skin infections) and numerous drugs (especially antibiotics), accounting for one of the names ("hypersensitivity vasculitis") given to this disorder. Release of endogenous antigens in the setting of an autoimmune response (eg, SLE; see below) may similarly initiate the vasculitic process.

Pathophysiology

Although immune complexes are generated in every antibody response, in the vast majority of cases they are not associated with pathologic effects. Their pathogenic potential is given effect when circulating immune complexes are deposited in the subendothelium, where they set in motion the complement cascade and activate myelomonocytic cells. This deposition of immune complexes in vessel walls depends on their physical characteristics, including size, and solubility. The solubility of immune complexes is not a fixed property, as it is profoundly influenced by the relative concentrations of antigen and antibody, which generally change as an immune response evolves. When antibody is in excess, immune complexes are rapidly cleared by the reticuloendothelial system. In contrast, when antigen is in excess, the soluble immune complexes gain access to the subendothelial space and cause injury. Thus, if the antigen is a drug, infectious organism, or foreign serum protein, the early antibody response occurs in the setting of large antigen excess, where complexes are soluble and potentially pathogenic. As the immune response progresses and titers of specific antibody rise, the size and solubility of these complexes decreases and they are more effectively cleared.

A classic example of the altered pathogenicity of immune complexes at various antigen:antibody ratios is serum sickness. (Penicillin-induced hypersensitivity vasculitis is a similar example.) When serum products from animals (eg, horses) are injected into humans for a therapeutic purpose (eg, as once used for passive immunization against snake venoms), the foreign serum proteins stimulate an immune response, with antibodies first appearing after approximately 1 week. Soon after antibody appears, patients develop fever, arthritis, vasculitis, and glomerulonephritis, consistent with deposition of soluble immune complexes and myelomonocytic cell activation at multiple sites. As the antibody titers rise, immune complexes are no longer formed at vast antigen excess but approach the zone of equivalence, and then antibody excess. They thus lose their pathogenicity as the immune response evolves. Provided that antigen administration is not sustained, the inflammatory disease will resolve spontaneously as those immune complexes that were deposited early (during the soluble phase) are cleared. Such significant clinical effects of immune complexes usually occur only when the initial antigen load is great—eg, due to a large bacterial load or drug ingestion.

Clinical Manifestations

Affected tissues are all highly enriched in small blood vessels, which are the target of injury in this syndrome.

A. Cutaneous Small Vessel Vasculitis: A frequent clinical presentation of immune complex-induced vasculitis in the skin is that of palpable purpura, which appear as red or violaceous papules. Cutaneous immune complex vasculitis seldom causes severe pain and only rarely leads to long-term injury.

B. Polyarthritis: The most common pattern of joint involvement with immune complex disease is an intense, self-limited symmetric polyarthritis. As the immune complexes are phagocytosed and cleared, the immune response remits unless further waves of immune complexes are deposited.

C. Glomerulonephritis: The nephrons are another extensive bed of small blood vessels where immune complexes are likely to be deposited. Acute immune complex glomerulonephritis causes proteinuria, hematuria, and the formation of red blood cell casts. In cases of extensive immune complex-mediated injury, immune complex vasculitis can cause oliguria and renal failure.

The most effective treatment for immune complex vasculitis is elimination of the inciting antigen (eg, by discontinuing an offending drug). Medications that reduce the degree of activation of myelomonocytic cells (eg, corticosteroids) are also helpful.

---

9. In what two immunologic settings does immune complex vasculitis occur?
10. What are the three most prominent organ systems affected by immune complex vasculitis? Describe the typical manifestations in each.
11. What three physical properties determine whether immune complexes will be deposited in vessel walls?
12. What happens once subendothelial deposition has occurred?
13. Why does pathogenicity of immune complexes generally decrease as antibody titers rise?

SYSTEMIC LUPUS ERYTHEMATOSUS

Clinical Presentation

Systemic lupus erythematosus (SLE), often referred to as "lupus," is the prototypical systemic autoimmune rheumatic disease, characterized by chronic inflammatory damage of multiple organ systems. A key feature of the disease is the unique adaptive immune response, driven by antigens contained in self tissues, which is apparently responsible for much of the widespread pathologic consequences of this disease. SLE is characteristically episodic, with a course characterized by flares and remissions. It is also highly variable in severity, ranging from mild to life-threatening. Tissues frequently affected include the skin, joints, kidneys, blood elements, and brain.

Epidemiology

The prevalence of SLE is approximately 30:100,000 in the general population in the United States. It occurs approximately nine times more frequently in women than in men and is most prevalent in blacks.

Etiology

SLE is a complex disease due to an interplay between inherited susceptibilities (over 20 different genetic loci) and poorly defined environmental factors. Genetic deficiencies of the proximal components of the classic complement pathway (eg, C1q, C1r, C1s, C4), while rare in most populations, are the strongest risk factors defined to date. Recent studies have demonstrated that the classic complement pathway is required for the efficient clearance of apoptotic cells by macrophages, and the development of lupus in individuals with these deficiencies may relate to impaired clearance of apoptotic cells in this setting (see below). The mechanisms whereby environmental factors (eg, drugs, viral infections) function to initiate or propagate lupus are not understood.

Pathophysiology

It is useful to view the pathogenesis of lupus in discrete kinetic phases even though the phases are not clearly separable clinically. Indeed, it is likely that events underlying initiation occur prior to the onset of clinically defined disease, which requires chronic amplification of the propagation phase to become clinically apparent.

A. Initiation: The exuberant autoantibody response in lupus targets a highly specific group of self antigens (see Table 24–2). Although this group of autoantigens does not share common features (eg, structure, distribution, or function) in healthy cells, these molecules are unified during apoptotic cell death, when they become clustered and structurally modified in apoptotic surface blebs (Figure 24–4). Indeed, recent studies suggest that the initiating event in lupus is a unique form of apoptotic cell death that occurs in a proimmune context (eg, viral infection).

A critical susceptibility defect for the development

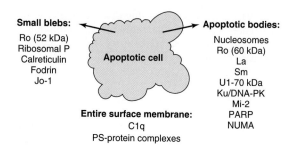

Figure 24–4. Autoantigens, while sharing no features in healthy cells, become unified in apoptotic cells. Here, they become clustered at the surface of the apoptotic cells, and this structure is modified.

and propagation of SLE appears to be impairment of normal clearance of apoptotic cells in tissues. Thus, in normal individuals, the fate of most apoptotic cells in tissues is rapid and efficient phagocytosis by macrophages, and antigens ingested in this way are rapidly degraded. Furthermore, phagocytosis of apoptotic cells inhibits secretion of proinflammatory cytokines from macrophages and induces secretion of several anti-inflammatory cytokines, contributing to the impaired ability of apoptotic cells to initiate a primary immune response. Lastly, the avid phagocytosis of apoptotic cells by normal macrophages prevents significant numbers from accessing dendritic cell populations (which are highly efficient initiators of primary immune responses). Together, these factors ensure that normal individuals do not efficiently immunize themselves with apoptotic material derived from their own tissues. In contrast, impaired clearance of apoptotic cells is observed in a subgroup of patients with SLE. Under conditions where apoptotic material is not efficiently cleared by macrophages (eg, in C1q deficiency), suprathreshold amounts of this material may gain access to potent antigen-presenting cell populations under proimmune conditions and initiate a response to molecules whose structure has been modified during apoptotic cell death.

B. Propagation: Autoantibodies in lupus can cause tissue injury by a variety of mechanisms:

1. The most frequent pathogenic mechanism is generation and deposition of immune complexes, in which antigen is derived from damaged and dying cells. When the concentration and size of the relevant complexes favors subendothelial deposition, these markedly proinflammatory complexes initiate inflammatory effector functions that result in tissue damage (see above). Of particular importance is the ability of immune complexes to ligate the Fcγ receptor, which activates myelomonocytic cell effector functions.

2. Autoantibodies bind to extracellular molecules in the target organs and activate inflammatory

Table 24–2. Autoantigens in systemic lupus erythematosus.

Nuclear	Nucleosomes (dsDNA and histone core)
	Ribonucleoprotein complexes
	  Sm
	  nRNP
	  Ro (60 kDa)
	  La

Cytoplasmic	Ribosomal protein P Ro (52 kDa)
Membrane-associated	Anionic phospholipids or phospholipid-binding proteins

effector functions at that site, with consequent tissue damage.

3. Autoantibodies directly induce cell death by ligating cell surface molecules or by penetrating into living cells and exerting functional effects.

It is important to note that the intracellular antigens which drive the immune response in lupus can be derived from damaged or apoptotic cells. Such damage or apoptosis occurs commonly in the course of immune effector pathways. Thus, these effector pathways can generate additional antigen, further stimulating the immune system and generating additional antigen. This autoamplification is a central feature of the propagation phase of lupus.

C. Flares: One of the characteristic features of an immune response is the establishment of immunologic memory, so that when it again encounters the antigen the immune system responds more rapidly and vigorously to lower concentrations than were required for the primary response. Flares in lupus appear to reflect immunologic memory, occurring in response to rechallenge of the primed immune system with antigen. Apoptosis not only occurs during cell development and homeostasis (particularly of hematopoietic and epithelial cells) but also in many disease states. Thus, numerous stimuli (eg, UV light exposure, viral infection, endometrial and breast epithelial involution) may provoke disease flares.

Clinical Manifestations

SLE is a multisystem autoimmune disease that affects predominantly women during the childbearing years (mean age at diagnosis is 30). It is characterized clinically by periodicity, and the numerous exacerbations that occur over the years are termed flares. The symptoms are highly variable but tend to be stereotyped in a given individual (ie, the prominent clinical features often remain constant over years). Production of specific autoantibodies is a universal feature. Several organ systems are frequently affected. Prominent among these is the skin, where photosensitivity and a variety of lupus-specific skin rashes (including a rash over the malar region) are frequent. Like those with other immune complex-mediated diseases, lupus patients may manifest a nonerosive symmetric arthritis. Renal disease, which takes the form of a spectrum of glomerulonephritides, is a frequent major cause of morbidity and mortality. Patients may manifest a variety of hematologic symptoms (including hemolytic anemia, thrombocytopenia, and leukopenia) as well as several neurologic syndromes (eg, seizures and organic brain syndrome).

---

14. What are the antigens against which antibodies are directed in SLE?
15. How many different genetic loci are believed to confer susceptibility to development of SLE? Which are the strongest ones?
16. What is believed to be the relationship of apoptosis to the initiation of SLE?
17. What prevents normal individuals from being immunized to apoptotic cell debris, and why does this host defense break down in patients with SLE?
18. What are three stimuli that typically provoke SLE flares?
19. What are the most prominently affected organ systems in SLE?

REFERENCES

General

Gallin JI et al (editors): *Inflammation: Basic Principles and Clinical Correlates,* 2nd ed. Raven, 1992.

Lanzavecchia A: How can cryptic epitopes trigger autoimmunity? J Exp Med 1995;181:1945.

Sercarz EE et al: Dominance and crypticity of T cell antigenic determinants. Ann Rev Immunol 1993;11:729.

Sneller MC, Fauci AS: Pathogenesis of vasculitis syndromes. Med Clin North Am 1997;81:221.

Gout

Kelley WN, Wortmann RL: Gout and hyperuricemia. In: *Textbook of Rheumatology,* 5th ed. Kelley WN et al (editors). Saunders, 1997.

Roubenoff R et al: Incidence and risk factors for gout in white men. JAMA 1991;266:3004.

Systemic Lupus Erythematosus

Botto M et al: Homozygous C1q deficiency causes glomerulonephritis associated with multiple apoptotic bodies. Nat Genet 1998;19:56.

Casciola-Rosen L, Rosen A: Ultraviolet light-induced keratinocyte apoptosis: A potential mechanism for the induction of skin lesions and autoantibody production in LE. Lupus 1997;6:175.

Klippel JH: Systemic lupus erythematosus: Demographics, prognosis, and outcome. J Rheum 1997;48:67.

Salmon JE et al: FcgammaRIIA alleles are heritable risk factors for lupus nephritis in African Americans. J Clin Invest 1996;97:1348.

25 Illustrative Case Studies

Eva M. Aagaard, MD

CASES & QUESTIONS
(Answers begin on page 593.)

CASE 1

A 4-year-old boy is brought in with pain and swelling of the right thigh after a fall in the home. An x-ray reveals an acute fracture of the right femur. Further questioning of the mother reveals that the boy has had two other known fractures—left humerus and left tibia—both with minimal trauma. The family history is notable for "a genetic bone problem" in the boy's father that got better as he grew into adulthood. A diagnosis of osteogenesis imperfecta is entertained.

Questions: Case 1
A. What are the four types of osteogenesis imperfecta? How are they genetically transmitted?
B. Which two types are most likely in this patient? How might they be distinguished clinically?
C. Further workup results in a diagnosis of type I osteogenesis imperfecta. What clinical features may the boy expect in adult life?
D. What is the pathogenesis of this patient's disease?

CASE 2

A young woman is referred for genetic counseling. She has a 3-year-old boy with developmental delay and small joint hyperextensibilty. The pediatrician has diagnosed fragile X-associated mental retardation. She is currently pregnant with her second child at 14 weeks of gestation. The family history is unremarkable. There is no family history of developmental delay.

Questions: Case 2
A. What is the genetic mutation responsible for fragile X-associated mental retardation? How does it cause the clinical syndrome of developmental delay, joint hyperextensibility, large testes, and facial abnormalities?
B. Which parent is the probable carrier of the genetic mutation? Explain the mechanism by which this parent and the grandparents are phenotypically unaffected.
C. What is the likelihood that the unborn child will be affected?

CASE 3

A 40-year-old woman, recently married and pregnant for the first time, comes to clinic with a question about the chances of having "a Down's baby."

Questions: Case 3
A. What is the rate of occurrence of Down's syndrome in the general population? What are some of the its common clinical features?
B. What major genetic abnormalities are associated with Down's syndrome? How might these abnormalities lead to the clinical features of the syndrome?
C. How might this woman's age contribute to her risk of having a child with Down's syndrome?

CASE 4

A newborn girl of Yemenite Jewish descent presents in pediatric clinic. A screening test for phenylketonuria was suggestive of the disease.

Questions: Case 4
A. What is the incidence of phenylketonuria in the general population? How does the risk differ among ethnic groups?
B. What is the primary defect in phenylketonuria?
C. What are the clinical manifestations of phenylketonuria? What is the pathophysiology underlying them?
D. How can phenylketonuria be treated?

E. When this child is of childbearing age, what should she be told about the risks to her fetus should she become pregnant?

CASE 5

A 2-month-old child is admitted to the intensive care unit with fever, hypotension, tachycardia, and lethargy. The past medical history is notable for a similar hospitalization at 2 weeks of age. Physical examination is notable for a temperature of 39 °C, oral candidiasis, and rales in the right lung field. Chest x-ray reveals multilobar pneumonia. Given the history of recurrent severe infection, the pediatrician suspects an immunodeficiency disorder.

Questions: Case 5
A. What is the most likely immunodeficiency in this child? Why?
B. What are the underlying genetic and cellular defects associated with this disease?
C. What is the overall prognosis for patients with this disorder?

CASE 6

An 18-year-old male presents with complaints of fever, facial pain, and nasal congestion consistent with a diagnosis of acute sinusitis. The past medical history is notable for multiple sinus infections, two episodes of pneumonia, and chronic diarrhea—all suggestive of primary immunodeficiency syndrome. Workup establishes a diagnosis of common variable immunodeficiency.

Questions: Case 6
A. What are the common infectious manifestations of common variable immunodeficiency?
B. What are the underlying immunologic abnormalities responsible for these infectious manifestations?
C. What other diseases is this patient at increased risk for?
D. What treatment is indicated?

CASE 7

A 31-year-old male injection drug user presents to the emergency department with a chief complaint of shortness of breath. He describes a 1-month history of intermittent fevers and night sweats associated with a nonproductive cough. He has become progressively more short of breath, initially only with exertion, but now he feels dyspneic at rest. He appears to be in moderate respiratory distress. His vital signs are abnormal with fever to 39 °C, heart rate of 112 bpm, respiratory rate of 20/min, and oxygen saturation of 88% on room air. Physical examination is otherwise unremarkable—but notable for the absence of abnormal lung sounds. Chest x-ray reveals a diffuse interstitial infiltrate characteristic of *Pneumocystis carinii* pneumonia, an opportunistic infection.

Questions: Case 7
A. What is the underlying disease most likely responsible for this man's susceptibility to pneumocystis pneumonia?
B. What is the pathogenesis of the immunosuppression caused by this underlying disease?
C. What is the natural history of this disease? What are some of the common clinical manifestations seen during its progression?

CASE 8

A 54-year-old man presents to the clinic for routine medical care. He is well, with no physical complaints. The history is remarkable only for a father with colon cancer at age 55. Physical examination is normal. Cancer screening is discussed, and the patient is sent home with fecal occult blood testing supplies. The results are positive. Colonoscopy reveals a villous adenoma as well as a 2 cm carcinoma.

Questions: Case 8
A. How are the two lesions thought to be related?
B. What are the two principal lines of evidence in favor of such a model?
C. What is the explanation for the presence of occult blood in stools of patients with even early colorectal cancer?

CASE 9

A 25-year-old man presents with complaints of testicular enlargement. Examination reveals a hard nodule on the left testicle, 2 cm in diameter. Biopsy is diagnostic of testicular cancer.

Questions: Case 9
A. From what cellular elements of the testes does testicular cancer generally arise? What is the normal development of these cells?
B. In addition to the testes, where else might testicular cancer arise? What is the explanation for this distribution?
C. What serum markers might be followed to evaluate disease progression and response to therapy?

CASE 10

A 28-year-old woman presents to her primary care physician with complaints of fatigue, intermittent fevers, and 5 lb. weight loss over a 6-week period. Her past medical history is remarkable for a renal transplant at age 15 performed for end-stage renal disease due to poststreptococcal glomerulonephritis. Physical examination reveals two enlarged, matted, nontender lymph nodes in the left anterior cervical chain; a firm, nontender, 1.5 cm lymph node in the right groin; and an enlarged liver. Biopsy of the lymph nodes in the cervical region reveals follicular, cleaved cell lymphoma.

Questions: Case 10
A. One theory states that chronic immune stimulation or modulation may be an early step in lymphomagenesis. What observations support this view?
B. How would one classify her lymphoma? What are some characteristics of this grade of lymphoma?
C. From which cell line do follicular lymphomas originate? What are some of the common genetic mutations seen with this type of lymphoma? How might one of these mutations contribute to the formation of lymphoma?
D. What is the pathophysiologic mechanism causing this patient's fever and weight loss?

CASE 11

A 65-year-old previously well man presents to the clinic with complaints of fatigue of 3 months' duration. Questioning reveals diffuse weakness and feeling "winded" when walking uphill or climbing more than one flight of stairs. All of the symptoms have slowly worsened over time. There are no other complaints, and the review of systems is otherwise negative. The patient has no significant past medical history, social history, or family history. On physical examination, he appears somewhat pale, with normal vital signs. The physical examination is unremarkable except for his rectal examination, which reveals brown, guaiac-positive stool. A blood test reveals anemia.

Questions: Case 11
A. What is the most likely form of anemia in this man? What is the probable underlying cause?
B. What is the mechanism by which this disorder results in anemia?
C. What might one expect to see in the peripheral blood smear?
D. What other tests might be ordered to confirm the diagnosis?
E. What is the pathophysiologic mechanism of the patient's fatigue, weakness, and shortness of breath? Why is he pale?

CASE 12

A 58-year-old black woman presents to the emergency room with complaints of progressive fatigue and weakness for the past 6 months. She is short of breath after walking several blocks. On review of systems she mentions mild diarrhea. She has noted intermittent numbness and tingling of her lower extremities and a loss of balance while walking. She denies other neurologic or cardiac symptoms and has no history of black or bloody stools or other blood loss. On physical examination she is tachycardiac to 110 bpm; other vital signs are within normal limits. Head and neck examination is notable for pale conjunctivas and a beefy red tongue with loss of papillae. Cardiac examination shows a rapid regular rhythm with a grade 2/6 systolic murmur at the left sternal border. Lung, abdominal, and rectal examinations are normal. Neurologic examination reveals decreased sensation to light touch and vibration in the lower extremities. The hematology consultant on call is asked to see this patient because of a low hematocrit.

Questions: Case 12
A. What vitamin deficiency is the probable cause of this woman's anemia? How does this result in anemia?
B. What might one expect the peripheral blood smear to look like? What other blood tests may be ordered, and what results are anticipated? What test might differentiate the various causes of this vitamin deficiency?
C. Workup reveals pernicious anemia. What is the pathogenesis of this disease? What is the evidence to support an autoimmune origin?
D. What is the pathophysiologic mechanism of this woman's symptoms of tachycardia, paresthesias, and impaired proprioception?

CASE 13

A 6-year-old boy presents to the pediatric emergency department. His mother states that he has had 3 days of general malaise and fevers to 38.5 °C.
He has no other localizing symptoms. The past medical history is remarkable for multiple febrile illnesses. His mother says, "It seems like he gets sick every month." Physical examination is notable for cervical lymphadenopathy and oral ulcers. Blood tests reveal a neutrophil count of 200/µL. The patient is admitted to the hospital. Blood, urine, and cerebrospinal fluid cultures are negative, and over 48 hours his neutrophil counts return to normal. He is then discharged.

He returns to the emergency department a few weeks later with the same presentation. The pediatric resident admits him to the hospital for further workup of his fevers and neutropenia. A diagnosis of cyclic neutropenia is entertained.

Questions: Case 13
A. What is the likely pathogenesis of cyclic neutropenia? What evidence supports this theory?
B. What aspects of this case presentation support the diagnosis of cyclic neutropenia? What is the expected clinical course?
C. Assuming that the diagnosis of cyclic neutropenia is correct, what would one expect the peripheral blood smear to look like? What would the bone marrow examination results be at this second admission? What would they be in 2 weeks?

CASE 14

A 36-year-old man was admitted to hospital 5 days ago after sustaining multiple fractures to the lower extremities by jumping from a three-story building in a suicide attempt. His fractures required surgical repair. He has no significant past medical history. Current medications include morphine for pain and subcutaneous heparin for prophylaxis against deep vein thrombosis. Consultation with a hematologist is requested because of a dropping platelet count. On physical examination, the patient has multiple bruises, and his lower extremities are casted bilaterally. Examination is otherwise normal. Laboratory tests from the last several days reveal a platelet count that has dropped from 170,000/µL on admission to 30,000/µL today.

Questions: Case 14
A. What is the most likely cause of this man's thrombocytopenia?
B. By what mechanisms does thrombocytopenia occur in patients with this disorder?
C. What are the possible clinical consequences of this patient's thrombocytopenia?

CASE 15

A 23-year-old woman presents to the emergency room with a chief complaint of shortness of breath of acute onset. It was associated with right-sided chest pain, which increased with inspiration. She denies fever, chills, cough, or other respiratory symptoms. She has had no lower extremity swelling. She has not been ill, bedridden, or immobile for prolonged periods. The past medical history is notable for an episode of deep vein thrombosis in the right lower extremity while taking oral contraceptives—about 2 years ago. She has been otherwise healthy and is currently taking no medications. The family history is notable for a father who died of a pulmonary embolism. On physical examination she appears anxious and in mild respiratory distress. She is tachycardic to 110 bpm, with a respiratory rate of 20/min. She has no fever, and blood pressure is stable. The remainder of the physical examination is normal. Chest x-ray is normal. Ventilation-perfusion scan reveals a high probability of pulmonary embolus. Given her prior history of deep vein thrombosis, a hypercoagulable state is suspected.

Questions: Case 15
A. What constitutes "Virchow's triad" of predisposing factors for venous thrombosis? Which components of the triad may be present in this patient?
B. What are some causes of inherited hypercoagulable states? How do they result in hypercoagulability?
C. How might this woman be evaluated for the presence of an inherited hypercoagulable state?

CASE 16

A 35-year-old woman presents to the clinic with a chief complaint of double vision. She reports intermittent and progressively worsening double vision for approximately 2 months—rarely at first, but now every day. She works as a computer programmer, and the symptoms increase the longer she stares at the computer screen. She has also noted a drooping of her eyelids that also seems to worsen with prolonged working at the screen. Both symptoms subside with rest. She is generally fatigued but has noted no other weakness or neurologic symptoms. The past medical history is unremarkable. Physical examination is notable only for the neurologic findings. Cranial nerve examination discloses a right sixth nerve palsy and bilateral ptosis which worsen with repetitive eye movements. Motor, sensory, and reflex examinations are otherwise unremarkable.

Questions: Case 16
A. What is the likely diagnosis? What is the pathogenesis of this disease?
B. What other neurologic manifestations might one expect to see?
C. What is the mechanism by which this patient's ocular muscle weakness increases with prolonged activity?
D. What associated conditions should be investigated in this patient?
E. What treatments should be considered?

CASE 17

A middle-aged man is transported to the emergency room unconscious and accompanied by a nurse from the medical floor. The nurse states that the patient was in line in front of her in the hospital cafeteria when he suddenly fell to the floor. He then had a "generalized tonic-clonic seizure." She called for assistance and accompanied him to the emergency room. No other historical information is available. On physical examination, the patient is confused and unresponsive to commands. He is breathing adequately and has oxygen in place via nasal prongs. His vital signs are as follows: temperature 38 °C, blood pressure 170/90 mm Hg, heart rate 105 bpm, and respiratory rate 18/min. Oxygen saturation is 99% on 2 L of oxygen. Neurologic examination is notable for reactive pupils of 3 mm, intact gag reflex, decreased movement of the left side of the body, and Babinski reflexes bilaterally. Examination is otherwise unremarkable.

Questions: Case 17
A. Describe what is meant by a generalized tonic-clonic seizure.
B. What are some of the underlying causes of seizure disorders? Which cause might you be most concerned about in this patient?
C. What is the pathophysiology of seizures?

CASE 18

A 72-year-old man presents to the emergency room with acute onset of right-sided weakness. The patient was eating breakfast when he suddenly lost strength in the right side of his body, such that he was unable to move his right arm or leg. He also noted a loss of sensation in the right arm and leg and difficulty in speaking. His wife called 911 and he was brought to the emergency room. His past medical history is remarkable for long-standing hypertension, hypercholesterolemia, and recently diagnosed coronary artery disease. On physical examination, his blood pressure is 190/100 mm Hg. Neurologic examination is notable for right facial droop and a dense right hemiparesis. The Babinski reflex is present on the right. CT scan of the brain shows no evidence of hemorrhage. He is admitted to the neurologic intensive care unit.

Questions: Case 18
A. What is the diagnosis? Which artery or vascular territory is apt to be involved?
B. What are some risk factors for this condition?
C. What are the possible mechanisms by which this man developed these focal neurologic deficits? Which are most likely in this patient? Why?
D. What underlying disorder may be responsible? How does it result in stroke?

CASE 19

A 25-year-old woman presents with the complaint of a rash that has developed over the last several weeks and seems to be progressing. On examination, she is noted to have several plaque-like lesions over the extensor surfaces of both upper and lower extremities as well as similar lesions on her scalp. The plaques are erythematous with silvery scales and are sharply marginated.

Questions: Case 19
A. What is the likely diagnosis? Is this skin disease genetic, environmental, or both? Based on what evidence?
B. What are the pathophysiologic mechanisms behind the development of the plaques, scale, and erythema characteristic of this disorder?
C. What immunologic defects have been implicated in patients with this skin disease?

CASE 20

A 35-year-old woman presents to clinic with complaints of a rash. She states that she recently returned from Africa. During her trip, she developed an itchy rash on both arms. She has an unremarkable past medical history. Medications recently taken include chloroquine for malaria prophylaxis. Examination discloses multiple small violaceous papules on the flexor surfaces of the arms. The lesions have angular borders and flat tops. Some of the lesions have white streaks on their surfaces.

Questions: Case 20
A. What is the likely diagnosis? What is the possible underlying cause?
B. What is the pathophysiologic mechanism by which these skin lesions are formed?
C. What histopathologic changes in the skin are responsible for the appearance of these lesions as violaceous papules with white striae?

CASE 21

A 27-year-old woman presents to the urgent care clinic with complaint of a red, itchy rash developing suddenly the day before on her arms and legs and then spreading to the trunk. She denies ulcers in the mouth or genital area. The past medical history is unremarkable except for occasional episodes of genital herpes. The most recent outbreak was approximately 2 weeks ago. She generally takes oral acyclovir on such occasions, but her prescription has run out and so she did not take any with her last bout. On physical examination, she has multiple thin, erythematous papules over the arms, legs, and trunk. Many of the papules have a central area of duskiness or clearing, such that the lesions resemble targets. She has no evidence of mucosal involvement.

Questions: Case 21
A. What is the likely diagnosis?
B. What is the pathophysiologic mechanism by which these skin lesions are formed? How is this disease similar to and different from lichen planus?

C. What factors may have triggered this rash? What evidence supports this link?
D. What is responsible for the target-like appearance of these lesions, and what does the histopathology show?

CASE 22

A 65-year-old man presents to the dermatology clinic with the complaint of "blisters" developing on his abdomen and extremities over the last week. Initially, the lesions were red patches, followed by the blister formation. The lesions are not painful, but they do itch. He has no other complaints and denies mucous membrane involvement. Examination shows only multiple large, tense blisters with an erythematous base over the lower trunk and extremities. The clinical picture is felt to be most consistent with bullous pemphigoid.

Questions: Case 22
A. What is the major differential diagnosis? How do these two diseases differ, and why is the distinction important?
B. Assuming the diagnosis of bullous pemphigoid is correct, what would one expect histologic examination to show?
C. What would one expect to find on direct immunofluorescence microscopy? To what are these autoantibodies bound?
D. What is the presumed mechanism by which blister formation occurs in bullous pemphigoid?

CASE 23

A 60-year-old man presents to the clinic with complaints of a recurring rash. He states that for the last 2–3 months he has had several episodes of a painless, nonpruritic rash over his distal lower extremities. The lesions are described as purple and raised. The past medical history is remarkable for hepatitis C—with no history of cirrhosis—and peripheral neuropathy. The patient has recently been treated for pneumonia with amoxicillin. He has taken no other medications. Physical examination is notable only for multiple reddish purple papules over the distal lower extremities, consistent with palpable purpura. The underlying skin is hyperpigmented. Biopsy reveals neutrophils, neutrophilic debris, and amorphous protein deposits involving the small blood vessels, consistent with fibrinoid necrosis.

Questions: Case 23
A. What is the likely dermatologic diagnosis? What are some possible precipitants of the disease in this patient?
B. What is the underlying pathogenetic mechanism by which the lesions are formed?

C. What histologic characteristics are responsible for the appearance of the lesions as papular and purpuric?
D. What additional symptoms should be inquired about in this patient? Should any laboratory tests be ordered?

CASE 24

A 55-year-old man who recently immigrated from China presents to the emergency department with fever. He states that he has had recurring fevers of 3 weeks' duration, associated with chills, night sweats, and malaise. Today he developed new painful lesions on the pads of his fingers, prompting him to come to the emergency room. His past medical history is remarkable for "being very sick as a child after a sore throat." He has recently had several teeth extracted for severe dental caries. He is taking no medications. On physical examination, he is febrile to 38.5 °C, blood pressure 120/80 mm Hg, heart rate 108 bpm, respiratory rate 16/min, with an oxygen saturation of 97% on room air. Skin examination is remarkable for painful nodules on the pads of several fingers and toes. He has multiple splinter hemorrhages in the nail beds and painless hemorrhagic macules on the palms of the hands. Funduscopic examination is remarkable for Roth spots. Chest examination is clear to auscultation and percussion. Cardiac examination is notable for a grade 3/6 holosystolic murmur heard loudest at the left lower sternal border, with radiation to the axilla. Abdominal and back examinations are unremarkable.

Questions: Case 24
A. What is the likely diagnosis? What are some common predisposing factors to this disease? Which is most likely in this patient?
B. Which infectious agents are most likely to be involved?
C. What hemodynamic factors predispose to this disease? How do these factors contribute to the establishment of this disease and resistance to normal host immune response?
D. What is the name given to the various lesions found on this man's hands and feet? What is the pathogenetic mechanism responsible for their formation?
E. What are some other common clinical manifestations of this disease? What is the most common cause of death in this disease?

CASE 25

A 25-year-old man presents to the emergency room with fever and altered mental status. He is accompanied by his wife, who provides the history. She states that her husband had been well until approximately 1 week ago, when he developed symptoms of an upper respiratory infection that were slow to improve. On the morning of admission, he complained of progressive severe headache and nausea. He vomited once. He became progressively lethargic as the day progressed, and she called for an ambulance to bring him to the hospital. He has no other medical problems and takes no medications. On examination, he is febrile to 39 °C, with a blood pressure of 95/60 mm Hg, heart rate of 100 bpm, and respiratory rate of 18/min. He is lethargic and confused, lying with his hand over his eyes. Funduscopic examination shows no papilledema. The neck is stiff, with a positive Brudzinski sign (flexion of the hip and knee with flexion of the neck). Heart, lung, and abdominal examinations are unremarkable. Neurologic examination is limited by his inability to cooperate but appears to be nonfocal. Kernig's sign (resistance to passive extension of the flexed leg with the patient lying supine) is negative.

Questions: Case 25
A. What diagnosis is suggested? What are the most likely etiologic agents in this patient? What would they be if he were a newborn? How about if he were a child?
B. What is the pathophysiologic sequence of events in the development of this disease? What features of the pathogens involved facilitate their ability to produce this disease?
C. What are the causes of cerebral edema in these patients?
D. What tests should be performed to confirm the diagnosis? What treatments should be started? Why?

CASE 26

A 68-year-old man presents to the hospital emergency department with fever and persistent cough. He has had cough productive of green sputum for 3 days, associated with shortness of breath, left-sided pleuritic chest pain, fever, chills, and night sweats. His past medical history is notable for COPD, requiring intermittent steroid use. His medications include albuterol, ipratropium bromide, and steroid inhalers. On examination, he is febrile to 38 °C, with a blood pressure of 110/50 mm Hg, heart rate of 98 bpm, and respiratory rate of 20/min. Oxygen saturation is 92% on room air. He is a thin man in moderate respiratory distress, speaking in sentences of three or four words. Lung examination is notable for rales in the left lung base and left axilla and diffuse expiratory wheezes. The remainder of the examination is unremarkable. Chest x-ray reveals a left lower lobe and left middle lobe infiltrate. A diagnosis of pneumonia is made, and the patient is admitted for administration of intravenous antibiotics.

Questions: Case 26
A. What are the four groups listed in the American Thoracic Society classification of patients with community-acquired pneumonia? To which group does this patient belong? Based on this classification, what are the likely pathogens involved in this case?
B. What are the mechanisms by which pathogens reach the lungs?
C. What are the normal host defenses against pneumonia?
D. What are some common host risk factors for pneumonia? What are the pathogenetic mechanisms by which they increase the risk of pneumonia? Which of these risk factors are present in this patient?

CASE 27

A 21-year-old woman presents with the complaint of diarrhea. She returned from Mexico the day prior to her visit. The day before that, she had an acute onset of profuse watery diarrhea. She denies blood or mucus in the stools. She has had no associated fever, chills, nausea, or vomiting. She has no other medical problems and is taking no medications. Examination is remarkable for diffuse, mild abdominal tenderness to palpation without guarding or rebound. Stool is guaiac-negative. A diagnosis of infectious diarrhea is suspected. A stool culture is performed.

Questions: Case 27
A. What are the different modes of spread of infectious diarrhea? Give an example of each.
B. What is the likely anatomic site of infection in this case? Why?
C. What is the most likely pathogen in this case? What is the pathogenetic mechanism by which it causes diarrhea?

CASE 28

A 65-year-old woman is admitted to the hospital with community-acquired pneumonia. She is treated with intravenous antibiotics for 2 days and switched to oral antibiotics on the third day in anticipation of discharge. On the evening of hospital day 3, she develops fever and tachycardia. Blood and urine cultures are ordered. The following morning, she is lethargic and difficult to arouse. Her temperature is 35 °C, blood pressure 85/40 mm Hg, heart rate 110 bpm, and respiratory rate 20/min. Oxygen saturation is 94% on room air. Head and neck examinations are unremarkable. Lung examination is unchanged from admission, with rales in the left base. Cardiac examination is notable for a rapid but regular rhythm, without murmurs, gallops, or rubs. Abdominal examination is normal. Extremities are warm. Neurologic examination is nonfocal. The patient is transferred to the intensive care unit for management of presumed sepsis and given intravenous fluids and antibiotics. Blood and urine cultures are positive for gram-negative rods.

Questions: Case 28
A. What factors contribute to hospital-related sepsis?
B. Which organisms most commonly cause gram-negative sepsis?
C. By what mechanism do gram-negative rods result in sepsis? What host mediators have been implicated in the pathogenesis of sepsis?
D. What organ systems are affected by these mediators? How do they result in septic shock?
E. What factors best predict outcome in patients with sepsis?

CASE 29

A 25-year-old black man presents complaining of rapid weight loss despite a voracious appetite. Physical examination reveals tachycardia (pulse rate 110 bpm at rest), fine moist skin, symmetrically enlarged thyroid, mild bilateral quadriceps muscle weakness, and fine tremor. The clinical findings strongly suggest hyperthyroidism.

Questions: Case 29
A. What other features of the history should be elicited?
B. What other physical findings should be sought?
C. Serum TSH and free thyroxine level are ordered. What results should be anticipated?
D. What are the possible causes of this patient's condition?
E. What is the most common cause of this patient's condition, and what is the pathogenesis of this disorder?
F. What is the pathogenesis of this patient's tachycardia, weight loss, skin changes, goiter, and muscle weakness?

CASE 30

A 45-year-old woman presents complaining of fatigue, 30 lb of weight gain despite dieting, constipation, and menorrhagia (excessive menstrual bleeding). On physical examination, the thyroid is not palpable; the skin is cool, dry, and rough; the heart sounds are quiet; and the pulse rate is 50 bpm. The rectal and pelvic examinations are normal and the stool is guaiac-negative. The clinical findings suggest hypothyroidism.

Questions: Case 30
A. What other features of the history should be elicited? What other findings should be sought on physical examination?
B. What is the pathogenesis of this patient's symptoms?
C. What laboratory tests should be ordered, and what results should be anticipated?
D. What are the possible causes of this patient's condition? Which is most likely?
E. What other conditions may be associated with this disorder?

CASE 31

A 40-year-old woman who has recently emigrated from Afghanistan comes to a practice office to establish medical care. She complains only of mild fatigue and depression. Physical examination reveals a prominent, symmetrically enlarged thyroid about twice normal size. The remainder of the examination is normal.

Questions: Case 31
A. What other features of the history should be elicited?
B. What is the most likely cause of the patient's thyroid enlargement? What is the pathogenetic mechanism of goiter formation in this disease?
C. What laboratory tests should be ordered and why?

CASE 32

A 47-year-old man presents complaining of nervousness, difficulty concentrating, restlessness, and insomnia. He has lost 25 lb over the past 6 weeks and complains of heat intolerance. Physical examination reveals a 1 cm nodule in the left lobe of the thyroid gland.

Questions: Case 32
A. What is the most likely explanation for the patient's condition?
B. What laboratory tests should be ordered to confirm the diagnosis?
C. What further evaluation of the nodule should be undertaken?
D. If a biopsy is done, what can be expected in the pathologist's report?

CASE 33

A 28-year-old woman returns for follow-up after routine laboratory tests show a markedly elevated total T_4 level. The patient is totally asymptomatic, and the physical examination is normal.

Questions: Case 33

A. What conditions and medications could be responsible for this presentation?
B. What further laboratory tests should be ordered?
C. If the patient is pregnant, how can the elevated total plasma T_4 level be explained?
D. If several asymptomatic family members have been told of similar laboratory test results, what is the most likely explanation of the patient's disorder?

CASE 34

A 35-year-old woman has hypertension of recent onset. Review of systems reveals several months of weight gain and menstrual irregularity. On examination she is obese, with a plethoric appearance. The blood pressure is 165/98 mm Hg. There are prominent purplish striae over the abdomen and multiple bruises over both lower legs. The patient's physician entertains a diagnosis of hypercortisolism (Cushing's syndrome).

Questions: Case 34

A. What other features of the history and physical examination should be sought?
B. Assuming that the diagnosis of hypercortisolism is correct, what is the underlying pathogenesis of her hypertension, weight gain, and skin striae?
C. List four causes of Cushing's syndrome and discuss the relationships between the hypothalamus, pituitary, and adrenal in each case. Which is the most likely cause in this patient?
D. How can the diagnosis of hypercortisolism be established in this patient?

CASE 35

A 38-year-old woman presents for annual follow-up of previously diagnosed Hashimoto's thyroiditis for which she has been receiving thyroid replacement therapy (levothyroxine, 0.15 mg/d). She reports a gradual onset of weakness, lethargy, and easy fatigability over the last 3 months. Review of systems reveals only recent menstrual irregularity, with no menses in 2½ months. Blood pressure is 90/50 mm Hg (compared with previous readings of 110/75 and 120/80 mm Hg) and her weight is down 13 lb since her last visit 11 months ago. The skin appears to be suntanned, but the patient denies sun exposure. The physician seeing her wonders if she has now developed adrenal insufficiency (Addison's disease).

Questions: Case 35

A. What other features of the history and physical examination should be sought?
B. If Addison's disease has developed, what should the serum electrolytes show, and why?
C. How can the diagnosis of adrenal insufficiency be established in this patient?
D. What is the pathogenesis of the hypotension, weight loss, and skin hyperpigmentation?

CASE 36

A 42-year-old man presents for evaluation of newly diagnosed hypertension. He is currently taking no medication and offers no complaints. A careful review of systems reveals symptoms of fatigue, loss of stamina, and frequent urination, particularly at night. Physical examination is normal except for a blood pressure of 168/100 mm Hg. Serum electrolytes are reported as follows: sodium 152 meq/L, potassium 3.2 meq/L, bicarbonate 32 meq/L, chloride 112 meq/L. The clinical picture is consistent with a diagnosis of primary hyperaldosteronism.

Questions: Case 36

A. What is the mechanism by which primary hyperaldosteronism causes the historical and physical examination findings in this patient?
B. What should the urinalysis and determination of urine electrolytes show, and why?
C. How can the diagnosis of hyperaldosteronism be established in this patient?

CASE 37

A 64-year-old man with a long history of gout and type 2 diabetes mellitus comes in for a routine checkup. Serum chemistries are as follows: sodium 140 meq/L, potassium 6.3 meq/L, bicarbonate 18 meq/L, BUN 43 mg/dL, creatinine 2.9 mg/dL, and glucose 198 mg/dL. Chart review shows previous potassium values of 5.3 meq/L and 5.7 meq/L. The patient is currently taking only colchicine, 0.5 mg daily, and glyburide, 5 mg twice daily.

Questions: Case 37

A. What is the most likely cause of this patient's hyperkalemia, and what is its pathogenesis?
B. What are other possible causes of hypoaldosteronism?
C. Plasma renin activity and aldosterone levels are sent to the laboratory. What results should be anticipated?

CASE 38

A 39-year-old woman comes to the office complaining of episodic anxiety, headache, and palpitations. She states that without dieting she has lost 15 lb over the past 6 months. Physical examination is normal except for a blood pressure of 200/100 mm

Hg and a resting pulse rate of 110 bpm. Chart review shows that prior blood pressures have always been normal, including one 6 months ago. A diagnosis of pheochromocytoma is entertained.

Questions: Case 38
A. What other features of the history should be elicited?
B. What laboratory tests should be ordered, and what results should be anticipated?
C. If pheochromocytoma is found, what is the pathogenesis of the symptoms of anxiety, headache, palpitations, and weight loss?

ANSWERS

Answers: Case 1
A. The four types of osteogenesis imperfecta are type I (mild), type II (perinatal, lethal), type III (progressive, deforming), and type IV (deforming with normal scleras). Types I, III, and IV are transmitted as autosomal dominant traits, though type III can occasionally be transmitted in an autosomal recessive manner. Type II, the most severe form, generally occurs as a sporadic dominant mutation.
B. Type II osteogenesis imperfecta presents at or before birth with multiple fractures and bony deformities, resulting in death in infancy and therefore is unlikely to be seen in a child of 4 years of age. Type III presents at birth or in early infancy with multiple fractures—often prenatal—and progressive bony deformities. The absence of prenatal fractures and early deformities in this patient's history is most suggestive of type I or type IV osteogenesis imperfecta. These individuals generally present in early childhood with one or a few fractures of long bones in response to minimal or no trauma, as seen in this case. Type I and type IV osteogenesis imperfecta are differentiated by their clinical severity and scleral hue. Type I tends to be less severe, with 10–20 fractures during childhood plus short stature but few or no deformities. These patients tend to have blue scleras. Patients with type IV osteogenesis imperfecta tend to have more fractures, resulting in significant short stature and mild to moderate deformities. Their scleras are normal or gray.
C. In patients with type I osteogenesis imperfecta, the fracture incidence decreases after puberty and the main features in adult life are short stature, conductive hearing loss, and occasionally dentinogenesis imperfecta (defective dentin formation in tooth development).
D. Type I osteogenesis imperfecta is caused by a single autosomal dominant mutation of the *COL1A1* gene. This mutation results in decreased or undetectable production of the proα1 mRNA needed to produce the α1 chain of type I collagen. This leads to a significant reduction in the synthesis of normal type I collagen, ultimately resulting in fragile bones.

Answers: Case 2
A. Fragile X-associated mental retardation is a syndrome caused by a genetic mutation of the X chromosome. The mutation leads to failure of the region between bands Xq27 and Xq28 to condense at metaphase, thereby increasing the "fragility" of the region. The mutation appears as an amplification of a $(CGG)_n$ repeat within the untranslated region of a gene named *FMR1*. The *FMR1* gene encodes an RNA-binding protein, named FMR1. However, in affected individuals amplification of the gene results in methylation of an area known as the CpG island, located at Xq27.3. This methylation prevents expression of the FMR1 protein.

The FMR1 protein is normally expressed in brain and testes. This protein resembles a group of proteins named hnRNPs (heterogeneous nuclear RNA-binding proteins) that function in the processing or transport of nuclear mRNA precursors. It is believed that the FMR1 protein plays a general role in the cellular metabolism of nuclear RNA but only in the tissues in which it is primarily expressed, ie, the central nervous system and testes. This would explain in part the symptoms of mental retardation and enlarged testes. It is not known why the absence of *FMR1* expression leads to joint laxity and hyperextensibilty and facial abnormalities.

B. Fragile X-associated mental retardation is an X-linked disease. Given that a male child inherits his X chromosome from his mother, she is clearly the carrier of the mutation.

The boy's mother and grandparents do not demonstrate the phenotype of fragile X-associated mental retardation because of the processes of premutation and parental imprinting. As mentioned above, the mutation in fragile X is associated with amplification of a segment of DNA containing the sequence $(CGG)_n$. This segment is highly variable in length. In individuals who are neither carriers nor affected, the number of repeats is generally less than 50. In transmitting males and unaffected carrier females, the number of repeats ranges from 52 to 193. Those with repeat numbers more than 52 but less than 200 are generally considered to carry the premutation. They are unaffected phenotypically, but the regions are unstable and when transmitted from generation to generation tend to undergo amplification into a full mutation. Full mutations, observed in all affected individuals, always have more than 200 amplifications.

The most important determinant of whether a premutation allele is subject to amplification is the sex of the parent who transmits the premutation allele. A premutation allele transmitted by a female expands to a full mutation with a likelihood proportionate to the length of the premutation. In contrast, a premutation allele transmitted by a male rarely expands to a full mutation regardless of the length of the premutation. This process is called parental imprinting. Thus, it is likely that the boy's mother and grandfather are carriers of a premutation allele and are therefore unaffected—and that this gene amplified to a full mutation on transmission to the boy.

C. The chance that her unborn child will be affected depends on its gender. If it is a boy, the chance that it will be affected is approximately 80%, whereas if it is a girl the chance is only 32%.

Answers: Case 3

A. Down's syndrome occurs approximately once in every 700 live births. Common features include developmental delay, growth retardation, congenital heart disease (50%), immunodeficiency, and characteristic major and minor facial and dysmorphic features, including upslanting palpebral fissures (82%), excess skin on the back of the neck (81%), brachycephaly (75%), hyperextensible joints (75%), flat nasal bridge (68%), epicanthal folds (59%), small ears (50%), and transverse palmar creases (53%).

B. There are two major genetic abnormalities associated with Down's syndrome. The most common abnormality occurs in children born to parents with normal karyotypes. It is caused by nondisjunction of chromosome 21 during meiotic segregation, resulting in one extra chromosome 21, or trisomy 21, with 47 chromosomes on karyotyping. Alternatively, Down's syndrome can be caused by DNA rearrangement resulting in fusion of chromosome 21 to another acrocentric chromosome via its centromere. This abnormal chromosome is called a Robertsonian translocation. Unlike those with trisomy 21, these individuals have 46 chromosomes on karyotyping. This type of translocation can sometimes be inherited from a carrier parent.

Both of these genetic abnormalities result in a 50% increase in gene dosage for nearly all genes on chromosome 21. In other words, the amount of protein produced by all or nearly all genes on chromosome 21 is approximately 150% of normal in Down's syndrome. The genes that have been shown to contribute to the Down's syndrome phenotype include the gene that encodes the amyloid protein found in the senile plaques of Alzheimer's disease and the one that encodes for the cytoplasmic form of superoxide dismutase, which plays an important role in free radical metabolism,

C. It is not known why advanced maternal age is associated with an increased risk of Down's syndrome. One theory suggests that biochemical abnormalities affect the ability of paired chromosomes to disjoin and that these abnormalities accumulate over time. Because germ cell development is completed in females before birth, these biochemical abnormalities are able to accumulate within the egg cells as the mother ages, thereby increasing the risk of nondisjunction. Another hypothesis is that structural, hormonal, and immunologic changes occur in the uterus as the woman ages, producing an environment less able to reject a developmentally abnormal embryo. Therefore, an older uterus would be more likely to support a trisomy 21 conceptus to term. Alternatively, it is possible that a combination of these and other genetic factors may contribute to the relationship between advanced maternal age and an increased incidence of Down's syndrome.

Answers: Case 4

A. The overall risk of phenylketonuria is approximately 1:10,000, though there is great geographic and ethnic variability. The highest risk occurs among Yemenite Jews (incidence of 1:5000), while Northern Europeans develop the disease at a rate of 1:10,000 and American blacks at a rate of 1:50,000.

B. The primary defect in phenylketonuria is a defect in phenylalanine hydroxylase. This enzyme is responsible for converting phenylalanine into tyrosine, a nonessential amino acid. Tyrosine is then used in multiple biosynthetic processes, including protein synthesis and metabolism, and the products of these processes, fumarate and acetoacetate, are used in gluconeogenesis. When hydroxylation of phenylalanine does not occur, phenylalanine accumulates and is transaminated to form phenylpyruvate and subsequently phenylacetate, both of which are detected in increased amounts in the blood and urine in individuals with phenylketonuria.

C. The primary manifestations of phenylketonuria are moderate to severe mental retardation, seizures, growth retardation, and eczematous skin.

Elevated phenylalanine levels have a direct effect on energy production, protein synthesis, and neurotransmitter homeostasis in the developing brain. Phenylalanine can also inhibit the transport of neutral amino acids across the blood-brain barrier, leading to a selective amino acid deficiency in the cerebrospinal fluid. These general effects on central nervous system metabolism lead to the neurologic manifestations of phenylketonuria.

The hypopigmentation in phenylketonuria is probably caused by an inhibitory effect of excess phenylalanine on the production of dopaquinone in melanocytes, the rate-limiting step in melanin production.

The pathophysiology of eczema is not well understood, but the disorder is seen in several other inborn errors of metabolism in which plasma concentrations of branched-chain amino acids are elevated.

D. Phenylketonuria is generally treated with a phenylalanine-restricted diet. This diet begins at birth with the use of a semisynthetic formula low in phenylalanine, combined with breast milk, and empirically titrated to a plasma phenylalanine level of ≤ 1 mmol/L. The diet must be continued indefinitely. Because this treatment results in persistent subtle neuropsychologic defects, researchers are examining alternative options, including somatic gene therapy.

E. When this child is herself of childbearing age, she must be counseled about the risks of maternal phenylketonuria. The syndrome, caused by in utero exposure to maternal hyperphenylalaninemia, is manifested by microcephaly, growth retardation, congenital heart disease, and severe developmental delay—regardless of fetal genotype. The incidence can be reduced by rigorous control of maternal phenylalanine concentrations from before conception until birth to levels much lower than generally required for phenylketonuria-affected individuals.

Answers: Case 5

A. The most likely cause of this child's recurrent infections is severe combined immunodeficiency disease (SCID). These patients have complete or near-complete failure of development of both cellular and humoral components of the immune system. Placental transfer of maternal immunoglobulin is insufficient to protect these children from infection, and for that reason they present at a very early age with severe infections.

B. SCID is a heterogeneous group of genetic and cellular disorders most often caused by defective maturation of a lymphoid stem cell. Two inheritance patterns have been identified. The most common is an X-linked form in which the maturation defect is mainly in the T lymphocyte lineage and is due to a point mutation in the gamma chain of the IL-2 receptor. The other form of inheritance is autosomal recessive and is also known as "Swiss type." The genetic defect for one type of the autosomally inherited form of SCID is a deficiency of ZAP-70, a tyrosine kinase important in normal T lymphocyte function. Deficiency of this tyrosine kinase results in total absence of CD8 T lymphocytes and functionally defective CD4 T lymphocytes. Other cases of the autosomal dominant form of SCID are due to defective recombinant activating gene *(RAG-1* and *RAG-2)* products. RAG-1 and RAG-2 initiate recombination of antigen-binding proteins, immunoglobulins and T cell receptors. The defect leads to both quantitative and qualitative (functional) deficiencies of T and B lymphocytes.

C. Without treatment, most patients with SCID die within the first year.

Answers: Case 6

A. Individuals with common variable immunodeficiency (CVI) commonly develop recurrent sinopulmonary infections such as sinusitis, bronchitis, and pneumonia. They may develop gastrointestinal malabsorption from bacterial overgrowth or chronic giardia infection in the small bowel.

B. CVI is a disorder of defective proliferation and differentiation response. The primary immunologic abnormality is a marked reduction in antibody production, with normal or reduced numbers of circulating B cells. This is most commonly caused by a defect in the terminal differentiation of B lymphocytes in response to T lymphocyte-dependent and -independent stimuli. However, defects in B lymphocyte development have been shown to occur at any stage of the maturation pathway.

Over half of patients with CVI also have some degree of T lymphocyte dysfunction. T lymphocyte dysfunction can be manifested as increased suppressor T lymphocyte activity, decreased cytokine production, defective synthesis of B lymphocyte growth factors, defective cytokine gene expression in T cells, decreased T cell mitogenesis, and deficient lymphokine-activated killer cell function.

C. Individuals with CVI are at increased risk of autoimmune disorders and malignancies. The autoimmune disorders most commonly seen in association with CVI include immune thrombocytopenic purpura, hemolytic anemia, and symmetric seronegative arthritis. The malignancies associated with CVI include lymphomas, gastric carcinoma, and skin cancers.

D. Treatment is mainly symptomatic along with replacement of immune globulin with monthly infusions of IGIV.

Answers: Case 7

A. Pneumocystis pneumonia is commonly seen in AIDS. An HIV-1 antibody test should be ob-

tained whenever the diagnosis of PCP is suspected.
B. AIDS is the consequence of infection with the human immunodeficiency virus (HIV-1), a retrovirus. HIV infection results in a marked decline in CD4 T lymphocytes, an increase in CD8 suppressor-cytotoxic T lymphocytes, and altered B cell function. The loss of CD4 cells seen in HIV infection is the result of multiple mechanisms, including (1) autoimmune destruction, (2) direct viral infection and destruction, (3) fusion and formation into multinucleated giant cells, (4) toxicity of viral proteins to CD4 T lymphocytes and the bone marrow, and (5) apoptosis (programmed cell death). HIV also infects monocytes, macrophages, and dendritic cells.
C. The clinical manifestations of HIV infection and AIDS are the direct consequence of progressive and severe immunosuppression and can be correlated with the degree of CD4 T lymphocyte destruction. HIV infection may present as an acute, self-limited febrile syndrome. This is often followed by a long clinically silent period, sometimes associated with generalized lymphadenopathy. The time course of disease progression may vary, with the majority of individuals remaining asymptomatic for 5–10 years. Approximately 70% of HIV-infected individuals will develop AIDS after a decade of infection. The reasons why AIDS develops and the fate of the other 30% are currently under investigation.

As the CD4 count declines, the incidence of infection increases. At CD4 counts between 200 and 500/µL, patients are at an increased risk for bacterial infections, including pneumonia and sinusitis. As CD4 counts continue to drop—generally below 250/µL—they are at high risk for opportunistic infections such as PCP, candidiasis, toxoplasmosis, cryptococcal meningitis, CMV retinitis, and *Mycobacterium avium* complex infection. HIV-infected individuals are also at increased risk for certain malignancies, including Kaposi's sarcoma, non-Hodgkin's lymphoma, primary central nervous system lymphoma, invasive cervical carcinoma, and anal squamous cell carcinoma. Other manifestations of AIDS include AIDS dementia complex, peripheral neuropathy, monarticular and polyarticular arthritides, unexplained fevers, and weight loss.

Answers: Case 8
A. Adenomas are thought to be related to colorectal carcinoma by means of stepwise genetic alterations, with adenomas representing a precancerous lesion that may ultimately progress to cancer. It is believed that stepwise genetic alterations result in phenotypic changes which progress to neoplasia. The first step is generally enhanced proliferation of cells, associated with mutation of the *ras* oncogene. This is followed by evasion of the immune system, invasion of tissue and stroma, ability to gain access to and exit from the lymphatics and bloodstream, establishment of metastatic foci, ability to recruit vascularization, and ultimately development of drug resistance. The ability of colon cancer cells to metastasize appears to be related to loss of all or part of the *DCC* gene (deleted in colon carcinoma), which codes for an adhesive protein.
B. Two principal lines of evidence support the model of stepwise genetic alterations in colon cancer: (1) Familial colon cancer syndromes are known to result from germline mutations, implicating a genomic cause. Familial adenomatous polyposis is the result of a mutation in the *APC* gene, while hereditary nonpolyposis colorectal carcinoma is associated with mutations in the DNA repair genes *hMSH2* and *hMLH1*. (2) Several factors linked to an increased risk of colon cancer are known to be carcinogenic. Substances derived from bacterial colonic flora, foods, or endogenous metabolites are known to be mutagenic. Levels of these substances can be decreased by taking a low-fat, high-fiber diet. Epidemiologic studies suggest that such a change in diet can reduce the risk of colon cancer.
C. Early in the progression of dysplasia, disrupted architecture results in the formation of fragile new blood vessels and destruction of existing blood vessels. These changes often occur prior to invasion of the basement membrane and, therefore, before progression to true cancer. These friable vessels can cause microscopic bleeding. This can be tested for by fecal occult blood testing, an important tool in the early detection of precancerous and cancerous colonic lesions.

Answers: Case 9
A. Testicular cancer arises from germinal elements within the testes. Germ cells give rise to spermatozoa and thus can theoretically retain the ability to differentiate into any cell type. The pluripotent nature of these cells is witnessed in the production of teratomas. These benign tumors often contain elements of all three germ cell layers, including hair and teeth.
B. During early embryogenesis, germline epithelium migrates along the midline of the embryo. This migration is followed by formation of the urogenital ridge and ultimately the aggregation of germline cells to form the testes and ovaries. The pattern of migration of the germline epithelium predicts the location of extragonadal testicular neoplasms. These neoplasms are found in the midline axis of the lower cranium, mediastinum, and retroperitoneum.

C. One can follow the serum concentrations of proteins expressed during embryonic or trophoblastic development to monitor tumor progression and response to therapy. These proteins include alpha-fetoprotein and human chorionic gonadotropin.

Answers: Case 10

A. The theory that chronic immune stimulation or modulation may play an early role in the formation of lymphoma is supported by several observations. Iatrogenic immunosuppression, as seen in this patient and in other transplant patients, can increase the risk of B cell lymphoma, possibly associated with Epstein-Barr virus infection. An increased risk of lymphoma is also seen in other immunosuppressed patients, such as those with AIDS and autoimmune diseases.

B. This patient has been diagnosed with a follicular cleaved cell lymphoma—a well-differentiated or low-grade lymphoma. Low-grade lymphomas retain the morphology and patterns of gene expression of mature lymphocytes, including cell surface markers such as immunoglobulin in the case of B lymphocytes. Their clinical course is generally more favorable, being characterized by a slow growth rate. Paradoxically, however, these lymphomas tend to present at a more advanced stage, as in this case.

C. Follicular lymphomas arise from lymphoblasts of the B cell lineage. Common chromosomal abnormalities include translocations of chromosome 14, including t(14;18), t(11;14), and t(14;19). The t(14;18) translocation results in a fusion gene known as IgH-*bcl-2*, which juxtaposes the immunoglobulin heavy chain enhancer on chromosome 14 in front of the *bcl-2* gene on chromosome 18. This results in enhanced expression of an inner mitochondrial protein encoded by *bcl-2*, which has been found to inhibit the natural process of cell death—apoptosis. Apoptosis is required to remove certain lymphoid clones whose function is not needed. Inhibition of this process probably contributes to proliferation of lymphoma cells.

D. This patient's symptoms of fever and weight loss are known as B symptoms. They are thought to be mediated by a variety of cytokines produced by lymphoma cells or may occur as a reaction of normal immune cells to the lymphoma. Two commonly implicated cytokines are IL-1 and TNF-α.

Answers: Case 11

A. The most likely cause of anemia in this patient is iron deficiency. Iron deficiency anemia is the most common form of anemia. In developed nations it is primarily the result of iron loss, almost always through blood loss. In men and in postmenopausal women, blood is most commonly lost from the gastrointestinal tract. In premenopausal women, menstrual blood loss is the major cause of iron deficiency.

In this man, there are no symptoms of significant bleeding from the gut as would be manifested by gross blood (hematochezia) or metabolized blood (melena) in the stool, and he has no gastrointestinal complaints. This makes some of the benign gastrointestinal disorders such as peptic ulcer, arteriovenous malformations, and angiodysplasias less likely. He has no symptoms of inflammatory bowel disease such as diarrhea or abdominal pain. Concern is thus aroused about possible malignancy, particularly colon cancer.

B. Blood loss results in anemia via a reduction in heme synthesis. With loss of blood comes loss of iron—the central ion in the oxygen-carrying molecule, heme. When there is iron deficiency, the final step in heme synthesis, during which ferrous iron is inserted into protoporphyrin IX, is interrupted. This results in inadequate heme synthesis, which causes inhibition of hemoglobin biosynthesis and therefore anemia.

C. In this man, because he is symptomatic, the peripheral blood smear is likely to be significantly abnormal. As the hemoglobin concentration of individual red blood cells falls, the cells take on the classic picture of microcytic (small), hypochromic (pale) erythrocytes. There is also apt to be anisocytosis (variation in size) and poikilocytosis (variation in shape), with target cells. The target cells occur because of the relative excess of red cell membrane compared with the amount of hemoglobin within the cell, leading to "bunching up" of the membrane in the center.

D. Laboratory tests may be ordered to confirm the diagnosis. The most commonly ordered test is serum ferritin, which, if low, is diagnostic of iron deficiency. Results may be misleading, however, in acute or chronic inflammation and significant illness. Because ferritin is an acute phase reactant, it can rise in these conditions, resulting in a normal ferritin level. Serum iron and transferrin levels can also be misleading, as these levels can fall not only in anemia but also in many other illnesses. Typically in iron deficiency, however, serum iron levels are low, while total iron-binding capacity (TIBC) is elevated. The ratio of serum iron to TIBC is less than 20% in uncomplicated iron deficiency.

Occasionally, when blood tests are misleading, a bone marrow biopsy is performed to examine iron stores. Iron is normally stored as ferritin in the macrophages of the bone marrow and is stained blue by Prussian blue stain. A decrease in the amount of iron stores on bone marrow biopsy is diagnostic of iron deficiency. More commonly, however, the response to an empiric trial of iron supplementation is used to determine the presence of iron deficiency in complicated cases.

E. Fatigue, weakness, and shortness of breath are the direct result of decreased oxygen-carrying capacity, which leads to decreased oxygen delivery to metabolically active tissues, causing his symptoms. He is pale because there is less oxygenated hemoglobin per unit of blood, and oxygenated hemoglobin is red, giving color to the skin. Pallor results also from a compensatory mechanism whereby superficial blood vessels constrict, diverting blood to more vital structures.

Answers: Case 12

A. The likely cause of this woman's anemia is vitamin B_{12} (cobalamin) deficiency, which is characterized by anemia, glossitis, and neurologic impairment. Vitamin B_{12} deficiency results in anemia via effects on DNA synthesis. Cobalamin is a crucial cofactor in the synthesis of deoxythymidine from deoxyuridine. Cobalamin accepts a methyl group from methyltetrahydrofolate, leading to the formation of methylcobalamin and reduced tetrahydrofolate. Methylcobalamin is required for the production of the amino acid methionine from homocysteine. Reduced tetrahydrofolate is required as the single-carbon donor in purine synthesis. Thus, cobalamin deficiency depletes stores of tetrahydrofolate, lowering purine production and impairing DNA synthesis. Impaired DNA synthesis results in decreased production of red blood cells. It also causes megaloblastic changes in the blood cells in the bone marrow. These cells are subsequently destroyed in large numbers by intramedullary hemolysis. Both processes result in anemia.

B. The peripheral blood smear varies depending on the duration of cobalamin deficiency. In this patient, because she is profoundly symptomatic, we would expect a full-blown megaloblastic anemia. The peripheral smear would have significant anisocytosis and poikilocytosis of the red cells as well as hypersegmentation of the neutrophils. In severe cases, morphologic changes in peripheral blood cells may be difficult to differentiate from those seen in leukemia.

Other laboratory tests that may be ordered include a lactate dehydrogenase (LDH) level and indirect bilirubin determination. Both should be elevated in cobalamin deficiency, reflecting the intramedullary hemolysis that occurs in vitamin B_{12} deficiency. Serum vitamin B_{12} would be expected to be low.

The various causes of megaloblastic anemia can often be differentiated by a Schilling test. This test measures the oral absorption of radioactively labeled vitamin B_{12} with and without added intrinsic factor, thereby directly evaluating the mechanism of the vitamin deficiency. It must be performed after cobalamin stores have been replenished.

C. Pernicious anemia is caused by autoimmune destruction of the gastric parietal cells, which are responsible for production of stomach acid and intrinsic factor. Autoimmune destruction of these cells leads to achlorhydria (loss of stomach acid), which is required for release of cobalamin from foodstuffs. The production of intrinsic factor decreases. Intrinsic factor is required for the effective absorption of cobalamin by the terminal ileum. Together these mechanisms result in vitamin B_{12} deficiency.

The evidence that parietal cell destruction is autoimmune in nature is strong. Pathologically, patients with pernicious anemia demonstrate gastric mucosal atrophy with infiltrating lymphocytes, predominantly antibody-producing B cells. Furthermore, over 90% of patients with this disease demonstrate antibodies to parietal cell membrane proteins, primarily to the proton pump. Over half of patients also have antibodies to intrinsic factor or to the intrinsic factor-cobalamin complex. These patients also have an increased risk of other autoimmune diseases.

D. The patient's tachycardia is probably a reflection of profound anemia. Unlike many other causes of anemia, pernicious anemia often leads to very severe decreases in the hemoglobin concentration. This results in a marked decrease in the oxygen-carrying capacity of the blood. The only way to increase oxygenation to metabolically active tissues is to increase cardiac output. This is accomplished by raising the heart rate. Over time, the stresses this puts on the heart can result in "high-output" congestive heart failure.

The neurologic manifestations—paresthesias and impaired proprioception—seen in this patient are caused by demyelination of the peripheral nerves and posterolateral spinal columns, respectively. The lack of methionine caused by vitamin B_{12} deficiency appears to be at least partly responsible for this demyelination, but the exact mechanism is unknown. Demyelination eventually results in neuronal cell death. Therefore, neurologic symptoms may not be improved by treatment of the vitamin B_{12} deficiency.

Answers: Case 13

A. The exact cause of cyclic neutropenia is not known. There appears to be a defect in the production of neutrophils as well as of the other cell lines, resulting in cyclic depletion of the storage pools. Because development of neutrophils from progenitor stage to maturity takes 2 weeks and the life span is only 12 days, depletion of the neutrophil cell line becomes clinically apparent. The other cell lines have longer life spans, and though they too undergo cyclic decreases in production this does not become clinically apparent.

The underlying defect is thought to be in an early progenitor cell type, possibly in growth factor receptor binding or receptor activity. Clinically, there is one report of transfer of the disease from an affected to an unaffected sibling via a stem cell bone marrow transplant, suggesting that the defect must be present in an early progenitor cell. When bone marrow cells from these individuals are placed in culture, there appears to be selective decreased responsiveness to G-CSF and GM-CSF, suggesting a defect in growth factor receptor binding or activity. Furthermore, when G-CSF is given in pharmacologic doses to patients with this disease, cycling of all cell lines continued but was decreased to 14 days, with mean numbers of neutrophils greater at each point in the cycle. This again suggests a defect in a progenitor cell.

B. The periodic neutropenia with spontaneous remission seen in this patient is characteristic of cyclic neutropenia. In this disease, patients develop a drop in neutrophil count approximately every 3 weeks (19–22 days), with nadirs (low neutrophil counts) lasting 3–5 days. Patients are generally well during periods when the neutrophil cell count is normal and become symptomatic as the counts drop below 250/µL. Neutrophils are responsible for a significant portion of the immune system's response to both bacterial and fungal infections. Thus, the primary clinical manifestation of cyclic neutropenia is recurrent infection. Each nadir is usually characterized by symptoms of fever and malaise. Cervical lymphadenopathy and oral ulcers, as seen in this patient, are also common. Life-threatening bacterial and fungal infections are uncommon but can occur, particularly as a result of infection from endogenous gut flora. More commonly, however, patients develop skin infections and chronic gingivitis.

C. The peripheral blood smear should be normal except for a paucity of neutrophils. Those neutrophils present would be normal in appearance. The bone marrow, however, would be expected to show increased numbers of myeloid precursors such as promyelocytes and myelocytes. Mature neutrophils would be rare. If marrow examination were repeated in 2 weeks, after neutrophil counts have improved, the results would be normal.

Answers: Case 14

A. The most likely diagnosis in this patient is drug-associated immune thrombocytopenia. Many drugs—but most commonly heparin—have been associated with this phenomenon.

B. Heparin leads to thrombocytopenia via two distinct mechanisms, both involving antibodies. It appears that heparin can bind to a platelet-produced protein, platelet factor 4 (PF4), which is released by platelets in response to activation. The heparin-PF4 complex acts as an antigenic stimulus, provoking the production of IgG. IgG can then bind to the complex, forming IgG-heparin-PF4. The new complex can bind to platelets via the Fc receptor of the IgG molecule or via the PF4 receptor. This binding can lead to two distinct phenomena. The first is platelet destruction by the spleen. Antibody adherence to the platelets changes their shape, causing the spleen to recognize them as abnormal and destroy them. This leads to simple thrombocytopenia, with few sequelae.

The second phenomenon is platelet activation, which can lead to more significant sequelae. Following formation of an IgG-heparin-PF4 complex, both IgG and PF4 can bind to platelets. The platelets can become cross-linked, leading to platelet aggregation. This decreases the number of circulating platelets, leading to thrombocytopenia. However, it may also lead to the formation of thrombus, or "white clot."

C. Even though the platelet count in drug-associated immune thrombocytopenia may be very low, significant bleeding is unusual. Most commonly, the primary manifestation is easy bruising, and, at platelet counts less than 5000/µL, petechiae may be seen on the skin or mucous membranes. When actual bleeding does occur, it is generally mucosal in origin, such as nosebleed, gingival bleeding, or gastrointestinal blood loss.

As noted above, when thrombocytopenia is due to heparin, paradoxical clotting may occur instead of bleeding. Thrombus formation often occurs at the site of previous vascular injury or abnormality and can present as either arterial or venous thrombosis.

Answers: Case 15

A. Virchow's triad describes three possible contributors to the formation of a clot: decreased blood flow, blood vessel injury or inflammation, and changes in the intrinsic properties of the blood. This patient has no history of immobility or other cause of decreased blood flow. She does, however, have a history of blood vessel injury, ie, deep vein thrombosis. Despite the absence of symptoms of a lower extremity thrombus, this is still the most likely site of origin of the pulmonary embolus. Finally, the recurrence now of thrombus formation along with the family history of clots is suggestive of a change in the intrinsic properties of the blood, as seen in the inherited hypercoagulable states.

B. The most common hypercoagulable states include

activated protein C resistance (factor V Leiden), protein C deficiency, protein S deficiency, antithrombin III deficiency, and hyperprothrombinemia (prothrombin gene mutation). Except for hyperprothrombinemia, each of these results in clot formation due to lack of adequate anticoagulation rather than overproduction of procoagulant activity; hyperprothrombinemia is caused by excess thrombin generation.

The most common site of the problem occurs at factor Va, which is required for activation of factor X, the central factor in the entire coagulation cascade. Protein C is the major inhibitor of factor Va. It acts by cleaving factor V into an inactive form, thereby slowing the activation of factor X. Protein C's negative effect is enhanced by protein S. Quantitative or qualitative reduction in either of these two proteins thus results in the unregulated procoagulant action of factor Xa.

Activated protein C resistance is the most common inherited hypercoagulable state. It results from a mutation in the factor V gene. This mutation alters the three-dimensional conformation of the cleavage site within factor Va, where protein C usually binds. Protein C is then unable to bind to factor Va and is therefore unable to inactivate it. Coagulation is not inhibited.

Antithrombin III (AT-III) inhibits the coagulation cascade at an alternative site. It inhibits the serine proteases, factors II, IX, X, XI, and XII. Deficiency of AT-III results in an inability to inactivate these factors, allowing the coagulation cascade to proceed unrestrained at multiple coagulation steps.

Hyperprothrombinemia is the second-most common hereditary hypercoagulable state and the only one so far recognized to be due to overproduction of procoagulant factors. It is caused by a mutation of the prothrombin gene that leads to elevated prothrombin levels. The increased risk of thrombosis is thought to be due to excess thrombin generation when the Xa-Va-PL-Ca^{2+} complex is activated.

C. This patient may be evaluated by various laboratory tests for the presence of an inherited hypercoagulable state. Quantitative evaluation of the relative amounts of protein C, protein S, and AT-III can all be performed. Qualitative tests that assess the ability of these proteins to inhibit the coagulation cascade can be measured via clotting assays. The presence of the specific mutation in factor V Leiden can be assessed via polymerase chain reaction.

Answers: Case 16

A. The most likely diagnosis in this patient is myasthenia gravis, a disease characterized by fluctuating fatigue and weakness of muscles with small motor units, particularly the ocular muscles. Myasthenia gravis is an autoimmune disorder resulting in simplification of the postsynaptic region of the neuromuscular end plate. Patients with this disease have lymphocytic infiltration at the end plate plus antibody and complement deposition along the postsynaptic membrane. The antibodies are directed at the acetylcholine receptor and bind to it, blocking acetylcholine binding and activation. The antibodies can cross-link the receptor molecules, leading to receptor internalization and degradation. They also activate complement-mediated destruction of the postsynaptic region, resulting in simplification of the end plate. Thus, patients with this disorder have impaired ability to respond to acetylcholine release from the presynaptic membrane.

B. Muscles with small motor units are most affected in myasthenia gravis. The ocular muscles are most frequently affected; oropharyngeal muscles, flexors and extensors of the neck and proximal limbs, and erector spinae muscles are next most commonly involved. In severe cases and without treatment, the disease can progress to involve all muscles, including the diaphragm and intercostal muscles, resulting in respiratory failure.

C. Normally, the number of quanta of acetylcholine released from the nerve terminal decreases with repetitive stimuli. There are usually no clinical consequences of this decrease because a sufficient number of acetylcholine receptor channels are opened despite the reduced amount of neurotransmitter. In myasthenia gravis, however, there is a deficiency in the number of acetylcholine receptors. Therefore, as the number of quanta released decreases, there is a decremental decline in neurotransmission at the neuromuscular junction. This is manifested clinically as muscle fatigue with sustained or repeated activity.

D. Myasthenia gravis is associated both with a family history of autoimmune disease and with the presence of coexisting autoimmune diseases. Hyperthyroidism due to Graves' disease occurs in 5% of patients. Rheumatoid arthritis, systemic lupus erythematosus, and polymyositis are all seen with increased frequency.

These patients also have a high incidence of thymic disease, with most demonstrating thymic hyperplasia and 10–15% having thymomas.

E. There are two basic strategies for treating this disease—decreasing the immune-mediated destruction of the acetylcholine receptors and increasing the amount of acetylcholine available at the neuromuscular junction. As noted previously, many patients with myasthenia gravis demonstrate disease of the thymus gland. The thymus is thought to play a role in the pathogenesis of myasthenia gravis by supplying helper T cells that are sensitized to thymic nicotinic receptors. Removal of the thymus in patients with generalized myasthenia gravis can improve symptoms and even induce remission. Plasmapheresis, corticosteroids, and immunosuppressant drugs can all be used to reduce the levels of antibody to acetylcholine receptors, thereby suppressing disease. Increasing the amount of acetylcholine available at the neuromuscular junction is accomplished by the use of cholinesterase inhibitors. Cholinesterase is responsible for the breakdown of acetylcholine at the neuromuscular junction. By inhibiting the breakdown of acetylcholine, cholinesterase inhibitors can compensate for the normal decline in released neurotransmitter during repeated stimulation and thus decrease symptoms.

Answers: Case 17
A. Generalized tonic-clonic seizures are characterized by sudden loss of consciousness followed rapidly by tonic contraction of the muscles, causing extension of the limbs and arching of the back. This phase lasts approximately 10–30 seconds and is followed by a clonic phase of limb jerking. The jerking builds in frequency, peaking after 15–30 seconds, and then gradually slows over another 15–30 seconds. The patient may remain unconscious for several minutes following the seizure. This is generally followed by a period of confusion lasting minutes to hours.
B. Recurrent seizures are in many cases idiopathic, particularly those seen in children. Seizures may also be due to brain injury from trauma, stroke, mass lesion, or infection. Finally, one must consider metabolic causes such as hypoglycemia, electrolyte abnormalities, or alcohol withdrawal. The cause of this patient's seizure is unknown because of the lack of an available history. However, because he has focal neurologic findings, with decreased movement of his left side, one must suspect an underlying brain lesion.
C. Seizures occur when neurons in a focal region or in the entire brain are activated synchronously. The kind of seizure depends on the location of the abnormal activity and the pattern of spread to different parts of the brain. The formation of a seizure focus in the brain may result from disruption of normal inhibitory circuits. This disruption may occur because of alterations in ion channels or from injury to inhibitory neurons and synapses. Alternatively, a seizure focus may be formed when groups of neurons become synchronized by reorganization of neural networks following brain injury. Following formation of a seizure focus, local discharge may then spread. This spread occurs by a combination of mechanisms. Following synchronous depolarization of abnormally excitable neurons—known as the paroxysmal depolarizing shift—extracellular potassium accumulates, depolarizing nearby neurons. Increased frequency of depolarization then leads to increased calcium influx into nerve terminals. This increases neurotransmitter release at excitatory synapses by a process known as posttetanic potentiation, whereby normally quiescent voltage-gated and N-methyl-D-aspartate (NMDA) receptor-gated excitatory synaptic neurotransmission is increased and inhibitory synaptic neurotransmission is decreased. The net effect of these changes is recruitment of neighboring neurons into a synchronous discharge, causing a seizure.

Answers: Case 18
A. The diagnosis in this patient is stroke, characterized by the sudden onset of focal neurologic deficits that persist for at least 24 hours. The focal symptoms and signs that result from stroke correlate with the area of the brain supplied by the affected blood vessel. In this case, the patient has weakness and sensory loss on the right side. These symptoms suggest involvement of the left middle cerebral artery—or at least its associated vascular territory. The vascular territory supplied by the middle cerebral artery includes the lateral frontal, parietal, occipital, and temporal cortex and adjacent white matter as well as the caudate, putamen, and internal capsule.
B. Risk factors for stroke include age, male sex, hypertension, hypercholesterolemia, diabetes, smoking, heavy alcohol consumption, and oral contraceptives.
C. Stroke is classified as either ischemic or hemorrhagic in origin. Ischemic stroke may result from thrombotic or embolic occlusion of the vessel. Hemorrhagic stroke may result from intraparenchymal hemorrhage, subarachnoid hemorrhage, subdural hemorrhage, epidural hemorrhage, or hemorrhage within an ischemic infarction. Given the CT scan result, it is likely that this man has sustained an ischemic rather than hemorrhagic stroke. Hemorrhagic and ischemic strokes can be difficult to differentiate on clinical grounds, but the former often produce a less predictable pattern of neurologic deficits. This is because the neurologic deficits in hemorrhagic stroke depend both on the location of the bleed and on factors that affect brain function at a distance from the hemorrhage, including increased intracranial pressure, edema, compression of neighboring brain tissue, and rupture of blood into the ventricles or subarachnoid space.
D. The most likely underlying cause of stroke in this patient is atherosclerosis. Atherosclerosis arises from vascular endothelial cell injury, of-

ten caused by chronic hypertension or hypercholesterolemia, both present in this man. Endothelial injury stimulates attachment of circulating monocytes and lymphocytes that migrate into the vessel wall and stimulate proliferation of smooth muscle cells and fibroblasts. This results in plaque formation. Damaged endothelium also serves as a nidus of platelet aggregation that further stimulates proliferation of smooth muscle and fibroblasts. The plaques formed may enlarge and occlude the vessel, leading to thrombotic stroke, or may rupture, releasing emboli and causing embolic stroke.

Answers: Case 19

A. The lesions described are characteristic of psoriasis vulgaris. Psoriasis is both a genetic and an environmental disorder. A genetic origin is supported by several lines of evidence. There is a high rate of concordance for psoriasis in monozygotic twins and an increased incidence of psoriasis in the relatives of affected individuals. Furthermore, overexpression of gene products of class I alleles of the major histocompatibility complex is seen in patients with psoriasis. However, psoriasis is unlikely to be completely genetic in nature since not all individuals with a genetic predisposition develop the disorder. Environmental triggers that appear to be necessary, at least in some individuals, include trauma, cold weather, infections, and various medications.

B. In psoriasis, there is shortening of the usual duration of the keratinocyte cell cycle and doubling of the proliferative cell population. This excessive epidermatopoiesis results in skin thickening and plaque formation. In addition to skin thickening, truncation of the cell cycle leads to an accumulation of cells within the cornified layer with retained nuclei. This pattern is known as parakeratosis and results in neutrophil migration into the cornified layer. Together these form the silvery scale characteristic of psoriasis. Finally, psoriasis induces endothelial cell proliferation, resulting in pronounced dilation, tortuosity, and increased permeability of the capillaries in the superficial dermis and causing erythema.

C. Many immunologic abnormalities have been implicated in psoriasis, but the exact pathophysiologic mechanism remains unclear. As mentioned above, psoriasis is associated with overexpression of MHC class I gene products. This suggests that CD8 T lymphocytes are involved, as the complex of MHC class I protein and antigen is the ligand of the T cell receptor of CD8 cells. Also seen in psoriasis is overexpression of a large number of cytokines, particularly IL-2.

Answers: Case 20

A. The lesions described are characteristic of the "pruritic polygonal purple papules" of lichen planus. Although the triggers of lichen planus are often obscure, several drugs have been implicated. Antimalarial agents (eg, chloroquine) and therapeutic gold are the most closely linked. It is believed that these drugs and other unknown triggers result in a cell-mediated autoimmune reaction leading to damage of the basal keratinocytes of the epidermis.

B. As mentioned above, the triggers leading to lichen planus formation are often idiopathic. However, it appears that some form of antigenic stimulation leads to infiltration and activation of CD4 T lymphocytes. These stimulated CD4 cells elaborate cytokines, leading to the recruitment of cytotoxic T lymphocytes. Cell-mediated cytotoxicity, cytokines, gamma interferon, and tumor necrosis factor combine to injure keratinocytes and contribute to vacuolization and necrosis of these cells. Injured, enucleated keratinocytes coalesce to form colloid bodies. Melanocytes are destroyed, and melanin is phagocytosed by macrophages.

C. The appearance of the lichen planus papules is a direct reflection of the underlying histopathologic features. The dense array of lymphocytes in the superficial dermis yields the elevated, flat-topped appearance of the papule. The whitish coloration—Wickman's striae—results from chronic inflammation and hyperkeratosis of the cornified layer of the epidermis. The purple hue of the lesions is caused by the macrophage phagocytosis of the released melanin, to form melanocytes. Although the melanin is brownish black in color, the melanophages are embedded in a colloid matrix. This causes extensive scattering of light by an effect known as the Tyndall phenomenon, resulting in interpretation of the lesion as dusky or violaceous by the human eye.

Answers: Case 21

A. The lesions described are characteristic of erythema multiforme. The lack of mucosal involvement suggests erythema multiforme minor.

B. Like lichen planus, erythema multiforme is an interface dermatitis. Both are caused by some inciting agent that results in lymphocyte migration to the epidermis and papillary dermis. Cytotoxic T cells then combine with elaborated cytokines, gamma interferon, and tumor necrosis factor to kill keratinocytes, resulting in enucleation, vacuolization, and coalescence to form colloid bodies.

Unlike lichen planus, with its dense dermal inflammatory infiltrate, the dermal infiltrate of lymphocytes in erythema multiforme is sparse. Thus, the vacuolated keratinocytes widely dis-

tributed in the epidermal basal layer are more conspicuous.
C. Many cases of erythema multiforme minor are triggered by herpes simplex virus, as seen in this patient. The evidence to support this association derives from both clinical and molecular data. Clinically, it has long been documented that erythema multiforme is often preceded by herpes simplex infection. Furthermore, antiherpetic therapy, such as acyclovir, can suppress the development of erythema multiforme in some individuals. Molecular studies have confirmed the presence of herpes simplex DNA within skin from erythema multiforme lesions. HSV DNA is also present in the peripheral blood lymphocytes and lesional skin after resolution of the rash but is not found in nonlesional skin.
D. The target-like lesions seen in erythema multiforme reflect zonal differences in the inflammatory response and its deleterious effects. At the periphery of the lesion, inflammation and vacuolization are sparse, resulting in the erythematous halo. The dusky bull's-eye in the center, on the other hand, is an area of dense epidermal vacuolization and necrosis.

Answers: Case 22
A. The major alternative diagnoses to consider are bullous pemphigoid and pemphigus, though other blistering diseases such as erythema multiforme and dermatitis herpetiformis should be considered as well. Bullous pemphigoid is characterized by subepidermal and pemphigus by intraepidermal vesiculation. The distinction is important because bullous pemphigoid has a more favorable prognosis.
B. Microscopically, bullous pemphigoid lesions show a subepidermal cleft containing lymphocytes, eosinophils, neutrophils, and eosinophilic material, representing extravasated proteins. An inflammatory infiltrate of eosinophils, neutrophils, and lymphocytes is also present in the dermis beneath the cleft.
C. Direct immunofluorescence microscopy demonstrates IgG and C3 bound in a linear distribution along the epidermal-dermal junction. These autoantibodies are bound to a 230 kDa protein within the lamina lucida, known as the "bullous pemphigoid antigen." This antigen has been localized to the hemidesmosomal complex of the epidermal basal cell. Its role is not established.
D. Blister formation is believed to begin with the binding of IgG to the bullous pemphigoid antigen, activating the complement cascade. Complement fragments then induce mast cell degranulation and attract neutrophils and eosinophils. The granulocytes and mast cells release multiple enzymes, resulting in enzymatic digestion of the epidermal-dermal junction and separation of the layers. It is also possible that the bullous pemphigoid antigen plays a vital structural role that is compromised when the autoantibodies bind, leading to cleavage of the epidermal-dermal junction.

Answers: Case 23
A. Palpable purpura over the distal lower extremities or other dependent areas—recurring over a period of months—and histologic study revealing fibrinoid necrosis are most consistent with leukocytoclastic vasculitis. Common precipitants include infections and medications. Bacterial, mycobacterial, and viral infections can all trigger leukocytoclastic vasculitis, with streptococcus and staphylococcus being the most common infectious precipitants. S pneumoniae is the most common cause of pneumonia in this age group and may have been the precipitant in this man. Hepatitis C is also associated with leukocytoclastic vasculitis. Many drugs have been associated with this disorder, including antibiotics, thiazides, and NSAIDs. Of the antibiotics, penicillins—such as the amoxicillin given to this man—are the most common offenders.
B. Eliciting factors such as microbial antigens or medications trigger the formation of immune complexes, consisting of antibodies bound to the exogenous antigen. For reasons not yet clear, these complexes are preferentially deposited in the small cutaneous vessels (venules). After becoming trapped in the tissue of the venules, the immune complexes activate the complement cascade, and localized production of chemotactic fragments and vasoactive molecules ensues. This attracts neutrophils, which release enzymes, resulting in destruction of the immune complexes, neutrophils, and vessel. Ultimately, erythrocytes and fibrin are able to exude through the vessel wall and enter the surrounding dermis, resulting in the classic finding of palpable purpura.
C. Leukocytoclastic vasculitis lesions are papular because of the intense neutrophilic inflammatory response in the vessels. The lesions are purpuric or erythematous because of the extravasated red blood cells that accumulate in the dermis.
D. Leukocytoclastic vasculitis may also involve small vessels in other portions of the body, including the joint capsules, soft tissues, kidneys, liver, and gastrointestinal tract. The most common systemic symptoms include arthralgias, myalgias, and abdominal pain. It would be important to evaluate for these symptoms and order laboratory tests to assess liver or renal involvement.

Answers: Case 24
A. This patient's presentation is characteristic of untreated infective endocarditis—an infection of

the interior of the heart, most commonly the valves. The most common predisposing factor is the presence of abnormal cardiac valves related to rheumatic heart disease, mitral valve prolapse with an audible murmur, congenital heart disease, prosthetic valve, or prior endocarditis. Injection drug use is an important risk factor for this disease. The patient's history of significant illness as a child after a sore throat suggests the possibility of rheumatic heart disease.

B. The most common infectious agents causing native valve endocarditis are gram-positive bacteria, including viridans streptococci, *S aureus,* and enterococci. Given the history of recent dental work, the most likely pathogen in this patient would be viridans streptococci, which are normal mouth flora.

C. The hemodynamic factors that predispose patients to the development of endocarditis include (1) a high-velocity jet stream, causing turbulent flow; (2) flow from a high- to a low-pressure chamber; and (3) a comparatively narrow orifice separating two chambers that creates a pressure gradient. The lesions of endocarditis tend to form on the surface of the valve in the lower-pressure cardiac chamber—or as satellite lesions, where the jet stream strikes the endocardium. The predisposed, damaged endothelium of an abnormal valve—or jet stream-damaged endothelium—promotes the deposition of fibrin and platelets, forming sterile vegetations. When bacteremia occurs such as after dental work, microorganisms can be deposited on these sterile vegetations. Once infected, the lesions continue to grow through further deposition of platelets and fibrin. These vegetations act as a sanctuary from host defense mechanisms such as phagocytosis and complement-mediated lysis. It is for this reason that prolonged administration of bactericidal antibiotics and possible operative intervention are required for cure.

D. The painful papules found on the pads of this man's fingers and toes are Osler's nodes. They are thought to be caused by deposition of immune complexes in the skin. The painless hemorrhagic macules (Janeway lesions) and splinter hemorrhages are thought to result from systemic embolization of the cardiac vegetations.

E. In addition to the symptoms described in this man (fever, chills, night sweats, malaise, Roth spots, Janeway lesions, splinter hemorrhages, and Osler nodes), patients with infective endocarditis can develop multisystem complaints, including headaches, back pain, focal neurologic symptoms, shortness of breath, edema, chest pain, cough, decreased urine output, hematuria, flank pain, abdominal pain, and others. These symptoms and signs reflect (1) hemodynamic changes from valvular damage, (2) end-organ damage by septic emboli (right-sided emboli to the lungs; left-sided emboli to the brain, spleen, kidney, gastrointestinal tract, and extremities), (3) immune complex deposition, and (4) persistent bacteremia and distal seeding of infection, resulting in abscess formation. Death is usually caused by hemodynamic collapse following rupture of the aortic or mitral valves or by septic emboli to the central nervous system, resulting in brain abscesses or mycotic aneurysms with resultant intracranial hemorrhage.

Answers: Case 25

A. The most likely diagnosis in this patient is meningitis. The acuity and severity of presentation are most consistent with a pyogenic bacterial cause, though viral, mycobacterial, and fungal causes should be considered as well. In adults, the most likely bacterial pathogens are *N meningitidis* and *S pneumoniae*. In newborns under 2 months of age, the most common pathogens are those to which the infant is exposed in the maternal genitourinary canal, including *E coli* and other gram negative bacilli, group B and other streptococci, and *L monocytogenes*. Between the ages of 2 months and 15 years, *N meningitidis* and *S pneumoniae* are the most common pathogens. *H influenzae,* previously the most common cause of meningitis in this age group, has become much less of a problem since the vaccine became available in 1988.

B. Bacterial meningitis begins with colonization of the host's nasopharynx. This is followed by local invasion of the mucosal epithelium and subsequent bacteremia. Cerebral endothelial cell injury follows and results in increased blood-brain barrier permeability, facilitating meningeal invasion. The resultant inflammatory response in the subarachnoid space causes cerebral edema, vasculitis, and infarction, ultimately leading to decreased cerebrospinal fluid flow, hydrocephalus, worsening cerebral edema, increased intracranial pressure, and decreased cerebral blood flow.

Bacterial pathogens responsible for meningitis possess several characteristics that facilitate the above steps. Nasal colonization is facilitated by pili on the bacterial surface of *N meningitidis* that assist in mucosal attachment. *N meningitidis, H influenzae,* and *S pneumoniae* also produce IgA proteases that cleave IgA, the antibody commonly responsible for inhibiting adherence of pathogens to the mucosal surface. By cleaving the antibody, the bacteria are able to evade this important host defense mechanism. In addition, *H influenzae* and *S pneumoniae* are often encapsulated, which can assist in nasopharyngeal colonization as well as systemic invasion. The capsule inhibits neutrophil phagocytosis and resists classic complement-mediated bactericidal activity, enhancing bacterial survival and replication.

It remains unclear how bacterial pathogens gain access to the central nervous system. It is thought that cells of the choroid plexus may contain receptors for them, facilitating movement into the subarachnoid space. Once the bacterial pathogen is in the subarachnoid space, host defense mechanisms are inadequate to control the infection. Subcapsular surface components of the bacteria, such as the cell wall and lipopolysaccharide, induce a marked inflammatory response mediated by IL-1 and TNF. Despite the induction of a marked inflammatory response and leukocytosis, there is a relative lack of opsonization and bactericidal activity such that the bacteria are poorly cleared from the cerebrospinal fluid. The inflammation produced, however, results in significant cerebral edema, contributing to many of the pathophysiologic consequences of this disease.

C. Cerebral edema may be vasogenic, cytotoxic, or interstitial in origin. Vasogenic cerebral edema is principally caused by the increase in the blood-brain barrier permeability that occurs when the bacteria invade the cerebrospinal fluid. Cytotoxic cerebral edema results from swelling of the cellular elements of the brain. This occurs because of toxic factors released by the bacteria and neutrophils. Interstitial edema is due to obstruction of cerebrospinal fluid flow.

D. Any patient suspected of having bacterial meningitis should have emergent lumbar puncture with Gram's stain and culture of the cerebrospinal fluid. If there is concern about a focal neurologic problem—such as may occur with abscess or of an increased intracranial pressure—CT or MRI of the brain may be performed prior to lumbar puncture. Antibiotics should be started immediately. Corticosteroids may be considered in patients with altered mental status or signs of increased intracranial pressure. Many of the clinical consequences of bacterial meningitis are due to the profound inflammatory response produced by bacterial invasion of the subarachnoid space. Rapid bacteriolysis, as may occur with administration of antibiotics, can release high concentrations of inflammatory bacterial fragments, thereby potentially exacerbating the inflammation and its clinical consequences. Corticosteroids may blunt this response.

Answers: Case 26

A. The American Thoracic Society has recommended classification of patients with community-acquired pneumonia into four groups based on comorbid disease and severity of illness. The four categories reflect changes in the spectrum of pathogens most commonly involved in pulmonary infection: (1) outpatients under 60 years of age without comorbid illness, (2) outpatients over 60 years of age or those with comorbid disease, (3) hospitalized patients not requiring intensive care unit admission, and (4) hospitalized patients requiring intensive care unit admission. The patient described in this case has a moderately severe infection, requiring hospitalization but not intensive care unit admission. The most likely pathogens are S pneumoniae, C pneumoniae, H influenzae, L pneumophila, S aureus, aerobic gram-negative bacilli, and respiratory viruses. Infection may be polymicrobial as well.

B. Pulmonary pathogens reach the lungs by one of four routes: (1) direct inhalation, (2) aspiration of upper airway contents, (3) spread along the mucosal membrane surface, and (4) hematogenous spread.

C. Normal pulmonary antimicrobial defense mechanisms include the following: (1) aerodynamic filtration by subjection of incoming air to turbulence in the nasal passages and then abrupt changes in the direction of the airstream as it moves through the pharynx and tracheobronchial tree; (2) the cough reflex to remove aspirated material, excess secretions, and foreign bodies; (3) the mucociliary transport system, moving the mucous layer upward to the larynx; (4) phagocytic cells, including alveolar macrophages and PMNs, as well as humoral and cellular immune responses, which help to eliminate the pathogens; and (5) pulmonary secretions containing surfactant, lysozyme, and iron-binding proteins, which further aid in bacterial killing.

D. Common host risk factors include the following: (1) an immunocompromised state, resulting in immune dysfunction and increased risk of infection; (2) chronic lung disease, resulting in decreased mucociliary clearance; (3) alcoholism, which increases the risk of aspiration; (4) injection drug abuse, which increases the risk of hematogenous spread of pathogens; (5) environmental or animal exposure, resulting in inhalation of specific pathogens; (6) residence in an institution, with its associated risk of microaspirations, and exposure via instrumentation (catheters and intubation); and (7) recent influenza infection, leading to disruption of respiratory epithelium, ciliary dysfunction, and inhibition of PMNs. This patient has a history of chronic lung disease, increasing his risk of pneumonia, and he may be partially immunocompromised by use of corticosteroids for his COPD.

Answers: Case 27

A. There are three primary modes of transmission of pathogens causing infectious diarrhea. Pathogens such as Vibrio cholerae are water-borne and transmitted via a contaminated water supply. Several pathogens, including *Staphylococcus aureus* and *Bacillus cereus,* are transmitted by contaminated food. Finally, some pathogens, such as shigella and rotavirus, are transmitted by person-to-person spread and are therefore commonly seen in institutional settings such as child care centers.

B. The description of this patient's diarrhea as profuse and watery suggests a small bowel site of infection. The small bowel is the site of significant electrolyte and fluid transportation. Disruption of this process leads to the production of profuse watery diarrhea, as seen in this patient.

C. The most likely cause of diarrhea in this patient, who has recently returned from Mexico, is enterotoxigenic *E coli* (ETEC), which causes up to 70% of cases of traveler's diarrhea. It is usually transmitted by fecal contamination of food. Diarrhea results from the production of two enterotoxins that "poison" the cells of the small intestine, causing watery diarrhea. ETEC produces both a heat-labile and a heat-stable enterotoxin. The heat-labile enterotoxin has two types of subunits, A and B. The B subunit binds to the intestinal cell membrane and facilitates entry of part of the A subunit. This results in activation of adenylyl cyclase and formation of cAMP, which stimulates water and electrolyte secretion by intestinal endothelial cells. The heat-stable toxin produced by ETEC results in guanylyl cyclase activation, also causing watery diarrhea.

Answers: Case 28
A. Factors that contribute to hospital-related sepsis are invasive monitoring devices, indwelling catheters, extensive surgical procedures, and the increased number of immunocompromised patients.
B. Gram-negative sepsis is most commonly caused by *P aeruginosa* and by *E coli* and other Enterobacteriacae.
C. Gram-negative bacteria contain an endotoxin, the lipid A component of the lipopolysaccharide-phospholipid-protein complex present in the outer cell membrane. When this endotoxin is released into the host's circulation, it induces several host mediators of sepsis. Endotoxin activates the coagulation cascade, the complement system, and the kinin system as well as the release of several host mediators such as cytokines, platelet-activating factor, endorphins, endothelium-derived relaxing factor, arachidonic acid metabolites, myocardial depressant factors, nitric oxide, and others.
D. These mediators have major effects on the myocardium and vasculature, ultimately leading to damage in multiple organs, including the kidney, liver, lung, and brain. The release of vasoactive substances, as described above, results in microcirculatory imbalances in blood flow, including regional shunting. This mismatch of blood flow with metabolic demand causes excessive blood flow to some areas with relative hypoperfusion of others, limiting optimal utilization of oxygen. Myocardial depression also occurs, with reduction in both left and right ventricular ejection fractions and increases in end-diastolic and end-systolic volumes. Refractory hypotension can ensue, resulting in end-organ hypoperfusion and injury.
E. The outcome in sepsis depends on the number of organs that fail, with mortality rates of 80–100% in patients who develop failure of three or more organ systems.

Answers: Case 29
A. Other historical features to be elicited include heat intolerance, excessive sweating, nervousness, irritability, emotional lability, restlessness, poor concentration, muscle weakness, palpitations, and increased frequency of bowel movements.
B. The examiner should evaluate the eyes for stare, lid lag, proptosis, or abnormal eye movements; the heart for irregular rhythm, flow murmur, or congestive failure; the breasts for gynecomastia; the nails for onycholysis; the pretibial area for dermopathy; and the deep tendon reflexes for a rapid relaxation phase.
C. The free thyroxine should be high; the TSH level should be low. Rarely, hyperthyroidism is caused by secondary or tertiary hyperthyroidism due to excessive TSH or TRH production, respectively. In these cases, TSH would be elevated.
D. Possible causes of this patient's condition include thyroid hormone overproduction (in Graves' disease, toxic multinodular goiter, autonomous hyperfunctioning follicular adenoma); thyroid gland destruction with release of stored hormone (in thyroiditis); or ingestion of excessive exogenous thyroid hormone.
E. Graves' disease is the most common cause of hyperthyroidism. Thyroid-stimulating immunoglobulins are present in the serum. These are autoantibodies of the IgG class, directed against TSH receptors on the follicular cell membrane. When they bind to the cell membrane TSH receptors, they stimulate hormone synthesis and secretion.
F. Tachycardia is thought to be related to direct effects of excess thyroid hormone on the cardiac conducting system. Weight loss results from an increase in the basal metabolic rate. Autoantibodies have been identified that stimulate the growth of thyroid epithelial cells and produce the goiter of Graves' disease. The muscle weak-

ness is related to increased protein catabolism and muscle wasting, decreased muscle efficiency, and changes in myosin.

Answers: Case 30

A. Other features to be elicited in the history include cold intolerance, mental slowing, forgetfulness, lethargy, muscle weakness or cramps, and hair loss. The examiner should also evaluate the body temperature, the musculature for weakness, the face and skin for puffiness and carotenemia, the extremities for edema, and the deep tendon reflexes for sluggishness and a slowed ("hung up") relaxation phase.

B. Weight gain is related to a decrease in the basal metabolic rate. Constipation is caused by decreased gastrointestinal motility. Menorrhagia results from anovulatory menstrual cycles. Thyroid atrophy and fibrosis may result from lymphocytic infiltration and destruction of thyroid follicles, destruction of the thyroid by surgery or radiation, or atrophy due to diminished TSH secretion. The skin changes of hypothyroidism are the result of accumulation of polysaccharides in the dermis. The quiet heart sounds may be related to development of pericardial effusion or of cardiomyopathy caused by deposition of mucopolysaccharides in the interstitium between myocardial fibers.

C. Serum TSH is the most sensitive test for detecting hypothyroidism. TSH is elevated in almost all cases of hypothyroidism—with the rare exceptions of pituitary and hypothalamic disease. Free thyroxine levels should be low.

D. In the adult, hypothyroidism may result from Hashimoto's (autoimmune) thyroiditis, lymphocytic thyroiditis, thyroid ablation (via surgery or radiation), hypopituitarism or hypothalamic disease, and drugs. The most common cause of this patient's hypothyroidism is Hashimoto's thyroiditis.

E. Other autoimmune disorders, including endocrine disorders such as diabetes mellitus and hypoadrenalism, and nonendocrine disorders such as pernicious anemia, systemic lupus erythematosus, and myasthenia gravis are all seen with increased frequency in patients with Hashimoto's thyroiditis.

Answers: Case 31

A. The physician should ask about causes of goiter such as increased intake of foods containing goitrogens (eg, cabbage), diminished intake of foods containing iodine (eg, fish), and use of medications associated with goiter (eg, lithium). Symptoms of thyroid encroachment on surrounding structures such as respiratory or swallowing difficulties should be elicited. Because of this patient's fatigue and depression, the physician should also probe for other symptoms of hypothyroidism.

B. The most common cause of goiter in developing nations is dietary iodine deficiency. Because this patient is 40 years old and recently emigrated from Afghanistan, iodine deficiency would be the most likely cause. A diet low in iodine (< 10 $\mu g/d$) hinders the synthesis of thyroid hormone, resulting in an elevated TSH level and thyroid hypertrophy.

C. The free thyroxine index or serum TSH should be determined to exclude hypothyroidism.

Answers: Case 32

A. This patient most likely has hyperthyroidism due to an autonomous hyperfunctioning follicular adenoma.

B. The free thyroxine index will be elevated and the serum TSH suppressed.

C. A radioactive iodine scan could be performed to confirm the diagnosis. Radioactive iodine uptake will be elevated in the region of the nodule and suppressed elsewhere. Thyroid scan will show a "hot" nodule.

D. Biopsy of the nodule will show normal follicles of varying size. Excisional biopsy will show compression of surrounding normal thyroid and areas of hemorrhage, fibrosis, and calcification or cystic degeneration.

Answers: Case 33

A. Although this patient has an elevated total T_4, she has no symptoms or signs of hyperthyroidism. An elevated total T_4 in clinically euthyroid individuals may be due to idiopathic or may be due to pregnancy, acute or chronic hepatitis, acute intermittent porphyria, estrogen-producing tumors, and hereditary disorders. Drugs that may cause elevated total T_4 are estrogens, oral contraceptives, methadone, heroin, perphenazine, and clofibrate.

B. The resin uptake of T_4 or T_3 (RT_4U or RT_3U) should be determined and the free thyroxine index calculated. The serum TSH level should be normal if the patient is euthyroid.

C. Elevated TBG levels in pregnancy lead to increased binding of free T_4. When the free T_4 falls, the pituitary secretes more TSH. This in turn leads to increased T_4 production by the gland and equilibration at a new equilibrium at which the total T_4 is elevated but the free T_4 is again normal.

D. A syndrome of familial euthyroid hyperthyroxinemia is most likely. These inherited syndromes may be caused by several mechanisms, including abnormal binding of T_4 (but not T_3) to albumin, an increased serum level of transthyretin, altered affinity of transthyretin for T_4, or pituitary and peripheral resistance to thyroid hormone.

Answers: Case 34

A. Additional features of Cushing's syndrome include hirsutism (82%), muscular weakness (58%) and muscle atrophy (70%), back pain (58%), acne (40%), psychologic symptoms (40%), edema (18%), headache (14%), polyuria and polydipsia (10%), and hyperpigmentation (6%).

B. The exact cause of hypertension in hypercortisolism remains unclear. It may be related to salt and water retention from the mineralocorticoid effects of the excess glucocorticoid, to increased secretion of angiotensinogen or deoxycorticosterone, or to a direct effect of glucocorticoids on blood vessels.

The cause of the obesity and redistribution of body fat seen in Cushing's syndrome is also somewhat unclear. It may be explained by the increase in appetite or by the lipogenic effects of the hyperinsulinemia caused by the cortisol excess. The striae result from increased subcutaneous fat deposition, which stretches the thin skin and ruptures the subdermal tissues. These striae are depressed below the skin surface because of loss of underlying connective tissue.

C. Major causes of Cushing's syndrome include Cushing's disease (ACTH-secreting pituitary adenoma), ectopic ACTH syndrome, functioning adrenocortical adenoma or carcinoma, and long-term high-dose exogenous glucocorticoid intake (iatrogenic Cushing's syndrome).

In Cushing's disease and in ectopic ACTH syndrome, production of both ACTH and cortisol is excessive. Adrenocortical adenomas or carcinomas are characterized by autonomous secretion of cortisol and suppression of pituitary ACTH. The most likely cause in this patient, a 38-year-old woman with gradual onset of symptoms, is Cushing's disease (ACTH-secreting pituitary adenoma).

D. The diagnosis of hypercortisolism can be established by measurement of free cortisol in a 24-hour urine specimen, demonstrating excessive excretion of cortisol (24-hour urinary free cortisol levels > 150 μg); or by performance of an overnight dexamethasone suppression test, demonstrating failure of 1 mg of dexamethasone to suppress morning cortisol secretion to < 5 μg/dL (0.14 μmol/L).

Answers: Case 35

A. Other symptoms of chronic adrenal insufficiency include anorexia, nausea, vomiting, hypoglycemia, and personality changes. The examiner should look also for orthostatic changes in blood pressure and pulse, hyperpigmentation of the mucous membranes and other areas, vitiligo, and loss of axillary and pubic hair.

B. The serum sodium is typically low and the serum potassium high. In Addison's disease, the deficiency of cortisol is associated with a deficiency of aldosterone, resulting in unregulated renal loss of sodium and retention of potassium. Additional blood chemistry findings suggesting Addison's disease include mild acidosis, azotemia, and hypoglycemia.

C. The diagnosis of hypoadrenocorticism can be established by performing an ACTH stimulation test. In Addison's disease, there is a low 8 AM plasma cortisol and virtually no increase in plasma cortisol 60 and 120 minutes after administration of 250 μg of synthetic ACTH (cosyntropin) intravenously or intramuscularly. The diagnosis can be confirmed by a second ACTH stimulation test, which measures the response of urinary 17-hydroxycorticosteroids to ACTH injected daily for 3 days.

D. Hypotension, including recumbent hypotension, occurs in about 90% of patients with Addison's disease and may cause orthostatic symptoms and syncope. These symptoms are related to the volume contraction resulting from unregulated renal losses of sodium.

Cortisol deficiency commonly results in loss of appetite and in gastrointestinal disturbances, including nausea and vomiting. Weight loss is common and, in chronic cases, may be profound (15 kg or more).

In primary adrenal insufficiency, the persistently low or absent plasma cortisol level results in marked hypersecretion of ACTH by the pituitary. ACTH has intrinsic melanocyte-stimulating hormone activity, causing a variety of pigmentary changes in the skin, including generalized hyperpigmentation.

Answers: Case 36

A. The major consequences of chronic aldosterone excess are sodium retention and potassium and hydrogen ion wasting by the kidney. Hypertension results from sodium retention and expansion of plasma volume. The prolonged potassium diuresis produces symptoms of potassium depletion, including muscle weakness, muscle cramps, nocturia (frequent nighttime urination), and lassitude. Blunting of baroreceptor function, manifested by postural falls in blood pressure without reflex tachycardia, may develop.

B. Prolonged potassium depletion damages the kidney (hypokalemic nephropathy), causing resistance to antidiuretic hormone (vasopressin). Patients may be unable to concentrate urine (nephrogenic diabetes insipidus), resulting in symptoms of thirst and polyuria and the finding of a low urine specific gravity (< 1.010). Urinary electrolytes show an inappropriately large amount of potassium in the urine.

C. The diagnosis of primary hyperaldosteronism is already suggested by finding hypokalemia in an untreated patient with hypertension. Since hypokalemia has been documented, the next step should be to assess the renin-angiotensin system by determining the random plasma renin activity. The plasma renin level is suppressed in primary hyperaldosteronism but increased in secondary hyperaldosteronism. Subsequent workup should include 24-hour urinary aldosterone excretion and plasma aldosterone determinations with the patient on a diet containing greater than 120 meq of sodium per day. A 24-hour urinary aldosterone exceeding 14 μg/d and a plasma aldosterone level of greater than 90 pg/mL confirm the diagnosis of primary hyperaldosteronism.

Answers: Case 37

A. This patient probably has hyporeninemic hypoaldosteronism (type IV renal tubular acidosis), a disorder characterized by hyperkalemia and acidosis in association with (usually mild) chronic renal insufficiency. The syndrome is thought to be due to impairment of renin production by the juxtaglomerular apparatus, associated with underlying renal disease. Chronic renal insufficiency is usually not severe enough by itself to account for the hyperkalemia. Impaired secretion of both potassium and hydrogen ion in the renal tubule causes the observed hyperkalemia and metabolic acidosis.

B. Other causes of hypoaldosteronism include (1) bilateral adrenalectomy; (2) acute or chronic adrenocortical insufficiency; (3) ingestion of exogenous mineralocorticoids (fludrocortisone) or inhibitors of the 11β-hydroxysteroid dehydrogenase type 2 enzyme (licorice), leading to sodium retention, volume expansion, and suppression of renin production; (4) long-standing hypopituitarism, resulting in atrophy of the zona glomerulosa; (5) congenital adrenal hypoplasia, caused by one or more enzymatic abnormalities in mineralocorticoid biosynthesis; and (6) pseudohypoaldosteronism, in which there is renal tubular resistance to mineralocorticoid hormones, presumably due to a deficiency of mineralocorticoid hormone receptors.

C. Plasma and urinary aldosterone levels and plasma renin activity are consistently low and unresponsive to stimulation by ACTH administration, upright posture, dietary sodium restriction, or furosemide administration.

Answers: Case 38

A. Other historical features to be elicited include chest pain (12%), flushing (14%), excessive sweating (50%), fainting (40%), and gastrointestinal symptoms such as nausea or vomiting (19%), abdominal pain (14%), and diarrhea (6%).

B. Pheochromocytoma is usually diagnosed by demonstrating abnormally high concentrations of catecholamines or their breakdown products in the urine or plasma. Epinephrine or norepinephrine levels can be measured in plasma, or their metabolites (metanephrines or vanillylmandelic acid [VMA]) can be measured in urine. For an outpatient, the 24-hour urinary metanephrines or VMA is probably the best screening test. If the patient has paroxysmal symptoms, it is best to sample blood during—or collect a timed urine directly after—a symptomatic episode.

While glucagon can be given to induce a paroxysm, this maneuver poses some risk to the patient and is not recommended. Administration of clonidine, 0.3 mg orally, to patients with pheochromocytomas has little or no effect on the blood pressure or plasma catecholamine level because these tumors behave autonomously, whereas in patients with other forms of hypertension clonidine reduces blood pressure.

C. Pheochromocytoma, as a tumor of adrenal medullary tissue, produces symptoms of catecholamine excess. Anxiety, headache, and palpitations are direct effects of the catecholamine discharge; the weight loss is secondary to one of the metabolic effects of excessive circulating catecholamines. These include an increase in basal metabolic rate and an increase in glycolysis and glycogenolysis, leading to hyperglycemia and glycosuria.

Subject Index

NOTE: Page numbers in bold face type indicate a major discussion. A *t* following a page number indicates tabular material and an *f* following a page number indicates a figure. Drugs are listed under their generic names. When a drug trade name is listed, the reader is referred to the generic name.

A–a DO$_2$ (A–a ΔPo$_2$/alveolar–arterial Po$_2$ difference), 198
 in chronic bronchitis, 207
 in emphysema, 207
 in noncardiogenic pulmonary edema, 214
 in pulmonary embolism, 217, 218
 wasted ventilation and, 196
A (α) cells, pancreatic, 432, 432t, 433f
 regulation of hormone release from, 434t, 437
 tumors of (glucagonomas), 456t, **457**
Aα fibers, 140
Aβ. *See* Amyloid β-peptide
Aβ fibers, 140
Aδ fibers, 137
 in pain sensation, 137, 139–140
a wave, 227, 228f
 in aortic stenosis, 242
Abdominal aorta, atherosclerosis involving, 271
Abdominal pain
 in acute pancreatitis, 368
 in chronic pancreatitis, 375
 gastrointestinal disease presenting with, 293, 294t
 in right ventricular failure, 240
Abdominal striae, in Cushing's syndrome, 515
Abdominal trauma, acute pancreatitis associated with, 365t, 366
Abducens nerve (cranial nerve VI), in control of eye movements, 142
Abetalipoproteinemia, histologic features of, 320t
Abnormal vaginal bleeding, 542, 545
 clinical manifestations of, 552
 etiology of, 545, 547t
 pathology and pathogenesis of, 550–551, 551t
Abortion, threatened, 544

Abscesses, 58
 in cyclic neutropenia, 117
 in hyper-IgE immunodeficiency, 44
 pancreatic, 370–371
Absence seizures, 154, 154t, 155f
Absorption, 294, 297
 in colon, 307
 disorders of, **308–309**
 in small intestine, 306–307, 307
Abulia, 148
ACA. *See* Adrenal cortex antibodies
Acanthosis nigricans, in Cushing's syndrome, 515
Accessory pancreatic duct (duct of Santorini), 362, 363f
Accessory pathways, in reentrant tachyarrhythmias, 233–234, 233f, 234f
ACE. *See* Angiotensin-converting enzyme
Acetoacetate, in diabetic ketoacidosis, 446, 446f
Acetone odor, in diabetic ketoacidosis, 446
Acetylcholine, in basal ganglia, 137, 137f
Acetylcholine receptor antibody, in myasthenia gravis, 153, 153f
Achalasia, esophageal, **309**, 311t
Achlorhydria, 304
 in iron deficiency anemia, 111
 in pernicious anemia, 111, 112f, 304
Acid, gastric secretion of, 298t, 302–304, 304f
 disorders of, 308, **312–314**, 314f
 in chronic renal failure, 397
 pancreatic insufficiency and, 377
Acid-mediated gastrointestinal injury, 308
 in chronic renal failure, 397
 reflux esophagitis, **309–312**, 311f
 regulation of acid secretion and, 302–304, 304f

Acid-peptic disease, 308, **312–314**, 314f
 in chronic renal failure, 397
Acidosis
 metabolic
  in acute pancreatitis, 370
  in chronic renal failure, 396
 renal tubular, 386t
  stone formation and, 403t
  type 4 (hyporeninemic hypoaldosteronism), 396, 509, 526
 respiratory
  in asthma, 203
  in chronic bronchitis, 207
  in emphysema, 207
Acinar protein (trypsinogen), in pancreatic juice, 364
 hypersecretion of in chronic pancreatitis, 373, 374f
Acini
 hepatic, 329, 330f
 pancreatic, 362–363, 363f
 pulmonary (terminal respiratory units), 186, 186f
 thyroid, 481, 482f
Acne, in Cushing's syndrome, 510f, 515, 516
Acoustic rhinometry, 38
Acquired factor inhibitors, 108
Acquired immunodeficiency. *See* Common variable immunodeficiency; HIV infection/AIDS
Acrocentric, definition of, 3t
Acrocentric autosomes, Down's syndrome and, 17
Acromegaly, 471, 473, 474t, 475t
ACTH (adrenocorticotropic hormone/corticotropin), 462–463, 464f, 502
 adrenal cortex affected by, 503
 cortisol levels affecting secretion of, 503, 504f, 506f

deficiency of
  in hypopituitarism, 473, 474, 475
  in secondary adrenocortical
    insufficiency, 520
  episodic and diurnal rhythm of
    secretion of, 502, 505f
excess of
  ectopic secretion causing, 413f, 509–510, 511t, 512f, 513, 514f
  clinical manifestations of, 515
  plasma ACTH and cortisol levels in, 505f, 513, 513f
  pituitary adenoma causing (Cushing's disease), 471, 473, 509, 511–513, 511t, 512f, 513f, 514f
  pituitary corticotroph hyperplasia causing, 509
glucocorticoid secretion regulated by, 502–503, 504f, 505f, 506f
hereditary adrenocortical unresponsiveness to, 519
mineralocorticoid secretion regulated by, 506–508
negative feedback regulation of, 502, 503, 504f, 506f
plasma levels of
  in Cushing's syndrome, 505f, 514f, 517
  in ectopic ACTH syndrome, 505f, 513, 513f
  in primary adrenocortical insufficiency, 520, 520f
  in secondary adrenocortical insufficiency, 520, 520f
stress response of, 502, 506f
ACTH stimulation test, in adrenocortical insufficiency diagnosis, 522, 523f
Actin
  in cardiac sarcomeres, 225, 226f
  in neoplasia, 83
Action potentials, 125, 126f
  in pacemaker cells, 229–231
  in ventricular and atrial myocytes, 229, 231f
Activated protein C resistance, 121, 122
Active transport
  in gastrointestinal tract, 297
  in liver, 329–340
Activin, ovarian production of, 530t
Acute adrenal crisis, 521
Acute infection, 58
Acute myelogenous/acute nonlymphocytic leukemia (AML/ANLL), 94–95, 94t
Acute phase reaction, 54
Acute (adult) respiratory distress syndrome, 213, 214, 280
  in acute pancreatitis, 370
  in septic shock, 77

Acute tubular necrosis, 390, 390–392, 393f
Adaptive immunity, **30–31**
ADCC. *See* Antibody-dependent cell-mediated cytotoxicity
Addison's disease (primary adrenocortical insufficiency), 509, 512f, 517
  etiology of, 517–520
  pathophysiology of, 520, 520f
  plasma ACTH and cortisol levels in, 505f
Adenomas
  adrenocortical
    Cushing's syndrome caused by, 510, 511t, 512f, 513, 513f, 514f
    primary aldosteronism (Conn's syndrome) caused by, 523, 523t, 524f, 525–526
  colonic, 87, 87f
    genetic alterations in, 86
  follicular, 496
  pituitary, **471–473**, 472f, 473t
    ACTH-secreting (Cushing's disease), 471, 473, 509, 511–513, 511t, 512f, 513f, 514f
    growth hormone-secreting, 471, 473, 474t, 475t
    prolactin-secreting (prolactinoma), 471, 472–473, 473t
    TSH-secreting, 487
  thyroid, 482f, 496
Adenomatous polyposis, familial, 87
Adenosine, as vasodilator, 264
Adenosine deaminase (ADA) deficiency, **42**, 43f
  SCID caused by, 40t, 42
Adenylyl cyclase, 127
  in adrenergic receptor function, 284
Adhesion molecules, in allergic airway disease, 37
Adhesion/adhesive proteins
  in neoplasia, **83**
  tumor suppressor genes encoding for, 81
Adhesions, gastrointestinal obstruction caused by, 293
Adipose tissue (fat)
  catecholamines affecting, 284t, 288t
  glucocorticoids affecting, 504, 507t
  redistribution of, in Cushing's syndrome, 510f, 514–515
  regulation of fuel homeostasis in, 436t
    insulin in, 435, 436t
  thyroid hormones affecting, 485t
Adrenal autoantibodies, adrenocortical insufficiency caused by, 518
Adrenal cortex, **500–528**
  ACTH affecting, 463, 503
  anatomy of, **500**, 501f

antibodies to, adrenocortical insufficiency caused by, 518
disorders of, 501t. *See also specific type*
  hyperfunction, 501t
  hyperplasia
    congenital
      hypertension and, 276
      plasma ACTH and cortisol levels in, 505f
    hypertension and, 276
    macronodular, 511, 513
    micronodular, 510–511, 513
    primary aldosteronism (Conn's syndrome) caused by, 523, 523t, 526
  hypofunction, 501t. *See also* Adrenocortical insufficiency
  hypoplasia, aldosterone deficiency in, 526
  tuberculosis, 518
  tumors
    Cushing's syndrome caused by, 510, 511t, 512f, 513, 513f, 514f
    primary aldosteronism (Conn's syndrome) caused by, 523, 523t, 524, 524f, 525–526
histology of, **500**, 502f
normal, **500–509**
physiology of, **501–509**. *See also* Glucocorticoids; Mineralocorticoids
Adrenal crisis, acute, 521
Adrenal disorders, 501t
  gastrointestinal manifestations of, 310t
  hypertension and, 275–277, 277f
Adrenal hemorrhage, acute adrenal insufficiency caused by, 518–519
Adrenal hyperplasia
  congenital
    hypertension and, 276
    plasma ACTH and cortisol levels in, 505f
    hypertension and, 276
    macronodular, 511, 513
    micronodular, 510–511, 513
    primary aldosteronism (Conn's syndrome) caused by, 523, 523t, 526
Adrenal medulla, **282–292**, 500
  anatomy of, **282**, 282f
  disorders of, **285–291**, 501t. *See also specific type and* Pheochromocytoma
  histology of, **282**
  hyperfunction of, 501t. *See also* Pheochromocytoma
  hypofunction of, **290–291**, 291t
  normal, **282–285**
  physiology of, **282–285**, 283f, 284t. *See also* Catecholamines

Adrenal metastases, adrenocortical insufficiency caused by, 519
Adrenalectomy, bilateral, effects of, 290
α-Adrenergic receptor blockade, for benign prostatic hyperplasia, 572, 572*t*
α-Adrenergic receptors
  catecholamine actions and, 283, 284*t*
  in prostatic smooth muscle, benign prostatic hyperplasia and, 572
β-Adrenergic receptors, catecholamine actions and, 283, 284*t*
Adrenocortical insufficiency, **517–522**, 518*t*
  diagnosis of, 522, 522*t*
  gastrointestinal manifestations of, 310*t*
  hyponatremia in, 478
  plasma electrolyte levels in, 522*t*
  primary (Addison's disease), 509, 512*f*, 517
    clinical manifestations of, 520–522, 521*t*
    etiology of, 517–520
    pathophysiology of, 520, 520*f*
    plasma ACTH and cortisol levels in, 505*f*
  secondary, 517
    clinical manifestations of, 520–522, 521*t*
    diagnosis of, 522
    etiology of, 520
    pathophysiology of, 520, 520*f*
Adrenocortical tumors, Cushing's syndrome caused by, 510, 511*t*, 512*f*, 513, 513*f*, 514*f*
Adrenocorticotropic hormone (ACTH), 462–463, 464*f*, 502
  adrenal cortex affected by, 503
  cortisol levels affecting secretion of, 503, 504*f*, 506*f*
  deficiency of
    in hypopituitarism, 473, 474, 475
    in secondary adrenocortical insufficiency, 520
  episodic and diurnal rhythm of secretion of, 502, 505*f*
  excess of
    ectopic secretion causing, 413*f*, 509–510, 511*t*, 512*f*, 513, 514*f*
      clinical manifestations of, 515
      plasma ACTH and cortisol levels in, 505*f*, 513, 513*f*
    pituitary adenoma causing (Cushing's disease), 471, 473, 509, 511–513, 511*t*, 512*f*, 513*f*, 514*f*
    pituitary corticotroph hyperplasia causing, 509
  glucocorticoid secretion regulated by, 502–503, 504*f*, 505*f*, 506*f*

hereditary adrenocortical unresponsiveness to, 519
  mineralocorticoid secretion regulated by, 506–508
  negative feedback regulation of, 502, 503, 504*f*, 506*f*
  plasma levels of
    in Cushing's syndrome, 505*f*, 514*f*, 517
    in ectopic ACTH syndrome, 505*f*, 513, 513*f*
    in primary adrenocortical insufficiency, 520, 520*f*
    in secondary adrenocortical insufficiency, 520, 520*f*
  stress response of, 502, 506*f*
Adrenogenital syndrome, 509
Adrenoleukodystrophy, X-linked, adrenal insufficiency in, 519–520
Adrenomedullary failure, 285, 291
Adrenomyeloneuropathy, adrenal insufficiency in, 519
Adult (acute) respiratory distress syndrome, 213, 214, 280
  in acute pancreatitis, 370
  in septic shock, 77
Advanced glycosylation end products, in diabetic microvascular disease, 449, 450*f*
Adventitia, 258, 259*f*
Afferent arteriole, glomerular, 382, 384*f*, 385*f*
Afibrinogenemia, 108*t*
Afterload, 227, 230*f*
Agammaglobulinemia, X-linked (Bruton's), 40*t*, **42**
  pathogens causing infection in, 41*t*, 56*t*
AGE. *See* Advanced glycosylation end products
Age
  blood pressure affected by, 262, 263*f*
  bone mass loss and, 425–426, 426*f*, 427. *See also* Osteoporosis
  maternal, Down's syndrome frequency and, 18, 18*f*, 19–20
  prostatic growth and, 568, 569
  testosterone levels affected by, 557, 560*f*
Age-dependent (reduced) penetrance, 5, 6
Agraphia, 149
AIDS. *See* HIV infection/AIDS
AIDS dementia complex, 48
Air embolism, 215*t*
AIRE gene, in autoimmune polyendocrinopathy-candidiasis-ectodermal dystrophy, 421
Airflow, 191–192, 193*f*. *See also* Ventilation
  distribution of, 193–194, 194*f*, 195*f*
  matching perfusion to, 194–198, 196*f*, 197*f*

resistance to, 186–187, 186*f*, 187*f*, 191–192, 193*f*
  in asthma, 186–187, 202–203
  in obstructive lung disease, 200–201
Airways
  allergic disease of
    asthma, **201–204**, 201*t*, 202*t*, 204*f*
    rhinitis, **36–39**, 37*t*
  anatomy of, 186–187, 186*f*, 187*f*, 188*f*
  caliber of, resistance and, 192
  hyperresponsiveness of
    in allergic rhinitis, 38
    in asthma, 201, 203–204
  obstruction of
    in asthma, 202–203
    in chronic bronchitis, 207
    resistance to airflow in, 186–187, 186*f*, 187*f*, 191–192, 193*f*
    in asthma, 186–187, 202–203
    in obstructive lung disease, 200–201
Alanine aminotransferase, in acute hepatitis, 350
Albright's hereditary osteodystrophy, 423
Albumin, 336*t*
Albuminuria, in diabetes mellitus, 452, 452*f*
Alcohol-induced dementia, 157
Alcohol use/abuse
  acute pancreatitis and, 365, 365*t*, 366, 371
  chronic pancreatitis and, 372
  cirrhosis and, 355, 356–357
  hepatitis and, 348, 349*t*, 352, 353*f*
  pneumonia and, 67, 67*t*
Alcoholic hepatitis
  acute, 348, 349*t*
  chronic, 352, 353*f*
Alcoholic hypoglycemia, liver dysfunction and, 338*t*
Alcoholic ketoacidosis, liver dysfunction and, 338*t*
Aldosterone. *See also* Mineralocorticoids
  disorders of secretion of. *See* Hyperaldosteronism; Hypoaldosteronism
  mechanism of action of, 508, 508*f*
  regulation of, 506–508, 507*f*
  synthesis/protein binding/metabolism of, 503*f*, 504–505
  zona glomerulosa secreting, 500, 502*f*, 503*f*
Aldosteronism. *See* Hyperaldosteronism
Alendronate, for osteoporosis prevention/management, 429
Alexia, 149
Alfuzosin, for benign prostatic hyperplasia, 572, 572*t*
Alkaline phosphatase, in acute hepatitis, 350
Alkalosis
  metabolic, in pheochromocytoma, 290
  in mineralocorticoid excess, 525

Alleles, 3*t*, 5
  dominant negative, 3*t*, 7–8
Allelic heterogeneity, 3*t*
  in osteogenesis imperfecta, 13
Allergen-specific IgE, measurement of, 39
Allergic airway disease
  asthma, **201–204**, 201*t*, 202*t*, 204*f*
  rhinitis, **36–39**, 37*t*
Allergic salute, 38
Allergic shiners, 36
Allergy/allergic reaction, 34
  IgE in, 34–35, 36
  new treatment methods based on, 35
  impaired health-related quality of life and, 39
  skin testing and, 39
Alpha-adrenergic receptor blockade, for benign prostatic hyperplasia, 572, 572*t*
Alpha-adrenergic receptors
  catecholamine actions and, 283, 284*t*
  in prostatic smooth muscle, benign prostatic hyperplasia and, 572
Alpha$_1$-antiprotease (alpha$_1$-protease inhibitor), 336*t*
  in chronic obstructive pulmonary disease, 205
  hepatic synthesis of, 336*t*
Alpha-blockers, for benign prostatic hyperplasia, 572, 572*t*
Alpha (A) cells, pancreatic, 432, 432*t*, 433*f*
  regulation of hormone release from, 434*t*, 437
  tumors of (glucagonomas), 456*t*, **457**
Alpha-fetoprotein, 336*t*
  hepatic synthesis of, 336*t*
  in testicular cancer, 91
Alpha fibers, 140
Alpha granules, in platelet activation, 102–103
17-Alpha-hydroxylase deficiency, hypertension and, 276
Alpha$_2$-macroglobulin, 336*t*
Alpha motor neurons, 129, 129*f*
Alpha$_1$-protease inhibitor (α_1-antiprotease), 336*t*
  in chronic obstructive pulmonary disease, 205
  hepatic synthesis of, 336*t*
Alpha-reductase
  in dihydrotestosterone synthesis, 560, 569, 571*f*
  in prostate gland, 569–570
Alpha-reductase inhibitors, for benign prostatic hyperplasia, 570–571, 570*t*, 571*f*
Alpha-tocopherol, in atherosclerosis prevention, 273
ALS. *See* Amyotrophic lateral sclerosis

ALT. *See* Alanine aminotransferase
Alternative pathway of complement activation, 54, 55*f*
Alveolar–arterial PO$_2$ difference (A–a DO$_2$/A–a ΔPO$_2$), 198
  in chronic bronchitis, 207
  in emphysema, 207
  in noncardiogenic pulmonary edema, 214
  in pulmonary embolism, 217, 218
  wasted ventilation and, 196
Alveolar dead space, 195–195, 196*f*
  in pulmonary embolism, 217
Alveolitis
  cryptogenic fibrosing (idiopathic pulmonary fibrosis), **208–210**, 208*f*, 209*t*, 210*f*, 211*f*
  in pneumonia, 66
Alzheimer's disease, **157–158**, 157*f*
  Down's syndrome and, 19, 158
Amacrine cells, retinal, 144
Amadori product, in diabetic microvascular disease, 449, 449*f*
Amantadine, for Parkinson's disease, 152
Amenorrhea, 545
  in adrenocortical insufficiency, 521
  clinical manifestations of, 551–552
  in Cushing's syndrome, 516
  etiology of, 545, 546*t*
  hypothalamic, 549
  ovarian failure causing, 545, 546–550, 546*t*, 551
  pathology and pathogenesis of, 545–550
  uterine disorders causing, 545, 546, 546*t*, 551
γ-Aminobutyric acid (GABA)
  in basal ganglia, 137, 137*f*
  glucagon release affected by, 437
  in hepatic encephalopathy, 360
  in seizure pathogenesis, 155, 156
Aminoglycoside antibiotics
  nephrotoxicity of, acute renal failure and, 390
  neuromuscular transmission affected by, 130*f*, 131
Aminotransferases, in acute hepatitis, 350
Amiodarone, hypothyroidism caused by, 491
AML. *See* Acute myelogenous/acute nonlymphocytic leukemia
Ammonia, hepatic metabolism of, 337
  liver dysfunction and, 342–344
Amniotic fluid embolism, 215*t*
Amorphic (loss-of-function) mutation, 3*t*, 6
  dominant inheritance and, 7
  recessive inheritance and, 6–7, 7*t*
Amphetamines, intraparenchymal hemorrhage associated with use of, 162

Amplification, genetic
  in fragile X-associated mental retardation syndrome, 14, 15*f*
  postzygotic, 16
  in oncogene activation, 80
Ampulla of Vater, 362, 363*f*
Amputations, for diabetic foot ulcers, 454
Amylase
  in pancreatic juice, 364
  serum levels of in acute pancreatitis, 369
Amylin (islet amyloid polypeptide), in type 2 diabetes, 444
Amyloid angiopathy, cerebral, 162
Amyloid β-peptide, in Alzheimer's disease, 158
Amyloid plaques, in Alzheimer's disease, 157, 157*f*
β-Amyloid precursor protein, in Alzheimer's disease, 158
Amyloidosis
  gastrointestinal manifestations of, 310*t*
  histologic features of, 320*t*
Amyotrophic lateral sclerosis
  clinical presentation of, 150
  pathology and pathogenesis of, 150–151, 151*f*
Anabolic effects, of androgens, 561
Anal canal, 295*f*
Anal dysplasia, in HIV infection/AIDS, 49
Anal sphincters, 295*f*
Anaphylactic (immediate/type I) hypersensitivity reaction, 34
Anaphylactic shock, 280
Anasarca, in right ventricular failure, 240
Anatomic dead space, 195
Androgen-binding protein, 560
Androgen deprivation, for benign prostatic hyperplasia, 569, 570*t*, 571*f*
Androgen receptor inhibitors, for benign prostatic hyperplasia, 570, 570*t*
Androgen receptors, in benign prostatic hyperplasia, 569–570, 571
Androgens
  adrenal, 500, 502*f*
    disorders of production of, **526–527**
    excess, 509, 527. *See also* Adrenogenital syndrome
  effects of, 561, 561*t*
  fetal-placental-maternal unit in production of, 538, 540*f*
  mechanism of action of, 560–561, 561*f*
  ovarian, 536–537
    postmenopausal production of, 542
  in polycystic ovary syndrome, 548, 549, 549*f*
  testicular
    in benign prostatic hyperplasia, 569–571, 570*f*

Androgens (cont.)
   effects of, 561, 561t
   mechanism of action of, 560–561, 561f
   regulation of, 558–560, 560f
   suppression of, for benign prostatic hyperplasia, 569, 570–571, 570t, 571f
   synthesis/protein binding/metabolism of, 557–558, 559f, 560f, 560t
Androstenedione
   adrenal, synthesis of, 503f
   disorders of, 526–527
   normal levels of, 560t
Anemia, 101, 105–106
   in adrenocortical insufficiency, 522
   aplastic, 105
   in chronic renal failure, 397
   erythropoietin levels in, 98
   hemolytic, 106f
      autoimmune, 105
   in hypothyroidism, 493
   iron deficiency, 105, **109–111**
   macrocytic, 105, 105t, 106f
      liver dysfunction and, 342
   megaloblastic, 105
      cell line changes in, 113, 114f
      pernicious anemia as, 111
   microcytic, 105, 105t, 106f
      iron deficiency, 109
   morphologic classification of, 105, 105t
   normocytic, 105t, 106f
   pernicious, **111–115**, 304
   sickle cell, 7t, 105
   thin blood smear appearance of erythrocytes in, 105, 106f
   in vitamin B_{12} deficiency, 105, 111
Aneuploidy, 2, 3t
   Down's syndrome and, 17
Aneurysms
   berry, 162
   Charcot-Bouchard, 162
Angelman's syndrome, 22t
Angina pectoris, 251, 253, 271
   in aortic stenosis, 241, 242
   in left ventricular failure, 238
   stable, 251, 252
   unstable, 251, 252
Angiography, pulmonary, in pulmonary embolism, 218
Angiomas, spider, in cirrhosis, 361
Angiomatosis, bacillary, in HIV infection/AIDS, 48
Angiopathy, cerebral amyloid, 162
Angiotensin I, 506, 507f
   in renal regulation of blood pressure, 386
Angiotensin II, 506, 507f
   ovarian production of, 530t
   in renal regulation of blood pressure, 386

Angiotensin-converting enzyme, 506, 507f
   in renal regulation of blood pressure, 386
Angiotensin-converting enzyme inhibitors, acute renal failure caused by, 390
Angiotensinogen, 506, 507f
   hepatic synthesis of, 336t
Anisocytosis, in anemia, 105, 106f
ANLL. *See* Acute myelogenous/acute nonlymphocytic leukemia
Anomia, 149
Anorexia, gastrointestinal disease presenting with, 293
Anorexia nervosa, amenorrhea in, 550
Anovulation, chronic, 547, 548t
ANP. *See* Atrial natriuretic peptide
Anterior lobe, cerebellar, 134, 134f
Antiacetylcholine-receptor antibody, in myasthenia gravis, 153, 153f
Antiadrenal antibodies, adrenocortical insufficiency caused by, 518
Antiandrogens, for benign prostatic hyperplasia, 569, 570–571, 570t, 571f
Antibody. *See also* Immunoglobulins
   antigen elimination by, 33
   antisperm, in infertility, 565
   deficiency of. *See also* Immunodeficiency diseases
      autoimmune phenomena and, 40
      infections associated with, 40, 41t, 56t
   structure and function of, 32–33, 33f
Antibody-dependent cell-mediated cytotoxicity, 29
   in inflammatory rheumatic diseases, 578
Antibody-heparin-PF4 complex
   in heparin-induced thrombocytopenia, 118, 118f
   in heparin-induced thrombocytopenia and thrombosis, 118–119
Antibody-mediated (humoral) immune response, 31, 32
   antigen elimination in, 33
   impairment of. *See also* Immunodeficiency diseases
      autoimmune phenomena and, 40
      infections associated with, 40, 41t, 56t
   microbial strategies against, 60t
Anticholinergic drugs, for Parkinson's disease, 152
Anticipation, genetic, 3t, 15
   in fragile X-associated mental retardation syndrome, 15–16, 15f
Anticoagulant, lupus, in adrenocortical insufficiency, 519
Anticoagulant factors, 104t. *See also* Thrombolytic system
   in hypercoagulable states, 120

Anticoagulant prophylaxis, pulmonary embolism and, 215, 216t
Anticonvulsants, 156, 156t
Antidiuretic hormone (ADH/vasopressin), 466–467, 467f
   deficiency of, in hypopituitarism, 473
   for differentiation of central from nephrogenic diabetes insipidus, 477
   ovarian production of, 530t
   receptors for, 467
   in renal regulation, 385, 386, 467
   syndrome of inappropriate secretion of, **478–479**, 478t
Antigen-antibody binding. *See also* Immune complexes
   in type II hypersensitivity reactions, 34
   in type III hypersensitivity reactions, 34
Antigen-antibody complexes. *See* Immune complexes
Antigen-presenting cells, 31
Antigens (immunogens), **31**
   humoral mechanisms of elimination of, 33
   processing and presentation of, 31
Anti-HBc, 350t
Anti-HBe, 350t
Anti-HBs, 350t
Antihemophilic factor (factor VIII), 104, 104t
   deficiency of, 108, 108t
Antihistamines, for early phase allergic symptoms, 38
Anti-IgE antibodies, in allergy treatment, 35
Anti-inflammatory agents, for late phase/chronic allergic symptoms, 38
Antimalarial agents, lichen planus (lichenoid reactions) caused by, 174t
Antimorphic (dominant negative) mutation, 3t, 7–8
Antioxidants, in atherosclerosis prevention, 273
Antiphospholipid antibody, in adrenocortical insufficiency, 519
Antiphospholipid syndrome, in adrenocortical insufficiency, 519
α_1-Antiprotease (alpha$_1$-protease inhibitor), 336t
   in chronic obstructive pulmonary disease, 205
   hepatic synthesis of, 336t
Antisperm antibodies, infertility and, 565
Antithrombin III, 104t, 105, 336t
   deficiency of, 121, 122
   hepatic synthesis of, 336t

Antmicrosomal antibody. *See* Thyroidal peroxidase antibody
Anus. *See also under* Anal
  cancer of, 86*t*
  in HIV infection/AIDS, 49
Aorta, 258, 259*f*
  coarctation of, hypertension caused by, 274
Aortic ejection sound, in aortic stenosis, 241, 242, 243*f*
Aortic valve, 222, 224*f*
  regurgitation/insufficiency of, **244–245**, 245*t*, 246*f*
  stenosis of, **241–244**, 242*t*, 243*f*
Apallic state, 148
APC gene, 82*t*
  in colon carcinoma, 87
APECED. *See* Autoimmune polyendocrinopathy-candidiasis-ectodermal dystrophy
Aphasia, 149
Apical impulse
  in aortic regurgitation, 244, 245
  in aortic stenosis, 241
  in left ventricular failure, 235, 238
  in mitral regurgitation, 247, 249–251
Aplastic anemia, 105
Apnea, sleep, in hypothyroidism, 493
Apocrine glands, catecholamines affecting, 284*t*, 288*t*
apoE4. *See* Apolipoprotein E
Apolipoprotein B, hepatic synthesis of, 336*t*
Apolipoprotein E, in Alzheimer's disease, 158
Apolipoproteins, in solubilization and transport of lipids, 335
Apoptosis
  in lymphoma, 93
  in male infertility, 563
  in spinal muscular atrophies, 150
  in systemic lupus erythematosus, 582, 582*f*, 583
APP. *See* β-Amyloid precursor protein
APP gene, in Alzheimer's disease, 158
Apparent mineralocorticoid excess, 276, 277*f*
Appendix, 295*f*
Apraxia, 148
Aquaporin-2 water channel, in diabetes insipidus, 476
ARDS. *See* Acute respiratory distress syndrome
Aromatase inhibitors, for benign prostatic hyperplasia, 571
Arousal
  anatomic basis of, 147
  physiology of, 147–148, 148*f*, 149*t*
Arrhythmias, **231–234**, 232*f*, 233*f*, 234*f*, 235*f*
Arterial blood gases, 198
  in chronic bronchitis, 207

  in emphysema, 207
  in idiopathic pulmonary fibrosis, 210
Arterial pressure. *See* Blood pressure
Arteries, 258, 259*f*
Arterioles, 258, 259*f*
  factors affecting, 266, 266*t*
  glomerular, 382, 384*f*, 385*f*
Arthritis
  gouty, 580
  psoriatic, 172
  rheumatoid, gastrointestinal manifestations of, 310*t*
  in systemic lupus erythematosus, 583
Ascertainment bias, 3*t*
  genetic anticipation caused by, 16
Ascites
  in cirrhosis, 355*f*, 357–359, 358*f*
  pancreatic, 366, 371
  in right ventricular failure, 240
Aseptic meningitis (lymphocyte-predominant), 62
Asherman's syndrome, 545, 546*t*
Aspartate aminotransferase, in acute hepatitis, 350
Aspirin, thromboxane/prostacyclin balance affected by, 264
Association areas, 149
Association cortex, parietal, 149
AST. *See* Aspartate aminotransferase
Asterixis
  in chronic renal failure, 397
  in hepatic encephalopathy, 360
Asthenospermia, in Kartagener's (immotile cilia) syndrome, 564, 566
Asthma, **201–204**, 201*t*, 202*t*, 204*f*
  airway hyperresponsiveness in, 201, 203–204
  airway resistance in, 186–187, 202–203
  "cardiac," 237
  gastrointestinal manifestations of, 310*t*
  impaired health-related quality of life and, 39
Astrocytes, 127–128, 127*f*
Astrocytosis, reactive, 128
Asymptomatic urinary abnormalities, 391*t*, 398, 399, 399*t*
AT-III. *See* Antithrombin III
Atamestane, for benign prostatic hyperplasia, 571
Ataxia, 136
Ataxia-telangiectasia, 40*t*
  pathogens causing infection in, 56*t*
Atheroma, 252, 252*f*
Atherosclerosis, **269–273**, 270*f*, 271*f*, 272*t*
  of cerebral circulation, in stroke, 160–162, 161*f*, 271
  in chronic renal failure, 397
  coronary artery, 251–253, 251*t*, 252*f*, 271

  in diabetes mellitus, 452–453, 453*f*
  hypertension affecting progression of, 274
Athetosis, in Huntington's disease, 137
Athyreotic cretins, 492
Atonic seizures, 155
Atopy, in asthma, 201
Atresia, ovarian follicle, 534, 535*f*
  amenorrhea and, 547
Atria, cardiac, 222, 223–224*f*
Atrial fibrillation, 235*f*
  in mitral stenosis, 247
Atrial flutter, 235*f*
Atrial myocytes, contraction of, 229, 231*f*, 232*f*
Atrial natriuretic peptide (ANP)
  blood pressure affected by, 277
  hyperthyroidism affecting, 490
  in mineralocorticoid excess, 525
  ovarian production of, 530*t*
  vascular smooth muscle affected by, 266
Atrial tachycardia, 235*f*
Atrioventricular heart block, 232, 232*f*, 233*f*
  in coronary artery disease, 253
Atrioventricular node, 222–224, 225*f*
  in coronary artery disease, 253
Atrophic gastritis, chronic/autoimmune, 112*f*, 113, **313**
Atrophic lichen planus, 175
Atypical hyperplasia, 85
Audiometry, 146
Auditory cortex, primary, 132*f*, 149
Auditory fibers, 146
Auer rods, 94
Auerbach's nerve plexus (myenteric nerve plexus), 294–296, 296*f*, 299
Aura, before seizure, 155
Austin Flint murmur, 244, 245
Autoantibodies
  in adrenocortical insufficiency, 518
  in diabetes mellitus, 442
  in systemic lupus erythematosus, 582–583, 582*f*, 582*t*
Autoimmune disorders, 577
  adrenocortical insufficiency caused by, 517, 518
  chronic atrophic gastritis and, 112*f*, 113, **313**
  chronic hepatitis and, 351*t*, 352
  chronic pancreatitis and, 373, 375
  Graves' disease and, 488, 488*t*
  Hashimoto's thyroiditis and, 488*t*
    gastrointestinal manifestations of, 310*t*
  hemolytic anemia and, 105
  polyendocrine/polyglandular failure and, 421–422, 492, 518
  premature ovarian failure in, 547
  type 1, 421, 422*f*, 518
  type 2, 422, 518

Autoimmune/chronic atrophic gastritis, 112*f*, 113, **313**
Autoimmune polyendocrinopathy-candidiasis-ectodermal dystrophy (APECED/autoimmune polyglandular failure, type 1), 421, 422*f*, 518
Autoimmune regulator gene, in autoimmune polyendocrinopathy candidiasis ectodermal dystrophy, 421
Automaticity, increased, in tachycardia, 233, 233*f*
Automatisms, in complex partial seizures, 155
Autonomic failure
  hypoglycemia-associated, 291
  with Parkinson's disease, 291
  primary (sympathetic neural failure), 285, 290–291
  pure, 291
Autonomic neuropathy, diabetic, 291, 448, 454, 454*t*
  hypoglycemia and, 448
Autoregulation, 264
Autosomal, definition of, 3*t*
Autosomal inheritance, dominant versus recessive, 6
Autosomes. *See also* Chromosomes
  acrocentric, Down's syndrome and, 17
AV node. *See* Atrioventricular node
Axon, 124, 125*f*
Azoospermia, 562, 563, 566
Azotemia, prerenal, 279, 392
  in adrenocortical insufficiency, 521, 522
  liver dysfunction and, 338*t*, 350

B cell lymphomas, in HIV infection/AIDS, 49
B (β) cells, pancreatic, 432, 432*t*, 433*f*
  autoimmune destruction of in diabetes, 440, 441–442
  catecholamines affecting, 284*t*, 288*t*
  regulation of hormone release from, 433, 434*f*, 434*t*
  tumors of (insulinomas), **455–456**, 456*t*
B lymphocytes, 29
  activation of, 32. *See also* Humoral (antibody-mediated) immune response
  impairment of function/deficiency of
    in common variable immunodeficiency, 44
    infections associated with, 40, 41*t*, 56*t*
  in lymph nodes, 30, 30*f*
  memory, 31
B vitamins, in atherosclerosis prevention,

272. *See also specific type under* Vitamin
Bacillary angiomatosis, in HIV infection/AIDS, 48
Bacillary dysentery, 72
Bacillus cereus, gastroenteritis caused by, 69
Background retinopathy, in diabetes mellitus, 449
Bacteremia
  in infective endocarditis, 60
  pulmonary edema and, 213, 214
  in sepsis, 74
Bacteria, hepatic clearance of, 337
  hepatic dysfunction and, 342
Bacterial infections
  in cyclic neutropenia, 116–117
  diarrhea, 69–73
  endocarditis, 59–61, 62*t*
  meningitis, 62–65, 63*t*, 64*f*
  peritonitis, in cirrhosis, 359
  pneumonia, 65–69, 66*t*, 67*t*, 68*f*
  sepsis, 73–77
Bacterial neurotropism, pathogenetic sequence of, 63–64, 63*t*, 64*f*
Balance, **145–146**
Balanced translocations, in hematologic neoplasms, 92
  leukemia, 94–95
Bands, 99*f*, 102
Baroreceptors, in vascular function regulation, 267–268, 267*f*, 268*f*
Barrett's esophagus, 312
Basal ganglia, **136–137**, 136*f*, 137*f*
Basal keratinocytes. *See* Keratinocytes
Basal layer of skin, 166, 166*f*
Basement membrane, of epidermis, 167, 169*f*
Basic fibroblast growth factor, in benign prostatic hyperplasia, 571
Basophils, 29, 101
  normal values for, 101*t*
bcl-2 gene, in lymphoma, 93
Beck's triad, 256
Bed-wetting, in diabetes insipidus, 476
Benign hyperphenylalaninemia, 23, 25
Benign prostatic hyperplasia, **568–574**
  clinical manifestations of, 573–574
  etiology of, 568
  pathogenesis of, 569–573, 570*f*, 572*t*, 573*t*
  pathology of, 568–569, 568*f*, 569*f*
Bentiromide test, in pancreatic insufficiency, 378
Bernheim effect, reversed, 239, 257
Bernoulli's principle, 261
Berry aneurysm, 162
Beta-adrenergic receptors, catecholamine actions and, 283, 284*t*
Beta-amyloid precursor protein, in Alzheimer's disease, 158
Beta-carotene, in atherosclerosis prevention, 273

Beta (B) cells, pancreatic, 432, 432*t*, 433*f*
  autoimmune destruction of in diabetes mellitus, 440, 441–442
  catecholamines affecting, 284*t*, 288*t*
  regulation of hormone release from, 433, 434*f*, 434*t*
  tumors of (insulinomas), **455–456**, 456*t*
Beta fibers, 140
Beta-hydroxybutyrate, in diabetic ketoacidosis, 446, 446*f*
11-Beta-hydroxylase deficiency, hypertension and, 276
bFGF. *See* Basic fibroblast growth factor
BH_4. *See* Tetrahydrobiopterin
Bias of ascertainment, 3*t*
  genetic anticipation caused by, 16
Bicalutamide, for benign prostatic hyperplasia, 570*t*
Bicarbonate
  in adrenocortical insufficiency, 522*t*
  in pancreatic juice, 363
  parathyroid hormone affecting excretion of, 408–410
Bile, 305
  enterohepatic circulation of, 334
  secretion/formation of, 331*f*
    disordered, 339–340, 340*f*, 341*t*. *See also* Cholestasis
Bile acids, enterohepatic circulation of, 334
Biliary system, 305*f*. *See also specific organ or structure*
  acute pancreatitis associated with disorders of, 365, 365*t*
  cancer of, 86*t*
Bilirubin, 339
  gallstones composed of, 316
  secretion of, 340*f*
Bilirubinuria, in acute pancreatitis, 370
Binding proteins, hepatic production of, 335–337
Binswanger's disease, 157
Biotransformation, hepatic, 334–335
  liver dysfunction and, 338*t*, 340–342, 343*t*
  phases of, 335
Bipolar cells, retinal, 144
Birth control pills, 537
Bisphosphonates, for osteoporosis prevention/management, 429
Bitemporal hemianopia, 145
  in pituitary adenoma, 472, 472*f*
Bladder
  cancer of, 86*t*
  catecholamines affecting, 284*t*, 288*t*
  obstruction-induced changes in, 573, 573*f*
  rupture of, in acute renal failure, 392*t*
Bladder outlet obstruction, in benign prostatic hyperplasia, 572
  androgen suppression relieving, 570–571, 570*t*, 571*f*

bladder response to, 573, 573f
clinical manifestations of, 573–574
mechanisms of, 572
prostatic capsule and, 569, 572
Bleeding
  abnormal vaginal. *See* Abnormal vaginal bleeding
  in drug-associated immune thrombocytopenia, 119
  gastrointestinal. *See* Gastrointestinal bleeding
  iron deficiency anemia caused by, 105, 109, 111
  during pregnancy, 543
Bleeding disorders, gastrointestinal manifestations of, 310t
Bleeding time, in drug-associated immune thrombocytopenia, 119
Blindness, in diabetes mellitus, 448, 449
Blood, **98–123**
  coagulation of. *See* Coagulation
  disorders of, **105–122**
  formed elements of, **98–103**
    anatomy of, 98–100
    development of, 98–100, 99f
    physiology of, 100–103
  normal structure and function of, **98–105**
Blood-brain barrier, 260
  in hypothalamus, 461
Blood cells, **98–103**. *See also specific type*
  anatomy of, 98–100
  development of, 98–100, 99f
  physiology of, 100–103
Blood clotting. *See* Coagulation
Blood flow
  factors determining, 261
  liver, **332**
  pulmonary
    distribution of, 193–194, 194f, 195f
    matching ventilation to, 194–198, 196f, 197f
  resistance to, 261–262
  catecholamines in, 285
  in septic shock, 76
Blood gases (arterial blood gases), 198
  in chronic bronchitis, 207
  in emphysema, 207
  in idiopathic pulmonary fibrosis, 210
Blood loss. *See* Bleeding
Blood pressure, 260, 262, 262f
  catecholamines affecting, 285
  in hypertension, 274
  measurement of, 262
  medullary control of, 267, 267f
  normal, 262, 263f
  renal regulation of, 385–386
Blood smear, 100, 100f, 101t, 106f
  in anemia, 106f, 109
    pernicious, 113, 114f
    in cyclic neutropenia, 116

in drug-induced immune thrombocytopenia, 119
erythrocytes on, 101, 106f
Blood urea nitrogen (BUN), in renal dysfunction, 388
acute renal failure and, 390, 392
Blood vessels, 258, 259f. *See also* Vascular system
catecholamines affecting, 284t, 288t
Blue scleras, in osteogenesis imperfecta, 9, 10
BMI. *See* Body mass index
BNP. *See* Brain natriuretic peptide
Body mass index, in obesity, 469
Body weight. *See also under* Weight
  physiology of control of, **468–469**, 468f
Bombesin, 298t
Bone, **410–413**, 411f, 412f
  brown tumors of, in hyperparathyroidism, 418
  calcium metabolism and, **410–413**
  disorders of
    in chronic renal failure, 396–397, 396f
    in osteogenesis imperfecta, 9–10
  loss of. *See* Osteoporosis
  mineralization of, 411
    defects in (osteomalacia), **429–430**, 429t
  remodeling of, 411–412, 412f
  resorption of, 411, 411f
    in Cushing's syndrome, 510f, 515
    in hyperparathyroidism, 418
    parathyroid hormone affecting, 410
    in postmenopausal osteoporosis, 426–427
  thyroid hormones affecting, 485t
Bone density
  decreased
    in hyperprolactinemia, 473
    in osteoporosis, 425–426, 427, 428
  measurement of, 428
Bone marrow, 29, 98–100
  in drug-induced immune thrombocytopenia, 119
  in immune system development, 102, 102f
  in pernicious anemia, 113–114, 114f
Bone marrow transplantation, pancreatic insufficiency after, 376
Bone mass, loss of. *See* Osteoporosis
Botulism, 130f, 131
Bowel alterations
  gastrointestinal disease presenting as, 293, 294t
  in hyperthyroidism, 490
  in hypothyroidism, 493
Bowman's capsule, 382, 384f
BPH. *See* Benign prostatic hyperplasia
Bradycardia, 231–232, 232f
  in coronary artery disease, 253
  in hypovolemia, 279

Bradykinin, vascular smooth muscle affected by, 265–266, 266f
Brain natriuretic peptide (BNP), vascular smooth muscle affected by, 266
Brain tumors, intraparenchymal hemorrhage caused by, 162
Brainstem lesions, sensory loss caused by, 142
BRCA1 gene, 82t, 88
BRCA2 gene, 82t, 88
Breast cancer, 86t, **88–89**
Breast feeding, 539–541, 542f
  oxytocin in, 467, 540, 542f
Breast milk, synthesis and secretion of, 466, 540–541, 542f
Breasts, 531, 533f
  development of, 539–540
  prolactin affecting, 466, 540
  disorders of, **544–545**
    benign disease, 544
  milk synthesis and secretion and, 540–541, 542f
  prolactin in, 466, 540–541, 542f
  structure of, 533f, 539–540
Breath sounds
  in emphysema, 207
  in left ventricular heart failure, 235
Breathing. *See also* Ventilation
  control of, 198–200
    in chronic hypercapnia, 200
    in chronic hypoxia, 200
    exercise and, 200
    integrated responses in, 199–200, 199f, 200f
    pulmonary embolism and, 216t
    sensory input in, 198–199, 198f
  Kussmaul, in diabetic ketoacidosis, 446
  resistance to, 186–187, 186f, 187f, 191–192, 193f
    in asthma, 186–187, 202–203
    in obstructive lung diseases, 200–201
  work of, 193, 193f
    flow and resistance and, 191–192, 193f
    in left ventricular failure, 237
    pulmonary embolism and, 216t
Bridging hepatic necrosis, 349
Broca's area, 148–149
Brodmann areas, 131, 132f
Bronchial hyperresponsiveness, in asthma, 201, 203–204
Bronchial provocation testing, in asthma, 203–204
Bronchial smooth muscle, catecholamines affecting, 284t
Bronchial vessels, 187, 188f, 189f
Bronchioles, 186, 186f
Bronchitis, chronic, **204–207**, 205f

Bronchoconstriction
 in asthma, 202–203
 resistance and, 192
Bronchopulmonary stretch receptors, 187, 188t
Brown-Séquard's syndrome, 141, 141f
Brown tumors of bone, in hyperparathyroidism, 418
Brudzinski's sign, in meningitis, 65
Bruising
 in Cushing's syndrome, 510f, 515
 in drug-associated immune thrombocytopenia, 119
Bruits, 261
 in renal hypertension, 274
Bruton's agammaglobulinemia. See X-linked agammaglobulinemia
BTK gene, in X-linked agammaglobulinemia, 42
Buffalo hump, in Cushing's syndrome, 514
Bulbourethral glands, Cowper's, 556, 557f, 558f
Bullae, 169
Bullous emphysema, 206
Bullous pemphigoid, **178–180**, 178f, 179f
Bullous pemphigoid antigen, 179
BUN. See Blood urea nitrogen
Bundle of His, 222–224, 225f
Burn shock, 280
Buserelin, for benign prostatic hyperplasia, 570, 570t

C3, 54, 55f. See also Complement
 in bullous pemphigoid, 179
 deficiency of, 54
C3 convertase, 54
C5–9, 54, 55f. See also Complement
 deficiency of, 54
C cells (parafollicular cells), **414–415**, 481, 482f
 in calcium metabolism, **414–415**
 neoplasm of (medullary carcinoma of thyroid), **424–425**, 496
C fibers
 in lungs, 187, 188t
 in control of breathing, 199
 in pain sensation, 139–140
c-mos, ovarian production of, 530t
C peptide, 433
 in hypoglycemia evaluation, 455, 456
C-reactive protein, hepatic synthesis of, 336t
C (constant) region, immunoglobulin, 32–33, 33f
Calcarine (primary visual) cortex, 132f, 142, 144
Calcitonin, 414–415, 415f, 481
 in calcium metabolism, 414–415
 serum levels of in medullary carcinoma of thyroid, 425
Calcitonin gene-related peptide, ovarian production of, 530t

Calcium
 in adrenergic receptor function, 283–284
 as coagulation factor (factor IV), 103f, 104, 104t
 dietary, osteoporosis and, 427, 427t
 hypersecretion of. See Hypercalcemia
 metabolism of, **405–415**
  disorders of, **415–430**. See also Hypercalcemia; Hypocalcemia
  in Cushing's syndrome, 515
  hyperparathyroidism and, **415–419**
  hypoparathyroidism and pseudohypoparathyroidism and, 420–424
  medullary carcinoma of thyroid and, **424–425**
  osteomalacia and, **429–430**
  osteoporosis and, **425–429**
  regulation of
   bone and, **410–413**
   parafollicular (C) cells in, **414–415**
   parathyroid gland/parathyroid hormone in, **405–410**
   parathyroid hormone-related peptide in, 410
   renal, 386–387, 408, 409f
    chronic renal failure and, 396–397, 396f
   vitamin D in, **413–414**
 in renal stones, 402, 403t
 in stroke, 163, 163f, 164
 supplementation of, in osteoporosis prevention, 427t, 428–429
Calcium receptor, parathyroid cell, 406, 407f
Calculi, renal. See Renal stones
Caloric responses, loss of in brain injuries, 145
cAMP. See Cyclic AMP
cAMP-dependent protein kinase, 127
Cancellous bone, 411
Cancer, **79–97**. See also specific type or structure or organ affected
 adhesive proteins in, 83
 cellular changes in, 83
 epithelial, **84–89**, 86t
  phenotypic transition in, 84–85, 84f, 85t
 gastrointestinal manifestations of, 310t
 genetic changes in, **79–80**
 germ cell, **89–91**, 89t
 growth factors in, **82–83**
 growth inhibitors in, **82–83**
 hematologic, **92–95**, 92f, 93t
 HIV-related, 48–49
 hormones in, **82–83**
 hypercalcemia and, 419t, **420**
 inherited susceptibility to, 80
 mesenchymal, **89–91**, 89t

 molecular and biochemical basis of, **79–83**
 neuroendocrine, **89–91**, 89t
 oncogenes in, **80–82**, 81t
 phenotypic changes in, 84–85, 84t, 85t
 preclinical phase of, 79
 proteolytic proteins in, 83
 renal stone formation and, 403t
 stromal proteins in, 83
 systemic effects of, **95**, 95t, 96t
 tumor suppressor genes in, **80–82**, 82t
Candidiasis
 chronic mucocutaneous, 40t
 in diabetes mellitus, 454
 esophageal and oral (thrush), in HIV infection/AIDS, 47
Capacitance vessels, 260
Capillaries, 259–260, 259f, 260f
 circulation in, 262–263, 263f
 dermal, in psoriasis, 170–171
Carbamazepine, 156t
Carbohydrate metabolism, **438–439**. See also Fuel homeostasis
 in fasting state, 438–439, 439t
 in fed state, 439, 439t
 glucagon in, 436t, 437, 438–439, 438f, 439t
 glucocorticoids in, 504
 hormonal control of, **438–439**, 438f, 439t
 in hyperthyroidism, 489–490
 insulin in, 434–435, 436t, 438–439, 438f, 439t
 in liver, 332–333, 332t, 333f, 436t
  glucagon in, 436t, 437
  insulin in, 435, 436t
  liver dysfunction and, 339
 stress affecting, 439
Carbon dioxide
 partial pressure of
  in asthma, 203
  in control of breathing, 198–200, 199f, 200f
  in idiopathic pulmonary fibrosis, 210, 211f
  in pulmonary embolism, 217
  ventilation/perfusion matching and, 196, 196f
 as vasodilator, 264
Carbon monoxide, diffusing capacity for (DLCO)
 in asthma, 203
 in chronic bronchitis, 207
 in emphysema, 207
 in idiopathic pulmonary fibrosis, 210
Carboxypeptidase, in pancreatic juice, 364
Carcinoembryonic antigen
 in colon carcinoma, 87–88
 in medullary carcinoma of thyroid, 425
Carcinogens, 80
Carcinoid syndrome, 90, 90t, 95

Carcinoid tumors, **90**, 91*t*
  peptide expression by, 90, 90*t*, 95, 96*t*
Carcinoma, 84–85, 86*t*. *See also specific type or structure or organ affected*
Carcinoma in situ (preinvasive carcinoma), 84, 84*f*, 85
"Cardiac asthma," 237
Cardiac cycle, 225–229
  pressure-time analysis of events in, 225–227, 228*f*
  pressure-volume analysis of events in, 227–229, 229*f*, 230*f*
Cardiac failure. *See* Heart failure
Cardiac function, in septic shock, 76–77
Cardiac murmurs. *See* Heart murmurs
Cardiac muscle, 224–225, 226*f*
  contraction of, 229, 231*f*, 232*f*
Cardiac output
  pressure-volume relationships and, 227
  in septic shock, 76
Cardiac tamponade, **255–257**
  obstructive shock and, 281
Cardiac valves, 222, 223–224*f*. *See also specific valve*
  in cardiac cycle, 227
  diseases of, **240–251**
Cardiogenic pulmonary edema, 212, 212–213, 214
Cardiogenic shock, 278, 278*t*, **280–281**
Cardiogram. *See* Electrocardiogram
Cardiovascular failure. *See* Heart failure
Cardiovascular system
  cardiac component of, **222–257**. *See also* Heart
    anatomy of, **222–224**, 223–224*f*, 225*f*
    coronary artery disease and, **251–253**, 251*t*, 252*f*
    disorders of, **231–251**
      in chronic renal failure, 397
      in Cushing's syndrome, 516–517
      in hyperthyroidism, 489
      in hypothyroidism, 493
      glucocorticoids affecting, 504, 507*t*
    histology of, **224–225**, 226*f*
    normal, **222–231**
    pericardial disease and, **254–257**, 254*f*, 254*t*, 255*f*
    physiology of, **225–231**, 228*f*, 229*f*, 230*f*, 231*f*, 232*f*
    thyroid hormones affecting, 485*t*
  vascular component of, **258–281**. *See also* Vascular system
    anatomy of, **258–260**, 258*f*, 259*f*, 260*f*
    disorders of, **269–281**
    glucocorticoids affecting, 507*t*
    histology of, **258–260**, 259*f*, 260*f*
    normal, **255–268**
    physiology of, **260–263**, 261*f*, 262*f*, 263*f*

  regulation of, **263–268**, 265*f*, 266*f*, 266*t*, 267*f*, 268*f*
Carney complex, 511
β-Carotene, in atherosclerosis prevention, 273
Carotenemia, in hypothyroidism, 494
Carotid bodies, in control of breathing, 198–199, 200*f*
Carrier state
  genetic, in fragile X-associated mental retardation syndrome, 14, 14*f*, 15, 15*f*
  in infection, 52
Catechol-*O*-methyltransferase, in pheochromocytoma, 290
Catecholamines. *See also specific type*
  effects of, 284*t*, 285
  excess of
    hypertension and, 276–277
    manifestations of, 287–290, 288*t*, 289*t*
  formation/secretion/metabolism of, 282–283, 283*f*
  in fuel homeostasis, 436*t*, 439
  glucose levels during stress and, 439
  in hypoglycemia, 447, 447*t*
  mechanism of action of, 283–285, 284*t*
  normal values for, 283
  pheochromocytoma releasing, 287–290, 288*t*, 289*t*
  regulation of secretion of, 283
Caudate nucleus, 136
CBG. *See* Corticosteroid-binding globulin
CCK-secretin test, 375, 376
CD4:CD8 T lymphocyte ratio, in HIV infection/AIDS, 45
CD4 T (helper T) lymphocytes, 32
  in allergic hypersensitivity, 35
  defective, in SCID, 41
  in erythema multiforme, 175
  in HIV infection/AIDS, 45–47, 46*t*
  in inflammatory rheumatic diseases, 577–578
  in lichen planus, 174
CD8 (cytotoxic) T lymphocytes, 31
  absence of, in SCID, 41
  activation of, 32. *See also* Cellular (cell-mediated) immune response
  in erythema multiforme, 175
  in HIV infection/AIDS, 45
  in inflammatory rheumatic diseases, 578
  in lichen planus, 174
  in psoriasis, 171
CD14, in sepsis, 74, 75*f*
CD40 ligand, 32
  defective expression of, in hyper-IgM immunodeficiency, 44
CD40 receptor, 32
CEA. *See* Carcinoembryonic antigen

Cecum, 295*f*
Celiac (nontropical) sprue, histologic features of, 320*t*
Cell adhesion molecules, vascular, 269
Cell body, neuronal, 124, 125*f*
Cell death
  in infection, 58, 58*f*
  programmed (apoptosis)
    in lymphoma, 93
    in male infertility, 563
    in spinal muscular atrophies, 150
    in systemic lupus erythematosus, 582, 582*f*, 583
Cellular (cell-mediated) immune response, 31, 32
  impairment of. *See also* HIV infection/AIDS; Immunodeficiency diseases
    infections associated with, 40, 41*t*, 56*t*
  microbial strategies against, 60*t*
  type IV (delayed) hypersensitivity reactions mediated by, 34
Cellular cytotoxicity
  antibody-dependent, 29
  in inflammatory rheumatic diseases, 578
  lymphocyte-mediated, in inflammatory rheumatic diseases, 578
Cellulitis, in cyclic neutropenia, 117
Central deafness, 146
Central diabetes insipidus, 476, 476*t*, 477
Central herniation, 147
Central nervous system. *See also* Nervous system
  catecholamines affecting, 284*t*
  disorders of
    in adrenocortical insufficiency, 521
    in chronic renal failure, 397
    gastrointestinal manifestations of, 310*t*
    HIV infection/AIDS manifestations in, 48
Central pontine myelinolysis, 479
Central (terminal) veins, 328–329, 330*f*
Centriacinar emphysema, 206
Centripetal obesity, in Cushing's syndrome, 510*f*, 514
Cerebellum, **134–136**, 134*f*, 135*f*
Cerebral adrenoleukodystrophy, adrenal insufficiency in, 519–520
Cerebral amyloid angiopathy, 162
Cerebral circulation
  dementia and, 157
  in strokes, 160–162, 161*f*, 271
Cerebral edema, in meningitis, 65
Cerebral hemorrhage, stroke caused by, 159*t*, 162, 162*f*
Cerebral ischemia
  focal, 160, 161*t*
  stroke caused by, 159–162, 159*f*, 159*t*, 160*f*, 161*f*, 161*t*

Cerebral vasculitis, in meningitis, 65
Cerebrospinal fluid analysis, in meningitis, 62–63
Cerebrovascular disease
  dementia and, 157
  in strokes, 160–162, 161f, 271
Ceruloplasmin, hepatic synthesis of, 336t
Cervical dysplasia, in HIV infection/AIDS, 49
Cervix, cancer of, 86t, 551
  human papillomavirus causing, 80, 551
  invasive, in HIV infection/AIDS, 49
CFTR gene, congenital absence of vas deferens and, 565
Challenge test, in assessment of neuroendocrine axis, 467
Chaotic atrial activity, in mitral stenosis., 247
Charcot-Bouchard aneurysms, 162
Chédiak-Higashi syndrome, 56
Chemokines
  in allergic airway disease, 37
  HIV binding to, 45
Chemoreceptors, in control of breathing
  central, 198f, 199
  peripheral, 198–199, 198f
Chemotherapy, spermatogenesis affected by, 564
Chest pain. See also Angina pectoris
  in aortic stenosis, 241, 242
  in coronary artery disease, 251, 253
  gastrointestinal disease presenting with, 293, 294t
  in left ventricular failure, 238
  in mitral regurgitation, 247
  in pericarditis, **254**
  pleuritic, in pulmonary embolism, 218
Chest radiographs
  in chronic bronchitis, 207
  in emphysema, 207
  in idiopathic pulmonary fibrosis, 210
  in pulmonary embolism, 218
Chest tightness, in asthma, 203
Chest wall, static properties of (compliance and elastic recoil), 190–191, 190f, 191f
  pathologic states and, 191, 192f
Chief cells
  gastric, 302
  parathyroid, 405
    adenomas of, hyperparathyroidism caused by, 415, 416t
Chlamydia pneumoniae, pneumonia caused by, 66t
Chloride, in adrenocortical insufficiency, 522t
Chloromas, 95
Cholangiopancreatography, endoscopic retrograde, in chronic pancreatitis, 376
Cholecalciferol. See Vitamin D

Cholecystitis, 317
Cholecystokinin (CCK), 298t, 305, 364
  in chronic pancreatitis, 375
  pancreatic juice secretion controlled by, 364
Cholelithiasis, **316–317**, 317f
  acute pancreatitis associated with, 365
  somatostatinoma causing, 457
Cholera, pathogenesis of, 71f, 72
Cholera toxin, 71f, 72
Cholestasis, 327, 328t, 331, 339–340, 340f, 341t
  cholesterol elevation in, 339, 342
  drugs causing, 343t
Cholesterol
  in atherosclerosis, 269
    lowering levels and, 272–273
  in cholestasis, 339, 342
  gallstones composed of, 316
  hepatic metabolism of, 332t, 333–334, 333f, 335f
  liver dysfunction and, 339, 342
  hyperthyroidism affecting levels of, 490
  hypothyroidism affecting levels of, 493
Cholesterol-side chain cleavage enzyme (P450-scc), in autoimmune polyendocrine syndrome, 518
Cholesteryl-[^{14}C]octanoate breath test, in pancreatic insufficiency, 378
Cholinergic crisis, 154
Cholinesterase inhibitors, for myasthenia gravis, 154
Chordee, infertility in, 565
Chorea, in Huntington's disease, 137
Choriocarcinoma, 544
Chorionic gonadotropin, human (hCG), 535–536, 536f
  in molar pregnancy, 544
  in testicular cancer, 91
Chorionic somatomammotropin, human (hCS/placental lactogen), 537
  fuel homeostasis in pregnancy and, 539, 541f, 543
Christmas factor (factor IX), 103f, 104, 104t, 336t
  deficiency of, 108, 108t
  hepatic synthesis of, 336t
Chromaffin cells, 282
  tumors of. See Pheochromocytoma
Chromaffin granules, 282
Chromaffin reaction, 282
Chromosomal deletion
  in leukemia, 94–95
  tumor suppressor gene function loss caused by, 80
Chromosomal duplications, in hematologic neoplasms, 92
  leukemia, 94–95

Chromosomal sex, 531
  disorders of, 545
Chromosomal translocations
  in hematologic neoplasia, 92, 93t
    leukemia, 94–95
  in oncogene activation, 80
  Robertsonian, 4t
    in Down's syndrome, 18, 18f, 20–21, 21f, 21t, 22
Chromosomes
  abnormalities of. See also specific type
    in hematologic malignancies, 92
    leukemia, 94–95
  acrocentric, Down's syndrome and, 17
  autosomal, 3t
Chronic bronchitis, **204–207**, 205f
Chronic granulomatous disease, **43**, 56
Chronic infection, 58
Chronic lymphocytic leukemia
  lymphocyte counts in, 107
  pathogens causing infection in, 56t
Chronic obstructive pulmonary disease, **204–207**
Chronic pulmonary thromboembolism, 219
Chvostek's sign, 370, 422
Chylomicron remnants, 269
Chylomicrons, 269
Chymotrypsin, in pancreatic juice, 364
  acute pancreatitis and, 367, 367f
Cigarette smoking. See Smoking
Cilia, respiratory, in defense against infection, 67, 68f
Circadian rhythm, of ACTH secretion, 502, 505f
Circulation. See also Vascular system
  capillary, 262–263, 263f
  enterohepatic, 334
  liver, **332**
  pulmonary
    distribution of, 193–194, 194f, 195f
    matching ventilation to, 194–198, 196f, 197f
  systemic, 258, 258f
Cirrhosis, 327, 328t, **355–361**, 355f, 357t
  alcohol abuse and, 355, 356–357
  alcoholic hepatitis and, 352, 353f
  nitric oxide and, 354
Citrate, in prevention of renal stone formation, 402
"Clasp knife" phenomenon, 134
Class I MHC molecules. See MHC class I molecules
Class II MHC molecules. See MHC class II molecules
Classic pathway of complement activation, 54, 55f. See also Complement
Claudication, intermittent, 272
Claustrum, 136
Clear cells, parathyroid, 405
Climacteric, 541

Clomiphene citrate, for ovulatory failure, 552
Clonal deletion, 29–30
Clonidine, for pheochromocytoma diagnosis, 290
Clonus, 134
Clostridium
 botulinum, toxins produced by, neuromuscular transmission affected by, 130*f*, 131
 difficile, diarrhea caused by, 69
Clotting, blood. *See* Coagulation
Clubbing, digital, in idiopathic pulmonary fibrosis, 210
CNP, vascular smooth muscle affected by, 266
Coagulation, **103–105**, 103*f*
 anatomic considerations in, 103–104
 disorders of, 108, 108*t*, **120–122**. *See also* Coagulopathies
  abnormal vaginal bleeding and, 551, 551*t*
  in acute hepatitis, 349–350
  in acute pancreatitis, 370
  in chronic renal failure, 397
  in cirrhosis, 360
  intraparenchymal hemorrhage caused by, 162
  liver dysfunction and, 338*t*, 349–350, 360
  disseminated intravascular. *See* Disseminated intravascular coagulation
  in heparin-induced thrombocytopenia and thrombosis, 119
 physiologic considerations in, 104–105
 platelets in, 102, 103*f*
Coagulation cascade, **103–105**, 103*f*
 disorders of, 108, 108*t*, **120–122**
 in cirrhosis, 360
Coagulation factors, **103–105**, 103*f*, 104*t*. *See also specific type under* Factor
 acquired inhibitors of, 108
 disorders of, **108**, 108*t*
 elevation of, in acute pancreatitis, 370
 hepatic synthesis of, 336*t*
  disorders of in cirrhosis, 360
Coagulopathies. *See also* Coagulation, disorders of
 in acute hepatitis, 349–350
 in acute pancreatitis, 370
 in cirrhosis, 360
 consumption, 108
 gastrointestinal manifestations of, 310*t*
 liver dysfunction and, 338*t*, 349–350, 360
Coarctation of aorta, hypertension caused by, 274
Cobalamin (vitamin B_{12})
 in atherosclerosis prevention, 272
 deficiency of

anemia and, 105, 111
liver dysfunction and, 342
pancreatic insufficiency and, 378
in pernicious anemia, 114–115, 304
in DNA synthesis, 112–113, 113*f*
Cocaine, intraparenchymal hemorrhage associated with use of, 162
Cochlea, 145, 146
Cognition
 anatomic basis of, 14, 147
 physiology of, 148–149
Coitus, technique and timing of, infertility and, 565
COL1A1
 α1 chains coded by, 10, 10*f*
 mutation in in osteogenesis imperfecta, 9, 11–13, 11*f*, 12*f*
COL1A2
 α2 chains coded by, 10, 10*f*
 mutation in in osteogenesis imperfecta, 9, 12–13
Collagen
 in hepatic fibrosis and cirrhosis, 355–356
 type I, in osteogenesis imperfecta, 10–13
 COL1A1 and *COL1A2* gene mutations and, 9, 11–13, 11*f*, 12*f*
Collagenous sprue, histologic features of, 320*t*
Collecting ducts, renal, 384*f*, 385, 385*f*
Collecting tubule, in renal regulation, 385
Colles' fracture, in osteoporosis, 428
Colloid, thyroid, 481, 482*f*
Colloid bodies, in lichen planus, 173–174, 174*f*
Colon, 295*f*, **307**
 disorders of, **318–325**
  carcinoma, **86–88**, 86*t*
 motility of, 307
 disorders of, 308
Colon cut-off sign, in acute pancreatitis, 369
Colonization, 52, 53, 57
Colony-forming units, 92
Color vision, cones in, 144
Colorectal cancer, hereditary nonpolyposis, 87
Coma, 147
 hyperosmolar, in diabetes, 446, 447
 myxedema, 494
 nonstructural causes of, 147–148, 148*t*
Coma vigil, 148
Commensals (normal flora), **52–53**, 52*t*
Common bile duct, obstruction of, in chronic pancreatitis, 376
Common variable immunodeficiency, 40*t*, **43–44**
 pathogens causing infection in, 41*t*, 56*t*
Compact bone, 410–411

Complement, 54, 55*f*, 578
 in bullous pemphigoid, 179
 classic and alternative pathways of activation of, 54, 55*f*
 in defense against infection, 54, 55*f*
 microbial strategies against, 60*t*
 disorders/deficiency of, 54
  pathogens causing infection in, 41*t*, 54
 in glomerulonephritis, 400, 400–401, 400*t*
 in gout, 579, 579*f*
 in inflammation, 53–54
 in inflammatory rheumatic diseases, **578**
 in leukocytoclastic vasculitis, 181, 181*f*
 in systemic lupus erythematosus, 582
Complex partial seizures, 154*t*, 155
Compliance, respiratory system, 190–191, 190*f*, 191*f*
 pathologic states and, 191, 192*f*
Compromised host. *See* Immunocompromised host
Computed tomography
 in acute pancreatitis, 368, 369*f*
 spiral, in pulmonary embolism, 218
COMT. *See* Catechol-*O*-methyltransferase
Concentric hypertrophy, in aortic stenosis, 242, 243*f*
Conducting airways, 186, 186*f*
Conduction
 cardiac, 222–224, 225*f*
 ephaptic, 140
 saltatory, 128
Conduction block, 232, 232*f*, 233*f*
 in coronary artery disease, 253
Conductive deafness, 146
Condylomas, cervical, 551
Cones, 142, 143–144
Confusion/confusional states, 147
 in left ventricular failure, 238
 in liver dysfunction (hepatic encephalopathy), 338, 338*t*, 339, 342–344, 350, 359–360, 360*t*
 nonstructural causes of, 147–148, 148*t*
 postictal, 154
Congenital adrenal hyperplasia, 527
 hypertension and, 276
 plasma ACTH and cortisol levels in, 505*f*
Congenital adrenal hypoplasia, aldosterone deficiency in, 526
Congenital infections, 57
Congenital thymic aplasia, 40*t*, **42**
 pathogens causing infection in, 41*t*, 56*t*
Congested shock
 cardiogenic, 281
 obstructive, 281

Congestion/stuffiness, nasal, in allergic rhinitis, 38
Congestive heart failure. *See* Heart failure
Conjugate eye movements, 145
Conn's syndrome (primary hyperaldosteronism), 509, 522
  diagnosis of, 525–526
  etiology of, 523–524, 523*t*, 524*f*
  hypertension and, 275–276, 525
  pathophysiology of, 524
  plasma electrolyte levels in, 522*t*
Consciousness, **147–149**
Constant (C) region, immunoglobulin, 32–33, 33*f*
Constipation
  in diverticular disease, 324
  gastrointestinal disease presenting with, 293, 294*t*
  in hypothyroidism, 493
Constitutive defenses against infection, **53–56**
  microbial strategies against, 60*t*
Constrictive pericarditis, 254, 254*f*, 255, 255*f*, 256*f*
Constructional tasks, 149
Consumption coagulopathy, 108
Contiguous gene syndromes, 22, 22*t*
Contraception, physiology of, **536–537**
Contractile proteins, in cardiac sarcomeres, 225
Contraction
  cardiac muscle, 229, 231*f*, 232*f*
  gastrointestinal smooth muscle, 296–297. *See also* Gastrointestinal motility
Convalescent phase, in hepatitis, 348*f*, 350
COPD. *See* Chronic obstructive pulmonary disease
Cor pulmonale, 239
  in chronic pulmonary thromboembolism, 219
Cornified layer of skin, 166, 166*f*
Coronary arteries, 222, 225*f*
  spasms of, 251, 251*t*
Coronary artery disease, **251–253**, 251*t*, 252*f*, 271
  in diabetes mellitus, 453*f*
Corpus luteum, 532*f*, 535, 535*f*
Corrigan's pulse, in aortic regurgitation, 245
Cortex
  association, parietal, 149
  cerebellar, **134–136**, 134*f*, 135*f*
  lymph node, 30, 30*f*
  motor, 128, 131–132, 132*f*
  parietal association, 149
  prefrontal, 148
  premotor, 131, 132*f*
  primary auditory, 132*f*, 149

  primary visual (calcarine), 132*f*, 142, 144
  sensory/somatosensory, 131, 132*f*, 139
Cortical-basal ganglionic-thalamic-cortical loop, 136, 136*f*
Cortical bone, 410–411
  remodeling of, 411–412, 412*f*
Cortical motor neurons, 131, 132*f*
Corticalism, hyperadrenal, 509. *See also* Cushing's syndrome
Corticobulbar tract, 129, 131
Corticospinal tract, 129, 131, 133*f*
Corticosteroid-binding globulin (CBG), 501
Corticosteroids. *See also* Glucocorticoids
  synthesis/secretion of, ACTH in, 462–463
Corticosterone
  adrenal cortical cells secreting, 500
  synthesis/protein binding/metabolism of, 501–502, 503*f*
Corticotroph cells, pituitary, Cushing's disease caused by hyperplasia of, 509
Corticotropin (ACTH), 462–463, 464*f*, 502
  adrenal cortex affected by, 503
  cortisol levels affecting secretion of, 503, 504*f*, 506*f*
  deficiency of
    in hypopituitarism, 473, 474, 475
    in secondary adrenocortical insufficiency, 520
  episodic and diurnal rhythm of secretion of, 502, 505*f*
  excess of
    ectopic secretion causing, 413*f*, 509–510, 511*t*, 512*f*, 513, 514*f*
    clinical manifestations of, 515
    plasma ACTH and cortisol levels in, 505*f*, 513, 513*f*
    pituitary adenoma causing (Cushing's disease), 471, 473, 509, 511–513, 511*t*, 512*f*, 513*f*, 514*f*
    pituitary corticotroph hyperplasia causing, 509
  glucocorticoid secretion regulated by, 502–503, 504*f*, 505*f*, 506*f*
  hereditary adrenocortical unresponsiveness to, 519
  mineralocorticoid secretion regulated by, 506–508
  negative feedback regulation of, 502, 503, 504*f*, 506*f*
  plasma levels of
    in Cushing's syndrome, 505*f*, 514*f*, 517
    in ectopic ACTH syndrome, 505*f*, 513, 513*f*
    in primary adrenocortical insufficiency, 520, 520*f*

    in secondary adrenocortical insufficiency, 520, 520*f*
  stress response of, 502, 506*f*
Corticotropin-releasing hormone (CRH), 462–463, 502, 504*f*
  ectopic secretion of, 510, 512*f*, 513
  response to in Cushing's disease, 511–513, 517
Cortisol. *See also* Glucocorticoids
  ACTH secretion affected by, 503, 504*f*, 506*f*
  adrenal cortical cells secreting, 500, 502*f*
  bound, 501–502
  deficiency of, 517–522. *See also* Adrenocortical insufficiency
  diurnal rhythm of secretion of, 502, 505*f*
  fetal, 538
  free, 501–502
    in Cushing's disease, 511, 514*f*, 517
  in fuel homeostasis, 436*t*, 439
  hypertension and, 276
  osteoporosis caused by excess of, 426
  regulation of, 502–503, 504*f*, 505*f*, 506*f*
  stress response of, 502, 506*f*
  glucose levels and, 439
  synthesis/protein binding/metabolism of, 501–502, 503*f*
Cosyntropin stimulation test, in adrenocortical insufficiency diagnosis, 522, 523*f*
Cotton wool spots, in diabetic retinopathy, 450
Cough
  in asthma, 203
  in chronic bronchitis, 206
  in idiopathic pulmonary fibrosis, 209
Countercurrent multiplier mechanism, in renal regulation, 385, 387
Counterregulatory hormones
  diabetes mellitus and, 445
  glucagon as, 437, 439
  glucose levels during stress and, 439
  growth hormone as, 465, 466*f*
  human chorionic somatomammotropin and, 539, 543
  pregnancy and, 539, 541*f*, 543
Courvoisier's law, 379–380
Cowper's bulbourethral glands, 556, 557*f*, 558*f*
CpG island, 3*t*
  in fragile X-associated mental retardation syndrome, 15*f*, 16
Crackles
  in chronic bronchitis, 206
  in idiopathic pulmonary fibrosis, 210
Cramps, menstrual. *See* Dysmenorrhea
Cranial nerve III (oculomotor nerve), in control of eye movements, 142

Cranial nerve IV (trochlear nerve), in control of eye movements, 142
Cranial nerve V, nucleus of spinal tract of, 139
Cranial nerve VI (abducens nerve), in control of eye movements, 142
Cranial nerve VIII, 146
Creatinine, serum levels of, in acute renal failure, 392
Cretinism, sporadic, 494
Cretins, athyreotic, 492
CRH. *See* Corticotropin-releasing hormone
Critical region, Down's syndrome, 22, 22*f*
Critical velocity, 261
Crohn's disease (regional enteritis), 321–322, 322, 323*t*
  histologic features of, 320*t*
Crush syndrome, 280
Cryptococcal meningitis, in HIV infection/AIDS, 48
Cryptogenic fibrosing alveolitis (idiopathic pulmonary fibrosis), **208–210**, 208*f*, 209*t*, 210*f*, 211*f*
Cryptorchism, infertility and, 564
Cryptosporidium, diarrhea caused by, 69
Cullen's sign, 370
Curettage, amenorrhea caused by scarring after, 546
Cushing's disease, 471, 473, 509, 511–513, 511*t*, 512*f*, 513*f*, 514*f*
Cushing's syndrome, 509, **509–517**, 510*f*, 511*t*
  clinical manifestations of, 510*f*, 513–517
  diagnosis of, 514*f*, 517
  etiology of, 509–511, 511*t*, 512*f*
  hypertension and, 276
  iatrogenic, 511*t*, 512*f*
  osteoporosis and, 426
  pathophysiology of, 511–513, 513*f*, 514*f*
  plasma ACTH and cortisol levels in, 505*f*, 514*f*, 517
Cutaneous sensory nerves, 137
Cutaneous small vessel vasculitis, 581
Cyanogens, in tropical pancreatitis, 372–373
Cyclic AMP, 127
  in adrenergic receptor function, 284
Cyclic GMP, vascular smooth muscle affected by, 266
Cyclic neutropenia, 106, **115–117**
Cyclins, 85
  in parathyroid tumor development, 417
Cyclooxygenase, aspirin affecting, 264

CYP11B genes, in glucocorticoid-remediable aldosteronism, 524
CYP21 gene, in congenital adrenal hyperplasia, 527
Cyproterone acetate, for benign prostatic hyperplasia, 570, 570*t*
Cystic fibrosis, 7*t*
  congenital absence of vas deferens and, 565, 566
  gastrointestinal manifestations of, 310*t*
  pancreatic insufficiency caused by, 376, 377
Cystine stones, 402, 403*t*
Cystinuria, renal stone formation and, 402
Cystometry, in benign prostatic hyperplasia, 574
Cystourethroscopy, in benign prostatic hyperplasia, 574
Cysts, dermoid, testicular, 91
Cytochrome P450
  altered hormone clearance in liver dysfunction and, 344
  in chronic pancreatitis, 375
Cytochrome P450c21, antibodies to, in adrenocortical insufficiency, 518
Cytochrome P450-scc, in autoimmune polyendocrine syndrome, 518
Cytokines
  in acute pancreatitis, 367, 368*f*
  in asthma, 202, 202*t*
  in atherosclerosis, 269, 270*f*
  defective response of, immunodeficiency diseases related to, 40*t*, **44–45**
  in glomerulonephritis and nephrotic syndrome, 399
  in hematopoiesis, 98, 99*f*, 100*t*
  in idiopathic pulmonary fibrosis, 209
  in inflammatory rheumatic diseases, 576, **577–578**
  proinflammatory, 54
  in psoriasis, 171
  in T lymphocyte activation/recognition, 32
Cytomegalovirus, retinitis caused by, in HIV infection/AIDS, 48
Cytoplasmic proteins, tumor suppressor genes encoding for, 81
Cytosolic copper-zinc superoxide dismutase (*SOD1*) gene, in amyotrophic lateral sclerosis, 150–151
Cytotoxic (type II) hypersensitivity reaction, 34
Cytotoxic (CD8) T lymphocytes, 31
  absence of, in SCID, 41
  activation of, 32. *See also* Cellular (cell-mediated) immune response

  in erythema multiforme, 175
  in HIV infection/AIDS, 45
  in inflammatory rheumatic diseases, 578
  in lichen planus, 174
  in psoriasis, 171
Cytotoxic cerebral edema, in meningitis, 65
Cytotoxicity, cell-mediated
  antibody-dependent, 29
  in inflammatory rheumatic diseases, 578
  lymphocyte-mediated, in inflammatory rheumatic diseases, 578
Cytotoxins, 58
Cytotrophoblast, 537, 538*f*

D (δ) cells, pancreatic, 432, 432*t*, 433*f*
  regulation of hormone release from, 434*t*, 437
  tumors of (somatostatinomas), 456*t*, **457**
D1 cyclin, in parathyroid tumor development, 417, 417*f*
D-dimer assay, in pulmonary embolism, 218
DAZ gene, azoospermia and, 563
DCC gene, 82*t*
  in colon carcinoma, 86
DCCT. *See* Diabetes Control and Complications Trial
Dead space
  alveolar, 195–195, 196*f*
  in pulmonary embolism, 217
  anatomic, 195
Deafness, 146
Deamination, oxidative, in liver, 332*t*, 333, 334*f*
Decidual layer, of placenta, 537, 538*f*
Deep venous thrombosis. *See also* Thrombosis
  in hypercoagulable states, 121–122
  pulmonary embolism and, 215–216, 215*t*, 216*t*, 218
  risk factors for, 215*t*, 216*t*
Defective glucose counterregulation, 291
Deficiency states. *See also specific type*
  bile secretion disorders and, 339
  gastrointestinal manifestations of, 310*t*
  liver dysfunction and, 338*t*, 339, 342
Degranulation, platelet, 102–103, 103*f*
Dehydration
  in diabetes insipidus, 477
  in diabetic ketoacidosis, 446
  in gastrointestinal disease, 293
  renal stone formation and, 402, 403*t*
Dehydroepiandrostenedione, disorders of adrenal production of, 526–527
Dehydroepiandrostenedione sulfate, disorders of cortical production of, 526–527

Dehydroepiandrosterone, adrenal cortical cells secreting, 500
　disorders of, 526–527
Delayed (type IV) hypersensitivity reaction, 34
Deletion
　in hematologic neoplasms, 92
　　leukemia, 94–95
　tumor suppressor gene function loss caused by, 80
Delta agent. *See* Hepatitis D virus
Delta (D) cells, pancreatic, 432, 432t, 433f
　regulation of hormone release from, 434t, 437
　tumors of (somatostatinomas), 456t, **457**
Delta fibers, 137
　in pain sensation, 137, 139–140
Delta wave, in reentrant tachyarrhythmias, 234, 234f
Delusions, 147
Demargination, 106
Dementia, 148, **156–158**
　causes of, 156–157, 157t
　depression presenting as, 157
　in HIV infection/AIDS, 48
　in hypothyroidism, 492
　in pernicious anemia, 115
DeMusset's sign, in aortic regurgitation, 245
Demyelination
　in pernicious anemia, 115
　　methionine deficiency and, 113, 113f
　in symmetric distal polyneuropathy, 453
Dendrites, 124, 125f
Dense granules, in platelet activation, 102–103
Dentate nucleus, 134
Dentinogenesis imperfecta, 9
Deoxycorticosterone, hypersecretion of, hypertension and, 276
Deoxyribonuclease, in pancreatic juice, 364
Depression, dementia and, 157
Dermal capillaries, in psoriasis, 170–171
Dermal papillae, 167, 168f
Dermatitis, 169
　interface, 170t, 171f
　　erythema multiforme, **175–177**, 176f, 177f
　　lichen planus, **173–175**, 173f, 174f, 174t
　nodular, 170t, 171f
　patterns of, 170t, 171f
　perioral, in Cushing's syndrome, 515
　perivascular, 170t, 171f
　psoriasiform, **170–173**, 170t, 171f, 172f, 172t
　　variants of, 173t

　spongiotic, 170t, 171f
　vesiculobullous, 170t, 171f, **178–180**, 178f, 179f
Dermatomes, 138, 138f
　sensory loss limited to, 141
Dermis, 166, 166f, 168, 169f
Dermoid cysts, testicular, 91
Dermopathy, thyrotoxic, 490–491
Desmoplastic reaction/response
　in breast cancer, 88–89
　in pancreatic carcinoma, 379
Desmosomes, 167, 167f
Desquamation, of vaginal epithelial cells, 533
Detrusor contractility, decreased, in benign prostatic hyperplasia, 573, 573f
Detrusor failure, in benign prostatic hyperplasia, 573, 573f
Detrusor overactivity/instability, in benign prostatic hyperplasia, 573, 573f
Dexamethasone suppression test, in Cushing's syndrome, 514f, 517
DHEA. *See* Dehydroepiandrostenedione
DHEAS. *See* Dehydroepiandrostenedione sulfate
DHT. *See* Dihydrotestosterone
DHT-receptor protein, 560–561, 561f
Diabetes Control and Complications Trial, 448
Diabetes insipidus, 473, **476–477**, 476t, 477t
Diabetes mellitus, 432, **439–455**
　adrenomedullary failure in, 291
　in chronic renal failure, 394, 395t, 396
　classification of, 440, 441t
　clinical presentation/manifestations of, 439–441, 445–454
　complications of
　　acute, 445–448
　　chronic, 448–454, 448t
　　glycemic control in prevention of, 447
　　macrovascular, 448, 448t, 452–453, 453f
　　microvascular, 448, 448–450, 448t, 449f, 450f
　in Cushing's syndrome, 510f, 514
　foot ulcers in, 454
　gastrointestinal manifestations of, 310t
　gestational, 440t, 441, 539, 543
　glucagonoma causing, 457
　hyperglycemia in, 439–440
　hyperosmolar coma in, 447
　hypoglycemia as complication of treatment of, 447–448, 447t
　infection in, 454
　ketoacidosis in, 440, 445–447, 446f
　management of, atherosclerosis development and, 272

　nephropathy in, 394, 395t, 448, 450–452, 451f, 452f
　neuropathy in, 448, 453–454, 454t
　　autonomic, 291, 448, 454, 454t
　　hypoglycemia and, 448
　pancreatic carcinoma and, 378
　pathology and pathogenesis of, 444–445
　pheochromocytoma and, 289
　pregestational, 543
　retinopathy in, 448, 449–450, 451f
　somatostatinoma causing, 457
　type 1, 440, 440t, 441t
　　etiology of, 441–443, 442f, 443f
　type 2, 440–441, 440t, 441t
　　etiology of, 443–444
　　obesity in, 441, 444, 470
Diabetic foot ulcers, 454
Diabetic ketoacidosis, 440, 445–447, 446f
Diacylglycerol, 127
　in adrenergic receptor function, 283–284
Diaphragm, control of, 198–200. *See also* Breathing, control of
Diarrhea, 318, **318–320**, 318t, 319t, 320t, 321t, 322t
　approach to, 69, 70t
　causes of, 318–319, 319t, 322t
　diagnosis of, 319t
　gastrointestinal disease presenting with, 293, 294t
　hemorrhagic, 72, 72f, 73f
　infectious, **69–73**, 319–320, 322t
　in HIV infection/AIDS, 48, 322t
　inflammatory, 72, 72f
　mechanisms of, 318t
　in pancreatic insufficiency, 378
　secretory, 71–72, 318, 318t
　　in medullary carcinoma of thyroid, 425
Diastole, 227, 228f
Diastolic dysfunction, 237, 237f
Diastolic pressure-volume relationship, 227, 229f
DIC. *See* Disseminated intravascular coagulation
Dictyotene stage, 3t
　nondisjunction in Down's syndrome in, 19–20
Diet
　osteoporosis and, 426
　in pancreatic carcinoma, 378
　in phenylketonuria management, 23
Diffusing capacity for carbon monoxide (D$_L$CO)
　in asthma, 203
　in chronic bronchitis, 207
　in emphysema, 207
　in idiopathic pulmonary fibrosis, 210
Diffusion, in gastrointestinal transport, 297

DiGeorge syndrome (congenital thymic aplasia), 40t, **42**
　hypoparathyroidism in, 421
　pathogens causing infection in, 41t, 56t
DiGeorge-velocardiofacial syndrome, 22t
Digestion, 294, 297
　in colon, 307
　disorders of, **308–309**
　　in pancreatic insufficiency, 376–378, 377t
　enzymes in. See Pancreatic juice
　in small intestine, 307
Digital clubbing, in idiopathic pulmonary fibrosis, 210
Dihydrotestosterone, 556, 560
　in benign prostatic hyperplasia, 569–571, 570f, 571f
　mechanism of action of, 560–562, 561f
　normal levels of, 557–558, 560t
　synthesis/protein binding/metabolism of, 557–558, 559f, 560t
Diiodotyrosine (DIT), 483–484, 483f
2,3-Diphosphoglycerate
　in iron deficiency anemia, 111
　in pernicious anemia, 115
Discriminative sensation, 140
Disequilibrium, linkage, 4t
　in fragile X-associated mental retardation syndrome, 17
Disequilibrium (loss of balance), vestibular system disease and, 146
Disse, space of, 330f, 331f
Disseminated intravascular coagulation, 108
　in acute pancreatitis, 370
　in cirrhosis, 360
Distal convoluted tubule, 384f, 385
　in renal regulation, 385, 386t
Distributive shock, 278, 278t, **280**
　sepsis and, 76, 280
DIT. See Diiodotyrosine
Diuresis, in mineralocorticoid excess, 525
Diurnal rhythm, of ACTH secretion, 502, 505f
Diverticular bleeding, 324, 325
Diverticular disease, 318, **324–325**, 325f
Diverticulitis, 324, 325
Diverticulosis, 324, 325f
Dizziness, vestibular system disease and, 146
D$_L$CO (diffusing capacity for carbon monoxide)
　in asthma, 203
　in chronic bronchitis, 207
　in emphysema, 207
　in idiopathic pulmonary fibrosis, 210
DNA methylation, in fragile X-associated mental retardation syndrome, 15f, 16
DNA synthesis, vitamin B$_{12}$ (cobalamin) and folic acid in, 112–113, 113f

DOC. See Deoxycorticosterone
"Doll's-eye" maneuver, 145
Dominant inheritance, 3t
　amorphic (loss-of-function) mutations and, 7
　dominant negative (antimorphic) alleles/mutations and, 3t, 7–8
Dominant negative (antimorphic) alleles/mutations, 3t, 7–8
Dopamine
　in basal ganglia, 137, 137f
　effects of, 285
　formation/secretion/metabolism of, 282–283, 283f
　normal values for, 283
　in Parkinson's disease, 152
　prolactin secretion regulated by, 466
Dopaminergic drugs, for Parkinson's disease, 152
Dopaminergic neurons, in Parkinson's disease, 152
Dorsal columns, 138, 138f
Dorsal root, 138, 138f
Dorsal root ganglia, 138
Dosage compensation, 3t
　lack of, loss-of-function mutations and, 6–7
Down's syndrome, 2, 7t, **17–22**
　Alzheimer's disease and, 19, 158
Down's syndrome critical region, 22, 22f
Doxazosin, for benign prostatic hyperplasia, 572, 572t
2,3-DPG. See 2,3-Diphosphoglycerate
Drug-associated/induced disorders
　acute pancreatitis, 365t, 366
　dementia, 157
　erythema multiforme, 175
　hepatic, 343t
　hepatitis, 343t, 347, 347t
　　time course of, 347, 348f
　hypothyroidism, 491
　immune thrombocytopenia, **117–119**, 117t
　leukocytoclastic vasculitis, 180
　lichen planus, 173, 174t
　male infertility, 564
　nephrogenic diabetes insipidus, 476
　osteoporosis, 426
　toxic epidermal necrolysis, 177, 177f
Drug metabolism and excretion, hepatic, 334–335
　liver dysfunction and, 338t, 340–342, 343t
Dual-energy x-ray absorptiometry (DXA), 428
Dual response, 37
Duchenne's muscular dystrophy, 7t
Duct of Santorini, 362, 363f
Duct of Wirsung, 362, 363f
Dumping syndrome, 302, 308
Duodenal stump syndrome, 366
Duodenal ulcer, 308, 312, **313–314**, 314f

Duodenum, 295f, 305
Duplication, chromosomal, in hematologic neoplasms, 92
　leukemia, 94–95
Dupuytren's contractures, in cirrhosis, 361
DVT. See Deep venous thrombosis
DXA. See Dual-energy x-ray absorptiometry
Dynorphin, ovarian production of, 530t
Dysalbuminemic hyperthyroxinemia, euthyroid, 496–497
Dysentery, 72
Dysesthesias, 140
Dysfibrinogenemia, 108t
Dyslipidemias
　gastrointestinal manifestations of, 310t
　liver dysfunction and, 342
Dysmenorrhea, 545, 546t
　clinical manifestations of, 552
　etiology of, 545, 546t
　pathology and pathogenesis of, 550
Dysmetria ("overshooting"), 136
Dysphagia
　gastrointestinal disease presenting with, 293, 294t
　in reflux esophagitis, 312
Dysplasia, 85
Dyspnea
　in aortic regurgitation, 244, 245
　in asthma, 203
　in coronary artery disease, 253
　in idiopathic pulmonary fibrosis, 209–210
　in left ventricular failure, 234–235, 237–238
　in mitral regurgitation, 247, 249
　in mitral stenosis, 247
　in pericardial tamponade, 256
　in pulmonary edema, 210–211
　in pulmonary embolism, 218
　in right ventricular failure, 239
Dysproteinemias, gastrointestinal manifestations of, 310t

E coli. See *Escherichia coli*
EAggEC. See Enteroaggregative *E coli*
Ear
　anatomy of, 1145–146
　physiology of, 146
Early phase response, in allergic airway disease, 36–37
Eccentric hypertrophy, in aortic regurgitation, 244–245
Ecchymoses
　in acute hepatitis, 349–350
　in Cushing's syndrome, 510f, 515
ECG. See Electrocardiogram
Ectopic ACTH syndrome, 509–510, 511t, 512f, 513, 514f
　plasma ACTH and cortisol levels in, 505f, 513, 513f
Ectopic CRH syndrome, 510, 512f, 513

Ectopic pregnancy, pelvic infection and, 550, 553
Edema
  cerebral, in meningitis, 65
  in cirrhosis, 359
  in glomerulonephritis and nephrotic syndrome, 400–401
  liver dysfunction and, 338t, 359
  pedal, in right ventricular failure, 240
  in preeclampsia-eclampsia, 553
  pulmonary. *See* Pulmonary edema
Edinger-Westphal nuclei, 142
EDRF (endothelium-derived relaxing factor). *See* Nitric oxide
Edrophonium, in myasthenia gravis diagnosis, 154
Effector cells, in immune response, 32
Efferent arteriole, glomerular, 382, 384f, 385f
Effort-independent flow, 192
Effusion
  parapneumonic, 66
  pericardial, **255**
  pleural
    in acute pancreatitis, 370
    in left ventricular failure, 238
EHEC. *See* Enterohemorrhagic *E coli*
EIEC. *See* Enteroinvasive *E coli*
Ejaculation
  premature, 565
  retrograde, in infertility, 565
Ejection sound, aortic, in aortic stenosis, 241, 242, 243f
Elastase, in pancreatic juice, 364
  acute pancreatitis and, 367, 367f
Elastic lamina, external and internal, 258, 259f
Elastic recoil of lungs, 190–191, 190f, 191f
  pathologic states and, 191, 192f
Electrocardiogram (ECG), 224
  in pulmonary embolism, 218
Electrolytes, plasma, mineralocorticoid secretion regulated by, 508
Elliptocytosis, hereditary, 105–106
Emboliform nucleus, 134
Embolism
  cerebral, stroke caused by, 159–162, 159f, 159t, 160f, 161f, 161t
  pulmonary, **215–219**, 215t, 216t, 217f, 219t
    chronic, 219
    in hypercoagulable states, 122
Emission, loss of, 565
Emphysema, **204–207**, 206f
  lung compliance in, 191, 192f
Empyema, 66
Encephalitis, von Economo's, parkinsonism caused by, 151
Encephalopathies
  hepatic, 338, 338t, 339, 342–344, 350, 359–360, 360t
  hypertensive, 274

metabolic, 148
  subcortical arteriosclerotic, 157
End-diastole, 227
End product deficiency, 3t
  in phenylketonuria, 27
End-systole, 227
Endocarditis
  infective, **59–61**, 61f, 62t
  nonbacterial thrombotic, 59, 61f
Endocrine disorders. *See also specific gland*
  in chronic renal failure, 398
  in male infertility, 564
Endocrine pancreas, 362, **432–458**
  anatomy and histology of, **432**, 432t, 433f
  catecholamines affecting, 284t, 288t
  disorders of, **439–457**. *See also specific type and* Diabetes mellitus
  normal, **432–439**
  physiology of, **433–439**
    regulation of fuel homeostasis and, 436t
  tumors of, **455–456**, 456t, **457**. *See also specific type*
Endocytosis
  in gastrointestinal transport, 297
  hepatocyte, 337
Endogenous infectious agent, 50
Endometriosis, 550
  dysmenorrhea in, 546t, 550
  infertility and, 553
Endometrium, 529–531, 531f
  cancer of, 551
    amenorrhea and, 551–552
  changes in in menstrual cycle, 532f, 535
  disorders of
    abnormal vaginal bleeding and, 551
    infertility and, 553
  endocrine and paracrine products of, 532t
Endopeptidases, in pancreatic juice, 364
Endoscopic retrograde cholangiopancreatography, in chronic pancreatitis, 376
Endosomes, in thyroid hormone secretion, 483
Endothelial cells
  damage to, in preeclampsia-eclampsia, 553, 554
  hepatic, 329
  vascular, 258, 259f
    vascular function regulated by substances secreted by, 264–265, 265f
Endothelins, 265, 265f
Endothelium-derived relaxing factor (EDRF). *See* Nitric oxide
Endotoxins, 58
  in acute pancreatitis, 367

impaired hepatic clearance of, 342
  in sepsis, 74
Energy generation. *See also* Glucose, metabolism of
  by liver, 332–334, 332t, 333f, 334f, 335f
  liver dysfunction and, 338t, 339
Enkephalins
  gastrointestinal secretion of, 298t
  ovarian production of, 530t
Enteric nervous system, 296–297, 299, 299f
Enteritis
  radiation, histologic features of, 320t
  regional (Crohn's disease), 321–322, 322, 323t
    histologic features of, 320t
Enteroaggregative *E coli*, diarrhea caused by, 70, 70t, 71f
Enterochromaffin cells, carcinoid tumors arising from, 90
Enterocytes, 305
  secretagogues acting from, 307
Enteroglucagon, 298t
Enterohemorrhagic *E coli*, diarrhea caused by, 70, 70t, 71f, 72, 72f, 73f
Enterohepatic circulation, 334
Enteroinvasive *E coli*, diarrhea caused by, 70, 70t, 71f, 72
Enterokinases, in trypsin formation, 364
Enteropathogenic *E coli*, diarrhea caused by, 70, 70t, 71f
Enteropathy, protein-losing, 322
Enteropeptidases, in trypsin formation, 364
Enterotoxigenic *E coli*, diarrhea caused by, 70, 70t, 71f, 72
Enterotoxins, diarrhea caused by, 71f, 72
Enuresis, in diabetes insipidus, 476
Enzyme defects, in primary immunodeficiency diseases, 40t, **43–44**
Enzyme induction, in hepatic drug detoxification, 340
Eosinophilia, nasal, in allergic airway disease, 38–39
Eosinophilic gastroenteritis, histologic features of, 320t
Eosinophils, 29, 101
  in allergic airway disease, 37, 38–39
  normal values for, 101t
EPEC. *See* Enteropathogenic *E coli*
Ephaptic conduction, 140
Epidermal-dermal junction, 166f, 167–168, 168f
Epidermal growth factor, in benign prostatic hyperplasia, 572
Epidermal growth factor-like factor, ovarian production of, 530t
Epidermis, 166, 166f
  proliferation of in psoriasis, 170
Epidermopoiesis, in psoriasis, 170

Epididymis, 556, 557f
Epidural hematomas, 162
Epigenetic effect, 3t, 17
   in fragile X-associated mental retardation syndrome, 17
Epilepsy, **154–156**
   drugs for treatment of, 156, 156t
   secondary, 156
Epinephrine. *See also* Catecholamines
   deficiency of (adrenomedullary failure), 285, 291
   effects of, 284t, 285
   formation/secretion/metabolism of, 282–283, 283f
   glucose levels during stress and, 439
   mechanism of action of, 283–285, 284t
   normal values for, 283
   pheochromocytoma releasing, 287, 289–290
Epispadias, infertility in, 565
Episteride, for benign prostatic hyperplasia, 570–571, 570t, 571f
Epithelial neoplasia, **84–89**, 86t. *See also specific type*
   phenotypic transition in, 84–85, 84f, 85f
Epithelium
   as defense against infection, 53
   immunologic functions of, 29
   pulmonary, anatomy of, 186–187, 186f, 187f
EPO. *See* Erythropoietin
Equal pressure point, 192, 193f
Equilibrium potential, neuronal, 124–125
ERCP. *See* Endoscopic retrograde cholangiopancreatography
Erectile dysfunction, 565
Erection, loss of, 565
Ergocalciferol (vitamin D_2), 413
Erosive lichen planus, 175
Erosive polyarthritis, chronic, in gout, 580
ERV (expiratory reserve volume), 185
Erythema
   multiforme, **175–177**, 176f, 177f
      major, 177
      minor, 177
   necrolytic migratory, in glucagonoma, 457
Erythrocytes (red blood cells), 98, 100–101
   development of, 98, 99f
   disorders of, **105–106**, 105t, 106f, **109–115**. *See also specific type and* Anemia
   normal values for, 101t
   physiology of, 100–101
Erythrodermic psoriasis, 173t
Erythropoiesis, 98, 99f
   renal regulation of, 387
Erythropoietin, 387
   in hematopoiesis, 98, 99f, 100t, 387
Escape phenomenon, in mineralocorticoid excess, 525

Escherichia coli
   diarrhea caused by, 70–72, 70t, 71f, 72f, 73f
   meningitis caused by, 63, 63t
Escherichia coli O157:H7, diarrhea caused by, 72, 72f, 73f
Esophageal achalasia, **309**, 311t
Esophageal candidiasis, in HIV infection/AIDS, 47
Esophageal motility, 300–301, 302f
   disorders of, 308
      achalasia, **309**, 311t
Esophageal sphincters, 300–301, 301t
   in achalasia, 309
   in reflux esophagitis, 311, 311f
Esophageal (gastroesophageal) varices, 338
   in cirrhosis, 359
Esophagitis, reflux, **309–312**, 311f
Esophagus, 295f, **300–301**, 301t
   Barrett's, 312
   disorders of, **309–312**. *See also specific type*
      carcinoma, 86t
      common presentations of, 294t
      functional obstruction, 309
Essential hypertension, 273, 273t
   of pregnancy, 552
Estradiol
   in benign prostatic hyperplasia, 571
   normal levels of in men, 560t
Estrogen receptors, in breast cancer, 83
Estrogen replacement therapy
   in atherosclerosis prevention, 272–273
   in osteoporosis prevention, 429
Estrogens
   in benign prostatic hyperplasia, 571
   changes in in menstrual cycle, 532f, 534–535
   decreased secretion of, menopause and, 541
   deficiency of
      in chronic renal failure, 398
      in osteoporosis, 426, 427
      in endometrial cancer, 551
   excess of
      in cirrhosis, 361
      liver dysfunction and, 344, 361
      ovaries producing, 536–537
      in pregnancy, disorders associated with, 543–544, 543t
   tissues dependent on
      maturation of, 533
      menopause affecting, 541
Estrone, normal levels of in men, 560t
ETEC. *See* Enterotoxigenic *E coli*
Ethanol. *See under* Alcohol
Ethosuximide, mechanism of action of, 156, 156t
Euploidy, deviations from. *See also specific type*
   in Down's syndrome, 17

Euthyroid hyperthyroxinemia
   dysalbuminemic, 496–497
   familial, 496–497
Excitatory neurotransmitters, 127
Excitatory postsynaptic potential, 127
Excitotoxicity, in neuronal ischemia/stroke, 162–164, 163f
Exercise, control of breathing and, 200
Exocrine pancreas, **362–381**
   anatomy of, **362**, 363f
   disorders of, **364–380**. *See also specific type*
   histology of, **362–363**, 363f
   normal, **362–364**
   physiology of, **363–364**. *See also* Pancreatic juice
Exocytosis, in gastrointestinal transport, 297
Exogenous infectious agent, 50
Exopeptidases, in pancreatic juice, 364
Expiratory reserve volume (ERV), 185
Expressivity, 3t, **5–6**, 6f
   in fragile X-associated mental retardation syndrome, 15, 15f
   variable, 6, 6f
External elastic lamina, 258, 259f
Extracellular membrane proteins, ovarian production of, 530t
Extraocular muscles, in control of eye movements, 142, 144f
Extrapyramidal neurons, 129
Extrinsic coagulation pathway, 103f, 104
Eye, anatomy of, 142–143, 143f, 144f
Eye fields, frontal, 142
Eye movements
   conjugate, 145
   control of, **142–145**
      anatomic structures in, 142, 144f
      physiology of, 145
   saccadic, 142

F cells (PP cells), pancreatic, 432, 432t
   pancreatic polypeptide produced by, 432, 432t, 438
   tumors of (PPomas), 456t
F(ab) fragments, 33, 33f
Facilitated diffusion, in gastrointestinal transport, 297
Factor I (fibrinogen), 103f, 104t, 336t
   deficiency of, 108t
   hepatic synthesis of, 336t
Factor II (prothrombin), 104, 104t, 336t
   elevated levels of, 121
   hepatic synthesis of, 336t
Factor IIa (thrombin), 103f, 104, 104t
   in platelet activation, 103
Factor III (tissue thromboplastin/tissue factor), 104, 104t
Factor IV. *See* Calcium
Factor V (proaccelerin), 103f, 104t, 120, 120f
   deficiency of, 108t

Factor Va, 103f, 104, 120, 120f
Factor V Leiden, 121, 122
Factor VII (proconvertin), 103f, 104, 104t, 336t
  deficiency of, 108t
  hepatic synthesis of, 336t
Factor VIIa, 103f
Factor VIII (antihemophilic factor), 104, 104t
  deficiency of, 108, 108t
Factor VIIIa, 103f, 104
Factor IX (Christmas factor), 103f, 104, 104t, 336t
  deficiency of, 108, 108t
  hepatic synthesis of, 336t
Factor IXa, 103f, 104
Factor X (Stuart-Prower factor), 103f, 104, 104t, 120, 336t
  deficiency of, 108t
  hepatic synthesis of, 336t
Factor Xa, 103f, 104, 120
Factor XI (plasma thromboplastin antecedent), 103f, 104, 104t
  deficiency of, 108t
Factor XIa, 103f, 104
Factor XII (Hageman factor), 103f, 104, 104t
  deficiency of, 108t
Factor XIIa, 103f, 104
Factor XIII (fibrin-stabilizing factor), 104, 104t
  deficiency of, 108t
Factor XIIIa, 103f, 104
Factors
  coagulation, **103–105**, 103f, 104t. *See also specific type*
    acquired inhibitors of, 108
    disorders of, **108**, 108t
    in neoplasia, **82–83**
Familial adenomatous polyposis, 87
Familial euthyroid hyperthyroxinemia, 496–497
Familial glucocorticoid deficiency, 519
Familial hyperaldosteronism
  type I (glucocorticoid-remediable aldosteronism), 276, 524
  type II, 524
Familial hypercholesterolemia, liver dysfunction and, 338t, 342
Familial (benign) hypocalciuric hypercalcemia, **419–420**, 419t
Familial malignancies, 80
Fas-Fas-ligand pathway, in lymphocyte-mediated cytotoxic rheumatic disease, 578
Fasciculations, 131, 150
Fasting hyperglycemia, 444
  in Cushing's syndrome, 516
Fasting hypoglycemia
  insulin-mediated vs. non-insulin-mediated, 455–456
  insulinoma causing, 455–456
Fasting pattern, of intestinal motility, 306

Fasting state, carbohydrate metabolism in, 438–439, 439t
Fat. *See* Adipose tissue
Fat cell hyperplasia, in obesity, 470
Fat cell hypertrophy, in obesity, 470
Fat embolism, 215t
Fatigue
  in left ventricular failure, 238
  in mitral regurgitation, 247, 249
  in mitral stenosis, 247
Fats. *See* Lipids
Fatty liver, 338t, 339
  drugs causing, 343t
Fatty streak, formation of, 269, 270f
Fc fragments/receptors, 33, 33f
  in inflammatory rheumatic diseases, 577, 578
Fcα receptor, in systemic lupus erythematosus, 582
Feeding pattern, of intestinal motility, 306
Felbamate, 156t
Female reproductive tract, **529–555**
  anatomy of, **529–531**, 531f, 532f, 533f
  contraception and, **536–537**
  disorders of, **542–555**. *See also specific type*
  endocrine and paracrine products of, 530t, 532t
  lactation and, **539–541**, 542f
  menopause and, **541–542**
  menstrual cycle and, **533–536**, 534f, 535f
    disorders of, **545–552**, 546t, 547t, 548t, 549f, 551t
  normal, **529–542**
  ovarian steroid physiology and, **536–537**
  pregnancy and, **537–539**, 538f, 539t, 540f, 541f
    disorders of, **543–544**
    preeclampsia-eclampsia and, **553–555**, 554t
  sexual differentiation and, **531–533**, 534f
    disorders of, **535**
Fenestrations, capillary, 259, 260f
  in glomerular endothelium, 383, 384f
  in hypothalamus, 461
  in portal system, 332
Ferritin, 109, 337
Fertilization, 535–536, 537
fes oncogene, 81t
α-Fetoprotein, 336t
  hepatic synthesis of, 336t
  in testicular cancer, 91
FEV$_1$, 185
  in asthma, 203
  in chronic bronchitis, 207
  in emphysema, 207
  in idiopathic pulmonary fibrosis, 210
FEV$_1$%, 185
  in asthma, 203

  in chronic bronchitis, 207
  in emphysema, 207
  in idiopathic pulmonary fibrosis, 210
Fever
  in acute pancreatitis, 369
  "glucose," in adrenocortical insufficiency, 521
FGF. *See* Fibroblast growth factors
FGF7. *See* Fibroblast growth factor 7
FH-I. *See* Familial hyperaldosteronism, type I
FH-II. *See* Familial hyperaldosteronism, type II
Fibrillation, atrial, 235f
  in mitral stenosis, 247
Fibrillations, muscle, 131
Fibrin, formation of, 103f, 104
Fibrin-stabilizing factor (factor XIII), 104, 104t
  deficiency of, 108t
Fibrinogen (factor I), 103f, 104t, 336t
  deficiency of, 108t
  hepatic synthesis of, 336t
Fibroblast growth factor 7, in benign prostatic hyperplasia, 571–572
Fibroblast growth factors, in benign prostatic hyperplasia, 571–572
"Fight or flight" response, catecholamines in, 283, 285
Filgrastim. *See also* Granulocyte colony-stimulating factor
  for cyclic neutropenia, 116
Final common pathway. *See* Lower motor neurons
Finasteride, for benign prostatic hyperplasia, 570–571, 570t, 571f
First heart sound (S$_1$), 227
Fitness (genetic), 3t, 5
  in fragile X–associated mental retardation syndrome, 17
  in phenylketonuria, 26
Flank pain, in renal stones, 401, 402–404
Flares
  in gout, 580
  in systemic lupus erythematosus, 583
"Flight or fight" response, catecholamines in, 283, 285
Flocculonodular lobe, 134, 134f
Flow. *See* Airflow; Blood flow
Fluid balance
  in adrenocortical insufficiency, 521
  in chronic renal failure, 395
  liver dysfunction and, 338t, 344, 344t
  renal dysfunction and, 388–389
  renal regulation of, 385, 387
Flutamide, for benign prostatic hyperplasia, 570t
Flutter, atrial, 235f
FMR. *See* Fragile X–associated mental retardation syndrome

FMR1 gene, in fragile X-associated mental retardation syndrome, 15f, 16
Foam cells, 269, 270f
Focal (partial) seizures, 154t, 155
Folic acid
 in atherosclerosis prevention, 272
 deficiency of
  liver dysfunction and, 342
  megaloblastic anemia caused by, 105
 in DNA synthesis, 112–113, 113f
Follicle regulatory protein, ovarian production of, 530t
Follicle-stimulating hormone (FSH), 464, 534
 changes in in menstrual cycle, 532f, 534–535
 deficiency of, in hypopituitarism, 474
 in male reproductive function, 558, 560, 560f
  infertility evaluation and, 566, 567f
  normal levels of in men, 560t
 ovarian response to, 534–535, 535f
 in polycystic ovary syndrome, 547, 548, 549f
Follicles
 ovarian, 529
  changes in in menstrual cycle, 532f, 534–535, 535f
 thyroid, 481, 481–482, 482f, 483f
Follicular adenoma, of thyroid, 496
Follicular carcinoma, of thyroid, 496
Follicular phase, of ovarian cycle, 534–535
Folliculitis, 170t, 171f
Follistatin, ovarian production of, 530t
Food poisoning, 73t. *See also* Diarrhea
Foot ulcers, diabetic, 454
Forced expiratory volume in 1 second (FEV_1), 185
 in asthma, 203
 in chronic bronchitis, 207
 in emphysema, 207
 in idiopathic pulmonary fibrosis, 210
 ratio of to forced vital capacity ($FEV_1\%$), 185
  in asthma, 203
  in chronic bronchitis, 207
  in emphysema, 207
  in idiopathic pulmonary fibrosis, 210
Forced vital capacity (FVC), 185
 in asthma, 203
 in chronic bronchitis, 207
 in emphysema, 207
 in idiopathic pulmonary fibrosis, 210
 ratio of to FEV_1 ($FEV_1\%$), 185
  in asthma, 203
  in chronic bronchitis, 207
  in emphysema, 207
  in idiopathic pulmonary fibrosis, 210

Foreign body, pulmonary embolism caused by, 215t
fos oncogene, 81t
Founder effect, 3t
 in fragile X-associated mental retardation syndrome, 17
 in phenylketonuria, 26
Fourth heart sound (S_4)
 in aortic stenosis, 241
 in coronary artery disease, 253
 in left ventricular failure, 238f, 239
Fractures
 in osteogenesis imperfecta, 9–10
 osteoporotic, 428, 428f
Fragile X-associated mental retardation syndrome, 2, 7t, **14–17**
Frameshift mutation, tumor suppressor gene function loss caused by, 80
Frank-Starling relationship, 229
FRC (functional residual capacity), 185
 in asthma, 203
 in emphysema, 207
Free cortisol, 501–502
 urinary, in Cushing's disease, 511, 514f, 517
Free radicals
 in amyotrophic lateral sclerosis, 150–151
 in emphysema, 205, 206f
Free thyroxine (FT_4), 486
 in hyperthyroidism, 487
Free thyroxine index (FT_4I), 486
 in hyperthyroidism, 487
Friction rub, pericardial, 254, 254–255
Frontal eye fields, 142
Frontal lobe syndrome, 148
FSH. *See* Follicle-stimulating hormone
FT_4. *See* Free thyroxine
FT_4I. *See* Free thyroxine index
Fuel homeostasis
 catecholamines in, 436t, 439
 cortisol in, 436t, 439
 glucagon in, 436t, 437
 growth hormone in, 436t, 439
 hormonal regulation of, 436t, 438–439, 438f, 439t
 human chorionic somatomammotropin in, pregnancy and, 539, 541f, 543
 insulin in, 434–435, 436t
 somatostatin in, 436t, 438
Functional residual capacity (FRC), 185
 in asthma, 203
 in emphysema, 207
Functional zonation of liver, 329, 330f, 338–339
Fungal infections
 endocarditis, 59–61, 62t
 pneumonia, 65–69
Furunculosis, in cyclic neutropenia, 117
Fusion gene, in cancer, 80
 in hematologic neoplasia, 92, 93t

Fusion protein, in cancer, 80
 in hematologic neoplasia, 92, 93t
FVC (forced vital capacity), 185
 in asthma, 203
 in chronic bronchitis, 207
 in emphysema, 207
 in idiopathic pulmonary fibrosis, 210
 ratio of to FEV_1 ($FEV_1\%$), 185
  in asthma, 203
  in chronic bronchitis, 207
  in emphysema, 207
  in idiopathic pulmonary fibrosis, 210

G cells, 302
G-CSF. *See* Granulocyte colony-stimulating factor
G protein-coupled receptor, for somatostatin, 438
G proteins
 in adrenergic receptor function, 283–284
 in multinodular goiter, 496
 in pituitary adenomas, 472
 ras oncogene as, 81, 81t
GABA (γ-aminobutyric acid)
 in basal ganglia, 137, 137f
 glucagon release affected by, 437
 in hepatic encephalopathy, 360
 in seizure pathogenesis, 155, 156
GABAergic neurons, in Parkinson's disease, 137
GAD. *See* Glutamic acid decarboxylase
Galactorrhea, 471
Gallbladder, **304–305**, 305f
 disorders of, **316–317**, 317f
  acute pancreatitis associated with, 365
  common presentations of, 294t
Gallstones, **316–317**, 317f
 acute pancreatitis associated with, 365
Gamete, 2, 3t
Gamma-aminobutyric acid (GABA)
 in basal ganglia, 137, 137f
 glucagon release affected by, 437
 in hepatic encephalopathy, 360
 in seizure pathogenesis, 155, 156
Gamma-carboxylase, in coagulation, 104
Gamma globulin, intravenous, for common variable immunodeficiency, 44
Gamma interferon, 32
 in allergic hypersensitivity, 34
Gamma motor neurons, 129, 130f
Gangliomas, 287
Ganglion cells, retinal, 144
Gangrene, atherosclerosis and, 272
Gas exchange. *See also* Ventilation
 impaired, in pulmonary embolism, 216t
Gastrectomy, pancreatic insufficiency caused by, 377
Gastric carcinoma, 86t

Gastric disorders
 cancer, 86t
 common presentations of, 294t
Gastric emptying, delayed (gastroparesis), 308, **314–316**, 315t
Gastric motility, 302
 disorders of, 308, **314–316**, 315t
Gastric secretion, 298t, 302–304, 304f
 disorders of, 308
  pancreatic insufficiency and, 377
Gastric ulcer, 308, **313**
Gastrin, 298t
 hypersecretion of, pancreatic insufficiency and, 377
Gastrinoma, 456t
 pancreatic insufficiency and, 377
Gastritis
 acute erosive, **313**
 chronic/autoimmune atrophic, 112f, 113, **313**
Gastrocolic reflex, 307
Gastroenteritis, 69–70, 73t. See also Diarrhea
 eosinophilic, histologic features of, 320t
 uremic, 397
Gastroesophageal (lower esophageal) sphincter, 300, 301t
 in achalasia, 309
 in reflux esophagitis, 311, 311f
Gastroesophageal (esophageal) varices, 338
 in cirrhosis, 359
Gastrointestinal bleeding, 293, 294t
 in cirrhosis, 359
 diverticular, 324, 325
 in iron deficiency anemia, 109, 111
Gastrointestinal infection. See also Diarrhea
 approach to, 69, 70t
 E coli causing, 70–72, 70t, 71f, 72f, 73f
Gastrointestinal motility, 293, 296–297
 colonic, 307
 disorders of, **308**
  in diabetic autonomic neuropathy, 454
  diarrhea and, 318t
  in hyperthyroidism, 490
  in hypothyroidism, 493
  esophageal, 300–301, 301t
  gastric, 302
  oropharyngeal, 300–301
  small intestinal, 306
Gastrointestinal secretion, 293–294, 297, 297f, 298t
 in colon, 307
 disorders of, **308**
  pancreatic insufficiency and, 377
  gastric, 298t, 302–304, 304f
  in small intestine, 306–307
Gastrointestinal smooth muscle
 catecholamines affecting, 284t

contraction of, 296–297. See also Gastrointestinal motility
Gastrointestinal tract, 293–326. See also specific organ or structure
 catecholamines affecting, 284t, 288t
 defense mechanisms of, 299–300, 300t, 301f
 disorders of, **308–325**
  in chronic renal failure, 397
  common presentations of, 294t
  digestion and absorption and, **308–309**
  in hyperthyroidism, 310t, 490
  in hypothyroidism, 493
  in iron deficiency anemia, 111
  motility and, **308**
  secretion and, **308**
 functions of, **296–297**, 297f, 298t. See also Gastrointestinal motility
 control of, 297–299, 299f
 histology of, 294, 296f
 obstruction of, 293
 secretory products of, 293–294, 297, 297f, 298t. See also Gastrointestinal secretion
 stenosis of, obstruction caused by, 293
 structure of, **293–296**, 295f, 296f
 systemic disease manifestations as, **309**
 thyroid hormones affecting, 485t
Gastroparesis, 308, **314–316**, 315t
Gaze centers, 142
Gender
 determination of, **531–533**, 534f. See also Sexual differentiation
 disorders associated with, **545**
 parental
  Down's syndrome and, 19, 20, 21t
  fragile X-associated mental retardation syndrome and, 14f, 15f, 17
Gene dosage, 3t
 in Down's syndrome, 18, 18f, 21–22, 22f
Generalization, secondary, of seizure, 155
Generalized tonic-clonic seizures, 154, 154t
Genes, 5
 cancer and, 79–80. See also Oncogenes; Tumor suppressor genes
Genetic amplification
 in fragile X-associated mental retardation syndrome, 14, 15f
 postzygotic, 16
 in oncogene activation, 80
Genetic anticipation, 3t, 15
 in fragile X-associated mental retardation syndrome, 15–16, 15f
Genetic counseling, 8
Genetic disease, **2–27**
 amenorrhea in, 547, 551

clinical issues at presentation of, **8**
 definition of terms related to, 3–4t
 inheritance patterns and, **6–8**
 mutations causing, 2, 5f, **6–8**. See also specific type
 penetrance and expressivity and, **5–6**, 6f
 prevalence of, 7t, **8**
 unique aspects of, 2–8
Genetic heterogeneity, 3t
 in osteogenesis imperfecta, 13
Geniculate nuclei, lateral, 142, 143f, 144
Genital tract infections
 in female
  dysmenorrhea and, 546t, 550
  ectopic pregnancy and, 550, 553
  infertility and, 553
 in male, infertility and, 564–565
Genitalia, development of, 531–533, 534f
Genitourinary smooth muscle, catecholamines affecting, 284t
Germ cells
 aplasia of, in male infertility, 563
 neoplasia of, **89–91**, 89t. See also specific type
 primordial, 4t
Germline mosaicism, 5f. See also Mosaicism
Gestational diabetes mellitus, 440t, 441, 539, 543
GH. See Growth hormone
GHRH. See Growth hormone-releasing hormone
Giardiasis, histologic features of, 320t
Gigantism, 471, 473, 474t
Gilbert's syndrome, 340, 341t
GIP, 298t
Glaucoma, in Cushing's syndrome, 516
Globose nucleus, 134
Globus pallidus, 136, 136f
Glomerular basement membrane, 382–383, 384f
Glomerular disease, 388
 in diabetes mellitus, 451–452, 451f, 452f
Glomerular filtration, 385
 regulation of, 387
Glomerular hyperfiltration, 387
Glomerular sclerosis, 395
Glomerulonephritis, **398–401**, 400t
 acute, 398, 398t, 399–400
 in acute renal failure, 392t
 chronic, 398, 399, 400
 in chronic renal failure, 394, 395t
 electron-dense deposits in, 400t
 hypertension and, 275
 immune complexes in, 399, 400t, 581
 membranoproliferative, 401t
 membranous, 400
 rapidly progressive, 398, 399, 399t, 400
 sclerosing, 400

Glomerulopathies, liver dysfunction and, 338*t*
Glomerulosclerosis
 in diabetes mellitus, 451, 451*f*
 focal and segmental, 401*t*
Glomerulus, 382, 382–385, 384*f*, 389*f*
Glossitis
 in iron deficiency anemia, 111
 in pernicious anemia, 115
Glove distribution, in symmetric distal polyneuropathy, 454
GLP-1(7–36). *See* Glucagon-like peptide-1(7–36)
Glucagon, 432, **436–437**
 A cells secreting, 432, 432*t*, 433*f*
  regulation of, 434*t*, 437
 in carbohydrate metabolism, 436*t*, 437, 438–439, 438*f*, 439*t*
  stress and, 439
 deficiency of, in adrenomedullary failure, 291
 effects of, 436*t*, 437, 439
 hypoglycemia in diabetics and, 447–448
 mechanism of action of, 437
 regulation of secretion of, 434*t*, 437
 synthesis and metabolism of, 436, 437*f*
Glucagon:insulin ratio
 carbohydrate metabolism and, 439*t*, 444
 in diabetes, 444
Glucagon-like peptide-1(7–36), 435, 437*t*
Glucagonoma, 456*t*, **457**
Glucocorticoid-remediable aldosteronism, 276, 524
Glucocorticoids, **501–504**
 adrenal cortical cells secreting, 500, 502*f*
 deficiency of, 509, **517–522**. *See also* Adrenocortical insufficiency
  familial, 519
  in panhypopituitarism, 473, 474
 effects of, 504, 507*t*
 excess of, 509. *See also* Cushing's syndrome
  hypertension and, 276
  osteoporosis and, 426, 427–428
 exogenous, secondary adrenocortical insufficiency caused by, 520
 free and bound, 501–502
 mechanism of action of, 504
 permissive action of, 504, 507*t*
 regulation of, 502–503, 504*f*, 505*f*, 506*f*
 synthesis/protein binding/metabolism of, 501–502, 503*f*
Glucokinase, 433
 in type 2 diabetes, 444
Gluconeogenesis, in liver, 332–333, 332*t*, 333*f*, 436*t*
 glucagon in, 436*t*, 437
 insulin in, 435, 436*t*

Glucose
 defective counterregulation of, 291
 elevated levels of. *See* Hyperglycemia
 glucagon secretion regulated by, 434*t*, 437
 insulin secretion regulated by, 433, 434*t*
 metabolism of. *See also* Carbohydrate metabolism; Glucose intolerance
  glucagon in, 436*t*, 437
  glucocorticoids in, 504
  hormonal control of, 438–439, 438*f*, 439*t*
  insulin in, 434–435, 436*f*
  in liver, 332–333, 332*t*, 333*f*, 436*t*
   glucagon in, 436*t*, 437
   insulin in, 435, 436*t*
   liver dysfunction and, 339
"Glucose fever," in adrenocortical insufficiency, 521
Glucose intolerance
 in Cushing's syndrome, 513–514
 in glucagonoma, 457
 in mineralocorticoid excess, 525
 in pheochromocytoma, 289
Glucose sensor, 433
Glucose transporters, 433, 435
Glucosuria
 in Cushing's syndrome, 516
 in diabetes mellitus, 445
Glucuronides, in thyroid hormone metabolism, 484
GLUT 2, 433
GLUT 4, 435
 in type 2 diabetes, 444
Glutamate
 in amyotrophic lateral sclerosis, 150, 151*f*
 in stroke, 163–164, 163*f*
Glutamic acid decarboxylase, in diabetes mellitus, 442
Glutathione, hepatocyte synthesis of, 337
Glycated HbA, in diabetes, 449, 449*f*
Glycemic control
 in diabetes complication prevention, 448
 during pregnancy, 543
Glycogen, synthesis of in liver, 332–333, 332*t*, 333*f*, 436*t*
 insulin in, 435, 436*t*
 liver dysfunction and, 339
Glycogen synthetase, in type 2 diabetes, 444
Glycogenolysis, in liver, 332–333, 332*t*, 333*f*, 436*t*
 glucagon in, 436*t*, 437
 insulin in, 435, 436*t*
Glycolysis, in liver, 332–333, 332*t*, 333*f*, 436*t*
 insulin in, 435, 436*t*
 liver dysfunction and, 339

Glycosylation end products, advanced, in diabetic microvascular disease, 449, 450*f*
GM-CSF. *See* Granulocyte-macrophage colony-stimulating factor
GnRH. *See* Gonadotropin-releasing hormone
Goblet cells, 305
Goiter, 485, 486, 486–487, **494–496**, 494*f*, 495*t*
 multinodular, 495, 495*f*
Goitrogens, 494, 495*t*
Gonadal dysfunction, in Cushing's syndrome, 516
Gonadal dysgenesis, 545, 546*t*
Gonadal mosaicism. *See also* Mosaicism
 in osteogenesis imperfecta, 13, 13*f*
Gonadal sex, 531
 disorders of, 545
Gonadal steroid-binding globulin. *See* Steroid hormone-binding globulin
Gonadotrophs, 534
Gonadotropin-releasing hormone (GnRH), 464, 534
 altered release of, in female reproductive tract disorders, 542
 amenorrhea and, 549–550
 in male reproductive function, 558, 560*f*
  infertility and, 563
 ovarian production of, 530*t*
 in polycystic ovary syndrome, 548
 prolactin affecting, 540–541
 stress-related amenorrhea and, 549
Gonadotropin-releasing hormone (GnRH) agonists, for benign prostatic hyperplasia, 570, 570*t*
Gonadotropin surge-inhibiting factor, ovarian production of, 530*t*
Gonadotropins, 464, 534. *See also* Follicle-stimulating hormone; Luteinizing hormone
 changes in, in menstrual cycle, 532*f*, 534–535
 human chorionic. *See* Human chorionic gonadotropin
 ovarian response to, 534–535, 535*f*
Goserelin, for benign prostatic hyperplasia, 570*t*
Gout, **578–580**, 579*f*, 580*t*
 renal stone formation and, 403*t*
gp39. *See also* CD40 ligand
 defective expression of, in hyper-IgM immunodeficiency, 44
gp120, in HIV binding to T cells, 45
GRA. *See* Glucocorticoid-remediable aldosteronism
Grand mal seizures. *See* Tonic-clonic seizures

Granulocyte colony-stimulating factor (G-CSF)
  in cyclic neutropenia, 116
  in hematopoiesis, 98, 99f, 100t
Granulocyte-macrophage colony-stimulating factor (GM-CSF)
  in cyclic neutropenia, 116
  in hematopoiesis, 98, 99f, 100t
Granulocytes, 101–102. *See also specific type and* Leukocytes
  development of, 98, 99f
  storage pool of, in cyclic neutropenia, 115–116
Granulomas, hepatic, drugs causing, 343t
Granulomatous disease, chronic, **43**, 56
Granulosa cells, 529
Granzymes, in lymphocyte-mediated cytotoxic rheumatic disease, 578
Graphesthesia, 140
Graves' disease, 482f, 486, 487–488
  TSH receptor-stimulating antibody in, 485, 486, 488, 488f
Graves' ophthalmopathy, 490, 490f
Grey Turner's sign, 370
Group B streptococci, meningitis caused by, 63, 63t
Growth factors
  in atherosclerosis, 269, 270f
  in benign prostatic hyperplasia, 571–572
  in neoplasia, **82–83**
  ovarian production of, 530t
Growth hormone (GH), 465, 465f, 465t, 466t
  factors affecting secretion of, 465, 465f, 466t
  in fuel homeostasis, 436t, 439
  glucose levels during stress and, 439
  pituitary adenoma secreting, 471, 473, 474t, 475t
Growth hormone-releasing hormone (GHRH), 465, 465f
Growth inhibitors, in neoplasia, **82–83**
Growth retardation, in Cushing's syndrome, 510f, 516
gsp gene, in multinodular goiter, 496
Gustatory sweating, in diabetic autonomic neuropathy, 454
Gut-associated lymphoid tissue, 30
Guttate psoriasis, 173t
Gynecomastia, in cirrhosis, 361

H+-K+ ATPase (proton pump), 297
  in gastric acid secretion, 302, 304f
  in pernicious anemia, 112, 112f
Haemophilus influenzae
  meningitis caused by, 63, 63t, 64, 65
  pneumonia caused by, 66t
Haemophilus influenzae vaccine, 63
Hageman factor (factor XII), 103f, 104, 104t
  deficiency of, 108t

Hageman trait, 108t
Hair cells, 145
Hairy leukoplakia, in HIV infection/AIDS, 47
Hallucinations, 147
Hampton's hump, 218
Haplotype, 3t
  phenylketonuria, 25–26, 25f, 25t, 26t
Haptoglobin, 336t
Hard exudates, in diabetic retinopathy, 450, 451f
Hashimoto's thyroiditis, 482f, 491, 492
  autoimmune disorders associated with, 488t, 492
HAV. *See* Hepatitis A virus
HbA, glycated, in diabetes, 449, 449f
HbA$_{1c}$, in diabetes, 449, 449f
HBcAg, 350, 350t
HBeAg, 350t
HbsAg, 350, 350t
HBV. *See* Hepatitis B virus
HBV-associated delta agent. *See* Hepatitis D virus
hCG. *See* Human chorionic gonadotropin
hCS. *See* Human chorionic somatomammotropin
HCV. *See* Hepatitis C virus
HDL. *See* High-density lipoproteins
HDV. *See* Hepatitis D virus
Head and neck cancer, 86t
Health-related quality of life, impaired, allergy and asthma and, 39
Hearing, **145–146**, 146
Heart, **222–257**
  anatomy of, **222–224**, 223–224f, 225f
  catecholamines affecting, 284t, 288t
  coronary artery disease and, **251–253**, 251t, 252f, 271
  disorders of, **231–251**
    in chronic renal failure, 397
    in Cushing's syndrome, 516–517
    in hyperthyroidism, 489
    in hypothyroidism, 493
  electrical activity of, electrocardiography for measurement of, 224
  histology of, **224–225**, 226f
  normal, **222–231**
  pericardial disease and, **254–257**, 254f, 254t, 255f
  physiology of, **225–231**, 228f, 229f, 230f, 231f, 232f
  thyroid hormones affecting, 485t
Heart attack. *See* Myocardial infarction
Heart block, 232, 232f, 233f
  in coronary artery disease, 253
Heart failure, **234–240**
  in acute renal failure, 392t
  in aortic stenosis, 241, 242
  in chronic renal failure, 396
  left ventricular, **234–239**, 235t, 236f, 237f, 238f

  in pernicious anemia, 115
  right ventricular, **239–240**, 239t, 240f
Heart murmurs, 240–241, 241f
  in aortic regurgitation, 244, 245, 246f
  in aortic stenosis, 241, 242, 243f
  in mitral regurgitation, 247, 249, 250f
  in mitral stenosis, 247, 248f
Heart rate, cardiac output affected by, 227
Heart sounds, 227
  in aortic regurgitation, 244, 245
  in left ventricular failure, 238–239, 238f
  in pericardial tamponade, 257
Heart valves, 222, 223–224f. *See also specific valve*
  in cardiac cycle, 227
  diseases of, **240–251**
Heartburn, in reflux esophagitis, 309–311, 312
Heat-labile toxin (LT), diarrhea caused by, 72
Heat-stable toxin (ST), diarrhea caused by, 72
Heavy chains, immunoglobulin, 32, 33f
Helicobacter pylori, 69
  acid-mediated gastrointestinal injury and, 304, 312–313, 314, 314f
  chronic atrophic gastritis and, 313
HELLP syndrome, 553
Helper (CD4) T lymphocytes, 32
  in allergic hypersensitivity, 35
  defective, in SCID, 41
  in erythema multiforme, 175
  in HIV infection/AIDS, 45–47, 46t
  in inflammatory rheumatic diseases, 577–578
  in lichen planus, 174
Hematemesis, 294t
Hematochezia, in iron deficiency anemia, 111
Hematocrit, normal, 101t
Hematologic disorders
  in chronic renal failure, 397
  gastrointestinal manifestations of, 310t
  neoplasms, **92–95**, 92f, 93t. *See also specific type*
Hematopoiesis, 98–100
  megaloblastic, 114f
Hematuria, in renal stones, 401, 404
Heme, 101, 109
  iron in synthesis of, 109, 110f
Hemianopia
  bitemporal, 145
    in pituitary adenoma, 472, 472f
  homonymous, 145
Hemizona assay, 567–568
Hemochromatosis, liver dysfunction and, 338t
Hemodialysis, neuromuscular disorders in patients receiving, 397

Hemodynamics
 in pulmonary embolism, 216t, 217
 in septic shock, 76–77
 vasopressin osmoregulation and, 467, 467f
Hemoglobin, 101
 in anemia, 105–106
  iron deficiency, 109, 110–111
 erythropoietin levels and, 98
 glycated, in diabetes, 449, 449f
 normal values for, 101t
 in polycythemia, 106
Hemoglobin A, glycated (HbA$_{1c}$), in diabetes mellitus, 449, 449f
Hemoglobin-oxygen dissociation curve, 196–197, 197f
Hemoglobinopathies, anemia and, 105
Hemolysis
 hyperbilirubinemia caused by, 340
 intramedullary, in pernicious anemia, 114
Hemolytic anemia, 106f
 autoimmune, 105
Hemopexin, 336t
 hepatic synthesis of, 336t
Hemophilia A, 108, 108t
Hemophilia B, 108, 108t
Hemoptysis
 in left ventricular failure, 235
 in mitral stenosis, 247
 in pulmonary embolism, 218
Hemorrhage. *See also* Bleeding
 during pregnancy, 543
Hemorrhagic diarrhea, 72, 72f, 73f
Hemorrhagic shock, 280
Hemorrhagic stroke, 159t, 162, 162f
Hemosiderin, 109
Hemostasis. *See also* Coagulation
 disorders of, in chronic renal failure, 397
Henle, loop of, 385, 385f
 in renal regulation, 385
Heparin-induced thrombocytopenia, 117–118, 118f
Heparin-induced thrombocytopenia and thrombosis, 118–119
Hepatic artery, 328, 330f
Hepatic disease, 327, 328t
 acute, 327
 cancer, 86t
  cirrhosis and, 360–361
 manifestations of, **339–344**
Hepatic encephalopathy, 338, 338t, 339, 342–344, 350, 359–360, 360t
Hepatic failure, fulminant, 327, 328t
Hepatic fibrosis, in cirrhosis, 355–356, 356f
Hepatic lobules, 329, 330f
Hepatic necrosis
 in acute hepatitis, 349
 bridging, 349

 in chronic hepatitis, 352–354, 353f
 drugs causing, 343t
 massive, 349
 piecemeal (periportal hepatitis), 352, 353f
Hepatic portal vein, 328–329, 330f
Hepatic regeneration, 331
Hepatitis
 acute, 327, 328t, **344–351**
  pathology of, 348–349
  time course of, 347, 348f
 alcoholic
  acute, 348, 349t
  chronic, 352, 353f
 chronic, 327, 328t, 345f, **351–355**, 351t
  active (aggressive), 351, 351t
   pathology of, 353f, 354
  alcoholic, 352, 353f
  idiopathic, 352, 353f
  persistent, 351, 351t
   pathology of, 354
  postviral, 352
 clinical syndromes associated with, 345
 periportal (piecemeal necrosis), 352, 353f
 toxic (drug-associated), 343t, 347, 347t
  time course of, 347, 348f
 viral
  characteristics of, 346t
  chronic, 352
  clinical manifestations of, 345, 345f, 349–350, 349–351, 350t
  etiology of, 345–347, 346t
  extrahepatic manifestations of, 348
  liver damage caused by, 347–348
  pathogenesis of, 327–328
  time course of, 347, 348f
Hepatitis A virus, 345
 antibodies produced in infection with, 350
 characteristics of infection with, 346t
 time course of infection with, 347, 348f
Hepatitis B virus, 345, 345–347
 antibodies produced in infection with, 350, 350t
 characteristics of infection with, 346t
 chronic infection caused by, 352
 hepatitis D virus infection and, 347
 time course of infection with, 347, 348f
Hepatitis C virus, 345, 347
 characteristics of infection with, 346t
 chronic infection caused by, 352
Hepatitis D virus, 345, 347
 characteristics of infection with, 346t
 chronic infection caused by, 352

Hepatitis E virus, 345
 characteristics of infection with, 346t
Hepatocellular carcinoma, cirrhosis and, 360–361
Hepatocytes, 327, 330–331, 331f
 dysfunction of, 338, 338t
 effects of, 331
 endocytic functions of, 337
 in glutathione synthesis, 337
 in hepatic regeneration, 331
 segregation of functions of, 330–331, 331f
Hepatojugular reflux, in right ventricular failure, 240
Hepatorenal syndrome, liver dysfunction and, 338t, 354, 357
HER2/neu oncogene, 81t, 82
 in breast cancer, 88, 89
Hereditary chronic pancreatitis, 373
Hereditary elliptocytosis, 105–106
Hereditary nonpolyposis colorectal cancer, 87
Hereditary spherocytosis, 105–106
Hering-Breuer reflex, 199
Herniation syndromes, 147, 148f
Herpes simplex virus infection
 cervical cancer and, 551
 erythema multiforme and, 175, 176
 in HIV infection/AIDS, 48
Herpes zoster infection, in HIV infection/AIDS, 48
Heterochromatin, 3t
Heterogeneity
 allelic, 3t
  in osteogenesis imperfecta, 13
 genetic, 3t
  in osteogenesis imperfecta, 13
 phenotypic, 4t
  in osteogenesis imperfecta, 13
Heterozygote advantage, 4t
 in fragile X-associated mental retardation syndrome, 17
 in phenylketonuria, 26
HEV. *See* Hepatitis E virus
5-HIAA. *See* 5-Hydroxyindoleacetic acid
High-density lipoproteins, 269
 metabolism of, in liver, 334, 335f
High-grade lymphoma, 93
Hip fractures, in osteoporosis, 428
Hirsutism
 in Cushing's syndrome, 516
 in polycystic ovary syndrome, 547, 548t, 549, 549f
His bundle, 222–224, 225f
Histamine, gastrointestinal secretion of, 298t
HIV infection/AIDS, **45–49**
 adrenocortical insufficiency in, 519
 criteria for definition and diagnosis of, 46t
 lymphoma in, 49, 93
 lymphopenia in, 107, 107t

HIV infection/AIDS (cont.)
  pathogens causing infection in, 47–48, 56t
  pneumonia in, 66, 67t
HLA See Human leukocyte antigens
HMG-CoA reductase inhibitors, in atherosclerosis prevention, 272
hMLH1 gene, 82t
  in colon carcinoma, 87
hMSH2 gene, 82t
  in colon carcinoma, 87
Hodgkin's disease, pathogens causing infection in, 56t
Homocysteine, in atherosclerosis, 272
Homocysteine thiolactone, in atherosclerosis, 272
Homonymous hemianopia, 144–145
Horizontal cells, retinal, 144
Hormonal feedback
  in ACTH regulation, 502, 503, 504f, 506f
  in male reproductive function, 558–560, 560f
    infertility and, 562, 563–564
  in menstrual cycle regulation, 533–534, 534f
    disorders of, 542, 547–549, 548t, 549t
    infertility and, 552–553
Hormones
  female reproductive tract producing, 530t, 532t, 539t
  gastrointestinal, 298t, 299
  hepatic clearance of, liver dysfunction and, 344
  in neoplasia, **82–83**
    systemic effects of tumor expression of, 95, 96t
  vascular smooth muscle affected by, 265–266
Horner's syndrome, 143
Host cell death, in infection, 58, 58f
Host defenses against infection, **52–59**
  constitutive, **53–56**
  gastrointestinal, 299–300, 300t, 301f
  induced, **56**, 56t. See also Immune response/immunity
  microbial strategies against, 60t
  pulmonary, 66–68, 67t, 68f, 189, 189t
hPL. See Placental lactogen
HSV. See Herpes simplex virus infection
hTR, 485
hTR-α1, 485
hTR-β1, 485
  mutations in gene for, in generalized resistance to thyroid hormone (Refetoff's syndrome), 485, 497
Human chorionic gonadotropin (hCG), 535–536, 536f, 537–538
  in molar pregnancy, 544
  in testicular cancer, 91

Human chorionic somatomammotropin (hCS/placental lactogen), 537
  fuel homeostasis in pregnancy and, 539, 541f, 543
Human Genome Project, **8**
Human immunodeficiency virus infection. See HIV infection/AIDS
Human leukocyte antigens (HLA)
  in autoimmune polyendocrine syndrome, 518
  in diabetes mellitus, 442
  in Graves' disease, 488
  in Hashimoto's thyroiditis, 492
  in psoriasis, 172
Human papillomavirus, 80
  in cancer of the cervix, 80, 551
Human T cell leukemia virus, 80
Human thyroid hormone receptors, 485
Humoral (antibody-mediated) immune response, 31, 32
  antigen elimination in, 33
  impairment of. See also Immunodeficiency diseases
    autoimmune phenomena and, 40
    infections associated with, 40, 41t, 56t
  microbial strategies against, 60t
Humoral secretagogues, 307
Huntington's disease, 137
Hürthle cells, 492
Hydatidiform mole, 544
Hydrochloric acid, gastric secretion of, 298t, 302–304, 304f
  disorders of, 308
  pancreatic insufficiency and, 377
Hydrogen ion concentration, in control of breathing, 199–200
Hydrophilic substances, in hepatic drug metabolism and excretion, 335
β-Hydroxybutyrate, in diabetic ketoacidosis, 446, 446f
5-Hydroxyindoleacetic acid, urinary, in carcinoid syndrome, 90
11β-Hydroxylase-aldosterone synthase gene, in glucocorticoid-remediable aldosteronism, 276, 524
11β-Hydroxylase deficiency
  adrenal androgen excess caused by, 527
  hypertension and, 276
17α-Hydroxylase deficiency, hypertension and, 276
21-Hydroxylase antibodies, adrenocortical insufficiency caused by, 518
21-Hydroxylase deficiency, adrenal androgen excess caused by, 527

11β-Hydroxysteroid dehydrogenase type 2, in apparent mineralocorticoid excess, 276, 277f
5-Hydroxytryptamine (serotonin), carcinoid tumor expression of, 90
25-Hydroxyvitamin D (25-[OH]D), 413, 413f, 414
  testing for in vitamin D deficiency, 413
Hyperadrenal corticalism, 509. See also Cushing's syndrome
Hyperaldosteronism (aldosteronism), **522–526**, 523t
  familial
    type I (glucocorticoid-remediable), 276, 524
    type II, 524
  glucocorticoid-remediable, 276, 524
  hypertension and, 275–276, 525
  primary (Conn's syndrome), 509, 522
    diagnosis of, 525–526
    etiology of, 523–524, 523t, 524f
    hypertension and, 275–276, 525
    pathophysiology of, 524
    plasma electrolyte levels in, 522t
  secondary, 506, 522
    diagnosis of, 526
    etiology of, 524
    pathophysiology of, 524
Hyperamylasemia, in acute pancreatitis, 369
Hyperbilirubinemia, 340
  in acute hepatitis, 349
  in acute pancreatitis, 370
Hypercalcemia
  in acute pancreatitis, 366
  calcitonin affected by, 414
  in chronic pancreatitis, 373
  differential diagnosis of, 418, 419t
  familial (benign) hypocalciuric, **419–420**, 419t
  in hyperparathyroidism, 418, 419t
  laboratory findings in, 419t
  of malignancy, 419t, **420**
  in pheochromocytoma, 290
Hypercalciuria
  in Cushing's syndrome, 515
  renal stone formation and, 402, 403t
Hypercapnia
  in asthma, 203
  chronic, 200
  in chronic bronchitis, 207
  in emphysema, 207
  in idiopathic pulmonary fibrosis, 210
  in noncardiogenic pulmonary edema, 214
  ventilatory response to, 199, 200
Hypercholesterolemia, familial, liver dysfunction and, 338t, 342
Hypercoagulable states
  gastrointestinal manifestations of, 310t

inherited, **120–122**, 120*f*
pregnancy as, 543–544, 543*t*
Hypercortisolism, 509. *See also*
Cushing's syndrome
Hyperdefecation, in hyperthyroidism, 490
Hyperdynamic pulses, in aortic regurgitation, 244, 245
Hyperemia, reactive, nitric oxide and, 264–265
Hyperestrogenism, liver dysfunction and, 338*t*
Hyperfiltration, glomerular, in diabetes mellitus, 452
Hypergammaglobulinemia, liver dysfunction and, 338*t*
Hyperglycemia, 439–440, 444, 445. *See also* Diabetes mellitus
  in acute pancreatitis, 370
  control of, in diabetes complication prevention, 448
  in Cushing's syndrome, 514, 516
  in diabetic ketoacidosis, 445
  fasting, 444
  liver dysfunction and, 338*t*, 339
  postprandial, 444
  rebound (Somogyi phenomenon), 448
Hypergonadotropic hypogonadism, 563–564
Hyperhomocyst(e)inemia, in atherosclerosis, 272
Hyper-IgE immunodeficiency, 40*t*, **44–45**
Hyper-IgM immunodeficiency, 40*t*, **44**
Hyperinflation
  in asthma, 203
  in chronic bronchitis, 207
  in emphysema, 207
Hyperinsulinemia
  hypertension and, 278, 453
  in polycystic ovary syndrome, 547–548, 548*t*, 549*f*
  in type II diabetes, 443, 453
Hyperkalemia
  in acute pancreatitis, 370
  in adrenocortical insufficiency, 521, 522, 522*t*
  in chronic renal failure, 395–396
Hyperkeratosis, in lichen planus, 174
Hyperlipasemia, in acute pancreatitis, 369–370
Hyperlipidemia
  acute pancreatitis associated with, 366, 370
  in glomerulonephritis and nephrotic syndrome, 401
Hypermagnesemia, in chronic renal failure, 396
Hypermorphic mutation, 4*t*, 6
Hypernatremia, diabetes insipidus and, 476–477, 477, 477*t*

Hyperosmolar coma, in diabetes mellitus, 446, 447
Hyperoxaluria, renal stone formation and, 403*t*
Hyperparathyroidism, **415–419**
  hypercalcemia in, 418, 419*t*
  primary, 415–416, 416*t*, 418, 418*t*, 419*t*
    gastrointestinal manifestations of, 310*t*
    neonatal severe, 419
    renal stone formation and, 402, 403*t*, 418
  secondary, 416, 418–419
    hypocalcemia in, 423, 424*t*
    laboratory findings in, 424*t*
    osteoporosis and, 427
Hyperphenylalaninemia, 23. *See also* Phenylketonuria
  benign, 23, 25
  incidence of, 23
Hyperphosphatemia
  in chronic renal failure, 396–397, 396*f*
  in hypoparathyroidism, 422
  1,25-(OH)$_2$D production affected by, 408
Hyperpigmentation
  in adrenocortical insufficiency, 520–521
  in Cushing's syndrome, 515
Hyperplasia, 84–85, 84*f*
  adrenal
    congenital, 527
      hypertension and, 276
      plasma ACTH and cortisol levels in, 505*f*
    hypertension and, 276
    macronodular, 511, 513
    micronodular, 510–511, 513
    primary aldosteronism (Conn's syndrome) caused by, 523, 523*t*, 526
  atypical, 85
  of breast epithelial cells, during pregnancy, 88
  in colon cancer, 87
  fat cell, in obesity, 470
  hepatic, 331
  parathyroid gland, 415–416
  prostatic. *See* Benign prostatic hyperplasia
Hyperprolactinemia, 472–473, 473*t*
  chronic anovulation and, 547, 548*t*
  in hypogonadotropic hypogonadism, 564
  in hypothyroidism, 494
Hyperprothrombinemia, 121
Hyperresponsiveness, airway
  in allergic rhinitis, 38
  in asthma, 201, 203–204
Hypersecretion, in allergic rhinitis, 37–38
Hypersensitivity immune responses, 34

Hypersensitivity (immune complex) vasculitis, 580–581
Hypersplenism
  in cirrhosis, 360
  platelet count affected in, 107
Hypertension, **273–278**, 273*t*, 275*t*, 277*f*
  in atherosclerosis, 272*t*, 273
  in chronic renal failure, 394, 395*t*, 397
  in Cushing's syndrome, 510*f*, 516
  in diabetes mellitus, 453
  diastolic dysfunction caused by, 237
  essential (primary), 273, 273*t*
    of pregnancy, 553
  in glomerulonephritis and nephrotic syndrome, 400–401
  hyperinsulinemia and, 278, 453
  insulin resistance and, 278, 453
  intracerebral hemorrhage caused by, 162, 162*f*
  malignant, 274
  in mineralocorticoid excess, 275–276, 277*f*, 525
  in pheochromocytoma, 287–288, 289*t*
  pill, 275
  portal, 338
    in cirrhosis, 357, 357*t*
  in preeclampsia-eclampsia, 553–555
  during pregnancy, 553–555
  pulmonary, 239
    in emphysema, 207
    in idiopathic pulmonary fibrosis, 210
  renal, 275
    bruits in, 274
    clinical and laboratory findings in, 391*t*
    renal stone formation and, 402
  renovascular, 271
  secondary, 273
  "white coat," 262
Hypertensive encephalopathy, 274
Hypertensive retinopathy, 274
Hyperthyroidism, 486, **486–491**, 487*t*
  chronic anovulation and, 547, 548*t*
  gastrointestinal manifestations of, 310*t*, 490
  goiter associated with, 494, 495, 495*t*
  male infertility and, 564
  secondary, 487
  subclinical, 498
  tertiary, 487*t*
Hyperthyroxinemia
  dysalbuminemic euthyroid, 496–497
  familial euthyroid, 496–497
Hypertriglyceridemia, in diabetes mellitus, 453
  ketoacidosis and, 446
Hypertrophic lichen planus, 175
Hypertrophy
  of breast epithelial cells, 88
  concentric, in aortic stenosis, 242, 243*f*
  eccentric, in aortic regurgitation, 244–245, 246*f*
  fat cell, in obesity, 470

Hyperuricemia
  in chronic renal failure, 396
  in gout, 579
Hyperuricosuria, renal stone formation and, 402, 403*t*
Hypoadrenal states, hyponatremia in, 478
Hypoalbuminemia
  in cirrhosis, 359
  hypocalcemia caused by, 421
  liver dysfunction and, 338*t*, 359
Hypoaldosteronism, **526**
  hyporeninemic (type 4 renal tubular acidosis), 396, 509, 526
  plasma electrolyte levels in, 522*t*
Hypocalcemia
  in acute pancreatitis, 370
  in chronic renal failure, 396–397, 396*f*
  clinical manifestations of, 422–424, 423*f*, 423*t*, 424*t*
  differential diagnosis of, 421, 421*t*, 423, 424*t*
  etiology of, 420–421
  hypoparathyroidism causing, 420–421, 421*t*
  in pancreatic insufficiency, 378
  parathyroid hyperplasia caused by, 406
  pathogenesis of, 422
Hypocalciuric hypercalcemia, familial (benign), **419–420**, 419*t*
Hypocapnia, in pulmonary embolism, 217
Hypogammaglobulinemia
  acquired/adult-onset (common variable immunodeficiency), 40*t*, **43–44**
    pathogens causing infection in, 41*t*, 56*t*
  histologic features of, 320*t*
Hypoglycemia
  in adrenocortical insufficiency, 520, 522, 522*t*
  catecholamine release and, 447, 447*t*
  as complication of insulin treatment in diabetes, 447–448, 447*t*
  fasting
    insulin-mediated vs. non-insulin-mediated, 455–456
    insulinoma causing, 455–456
  insulinoma causing, 455–456
  liver dysfunction and, 338*t*, 339
  neuroglycopenic, 447, 447*t*
    insulinoma causing, 455
  nocturnal, 447
  symptoms and signs of, 447*t*
Hypoglycemia-associated autonomic failure, 291
Hypoglycemia unawareness, 291
Hypogonadism
  hypergonadotropic, 563–564
  hypogonadotropic, 563, 565–566
  liver dysfunction and, 338*t*
Hypokalemia
  in acute pancreatitis, 370

  in mineralocorticoid excess/hyperaldosteronism, 525
Hypokalemic nephropathy, in mineralocorticoid excess, 525
Hypomorphic mutation, 4*t*, 6
Hyponatremia
  in adrenocortical insufficiency, 521, 522, 522*t*
  in syndrome of inappropriate vasopressin secretion, 478
Hypoparathyroidism, **420–424**, 421*t*
  laboratory findings in, 424*t*
Hypophosphatemia, 1,25-$(OH)_2$D production affected by, 408
Hypopituitarism, **473–475**, 475*t*
  hypoaldosteronism and, 526
  plasma ACTH and cortisol levels in, 505*f*
Hypoplasia, adrenal, congenital, aldosterone deficiency in, 526
Hyporeninemic hypoaldosteronism (type 4 renal tubular acidosis), 396, 509, 526
Hyposensitization, for late phase/chronic allergic symptoms, 38
Hypospadias, infertility in, 565
Hypospermatogenesis, 563
Hypotension
  in adrenocortical insufficiency, 521
  in aortic regurgitation, 241
  orthostatic, in diabetic autonomic neuropathy, 454
  in pericardial tamponade, 256
  refractory, in septic shock, 77
Hypothalamic amenorrhea, 549
Hypothalamic nuclei, 459, 460*f*
  functions of, 459, 461*t*
Hypothalamic-pituitary function, female reproductive disorders and, **542**
Hypothalamic-pituitary-testicular axis, in male reproductive function, 558, 558–560, 560*f*
Hypothalamic-pituitary-thyroid axis, 484–485, 484*f*
Hypothalamus, **459–480**
  anatomy/histology/cell biology of, 459–462, 460*f*
  in body weight control, 468–469, 468*f*
  disorders of, **469–479**
    amenorrhea/infertility in, 545, 546*t*, 549
    hypothyroidism and, 491, 492
  hormones secreted by, 462
  normal, **459–462**
  physiology of, **462–469**
Hypothermia, in hypothyroidism, 492
Hypothyroidism, 486, **491–494**, 491*t*, 493*t*, 494*f*
  chronic anovulation and, 547, 548*t*

  gastrointestinal manifestations of, 310*t*
  goiter associated with, 494, 495, 495*t*
  hyponatremia in, 478
  male infertility and, 564
  subclinical, 497–498
Hypotonia, 136
Hypotonic syndromes, 478*t*
  syndrome of inappropriate vasopressin secretion as, 478
Hypovolemia, in acute renal failure, 392*t*
Hypovolemic shock, 278, 278*t*, **279–280**, 279*t*
Hypoxemia
  in asthma, 203
  in chronic bronchitis, 207
  in emphysema, 207
  in idiopathic pulmonary fibrosis, 210
  in noncardiogenic pulmonary edema, 214
  in pulmonary embolism, 217–218, 217*f*, 218
  ventilatory response to, 199, 200
Hypoxia
  in acute renal failure, 391, 393*f*, 393*t*
  chronic, 200
  in idiopathic pulmonary fibrosis, 210
  ventilatory response to, 199, 200, 200*f*
Hypoxic pulmonary vasoconstriction, 194
HZV. *See* Herpes zoster infection

IAA. *See* **Insulin autoantibody**
IAPP. *See* Islet amyloid polypeptide
Iatrogenic Cushing's syndrome, 511*t*, 512*f*
IC (inspiratory capacity), 185
ICA. *See* Islet cell antibodies
Icteric phase, in viral hepatitis, 348*f*, 349–350
Icterus (jaundice), 339, 341*t*
  in acute pancreatitis, 370
  in hepatitis, 347, 348*f*, 349
Idiopathic chronic hepatitis, 352, 353*f*
Idiopathic (interstitial) pulmonary fibrosis, **208–210**, 208*f*, 209*f*, 210*f*, 211*f*
Idiopathic stone disease, 403*t*
IDL. *See* Intermediate-density lipoproteins
IFN-γ. *See* Gamma interferon
IgA, 33
  in breast milk, 540
  selective deficiency of, 40*t*, **44**
    pathogens causing infection in, 56*t*
IgA nephropathy, 399
IgD, 33
IgE, 33
  allergen-specific, measurement of, 39
  in allergic reactivity, 34–35
  in allergic rhinitis, 36, 39
  in asthma, 201, 202
  elevated levels of (hyper-IgE

immunodeficiency), 40t, **44–45**
neutralization of, in allergy treatment, 35
in type I (anaphylactic/immediate) hypersensitivity reaction, 34
IgG, 33
  in acute hepatitis, 350, 350t
  in antigen elimination, 33
  in bullous pemphigoid, 178f, 179
  in heparin-induced thrombocytopenia, 118–119, 118f
  structure of, 33f
  in type II (cytotoxic) hypersensitivity reactions, 34
IgG-heparin-PF4 complex
  in heparin-induced thrombocytopenia, 118, 118f
  in heparin-induced thrombocytopenia and thrombosis, 118–119
IGIV. *See* Intravenous gamma globulin
IgM, 33
  in acute hepatitis, 350, 350t
  elevated levels of (hyper-IgM immunodeficiency), 40t, **44**
  selective deficiency of, pathogens causing infection in, 56t
  in type II (cytotoxic) hypersensitivity reactions, 34
IL. *See specific type under* Interleukin
Ileocecal valve, 295f
Ileum, 295f, 305
Ileus, in acute pancreatitis, 368–369
Imaging
  in chronic bronchitis, 207
  in emphysema, 207
  in idiopathic pulmonary fibrosis, 210
  in pulmonary embolism, 218
Immediate (anaphylactic/type I) hypersensitivity reaction, 34
Immobility, osteoporosis associated with, 428
Immotile cilia (Kartagener's) syndrome, male infertility and, 564, 566
Immune complex-mediated (type III) hypersensitivity reaction, 34
Immune complexes
  in glomerular disease, 388, 389f, 581
  in glomerulonephritis, 399, 400t, 581
  in inflammatory rheumatic diseases, 577, 577f
  in systemic lupus erythematosus, 582
  in vasculitis, **580–581**
  leukocytoclastic, 180–181, 181f
Immune response/immunity, 31–35, 31f
  antibody-mediated (humoral), 31, 32
    antigen elimination in, 33
    impairment of. *See also* Immunodeficiency diseases
      autoimmune phenomena and, 40
      infections associated with, 40, 41t, 56t

microbial strategies against, 60t
cellular (cell-mediated), 31, 32
  impairment of. *See also* HIV infection/AIDS; Immunodeficiency diseases
    infections associated with, 40, 41t, 56t
    microbial strategies against, 60t
  type IV (delayed) hypersensitivity reactions mediated by, 34
  gastrointestinal tract in, 299, 300t, 301f
  glucocorticoids affecting, 507t
  hypersensitivity, 34
  innate and adaptive, **30–31**
  lungs in, 189, 189t
  passive, 57
  in viral hepatitis, 347–348
Immune system, **28–49**
  abbreviations and acronyms used in association with, 28t
  anatomy of, **28–30**
  cells of, 28–29
  development of from stem cells, 102, 102f
  disorders of, **36–49**. *See also specific disorder*
  glucocorticoids affecting, 507t
  organs of, 29–30
  physiology of, **30–35**. *See also* Immune response/immunity
Immune thrombocytopenia, drug-associated, **117–119**, 117t
Immunocompromised host. *See also* HIV infection/AIDS
  opportunistic infections in, 52
  pneumonia in, 66, 67t
Immunodeficiency diseases. *See also specific type*
  acquired. *See* HIV infection/AIDS; Immunodeficiency diseases, common variable
  autoimmune phenomena and, 40
  common variable, 40t, 41t, **43–44**, 56t
  hyper-IgE, 40t, **44–45**
  hyper-IgM, 40t, **44**
  infection and, 40, 41t, 56t
  pneumonia in patient with, 67t
  primary, **39–45**, 40t. *See also specific type*
  severe combined, 40t, **41**, 41t, 56t
Immunogens (antigens), **31**
  humoral mechanisms of elimination of, 33
  processing and presentation of, 31
Immunoglobulins. *See also specific type under* Ig
  isotypes of, 33
  structure and function of, 32–33, 33f
Immunologic memory, 31
  in systemic lupus erythematosus, 582
Implantation, 535–536, 536f
  faulty, in preeclampsia-eclampsia, 553

Impotence, 565
  in diabetes mellitus, 454
Imprinting, 4t
  in fragile X-associated mental retardation syndrome, 17
Incontinence, urinary, in diabetic autonomic neuropathy, 454
Increased-permeability (noncardiogenic) pulmonary edema, 212, 213, 214
Indifferent phase, of sexual development, 531
Induced defenses against infection, **56**, 56t. *See also* Immune response/immunity
  microbial strategies against, 60t
Infantile spinal muscular atrophy (Werdnig-Hoffman disease), 150
Infection/infectious diseases, **50–78**
  acute pancreatitis associated with, 365–366, 365t
  chemical barriers to, 53
  complement system and, 54, 55f
  congenital, 57
  in Cushing's syndrome, 515–516
  in cyclic neutropenia, 116–117
  in diabetes mellitus, 454
  establishment of, **56–59**, 57t, 58f
  glomerulonephritis after, 398, 398t, 399–400, 401
  history in diagnosis of, 51t
  in HIV infection/AIDS, 47–48, 56t
  host-agent-environment paradigm in study of, 50
  host defenses against, **52–59**
    constitutive, **53–56**
    gastrointestinal, 299–300, 300t, 301f
    induced, 56, 56t. *See also* Immune response/immunity
    microbial strategies against, 60t
    pulmonary, 66–68, 67t, 68f, 189, 189t
  inflammatory response and, 53–54
  opportunistic, 52
    in HIV infection/AIDS, 48
  outcomes of, 58–59, 58f
  phagocytosis and, 54–56
  physical barriers to, 53
  in primary immunodeficiency diseases, 40, 41t, 56t
  resolution of, 58–59
  time course of, 58
  in uremia, 397
Infectious agents, 50, 50f. *See also specific type and* Infection/infectious diseases
Infectious diarrhea, **69–73**, 319–320, 322t
  in HIV infection/AIDS, 48
Infectious enterocolitis, in HIV infection/AIDS, 48
Infective endocarditis, **59–61**, 61f, 62t
Inferior quadrantanopia, 145

Infertility
  female, 529, **552–553**, 552t
    amenorrhea and, 551
    in Cushing's syndrome, 510f, 516
    ovulatory causes of, 552–553
    in polycystic ovary syndrome, 547, 548t
    tubal and pelvic causes of, 553
  in hyperthyroidism, 490
  in hypothyroidism, 494
  male, **562–568**, 562t
    clinical manifestations of, 565–568
    laboratory tests and evaluation of, 566–568, 567f, 568t
    posttesticular causes of, 562–563, 562t
    pretesticular causes of, 562, 562t
    symptoms and signs in, 565–566
    testicular causes of, 562, 562t
Inflammation (inflammatory response), 53–54
  in acute renal failure, 390
  atherosclerotic plaques and, 270
  in asthma, 202, 202t
  in Cushing's syndrome, 515–516
  in gout, 579–580, 580t
  infection causing, 58
    host defenses and, 53–54
  mechanisms of, 34
  in meningitis, 64–65
  systemic, sepsis and, 74, 74t
Inflammatory bowel disease, 318, **320–324**, 323t
Inflammatory demyelinating polyneuropathy, in HIV infection/AIDS, 48
Inflammatory diarrhea, 72, 72f
Inflammatory mediators, 34, 54
  in acute pancreatitis, 367, 368f
  in asthma, 202, 202t
  in early response, 36–37
  in late response, 37
  in sepsis, 74–76, 75f, 76f
Inflammatory rheumatic diseases, **576–583**. See also specific type
  acute, **576**, 576f
  chronic, **576–577**, 576f, 577f
  pathogenesis of inflammation in, **577–578**
Ingression, by microorganisms, 57, 57t
Inhalation injury, pulmonary edema and, 213
Inheritance, **6–8**
  dominant, loss-of-function (amorphic) mutation and, 7
  multifactorial, 8
  recessive, 4t
    amorphic (loss-of-function) mutations and, 6–7, 7t
  semi-dominant, 7

Inhibin
  in male reproductive function, 560, 560f
  ovarian production of, 530t
Inhibitory neurotransmitters, 127
Inhibitory postsynaptic potential, 127
Injection drug abuse, pneumonia and, 67t
Innate immunity, **30–31**
Inositol-1,4,5-trisphosphate, 127
  in adrenergic receptor function, 283–284
Inspiratory capacity (IC), 185
Inspiratory reserve volume (IRV), 185
Insulin, 432, **433–435**, 436t
  antibodies against, in diabetes mellitus, 442
  B cells secreting, 432, 432t, 433f
    regulation of, 433, 434f, 434t
  in carbohydrate metabolism, 434–435, 436t, 438–439, 438f, 439t
  chronic renal failure affecting metabolism of, 398
  deficiency of, 440. See also Diabetes mellitus
  for diabetes mellitus. See Insulin therapy
  effects of, 434–435, 436t
  first phase release of, impairment of in type 2 diabetes, 443
  mechanism of action of, 433–434, 435f
  regulation and secretion of, 433, 434f, 434t
  synthesis and metabolism of, 433, 433f
Insulin antagonism, glucocorticoids and, 504, 507t
Insulin autoantibody, 442
  insulin-mediated hypoglycemia caused by, 456
Insulin-dependent diabetes mellitus (IDDM), adrenomedullary failure in, 291
Insulin-like growth factor-1, 336t, 465
  in benign prostatic hyperplasia, 572
  hepatic synthesis of, 336t
  ovarian production of, 530t
  in polycystic ovary syndrome, 548, 549f
Insulin-like growth factor-1 receptors, 434
Insulin receptors, 433–434, 435f
  defects of, in diabetes mellitus, 444
Insulin resistance, 440, 441, 443–444
  in Cushing's syndrome, 514
  hepatic, in chronic pancreatitis, 375
  hypertension and, 278, 453
  obesity and, 470
  in polycystic ovary syndrome, 547–548, 548t, 549f
Insulin resistance syndrome (syndrome X), 453
Insulin therapy, hypoglycemia as complication of, 447–448, 447t
  surreptitious administration and, 456

Insulinoma, **455–456**, 456t
int-2 oncogene, 81t
Integrins
  in breast cancer, 89
  in neoplasia, 83
Integumentary system. See Skin
Intention tremor, 136
Interface dermatitis, 170t, 171f
  erythema multiforme, **175–177**, 176f, 177f
  lichen planus, **173–175**, 173f, 174f, 174t
Interferon, gamma, 32
  in allergic hypersensitivity, 34
Interleukin-1
  in acute pancreatitis, 367, 368f
  in hematopoiesis, 99f, 100t
  in meningitis, 64–65
  in sepsis, 74, 75f, 76f
  in T lymphocyte activation/recognition, 32
Interleukin-2
  in asthma, 202
  in inflammatory rheumatic diseases, 577
  overexpression of, in psoriasis, 171
  receptors for
    defect in in SCID, 41
    in T lymphocyte activation/recognition, 32
  in T lymphocyte activation/recognition, 32
  ulcerative colitis and, 321
Interleukin-3
  in asthma, 202
  in hematopoiesis, 98, 99f, 100t
Interleukin-4
  in allergic hypersensitivity, 34–35
  in asthma, 202
  in hematopoiesis, 99f, 100t
  in inflammatory rheumatic diseases, 577
Interleukin-5
  in asthma, 202
  in hematopoiesis, 99f, 100t
  in inflammatory rheumatic diseases, 577
Interleukin-6
  in acute pancreatitis, 367, 368f
  in asthma, 202
  in hematopoiesis, 99f, 100, 100t
  in inflammatory rheumatic diseases, 577
Interleukin-8
  in acute pancreatitis, 367, 368f
  in asthma, 202
Interleukin-10
  in asthma, 202
  in inflammatory rheumatic diseases, 577
  in ulcerative colitis, 321
Interleukin-11, in hematopoiesis, 99f, 100, 100t

Interleukin-12, in inflammatory rheumatic diseases, 577
Interleukin-13, in allergic hypersensitivity, 34
Intermediate-density lipoproteins, 269
Intermittent claudication, 272
Internal elastic lamina, 258, 259f
Interstitial (Leydig) cells, 556, 557f
Interstitial cerebral edema, in meningitis, 65
Interstitial pulmonary edema, 211, 212f
Interstitial (idiopathic) pulmonary fibrosis, **208–210**, 208f, 209t, 210f, 211f
Intestinal disorders. *See also* Gastrointestinal tract, disorders of
common presentations of, 294t
Intestinal motility, 306. *See also* Gastrointestinal motility
disorders of, 308
Intestinal secretion, 306–307. *See also* Gastrointestinal secretion
Intestinal smooth muscle
catecholamines affecting, 284t
contraction of, 296–297. *See also* Gastrointestinal motility
Intima, 258, 259f
Intracellular second messengers, 127
Intramedullary hemolysis, in pernicious anemia, 114
Intraocular pressure, in Cushing's syndrome, 516
Intraparenchymal hemorrhage, 162
Intravenous gamma globulin, for common variable immunodeficiency, 44
Intravenous pyelography, in benign prostatic hyperplasia, 574
Intrinsic coagulation pathway, 103f, 104
Intrinsic factor
gastrointestinal secretion of, 298t, 304
loss of, in pernicious anemia, 111, 112f, 304
Invasive carcinoma, 84, 84f, 85
Inverse psoriasis, 173t
Iodide, in thyroid hormone formation and secretion, 482
Iodide trapping (iodide pump), 482
Iodine
deficiency of, goiter caused by, 494, 495–496, 495t
in thyroid hormone formation and secretion, 482
Ion channels, 125
anticonvulsant mechanism of action and, 156, 156t
Iron
in heme, 109, 110f
total binding capacity of, in iron deficiency anemia, 109–110
Iron-associated proteins, 109, 110t

Iron deficiency anemia, 105, **109–111**
heme synthesis and, 108, 110f
Irreversible (refractory) shock, 279–280
Irritable bowel syndrome, 306, 308
Irritant receptors, pulmonary, 187, 188t
IRV (inspiratory reserve volume), 185
Ischemia
in acute renal failure, 391, 392t, 393f, 393t
myocardial
in coronary artery disease, 251–252, 251t
diastolic dysfunction caused by, 237
Ischemic stroke, 159–162, 159f, 159t, 160f, 161f, 161t
Islet amyloid polypeptide, in type II diabetes, 444
Islet cell antibodies, in diabetes mellitus, 442
Islets of Langerhans (pancreatic islets), 362, 432, 432t. *See also* Endocrine pancreas
tumors of, **455–456**, 456t, **457**. *See also specific type*
Isotype switching, in allergic hypersensitivity, 34
Isovolumic contraction, 227, 228f
Isovolumic relaxation, 227, 228f
Isovolumic systolic pressure-volume curve, 227, 229f, 230f
IVP. *See* Intravenous pyelography

J (juxtacapillary) receptors, pulmonary, 188t
in control of breathing, 199
Jaundice (icterus), 339, 341t
in acute pancreatitis, 370
in hepatitis, 347, 348f, 349
JC virus, progressive multifocal leukoencephalopathy caused by, 48
Jejunum, 295f, 305
Jerk nystagmus, 145, 146
Job's syndrome (hyper-IgE immunodeficiency), 40t, **44–45**
Jodbasedow phenomenon, 487
Joints, gout involving, 578, 579
Jugular venous pressure/waveforms
in constrictive pericarditis, 255, 255f
in pericardial tamponade, 256
in right ventricular failure, 239, 239–240, 240f
Juvenile onset diabetes, 440. *See also* Diabetes mellitus, type 1
Juxtacapillary (J) receptors, pulmonary, 188t
in control of breathing, 199
Juxtaglomerular apparatus
catecholamines affecting, 284t
in renal regulation of blood pressure, 386
K-*ras* gene, in pancreatic carcinoma, 379

Kalig-2 gene, in Kallmann's syndrome, 566
Kallikreins, 266
Kallmann's syndrome, 566
Kaposi's sarcoma, in HIV infection/AIDS, 48–49
Kartagener's (immotile cilia) syndrome, male infertility and, 564, 566
Karyotype, parental, Down's syndrome risk and, 20, 21t
Kennedy's disease, 150
Keratin filaments, 167
Keratinocyte growth factor, in benign prostatic hyperplasia, 571–572
Keratinocytes, 166–167, 166f, 167f, 169f
in erythema multiforme, 175–176, 177f
in lichen planus, 173–174, 174f
Kernicterus, 339
Kernig's sign, in meningitis, 65
Keto acids, hepatic production of, 333
Ketoacidosis
alcoholic, liver dysfunction and, 338t
diabetic, 440, 445–447, 446f
Ketogenesis, in diabetic ketoacidosis, 445, 446, 446f
Ketone bodies
in diabetes, 440
interconversion of, in diabetic ketoacidosis, 446, 446f
Ketosis, in diabetes, 445
KFG. *See* Keratinocyte growth factor
Kidney stones. *See* Renal stones
Kidneys, **382–404**. *See also under Renal*
anatomy/histology/cell biology of, **382–385**, 383f, 384f, 385f
in blood pressure regulation, 385–386
in calcium metabolism, 386–387, 408, 409f
cancer of, 86t
catecholamines affecting, 284t
disorders of, **388–404**, 390t. *See also specific type*
adaptations to, 387
gastrointestinal manifestations of, 310t
hypertension and, 275
liver dysfunction and, 338t, 344, 344t, 350, 354
manifestations of altered function in, **388–390**
structure and function alterations in, 368, 390t
in erythropoiesis, 387
glucocorticoids affecting, 507t
liver dysfunction affecting, 338t, 350
normal, **382–388**
physiology of, **385–387**, 386t, 387t
regulation of, 387, 387t
transplantation of, gastrointestinal manifestations in, 310t
vitamin D synthesis in, 413–414, 413f

Killer cells, natural, 29
Kimmelstiel-Wilson nodules, 451, 451f
Kininogens, 266
Kinins
  in gout, 579
  vascular smooth muscle affected by, 265–266, 266f
Klinefelter's syndrome, spermatogenesis defects in, 563
Korotkoff sounds, 261, 262
Kugelberg-Welander disease, 150
Kupffer cells, 329, 330f, 337
Kussmaul breathing, in diabetic ketoacidosis, 446
Kussmaul's sign, 254, 255, 256f

Lactate dehydrogenase, in pernicious anemia, 114
Lactation, **539–541**, 542f
  prolactin in, 466, 540–541, 542f
Lactic acidosis, in acute pancreatitis, 370
Lactiferous ducts, 533f, 539, 540
Lactogen, placental (hPL/chorionic somatomammotropin), 537
  fuel homeostasis in pregnancy and, 539, 541f, 543
Lactulose, for altered ammonia metabolism, 342
Lacunar infarctions, 160
Lacunar state, 157
Lambert-Eaton myasthenic syndrome, 130f, 131
Lamina densa, 167–168, 169f
Lamina lucida, 167–168, 169f
Lamina propria, 294, 296f
Laminar flow
  in blood vessels, 260–261
  resistance and, 192
Lamotrigine, 156t
Langer-Gideon syndrome, 22t
Langerhans, islets of (pancreatic islets), 362, 432, 432t. *See also* Endocrine pancreas
  tumors of, **455–456**, 456t, **457**. *See also specific type*
Langerhans cells, 167
Language, 148–149
Laplace's law, 261
  in aortic regurgitation, 244
  in aortic stenosis, 242
Large intestine, 295f
  disorders of, common presentations of, 294t
Late phase response, in allergic airway disease, 37
Latent infection, 59
Lateral gaze center, 142
Lateral geniculate nuclei, 142, 143f, 144
Lateral spinothalamic tracts, 138f, 139, 139f

LATS (long-acting thyroid stimulator). *See* TSH receptor-stimulating antibody
Law of Laplace, 261
  in aortic regurgitation, 244
  in aortic stenosis, 242
LDH. *See* Lactate dehydrogenase
LDL. *See* Low-density lipoproteins
LDL receptor, on hepatocytes, 333–334, 342
Left shift, of granulocyte lineage, 102
Left ventricular heart failure, **234–239**, 235t, 236f, 237f, 238f
Legionella, pneumonia caused by, 66t
Leiden (factor V) mutation, 121, 122
Lemniscus
  medial, 138, 139f
  trigeminal, 139, 139f
Leptin
  in body weight control, 468–469, 468f
  in Cushing's syndrome, 514–515
  in obesity, 471
Lesch-Nyhan syndrome, renal stone formation and, 403t
Leukemias
  acute myelogenous/acute nonlymphocytic (AML/ANLL), **94–95**, 94t
  chromosomal translocations in, 93t
  chronic lymphocytic
    lymphocyte counts in, 107
    pathogens causing infection in, 56t
  classification of, 92f
Leukocytes (white blood cells), 101–102. *See also specific type*
  development of, 98, 99f
  disorders of, **106–107**, 107t, **115–117**. *See also specific type*
  normal values for, 101t
  polymorphonuclear. *See* Neutrophils
  suppression of in uremia, 397
Leukocytoclastic vasculitis, **180–182**, 180f, 181f
Leukocytosis, 106
Leukoencephalopathy, progressive multifocal, 48
Leukoplakia, hairy, in HIV infection/AIDS, 47
Leukospermia, 566, 567t
Leukostasis, 95
Leukotriene B4, in gout, 579, 579f
Leuprolide, for benign prostatic hyperplasia, 570, 570t
Levodopa, for Parkinson's disease, 152
Lewy bodies, 152
Leydig cell axis, in male reproductive function, 558, 560f
Leydig (interstitial) cells, 556, 557f
LH. *See* Luteinizing hormone
Li-Fraumeni syndrome, 81
Libido, loss of, 565
Lichen planus, **173–175**, 173f, 174f, 174t

Liddle's syndrome, hypertension and, 275
Ligand-gated ion channels, 125
Light chains, immunoglobulin, 32, 33f
Light reflex, pupillary, 145, 145f
Limiting plate, 329
Linkage analysis, in breast cancer, 88
Linkage disequilibrium, 4t
  in fragile X-associated mental retardation syndrome, 17
  in phenylketonuria, 25, 25f, 25t, 26
Lipase
  pancreatic, 364
    acute pancreatitis and, 367, 367f
  insufficiency of, 376–378
  serum levels of in acute pancreatitis, 369–370
Lipid A, in endotoxins, 74, 75f
Lipids
  accumulation of in foam cells, 269, 270f
  malabsorption of. *See* Steatorrhea
  metabolism of
    atherosclerosis and, 269–270, 271f
    in liver, 332t, 333–334, 333f, 335f, 436t
    insulin in, 435, 436t
    liver dysfunction and, 339, 342
Lipocytes, 329, 337
  in cirrhosis, 356, 356f
Lipogenesis, in liver, 436t
  insulin in, 435, 436t
Lipohyalinosis, in ischemic stroke, 160
Lipolysis, in diabetes, 445
Lipophilic substances, in hepatic drug metabolism and excretion, 335
Lipopolysaccharide, in sepsis, 74, 75f
Lipoproteins
  high-density, 269
  intermediate-density, 269
  low-density, 269
  metabolism of in liver, 333–334, 335f, 436t
    insulin in, 435, 436t
    liver dysfunction and, 339, 342
  thyroid hormones affecting, 485t
  very low density, 269
Listeria monocytogenes, meningitis caused by, 63, 63t
Lithium, hypothyroidism caused by, 491
  goiter and, 494, 495t
Lithostathines, in chronic pancreatitis, 373, 375
Liver, **327–361**. *See also under* Hepatic
  anatomy/histology/cell biology of, **328–332**, 329f, 331f
  blood supply of, **332**
  carbohydrate metabolism in, 332–333, 332t, 333f, 436t
  glucagon in, 436t, 437

insulin in, 435, 436*t*
liver dysfunction and, 339
carcinoid metastasis to, 90
catecholamines affecting, 284*t*, 288*t*
cirrhosis of. *See* Cirrhosis
diseases of, 327, 328*t*
   acute, 327
   cancer, 86*t*
      cirrhosis and, 360–361
      manifestations of, **339–344**
energy generation/substrate interconversion by, 332–334, 332*t*, 333*f*
   liver dysfunction and, 338*t*, 339
fatty, 338*t*, 339
   drugs causing, 343*t*
fibrosis of, in cirrhosis, 355–356, 356*f*
functional zonation of, 329, 330*f*
glucocorticoids affecting, 504, 507*t*
hepatitis-induced damage to, 347–348
hepatocyte dysfunction and, 331
lipid metabolism in, 332*t*, 333–334, 333*f*, 335*f*, 436*t*
   insulin in, 435, 436*t*
   liver dysfunction and, 339, 342
lobules of, 329, 330*f*
necrosis of
   in acute hepatitis, 349
   bridging, 349
   in chronic hepatitis, 352–354, 353*f*
   drugs causing, 343*t*
   massive, 349
   piecemeal (periportal hepatitis), 352, 353*f*
organization of, 329–330, 330*f*
physiology of, **332–337**, 332*t*
plasma protein synthesis/secretion by, 332*t*, 334, 336*t*
   liver dysfunction and, 338*t*, 339, 342
protection/clearance functions of, 332*t*, 337
   liver dysfunction and, 338*t*, 342–344
protein metabolism in, 332*t*, 333, 334, 334*f*, 336*t*
   liver dysfunction and, 338*t*, 339, 342
regeneration and, 331
regulation of fuel homeostasis in, 436*t*
   insulin in, 435, 436*t*
solubilizing/transport/storage functions of, 332*t*, 334–337
   liver dysfunction and, 338*t*, 339–342, 340*f*, 341*t*
structure and function of, **328–337**
vitamin D synthesis in, 413, 413*f*
Liver acinus, 329, 330*f*
"Liver function tests," 350
Lobules
   hepatic, 329, 330*f*
   pancreatic, 362–363, 363*f*

Locus (gene), 5
Long-acting thyroid stimulator. *See* TSH receptor-stimulating antibody
Loop of Henle, 385, 385*f*
   in renal regulation, 385
Loss-of-function (amorphic) mutation, 3*t*, 6
   dominant inheritance and, 7
   recessive inheritance and, 6–7, 7*t*
Low-density lipoproteins, 269
   metabolism of
      diabetes mellitus and, 453
      in liver, 333–334, 335*f*
      liver dysfunction and, 342
Low-grade lymphoma, 93
Low-resistance (distributive) shock, 278, 278*t*, **280**
   sepsis and, 76, 280
Lower esophageal (gastroesophageal) sphincter, 300, 301*t*
   in achalasia, 309
   in reflux esophagitis, 311, 311*f*
Lower motor neurons, 129, **129–131**, 129*f*, 130*f*
LPB. *See* LPS-binding protein
LPS. *See* Lipopolysaccharide
LPS-binding protein, in sepsis, 74, 74*f*
LT. *See* Heat-labile toxin
Luminal secretagogues, 307
Lung cancer, 86*t*
Lung capacities, 185
Lung infection
   defense mechanisms against, 66–68, 67*t*, 68*f*, 189, 189*t*
   in HIV infection/AIDS, 47
   pneumonia, **65–69**, 66*t*, 67*t*, 68*f*
Lung sounds, in emphysema, 207
Lung volumes, 185
   ventilation distribution and, 194, 194*f*
Lungs. *See also under* Pulmonary; Respiratory
   anatomy of, **184–190**
   catecholamines affecting, 284*t*
   components of, 184, 185*t*
   defense mechanisms of, 66–68, 67*t*, 68*f*, 189, 189*t*
   diseases of, **184–221**
      chronic, pneumonia and, 67, 67*t*
      obstructive, **200–207**
      restrictive, **208–210**
   distribution of airflow in, 193–194, 194*f*, 195*f*
   dynamic properties of (flow and resistance), 186–187, 186*f*, 187*f*, 191–192, 193*f*
   immune structure and function of, 189, 189*t*
   innervation of, 187, 188*f*, 188*t*
   normal, **184–200**
   physiology of, **190–200**

static properties of (compliance and elastic recoil), 190–191, 190*f*, 191*f*
   pathologic states and, 191, 192*f*
   vascular system of, 187, 188*f*, 189*f*
Lupus anticoagulant, in adrenocortical insufficiency, 519
Lupus erythematosus, systemic, **581–583**, 582*f*, 582*t*
   gastrointestinal manifestations of, 310*t*
Luteal phase, of ovarian cycle, 535
Luteinization inhibitor, ovarian production of, 530*t*
Luteinization stimulator, ovarian production of, 530*t*
Luteinizing hormone (LH), 464, 534
   changes in in menstrual cycle, 532*f*, 534–535
   deficiency of, in hypopituitarism, 474
   in male reproductive function, 558, 560, 560*f*
      infertility evaluation and, 566, 567*f*
      normal levels of in men, 560*t*
   ovarian response to, 534–535, 535*f*
   in polycystic ovary syndrome, 547, 548, 549, 549*f*
Luteinizing hormone receptor-binding inhibitor, ovarian production of, 530*t*
Lymph nodes, 30, 30*f*
Lymphangiectasia, histologic features of, 320*t*
Lymphatics, 260
   pulmonary, 187–189, 188*f*
Lymphocyte count
   abnormalities in, 106–107, 107*t*
   normal, 101*t*
Lymphocyte-mediated cytotoxicity, in inflammatory rheumatic diseases, 578
Lymphocyte-predominant meningitis (aseptic meningitis), 62
Lymphocytes, 29, 102. *See also* B lymphocytes; T lymphocytes
   disorders of, 106–107, 107*t*
   normal values for, 101*t*
Lymphocytic thyroiditis, 491
Lymphocytosis, 106–107, 107*t*
Lymphoma, **93–94**
   chromosomal translocations in, 93*t*
   intestinal, histologic features of, 320*t*
   non-Hodgkin's, in HIV infection/AIDS, 49, 93
   REAL (Revised European and American Lymphoma) classification of, 93, 93*t*
Lymphopenia, 107, 107*t*
Lysosomal enzymes, in acute pancreatitis, 366
Lysylbradykinin, vascular smooth muscle affected by, 265–266, 266*f*

M-CSF. *See* **Macrophage colony-stimulating factor**
MAC. *See Mycobacterium, avium-intracellulare*
Macroadenomas, pituitary, 471
   Cushing's disease caused by, 509
   mass effects caused by, 471, 472f, 473
Macrocytic anemia, 105, 105t, 106f
   liver dysfunction and, 342
α_2-Macroglobulin, 336t
   hepatic synthesis of, 336t
Macronodular cirrhosis, 357
Macronodular hyperplasia, adrenal, 511, 513
Macro-ovalocytes, in pernicious anemia, 113
Macrophage colony-stimulating factor (M-CSF)
   in atherosclerosis, 269, 270f
   in hematopoiesis, 99f, 100t
Macrophages, 29
   development of, 98, 99f
   in gout, 579
   in inflammatory rheumatic diseases, **578**
Macrosomia, gestational diabetes and, 543
Macrovascular disease, in diabetes mellitus, 448, 448t, 452–453, 453f
Macula densa, 384f
   in regulation of blood pressure, 385–386
   in regulation of glomerular filtration, 387
Macules, 169
Magnesium depletion, in hypocalcemia, 422, 423, 424t
   laboratory findings in, 423, 424t
Major basic protein, in allergic airway disease, 37
Major histocompatibility complex, 32. *See also under MHC*
   diabetes mellitus and, 442
Malabsorption, 293
   bile secretion disorders and, 339
   diarrhea and, 318, 318t
   fat, in pancreatic insufficiency, 376, 377, 377–378, 377t
   signs and symptoms and, 321t
   small intestinal diseases causing, histologic features of, 320t
Maldigestion, pancreatic insufficiency and, 376–378, 376t, 377t
Male reproductive tract, **556–575**
   accessory glands of, 556, 557f, 558f
   anatomy and histology of, **556**, 557f, 558f
   disorders of, **562–574**
   normal, **556–561**
   physiology of, **557–561**, 559f, 560f, 560t, 561f. *See also* Androgens
   sexual differentiation and, 531–533, 534f
   disorders associated with, 545
Male sexual dysfunction
   in Cushing's syndrome, 516
   in diabetes mellitus, 454
   infertility and, 565
Malignancies. *See* Cancer
Malignant hypertension, 274
Malignant otitis externa, in diabetes mellitus, 454
Malignant teratomas, testicular, 91
Masculinization, adrenal androgen excess and, 509, 527
Mass effects, in pituitary adenoma, 471, 472f, 473
Maternal age, Down's syndrome frequency and, 18, 18f, 19–20
Maternal phenylketonuria, 23
Maturation arrest, 563
Mature teratomas, testicular, 91
Maturity-onset diabetes of the young (MODY), 444
MC-4 receptor, in body weight control, 469
MCC gene, 82t
MCV. *See* Mean corpuscular volume
MDR-1 protein/gene product, 83
   in colon carcinoma, 87–88
Mean corpuscular volume
   in anemia, 105, 105t
   normal, 101t, 105
Media, 258, 259f
Medial lemniscus, 138, 139f
   sensory loss caused by lesions of, 142
Medial longitudinal fasciculus, 142
Mediators. *See* Inflammatory mediators
Medulla
   adrenal. *See* Adrenal medulla
   lymph node, 30, 30f
   sensory loss caused by lesions of, 142
Megakaryocytes, 98–100, 99f, 102
   in drug-associated immune thrombocytopenia, 119
Megaloblastic anemia, 105
   cell line changes in, 113, 114f
   pernicious anemia as, 111
Megaloblastic hematopoiesis, 114f
Meissner nerve plexus (submucosal nerve plexus), 294, 296f, 299
Melanocortin receptors, in body weight control, 469
Melanocytes, 167, 168f
Melena, 294t
   in iron deficiency anemia, 111
Membrane attack complex, 54, 55f
Membrane potential, 125
Membrane proteins, extracellular, ovarian production of, 530t
Membranoproliferative glomerulonephritis, 401t
Membranous glomerulonephritis, 400
Membranous nephropathy, 401t
Memory, 149
   immunologic, 31, 32
Memory cells, 31
MEN. *See* Multiple endocrine neoplasia
MEN1 gene, 417–418
Menarche, 533
Mendelian conditions, 2
Menin, parathyroid tumor formation and, 417–418
Meningismus, in meningitis, 62
Meningitis, **62–65**, 63t, 64f
   cryptococcal, in HIV infection/AIDS, 48
Menopause, **541–542**
   amenorrhea and, 545, 546t
Menorrhagia, 545
   in hypothyroidism, 494
Menstrual cramps. *See* Dysmenorrhea
Menstrual cycle (menstruation/menstrual bleeding), 529, 532f, **533–536**, 534f, 535f
   altered/disorders of, 529, **545–552**
   in Cushing's disease, 510f, 516
   in hyperthyroidism, 490
   in hypothyroidism, 494
   cessation of (menopause), **541–542**
   iron deficiency anemia and, 109
Mental retardation
   in Down's syndrome, 18, 19
   fragile X-associated, 2, 7t, **14–17**
   in hypothyroidism, 492
   in phenylketonuria, 23
Mental status changes
   in Cushing's syndrome., 510f, 516
   in liver dysfunction (hepatic encephalopathy), 338, 338t, 339, 342–344, 350, 359–360, 360t
Mesangium, 382, 383, 384f
Mesencephalic nuclei of trigeminal nerve, 139
Mesencephalic reticular nuclei, 136
Mesenchymal neoplasia, **89–91**, 89t. *See also specific type*
Metabolic acidosis
   in acute pancreatitis, 370
   in chronic renal failure, 396
Metabolic alkalosis, in pheochromocytoma, 290
Metabolism
   catecholamines affecting, 285
   disorders of
     in chronic renal failure, 398
     gastrointestinal manifestations of, 310t
   in hyperthyroidism, 489
   in hypothyroidism, 493

Metanephrine, 283
  in pheochromocytoma, 290
Metaplasia, 85
Metastatic disease, 84, 84f, 85
  adrenal, adrenocortical insufficiency caused by, 519
Methimazole, hypothyroidism caused by, 491
  goiter and, 494, 495t
Methionine, deficiency of, demyelination and, 113, 113f
3-Methoxy-4-hydroxymandelic acid (vanillylmandelic acid/VMA), 283
N-Methyl-D-aspartate (NMDA) receptor-gated channels, in seizure pathogenesis, 155–156
Methylation, 16–17
  DNA, in fragile X-associated mental retardation syndrome, 15f, 16
1-Methyl-4-phenyl-1,2,3,6-tetrahydropyridine (MPTP), parkinsonism caused by, 152, 152f
Metrorrhagia, 545
MHC (major histocompatibility complex), 32
  diabetes mellitus and, 442
MHC class I molecules, 32
  in psoriasis, 170, 171
MHC class II molecules, 32
  in diabetes mellitus, 442
MHC restriction, 32
Microadenomas, pituitary, 471
  Cushing's disease caused by, 509
  hormonal effects of, 471, 472
Microalbuminuria, in diabetes mellitus, 452, 452f
Microaneurysms, in diabetic retinopathy, 449, 451f
Microbes. See Normal microbial flora; Pathogens
Microcytic anemia, 105, 105t, 106f
  iron deficiency, 109
Microglia, 127f, 128
Micronodular cirrhosis, 357
Micronodular hyperplasia, adrenal, 510–511, 513
Microsomal P450, altered hormone clearance in liver dysfunction and, 344
Microvascular disease, in diabetes mellitus, 448, 448–450, 448t, 449f, 450f
Microvilli, intestinal, 294, 305
Middle ear, anatomy of, 145–146
Migrating motor complex, 306
Milk synthesis and secretion, 540–541, 542f
  prolactin affecting, 466, 540–541, 542f
Miller-Dieker syndrome, 22t

Mineral metabolism, in chronic renal failure, 396–397, 396f
Mineralization, bone, 411
  defects in (osteomalacia), **429–430**, 429t
Mineralocorticoids, **504–509**. See also Aldosterone
  deficiency of, 509, **526**. See also Hypoaldosteronism
  effects of, 508f, 509
  excess of, 509, **522–526**. See also Conn's syndrome; Hyperaldosteronism
    apparent, 276, 277f
    clinical consequences of, 524–525
    in diabetes insipidus, 478–479
    hypertension and, 275–276, 277f, 525
  mechanism of action of, 508, 508f
  regulation of, 506–508, 507f
  synthesis/protein binding/metabolism of, 503f, 504–505
  zona glomerulosa secreting, 500, 502f
Minimal change disease, 399, 401t
Minute ventilation, exercise affecting, control of breathing and, 200
MIT. See Monoiodotyrosine
Mitral valve, 222, 224f
  prolapse of, mitral regurgitation caused by, 247–249
  regurgitation/insufficiency of, **247–251**, 249t, 250f
  stenosis of, **247**, 248f, 249t
MODY. See Maturity-onset diabetes of the young
Molar pregnancies, 544
Molecular mimicry, in diabetes mellitus, 442
Monocyte-macrophage line, in hematopoiesis, 98, 99f
Monocytes, 29, 102
  development of, 98, 99f
  normal values for, 101t
Monoiodotyrosine (MIT), 483–484, 483f
Mononeuropathy, 141
  in diabetes mellitus, 454
  multiplex, 141
    in diabetes mellitus, 454
Monosodium urate crystals, in gout, 579, 579f
Monosomy, 4t
Moon facies, in Cushing's syndrome, 510f, 514
Moraxella catarrhalis, pneumonia caused by, 66t
Mosaicism, 2, 4t, 5f
  in Down's syndrome, 21
  gonadal, in osteogenesis imperfecta, 13, 13f
  ovarian failure/amenorrhea in, 547
  somatic, in fragile X-associated mental retardation syndrome, 16

Motilin, 298t, 306
Motility, gastrointestinal, 293, 296–297
  colonic, 307
  disorders of, **308**
    in diabetic autonomic neuropathy, 454
    diarrhea and, 318t
    in hyperthyroidism, 490
    in hypothyroidism, 493
  esophageal, 300–301, 301t
  gastric, 302
  oropharyngeal, 300–301
  small intestinal, 306
Motor cortex, 128, 131–132, 132f
Motor neurons, 125f, 129f
  alpha, 129, 129f
  cortical, 131, 132f
  diseases associated with lesions of, **149–151**. See also specific type
  gamma, 129, 130f
  lower, 120f, 129, **129–131**, 129f
  upper, 129, **131–134**, 132f, 133f
Motor system, **129–137**
  basal ganglia, **136–137**, 136f, 137f
  cerebellum, **134–136**, 134f, 135f
  lower motor neurons and skeletal muscles, 129, **129–131**, 129f, 130f
  upper motor neurons, 129, **131–134**, 132f, 133f
Motor unit, 129, 129f
Mouth, 295f
Movement disorders, 136–137
MPTP (1-methyl-4-phenyl-1,2,3,6-tetrahydropyridine), parkinsonism caused by, 152, 152f
Mucin, gastrointestinal secretion of, 298t, 307
Mucocutaneous candidiasis, chronic, 40t
Mucormycosis, in diabetes mellitus, 454
Mucous membranes, as defense against infection, 53
Mucoviscidosis. See Cystic fibrosis
Mucus, hypersecretion of, in allergic rhinitis, 37–38
Müllerian-inhibiting substance, 531
  ovarian production of, 530t
Müller's sign, in aortic regurgitation, 245
Multifactorial inheritance, 8
Multi-infarct dementia, 157
Multinodular goiter, 495, 495f
Multiple endocrine neoplasia (MEN), 416, 416t
  hyperparathyroidism in, 416, 416t
  islet cell tumors in, 456t
  type 1, 416, 416t
    gene responsible for, 417–418
    insulinoma in, 455, 456t
  type 2, oncogene inheritance and, 80

Multiple endocrine neoplasia (*cont.*)
   type 2a (Sipple's syndrome), 416, 416*t*
      medullary carcinoma of thyroid in, 424, 425
      pheochromocytoma in, 286, 286*t*
   type 2b, 416, 416*t*
      medullary carcinoma of thyroid in, 424, 425
      pheochromocytoma in, 286, 286*t*
Multiple myeloma, pathogens causing infection in, 56*t*
Multiple organ failure, in septic shock, 76*f*, 77
Multiple system atrophy, 291
Mumps orchitis, infertility and, 564–565
Murmurs
   heart. *See* Heart murmurs
   vascular, 261
Muscles
   cardiac, 224–225, 226*f*
      contraction of, 229, 231*f*, 232*f*
   disorders of
      in Cushing's syndrome, 510*f*, 514
      in hyperthyroidism, 489
      in hypothyroidism, 492–493
   extraocular, in control of eye movements, 142, 144*f*
   glucocorticoids affecting, 504, 507*t*
   regulation of fuel homeostasis in, 436*t*
      insulin in, 435, 436*t*
   of respiration, control of, 198–200. *See also* Breathing, control of
   skeletal
      catecholamines affecting, 284*t*
      lower motor neurons and, **129–131**
   smooth
      bronchial, catecholamines affecting, 284*t*
      genitourinary, catecholamines affecting, 284*t*
      intestinal
         catecholamines affecting, 284*t*
         contraction of, 296–297. *See also* Gastrointestinal motility
      prostate gland, alpha-adrenergic receptors in, benign prostatic hyperplasia and, 572
      vascular
         catecholamines affecting, 284*t*
         hormones affecting, 265–266
   thyroid hormones affecting, 485*t*
Muscular dystrophy, Duchenne's, 7*t*
Muscularis externa, 294, 296*f*
Muscularis mucosae, 294, 296*f*
Mutation, 2, 5, 5*f*, **6–8**. *See also specific type*
   amorphic (loss-of-function), 3*t*, 6
      dominant inheritance and, 7
      recessive inheritance and, 6–7, 7*t*
   antimorphic (dominant negative), 3*t*, 7–8

   frameshift, tumor suppressor gene function loss caused by, 80
   hypermorphic, 4*t*, 6
   hypomorphic, 4*t*, 6
   mechanisms of, **6–8**
   neomorphic, 4*t*, 6
   point
      in oncogene activation, 80
      tumor suppressor gene function loss caused by, 80
   rate of, in fragile X-associated mental retardation syndrome, 17
Myasthenia gravis, 130*f*, 131, **153–154**, 153*f*
Myasthenic syndrome, Lambert-Eaton, 130*f*, 131
myb oncogene, 81*t*
myc oncogene, 81*t*
Mycobacterium
   avium-intracellulare, infection in HIV/infection caused by, 47
   pneumoniae, pneumonia caused by, 66*t*
   tuberculosis, infection in HIV/infection caused by, 47
Myelin, methionine and, 113, 113*f*
Myelin sheath, formation of, 128, 128*f*
Myelination, 128, 128*f*
Myelinolysis, central pontine, 479
Myelodysplastic (preleukemic) syndrome, 94, 95
Myeloma, pathogens causing infection in, 56*t*
Myelomonocytic cells. *See also* Macrophages; Neutrophils
   in inflammatory rheumatic diseases, **578**
Myeloperoxidase
   deficiency of, 56
   in neutrophils, 101
Myelopoiesis, 98, 99*f*
Myeloproliferative disorder, polycythemia as, 106
Myenteric nerve plexus (Auerbach's nerve plexus), 294–296, 296*f*, 299
Myocardial depression, in septic shock, 76–77
Myocardial infarction, 251, 253, 271
Myocardial ischemia
   in coronary artery disease, 251–252, 251*t*
   diastolic dysfunction caused by, 237
Myocardium. *See also* Heart
   catecholamines affecting, 284*t*
Myoclonic epilepsy, 155
Myoclonic seizures, 155
Myocytes, cardiac, 224–225, 226*f*
   contraction of, 229, 231*f*, 232*f*
Myofibrils, cardiac, 224–225, 226*f*
Myoglobin, 109
Myopathy, thyrotoxic, 489

Myosin, in cardiac sarcomeres, 226*f*
Myotactic stretch reflex, 129, 130*f*
Myotonic dystrophy, gastrointestinal manifestations of, 310*t*
Myxedema, 486, 493, 493*t*, 494*f*. *See also* Hypothyroidism
   pretibial, 490–491
Myxedema coma, 494
Myxedema madness, 492

N-methyl-D-aspartate (NMDA) receptor-gated channels, in seizure pathogenesis, 155–156
N-ras oncogene, in hematologic neoplasia, 92
Na^+-H^+ exchange, facilitation of, hypertension and, 278
Na^+-K^+ ATPase (sodium-potassium pump), 297
   in intestinal secretion, 307
   in signal propagation, 124
NADPH oxidase, 101
Nafarelin, for benign prostatic hyperplasia, 570, 570*t*
NANC. *See* Nonadrenergic, noncholinergic (NANC) system
Nasal eosinophilia, in allergic airway disease, 38–39
Nasal stuffiness/congestion, in allergic rhinitis, 38
Natriuretic hormones
   hypertension and, 277
   vascular smooth muscle affected by, 266
Natural killer cells, 29
Nausea
   in acute pancreatitis, 368
   gastrointestinal disease presenting with, 293, 294*t*
   in myocardial infarction, 253
Necrolysis, toxic epidermal, 177, 177*f*
Necrolytic migratory erythema, in glucagonoma, 457
Necrosis-fibrosis sequence, in chronic pancreatitis, 374–375, 374*f*
Necrotizing papillitis, in diabetes mellitus, 454
Neisseria meningitidis, meningitis caused by, 63, 63*t*, 64
Nelson's syndrome, 473, 515
Neomorphic mutation, 4*t*, 6
Neonatal severe primary hyperparathyroidism, 419
Neoplasia. *See* Cancer
Neovascularization, in diabetic retinopathy, 450
Nephritic disorders, 388, 389*f*
Nephritis
   acute, clinical and laboratory findings in, 391*t*
   interstitial, in acute renal failure, 392*t*

Nephrogenic diabetes insipidus, 476, 476t, 477
Nephrolithiasis (renal stones), **401–404**, 402t, 403t
  in acute renal failure, 390, 391t
  clinical and laboratory findings in, 391t
  in Cushing's syndrome, 515
  in hyperparathyroidism, 402, 403t, 418
  in pancreatic insufficiency, 378
Nephrons, 382, 384f, 385f
  number of, hypertension and, 386
Nephropathy
  diabetic, 394, 395t, 448, 450–452, 451f, 452f
  hypokalemic, in mineralocorticoid excess, 525
  IgA, 399
  membranous, 401t
Nephrotic disorders, 388, 389f
Nephrotic syndrome, **398–401**, 401t
  clinical and laboratory findings in, 391t, 398, 401, 401t
Nephrotoxic drugs, acute renal failure caused by, 390
Nernst equation, 124–125
Nerve growth factor, ovarian production of, 530t
Nerve impulse, conduction of, 125, 126f
Nervous system, **124–165**
  catecholamines affecting, 284t
  cell biology of, **124–128**
  disorders of, **149–164**. See also specific type
    gastrointestinal manifestations of, 310t
    hypertension and, 277–278
  enteric, 296–297
  functional anatomy of
    hearing/balance and, **145–146**
    vision/control of eye movements and, **142–145**
  functional neuroanatomy of, **129–149**
    consciousness/arousal/cognition and, **147–149**
    motor system and, **129–137**
    somatosensory system and, **137–142**
  in gastrointestinal function regulation, 296–297, 299, 299f
  histology of, **124–128**
  hypertension and, 277–278
  mitral stenosis and, 247
  normal structure and function of, **124–128**
  pulmonary, 187, 188f, 188t
  thyroid hormones affecting, 485t
  in vascular function regulation, 266–268, 266t, 267f, 268f
Neural failure, sympathetic (primary autonomic failure), 285, 290–291

Neuritic plaques, in Alzheimer's disease, 157, 157f
Neuroanatomy, functional, **129–149**
  consciousness/arousal/cognition and, **147–149**
  hearing/balance and, **145–146**
  motor system and, **129–137**
  somatosensory system and, **137–142**
  vision/control of eye movements and, **142–145**
Neurocrines, gastrointestinal secretion of, 298t
Neuroendocrine axis, 459
  female reproductive, 533–534, 534f. See also Menstrual cycle
  disorders of, 542–543, 547–549, 548t, 549t
  infertility and, 552–553
  male reproductive, 558–560, 560f
  infertility and, 562, 563–564
  physiology of, **467–468**
  reproductive system, gonadotropins in regulation of, 464
Neuroendocrine neoplasia, **89–91**, 89t. See also specific type
Neurofibrillary tangles
  in Alzheimer's disease, 157f
  in Down's syndrome, 19
Neurofibromas, 91
Neurofibromatosis, 7t, 91
  type I (Recklinghausen's disease), pheochromocytoma in, 286, 286t
Neurofibrosarcomas, 91
Neurofilament protein dysfunction, in amyotrophic lateral sclerosis, 151
Neurogenic bladder, in diabetic autonomic neuropathy, 454
Neurogenic shock, 280
Neuroglycopenic hypoglycemia, 447, 447t
  insulinoma causing, 455
Neurologic disorders, **149–164**. See also specific type
  gastrointestinal manifestations of, 310t
  hypertension and, 277–278
Neuromuscular disorders, in chronic renal failure, 397
Neuromuscular junction, 129–131, 130f
Neuromuscular transmission, disorders of, 130f, 131
  myasthenia gravis, 130f, 131, **153–154**, 153f
Neuronal pathways, in inflammation, 30
Neurons, 124–127, 125f. See also Motor neurons
  sensory, 138
Neuropathic pain, 140
Neuropathies
  in chronic renal failure, 397
  diabetic, 448, 453–454, 454t
    autonomic, 291, 448, 454, 454t

hypoglycemia and, 448
in HIV infection/AIDS, 48
Neuropeptide Y
  in body weight control, 468f, 469
  in obesity, 471
  ovarian production of, 530t
Neuropeptides, in inflammation, 30
Neurotoxins, 58
  gastroenteritis caused by, 69–70
Neurotransmitters, 125, 125–127
Neurotropism, bacterial, pathogenetic sequence of, 63–64, 63t, 64f
Neutropenia, 55, 106, 107t, 115
  cyclic, 106, **115–117**
Neutrophil count
  abnormalities in, 106, 107t
  in neutropenia, 107t, 115–116, 116f
  normal, 101t
Neutrophil-predominant meningitis, 62
Neutrophilia, 107t
Neutrophilic pleocytosis, in meningitis, 62, 64
Neutrophils (polymorphonuclear leukocytes), 29, 54–56, 101–102
  deficiency/defects in, 55–56
  development of, 98, 99f
  disorders of, 106, 107t
  in gout, 579, 579f
  in inflammatory rheumatic diseases, **578**
  normal values for, 101t
  phagocytosis by, 54–56
NF-1 gene, 82t
  in sarcomas, 91
NF-2 gene, 82t
Niacin, deficiency of, gastrointestinal manifestations of, 310t
Night vision, poor, in retinitis pigmentosa, 143
Nitric oxide
  in cirrhosis and hepatorenal syndrome, 354
  hypertension and, 278
  in vascular function regulation, 264–265, 265f
Nitric oxide synthase, 264, 265f
Nitroprusside, hypothyroidism caused by, goiter and, 494, 495t
NK cells. See Natural killer cells
nm23 gene, 82t
  in breast cancer, 89
NMDA (N-methyl-D-aspartate) receptor-gated channels, in seizure pathogenesis, 155–156
NO. See Nitric oxide
Nocturia
  in diabetes insipidus, 476
  in diabetes mellitus, 445
  in left ventricular failure, 238
Nocturnal hypoglycemia, 447, 447t
Nodes of Ranvier, 128, 128f
Nodule, 169

Non-A/non-B hepatitis. *See* Hepatitis C virus; Hepatitis E virus
Non-Hodgkin's lymphoma. *See also* Lymphoma
  in HIV infection/AIDS, 49, 93
Nonadrenergic, noncholinergic (NANC) system, lungs supplied by, 187
Nonbacterial thrombotic endocarditis, 59, 61*f*
Noncardiogenic pulmonary edema, 212, 213, 214
Nondisjunction, 4*t*
  in Down's syndrome, 18, 19, 20*f*
Nonproliferative retinopathy, in diabetes, 449–450
Nonsteroidal anti-inflammatory drugs (NSAIDs)
  acute renal failure caused by, 390
  gastric ulcers and, 313
Nontropical (celiac) sprue, histologic features of, 320*t*
Noradrenergic stimulation, in vascular function regulation, 266–268, 266*t*, 267*f*, 268*f*
Norepinephrine. *See also* Catecholamines
  effects of, 284*t*, 285
  formation/secretion/metabolism of, 282–283, 283*f*
  mechanism of action of, 283–285, 284*t*
  normal values for, 283
  pheochromocytoma releasing, 287
Normal microbial flora, **52–53**, 52*t*
Normetanephrine, 283
Normocytic anemia, 105*t*, 106*f*
NOS. *See* Nitric oxide synthase
Nosocomial organisms, 52
NPY. *See* Neuropeptide Y
NSAIDs. *See* Nonsteroidal anti-inflammatory drugs
Nuclei of Edinger-Westphal, 142
Nucleus of the spinal tract of cranial nerve V, 139
"Null cells," 29
Nystagmus, jerk, 145, 146

O side chain, in endotoxins, 74, 75*f*
Obesity, **469–471**
  chronic anovulation and, 548*t*
  in Cushing's syndrome, 510*f*, 514–515
  disorders associated with, 469, 469*t*, 470*f*
  genetics of, 471
  in type II diabetes mellitus, 441, 444, 470
  visceral (central) vs. subcutaneous (peripheral), 470–471
Obligate pathogen, 52*t*
Oblique muscles, 142, 144*f*
Obstructive lung disease, **200–207**
Obstructive shock, 278, 278*t*, **281**
Octreotide, 437

Ocular dominance columns, 144
Oculomotor nerve (cranial nerve III), in control of eye movements, 142
Oculosympathetic pathways, 142–143, 144*f*
Oddi, sphincter of, 305, 305*f*
ODF. *See* Osteoclast differentiation factor
ODF receptor, 411
Odynophagia, gastrointestinal disease presenting with, 293
$1,25\text{-}(OH)_2D$, 413–414
  in age-related bone loss, 427
  in calcium and phosphate homeostasis, 408–410, 409*f*, 414
  in hypoparathyroidism, 422
$25\text{-}(OH)D$, 413, 413*f*, 414
  in hypocalcemia, 423, 424*t*
  testing for in vitamin D deficiency, 413
Oil embolism, 215*t*
Oligodendrocytes, 127*f*, 128, 128*f*
Oligospermia, 563, 566
  varicocele causing, 564
Olivopontocerebellar degeneration, sporadic, 291
Oncogenes, 80, **80–82**, 81*t*
  activation of, 80
  inheritance of, 80
Oocyte meiosis inhibitor, ovarian production of, 530*t*
Oocytes, 529
  maturation of, 534, 535*f*
Opening snap, in mitral stenosis, 247, 248*f*
Ophthalmopathy, Graves,' 490, 490*f*
Opportunistic infections, 52
  in HIV infection/AIDS, 48
  intestinal, histologic features of, 320*t*
Opsonins, 54
Opsonization, 33
Optic chiasm, 142, 143*f*
  lesions affecting, 144–145
Optic radiations, 142, 143*f*
Optic tracts, 142, 143*f*
Oral candidiasis (thrush), in HIV infection/AIDS, 47
Oral contraceptives, 537
Orchidometry, in infertility evaluation, 566
Orchiopexy, for cryptorchism, 564
Orchitis, mumps, infertility and, 564–565
Orexins, in body weight control, 469
Organ failure, in septic shock, 76*f*, 77
Orgasm, loss of, 565
Oropharyngeal motility, 300–301
Oropharynx, **300–301**
Orosomucoid, 336*t*
Orthopnea
  in left ventricular failure, 235, 237–238
  in mitral regurgitation, 247, 249
  in mitral stenosis, 247

Orthostatic hypotension, in diabetic autonomic neuropathy, 454
Ortner's syndrome, 247
Osmotic diarrhea, 318–319, 318*t*
Osmotic diuresis, diabetes insipidus differentiated from, 477
Osteoblasts, 411
  in bone remodeling, 412, 412*f*
  $1,25\text{-}(OH)_2D$ affecting, 414
Osteocalcin, 411
Osteoclast differentiation factor, 411, 412
Osteoclasts, 411, 411*f*
  in bone remodeling, 412*f*
  $1,25\text{-}(OH)_2D$ affecting, 414
Osteocytes, 411
Osteodystrophy, Albright's hereditary, 423
Osteogenesis imperfecta, 2, 7*t*, **9–13**
  penetrance and expressivity in, 6*f*
  subtypes of, 9–10, 9*t*
Osteomalacia, **429–430**, 429*t*
Osteopenia, in hyperparathyroidism, 418
Osteoporosis, **425–429**, 426*f*, 426*t*, 427*t*, 428*f*, 529, 542
  amenorrhea/estrogen deficiency and, 551
  in Cushing's syndrome, 510*f*, 515
Osteosarcoma, 91
Osteosclerosis, in hyperparathyroidism, 418
Otitis externa, malignant, in diabetes mellitus, 454
Otitis media, serous, 39
Ouabain
  hypertension and, 277
  vascular smooth muscle affected by, 266
Ovarian cancer, 86*t*
Ovarian failure
  amenorrhea caused by, 545, 546–550, 546*t*, 551
  chronic anovulation and, 548*t*
  infertility caused by, 552–553
  premature, 546*t*, 547
Ovarian follicles, 529
  changes in in menstrual cycle, 532*f*, 534–535, 535*f*
Ovaries, 529, 531*f*
  changes in in menstrual cycle, 532*f*, 534–535, 535*f*
  disorders of, **542**
    amenorrhea caused by, 545, 546–550, 546*t*
    infertility caused by, 552–553
  endocrine and paracrine products of, 530*t*
  polycystic, 546*t*, 547–549, 548*t*, 549*f*
  steroid hormones produced by, 532*f*, 534–535, 536
    gonadotropins affecting, 464
Overshooting (dysmetria), 136

Ovulation, 532f, 534, 535f, 536f
  disorders of, infertility and, 552–553
Oxalate, in renal stones, 402
Oxidants, in emphysema, 205, 206f
Oxidative deamination, in liver, 332t, 333, 334f
Oxidative stress, in chronic pancreatitis, 375
Oximetry, in pulmonary embolism, 217, 217f
Oxygen, partial pressure of
  in control of breathing, 198–200, 199f, 200f
  hypoxic pulmonary vasoconstriction and, 194
  in pulmonary embolism, 217, 217f
  ventilation/perfusion matching and, 196, 196f
Oxygen-carrying capacity, decreased
  in iron deficiency anemia, 110–111
  in pernicious anemia, 115
Oxygen-hemoglobin dissociation curve, 196–197, 197f
Oxyphil cells, parathyroid, 405
Oxytocin, 467
  in breast feeding, 467, 540, 542f
  ovarian production of, 530t

p16 gene, in pancreatic carcinoma, 379
p53 gene, 81, 82t
  in breast cancer, 88
  in hematologic neoplasia, 92
  in Li-Fraumeni syndrome, 80
  in pancreatic carcinoma, 379
  in sarcomas, 91
P450
  altered hormone clearance in liver dysfunction and, 344
  in chronic pancreatitis, 375
P450c21, antibodies to, in adrenocortical insufficiency, 518
P450-scc, in autoimmune polyendocrine syndrome, 518
P wave, of electrocardiogram, 224, 225f
Pacemaker cells, cardiac, 222–224, 225f
  action potential of, 229–231
$PaCO_2$ (partial pressure of carbon dioxide in arterial blood)
  in asthma, 203
  in control of breathing, 198–200, 199f, 200f
  in idiopathic pulmonary fibrosis, 210, 211f
  in pulmonary embolism, 217
  ventilation/perfusion matching and, 196
PAF. *See* Platelet-activating factor
Pain
  abdominal
    in acute pancreatitis, 368
    in chronic pancreatitis, 375
    gastrointestinal disease presenting with, 293, 294t
    in right ventricular failure, 240
  chest. *See also* Angina pectoris
    in aortic stenosis, 241, 242
    in coronary artery disease, 251, 253
    gastrointestinal disease presenting with, 293, 294t
    in left ventricular failure, 238
    in mitral regurgitation, 247
    in pericarditis, **254**
    in pulmonary embolism, 218
  flank, in renal stones, 401, 402–404
  leg, in pulmonary embolism, 218
  neuropathic, 140
  sensation of, 139, 139–140, 139f
    Aδ fibers in, 137, 139–140
    C fibers in, 139–140
    circuits modulating, 140, 140f
Pain modulating circuits, 140, 140f
Palatal clicking, in allergic rhinitis, 38
Palmar crease, transverse, in Down's syndrome, 19
Palpable purpura, in leukocytoclastic vasculitis, 180, 180f
Palpitations
  in mitral regurgitation, 247, 249
  in mitral stenosis, 247
Panacinar emphysema, 206
Pancreas
  divisum, 372
  endocrine, 362, **432–458**
    anatomy and histology of, **432**, 432t, 433f
    catecholamines affecting, 284t, 288t
    disorders of, **439–457**. *See also* specific type and Diabetes mellitus
    normal, **432–439**
    physiology of, **433–439**
      regulation of fuel homeostasis and, 436t
    tumors of, **455–456**, 456t, **457**. *See also specific type*
  exocrine, **362–381**
    anatomy of, **362**, 363f
    disorders of, **364–380**. *See also specific type*
    histology of, **362–363**, 363f
    normal, **362–364**
    physiology of, **363–364**. *See also* Pancreatic juice
Pancreatic abscesses, 370–371
Pancreatic ascites, 366, 371
Pancreatic calculi, in chronic pancreatitis, 373, 374, 374f, 375
Pancreatic carcinoma, 86t, **378–380**, 379t
  chronic pancreatitis and, 376, 378
Pancreatic ducts, 362, 363f
  accessory (duct of Santorini), 362, 363f
  obstruction of, in chronic pancreatitis, 372, 375, 376
Pancreatic insufficiency, **376–378**, 376t, 377t
Pancreatic islets (islets of Langerhans), 362, 432, 432t. *See also* Pancreas, endocrine
  tumors of, **455–456**, 456t, **457**. *See also specific type*
Pancreatic juice, 362
  in acute pancreatitis, 366–367, 367f, 368f
  CCK-secretin test of, 375, 376
  composition of, 363–364
  digestive functions of, 364
  regulation of secretion of, 364
Pancreatic necrosis, infected, 370–371
Pancreatic phlegmon, 370
Pancreatic polypeptide, 298t, **438**
  in chronic pancreatitis, 375
  F cells (PP cells) secreting, 432, 432t, 438
Pancreatic pseudocysts
  in acute pancreatitis, 370, 371, 371f
  in chronic pancreatitis, 373, 376
Pancreatic stone proteins. *See* Lithostathines
Pancreatic tail syndrome, 366
Pancreatitis
  acute, **364–371**, 365t, 367f, 368f, 368t, 369f, 372t
    in chronic pancreatitis pathogenesis, 374–375, 374f
  chronic, **372–376**, 372t, 373t, 374f, 375t
    pancreatic carcinoma and, 376, 378
    pancreatic insufficiency caused by, 376, 377
    hereditary, 373
    tropical, 372–373
Pancreolauryl test, in pancreatic insufficiency, 378
Paneth cells, 305–306
Panhypopituitarism, 466, **473–475**, 475t
  hypoaldosteronism and, 526
Panniculitis, 170t, 171f
PaO_2 (partial pressure of oxygen in arterial blood)
  in control of breathing, 198–200, 199f, 200f
  in pulmonary embolism, 217, 217f
  ventilation/perfusion matching and, 196
Papanicolaou smear, 529, 551
Papillary carcinoma, of thyroid, 496
Papillitis, necrotizing, in diabetes mellitus, 454
Papillomavirus, human, 80
  in cancer of the cervix, 80, 551
Papules, 169

Paracrines
  female reproductive tract producing, 530t, 532t, 539t
  gastrointestinal, 298t, 299
Paradoxic pulse
  in asthma, 203
  in pericardial tamponade, 256, 256–257
Parafollicular cells (C cells), **414–415**, 481, 482f
  in calcium metabolism, **414–415**
  neoplasm of (medullary carcinoma of thyroid), **424–425**, 496
Paraganglioma, 287
Parahemophilia, 108t
Parakeratosis, in psoriasis, 170
Paralysis
  pseudobulbar, 134
  upper motor lesions causing, 134
Paralytic ileus, in acute pancreatitis, 368–369
Paranasal sinusitis, 39
Paraneoplastic syndromes, 95, 96t
Parapneumonic effusion, 66
Parasite eggs, pulmonary embolism caused by, 215t
Parasitic infections, 59
  pneumonia, 65–69
Parasympathetic nervous system, lungs supplied by, 187
Parathyroid glands, **405–410**
  anatomy of, 405
  carcinoma of, 416
  disorders of, gastrointestinal manifestations of, 310t
  histology of, 405
  hyperplasia of, 415–416
  physiology of, 405–407, 406f, 407f. *See also* Parathyroid hormone
  in regulation of calcium metabolism, **405–410**
Parathyroid hormone, 405
  assays for, 406–407, 407f
  in calcium metabolism, 109f, 406–407, 406f, 407f, 408–410
    kidney as site of action of, 386, 408, 409f
  deficiency of, 420–424, 421t. *See also* Hypoparathyroidism
  effects of, 408–410, 409f
  excess of, 416–419, 419t. *See also* Hyperparathyroidism
  in familial (benign) hypocalciuric hypercalcemia, 419, 419t
  mechanism of action of, 408, 408f
  osteoporosis and, 427
  in pseudohypoparathyroidism, 422
  serum levels of, in hypocalcemia, 423, 424t
Parathyroid hormone-related peptide, 408, **410**, 410f

hypercalcemia of malignancy caused by, 419t, 420
Paratonia, 148
Parenchyma, hepatic, 329, 330f
Parental gender
  Down's syndrome and, 19, 20, 21t
  fragile X-associated mental retardation syndrome and, 14f, 15f, 17
Parental imprinting, 4t
  in fragile X-associated mental retardation syndrome, 17
Paresthesia, in pernicious anemia, 115
Parietal association cortex, 149
Parietal cells, 302
  gastric acid secretion and, 302, 304f
Parietal lobe, sensory loss caused by lesions of, 142
parkin gene, in Parkinson's disease, 152
Parkinsonism, 151–152
Parkinson's disease, 137, **151–152**, 152f
  with autonomic failure, 291
Paroxysmal depolarizing shift, 155
Paroxysmal nocturnal dyspnea
  in left ventricular failure, 235, 238
  in mitral regurgitation, 249
Partial mole, 544
Partial pressures. *See* Carbon dioxide, partial pressure of; Oxygen, partial pressure of
Partial seizures, 154t, 155
Parturition, oxytocin in, 467
Passive immunity, 57
Patches, 169
Pathogens. *See also* Infection/infectious diseases
  nosocomial, 52
  obligate, 52t
  strategies of against host defenses, 60t
Pathophysiology
  definition and importance of, **1**
  genetic, unique aspects of, **2–8**
P_{CO_2} (partial pressure of carbon dioxide)
  in asthma, 203
  control of breathing and, 198–200, 199f, 200f
  in idiopathic pulmonary fibrosis, 210, 211f
  ventilation/perfusion matching and, 196, 196f
PDGF. *See* Platelet-derived growth factor
Pedal edema, in right ventricular failure, 240
Pelvic inflammatory disease
  dysmenorrhea in, 546t, 550
  ectopic pregnancy and, 550, 553
  infertility and, 553
Pemphigoid, bullous, **178–180**, 178f, 179f
Penetrance, 4t, **5–6**, 6f
  breast cancer genetic testing and, 88
  in fragile X-associated mental retardation syndrome, 14, 14f, 15, 15f
  reduced (age-dependent), 5, 6
Penetration, by microorganisms, 57, 57t
Penis, anatomic defects of, infertility and, 565, 566
Peptic ulcers, 308, **312–314**, 314f. *See also* Acid-mediated gastrointestinal injury
  in chronic renal failure, 397
Peptide histidine methionine, ovarian production of, 530t
Peptides/peptide hormones
  hypothalamic, 462
  tumor expression of
    carcinoid, 90, 90t, 95, 96t
    systemic effects of, 96t
Perforin, in lymphocyte-mediated cytotoxic rheumatic disease, 578
Perfusion, pulmonary. *See also under* Ventilation/perfusion
  distribution of, 193–194, 194f, 195f
  matching ventilation to, 194–198, 196f, 197f
Pericardial disease, **254–257**, 254f, 254t, 255f
Pericardial effusion, **255**
Pericardial friction rub, 254, 254–255
Pericardial knock, 254, 255, 255f
Pericardial sac, 222
Pericardial tamponade, **255–257**
  obstructive shock and, 281
Pericarditis, **254–255**, 254f, 254t, 255f, 256f
  in chronic renal failure, 397
Pericytes, 259, 260f
Periodontal disease, in diabetes mellitus, 454
Perioral dermatitis, in Cushing's syndrome, 515
Peripheral blood smear. *See* Blood smear
Peripheral edema. *See* Edema
Peripheral nervous system
  catecholamines affecting, 284t
  disorders of. *See also* Neuropathies
    sensory loss and, 141, 141f
  HIV infection/AIDS manifestations in, 48
Periportal hepatitis (piecemeal necrosis), 352, 353f
Peristaltic response, 297
Peritonitis, bacterial, in cirrhosis, 359
Permissive action, of glucocorticoids, 504, 507t
Pernicious anemia, **111–115**, 304
Petechiae, in drug-associated immune thrombocytopenia, 119
Petit mal seizures. *See* Absence seizures
Peyronie's disease, 566
PF4. *See* Platelet factor 4

pH
  in chronic hypercapnia, 200
  in chronic renal failure, 396
  in control of breathing, 199–200
  of pancreatic juice, 363
Phagocytes
  defective function of
    in chronic granulomatous disease, 43
    pathogens causing infection in, 41*t*
  microbial strategies against, 60*t*
Phagocytosis, 54–56, 102
  monocytes in, 102
Phagosome, 54
Pharynx, 295*f*
Phase I reactions, in biotransformation, 335, 340–342
Phase II reactions, in biotransformation, 335, 340–342
Phenobarbital, 156*t*
Phenotype, 5
  malignant, 79. *See also* Cancer
    progression of changes and, 84–85, 84*f*, 85*t*
Phenotypic heterogeneity, 4*t*
  in osteogenesis imperfecta, 13
Phenotypic sex, 531
  disorders of, 545
Phenoxybenzamine, for benign prostatic hyperplasia, 572*t*
Phenylalanine
  metabolism of, 24, 24*f*
  newborn screening for levels of, 23
Phenylalanine hydroxylase, defective, in phenylketonuria, 26, 26*f*, 26*t*
Phenylketonuria, 2, 7*t*, **23–27**
  maternal, 23
Phenytoin, 156*t*
Pheochromocytoma, 285, **286–290**, 286*t*, 287*f*, 288*t*, 289*t*
  hypertension and, 276–277, 287
Phlegmon, pancreatic, 370
Phosphate
  deficiency of, in osteomalacia, 429
  metabolism of
    parathyroid hormone in regulation of, 408–410, 409*f*
    renal regulation of, 386–387
      chronic renal failure and, 396–397, 396*f*
    replacement, in diabetic ketoacidosis treatment, 446
    serum levels of, in hypocalcemia, 423, 424*t*
Phospholipase A_2, in pancreatic juice, 364
  acute pancreatitis and, 367, 367*f*
Phospholipase C, 127
  in adrenergic receptor function, 283
Phospholipids, in coagulation, 103*f*, 104
Phosphorylation, in ion channel regulation, 127

Photoreceptors/photoreceptor cells, 142, 143–144
Pica, in iron deficiency anemia, 111
Pili, bacterial, colonization in meningitis and, 64
Pill hypertension, 275
Pituitary gland, **459–480**
  anatomy/histology/cell biology of, 459–462, 461*f*, 462*f*
  anterior, 461, 461*f*, 462*f*
    hormones secreted by, 462, **462–466**
    blood circulation in, 462, 463*f*
  disorders of, **469–479**. *See also specific type*
    adenomas, **471–473**, 472*f*, 473*t*
      ACTH-secreting (Cushing's disease), 471, 473, 509, 511–513, 511*t*, 512*f*, 513*f*, 514*f*
      growth hormone-secreting, 471, 473, 474*t*, 475*t*
      prolactin-secreting (prolactinoma), 471, 472–473, 473*t*
      TSH-secreting, 487
    amenorrhea/infertility in, 545, 546*t*, 549
    hypothyroidism and, 491, 492
  normal, **459–462**
  physiology of, **462–469**
  posterior, 461, 461*f*, 462*f*
    hormones secreted by, 462, **466–467**
Pituitary insufficiency (hypopituitarism), **473–475**, 475*t*
  hypoaldosteronism and, 526
  postpartum, 474
Pituitary portal system, 462, 463*f*
Placenta, 537, 538*f*
  abruption (premature separation) of, 543, 544
  in essential hypertension of pregnancy, 553, 554
  hormones produced by, 535–536
  in preeclampsia-eclampsia, 554
  previa, 544
Placental insufficiency, essential hypertension of pregnancy and, 553
Placental lactogen (hPL/chorionic somatomammotropin), 537
  fuel homeostasis in pregnancy and, 539, 541*f*, 543
Plaque-type psoriasis (psoriasis vulgaris), 173*t*
Plaques, 169
Plasma cells, in lymph nodes, 30, 30*f*
Plasma electrolytes
  in adrenocortical disease, 522, 522*t*
  mineralocorticoid secretion regulated by, 508
Plasma proteins
  in glomerulonephritis and nephrotic syndrome, 401

  hepatic synthesis/secretion of, 332*t*, 334, 336*t*
  liver dysfunction and, 338*t*, 339, 342
Plasma renin activity
  in hyperaldosteronism, 525
  in hypertension, 274
Plasma thromboplastin antecedent (factor XI), 103*f*, 104*t*
  deficiency of, 108*t*
Plasmin, 103*f*, 105
Plasminogen, 103*f*, 104*t*, 105
Plasminogen activator, ovarian production of, 530*t*
Platelet-activating factor, 103
Platelet adhesion, 102, 103*f*
Platelet count
  abnormalities in, 107–108, 107*t*
  in drug-associated immune thrombocytopenia, 119
  normal, 101*t*
Platelet-derived growth factor
  in breast cancer, 88–89
  in glomerulonephritis and nephrotic syndrome, 399
  ovarian production of, 530*t*
Platelet factor 4
  in heparin-induced thrombocytopenia, 117–118, 118*f*
  in heparin-induced thrombocytopenia and thrombosis, 119
Platelet plug, 103
Platelets, 102–103
  catecholamines affecting, 284*t*
  development of, 98–100, 99*f*
  disorders of, **107–108**, 107*t*, **117–120**. *See also specific type*
    functional/qualitative, 107*t*, 108
    intraparenchymal hemorrhage caused by, 162
    quantitative, 107, 107*t*
  normal values for, 101*t*
Pleocytosis, neutrophilic, in meningitis, 62, 64
Pleural effusion
  in acute pancreatitis, 370
  in left ventricular failure, 238
Pleural pressure, ventilation distribution and, 193–194, 194*f*
Pleurisy, 66
Pleuritic chest pain, in pulmonary embolism, 218
Pleuropulmonary disorders, in acute pancreatitis, 370
Plummer's disease, 496
Pluripotential stem cells, immune system development from, 102, 102*f*
PML gene, in leukemia, 94–95
Pneumocystis carinii pneumonia, in HIV infection/AIDS, 47
Pneumonia, **65–69**, 66*t*, 67*t*, 68*f*
  in HIV infection/AIDS, 47

PNP deficiency. *See* Purine nucleoside phosphorylase (PNP) deficiency
Po$_2$ (partial pressure of oxygen)
 control of breathing and, 198–200, 199f, 200f
 hypoxic pulmonary vasoconstriction and, 194
 ventilation/perfusion matching and, 196, 196f
Podagra, 580
Podocytes, 383, 384f
Poikilocytosis, in anemia, 105, 106f
Point mutation
 in oncogene activation, 80
 tumor suppressor gene function loss caused by, 80
Poiseuille-Hagen formula, 261
Polyarthritis
 chronic erosive, in gout, 580
 in immune complex vasculitis, 581
Polycystic ovary syndrome, 546t, 547–549, 548t, 549f
Polycythemia, 106
 in chronic bronchitis, 207
 in emphysema, 207
Polydipsia
 in diabetes mellitus, 445
 primary, diabetes insipidus differentiated from, 477
Polyglandular failure/polyendocrine syndrome, autoimmune, 421–422, 492, 518
 premature ovarian failure in, 547
 type 1, 421, 422f, 518
 type 2, 422, 518
Polyglutamation, in DNA synthesis, 113, 113f
Polymerase chain reaction, in hypercoagulable states, 121
Polymorphism, 4t, 5
 restriction fragment length (RFLP), 4t, 5
 in phenylketonuria, 25
Polymorphonuclear leukocytes (neutrophils), 29, 54–56, 101–102
 deficiency/defects in, 55–56
 development of, 98, 99f
 disorders of, 106, 107t
 in gout, 579, 579f
 in inflammatory rheumatic diseases, **578**
 normal values for, 101t
 phagocytosis by, 54–56
Polyneuropathy, 141
 in HIV infection/AIDS, 48
 symmetric distal, in diabetes mellitus, 453–454, 454t
Polyol pathway
 in diabetic microvascular disease, 449, 450f
 in symmetric distal polyneuropathy, 454
Polyphagia, in diabetes mellitus, 445
Polyposis, adenomatous familial, 87
Polyuria
 in diabetes insipidus, 476, 477
 in diabetes mellitus, 445
POMC. *See* Pro-opiomelanocortin
Pontine myelinolysis, central, 479
Portal blood flow, 332
Portal hypertension, 338
 in cirrhosis, 357, 357t
Portal system, pituitary, 462, 463f
Portal-to-systemic shunting, 327, 338, 338t
 altered hormone clearance and, 344
 in ascites formation, 358
 transhepatic intrajugular (TIPS), for ascites, 359
Portal triads (spaces), 329, 330f
Portal vein, hepatic, 328–329, 330f
Positional cloning, in breast cancer, 88
Postcoital test, 566–567
Posterior lobe, cerebellar, 134, 134f
Postictal confusion, 154
Postinfectious acute glomerulonephritis, 398, 398t, 399–400, 401
Postprandial hyperglycemia, 444
 in Cushing's syndrome, 516
Posttetanic potentiation, 155–156
Postural sensation, 139
Postural syncope, 280
Postzygotic amplification, in fragile X-associated mental retardation syndrome, 16
Postzygotic event, 4t
Potassium
 in adrenocortical insufficiency, 521, 522, 522t
 aldosterone secretion regulated by, 508
 in chronic renal failure, 395–396
 metabolism of, liver dysfunction and, 338t
 in stroke, 163, 163f
 supplementary, in diabetic ketoacidosis treatment, 446
 as vasodilator, 264
Potassium citrate, in prevention of renal stone formation, 402
Pounding pulses, in aortic regurgitation, 244, 245
PP. *See* Pancreatic polypeptide
PP cells (F cells), pancreatic, 432, 432t
 pancreatic polypeptide produced by, 432, 432t, 438
 tumors of (PPomas), 456t
PPoma, 456t
PR interval, of electrocardiogram, 224, 225f
PRAD1 gene, 81t, 417, 417f
Prader-Willi syndrome, 22t
Prazosin, for benign prostatic hyperplasia, 572, 572t
Prealbumin, thyroid-binding. *See* Transthyretin
Precapillary sphincters, 259, 259f
 in refractory shock, 279
Prechiasmal lesions, 144
Preclinical phase of cancer, 79
Preeclampsia-eclampsia, 529, **553–555**, 554t
 gestational and pregestational diabetes and, 543
Preexcitation, in reentrant tachyarrhythmias, 234, 234f
Prefrontal cortex, 148
Pregestational diabetes mellitus, 543
Pregnancy, **537–539**, 538f, 539t, 540f, 541f
 amenorrhea caused by, 545, 546t
 as counterregulatory state, 539, 541f, 543
 diabetes insipidus during, 477
 diabetes mellitus during, 440t, 441, 539, 543
 disorders of, **543–544**
  preeclampsia-eclampsia, 529, **553–555**, 554t
 ectopic, pelvic infection and, 550, 553
 fuel homeostasis in, 539, 541f
 gastrointestinal manifestations of, 310t
 hypertension in, 553–555
 molar, 544
 pathogens causing infection in, 56t
 spontaneous termination of, 544
 steroids in, 539
 successful, prerequisites for, 537, 538f, 539t, 540f
Preinvasive carcinoma (carcinoma in situ), 84, 84f, 85
Preleukemic (myelodysplastic) syndrome, 94, 95
Preload, 227–229, 230f
Premature ejaculation, 565
Premature ovarian failure, 546t, 547
Premenstrual syndrome, 546t, 550, 552
Premotor cortex, 131, 132f
Premutation, 4t
 in fragile X-associated mental retardation syndrome, 14, 15f, 16
Preproglucagon, 436, 437f
Preproinsulin, 433
Preproliferative retinopathy, in diabetes mellitus, 450
Prepro-opiomelanocortin, 464f
PreproPTH, 406, 407f
Preprosomatostatin, 437
Prerenal azotemia, 279, 392
 in adrenocortical insufficiency, 521, 522
 liver dysfunction and, 338t, 350
Presenilins, in Alzheimer's disease, 158

Pressure. *See also* Blood pressure
  in cardiovascular system, 260, 262, 262*f*
  sensation of, 139, 139*f*
Pressure-flow studies, in benign prostatic hyperplasia, 574
Pressure-time analysis, of events in cardiac cycle, 225–227, 228*f*
Pressure-volume analysis, of events in cardiac cycle, 227–229, 229*f*, 230*f*
  in aortic regurgitation, 245, 246*f*
  in aortic stenosis, 242, 243*f*
Pretibial myxedema, 490–491
Primary auditory cortex, 132*f*, 149
Primary autonomic failure (sympathetic neural failure), 285, 290–291
Primary (essential) hypertension, 273, 273*t*
  of pregnancy, 553
Primary immunodeficiency diseases, **39–45**, 40*t*
  defective cytokine response and, 40*t*, **44–45**
  defective proliferation and differentiation responses and, 40*t*, **43–44**
  early defects in cellular maturation and, 40*t*, **41–42**
  enzyme defects and, 40*t*, **42–43**
  infection and, 40, 41*t*, 56*t*
Primary motor area, 131, 132*f*
Primary ovarian failure, chronic anovulation and, 548*t*
Primary sensory cortex, 131, 132*f*
Primary visual cortex, 132*f*, 142, 144
Primordial germ cells, 4*t*
  in fragile X-associated mental retardation syndrome, 16
Proaccelerin (factor V), 103*f*, 104*t*, 120, 120*f*
  deficiency of, 108*t*
Procoagulant factors, 104, 104*t*
Procoagulant pathways, 103*f*, 104
Procollagen, molecular assembly of, 10–11, 10*f*
Proconvertin (factor VII), 103*f*, 104, 104*t*, 336*t*
  deficiency of, 108*t*
  hepatic synthesis of, 336*t*
Prodrome, in viral hepatitis, 348*f*, 349
Progesterone
  changes in in menstrual cycle, 532*f*, 535
  ovaries producing, 536–537
  placenta producing, 536, 536*f*, 538
Progestins, for benign prostatic hyperplasia, 570, 570*t*
Programmed cell death (apoptosis)
  in lymphoma, 93
  in male infertility, 563
  in spinal muscular atrophies, 150

  in systemic lupus erythematosus, 582, 582*f*, 583
Progressive multifocal leukoencephalopathy, 48
Progressive proximal spinal and bulbar muscular atrophy of late onset (Kennedy disease), 150
Proinflammatory cytokines, 54
  in gout, 579
Proinsulin, 433
Prolactin, 466
  elevated levels of (hyperprolactinemia), 472–473, 473*t*
    chronic anovulation and, 547, 548*t*
    in hypogonadotropic hypogonadism, 564
    in hypothyroidism, 494
    in lactation/milk synthesis and secretion, 466, 540–541, 542*f*
  normal levels of in men, 560*t*
  pituitary adenoma secreting (prolactinoma), 471, 472–473, 473*f*
Prolactinoma, 471, 472–473, 473*t*
Proliferative retinopathy, in diabetes, 448, 450
Pro-opiomelanocortin (POMC), 462
  ovarian production of, 530*t*
Proprioception, 139*f*, 140
  impaired, in pernicious anemia, 115
Proprioceptors, in control of breathing, 198*f*, 199
Proptosis, in Graves' disease, 490, 490*f*
Propylthiouracil, hypothyroidism caused by, 491
  goiter and, 494, 495*t*
Prorenin, 506
Prostacyclin, in vascular function regulation, 264
Prostaglandins, 298*t*
  in dysmenorrhea, 550
  gastrointestinal secretion of, 298*t*
  in vascular function regulation, 264
Prostate gland, 556, 558*f*, 568*f*
  alpha-adrenergic receptors in smooth muscle of, benign prostatic hyperplasia and, 572
  benign hyperplasia of, **568–574**
    clinical manifestations of, 573–574
    etiology of, 568
    pathogenesis of, 569–573, 570*f*, 572*t*, 573*t*
    pathology of, 568–569, 568*f*, 569*f*
  cancer of, 86*t*
  growth of
    age-related, 568, 569
    hormonal regulation of, 569–571, 570*f*

Prostatic capsule, benign prostatic hyperplasia and, 569, 572
Prostatic fluid, 556
Protease inhibitors, deficiency of, in emphysema, 205, 206*f*
Protein C, 104, 104*t*, 105, 120, 120*f*, 336*t*
  activated, resistance to, 121, 122
  deficiency of, 121, 122
  hepatic synthesis of, 336*t*
Protein-losing enteropathy, 322
Protein S, 104, 104*t*, 105, 120, 120*f*
  deficiency of, 121, 122
Proteins
  dietary, renal stone formation and, 402
  iron-associated, 109, 110*t*
  membrane, extracellular, ovarian production of, 530*t*
  metabolism of, in liver, 332*t*, 333, 334, 334*f*, 336*t*
    liver dysfunction and, 338*t*, 339, 342
  in neoplasia, **83**
  in pancreatic juice, 363
  plasma, synthesis/secretion of, in liver, 332*t*, 334, 336*t*
    liver dysfunction and, 338*t*, 339, 342
  tumor suppressor genes encoding for, 81
Proteinuria
  in diabetes mellitus, 452, 452*f*
  in preeclampsia-eclampsia, 553
Proteolytic proteins, in neoplasia, **83**
Prothrombin (factor II), 104, 104*t*
  elevated levels of, 121
Prothrombin 20210 AG mutation, 122
Proto-oncogenes, 80
Proton pump (H^+-K^+ ATPase), 297
  in gastric acid secretion, 302, 304*f*
  in pernicious anemia, 112, 112*f*
Proximal convoluted tubule, 384*f*, 385
  in renal regulation, 385, 386*t*
Pruritus
  in allergic rhinitis, 37–38
  in liver dysfunction, 339
Pseudobulbar paralysis, 134
Pseudocapsule, of sarcoma, 91
Pseudo-Cushing's syndrome, 517
Pseudocysts, pancreatic
  in acute pancreatitis, 370, 371, 371*f*
  in chronic pancreatitis, 373, 376
"Pseudodementia," 157
Pseudohermaphroditism, 545
Pseudohypoaldosteronism, 526
Pseudohyponatremia, 478–479, 479*t*
Pseudohypoparathyroidism, **420–424**
  clinical manifestations of, 423, 424*t*
  definition of, 421
  pathogenesis of, 422
Psoriasis (psorasiform dermatitis), **170–173**, 170*t*, 171*f*, 172*f*, 172*t*
  variants of, 173*t*

Psoriatic arthritis, 172
PSPs (pancreatic stone proteins). *See* Lithostathines
Psychiatric illness, in Cushing's syndrome., 510*f*, 516
PTH. *See* Parathyroid hormone
PTH receptor, 408, 408*f*
PTH/PTHrP receptors, 408, 408*f*
PTHrP. *See* Parathyroid hormone-related peptide
Puberty, in female, 533
Pulmonary angiography, in pulmonary embolism, 218
Pulmonary arteries, 187, 188*f*, 189*f*
Pulmonary disease, **184–221**
  in chronic renal failure, 397
  gastrointestinal manifestations of, 310*t*
  lung anatomy and, **184–190**
  lung physiology and, **190–200**
  obstructive, **200–207**
  restrictive, **208–210**
Pulmonary edema, **210–214**, 211*t*, 212*f*, 213*f*
  in acute pancreatitis, 370
  in aortic regurgitation, 244, 245
  in chronic renal failure, 397
  in left ventricular failure, 237, 237*f*
  in mitral regurgitation, 249
  in right ventricular failure, 239
Pulmonary embolism, **215–219**, 215*t*, 216*t*, 217*f*, 219*t*
  chronic, 219
  in hypercoagulable states, 122
Pulmonary fibrosis
  idiopathic (interstitial), **208–210**, 208*f*, 209*t*, 210*f*, 211*f*
  lung compliance in, 191, 192*f*
Pulmonary function tests
  in asthma, 203, 204*f*
  in chronic bronchitis, 207
  in emphysema, 207
  in idiopathic pulmonary fibrosis, 210, 210*f*
Pulmonary hypertension, 239
  in emphysema, 207
  in idiopathic pulmonary fibrosis, 210
Pulmonary infarction, pulmonary embolism and, 218
Pulmonary infection
  defense mechanisms against, 66–68, 67*t*, 68*f*, 189, 189*t*
  in HIV infection/AIDS, 47
  pneumonia, **65–69**, 66*t*, 67*t*, 68*f*
Pulmonary lymphatics, 187–189, 188*f*
Pulmonary nervous system, 187, 188*f*, 188*t*
Pulmonary perfusion. *See also under* Ventilation/perfusion
  distribution of, 193–194, 194*f*, 195*f*
  matching ventilation to, 194–198, 196*f*, 197*f*
Pulmonary stretch receptors, 187, 188*t*

Pulmonary surfactant, 185, 191
  pathologic states and, 191
Pulmonary valve, 222, 223–224*f*
Pulmonary vascular system, 187, 188*f*, 189*f*
Pulmonary vasoconstriction, hypoxic, 194
Pulmonary veins, 188*f*, 189*f*, 222, 223–224*f*
Pulmonary ventilation. *See also under* Ventilation/perfusion
  distribution of, 193–194, 194*f*, 195*f*
  matching perfusion to, 194–198, 196*f*, 197*f*
Pulses, hyperdynamic (pounding), in aortic regurgitation, 244, 245
Pulsus alternans, in left ventricular heart failure, 235
Pulsus paradoxus
  in asthma, 203
  in pericardial tamponade, 256, 256–257
Pulsus parvus, in aortic stenosis, 241, 242
Pulsus tardus, in aortic stenosis, 241, 242
Pupillary light reflex, 145, 145*f*
Pupils, control of size of, 142–143, 144*f*, 145, 145*f*
Pure autonomic failure, 291
Purine nucleoside phosphorylase (PNP) deficiency, 40*t*, **42–44**, 43*f*
Purkinje fibers/system, 222–224, 225*f*
Purpura
  in acute pancreatitis, 370
  palpable, in leukocytoclastic vasculitis, 180, 180*f*
Pursuit eye movements, 142
Pustular psoriasis, generalized and localized, 173*t*
Pustule, 169
Putamen (corpus striatum), 136, 136*f*
Pyelography, intravenous, in benign prostatic hyperplasia, 574
Pyloroplasty, 308
Pyramidal neurons/tract, 129, 131
  lesions of, 134

QRS complex, of electrocardiogram, 224, 225*f*
  in reentrant tachyarrhythmias, 234, 234*f*
Quadrantanopia, superior and inferior, 145
Quality of life, impaired, allergy and asthma and, 39
Quincke's pulse, in aortic regurgitation, 245

Rachitic rosary, 429
Radiation enteritis, histologic features of, 320*t*
Radiation therapy, spermatogenesis affected by, 564

Radiculopathy, 141
Radioactive iodine uptake, in hyperthyroidism, 487
RAG-1/RAG-2, deficiency of, in SCID, 41
RAI. *See* Radioactive iodine uptake
Rales
  in left ventricular failure, 235, 238
  in mitral stenosis, 247
Raloxifene, for osteoporosis prevention/management, 429
RANK, 411
RANKL (receptor activator of NF-kappa B ligand), 411
Ranson's criteria, 371, 372*t*
Ranvier, nodes of, 128, 128*f*
Rapidly progressive glomerulonephritis, 398, 399, 399*t*, 400
*RAR*α gene, in leukemia, 94–95
ras oncogene, 81, 81*t*
  in colon carcinoma, 86
  in hematologic neoplasia, 92
Rb gene, 82*t*
  in hematologic neoplasia, 92
RBM gene, azoospermia and, 563
Reabsorption lacunae, 481, 482*f*
Reactive astrocytosis, 128
Reactive hyperemia, nitric oxide and, 264–265
REAL (Revised European and American Lymphoma) classifications for lymphoma, 93, 93*t*
Receptive relaxation, in gastric motility, 302
Receptor activator of NF-kappa B ligand (RANKL), 411
Receptor-mediated uptake, in liver, 329
Recessive inheritance, 4*t*
  amorphic (loss-of-function) mutations and, 6–7, 7*t*
Recklinghausen's disease (type I neurofibromatosis), pheochromocytoma in, 286, 286*t*
Rectum, 295*f*
Rectus muscles, 142, 144*f*
Red blood cells. *See* Erythrocytes
Red cell count, normal, 101*t*
Red nuclei, 135*f*, 136
Reduced penetrance, 5, 6
5α-Reductase
  in dihydrotestosterone synthesis, 560, 569, 571*f*
  in prostate gland, 569–570
5α-Reductase inhibitors, for benign prostatic hyperplasia, 570–571, 570*t*, 571*f*
Reentrant tachyarrhythmias, 233–234, 233*f*, 234*f*, 235*f*
Refetoff's syndrome (generalized resistance to thyroid hormone), 485, 497

Reflex withdrawal, 130f, 137
Reflexes, pupillary light, 145, 145f
Reflux, hepatojugular, in right ventricular failure, 240
Reflux esophagitis, **309–312**, 311f
Refractory (irreversible) shock, 279–280
Regeneration, hepatic, 331
Regional enteritis (Crohn's disease), 321–322, 322, 323t
  histologic features of, 320t
Regulatory proteins, tumor suppressor genes encoding for, 81
Relaxation, receptive, in gastric motility, 302
Relaxin, ovarian production of, 530t
Remodeling, bone, 411–412, 412f
Renal acidification, impaired, liver dysfunction and, 338t
Renal artery, constriction of, renal hypertension and, 275
Renal blood flow, regulation of, 387, 387t
Renal cancer, 86t
Renal disease, **388–404**. *See also specific type and* Renal failure
  adaptations to, 387
  gastrointestinal manifestations of, 310t
  hypertension and, 275
  liver dysfunction and, 338t, 344, 344t, 350, 354
  manifestations of altered function in, **388–390**
  structure and function alterations in, **368**, 390t
Renal failure
  acute, **389–394**, 391t, 392f, 392t
    clinical and laboratory findings in, 391t
    liver dysfunction and, 338t
  chronic, 391t, **394–398**, 394t, 395t, 396f
    clinical and laboratory findings in, 391t, 394, 394t
    gastrointestinal manifestations of, 310t
  in diabetes mellitus, 394, 395t, 448, 450–452, 451f, 452f
  intrarenal causes of, 388, 390, 390t
  postrenal causes of, 388, 390, 390t
  prerenal causes of, 388, 390, 390t
Renal function, **385–387**, 386t, 387t. *See also* Kidneys
  glucocorticoids affecting, 507t
  regulation of, 387, 387t
Renal hypertension, 275
  bruits in, 274
  clinical and laboratory findings in, 391t
Renal stones (nephrolithiasis), **401–404**, 402t, 403t
  in acute renal failure, 390, 391t
  clinical and laboratory findings in, 391t

  in Cushing's syndrome, 515
  in hyperparathyroidism, 402, 403t, 418
  in pancreatic insufficiency, 378
Renal transplantation, gastrointestinal manifestations in, 310t
Renal tubular acidosis, 386t
  stone formation and, 403t
  type 4 (hyporeninemic hypoaldosteronism), 396, 509, 526
Renal tubular defects, clinical and laboratory findings in, 391t
Renal tubules, 382, 384f, 385
  acute necrosis of, 390, 390–392, 393f
  in renal regulation, 385, 386t
Renal vessels, atherosclerosis involving, 271
Renin, 506, 507f
  deficiency of, in hypoaldosteronism, 526
  ovarian production of, 530t
  plasma activity of
    in hyperaldosteronism, 525
    in hypertension, 274
  in renal regulation of blood pressure, 386
Renin-angiotensin system
  abnormality of, hypertension and, 275
  in aldosterone regulation, 506, 507t
Renovascular hypertension, 271
Reperfusion-induced injury, 280
Reproductive systems. *See also* Female reproductive tract; Male reproductive tract
  disorders of, in hyperprolactinemia, 472–473, 547, 548t, 564
Reserve volume, expiratory (ERV), 185
Residual capacity, functional (FRC), 185
Residual volume (RV), 185
  in asthma, 203
  in emphysema, 207
Resistance
  airflow, 186–187, 186f, 187f, 191–192, 193f
    in asthma, 186–187, 202–203
    in obstructive lung diseases, 200–201
  vascular, 261–262
    catecholamines in, 285
    in septic shock, 76
Resistance vessels, 258
Respiration. *See* Breathing; Ventilation
Respiratory acidosis
  in asthma, 203
  in chronic bronchitis, 207
  in emphysema, 207
Respiratory distress, acute, 213, 214, 280
  in acute pancreatitis, 370
  in septic shock, 77
Respiratory muscles, control of, 198–200. *See also* Breathing, control of

Resting membrane potential, 125
Restriction fragment length polymorphism (RFLP), 4t, 5
  in phenylketonuria, 25
Restrictive lung disease, **208–210**
RET gene/mutation, 81t
  in multiple endocrine neoplasia, 418
  medullary carcinoma of thyroid and, 424, 425
  pheochromocytoma and, 286–287
Retardation. *See* Mental retardation
Rete ridges, 167, 168f
  in psoriasis, 170, 171f, 172f
Reticular activating system, 147
Reticulocytes, 101
Reticuloendothelial cells, hepatic, 329
  in cirrhosis, 356
Retina, 142, 143–144
  visual processing in, 144
Retinal detachment, in diabetic retinopathy, 450
Retinitis, cytomegalovirus, in HIV infection/AIDS, 48
Retinitis pigmentosa, 143–144
Retinoblastoma gene, 82t
  in hematologic neoplasia, 92
Retinopathy
  diabetic, 448, 449–450, 451f
  hypertensive, 274
Retrochiasmal lesions, 145
Retrograde ejaculation, in infertility, 565
Retropulsion, in Alzheimer's disease, 157
Reverse triiodothyronine (RT_3), 484
Reversed Bernheim effect, 239, 257
Revised European and American Lymphoma (REAL) classifications for lymphoma, 93, 93t
RFLP (restriction fragment length polymorphism), 4t, 5
  in phenylketonuria, 25
Rhabdomyolysis, in acute renal failure, 390
Rhabdomyosarcoma, 91
Rheumatic diseases, inflammatory, **576–583**. *See also specific type*
  acute, **576**, 576f
  chronic, **576–577**, 576f, 577f
  pathogenesis of inflammation in, **577–578**
Rheumatic heart disease, mitral stenosis caused by, 247, 249t
Rheumatoid arthritis, gastrointestinal manifestations of, 310t
Rheumatologic disorders, gastrointestinal manifestations of, 310t
Rhinitis, allergic, **36–39**, 37t
Rhinometry, acoustic, 38
Ribonuclease, in pancreatic juice, 364
"Rice-water stools," in cholera, 72

Rickets, 429
Right ventricular heart failure, **239–240**, 239*t*, 240*f*
Rinne test, 146
RNA-binding motif, azoospermia and, 563
Robertsonian translocation, 4*t*
  in Down's syndrome, 18, 18*f*, 20–21, 21*f*, 21*t*, 22
Rods, 142, 143
Rosenthal's syndrome, 108*t*
Rotavirus, diarrhea caused by, 69
RT_3. *See* Reverse triiodothyronine
RT_3U. *See* T_3 resin uptake
RT_4U. *See* T_4 resin uptake
Ruffled border, 411, 411*f*
RV (residual volume), 185
  in asthma, 203
  in emphysema, 207

S_1 **(first heart sound), 227**
S_2 (second heart sound), 227
S_3 (third heart sound)
  in aortic regurgitation, 244, 245
  in left ventricular failure, 238, 238*f*
  in mitral regurgitation, 247, 249
  in right ventricular failure, 239
S_4 (fourth heart sound)
  in aortic stenosis, 241
  in coronary artery disease, 253
  in left ventricular failure, 238*f*, 239
S182 (presenilin 1) gene, in Alzheimer's disease, 158
SA node. *See* Sinoatrial node
Saccadic eye movements, 142
Saccule, 145
Salmonella, diarrhea caused by, 69, 72
Salt. *See* Sodium
Salt sensitivity, hypertension and, 275, 275*t*
Saltatory conduction, 128
Santorini, duct of, 362, 363*f*
Saprophytic infection, 59
Sarafatoxins, endothelins and, 265, 265*f*
Sarcoidosis
  gastrointestinal manifestations of, 310*t*
  pathogens causing infection in, 56*t*
Sarcomas, 89*t*, **91**
  Kaposi's, in HIV infection/AIDS, 48–49
Sarcomeres, 225, 226*f*
Satiety, 468
Scavenger receptor, 269
Schilling test, in pernicious anemia, 114–115
Schmidt's syndrome (autoimmune polyglandular failure/polyendocrine syndrome, type 2), 422, 518
Schwann cells, 128, 128*f*
  tumors of (schwannomas)
    benign (neurofibromas), 91
    malignant (neurofibrosarcomas), 91

SCID-ADA, 40*t*, 42
Scleras, blue, in osteogenesis imperfecta, 9, 10
Scleroderma, gastrointestinal manifestations of, 310*t*
Sclerosing chronic glomerulonephritis, 400
Scrotum, 556, 557*f*
Second heart sound (S_2), 227
Second messengers, 127
  in adrenergic receptor function, 283–284
Secondary generalization, of seizure, 155
Secondary hyperaldosteronism, 506
Secondary hypertension, 273
Secondary sex characteristics, male, androgens in development of, 561, 561*t*
Secretagogues, 307
Secretin, 298*t*, 364
  pancreatic juice secretion controlled by, 364
Secretory diarrhea, 71–72, 318, 318*t*
  in medullary carcinoma of thyroid, 425
Segmental response, 297
Seizures, **154–156**
  classification of, 154*t*
  drugs for management of, 156, 156*t*
Selective IgA deficiency, 40*t*, **44**
  pathogens causing infection in, 56*t*
Selective IgM deficiency, pathogens causing infection in, 56*t*
Selegiline, for Parkinson's disease, 152
Semen, 556
Semen analysis, 566, 567*f*, 567*t*
Semi-dominant inheritance, 7
Semicircular canals, 145
Seminal plasma, antibodies to, infertility and, 565
Seminal vesicles, 556, 557*f*
Seminiferous tubule axis, in male reproductive function, 558, 558–560, 560*f*
Seminiferous tubules, 556, 557*f*
Senile osteoporosis. *See* Osteoporosis
Senile plaques, Down's syndrome and, 19
Sensorimotor nerves, 138
Sensorineural deafness, 146
Sensory (somatosensory) cortex, 131, 132*f*, 139
Sensory loss, anatomy of, 140–142, 141*f*
Sensory nerves. *See* Somatosensory system
Sensory neurons, 138
Sensory nuclei of trigeminal nerve, 139
Sentinel loop, in acute pancreatitis, 369
Sepsis, **73–77**, 74*t*, 75*f*, 76*f*
  acute renal failure caused by, 390
  definition of, 74, 74*t*
  in gastrointestinal disease, 293
  severe, 74, 74*t*, 75*f*

Septic embolism, 215*t*
Septic shock, **73–77**, 74*t*, 75*f*, 76*f*, 280
  definition of, 74, 74*t*
Serosa, 296, 296*f*
Serotonin (5-hydroxytryptamine), carcinoid tumor expression of, 90
Serous otitis media, 39
Sertoli-cell-only syndrome, 563
Sertoli cells, 556
Serum sickness, 581
Severe combined immunodeficiency disease (SCID), 40*t*, **41**
  ADA deficiency causing, 40*t*, 42
  pathogens causing infection in, 41*t*, 56*t*
Sex (gender)
  determination of, **531–533**, 534*f*. *See also* Sexual differentiation
  disorders associated with, **545**
  parental
    Down's syndrome and, 19, 20, 21*t*
    fragile X-associated mental retardation syndrome and, 14*f*, 15*f*, 17
Sex hormone-binding globulin. *See* Steroid hormone-binding globulin
Sex hormones. *See* Steroids/steroid hormones
Sexual differentiation, **531–533**, 534*f*
  disorders of, **535**
  embryonic, 531–533, 534*f*
  of estrogen dependent tissues, 533
  in puberty, 533
Sexual dysfunction
  in Cushing's syndrome, 516
  in diabetes mellitus, 454
  male infertility and, 565
SHBG. *See* Steroid hormone-binding globulin
Shear stress, in atherosclerosis, 269
Sheehan's syndrome, 474, 549
Shiga toxin, 72, 72*f*, 73*f*
Shigella, diarrhea caused by, 69, 72, 72*f*, 73*f*
Shiners, allergic, 36
Shock, **278–281**, 278*t*
  in acute pancreatitis, 369
  anaphylactic, 280
  burn, 280
  cardiogenic, 278, 278*t*, **280–281**
  congested, 281
  in coronary artery disease, 253
  distributive (vasogenic/low-resistance), 278, 278*t*, **280**
  sepsis and, 76, 280
  hemorrhagic, 280
  hypovolemic, 278, 278*t*, **279–280**, 279*t*
  neurogenic, 280
  obstructive, 278, 278*t*, **281**
  refractory (irreversible), 279–280

septic, **73–77**, 74*t*, 75*f*, 76*f*, 280
surgical, 280
traumatic, 280
Shortness of breath. *See* Dyspnea
Shunts
in chronic bronchitis, 207
in pulmonary embolism, 217
ventilation/perfusion ratios and, 195, 196, 196*f*
Shy-Drager syndrome, 291
SIADH. *See* Syndrome of inappropriate vasopressin (ADH) secretion
Sickle cell anemia, 7*t*, 105
Simple partial seizures, 154*t*, 155
Sinoatrial node, 222–224, 225*f*
Sinusitis, 39
Sinusoids, hepatic, 329, 330*f*
Sipple's syndrome (MEN 2a), 416, 416*t*
medullary carcinoma of thyroid in, 424, 425
pheochromocytoma in, 286, 286*t*
SIRS. *See* Systemic inflammatory response syndrome
Skeletal muscle
catecholamines affecting, 284*t*
lower motor neurons and, **129–131**
Skin, **166–183**
anatomy of, 166
catecholamines affecting, 284*t*, 288*t*
in Cushing's syndrome, 510*f*, 515
as defense against infection, 53
diseases/lesions of, **169–182**. *See also specific type and* Dermatitis
cancer, 86*t*
in chronic renal failure, 398
in HIV infection/AIDS, 48
infections, in cyclic neutropenia, 117
inflammatory, 169, 170*t*, 171*f*
types of, 169
histology of, 166–168, 166*f*, 167*f*, 168*f*, 169*f*
in hyperthyroidism, 490–491
in hypothyroidism, 493–494
in left ventricular failure, 239
normal, **166–168**, 169*f*
vitamin D synthesis in, 413, 413*f*
Skin tests, allergy, 39
SLE. *See* Systemic lupus erythematosus
Sleep, 148
Sleep apnea, in hypothyroidism, 493
Small intestine, 295*f*, **305–307**. *See also under* Intestinal
absorption in, 306–307, 307
anatomy and histology of, 305–306, 306*f*
digestion in, 307
disorders of, **318–325**
common presentations of, 294*t*
motility of, 306
disorders of, 308
secretion in, 306–307
Small vessel vasculitis, cutaneous, 581

SMN gene, in spinal muscular atrophies, 150
Smoking
in atherosclerosis, 272*t*, 273
in chronic obstructive pulmonary disease, 205
pancreatic carcinoma and, 378
Smooth muscle
bronchial, catecholamines affecting, 284*t*
gastrointestinal
catecholamines affecting, 284*t*
contraction of, 296–297. *See also* Gastrointestinal motility
genitourinary, catecholamines affecting, 284*t*
prostate gland, alpha-adrenergic receptors in, benign prostatic hyperplasia and, 572
vascular
catecholamines affecting, 284*t*
hormones affecting, 265–266
Sneezing, in allergic rhinitis, 37–38
SOD1 (cytosolic copper-zinc superoxide dismutase) gene, in amyotrophic lateral sclerosis, 150–151
Sodium
in adrenocortical insufficiency, 521, 522, 522*t*
aldosterone secretion regulated by, 508
dietary, renal stone formation and, 402
mineralocorticoids in regulation of excretion of, 504
renal dysfunction affecting balance of, 388–389
retention of
in acute renal failure, 392–394, 393*t*
in chronic renal failure, 395
in Liddle's syndrome, hypertension and, 275
liver dysfunction and, 338*t*, 344, 344*t*
ascites formation and, 358–359
in mineralocorticoid excess, 524–525
sensitivity to, hypertension and, 275, 275*t*
in stroke, 163, 163*f*, 164
Sodium co-transporters, in intestinal secretion, 307
Sodium-hydrogen exchange, facilitation of, hypertension and, 278
Sodium-potassium pump (Na^+-K^+ ATPase), 297
in intestinal secretion, 307
in signal propagation, 124
Soft exudates, in diabetic retinopathy, 450
Somatic mosaicism, 5*f*. *See also* Mosaicism

in fragile X-associated mental retardation syndrome, 16
Somatosensory (sensory) cortex, 131, 132*f*, 139
Somatosensory system, **137–142**
anatomy of, 137–139, 138*f*, 139*f*
physiology of, 139–142
Somatostatin, 298*t*, **437–438**
D cells secreting, 432, 432*t*, 433*f*
regulation of, 434*t*, 437
growth hormone secretion affected by, 465, 465*f*
mechanism of action and effects of, 436*t*, 438
ovarian production of, 530*t*
receptors for, 438
synthesis/metabolism/regulation of secretion of, 434*t*, 437
Somatostatin-14, 437
Somatostatin-28, 437
Somatostatinoma, 456*t*, **457**
Somogyi phenomenon, 448
Sorbitol pathway, in diabetic microvascular disease, 449, 450*f*
Sounds of Korotkoff, 261, 262
Space of Disse, 330*f*, 331*f*
Spasticity, 132
Specificity, immunologic, 31
Sperm motility
normal, 566
poor, in Kartagener's (immotile cilia) syndrome, 564, 566
Sperm mucus-penetration test, 567
Sperm penetration assay, 567
Sperm-zona interactions, laboratory evaluation of, 567–568
Spermatogenesis, 556
defective, 563–564
varicocele-impaired, 564
Spermatozoa, 556
antibodies to, infertility and, 565
laboratory evaluation of, 566, 567*f*, 567*t*
Spherocytosis, hereditary, 105–106
Sphincters
anal, 295*f*
gastrointestinal, 296
lower esophageal (gastroesophageal), 300, 301*t*
in achalasia, 309
in reflux esophagitis, 311, 311*f*
of Oddi, 305, 305*f*
precapillary, 259, 259*f*
in refractory shock, 279
Spider angiomas, in cirrhosis, 361
Spinal cord, 138, 138*f*
injury/lesions of
gastrointestinal manifestations of, 310*t*
sensory loss caused by, 141
subacute combined degeneration of, 114

Spinal muscular atrophies, 150
Spinal root lesions, sensory loss caused by, 141
Spinal shock, 132
Spindle receptors, in control of breathing, 198f, 199
Spinothalamic tracts, 138f, 139, 139f
  sensory loss caused by lesions of, 142
Spinous layer of skin, 166, 166f, 167, 167f
Spiral CT, in pulmonary embolism, 218
Spirogram, normal, 185
Spleen, 30
Splenectomy, acute pancreatitis after, 366
Splenomegaly, in cirrhosis, 360
Spontaneous bacterial peritonitis, in cirrhosis, 359
Sporadic cretinism, 494
Sporadic olivopontocerebellar degeneration, 291
Sprue
  celiac (nontropical), histologic features of, 320t
  collagenous, histologic features of, 320t
  tropical, histologic features of, 320t
Squamous cell carcinoma, anal, in HIV infection/AIDS, 49
SS-14. *See* Somatostatin-14
SS-28. *See* Somatostatin-28
ST. *See* Heat-stable toxin
Stable angina, 251, 252
Staphylococcus aureus
  diarrhea caused by, 69, 73t
  food poisoning caused by, 73, 73t
  pneumonia caused by, 66t
Steatorrhea
  in chronic pancreatitis, 376
  gastrointestinal disease presenting with, 294t
  liver dysfunction and, 338t
  in pancreatic insufficiency, 376, 377, 377–378, 377t
  somatostatinoma causing, 457
Stem cells
  blood cells formed from, 98, 99f
  immune system development from, 102, 102f
Stereognosis, 140
Steroid acne, in Cushing's syndrome, 510f, 515, 516
Steroid hormone-binding globulin (sex hormone-binding globulin/gonadal steroid-binding globulin), 336t, 557
  hepatic synthesis of, 335–336, 336t
  in polycystic ovary syndrome, 548, 549f
Steroids/steroid hormones
  adrenal cortical cells secreting, 500, 502f
  disorders of, 526–527

changes in in menstrual cycle, 532f, 534–535
fetal-placental-maternal synthesis of, 537–538, 540f
in neoplasia, 83
ovarian, 532f, 534–535, 536
  gonadotropins affecting synthesis/secretion of, 464
  physiology of, **536–537**
  in pregnancy, 539, 540f
  disorders associated with, 543–544, 543t
testicular
  gonadotropins affecting synthesis/secretion of, 464
  synthesis/protein binding/metabolism of, 557–558, 559f, 560f, 560t
Stevens-Johnson syndrome, 177
STM2 (presenilin 2) gene, in Alzheimer's disease, 158
Stocking distribution, in symmetric distal polyneuropathy, 453
Stomach, 295f, **302–304**, 303f, 304f
  anatomy and histology of, 302, 303f
  disorders of, **312–316**
    cancer, 86t
    in chronic renal failure, 397
    common presentations of, 294t
  motility of, 302
    disorders of, 308, **314–316**, 315t
  secretion by, 298t, 302–304, 304f
    disorders of, 308
      pancreatic insufficiency and, 377
  ulcer in, 308, **313**
Stool, blood in, 294t
  in iron deficiency anemia, 111
Storage pool (granulocyte), in cyclic neutropenia, 115–116
Stratum corneum, 166, 166f
Stratum granulosum, 166, 166f
Streak gonads, 545
Streamlined flow, resistance and, 192
Streptococcus, group B
  glomerulonephritis after infection with, 398, 398t, 399–400, 401
  meningitis caused by, 63, 63t
Streptococcus pneumoniae
  meningitis caused by, 63, 63t, 64
  pneumonia caused by, 66t
Stress
  ACTH and cortisol secretion and, 502, 504, 506f, 507t
  amenorrhea and, 549
  carbohydrate metabolism affected by, 439
  diabetes and, 445
  lack of response to, in hypopituitarism, 473, 474

Stretch receptors, in control of breathing, 199
Stretch reflex, 129, 130f
Striae, in Cushing's syndrome, 510f, 514, 515
Striatonigral degeneration, 291
Stroke, **158–164**
  classification of, 159, 159t
  hemorrhagic, 159t, 162, 162f
  ischemic, 159–162, 159f, 159t, 160f, 161f, 161t
Stroke volume, cardiac output affected by, 227
Stromal proteins, in neoplasia, **83**
Stromolysin 3, in breast cancer, 89
Structural proteins, in neoplasia, 83
Struvite stones, 402, 403t
Stuart-Prower factor (factor X), 103f, 104, 104t, 120, 336t
  hepatic synthesis of, 336t
Stuffiness/congestion, nasal, in allergic rhinitis, 38
Stx1 toxin, 72
Stx2 toxin, 72
Subacute combined degeneration, of spinal cord, 114
Subacute infection, 58
Subarachnoid hemorrhage, 162
Subcortical arteriosclerotic encephalopathy, 157
Subcutis, 166
Subdural hematoma, 162
Subepidermal cleft, in bullous pemphigoid, 178, 178f
Submucosa, 294, 296f
Submucosal nerve plexus (Meissner nerve plexus), 294, 296f, 299
Substance P, 530f
Substantia nigra, 136
  dopaminergic neurons in, in Parkinson's disease, 152
Substrate accumulation, 4t
  in phenylketonuria, 27
Substrate interconversion, in liver, 332–334, 332t, 333f, 334f, 335f
  aberrant function in disease and, 338t, 339
Subthalamic nuclei, 136
Sulfonylureas
  hypothyroidism caused by, goiter and, 494, 495t
  insulin-mediated hypoglycemia caused by, 456
Superior quadrantanopia, 145
Supraclavicular fat pads, in Cushing's syndrome, 514
Supraventricular tachycardia, 234, 235f
Surface tension, of lungs, 190–191, 191f
Surfactant, 185, 191
  pathologic states and, 191
  pulmonary embolism, 217

Surgical shock, 280
Survival motor neuron (*SMN*) gene, in spinal muscular atrophies, 150
SVR. *See* Systemic vascular resistance
Swallowing disorders. *See* Dysphagia; Odynophagia
Sweating
 gustatory, in diabetic autonomic neuropathy, 454
 in left ventricular failure, 239
Swiss-type severe combined immunodeficiency disease (SCID), 40*t*, 41
Sympathetic nervous system
 lungs supplied by, 187
 vasodilator, 268
 vasomotor, 266–268, 266*t*, 267*f*, 268*f*
Sympathetic neural failure (primary autonomic failure), 285, 290–291
Synapses, 124, 125–127, 126*f*
Synaptic cleft, 125, 126*f*
Syncope, 280
 in aortic stenosis, 241, 242
 postural, 280
 in pulmonary embolism, 218
Syncytiotrophoblast, 537
Syndrome of inappropriate vasopressin (ADH) secretion (SIADH), **478–479**, 478*t*
Syndrome X, 453
Syringomyelia, 141, 141*f*
Systemic inflammatory response syndrome, 74, 74*t*
Systemic lupus erythematosus, **581–583**, 582*f*, 582*t*
 gastrointestinal manifestations of, 310*t*
Systemic vascular resistance, in septic shock, 76
Systole, 227, 228*f*
Systolic dysfunction, 235–237, 236*f*
Systolic heave, in right ventricular failure, 239

T_3. *See* Triiodothyronine
T_3 resin uptake (RT_3U), 486
T_3 toxicosis, 487
T_4. *See* Thyroxine
T_4 resin uptake (RT_4U), 486
T cell receptors, 32
 ulcerative colitis and, 321
T lymphocytes, 29. *See also* Cellular (cell-mediated) immune response
 in atherosclerosis, 269, 270*f*
 cytotoxic (CD8), 31
  absence of, in SCID, 41
  activation of, 32
  in erythema multiforme, 175
  in HIV infection/AIDS, 45
  in inflammatory rheumatic diseases, 578

 in lichen planus, 174
 in Graves' disease, 488, 488*f*
 helper (CD4), 32
  in allergic hypersensitivity, 35
  defective, in SCID, 41
  in erythema multiforme, 175
  in HIV infection/AIDS, 45–47, 46*t*
  in inflammatory rheumatic diseases, 577–578
  in lichen planus, 174
 in hypothyroidism, 492
 impairment of function/deficiency of. *See also* HIV infection/AIDS; Immunodeficiency diseases
  in common variable immunodeficiency, 44
  in DiGeorge syndrome, 42
  infections associated with, 40, 41*t*, 56*t*
  in PNP deficiency, 42–43
  in SCID, 41
 in lymph nodes, 30, 30*f*
 receptors for, 32
 recognition and activation of, 32
 in type IV (delayed) hypersensitivity reactions, 34
t-PA. *See* Tissue plasminogen activator
T ("transient") currents, in absence seizures, 156
T wave, of electrocardiogram, 224, 225*f*
Tachycardia, 233–234, 233*f*, 234*f*, 235*f*
 in asthma, 203
 in chronic bronchitis, 206–207
 in diabetic autonomic neuropathy, 454
 in emphysema, 207
 in hypovolemia, 279
 in myocardial infarction, 253
Tachypnea
 in asthma, 203
 in idiopathic pulmonary fibrosis, 209–210
Tamponade, **255–257**
 obstructive shock and, 281
Tamsulosin, for benign prostatic hyperplasia, 572*t*
Target cells, in iron deficiency anemia, 109
TBG. *See* Thyroxine-binding globulin
TBPA (thyroxine-binding prealbumin). *See* Transthyretin
Temperature, sensation of, 139, 139*f*
 Aδ fibers in, 137, 139
Teratomas, testicular
 malignant, 91
 mature, 91
Terazosin, for benign prostatic hyperplasia, 572, 572*t*
Terminal respiratory units (acini), 186, 186*f*
Terminal (central) veins, 328–329, 330*f*

Testes, 556, 557*f*
 disorders of, in infertility, 562, 564
 regulation of function of, 558–560, 560*f*
 steroid hormones produced by, 557–561, 559*f*, 560*f*, 560*t*, 561*f*. *See also* Androgens; Testosterone
 gonadotropins affecting, 464
 undescended, infertility and, 564
Testicular atrophy, 562, 563*t*, 566
Testicular biopsy, in male infertility evaluation, 568
Testicular cancer, **90–91**
 treatment for, infertility after, 564
Testicular fluid, 558–560
Testosterone, 556, 557, 559*f*
 in benign prostatic hyperplasia, 569–571, 570*f*, 571*f*
 deficiency of, in chronic renal failure, 398
 effects of, 561, 561*t*
 infertility evaluation and, 566, 567*f*
 mechanism of action of, 560–561, 561*f*
 normal levels of, 557, 560*f*, 560*t*
 regulation of, 558–560, 560*f*
 synthesis/protein binding/metabolism of, 557, 559*f*, 560*t*
Testosterone-receptor protein, 560–561, 561*f*
Tetany, 422
Tetrahydrobiopterin, defects in metabolism of, in phenylketonuria, 24*f*, 25
Tg Ab. *See* Thyroglobulin antibody
TGF. *See* Transforming growth factors
TGFα. *See* Transforming growth factors, α
TGFβ. *See* Transforming growth factors, β
T_H1 cells
 in allergic hypersensitivity, 35
 in inflammatory rheumatic diseases, 577–578
T_H2 cells
 in allergic hypersensitivity, 35
 in inflammatory rheumatic diseases, 577–578
Thalamic nuclei, 139, 139*f*
Thalamus, sensory loss caused by lesions of, 142
Thalassemias, 105
Therapeutic gold, lichen planus (lichenoid reactions) caused by, 173, 174*t*
Thin blood smear, 100, 100*f*, 101*t*, 106*f*. *See also* Blood smear
 in anemia, 106*f*
Thioamides, hypothyroidism caused by, 491
 goiter and, 494, 495*t*

Thiocyanates, hypothyroidism caused by, goiter and, 494, 495*t*
Third heart sound (S$_3$)
 in aortic regurgitation, 244, 245
 in left ventricular failure, 238, 238*f*
 in mitral regurgitation, 247, 249, 250*f*
 in right ventricular failure, 239
Third spacing, in septic shock, 280
Threatened abortion, 544
Thrombin (factor IIa), 103*f*, 104, 104*t*
 in platelet activation, 103
Thrombocythemia, essential, 108
Thrombocytopenia, 102, 107, 107*t*
 heparin-induced, 117–118, 118*f*
 immune, drug-associated, **117–119**, 117*t*
 and thrombosis, heparin-induced, 118–119
Thrombocytosis, 107*t*, 108
Thromboembolism. *See also* Thrombosis
 in hypercoagulable states, 121–122
 pulmonary, **215–219**, 215*t*, 216*t*, 217*f*, 219*t*
 chronic, 219
Thrombolytic system/pathway, 103*f*, 104–105
Thromboplastin, tissue (tissue factor/factor III), 104, 104*t*
Thromboplastin antecedent, plasma (factor XI), 103*f*, 104*t*
 deficiency of, 108*t*
Thrombopoiesis, 98–100, 99*f*
Thrombopoietin, in hematopoiesis, 99*f*, 100, 100*t*
Thrombosis, 120
 cerebral, stroke caused by, 159–162, 159*f*, 159*t*, 160*f*, 161*f*, 161*t*, 271
 deep venous
  in hypercoagulable states, 121–122
  pulmonary embolism and, 215–216, 215*t*, 216*t*, 218
 in heparin-induced thrombocytopenia and thrombosis, 119
 in hypercoagulable states, 121–122
 in mitral stenosis, 247
 during pregnancy, 543–544, 543*t*
Thrombotic stroke, 159–162, 159*f*, 159*t*, 160*f*, 161*f*, 161*t*, 271
Thromboxanes, in vascular function regulation, 264
Thrush (oral candidiasis), in HIV infection/AIDS, 47
Thymectomy, for myasthenia gravis, 154
Thymic aplasia, congenital (DiGeorge syndrome), 40*t*, **42**
 hypoparathyroidism in, 421
 pathogens causing infection in, 41*t*, 56*t*
Thymoma, in myasthenia gravis, 154
Thymus, 29–30
 in myasthenia gravis, 154
Thyroglobulin, 481
 formation and secretion of, 483–484

Thyroglobulin antibody (Tg Ab), 486
 in Hashimoto's thyroiditis, 492
Thyroid autoantibodies, 486
 in Hashimoto's thyroiditis, 492
Thyroid-binding prealbumin. *See* Transthyretin
Thyroid function tests, 486
 abnormal, in clinically euthyroid patient, 486, **496–498**, 497*t*
Thyroid gland, **481–499**
 ablation of, hypothyroidism and, 491
 anatomy of, **481**, 482*f*
 disorders of, **486–498**. *See also* Hyperthyroidism; Hypothyroidism
  adenoma, 482*f*, 496
  chronic anovulation and, 547, 548*t*
  enlargement (goiter), 485, 486, 486–487, **494–496**, 494*f*, 495*t*
  gastrointestinal manifestations of, 310*t*
  medullary carcinoma, **424–425**, 496
  nodules, 486, **496**
   in goiter, 496
  papillary or follicular carcinoma, 496
  subclinical, 497–498
  tumors, **496**
 histology of, **481–482**, 483*f*
 normal, **481–486**
 parafollicular cells of. *See* Parafollicular cells
 physiology of, **482–485**, 483*f*, 484*f*, 485*t*. *See also* Thyroid hormones
Thyroid hormone-binding proteins, 484
 increases and decreases in, 496, 497*t*
Thyroid hormones, 463–464. *See also* Thyroxine; Triiodothyronine
 effects of, 485, 485*t*
 formation and secretion of, 482–484, 483*f*
 regulation of, 484–485
 generalized resistance to (Refetoff's syndrome), 485, 497
 mechanism of action of, 485
 plasma levels of
  in goiter, 495
  in hyperthyroidism, 487
  in hypothyroidism, 491
  measurement of, 486
  normal, 484
 transport and metabolism of, 484
Thyroid nodules, 486, **496**
 in goiter, 496
Thyroid-stimulating hormone (thyrotropin/TSH), 463–464, 484–485, 484*f*
 deficiency of
  in hypopituitarism, 474
  in hypothyroidism, 491
 in goiter, 494, 495, 496

iodide pump stimulated by, 482
 plasma levels of
  in goiter, 495
  in hyperthyroidism, 486, 487
  in hypothyroidism, 486, 491
  measurement of, 486
 receptor for, 485
  antibodies to, 485, 486
Thyroid-stimulating immunoglobulin. *See* TSH receptor-stimulating antibody
Thyroid storm, 491
Thyroid surgery
 hypoparathyroidism after, 421
 hypothyroidism after, 493
Thyroidal peroxidase antibody (TPO Ab/antimicrosomal antibody), 486
 in Hashimoto's thyroiditis, 492
Thyroidectomy
 hypoparathyroidism after, 421
 hypothyroidism after, 493
Thyroiditis
 autoimmune, gastrointestinal manifestations of, 310*t*
 Hashimoto's, 482*f*, 491, 492
  autoimmune disorders associated with, 488*t*, 492
 lymphocytic, 491
Thyrotoxic dermopathy, 490–491
Thyrotoxic myopathy, 489
Thyrotoxicosis. *See* Hyperthyroidism
Thyrotropin (TSH), 463–464, 484–485, 484*f*
 deficiency of
  in hypopituitarism, 474
  in hypothyroidism, 491
 in goiter, 494, 495, 496
 iodide pump stimulated by, 482
 plasma levels of
  in goiter, 495
  in hyperthyroidism, 486, 487
  in hypothyroidism, 486, 491
  measurement of, 486
 receptor for, 485
  antibodies to, 485, 486
Thyrotropin-releasing hormone (TRH), 463–464, 484
 for hypothyroidism, 491
Thyrotropin-releasing hormone (TRH) test
 in hyperthyroidism, 487
 in hypothyroidism, 492
Thyroxine (T$_4$), 463–464, 481, 483*f*
 abnormal binding of, 496–497
 effects of, 485, 485*t*
 formation and secretion of, 482–484, 483*f*
 regulation of, 484–485
 free (FT$_4$), 486
  in hyperthyroidism, 487
 mechanism of action of, 485

plasma levels of
   in goiter, 495
   in hyperthyroidism, 487
   in hypothyroidism, 491
   normal, 484
resin uptake of (RT_4U), 486
total plasma (TT_4), 486
transport and metabolism of, 484
Thyroxine-binding globulin, 484
   hepatic synthesis of, 336*t*
   increases and decreases in, 496, 497*t*
Thyroxine-binding prealbumin. *See* Transthyretin
Tiagabine, 156*t*
TIAs. *See* Transient ischemic attacks
TIBC. *See* Total iron-binding capacity
Tidal volume (VT), 185
Tight junctions, hepatic, 331
Tinnitus, 146
TIPS. *See* Transhepatic intrajugular portal-to-systemic shunting
Tissue factor/thromboplastin (factor III), 104, 104*t*
Tissue plasminogen activator (t-PA), 105
TLC (total lung capacity), 185
   in asthma, 203
   in emphysema, 207
   in idiopathic pulmonary fibrosis, 210
TNF-related activation-induced cytokine (TRANCE), 411
α-Tocopherol, in atherosclerosis prevention, 273
Tonic-clonic seizures, 154, 154*t*
Tophi, in gout, 578, 580
Total iron-binding capacity, in iron deficiency anemia, 109–110
Total lung capacity (TLC), 185
   in asthma, 203
   in emphysema, 207
   in idiopathic pulmonary fibrosis, 210
Total plasma thyroxine (TT_4), 486
Touch, sensation of, 139, 139*f*
Toxic epidermal necrolysis, 177, 177*f*
Toxic/drug-associated hepatitis, 343*t*, 347, 347*t*
   time course of, 347, 348*f*
Toxoplasmosis, in HIV infection/AIDS, 48
TPO Ab. *See* Thyroidal peroxidase antibody
Trabecular bone, 411
   remodeling of, 412, 412*f*
"Tram track lines," in chronic bronchitis, 207
TRANCE. *See* TNF-related activation-induced cytokine
Transamination, in liver, 332*t*, 333, 334*f*
Transcortin, 501
Transcription factor, aberrant, in hematologic neoplasms, 92
Transferrin, 109, 336*t*, 337

hepatic secretion/synthesis of, 336*t*, 337
receptor for, 337
Transforming growth factors
   α, ovarian production of, 530*t*
   β, 83
      in benign prostatic hyperplasia, 571–572
      in breast cancer, 88–89
      ovarian production of, 530*t*
      in benign prostatic hyperplasia, 571–572
      in glomerulonephritis and nephrotic syndrome, 399
Transhepatic intrajugular portal-to-systemic shunting (TIPS), for ascites, 359
Transient (T) currents, in absence seizures, 156
Transient ischemic attacks, 160
Translocations, chromosomal
   in hematologic neoplasia, 92, 93*t*
   leukemia, 94–95
   in oncogene activation, 80
   Robertsonian, 4*t*
      in Down's syndrome, 18, 18*f*, 20–21, 21*f*, 21*t*, 22
Transmembrane conductance regulator gene, congenital absence of vas deferens and, 565
Transmural pressure
   in law of Laplace, 261
   pulmonary edema and (cardiogenic pulmonary edema), 212, 212–213, 214
Transplantation
   bone marrow, pancreatic insufficiency after, 376
   pneumonia after, 67*t*
   renal, gastrointestinal manifestations in, 310*t*
Transrectal ultrasonography, in male infertility evaluation, 568
Transthyretin (thyroid-binding prealbumin), 484
   changes in serum concentrations of, 496–497
   hepatic synthesis of, 336*t*
Transurethral needle ablation of prostate (TUNA), for benign prostatic hyperplasia, 572
Transurethral resection of prostate, for bladder outlet obstruction in benign prostatic hyperplasia, 572
Transverse palmar crease, in Down's syndrome, 19
Trauma, acute pancreatitis associated with, 365*t*, 366
Traumatic shock, 280
Traveler's diarrhea, 322*t*
Trefoil peptides, in gastrointestinal defenses, 300

Tremor, intention, 136
Tricuspid valve, 222, 223–224*f*
Trigeminal lemniscus, 139, 139*f*
Trigeminal nerve, main sensory and mesencephalic nuclei of, 139
Trigeminal system, 139, 139*f*
   sensory loss caused by lesions of, 142
Trigeminothalamic tract, sensory loss caused by lesions of, 142
Triggered activity, in tachycardia, 233, 233*f*
Triglycerides. *See also* Hypertriglyceridemia
   hepatic metabolism of, 333–334, 333*f*, 335*f*, 436*t*
   insulin in, 435, 436*t*
   liver dysfunction and, 342
Triiodothyronine (T_3), 463–464, 481, 483*f*
   effects of, 485, 485*t*
   formation and secretion of, 482–484, 483*f*
   regulation of, 484–485
   mechanism of action of, 485
   nonthyroidal illness and drugs affecting, 497
   plasma levels of
      in goiter, 495
      in hyperthyroidism, 487
      in hypothyroidism, 491
      measurement of, 486
      normal, 484
   receptors for, 485
      abnormal, 485, 497
   resin uptake of (RT_3U), 486
   reverse (RT_3), 484
   transport and metabolism of, 484
Triplet repeat, 4*t*
   amplification of in fragile X-associated mental retardation syndrome, 14, 15*f*, 16
   postzygotic, 16
Trisomy, 4*t*
Trisomy 21, 17. *See also* Down's syndrome
   Alzheimer's disease and, 19, 158
   critical region in, 22, 22*f*
   extra chromosome donor and, 19, 19*f*
   gene dosage and, 21–22, 22*f*
   nondisjunction in, 18, 19, 20*f*
   phenotypic features of, 18–19, 19*t*
   recurrence risk for, 20, 21*t*
      Robertsonian translocation and, 20, 21*f*, 21*t*
Trochlear nerve (cranial nerve IV), in control of eye movements, 142
Trophoblastic malignancies, 544
Tropical pancreatitis, 372–373
Tropical sprue, histologic features of, 320*t*
Tropomyosin, 225

Trousseau's sign, 370, 422, 423f
Trypsin, in pancreatic juice, 364
  acute pancreatitis and, 367, 367f
Trypsinogen, in pancreatic juice, 364
  hypersecretion of in chronic pancreatitis, 373, 374f
TSH. See Thyrotropin
TSH-R. See TSH receptor
TSH-R [block] Ab. See TSH receptor-blocking antibody
TSH-R [stim] Ab. See TSH receptor-stimulating antibody
TSH receptor, 484
TSH receptor antibody, 486
TSH receptor-blocking antibody (TSH-R [block] Ab), 486
  in Hashimoto's thyroiditis, 492
TSH receptor-stimulating antibody (TSH-R [stim] Ab), 485, 486
  in Graves' disease, 485, 486, 488, 488f
TSI (thyroid-stimulating immunoglobulin). See TSH receptor-stimulating antibody
TT_4. See Total plasma thyroxine
Tuberculosis
  adrenal, 518
  pneumocystic, 47
Tubular acidosis, 386t
  stone formation and, 403t
  type 4 (hyporeninemic hypoaldosteronism), 396, 509, 526
Tubular necrosis, acute, 390, 390–392, 393f
Tubular resorption, 385, 386t
Tubuloglomerular feedback, 387
Tumor embolism, 215t
Tumor necrosis factor
  in acute pancreatitis, 367, 368f
  in meningitis, 64–65
  in sepsis, 74, 75f, 76f
Tumor suppressor genes, 80, **80–82**, 81t
  loss of function of, 80
TUNA. See Transurethral needle ablation of prostate
Tuning fork tests of hearing, 146
Turbulent flow
  noise caused by, 262
  resistance and, 192
Turner's syndrome, 545, 547
TURP. See Transurethral resection of prostate
Twenty four-hour urine free cortisol, in Cushing's disease, 511, 514f, 517
Two-point discrimination, 140
Tyndall phenomenon, in lichen planus, 175
Type 1 diabetes mellitus, 440, 440t, 441t. See also Diabetes mellitus
  etiology of, 441–443, 442f, 443f

Type I (anaphylactic/immediate) hypersensitivity reaction, 34
Type 2 diabetes mellitus, 440–441, 440t, 441t. See also Diabetes mellitus
  etiology of, 443–444
Type II (cytotoxic) hypersensitivity reaction, 34
Type III (immune complex-mediated) hypersensitivity reaction, 34
Type IV (delayed) hypersensitivity reaction, 34
Tyrosine, phenylalanine in production of, 24, 24f

Ulcerative colitis, 321–322, 323t, 324
Ulcers
  diabetic, of foot, 454
  peptic, 308, **312–314**, 314f. See also Acid-mediated gastrointestinal injury
  in chronic renal failure, 397
Ultrasonography
  in benign prostatic hyperplasia, 574
  transrectal, in male infertility evaluation, 568
Uncal herniation, 147, 148f
Unstable angina, 251, 252
Upper motor neurons, 129, **131–134**, 132f, 133f
Urate crystals, in gout, 578, 579
Urea, renal dysfunction affecting excretion of, 388
Urea cycle, 333, 334f
Urea nitrogen, blood (BUN), in renal dysfunction, 388
  acute renal failure and, 390, 392
Uremia, 388, 394, 394t, 395. See also Renal failure
  platelet disorders in, 108
Uremic fetor, 397
Uremic frost, 398
Uremic gastroenteritis, 397
Ureter, cancer of, 86t
Ureteral obstruction, hypertension and, 275
Urethral glands, 556
Uric acid, increased serum levels of
  in chronic renal failure, 396
  in gout, 579
Uric acid crystals, in gout, 579
Uric acid stones, 402, 403t
Urinalysis, in acute renal failure, 392
Urinary free cortisol, in Cushing's disease, 511, 514f, 517
Urinary incontinence, in diabetic autonomic neuropathy, 454
Urinary retention, in benign prostatic hyperplasia, 573, 573f
Urinary tract
  asymptomatic abnormalities of, 391t, 398, 399, 399t

  infection of
    clinical and laboratory findings in, 391t
  renal stone formation and, 402
  obstruction of. See also Renal stones
    in acute renal failure, 390
    in benign prostatic hyperplasia, 572
    androgen suppression relieving, 570–571, 570t, 571f
    bladder response to, 573
    clinical manifestations of, 573–574
    mechanisms of, 572
    prostatic capsule and, 569, 572
    clinical and laboratory findings in, 391t
    mechanical causes of, 402t
Urine
  acidification of, impaired, liver dysfunction and, 338t
  concentration of, 385, 386
  lack of in diabetes insipidus, 476
Urodynamic evaluation, in benign prostatic hyperplasia, 574
Uroflowmetry, in benign prostatic hyperplasia, 574
Uterine tubes, 531, 531f
  disorders of, **542–543**
  infertility and, 553
Uterus, 529–531, 531f
  catecholamines affecting, 284t
  disorders of, **542–543**
    abnormal vaginal bleeding caused by, 551
    amenorrhea caused by, 545, 546, 546t, 551
    cancer, 86t, 551
  oxytocin affecting, 467
Utricle, 145

V_{1A} receptors, 467
V_{1B} receptors, 467
V_2 receptors, 467
  in diabetes insipidus, 476
V (variable) region, immunoglobulin, 32, 33f
v wave, 227, 228f
  in mitral regurgitation, 249, 250f
  in pericarditis, 255, 255f
$\dot{V}/\dot{Q}$ mismatching, 194, 197–198, 197f
  in asthma, 203
  in chronic bronchitis, 207
  in emphysema, 207
  in left ventricular failure, 237
  in noncardiogenic pulmonary edema, 214
$\dot{V}/\dot{Q}$ ratios, 195, 196f, 197–198, 197f
  in asthma, 203
  in chronic bronchitis, 207
  in emphysema, 207
  high, 195, 197f, 198
  in idiopathic pulmonary fibrosis, 210

low, 197–198, 197f
  in pulmonary embolism, 217
Vagal sensory fibers, pulmonary, 187, 188t
Vagina, 531, 531f
  disorders of, **542–543**
Vaginal bleeding, abnormal, 542, 545
  clinical manifestations of, 552
  etiology of, 545, 547t
  pathology and pathogenesis of, 550–551, 551t
Vagotomy, gastric motility disorders associated with, 308
Valproate, 156t
Valves, heart, 222, 223–224f. *See also specific valve*
  in cardiac cycle, 227
  diseases of, **240–251**
Vanillylmandelic acid (VMA), 283
Variable expressivity, 6, 6f
Variable (V) region, immunoglobulin, 32, 33f
Varices, esophageal (gastroesophageal), 338
  in cirrhosis, 359
Varicocelectomy, 564
Varicoceles, 564, 566
Vas deferens, 556, 557f
  bilateral congenital absence of, 565, 566
Vascular cell adhesion molecules, 269
Vascular malformations, intraparenchymal hemorrhage caused by, 162
Vascular resistance, 261–262
  catecholamines in, 285
  in septic shock, 76
Vascular smooth muscle. *See also Vascular system*
  catecholamines affecting, 284t
  hormones affecting, 265–266
Vascular system, **258–281**
  anatomy of, **258–260**, 258f, 259f, 260f
  biophysical considerations and, 260–262, 261f, 262f
  catecholamines affecting, 284t, 288t
  disorders of, **269–281**. *See also specific type*
    in acute renal failure, 392t
    in diabetes mellitus, 448, 448–453, 448t
  failure of, in septic shock, 77
  histology of, **258–260**, 259f, 260f
  normal, **255–268**
  physiology of, **260–263**, 261f, 262f, 263f
  pressures in, 260, 262, 262f
  in psoriasis, 170–171
  pulmonary, 187, 188f, 189f
  regulation of, **263–268**, 265f, 266f, 266t, 267f, 268f

Vasculitis, 170t, 171f, **180–182**
  cerebral, in meningitis, 65
  cutaneous small vessel, 581
  immune complex, **580–581**
  leukocytoclastic, **180–182**, 180f, 181f
Vasoactive intestinal polypeptide (VIP), 298t
  ovarian production of, 530t
Vasoconstriction
  in hypovolemia, 279
  hypoxic pulmonary, 194
  in left ventricular failure, 239
  norepinephrine causing, 285
  in pheochromocytoma, 288
  sympathetic control of, 266–268, 266t, 267f, 268f
Vasodilation
  epinephrine causing, 285
  sympathetic control of, 266t, 268
Vasodilator metabolites, in cardiovascular regulation, 264
Vasogenic cerebral edema, in meningitis, 65
Vasogenic (distributive) shock, 278, 278t, **280**
  sepsis and, 76, 280
Vasomotor symptoms, in menopause, 541
Vasomotor system, sympathetic, in vascular function regulation, 266–268, 266t, 267f, 268f
Vasopressin (antidiuretic hormone/ADH), 466–467, 467f
  deficiency of, in hypopituitarism, 473
  for differentiation of central from nephrogenic diabetes insipidus, 477
  ovarian production of, 530t
  receptors for, 467
  in renal regulation, 385, 386, 467
  syndrome of inappropriate secretion of, **478–479**, 478t
Vater, ampulla of, 362, 363f
VC (vital capacity), 185
  forced (FVC). *See Forced vital capacity*
VCAMs. *See Vascular cell adhesion molecules*
Vectors, in disease transmission, 50, 50f
Vegetations, endocarditic, 59, 61f
Veins, 259f, 260
Vena cava, 259f
Venography, in male infertility evaluation, 568
Venous pressure/waveforms, jugular
  in constrictive pericarditis, 255, 255f
  in pericardial tamponade, 256
  in right ventricular failure, 239, 239–240, 240f

Venous thrombosis
  pulmonary embolism and, 215–216, 216t, 218
  risk factors for, 215t, 216t
Ventilation. *See also* Breathing
  distribution of, 193–194, 194f, 195f
  matching perfusion to, 194–198, 196f, 197f
  wasted (alveolar dead space), 195–195, 196f
  in pulmonary embolism, 217
Ventilation/perfusion matching, 194–198, 196f, 197f
Ventilation/perfusion mismatching, 194, 197–198, 197f
  in asthma, 203
  in chronic bronchitis, 207
  in emphysema, 207
  in left ventricular failure, 237
  in noncardiogenic pulmonary edema, 214
Ventilation/perfusion ratios, 195, 196f, 197–198, 197f
  in asthma, 203
  in chronic bronchitis, 207
  in emphysema, 207
  high, 195, 197f, 198
  in idiopathic pulmonary fibrosis, 210
  low, 197–198, 197f
  in pulmonary embolism, 217
Ventilation/perfusion scanning, in pulmonary embolism, 218, 219t
Ventricles, cardiac, 222, 223–224f
Ventricular myocytes, contraction of, 229, 231f, 232f
Ventricular relaxation, 227, 228f
Venules, 259f, 260
Vertebral fractures, osteoporotic, 428, 428f
Vertical gaze center, 142
Vertigo, 146
Very low density lipoproteins, 269
  metabolism of
    in diabetes mellitus, 445, 453
      ketoacidosis and, 446
    in liver, 333, 335f
      insulin and, 435
      liver dysfunction and, 339
Vesicles, 169
Vesicular transport, 259
Vesiculobullous dermatitis, 170t, 171f, **178–180**, 178f, 179f
Vesiculobullous lichen planus, 175
Vestibular function, 146
Vestibular nuclei, 146
VHL gene, 82t
  mutations of, pheochromocytoma and, 286
Vibratory sense, 139f, 140
Vibrio cholerae, diarrhea caused by, 71–72, 71f

Vigabatrin, 156t
Villi, intestinal, 294, 296f, 305, 306f
VIPoma, 456t
Viral infections
in carcinogenesis, 80
gastroenteritis, 69. *See also* Diarrhea
hepatitis. *See* Hepatitis, viral
meningitis, 62–65
pneumonia, 65–69
Virchow's triad, 120, 215
Vision (visual system), **142–145**
anatomy of, 142–143, 143f, 144f
physiology of, 143–145, 145f
Visual cortex, primary, 132f, 142
Visual field defects, 143f, 144–145
in Cushing's syndrome, 516
in pituitary adenoma, 472, 472f
Visual fields, 142, 143f, 144
Visuomotor integration, 149
Vital capacity (VC), 185
forced (FVC). *See* Forced vital capacity
Vitamin B_6, in atherosclerosis prevention, 272
Vitamin B_{12} (cobalamin)
in atherosclerosis prevention, 272
deficiency of
anemia and, 105, 111
liver dysfunction and, 342
pancreatic insufficiency and, 378
in pernicious anemia, 114–115, 304
in DNA synthesis, 112–113, 113f
Vitamin D, **413–414**, 413f
in calcium metabolism, **413–414**
deficiency of, in osteomalacia, 429
in hypocalcemia, 423, 424t
in osteoporosis, 427, 427t
supplementary, for osteoporosis prevention/management, 429
Vitamin D_2, 413
Vitamin D receptor, 414
Vitamin E, in atherosclerosis prevention, 273
Vitamin K, in coagulation, 104
acute hepatitis and, 349–350
cirrhosis and, 360
Vitamins, deficiency of. *See also* Deficiency states
liver dysfunction and, 338t, 339, 342
Vitiligo, in adrenocortical insufficiency, 520–521
Vitreous hemorrhage, in diabetic retinopathy, 450
VLDL. *See* Very low density lipoproteins
VMA. *See* Vanillylmandelic acid
Voltage-gated ion channels, 125
anticonvulsant mechanism of action and, 156, 156t

Volume status, in chronic renal failure, 395
Vomiting
in acute pancreatitis, 368
gastrointestinal disease presenting with, 293, 294t
in myocardial infarction, 253
von Economo's encephalitis, parkinsonism caused by, 151
von Hippel-Lindau disease, pheochromocytoma in, 286, 286t
von Willebrand disease, 108, 108t
von Willebrand factor, 104
deficiency of, 108, 108t
V_T (tidal volume), 185
vWF. *See* von Willebrand factor

WAGR syndrome, 22t
Warfarin, 104
Wasted ventilation (alveolar dead space), 195–195, 196f
in pulmonary embolism, 217
Water balance
in adrenocortical insufficiency, 521
in chronic renal failure, 395
liver dysfunction and, 338t, 344, 344t
renal dysfunction and, 388–389
renal regulation of, 385, 387
Water-hammer pulse, in aortic regurgitation, 245
Water intoxication, in adrenocortical insufficiency, 521
Waterhouse-Friderichsen syndrome, 519
Weber test, 146
Weight, physiology of control of, **468–469**, 468f
Weight gain
in Cushing's syndrome, 514
in hypothyroidism, 492
Weight loss
in adrenocortical insufficiency, 521
in hyperthyroidism, 489
in pancreatic insufficiency, 378
Werdnig-Hoffman disease, 150
Wernicke's area, 149
Westermark's sign, 218
Wheezing
in asthma, 203
in chronic bronchitis, 206
in left ventricular failure, 237
Whipple's disease, histologic features of, 320t
Whipple's triad, 455
White blood cell count, 101t
abnormalities of, 107–108, 107t
White blood cells. *See* Leukocytes
"White coat hypertension," 262
Wickham's striae, in lichen planus, 174

Williams' syndrome, 22t
Wilms tumor suppressor gene, in hematologic neoplasia, 92
Wirsung, duct of, 362, 363f
Wiskott-Aldrich syndrome, pathogens causing infection in, 56t
Withdrawal reflex, 130f, 137
Wolff-Chaikoff block, 491
Wolff-Parkinson-White syndrome, 233–234, 234f
Work of breathing, 193, 193f
flow and resistance and, 191–192, 193f
in left ventricular failure, 237
pulmonary embolism and, 216t
Wormian bones, in osteogenesis imperfecta, 9
WT-1 gene, 82t
in hematologic neoplasia, 92

X chromosome, fragile, mental retardation and, 2, 7t, 14–17
X-linked adrenoleukodystrophy, adrenal insufficiency in, 519–520
X-linked agammaglobulinemia, 40t, **42**
pathogens causing infection in, 41t, 56t
X-linked inheritance, 6
X-linked severe combined immunodeficiency disease, 41
Xanthomas, 339, 361

Y chromosome, microdeletions causing infertility and, 563
Y chromosome RNA recognition motif. *See* RNA-binding motif
Young syndrome, 566
Yq6 deletion interval, azoospermia and, 563
YRRM gene. *See* *RBM* gene

Zanoterone, for benign prostatic hyperplasia, 570t
ZAP-70, deficiency of, in SCID, 41
Zinc, deficiency of, gastrointestinal manifestations of, 310t
Zona fasciculata, 500, 502f, 503f
Zona glomerulosa, 500, 502f, 503f
hyperplasia of, hypertension and, 276
Zona pellucida glycoprotein 3, in sperm-zona binding, 568
Zona reticularis, 500, 502f, 503f
Zoonotic hosts, in disease transmission, 50, 50f
ZP3. *See* Zona pellucida glycoprotein 3
Zymogen granules, 363, 363f
Zymogens, in pancreatic juice, 363–364